Abbreviated Table of Contents (Continued)

MAYO CLINIC CARDIOLOGY REVIEW

SECOND EDITION

MAYO CLINIC CARDIOLOGY REVIEW

SECOND EDITION

JOSEPH G. MURPHY

M.D., F.R.C.P.I., F.A.C.C., F.E.S.C.

EDITOR-IN-CHIEF

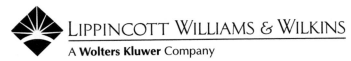

LIPPINCOTT WILLIAMS & WILKINS

A **Wolters Kluwer** Company

Philadelphia • Baltimore • New York • London
Buenos Aires • Hong Kong • Sydney • Tokyo

Acquisitions Editor: Ruth W. Weinberg
Developmental Editor: Keith Donnellan
Production Editor: Robert Pancotti
Manufacturing Manager: Tim Reynolds
Cover Designers: Jeffrey A. Satre, Diana Andrews
Marketing Manager: Melissa Fox
Printer: R. R. Donnelley Willard

The triple-shield Mayo logo and the words MAYO and MAYO CLINIC are registered marks of Mayo Foundation for Medical Education and Research.

© 2000, 1997 by Mayo Foundation for Medical Education and Research
Published by
Lippincott Williams & Wilkins
530 Walnut Street
Philadelphia, PA 19106
LWW.com

Printed in the USA

Library of Congress Cataloging-in-Publication Data

Mayo Clinic cardiology review/editor, Joseph G. Murphy.—2nd ed.
    p.   cm.
  Includes bibliographical references and index.
  ISBN 0-7817-2326-4
  1. Cardiology Outlines, syllabi, etc. 2. Cardiology Examinations, questions, etc. I. Murphy, Joseph G. II. Mayo Clinic. III. Title: Cardiology review.
  [DNLM: 1. Heart Diseases Examination Questions. 2. Heart Diseases Outlines. WG 18.2 M473 2000]
  RC669.M39 2000
  616.1'20076—dc21
DNLM/DLC
for Library of Congress
                                                      99-32851
                                                     CIP

10 9 8 7 6 5 4 3

Dedication

This book is dedicated to my parents, my wife Marian, without whose support and encouragement this textbook would not have been possible, and my children Owen, Sinéad and Aidan, without whose help the book may have been completed somewhat sooner.

Table of Contents

Foreword to the First Edition

I am delighted to have this opportunity to introduce the *Mayo Clinic Cardiology Review*. The tremendous amount of work and dedication required to accomplish this summary of the current state of the art reflects a long-standing tradition of the medical profession and one that Mayo has always taken seriously, namely, the sharing of knowledge and experience with others. The authors have concisely presented material that should not only be of value in preparing for the board examination but also serve as a source of reference for many who desire specific practical information in both the clinical realities of practice and the basic science that is fundamental to our current and future success in helping patients with cardiovascular diseases.

While the pressures in medicine mount with efforts to deal with the escalating cost of medical care, it is refreshing to review a text that remains focused on the individual patient. My personal bias is that this should continue to be the focus of our profession.

This year marks the 50th anniversary of cardiac catheterization at the Mayo Clinic. The advances in our knowledge and ability to help patients with cardiovascular disease have been astounding over the past 5 decades. The future promises to be equally exciting.

Robert L. Frye, M.D.
Chair, Department of Internal Medicine
Mayo Clinic and Mayo Foundation
Professor of Medicine
Mayo Medical School
Rochester, Minnesota

Foreword to the Second Edition

It is a pleasure to be asked to write this Foreword for the second edition of the *Mayo Clinic Cardiology Review*.

Fellows and clinicians in cardiology are faced with a rapidly expanding body of information and a shrinking amount of free time that can be devoted to reading and the acquisition of new knowledge. This book provides a contemporary and succinct distillation of the current status of clinical cardiovascular disease. In addition, it presents a wonderfully integrated clinical approach based on the extensive experience at Mayo Clinic.

The genesis of this book is the syllabus for the Mayo Cardiovascular Review Course. The book is written specifically for cardiology fellows, busy clinicians in cardiology or internal medicine practice, candidates for cardiology boards or recertification, and candidates for examination in general internal medicine both in North America and abroad. It is designed to be read in about 6 months, and the 1348 pages of text are accompanied by 111 pages of superb color photographs. The principles of cardiovascular disease and its treatment are comprehensively but precisely presented and are supplemented by more than 600 multiple-choice questions with explanatory answers, teaching points, and examination points.

The emphasis of this book is on the patient, and the objectives extend way beyond the passing of an examination. In this respect, appropriate emphasis on the cellular pathophysiologic basis of diseases is provided by chapters on essential molecular biology, cellular electrophysiology, atherosclerosis and endothelial function, lipid metabolism, and the coagulation system. Advances in basic science and the era of molecular cardiology have radically altered our basic concepts of physiology and pathophysiology, and it is incumbent on all of us, irrespective of the length of time we have been in practice, to renew our understanding of the basic concepts of cardiovascular disease. This book meets this objective admirably.

As we struggle with cost containment and other aspects of a changing health care environment, it is refreshing and stimulating to see how far cardiology has progressed during the past 30 years. We are now on the threshold of the scientific revolution as this century comes to an end and the Human Genome Project approaches completion. This book, which reflects the commitment and the contributions of Mayo Clinic to education, will continue to provide an insightful perspective of the constantly changing practice of cardiovascular diseases in the years to come.

Bernard J. Gersh, M.B., Ch.B., D. Phil.
Consultant, Division of Cardiovascular
Diseases and Internal Medicine
Mayo Clinic and Mayo Foundation
Professor of Medicine
Mayo Medical School
Rochester, Minnesota

Preface

This textbook is designed to present the field of cardiology in a reader-friendly format in a reasonable length text that can be read in about 6 months. Many small cardiology textbooks are bare-bones compilations of facts that do not explain the fundamental concepts of cardiovascular disease, and many large cardiology textbooks are voluminous and describe cardiology in detail from basic cellular concepts to clinical practice. The *Mayo Clinic Cardiology Review* is designed to be a bridge between these approaches. We seek to present a solid framework of ideas with sufficient depth to make the matter interesting yet concise, aimed specifically toward busy fellows in training or practicing clinicians wanting to update their knowledge. Attractive color photographs have been added to supplement, but not replace, the basic text. Teaching points, clinical pearls, and multiple-choice questions have been added to make the textbook come alive and challenge the reader.

The concept for this textbook originated from the first syllabus for the Mayo Cardiovascular Review Course, a function the textbook continues to fulfill. The impetus to produce this textbook owes much to the encouragement of Rick A. Nishimura, M.D., the director of the Mayo Cardiovascular Review Course.

The second edition of the textbook has been expanded at the suggestion of cardiology fellows and now includes 14 new chapters on cardiac pharmacology and atlas chapters of electrophysiologic tracings, angiographic images, radiographs of congenital heart defects, and hemodynamic tracings.

The text is intended primarily for cardiology fellows studying for cardiology board certification and practicing cardiologists studying for board recertification. It will also be useful for physicians studying for memberships and fellowships of the Royal Colleges of Physicians, internists and general physicians with a special interest in cardiology, and coronary care and critical care nurses. The book follows the format of the 45 lectures for the Mayo Cardiovascular Review Course but has an additional 41 chapters. More than 600 new multiple-choice questions and explanatory answers have been added to the text.

I thank all my colleagues in the Division of Cardiovascular Diseases who have generously contributed to this work. I also thank William D. Edwards, M.D., and Robert Schwartz, M.D., for permission to use slides from the Mayo Clinic cardiology pathologic image database. LeAnn Stee and O. E. Millhouse, Ph.D., at Mayo Clinic, contributed enormously through their expert substantive editing. Ruth W. Weinberg at Lippincott Williams & Wilkins patiently guided this project through countless tribulations. I thank both the Mayo and the Lippincott Williams & Wilkins production teams: at Mayo— Roberta Schwartz (production editor), Sharon Wadleigh (editorial assistant), Jeffrey A. Satre (art director), and Barbara McLeod (Continuing Medical Education); at Lippincott Williams & Wilkins—Tim Reynolds (manufacturing manager), Dennis Teston (associate director of production), Robert Pancotti (production editor), Keith Donnellan (developmental editor), Melissa Fox (marketing manager), and Diana Andrews (creative director).

The editorial staff and I have made strenuous efforts to avoid any errors in this text, but as editor-in-chief I accept responsibility for any errors that may have eluded us. I would appreciate comments from our readers about how we might improve this textbook or, specifically, about any errors that you find. Our intentions are to update this textbook every 2 years and to produce multiple foreign versions, in addition to the current Spanish and Chinese versions of the first edition.

Joseph G. Murphy, M.D.
Consultant, Division of Cardiovascular
  Diseases and Internal Medicine and
Chair, Section of Scientific Publications
Mayo Clinic and Mayo Foundation
Associate Professor of Medicine
Mayo Medical School
Rochester, Minnesota
murphy.joseph@mayo.edu

Acknowledgments

We would like to acknowledge the following people, without whose help this project would not have been possible:

Editorial Production	O. Eugene Millhouse, Ph.D.
	LeAnn M. Stee
Production Editor	Roberta J. Schwartz
Art Director	Jeffrey A. Satre
Editorial Assistant	Sharon L. Wadleigh
Scientific Illustrators	Paul W. Honermann
	Diane Knight
	Jason T. Robinson
	Jim Tidwell
Digital Image Specialists	Peggy Chihak
	Thomas F. Flood
	Sandy Gaspar
Image Librarians	Kristi L. Hunter
	Nancy Moltaji

List of Contributors

Christopher P. Appleton, M.D.
Chair, Division of Cardiovascular Diseases, Mayo Clinic Scottsdale, Scottsdale, Arizona; Associate Professor of Medicine

Thomas Behrenbeck, M.D., Ph.D.
Consultant, Division of Cardiovascular Diseases and Internal Medicine; Associate Professor of Medicine

Peter B. Berger, M.D.
Consultant, Division of Cardiovascular Diseases and Internal Medicine; Associate Professor of Medicine

Peter A. Brady, M.D.
Fellow in Cardiovascular Diseases; Instructor in Medicine

Jerome F. Breen, M.D.
Consultant, Department of Diagnostic Radiology; Assistant Professor of Radiology

John F. Bresnahan, M.D.
Consultant, Division of Cardiovascular Diseases and Internal Medicine; Associate Professor of Medicine

John C. Burnett, Jr., M.D.
Consultant, Division of Cardiovascular Diseases and Internal Medicine; Professor of Medicine and of Physiology

Mark J. Callahan, M.D.
Consultant, Division of Cardiovascular Diseases and Internal Medicine; Assistant Professor of Medicine

Yong-Mei Cha, M.D.
Fellow in Cardiovascular Diseases

Timothy F. Christian, M.D.
Consultant, Division of Cardiovascular Diseases and Internal Medicine; Associate Professor of Medicine

Alfredo L. Clavell, M.D.
Senior Associate Consultant, Division of Cardiovascular Diseases and Internal Medicine; Assistant Professor of Medicine

Heidi M. Connolly, M.D.
Consultant, Division of Cardiovascular Diseases and Internal Medicine; Assistant Professor of Medicine

Leslie T. Cooper, Jr., M.D.
Senior Associate Consultant, Division of Cardiovascular Diseases and Internal Medicine; Assistant Professor of Medicine

William F. Dunn, M.D.
Consultant, Division of Pulmonary and Critical Care Medicine and Internal Medicine; Assistant Professor of Medicine

William D. Edwards, M.D.
Consultant, Division of Anatomic Pathology; Professor of Pathology

Maurice Enriquez-Sarano, M.D.
Consultant, Division of Cardiovascular Diseases and Internal Medicine; Associate Professor of Medicine

William K. Freeman, M.D.
Consultant, Division of Cardiovascular Diseases and Internal Medicine; Assistant Professor of Medicine

Paul A. Friedman, M.D.
Senior Associate Consultant, Division of Cardiovascular Diseases and Internal Medicine; Assistant Professor of Medicine

Gerald T. Gau, M.D.
Consultant, Division of Cardiovascular Diseases and Internal Medicine; Professor of Medicine

Martha Grogan, M.D.
Consultant, Division of Cardiovascular Diseases and Internal Medicine; Assistant Professor of Medicine

Stephen C. Hammill, M.D.
Consultant, Division of Cardiovascular Diseases and Internal Medicine; Professor of Medicine

David L. Hayes, M.D.
Consultant, Division of Cardiovascular Diseases and Internal Medicine; Professor of Medicine

Sharonne N. Hayes, M.D.
Consultant, Division of Cardiovascular Diseases and Internal Medicine; Assistant Professor of Medicine

Stuart T. Higano, M.D.
Consultant, Division of Cardiovascular Diseases and Internal Medicine; Assistant Professor of Medicine

Michael J. Hogan, M.D.
Consultant, Division of Hypertension and Internal Medicine; Assistant Professor of Medicine

Arshad Jahangir, M.D.
Special Clinical Fellow, Division of Cardiovascular Diseases and Internal Medicine; Instructor in Medicine

Donald L. Johnston, M.D.
Consultant, Division of Cardiovascular Diseases and Internal Medicine; Associate Professor of Medicine

Aleksandar Jovanovic, Ph.D.
Research Fellow in Cardiovascular Diseases; Instructor in Medicine

Sofija Jovanovic, D.V.M., Ph.D.
Research Fellow in Cardiovascular Diseases

Barry L. Karon, M.D.
Consultant, Division of Cardiovascular Diseases and Internal Medicine; Assistant Professor of Medicine

Stephen L. Kopecky, M.D.
Consultant, Division of Cardiovascular Diseases and Internal Medicine; Associate Professor of Medicine

Thomas E. Kottke, M.D.
Consultant, Division of Cardiovascular Diseases and Internal Medicine; Professor of Medicine

Iftikhar J. Kullo, M.D.
Senior Associate Consultant, Division of Cardiovascular Diseases and Internal Medicine; Instructor in Medicine

André C. Lapeyre III, M.D.
Consultant, Division of Cardiovascular Diseases and Internal Medicine; Assistant Professor of Medicine

Amir Lerman, M.D.
Consultant, Division of Cardiovascular Diseases and Internal Medicine; Associate Professor of Medicine

Margaret A. Lloyd, M.D.
Consultant, Division of Cardiovascular Diseases and Internal Medicine; Assistant Professor of Medicine

Robert D. McBane, M.D.
Senior Associate Consultant, Division of Cardiovascular Diseases and Internal Medicine; Instructor in Medicine

Marian T. McEvoy, M.D.
Consultant, Department of Dermatology; Associate Professor of Dermatology

Michael D. McGoon, M.D.
Consultant, Division of Cardiovascular Diseases and Internal Medicine; Professor of Medicine

Fletcher A. Miller, Jr., M.D.
Consultant, Division of Cardiovascular Diseases and Internal Medicine; Professor of Medicine

Victor M. Montori, M.D.
Chief Medical Resident in Internal Medicine

Brian P. Mullan, M.D.
Consultant, Department of Diagnostic Radiology; Assistant Professor of Radiology

Thomas M. Munger, M.D.
Consultant, Division of Cardiovascular Diseases and Internal Medicine; Assistant Professor of Medicine

Joseph G. Murphy, M.D.
Consultant, Division of Cardiovascular Diseases and Internal Medicine; Associate Professor of Medicine

Rick A. Nishimura, M.D.
Consultant, Division of Cardiovascular Diseases and Internal Medicine; Professor of Medicine

Thomas P. Nobrega, M.D.
Senior Associate Consultant, Division of Cardiovascular Diseases and Internal Medicine; Instructor in Medicine

Jae K. Oh, M.D.
Consultant, Division of Cardiovascular Diseases and Internal Medicine; Professor of Medicine

James H. O'Keefe, M.D.
Clinical Nuclear Cardiologist, Mid America Heart Institute; Associate Professor of Medicine, University of Missouri, Kansas City Medical School; Kansas City, Missouri

Lance J. Oyen, Pharm.D.
Pharmacist

Douglas L. Packer, M.D.
Consultant, Division of Cardiovascular Diseases and Internal Medicine; Professor of Medicine

John G. Park, M.D.
Fellow in Pulmonary Medicine

Robin Patel, M.D.
Senior Associate Consultant, Division of Infectious Diseases and Internal Medicine; Assistant Professor of Medicine

Udaya B. S. Prakash, M.D.
Consultant, Division of Pulmonary and Critical Care Medicine and Internal Medicine; Professor of Medicine

Nalini Rajamannan, M.D.
Fellow in Cardiovascular Diseases; Instructor in Medicine

Robert F. Rea, M.D.
Consultant, Division of Cardiovascular Diseases and Internal Medicine; Associate Professor of Medicine

Margaret M. Redfield, M.D.
Consultant, Division of Cardiovascular Diseases and Internal Medicine; Associate Professor of Medicine

Guy S. Reeder, M.D.
Consultant, Division of Cardiovascular Diseases and Internal Medicine; Professor of Medicine

Charanjit S. Rihal, M.D.
Consultant, Division of Cardiovascular Diseases and Internal Medicine; Associate Professor of Medicine

Richard J. Rodeheffer, M.D.
Consultant, Division of Cardiovascular Diseases and Internal Medicine; Professor of Medicine

John A. Rumberger, Ph.D., M.D.
Consultant, Division of Cardiovascular Diseases and Internal Medicine; Professor of Medicine

Paula J. Santrach, M.D.
Consultant, Division of Transfusion Medicine; Assistant Professor of Laboratory Medicine

Robert S. Schwartz, M.D.
Consultant, Division of Cardiovascular Diseases and Internal Medicine; Professor of Medicine

Win-Kuang Shen, M.D.
Consultant, Division of Cardiovascular Diseases and Internal Medicine; Associate Professor of Medicine

Clarence Shub, M.D.
Consultant, Division of Cardiovascular Diseases and Internal Medicine; Professor of Medicine

Robert D. Simari, M.D.
Consultant, Division of Cardiovascular Diseases and Internal Medicine; Associate Professor of Medicine

Hugh C. Smith, M.D.
Consultant, Division of Cardiovascular Diseases and Internal Medicine; Professor of Medicine

Peter C. Spittell, M.D.
Consultant, Division of Cardiovascular Diseases and Internal Medicine; Assistant Professor of Medicine

Marshall S. Stanton, M.D.
Consultant, Division of Cardiovascular Diseases and Internal Medicine; Associate Professor of Medicine

James M. Steckelberg, M.D.
Consultant, Division of Infectious Diseases and Internal Medicine; Professor of Medicine

Naeem K. Tahirkheli, M.D.
Fellow in Cardiovascular Diseases

A. Jamil Tajik, M.D.
Chair, Division of Cardiovascular Diseases and Internal Medicine; Professor of Medicine and of Pediatrics

Andre Terzic, M.D., Ph.D.
Consultant, Division of Cardiovascular Diseases and Internal Medicine and Department of Pharmacology; Associate Professor of Medicine and of Pharmacology

Daniel J. Tiede, M.D.
Senior Associate Consultant, Division of Cardiovascular Diseases and Internal Medicine; Instructor in Medicine

Carole A. Warnes, M.D.
Consultant, Division of Cardiovascular Diseases and Internal Medicine; Professor of Medicine

Sze-Man J. Wong, M.D.
Fellow in Cardiovascular Diseases

R. Scott Wright, M.D.
Senior Associate Consultant, Division of Cardiovascular Diseases and Internal Medicine; Assistant Professor of Medicine

MAYO CLINIC CARDIOLOGY REVIEW

SECOND EDITION

Chapter 1

The Cardiology Boards

Joseph G. Murphy, M.D.
Naeem Tahirkheli, M.D.

The function of the American Board of Internal Medicine (ABIM) is to enhance the quality of health care by maintaining standards for certifying internists and subspecialists.

The ABIM certification and recertification subspecialty examination in cardiovascular diseases is held annually in November.

Studying Cardiology

In the study of cardiology, it is important to fully understand normal cardiac physiology before learning the pathophysiology of cardiac diseases. Learning is greatly facilitated by incorporating new information into a preexisting framework of knowledge rather than memorizing the extraneous "facts of cardiology."

Several methods can make the study of cardiology more interactive and interesting and, in the end, more productive. A useful study method is to devise examination type multiple choice questions and then formulate in your mind the framework and logic behind the answer. This method will help to identify holes in your knowledge which can be filled in by consulting textbooks, journals, and colleagues. The advantage of this method is that you develop a "questioning attitude" that makes your reading of material an active, searching process rather than a passive, absorptive one.

Another useful study technique is to write all you know from memory about a specific topic in 30 minutes (time yourself). Although this is an old-fashioned way of learning, you will identify areas of ignorance and hone your powers of planning answers and organizing the material.

Another interactive way of learning is to select a question and to explain the answer to a friend, figuratively or literally. This will hone your skills at thinking through an answer in a logical way.

The Cardiology Boards

This examination consists of several hundred questions answered over a 2-day period. Topics covered on the examination are listed in Table 1. The examination is administered in several modules, with 60 questions per test book to be completed in 2 hours each. The examinations contain multiple-choice questions that test clinical judgment, decision making, and factual cardiovascular knowledge. In addition to multiple-choice questions, there are testing sessions in electrocardiographic (ECG) tracings and cardiac motion imaging studies (echocardiograms, ventriculograms, coronary arteriograms, and angiograms) presented in a still image print format. Each session is 2 hours.

Answers for all questions must be recorded on separate answer sheets. Credit is given only for answers recorded on the answer sheet within the time allowed for the examination session. After time has expired for a session, no extra time will be permitted for transferring answers to answer sheets.

Table 1.—Topics Tested on the Cardiology Board Examination*

Basic sciences
    Anatomy
    Pathology
    Physiology
    Pharmacology
Cardiac arrhythmias
Coronary artery disease
Primary myocardial disease and congestive heart failure
Pericardial disease
Valvular disease
Diseases of the aorta and peripheral vessels and lipid
  disorders
Hypertensive and pulmonary disease
Preventive and rehabilitative cardiology

*The examination includes questions on general internal medicine, critical care medicine, and cardiovascular surgery that pertain to the practice of cardiology.

To become certified in cardiovascular disease, a passing score must be achieved on two components: the ECG section and the multiple-choice questions and motion studies. Most questions are based on the presentation of clinical vignettes in outpatient, emergency room, and coronary care settings. The presentations are meant to simulate real-life situations and may be very detailed. A list of normal laboratory values is provided as needed. Refer to this list to interpret values given in an examination. These values could differ from those to which you are accustomed.

Also included on the examination are questions on basic cardiac and vascular physiology and pharmacology. These questions are usually directly applicable to clinical management of patients, such as the mode of action of antiarrhythmic agents, cholesterol metabolism, and vascular wall biology. Disease diagnosis, pathophysiology, and patient management—rather than isolated facts about cardiology—are stressed. The indications for and potential complications associated with cardiac procedures are emphasized rather than the technical aspects of the procedures.

The clinical applications of lessons learned from the major cardiology trials are important. Correct management of emergency situations is frequently tested and, in many cases, is considered a core competence.

In general, a moderately conservative approach to invasive investigations and treatments is appropriate. The guidelines of the American College of Cardiology/American Heart Association for specific cardiology investigations and treatments should be known in detail.

Candidates are expected to be able to interpret complex ECGs and pacemaker rhythm strips, hemodynamic recordings, coronary angiograms, ventriculograms, chest radiographs, and echocardiograms (including Doppler examinations). Basic electrophysiologic recordings, including His bundle electrograms, may be tested. Basic computed tomographic scans, positron emission tomographic scans, nuclear scans, and classic endomyocardial biopsy specimens may also be shown as part of the clinical vignette. Several weeks before the examination, candidates receive an information booklet that provides a detailed description of all question types and any new changes the Board has made in the examination format. It is extremely important to study the ECG answer sheet supplied with the booklet, because the ABIM may change the ECG answer codes in minor ways from year to year.

Example of a Board-Type Question

As mentioned above, the examination consists of only single-best-answer type questions, excluding K-type questions (e.g., A and C are correct or B and D are correct). Single-best-answer questions consist of a question stem (statement), which frequently is a patient case history that may incorporate laboratory data, diagnostic imaging, or pathologic slides, and a specific question and list of possible options. Each of the options is lettered (A, B, C, etc.). You are to choose the one best answer and blacken completely the appropriate lettered circle on the answer sheet, which is numbered to correspond to the items in the test book. Options other than the single best (correct) answer may be partially correct, but you must choose the one answer that is better than the others. An example follows:

A 75-year-old black man has a 6-month history of increasing dyspnea on effort. He denies orthopnea and paroxysmal nocturnal dyspnea. He had an episode of dizziness while lifting his 5-year-old grandchild at a family reunion last fall. He also has recently noted chest-tightness pain when he walks up a hill near his house. He does not report any palpitations. Several years ago his local physician noted a systolic murmur, but this was not investigated further at the time.

His medical history includes a shrapnel wound to his left leg in World War II, cholecystectomy 10 years ago for cholelithiasis complicated by postoperative septicemia, and recent cataract surgery on the left eye. He has had non-insulin-dependent diabetes mellitus for 5 years and takes an oral hypoglycemic agent. He has a 40-pack-year smoking history but stopped 10 years ago. He has a remote history of excess alcohol use.

On physical examination, the patient is about 40 pounds overweight. He has a loud ejection systolic murmur at the heart base that radiates to the neck but no diastolic murmur. The brachial pulse is normal in character. The apex beat is difficult to appreciate because of the patient's obesity. The first and second heart sounds are distant in intensity and no added sounds are heard. The murmur does not vary appreciably with the Valsalva maneuver. Jugular venous pressure is normal. The patient has a right femoral bruit but no carotid or abdominal bruits.

The results of laboratory studies are normal except for a moderate increase in the serum concentration of creatinine (1.3), a moderate increase in the serum level of glucose (148), and the presence of mild hematuria and proteinuria on urinalysis.

What investigation should you order next?
   a. Doppler flow studies of the carotid arteries
   b. Exercise sestamibi stress test
   c. Imatron (electron beam computed tomography) scan of the heart
   d. Coronary angiography
   e. Transthoracic echocardiography with Doppler studies

The logic behind this question is that the examination candidate is required first to make a probable diagnosis and then to choose the best imaging modality to confirm the diagnosis. This question requires a combination of knowledge and judgment about the most likely diagnosis in order to select the correct answer. A reasonable argument can be made for any of the imaging modalities and many are partially correct. However, one answer is more correct than the others.

This history is typical of a patient history with which all practicing cardiologists should be familiar. The initial part of the history suggests the diagnosis of aortic stenosis, but this is not fully supported by the normal brachial pulse. The other physical signs are deliberately vague (the nonpalpable apex, the distant heart sounds, etc.)
Possible answers:

a. Although it is possible that the patient has significant cerebrovascular disease and has had at least one possible cerebrovascular symptom (dizziness), the rest of the history and examination does not strongly suggest this as the primary diagnosis. However, the femoral bruit and the history of diabetes and smoking are consistent with the diagnosis of vascular disease.

b. The patient may also have severe coronary artery disease, which is supported by the history of mild angina and strong risk factors. In a hemodynamically stable patient, the examination board generally likes to see a progression from noninvasive to invasive studies and from less expensive to more expensive studies. Thus, although an exercise sestamibi stress test would be appropriate if the patient's primary problem were coronary artery disease, it would be problematic if the correct diagnosis was critical aortic stenosis. The old leg injury may be a problem with an exercise test, but there is insufficient information to make a definitive judgment about whether the patient has a good exercise capacity.

c. Electron beam computed tomography is likely to show coronary calcification, but this information is likely to be of little clinical value in an elderly patient.

d. If the patient's condition were hemodynamically unstable, an argument could be made for coronary angiography and aortic valve assessment. This would not be the best initial investigation at this stage but may be indicated if the patient required aortic valve surgery for critical aortic stenosis or if the severity of the patient's aortic valve disease as assessed echocardiographically was not concordant with his symptoms.

e. Transthoracic echocardiography appears to be the imaging modality likely to give the most useful clinical information without significant risk to the patient. Although a normal brachial pulse does not support the diagnosis of aortic stenosis, neither does it exclude the possibility in an elderly patient with likely noncompliant arterial vessels.

Note that the history contains a significant amount of "distracting" material, as do histories in real clinical situations: ethnic status, history of cholecystectomy and cataract surgery, and urinary tract infection.

The core question is "Does the candidate understand the correct management of an elderly, hemodynamically stable patient with increasing dyspnea on exertion, mild angina, and a possible presyncopal episode, with physical findings compatible with aortic stenosis?"

Candidates should approach this convoluted question by understanding that each question on the examination tests a core competence that generally can be stated in one sentence.

Data About Results of Cardiology Board Examinations

The average overall pass rate for candidates taking the Internal Medicine Board Examination for 1994 to 1997 was 51% to 69%: for first-time candidates, 65% to 85%; for repeat candidates, 34% to 52%. The results for the 1997 cardiology subspecialty board examination were 66% overall, 71% for first-time candidates, and 45% for repeat candidates. For candidates recertifying in internal medicine and cardiology, the pass rates were 91% and 82%, respectively.

Cardiovascular disease will be the single largest area tested in the 1999 ABIM Internal Medicine Examination, accounting for 14% of the questions. Most of the examination questions (about 75%) are based on patient presentations. The settings of the encounters reflect current medical practice, so most occur in an outpatient or emergency room setting; the rest occur in an inpatient setting, from an intensive care unit to a long-term-care facility. The majority of questions require the integration of information from several sources, the prioritization of alternatives, and clinical judgment to reach a correct conclusion. Few questions require simple recall of medical facts.

Interventional Cardiology Board Examination
The Interventional Cardiology Board Examination is a proctored 1-day test consisting of single-best-answer, multiple-choice questions designed to assess the candidate's knowledge and clinical judgment in aspects of interventional cardiology required to perform at a high level of competence. The areas tested are listed in Table 2.

Clinical Cardiac Electrophysiology Examination
The Clinical Cardiac Electrophysiology Examination is a proctored 1-day written test consisting of multiple-choice questions of the single-best-answer type. It assesses the candidate's knowledge and clinical judgment in aspects of cardiac electrophysiology required to perform at a high level of competence. These areas are listed in Table 3.

Tips for the Cardiology Board Examination

In the ECG and imaging sections of the Cardiology Board examination, pay special attention to the clinical descriptors that accompany the tracings and images. It's often here that the key to the correct diagnosis will be found.

Clinical Clues to the ECG Tracing Diagnosis

Metabolic ECGs
- A history of recent vomiting, pancreatitis, thyroid surgery, or multiple blood transfusions in a patient should suggest

a diagnosis of hypocalcemia and prolongation of the QT interval.
- A clinical history of renal failure or dialysis should alert the candidate to the classical ECG findings of both hyperkalemia and hypocalcemia.

The Healthy Patient
- Frequently, the examination ECG is of a healthy person who has had an incidental ECG as a requirement for life insurance or employment. This question is geared to

Table 2.—Areas Tested in the Interventional Cardiology Board Examination

Case selection (25%)
- Indications for angioplasty and related catheter-based interventions in management of ischemic heart disease, including factors that differentiate patients who require interventional procedures rather than coronary artery bypass surgery or medical therapy
- Indications for urgent catheterization in management of acute myocardial infarction, including factors that differentiate patients who require angioplasty, intracoronary thrombolysis, or coronary artery bypass surgery
- Indications for mitral, aortic, and pulmonary valvuloplasty in management of valvular disorders, including factors that differentiate patients who require surgical commissurotomy or valve repair or replacement
- Indications for catheter-based interventions in management of congenital heart disease in adults
- Indications for interventional approaches to management of hemodynamic compromise in patients who have acute coronary symptoms, including the use of pharmacologic agents, balloon counterpulsation, emergency pacing, and stent placement

Procedural techniques (25%)
- Planning and execution of interventional procedures, including knowledge of options, limitations, outcomes, and complications as well as alternatives to be used if an initial approach fails
- Selection and use of guiding catheters, guidewires, balloon catheters, and other FDA-approved interventional devices, including atherectomy devices and coronary stents
- Knowledge of intravascular catheter techniques and their risks
- Use of antithrombotic agents in interventional procedures
- Management of hemorrhagic complications

Table 2 (continued)

Basic science (15%)

    Vascular biology, including the processes of plaque formation, vascular injury, vasoreactivity, vascular healing, and restenosis

    Hematology, including the clotting cascade, platelet function, thrombolysis, and methods of altering clot formation

    Coronary anatomy and physiology, including angiographic data such as distribution of vascular segments, lesion characteristics, and their importance in interventions; alterations in coronary flow due to obstructions in vessels; the assessment and effect of flow dynamics on myocardial perfusion; the function of collateral circulation; and the effect of arterial spasm or microembolization on coronary flow

Pharmacology (20%)

    Biologic effects and appropriate use of vasoactive drugs, antiplatelet agents, thrombolytics, anticoagulants, and antiarrhythmics

    Biologic effects and appropriate use of angiographic contrast agents

Imaging (10%)

    Specific applications of imaging to interventional cardiology, including identification of anatomical features and visualization of lesion morphology by angiography and intravascular ultrasonography

    Radiation physics, radiation risks and injury, and radiation safety, including methods to control radiation exposure for patients, physicians, and technicians

Miscellaneous (5%)

    Ethical issues and risks associated with diagnostic and therapeutic techniques

    Statistics, epidemiologic data, and economic issues related to interventional procedures

Table 3.—Areas Tested in the Clinical Cardiac Electrophysiology Examination

Basic electrophysiology, including formation and propagation of normal and abnormal impulses, autonomic nervous control of cardiac electrical activity, and mechanisms of clinically significant arrhythmias and conduction disturbances

Evaluation and management of patients, both ambulatory and hospitalized, who have clinical syndromes resulting from bradyarrhythmias or tachyarrhythmias

Indications for and interpretation of noninvasive diagnostic studies, including esophageal, scalar, and signal-averaged electrocardiography, ambulatory electrocardiography, continuous in-hospital cardiac monitoring, exercise testing, tilt testing, and relevant imaging studies

Indications for and interpretation of diagnostic intracardiac electrophysiologic studies, and techniques of performing these studies

Indications for and effects of noninvasive therapeutic techniques, including esophageal and transcutaneous pacing, cardioversion, defibrillation, and cardiopulmonary resuscitation

Indications for and effects of invasive therapeutic techniques, including pacemaker and cardioverter-defibrillator implantation and catheter and surgical ablation of/for arrhythmias

Pharmacology, pharmacokinetics, and use of antiarrhythmic agents and other drugs that affect cardiac electrical activity

Some questions test an understanding of ethical issues and of the risks associated with diagnostic and therapeutic techniques and knowledge of the sensitivity and specificity of diagnostic studies

test the candidate's knowledge of ECG variants such as juvenile T waves, repolarization changes, and so forth. The ECG may also show features that suggest previously undiagnosed cardiac disease such as hypertrophic cardiomyopathy, congenital heart disease, atrial septal defect, mitral valve disease, long QT syndrome, or Wolff-Parkinson-White syndrome. Be alert for whether the patient is asymptomatic with a normal cardiac examination or is asymptomatic with a systolic murmur.

The Postoperative Patient

- Immediately after heart surgery—look for

hypothermia (Osborne wave), pericarditis (PR-segment depression and concave ST-segment elevation), pericardial effusion (low-voltage ECG), and pericardial tamponade (electrical alternans). If new Q waves are present after surgery, be extremely careful about diagnosing a perioperative myocardial infarction as sternotomy; cardiac manipulation at surgery may simulate infarction. In general, the diagnosis of myocardial infarction following cardiac surgery should not be made solely on the basis of an ECG tracing but should be supported by other clinical, enzyme, and echocardiographic evidence.

- In all postoperative patients who develop dyspnea or pleuritic chest pain or who are hemodynamically unstable, always consider pulmonary embolus ($S_1Q_3T_3$, right ventricular strain pattern, etc.).

Arrhythmias

- A history of aborted sudden death or recurrent syncope in a young patient or a strong family history of sudden death should suggest hypertrophic cardiomyopathy, long QT syndrome, or Brugada syndrome.
- Wide complex tachycardia in the setting of structural heart disease is ventricular tachycardia until proved otherwise.
- In patients with atrial fibrillation, look carefully at the ventricular response to determine whether it is regular— this may signify complete heart block, whereas an excessively fast ventricular response may suggest the possibility of Wolff-Parkinson-White syndrome.
- The presence of sinus bradycardia or the Wenkebach phenomenon may be a normal finding in an athletic patient but should be scored for examination purposes.
- Digoxin toxicity is an important clinical and ECG diagnosis; be aware of it. Digoxin toxicity is always tested in some form in most cardiology and internal medicine examinations. Paroxysmal atrial tachycardia with atrioventricular block and bidirectional ventricular tachycardia (originates from both left and right ventricles) are the two cardiac rhythms that strongly suggest the diagnosis. Instead of specifically stating that the patient was taking digoxin, the clinical history may state that the patient was taking cardiac medications. Be alert for patients taking heart failure medications who develop hypokalemia, because this can precipitate digoxin toxicity.

Chest Pain

- When coding myocardial infarctions, ST-segment elevation is acute myocardial injury and Q waves are infarction. Watch for posterior infarcts.
- Positional or pleuritic chest pain is pericarditis or pulmonary embolus until proved otherwise.
- The best examination strategy for the ECG section of the cardiology boards is a conservative approach, with careful coding of significant abnormalities, whereas debatable answers are best left uncoded. In patients with wide complex tachycardia, err on the side of coding ventricular tachycardia rather than supraventricular tachycardia with abberant conduction, because coding of the latter may lead to inappropriate and dangerous clinical

care. When in doubt, assume, for the purposes of the boards, that the patient has the more dangerous condition. Look carefully for diagnostic clues that will clinch the diagnosis of ventricular tachycardia such as fusion beats and capture beats. It is quite unlikely that the cardiology boards will show a truly ambiguous ECG.

- The best way to prepare for the ECG section of the examination is to code a large number of patient ECGs using examination-type scoring criteria. The ECG criteria listed in the ECG criteria chapter in this book are similar to the criteria used by the Boards but minor changes are made from year to year in the examination scoring criteria. These changes are announced in the instructions to candidates several weeks before the examination and may not be completely reflected in the chapter in this book.

Clinical Clues to Identification of Aortograms and Ventriculograms

- On the examination, aortograms typically show aortic incompetence, coarctation of the aorta, aortic dissection, patent ductus arteriosus, abberant subclavian vessels, or an aortic root perivalvular abscess. Clinical clues to the above diagnoses are, respectively, diastolic murmur, differential hypertension between arms and legs, severe back pain, continuous murmur, difficulty swallowing, and recent infective endocarditis or septicemia.
- In left ventriculograms and coronary angiograms in young patients, look for coronary artery anomalies, patent ductus arteriosus, and intraventricular shunt.
- In a right ventricular angiogram, look for interventricular shunt (ventricular septal defect) and pulmonary stenosis.
- In a left ventricular angiogram of a patient with Down syndrome, look for ostium primum/endocardial cushion defect (goose-neck abnormality of left ventricular outflow tract).
- For an unusual catheter path/position shown with an angiogram, look for persistent left superior vena cava, catheter crossing a patent foramen ovale, or patent ductus arteriosis.
- Be familiar with the appearance of mitral valve prolapse on a left ventriculogram.
- Always examine a left ventriculogram for the presence of mitral regurgitation on both RAO and LAO projections.
- Examine for a perivalvular leak in an aortic prosthetic valve on an aortogram. Note that a small amount of

regurgitation through a prosthetic valve is normal and is designed to "wash" the valve leaflet and to inhibit thrombosis.

- Coding of regional wall abnormalities on static ventriculogram images is difficult and should be practiced before the examination.

Important Angiographic Images

- Coronary anomalies, especially an anomalous right coronary artery taking origin from the left aortic cusp and an anomalous left circumflex coronary artery taking origin from the right aortic cusp
- Patent ductus arteriosus
- Pulmonic stenosis/tetralogy of Fallot on a right ventriculogram
- Persistent left superior vena cava
- Intracoronary dissection after percutaneous transluminal coronary angioplasty (PTCA)
- Intracoronary thrombus
- Coronary ectasia and aneurysmal disease
- Specifically look at the left main coronary artery in all coronary angiograms.
- If two identical coronary angiographic projections are shown for comparison, look for coronary vasospasm (before and after nitroglycerin infusion) or myocardial bridging (systolic vs diastolic).
- On a coronary angiogram after coronary intervention, look for dissection and /or thrombus.
- In an angiogram of a patient with acute myocardial infarction/unstable angina, look for intracoronary thrombus.

Important Electrophysiology and Pacemaker Tracings

- His bundle electrograms for *suprahisian* (atrioventricular nodal) and *infrahisian* block
- His bundle electrograms in atrioventricular dissociation/complete atrioventricular block
- Sudden AH prolongation before initiation of tachycardia is diagnostic of atrioventricular nodal reentrant tachycardia
- If the His bundle deflection (H spike) cannot be recognized or the HV spike is negative, the diagnosis is ventricular tachycardia or preexcited tachycardia.
- Atrioventricular nodal blocking agents are *not necessarily contraindicated* for regular (atrioventricular reentrant tachycardia) or rhythm (narrow or wide complex) tachycardia associated with an accessory bypass tract

(Wolff-Parkinson-White syndrome). However, they are *strongly contraindicated* for atrial fibrillation (irregular rhythm) in such a patient.
- If a narrow complex tachycardia becomes a wide complex tachycardia and the cycle length increases (rate slows) when the tachycardia becomes wide complex, the diagnosis is atrioventricular reentrant tachycardia via a bypass tract.
- In pacemaker rhythms, even when there is no atrial spike, the patient has a dual chamber pacemaker if the ventricular spike always follows the p wave at a fixed interval.
- Be familiar with pacemaker-mediated tachycardia, safety pacing, pacemaker syndrome, and upper rate limit pacemaker behavior (mode switching, etc).

Important Echocardiographic Images

- Infective endocarditis (vegetations, abscess, leaflet perforation)
- Atrial thrombus or myxoma
- Dilated cardiomyopathy
- Hypertrophic cardiomyopathy with or without dynamic obstruction
- Restrictive cardiomyopathy, including eosinophilia syndromes and obliterative cardiomyopathy
- Amyloid heart disease (marked increase in left ventricular thickness, with relatively low-voltage ECG), which is in contrast to left ventricular hypertrophy or hypertrophic cardiomyopathy, which exhibit an increase in left ventricular thickness with large voltages on the ECG.
- Tricuspid valve disease, including Ebstein anomaly (large right atrium and apical descent of tricuspid leaflets) and carcinoid syndrome
- Mitral valve disease, including mitral valve prolapse (must see prolapse in more than one plane), mitral stenosis, and mitral incompetence (know the basis for proximal isovelocity surface area [PISA] estimation of mitral regurgitation)
- Aortic valve disease, including aortic stenosis, bicuspid nonstenotic aortic valve, aortic incompetence
- Simple congenital heart defects, including atrial septal defect, ventricular defect, pulmonary stenosis, tetralogy of Fallot, patent ductus arteriosus, and coarctation of the aorta
- Pericardial disease, including pericardial effusion and constrictive pericarditis
- M-mode echocardiographic images may also be shown

on the board examination. Look specifically for mitral valve prolapse, fluttering of the anterior mitral leaflet associated with aortic regurgitation, and systolic anterior motion of the mitral leaflet in hypertrophic cardiomyopathy.

Physical Signs

> All cardiology and internal medicine examinations contain physical examination questions or clinical vignettes that rely on clues from the physical examination.

The following physical signs are particularly important:
1. Jugular venous pulsations
   - Large "V" wave—think of tricuspid regurgitation, especially if it is associated with a pulsating liver.
   - Rapid "Y" descent is usually associated with constrictive pericarditis.
   - Cannon "A" waves with tachycardia suggest ventricular tachycardia.
2. Arterial pulses
   - Bifid arterial pulse of aortic regurgitation and aortic stenosis combined, the characteristic pulse of hypertrophic cardiomyopathy (spike-and-dome pattern), or the dicrotic pulse seen in advanced heart failure
   - Pulsus parvus et tardus for severe aortic stenosis
   - Pulsus alternans for severe heart failure
   - Pulsus paradoxus of cardiac tamponade or severe lung disease
3. Apex beat palpation
   - Bifid or trifid apex beat impulse is usually associated with hypertrophic cardiomyopathy.
   - Palpable fourth heart sound is frequently associated with left ventricular hypertrophy.
   - Palpable third heart sound is associated with heart failure and severe mitral regurgitation.
4. Auscultation
   - Loud first heart sound of mitral stenosis; however, a soft first heart sound does not exclude severe mitral

stenosis and may reflect fixed, nonmobile calcified mitral valve leaflets (probably not a good candidate for mitral valve balloon valvuloplasty).
- If a widely split first heart sound occurs, consider Ebstein anomaly.
- Wide fixed splitting of the second heart sound is synonymous with atrial septal defect.
- If paradoxical splitting of the second heart sound occurs, consider paced rhythms in addition to severe aortic stenosis or left bundle branch block.
- Absent aortic second heart sound indicates severe aortic stenosis.
- The only right-sided sound (murmur, click, or heart sound) that decreases with inspiration is the pulmonary ejection click.
- If opening snap (OS) is present, remember that left atrial pressure, and thus the severity of mitral stenosis, can be gauged by the interval between the second heart sound and the opening snap (similarly for the opening sound associated with some mechanical prosthetic heart valves in the mitral position, e.g., Starr-Edwards valve). The shorter the second heart sound–OS timing, the higher the left atrial pressure.
- A third heart sound in the absence of overt heart failure may reflect severe mitral regurgitation even if the mitral murmur is soft or even absent. A murmur is frequently absent in acute mitral regurgitation. Color Doppler studies may also rarely be negative in the presence of severe mitral regurgitation if no turbulence is present.
- If on physical examination there are cannon "A" waves or variable splitting or intensity of the first or second heart sound in association with a regular wide complex tachycardia on the ECG, think of ventricular tachycardia. Look for flutter waves in the jugular venous waveform (JVP) in cases of suspected atrial flutter.
- Examination candidates should be conversant with the effects of various maneuvers on heart murmurs: especially amyl nitrite, the Valsalva maneuver, squatting and sudden standing, and the effect following an extrasystolic beat (PVC) (Tables 4 and 5).

Table 4.—Interventions Used to Alter the Intensity of Cardiac Murmurs

Respiration

Right-sided murmurs generally increase with inspiration. Left-sided murmurs usually are louder during expiration

Valsalva maneuver

Most murmurs decrease in length and intensity. Two exceptions are the systolic murmur of HCM, which usually becomes much louder, and that of MVP, which becomes longer and often louder. Following release of the Valsalva maneuver, right-sided murmurs tend to return to baseline intensity earlier than left-sided murmurs

Exercise

Murmurs caused by blood flow across normal or obstructed valves (e.g., PS, MS) become louder with both isotonic and submaximal isometric (handgrip) exercise. Murmurs of MR, VSD, and AR also increase with handgrip exercise. However, the murmur of HCM often decreases with near-maximum handgrip exercise

Positional changes

With standing, most murmurs diminish; 2 exceptions are the murmur of HCM, which becomes louder, and that of MVP, which lengthens and often is intensified. With prompt squatting, most murmurs become louder, but those of HCM and MVP usually soften and may disappear. Passive leg raising usually produces the same results as prompt squatting

Postventricular premature beat or atrial fibrillation

Murmurs originating at normal or stenotic semilunar valves increase in intensity during the cardiac cycle following a VPB or in the beat after a long cycle length in AF. By contrast, systolic murmurs due to atrioventricular valve regurgitation do not change, diminish (papillary muscle dysfunction), or become shorter (MVP)

Pharmacologic interventions

During the initial relative hypotension following amyl nitrite inhalation, murmurs of MR, VSD, and AR decrease, whereas those of AS increase because of increased stroke volume. During the later tachycardia phase, murmurs of MS and right-sided lesions also increase. This intervention may thus distinguish the murmur of the Austin Flint phenomenon from that of MS. The response in MVP often is biphasic (softer, then louder than control)

Transient arterial occlusion

Transient external compression of both arms by bilateral cuff inflation to 20 mm Hg greater than peak systolic pressure augments the murmurs of MR, VSD, and AR but not murmurs due to other causes

AF, atrial fibrillation; AR, aortic regurgitation; AS, aortic stenosis; HCM, hypertrophic cardiomyopathy; MR, mitral regurgitation; MS, mitral stenosis; MVP, mitral valve prolapse; PS, pulmonic stenosis; VPB, ventricular premature beat; VSD, ventricular septal defect.

From *J Am Coll Cardiol* 32:1486-1588, 1998. By permission of the American College of Cardiology.

Table 5.—Factors That Differentiate the Various Causes of Left Ventricular Outflow Tract Obstruction

	Valvular	Supravalvular	Discrete subvalvular	HOCM
Valve calcification	Common after age 40 yr	No	No	No
Dilated ascending aorta	Common	Rare	Rare	Rare
PP after VPB	Increased	Increased	Increased	Decreased
Valsalva effect on SM	Decreased	Decreased	Decreased	Increased
Murmur of AR	Common	Rare	Sometimes	No
Fourth heart sound	If severe	Uncommon	Uncommon	Common
Paradoxic splitting	Sometimes*	No	No	Rather common*
Ejection click	Most (unless valve calcified)	No	No	Uncommon or none
Maximal thrill and murmur	2nd RIS	1st RIS	2nd RIS	4th LIS
Carotid pulse	Normal to anacrotic* (parvus et tardus)	Unequal	Normal to anacrotic	Brisk, jerky, systolic rebound

AR, aortic regurgitation; HOCM, hypertrophic obstructive cardiomyopathy; LIS, left intercostal space; PP, pulse pressure; RIS, right intercostal space; SM, systolic murmur; VPB, ventricular premature beat.

*Depends on severity.

Modified from Marriott HJL: *Bedside Cardiac Diagnosis.* JB Lippincott Company, 1993, p 116. By permission of the publisher.

Summary of Physical Signs in Cardiovascular Disease

Left Ventricular Failure

1. Breathing:
    Tachypnea (secondary to hypoxia and increased intrapulmonary pressures)
    Cheyne-Stokes breathing, in severe heart failure
    Central cyanosis secondary to hypoxia in pulmonary edema
    Peripheral cyanosis with low cardiac output
2. Arterial pulse:
    Hypotension in cardiogenic shock and end-stage heart failure
    Sinus tachycardia due to increased sympathetic tone
    Pulsus alternans (alternate strong and weak beats in end-stage heart failure with regular heart rhythm) — differentiated from bigeminal rhythm, which is alternating regular and ectopic beats (atrial, junctional, or ventricular)
3. JVP:
    Normal in pure left heart failure, but may be increased in right heart failure secondary to left heart failure
4. Apex beat:
    Displaced to the left and inferiorly with left ventricular dilatation of any cause
    Dyskinesia of anterior wall after a large anterior wall myocardial infarction
    Palpable third or fourth heart sound
5. Auscultation:
    Left ventricular third heart sound and/or fourth heart sound
    Functional mitral incompetence murmur (due to valve ring dilatation and central mitral regurgitation)
6. Lung fields:
    Coarse rales of pulmonary edema (due to pulmonary venous hypertension)

Right Ventricular Failure

1. Breathing:
    Peripheral cyanosis due to low cardiac output
2. Arterial pulse:
    Low volume due to low cardiac output
3. JVP:
    Elevated because of increased systemic venous pressure (right heart preload)
    Positive hepatojugular reflex (increase in JVP with hepatic/abdominal compression)
    Kussmaul sign (a paradoxical increase in the height of the JVP due to the inability of the dilated right ventricle to stretch further to accommodate the increased venous return to the right heart that occurs during inspiration). This decreased right ventricular compliance typically occurs with right ventricular myocardial infarction but is also characteristic of tricuspid stenosis and constrictive pericarditis
    Large "V" waves (functional tricuspid regurgitation due to valve ring dilatation) and central mitral regurgitation
4. Precordium:
    Right ventricular lift (heave) at the left sternal border
5. Auscultation:
    Right ventricular third heart sound and/or fourth heart sound, pansystolic murmur of functional tricuspid regurgitation (absence of a murmur does not exclude tricuspid regurgitation)
6. Lung field:
    Pleural effusions (right > left)
7. Abdomen:
    Tender hepatomegaly due to increased venous back pressure transmitted via the hepatic veins; pulsatile liver, if tricuspid regurgitation is present
8. Peripheral edema:
    Due to a combination of fluid retention and increased venous pressure
    Ankle and sacral edema, ascites, or pleural effusions

Acute Pericarditis

Signs:
    Fever
    Three-component pericardial friction rub that may disappear when pericardial fluid accumulates

Chronic Constrictive Pericarditis

1. General signs:
    Cachexia, jaundice if there is significant liver dysfunction
2. Pulse and blood pressure:
    Pulsus paradoxus (more than the normal 10-mm Hg decrease in arterial pulse pressure on inspiration, because increased right ventricular filling reduces left ventricle filling and cardiac output)
    Chronic hypotension
3. JVP:
    Increased JVP

Kussmaul sign (rare)

Prominent "X" and "Y" descents

4. Apex beat:

Frequently impalpable because of thickened pericardium

5. Auscultation:

Distant heart sounds

Diastolic pericardial knock (rapid ventricular filling abruptly halted by constricted pericardium) occurs later than the third heart sound

6. Abdomen:

Hepatomegaly due to increased venous pressure

Splenomegaly due to increased venous pressure

Ascites

7. Periphery:

Peripheral edema

Cardiac Tamponade

1. General signs:

Tachypnea

Severe anxiety

Pallor

Syncope or near syncope

2. Pulse and blood pressure:

Tachycardia

Pulsus paradoxus

Hypotension

3. JVP:

Markedly increased JVP

Kussmaul sign (common)

Prominent "X" but absent "Y" descent

4. Apex beat:

Usually impalpable because of fluid in pericardial space

5. Auscultation:

Soft heart sounds

6. Lung fields:

Dullness and bronchial breathing at left base because of compression of the lingula of the lung by the distended pericardial sac (Ewart sign)

Infective Endocarditis

1. General signs:

Fever

Arthropathy (especially metacarpophalangeal joints, wrists, elbows, knees, ankles)

2. Hands:

Splinter hemorrhages

Finger clubbing (late sign)

Osler nodes (rare), painful skin lesions

Janeway lesions (very rare), painless skin lesions

3. Arms:

Evidence of intravenous drug use, especially in right heart endocarditis

4. Eyes:

Pale conjunctiva (anemia), retinal or conjunctival hemorrhages

Roth spots (fundal vasculitic lesions with a yellow center surrounded by red ring)

5. Heart:

Signs of underlying valvular or congenital heart disease

6. Abdomen:

Hepatomegaly

Splenomegaly

Hematuria

7. Periphery:

Evidence of embolization to abdominal viscera, limbs, or central nervous system

Acute Pulmonary Hypertension

The right ventricle has a limited ability to increase pulmonary artery pressure acutely. Acute pulmonary hypertension usually occurs in the setting of an acute pulmonary embolus and is manifested by acute right ventricular failure. Acute systemic hypotension, hypoxia, and shock may dominate the clinical picture.

Chronic Pulmonary Hypertension

1. General signs:

Dyspnea

Tachypnea

Central cyanosis due to arterial desaturation

Peripheral cyanosis and cold extremities due to low cardiac output at end-stage disease

Hoarseness (rare) due to compression of the left recurrent laryngeal nerve by the pulmonary artery

2. Arterial pulse:

May be low volume because of the low cardiac output at end-stage disease

3. JVP:

Prominent "A" wave as long as sinus rhythm is maintained because of forceful right atrial contraction required to fill hypertrophied right ventricle

4. Precordium:

Right ventricular heave

Palpable second pulmonic sound
Palpable dilated pulmonary artery

5. Auscultation:
   Systolic ejection click due to dilatation of the pulmonary artery
   Loud second pulmonic sound because of forceful pulmonary valve closure due to high pulmonary artery pressure
   Right ventricular fourth and/or third heart sound if right ventricular failure is present
   Pulmonary ejection systolic murmur due to turbulent blood flow in dilated pulmonary artery
   Diastolic pulmonary incompetence murmur if the pulmonary valve ring is significantly dilated and functional pulmonary valve regurgitation occurs

6. Note:
   Additional signs of right ventricular failure will occur in end-stage pulmonary hypertension (cor pulmonale)

Mitral Stenosis

1. General signs:
   Tachypnea
   Mitral facies (combination of vasodilatation and peripheral cyanosis, in severe end-stage mitral stenosis)

2. Arterial pulse and blood pressure:
   Normal or reduced pulse volume due to decreased cardiac output at late stages
   Atrial fibrillation may be present because of left atrial enlargement
   Low blood pressure at late stages of disease

3. JVP:
   Usually normal
   Prominent "A" wave if pulmonary hypertension is present
   Loss of the "A" wave if atrial fibrillation supervenes

4. Precordium:
   Tapping apex beat (due to palpable first heart sound)
   Right ventricular heave
   Palpable second pulmonic sound if pulmonary hypertension is present
   Diastolic thrill (rarely present)

5. Auscultation:
   Loud first heart sound (indicates that the mitral valve leaflets are widely separated, yet mobile at the onset of systole)
   Loud second pulmonic sound if pulmonary hypertension is present

Opening snap (high left atrial pressure forcefully opens the valve leaflets)
Low-pitched rumbling diastolic murmur
Late diastolic accentuation of the diastolic murmur may occur with atrial contraction if the patient is in sinus rhythm, but is usually absent in atrial fibrillation

---

Signs indicating severe mitral stenosis (valve area less than 1 cm^2):
   Low pulse pressure
   Soft first heart sound (immobile valve leaflets)
   Early opening snap (short time from aortic second sound to opening snap because of increased left atrial pressure)
   Long diastolic murmur (persists as long as there is a gradient)
   Diastolic thrill at the apex
   Signs of pulmonary hypertension

Mitral Regurgitation (Chronic)

1. General signs:
   Tachypnea

2. Arterial pulse:
   Usually normal
   Atrial fibrillation is common

3. JVP:
   Normal unless right ventricular failure has occurred
   Loss of "A" wave in atrial fibrillation

4. Palpation:
   Apex beat may be displaced laterally, diffuse, greater than 3 cm in diameter, or hyperdynamic, depending on the extent of ventricular dilatation
   Pansystolic apical thrill
   Parasternal impulse (due to left atrial enlargement behind the right ventricle)

5. Auscultation:
   Soft or absent first heart sound (by the end of diastole, atrial and ventricular pressures have equalized and the valve leaflets have drifted back together)
   Left ventricular third heart sound even in the absence of heart failure, due to rapid left ventricular filling in early diastole
   Pansystolic murmur maximal at the apex (usually radiating toward the axilla)

> Signs indicating severe chronic mitral regurgitation:
> Small volume pulse
> Enlarged left ventricle
> Third heart sound
> Soft first heart sound
> Early aortic second sound because rapid left ventricular emptying into the left atrium in addition to the aorta causes the aortic valve to close early
> Early diastolic rumble (flow murmur due to increased diastolic flow across the mitral valve)
> Signs of pulmonary hypertension
> Signs of left ventricular failure

Acute Mitral Regurgitation

Patients can present with pulmonary edema and cardiovascular collapse. A loud apical ejection murmur is usually present (it is frequently short in duration because atrial pressure is markedly increased). With rupture of anterior leaflet chordae, the murmur radiates to the axilla and back; with rupture of the posterior leaflet, the murmur radiates to the anterior chest wall.

Mitral Valve Prolapse

1. Auscultation:
   Systolic click (usually mid-systolic) may be the only audible abnormality; note that the click is not always audible in patients with documented mitral valve prolapse
   Systolic murmur—high-pitched late peaking systolic murmur commencing with the click and extending throughout the rest of systole
2. Dynamic auscultation:
   Murmur and click occur earlier and may be louder with the Valsalva maneuver and with standing, but both occur later and may be softer with squatting and isometric exercise

Aortic Stenosis

1. General signs:
   Usually nothing specific
2. Pulse:
   There may be a plateau pulse or the pulse may be late peaking (tardus). The pulse is frequently of small volume (parvus) and the pulse pressure is reduced
3. Palpation:
   The apex beat is hyperdynamic (pressure overload) and may be slightly displaced laterally

Systolic thrill at the base of the heart (aortic area)
Carotid shudder
4. Auscultation:
   Narrowly split or reversed split second heart sound because of prolonged left ventricular ejection
   Soft or absent second heart sound
   Rough mid-systolic ejection murmur, maximal over the aortic area and extending into the carotid arteries, is characteristic but may also be heard well at the apex (the murmur is loudest with the patient sitting up in full expiration)
   Associated aortic regurgitation is common
   In congenital aortic stenosis in which the valve cusps remain mobile and the dome of the valve comes to a sudden halt, an ejection click may precede the murmur (the ejection click is absent if the valve is calcified or if the stenosis is not at the valve level)

> Signs indicating severe aortic stenosis (valve area < 0.75 cm^2):
> Plateau pulse
> Thrill in the aortic area
> Prolonged murmur length and lateness of the peak in the systolic murmur
> Fourth heart sound
> Paradoxical splitting of the second heart sound because of greatly delayed aortic valve closure
> Absent aortic second sound
> Left ventricular failure (very late sign)
> Right ventricular failure is preterminal

Named Signs of Aortic Regurgitation

Quincke sign—marked capillary pulsation in the nailbeds, with blanching during diastole with mild nail pressure

Corrigan sign—forceful carotid upstroke with rapid decline

De Musset sign—head nodding in time with the heartbeat

Hill sign—increased blood pressure in the legs compared with the arms (≥ 30 mm Hg discrepancy)

Müller sign—pulsation of the uvula in time with the heartbeat

Duroziez sign—systolic and diastolic bruit over the femoral artery on gradual compression of the vessel by the stethoscope bell

Traube sign—a double sound heard over the femoral artery on

compressing the vessel distally; this is the "pistol-shot" sound that may be heard with very severe aortic regurgitation

Note—these signs are present only in severe chronic aortic incompetence and usually not clinically helpful.

Aortic Regurgitation

1. General signs:
   Marfan syndrome in a small number of patients
   Ankylosing spondylitis or other seronegative arthropathy
2. Pulse and blood pressure:
   The pulse is characteristically collapsing, rapid upstroke followed by a rapid decline
   Wide pulse pressure
3. Neck:
   Prominent carotid pulsations (Corrigan sign)
4. Palpation:
   Apex beat is characteristically displaced laterally and hyperkinetic
   A diastolic thrill may be felt at the left sternal edge when the patient sits forward in expiration
5. Auscultation:
   Aortic second sound may be soft
   A decrescendo high-pitched diastolic murmur beginning immediately after the second heart sound and extending into diastole (it is loudest at the third and fourth left intercostal spaces)
   A systolic ejection murmur is usually present (due to associated aortic stenosis or to torrential flow across a nonstenotic aortic valve)
   Aortic stenosis is distinguished from an aortic flow murmur by the presence of the peripheral signs of significant aortic stenosis, such as a plateau pulse
   Listen for the Austin Flint murmur (a low-pitched rumbling mid-diastolic murmur audible at the apex—the regurgitant jet from the aortic valve causes the anterior mitral valve leaflet to shudder); the murmur is similar to that of mitral stenosis but can be distinguished from mitral stenosis because the first heart sound is not loud and there is no opening snap

> Signs indicating severe chronic aortic regurgitation:
> Collapsing pulse
> Wide pulse pressure
> Long decrescendo diastolic murmur
> Left ventricular third heart sound
> Soft aortic second sound
> Austin Flint murmur
> Signs of left ventricular failure

Tricuspid Stenosis

1. JVP:
   Increased giant "A" waves with a slow "Y" descent may be seen
2. Auscultation:
   Diastolic murmur audible at left sternal edge, accentuated in inspiration, very similar to the murmur of mitral stenosis except for the site of maximal intensity
   Tricuspid stenosis is rare, usually rheumatic in etiology, and is frequently accompanied by mitral stenosis
   No signs of pulmonary hypertension
3. Abdomen:
   Presystolic pulsation of the liver caused by forceful atrial systole

Tricuspid Regurgitation

1. JVP:
   Large "V" waves
   JVP is increased if right ventricular failure has occurred
2. Palpation:
   Right ventricular heave
3. Auscultation:
   A pansystolic murmur maximal at the lower end of the sternum that increases on inspiration is classic but may be absent, and the diagnosis must be made on the basis of peripheral signs alone
4. Abdomen:
   Pulsatile, large, tender liver is usually present
   Ascites, peripheral edema, and pleural effusions may occur
5. Legs:
   Dilated pulsatile veins

Pulmonary Stenosis

1. General signs:
   Peripheral cyanosis (due to low cardiac output)
2. Pulse:
   Normal or reduced (because of a low cardiac output)
3. JVP:
   Giant "A" waves because of right atrial hypertrophy; JVP may be increased because of right heart failure
4. Palpation:
   Right ventricular heave
   Thrill over the pulmonary area
5. Auscultation:
   Murmur may be preceded by an ejection click

Harsh ejection systolic murmur heard best in the pulmonary area and typically present with inspiration

Right ventricular fourth heart sound may be present (because of right atrial hypertrophy)—augments with inspiration

6. Abdomen:

Presystolic pulsation of the liver may be present

Signs of severe pulmonary stenosis:
  Ejection systolic murmur peaking late in systole
  Absence of an ejection click (also absent when the pulmonary stenosis is infundibular, i.e., below the valve level)
  Presence of a fourth heart sound
  Signs of right ventricular failure

Pulmonary Regurgitation

1. Auscultation:

A decrescendo diastolic murmur that is high-pitched and audible at the left sternal edge is characteristic; the murmur increases on inspiration

The "Graham Steell murmur" is functional pulmonary incompetence due to severe mitral stenosis

Signs of pulmonary hypertension may also be present

2. Note:

If there is no sign of pulmonary hypertension, a decrescendo diastolic murmur at the left sternal edge is more likely to be due to aortic regurgitation than to pulmonary regurgitation.

Hypertrophic Cardiomyopathy

1. Pulse:

Sharp-rising and jerky

Rapid ejection by the hypertrophied ventricle early in systole is followed by obstruction caused by the displacement of the mitral valve into the outflow tract. This is very different from the pulse of aortic stenosis

2. JVP:

There usually is a prominent "A" wave, because of forceful atrial contraction against a noncompliant right ventricle

3. Palpation:

Double or triple apical impulse due to presystolic expansion of the ventricle caused by atrial contraction

4. Auscultation:

Late systolic murmur at the lower left sternal edge and apex (due to ventricular obstruction) in late systole

Pansystolic murmur at the apex (due to mitral regurgitation)

Fourth heart sound

5. Dynamic maneuver:

The outflow murmur is increased by the Valsalva maneuver, by standing, and by isotonic exercise; it is decreased by squatting and isometric exercise

Ventricular Septal Defect

1. Palpation:

Hyperkinetic, laterally displaced apex if the defect is large

Thrill at the sternal edge

2. Auscultation:

Harsh pansystolic murmur maximal at lower left sternal edge with a third or fourth heart sound (the murmur is louder on expiration; sometimes a mitral regurgitation murmur is associated); the murmur is often louder and more harsh when the defect is small

Atrial Septal Defect

1. Precordium:

Normal or right ventricular lift

2. Auscultation:

Fixed splitting of the second heart sound

The defect produces no murmur directly, but increased flow through the right side of the heart can produce a low-pitched diastolic flow murmur across the tricuspid valve and a pulmonary systolic ejection murmur (both are louder on inspiration)

The signs of an ostium primum defect are the same as for an ostium secundum defect, but associated mitral regurgitation, tricuspid regurgitation, or a ventricular septal defect may be present

The physical signs of a sinus venosus atrial septal defect are the same as those of a secundum atrial septal defect

Patent Ductus Arteriosus

1. Pulse and blood pressure:

A collapsing pulse with a sharp upstroke (due to ejection of a large volume of blood into the aorta during systole); there is rapid run-off of blood from the aorta into the pulmonary artery

Low diastolic blood pressure (due to rapid run-off from the aorta)

2. Precordium:

Hyperkinetic apex beat

3. Auscultation:

If the shunt is of moderate size, a single second heart sound is heard, but if the shunt is of large size, reversed splitting of the second heart sound occurs (a delayed aortic second sound occurs because of the increased left ventricular stroke volume)

A continuous loud "machinery" murmur maximal at the first left intercostal space is usually present

Eisenmenger Syndrome (Right-to-Left Shunt)

Clinical signs:

Central cyanosis due to the right-to-left shunting

Finger and toe clubbing

Polycythemia

Signs of pulmonary hypertension

It may be possible to decide at what level the right-to-left shunt occurs by listening to the second heart sound. A wide fixed splitting of the second heart sound suggests an atrial septal defect. The presence of a single second heart sound suggests truncus arteriosus or a ventricular septal defect. A normal or reversed second heart sound suggests patent ductus arteriosus.

> The onset of Eisenmenger syndrome is often heralded by a softening of the patient's original left-to-right murmur, a decrease in left heart size, and an increase in the second pulmonic sound.

Tetralogy of Fallot

1. Clinical signs:

Central cyanosis is common and occurs because of a large right-to-left shunt at the ventricular level, where right and left ventricular pressures are equalized. In addition, the aorta overrides both ventricular outflow tracts and receives a combination of saturated and desaturated blood

Finger and toe clubbing and polycythemia

Signs of right ventricular enlargement, including a parasternal right ventricular lift and a thrill at the left sternal edge

Normal left ventricular impulse

Aortic click

Second heart sound is single (absent second pulmonic sound)

Pulmonary systolic ejection murmur—the louder and longer the pulmonary murmur the better, because this indicates better blood flow through the pulmonary

circulation

No significant murmur across the ventricular septal defect (no gradient)

Continuous murmur from bronchial collaterals or associated patent ductus arteriosus

The lungs are protected from pulmonary hypertension by the pulmonary stenosis (valvular and infundibular)

Named Murmurs in Cardiology

Graham Steell murmur—Functional pulmonary regurgitation murmur due to severe pulmonary hypertension usually associated with severe mitral stenosis

Austin Flint murmur—Functional mitral stenosis murmur due to incomplete mitral valve opening because of severe aortic incompetence

Rytand murmur—Mid-diastolic mitral flow murmur that occurs in patients with complete heart block

Carey Coombs murmur—Acute mitral valvulitis due to acute rheumatic fever that causes a short diastolic rumbling-type murmur

Dock murmur—Very localized high-pitched diastolic murmur heard in the 2nd-3rd left intercostal interspaces; due to high-grade stenosis of the left anterior descending coronary artery

Frequently Asked Questions About the Cardiovascular Subspecialty Examination

What is the question blueprint for the Cardiology Board Examination?

The ABIM published the examination question blueprint for the 1999 cardiovascular examination (Table 6).

As indicated in Table 6, more than 90% of the examination is based on clinical cardiology and less than 10% on the underlying physiology and biochemistry. Although most clinical cardiology questions relate to ischemic heart disease, valvular heart disease, heart failure, and so forth, approximately 20% of the questions are related areas of cardiology that are less emphasized, including congenital heart disease, vascular disease, and hypertension.

Is There an Oral or Clinical Component to the Examination?

No. The Cardiology Boards is a comprehensive, multiple-choice, written examination. The ABIM determined that it would be logistically difficult to schedule oral or clinical examinations and that the fairness and reliability of oral examinations could not be guaranteed.

> Oral questions, essay-type questions, and performance of a clinical examination are not part of the Cardiology Board examination but are required in many of the examinations of the Royal College of Physicians.

How Is the Passing Grade Set in the Examination?

The ABIM board members discuss the minimal acceptable knowledge base for a candidate to be competent in each area of cardiology. These judgments are combined to derive a minimum overall passing score. The standard for passing is maintained constant between examinations by comparing the scores from similar questions in current and previous examinations. Scores are adjusted to ensure a common examination standard regardless of the year the examination is taken.

● The standard for passing the Cardiology Boards is not dependent on the year the test is taken.

What Are Core and Noncore Questions and How Can They Be Differentiated?

The Cardiology Boards has both core and noncore components, with separate standards for each component. A candidate must pass both components to pass the examination. Generally, core questions are ones that test an important area of cardiology competence or require management of a frequently encountered clinical situation and are questions that a proficient cardiologist would be expected to answer correctly. Most candidates who fail the core questions also fail the noncore ones. The core questions are distributed throughout the test. It is not possible for candidates to reliably distinguish between core and noncore questions. From a practical point, candidates should concentrate on answering all questions and not try to identify likely core questions, because it only wastes time. Candidates cannot compensate for a poor score on the core questions by a good performance on the noncore questions.

● Most candidates who fail the core questions also fail the noncore ones.

Table 6.—Blueprint for the American Board of Internal Medicine Subspecialty Examination in Cardiovascular Disease

Primary category	% of questions
Valvular heart disorders	12
Cardiac pharmacology	12
Cardiac arrhythmias	11.5
Acute myocardial infarction	10.5
Coronary artery disease	9
Aorta-peripheral vascular disorders	9
Congestive heart failure	8
Physiology/biochemistry	7.5
Congenital heart disorders	7
Hypertension/pulmonary disorders	4.7
Pericardial disease	3.3
Cardiomyopathy	3
Miscellaneous	2.5

> Candidates should try to answer all questions and not waste time attempting to distinguish between core and noncore questions.

Are There Negative Grades for Wrong Answers?

In the multiple-choice section, wrong answers are not subtracted from correct ones; therefore, if you do not know the answer, guess. However, in the ECG and cardiovascular imaging sections of the examination, a negative marking system is used, and guessing answers in these sections is not advised.

> In the ECG and cardiovascular imaging sections, a negative marking system is used, and guessing answers in these sections is not advised.

Does the ABIM Provide or Endorse Any Courses or Textbooks for Candidates?

The ABIM does not participate in or endorse any specific cardiovascular board course or textbook.

What Is the Question Format Used on the Cardiology Boards?

The question format is single best answer. Questions with

double negatives and K-type questions (1 and 3 correct, 2 and 4 correct, etc.) are no longer used on the examination.

What Is the Cardiovascular Imaging Component of the Cardiology Boards?

This component is misnamed because it uses still-frame echocardiograms, ventriculograms, and angiograms to test competence in cardiovascular imaging. This section is a source of complaint by many cardiology fellows. To prepare for this section, candidates should accustom themselves to looking at still-frame images of common cardiovascular conditions. Generally, most of the images that are shown have obvious abnormalities and have the "classic" attributes of the condition featured. The assessment of regional wall motion abnormalities from still-frame ventriculograms has proved difficult on previous examinations.

> Candidates should practice making the diagnosis of regional wall motion abnormalities on still-frame diastolic and systolic images from ventriculograms and echocardiograms.

How Are Cardiology Board Questions Set?

The ABIM maintains a large bank of cardiology questions that are updated regularly. Board-certified cardiologists are invited to submit questions to the data bank. Submitted questions are reviewed by the ABIM for scientific accuracy, clarity of meaning, and clinical importance. There needs to be broad agreement by a panel of experts about the correctness of an answer. Before a question is included in the examination, it is reviewed both by clinicians and by ABIM examination reviewers.

> It is useful for candidates to imagine a question being discussed at an ABIM question review session and the need for a consensus opinion about the correct answer. The consensus answer that the candidate thinks a panel of senior clinicians would give is likely to be the correct answer, rather than an obtuse idiosyncratic answer.

What Is the Ideal Cardiology Board Question?

The ideal examination question should have a clear scientific answer, be written in unambiguous language, be clinically important, and differentiate between stronger and weaker candidates. If the question is either obvious or too difficult, it will be rejected.

Can Cardiology Board Questions Be Answered by "Gaming Techniques"?

The answer is probably not. By gaming, I mean using strategies that require no medical knowledge but depend on finding clues to the answer in the question itself. One of the assignments of the ABIM examination reviewers is to eliminate any nonmedical clues to the correct answer.

What Are the "Lethal" Errors That May Befall Cardiology Board Candidates?

Lethal errors include "time errors," when a candidate does not complete a significant portion of the examination, and "out-of-sequence errors," in which a candidate mismatches the question number and the answer number. This usually occurs when a candidate skips from question to question. All questions should be answered *sequentially* to avoid the possibility of out-of-sequence errors. In general, there is a mild time pressure on the Cardiology Boards: it is perilous to ignore the time factor.

Should Unknown Questions Be Guessed Immediately or Left Until Last?

Candidates have many strategies in examinations, and there is no best option. If questions are left to be answered at the end of the examination, no more than 10% should remain for the last round.

Are All Questions Graded Equally?

The scheme of the ABIM is confidential, but the principle of equal grades for equal question time applies.

Are All Questions Graded?

The performance of individual questions as well as candidate performance is assessed by the ABIM. A question with a very high number of correct answers or incorrect answers may be discarded after the examination and not graded. A question with a high dispersion score (i.e., all possible answers are selected in nearly equal amounts) may suggest that candidates are guessing the answer to that question. The correlation between the overall performance of candidates and their performance on a specific question is examined. If candidates with high overall scores consistently fail to answer correctly a specific question, it suggests that the question is worded unfairly or ambiguously.

How Should Ethical Questions Be Answered?

Frequently, candidates think ethical questions are ambiguous and difficult to answer. The ABIM does not endorse the ethical standards of a particular culture or religion but asks questions that require knowledge of the acceptable standards of ethical behavior. Important areas for ethical questions are decisions about resuscitation, withdrawal of life support, and consent for clinical trials. Generally, the answer that respects the independence of a competent patient is usually correct.

> In ethical questions, the answer that respects the independence of a competent patient is usually correct.

How Should Long Questions Be Answered?
Long questions may be more than one page in length and take up to 5 minutes to read. Long questions usually encompass the patient's history, physical examination findings, and results of numerous investigations. These questions are meant to evaluate a candidate's ability to find the "needle in the haystack."

A strategy for long questions is to read the last paragraph of the question and the possible answer choices. This may obviate reading the question in its entirety and save time. If the thrust of the question is not obvious at this stage, the entire question must be read. Frequently, the "heart" of the question is in the last paragraph.

Watch for clinical clues to the cardiac diagnosis.

> A strategy for long questions is first to read the last paragraph of the question and the possible answers.

What Procedural Skills Are Required for Cardiovascular Subspecialty Certification?
The following procedural skills are required for cardiology board certification: advanced cardiac life support (ACLS), including cardioversion; ECG, including ambulatory monitoring and exercise testing; echocardiography; insertion of arterial catheters; and catheterization of the right side of the heart, including insertion and management of temporary pacemakers.

> The ABIM expects candidates to know the procedural details, indications, and possible complications of ACLS, ECG, echocardiography, insertion of arterial catheters, and catheterization of the right side of the heart. For nonmandatory procedures such as angioplasty and electrophysiologic testing, the underlying science, indications, and potential complications should be known but not the procedural details. For example, catheter selection, stent size, and PTCA balloon type are unimportant for this examination.

What Information Does the ABIM Provide to Program Directors?
The ABIM forwards the individual pass/fail results to the program director of the candidates taking the examination for the first time. A report of the complete examination score is provided to the program director if the candidate authorizes it.

What Is Board Eligibility?
Effective July 1, 1997, the ABIM no longer will use, define, or recognize the term "Board Eligible."

What Is Cardiology Board Recertification?
Since 1990, Cardiovascular Board certification has been limited to 10 years. The requirements for recertification are
1) Valid, unrestricted medical licensure
2) Initial certification in cardiovascular medicine
3) Verification of clinical competence
4) Successful performance on the "self-evaluation process"
5) Successful performance on the final examination

Recertification in cardiology does not require recertification in internal medicine. There are three steps for recertification: a self-evaluation process, an assessment of clinical competence, and a final examination.

The self-evaluation process is an at-home, open-book, self-evaluation examination. Each module comprises 60 questions that emphasize problem-solving rather than knowledge recall. Candidates are required to take and to pass a minimum of three modules in cardiology, one module in general internal medicine, and one elective module. The Board requires peer assessment of clinical performance at the local level for recertification. Diplomates need a valid and unrestricted license and a current basic life-saving or advanced cardiac life-support certificate.

The last step in the recertification program is a 1-day, supervised, multiple-choice examination to be administered annually.

Notes

Chapter 2

Cardiovascular Reflex and Humoral Control of the Circulation

Alfredo L. Clavell, M.D.
John C. Burnett, Jr., M.D.

> Cardiology Board candidates are expected to understand the normal reflex and humoral control mechanisms of the circulation and their derangement in heart failure.

Optimal regulation of the circulation is dependent on an integration of cardiovascular reflexes with local and circulating humoral factors that regulate myocardial contractility, vascular tone, and intravascular volume (the intravascular volume is regulated primarily through renal sodium excretion). Under physiologic conditions, cardiovascular reflexes function in short-term cardiovascular control, whereas humoral mechanisms function as more long-term modulators of cardiovascular homeostasis.

Cardiovascular Reflexes

Two principal cardiovascular reflex arcs are involved in the regulation of blood pressure:

1. Arterial baroreceptors are located in the carotid sinus and aortic arch and respond with increasing neural discharge in response to stretch caused by increases in arterial blood pressure.

2. Cardiopulmonary baroreceptors are located in the ventricular myocardia and also in the atria and venoatrial junctions.

Normal Cardiac Function

The arterial and cardiopulmonary reflexes discharge during cardiac systole, their rate of discharge being directly related to the force of myocardial contraction and to cardiac filling pressure. Afferent signals from both arterial and cardiopulmonary receptors signal to the nucleus solitarius in the brain stem.

The principal functions of these receptors are twofold: 1) to inhibit efferent sympathetic neural outflow to the heart and circulation, resulting in decreases in arterial blood pressure and systemic vascular resistance, and 2) to augment efferent parasympathetic neural outflow to the heart, resulting in sinus node slowing and prolongation of atrioventricular conduction.

During reductions in arterial pressure and cardiac filling pressures under physiologic conditions, the inhibitory discharge of these receptors declines. Efferent sympathetic neural outflow increases, resulting in an increase in systemic vascular resistance, and efferent parasympathetic outflow decreases, resulting in tachycardia. Conversely, during increases in arterial blood pressure and cardiac filling pressures, the inhibitory discharge of these receptors is enhanced. Efferent sympathetic neural outflow decreases, resulting in a decrease in systemic vascular resistance, and parasympathetic outflow increases, resulting in bradycardia.

Congestive Heart Failure

In chronic congestive heart failure (CHF), a chronic reduction in arterial filling results in a decrease in inhibitory signaling to the cardiovascular reflex center, causing a significant increase in systemic vascular resistance. Despite high cardiac filling pressures due to ventricular dysfunction, an attenuation in the inhibitory action of the cardiopulmonary baroreceptors occurs. The dysfunction of cardiovascular reflexes in CHF results in enhanced adrenergic activity with systemic vasoconstriction. Additionally, sympathetic activation may have secondary actions and lead to activation of local and neurohumoral systems (such as the renin-angiotensin system) and to avid sodium retention due to increased sodium resorption by the kidney.

- Arterial baroreflexes are located in the carotid sinus and aortic arch and respond to increases in arterial blood pressure.
- Dysfunction of cardiovascular reflexes in congestive heart failure results in enhanced adrenergic activity with systemic vasoconstriction.

Local and Circulating Humoral Systems

Vasodilatory, Natriuretic, and Antimitogenic Systems

Natriuretic Peptides
The natriuretic peptide system encompasses a family of cardiovascular peptides: atrial (ANP) and brain (BNP) natriuretic peptides are of cardiac myocyte origin, whereas C-type natriuretic peptide (CNP) is of endothelial cell origin. These peptides are released in response to both acute and chronic atrial stretch (ANP and BNP) and in response to numerous other humoral stimuli (CNP). They have important actions on the heart, functioning through autocrine and paracrine mechanisms, and on other organ systems such as the kidney, adrenal gland, and the vascular wall. Important biologic actions include modulation of myocardial function and structure, natriuresis, inhibition of the renin-angiotensin-aldosterone system, vasodilatation, and an antimitogenic effect on vascular smooth muscle cells. CNP is devoid of natriuretic actions but is a powerful vasodilatory and antimitogenic peptide. The biologic actions of this important cardiovascular humoral system are via activation of specific particulate guanylate cyclase receptors, which function via the second messenger cyclic guanosine monophosphate. Importantly, the activity of this system is modulated by two pathways responsible for clearance and degradation of the

natriuretic peptides, including neutral endopeptidase and a unique receptor-based clearance mechanism.

In chronic CHF, ANP and BNP circulating levels are increased. They have functional significance in the overall regulation of the cardiovascular system in CHF because their inhibition with unique receptor antagonists results in a rapid deterioration in experimental animal models of heart failure, as manifested by rapid activation of the renin-angiotensin-aldosterone system together with vasoconstriction and sodium retention (Table 1). Because of this functional importance, therapeutic strategies have emerged to potentiate the endogenous natriuretic peptides through inhibition of their degradation by neutral endopeptidase and by exogenous administration of natriuretic peptides via the subcutaneous route. The increase in the values of the natriuretic peptides in heart failure has significance for both prognosis and diagnosis of early asymptomatic left ventricular dysfunction. In particular, BNP has recently been recognized as a marker for left ventricular dysfunction and hypertrophy.

- In chronic CHF, ANP and BNP levels are increased.

Endothelium-Derived Relaxing Factor (Nitric Oxide)
In addition to the natriuretic peptides, an endothelial cell-derived relaxing factor, nitric oxide (NO), also functions via activation of cyclic guanosine monophosphate through stimulation of soluble guanylate cyclase. The functional role of this endogenous factor is to cause vasodilatation and natriuresis and to inhibit vascular proliferation. Indeed,

Table 1.—Neurohumoral Mechanisms in Congestive Heart Failure

Vasodilatory, natriuretic, and antimitogenic factors	Vasoconstrictive, antinatriuretic, and mitogenic factors
Natriuretic peptides	Renin-angiotensin-aldosterone system
Kallikrein, kinins	
Prostaglandin	Sympathetic nervous system
Dopamine	Vasopressin
Endothelium-derived relaxing factor—nitric oxide	Thromboxane
	Endothelin
	Cytokines
Adrenomedullin	

Modified from Giuliani ER, Gersh BJ, McGoon MD, Hayes DL, Schaff HV (editors): *Mayo Clinic Practice of Cardiology.* Third edition. Mosby, 1996, p 560. By permission of Mayo Foundation.

inhibition of endogenous NO by unique inhibitors results in systemic, renal, and pulmonary vasoconstriction and sodium retention. Long-term inhibition of the endogenous NO system results in hypertension and ventricular and vascular remodeling.

Overt CHF is characterized by peripheral vasoconstriction, abnormalities of vascular tone, and sodium retention, but studies conflict with regard to NO activity in CHF. Some studies suggest that NO activity is enhanced in human and experimental animal heart failure, because inhibition of its generation in heart failure results in further ventricular dysfunction and systemic vasoconstriction.

- Nitric oxide (NO) functions via activation of cyclic guanosine monophosphate through stimulation of soluble guanylate cyclase.

Vasoconstrictor, Antinatriuretic, and Mitogenic Systems

Endocrine mechanisms exist to modulate vascular tone, growth of cardiac myocytes and vascular smooth muscle, and sodium excretion by the kidney. The sympathetic, renin-angiotensin-aldosterone, and endothelin systems emerge as three important vasoconstrictor, antinatriuretic, and mitogenic systems that control cardiovascular homeostasis and play a role in the pathophysiology of CHF.

Sympathetic Nervous System

Plasma catecholamines (norepinephrine and epinephrine) are the circulating humoral counterparts of the sympathetic nervous system. Norepinephrine is released locally from sympathetic nerve endings adjacent to myocardium and modulates myocardial contractility. The adrenal medulla also releases both catecholamines in response to diverse stimuli and amplifies the cardiovascular response to sympathetic nervous system activation. The myocardium is rich in β receptors, which are the target of these important cardiovascular hormones.

In chronic CHF there is activation of the sympathetic nervous system as a response to the reduction in myocardial contractility and cardiac output. Although the resultant vasoconstriction and increase in myocardial contractility are essential for maintaining blood pressure, eventually this response becomes deleterious and contributes to a further decline in myocardial function. In the presence of chronically increased serum norepinephrine levels, there is down-regulation of myocardial β receptors, perhaps as a protective mechanism. Circulating levels of norepinephrine correlate

with patient mortality in CHF.

β-Adrenergic blockade is an important new strategy in the therapeutic neurohumoral modulation of CHF. Recent studies demonstrate a paradoxic increase in left ventricular function with β-blockers, improved clinical symptoms, and better prognosis in heart failure, regardless of the cause of the CHF and in addition to angiotensin-converting enzyme inhibition.

- In CHF there is chronic activation of norepinephrine and down-regulation of myocardial β receptors.

Renin-Angiotensin-Aldosterone System

Angiotensin II is one of the most potent vasoconstrictor and mitogenic peptides that is produced both systemically and locally in the heart, lung, kidney, and vascular endothelium as a result of the abundant presence of angiotensin-converting enzyme (Table 2). Angiotensin II, which functions via specific receptor subtypes, also is responsible for stimulation of norepinephrine release and sympathetic activation. Metabolism and growth in myocyte and non-myocyte cells also are altered by circulating and locally generated angiotensin II, which increases cellular proliferation and impairs myocyte contractile activity. Additionally, aldosterone produced by the adrenal gland is activated by angiotensin II and has effects on non-myocytes in addition to its sodium-retaining action in the kidney. Most recently, studies have suggested that aldosterone may be responsible for cardiac fibrosis via specific receptors within the heart. These two important hormones, angiotensin II and aldosterone, have emerged as the targets for pharmacologic inhibition in the treatment of CHF; in severe

Table 2.—Angiotensin II: Sites and Actions

Targets	Actions
Heart	Positive inotropism, hypertrophy
Kidney	Renin release, mesangial contraction, sodium resorption
Adrenal body	Aldosterone release
Brain	Vasopressin release, thirst, increased sympathetic outflow
Sympathetic nervous system	Norepinephrine release
Vascular smooth muscle	Vasoconstriction, hypertrophy

From Giuliani ER, Gersh BJ, McGoon MD, Hayes DL, Schaff HV (editors): *Mayo Clinic Practice of Cardiology.* Third edition. Mosby, 1996, p 562. By permission of Mayo Foundation.

human CHF, inhibition of angiotensin II generation has resulted in improvement in mortality and morbidity. However, escape from angiotensin-converting enzyme inhibition is noted chronically, and newer strategies relying on angiotensin II receptor and aldosterone antagonists in combination with angiotensin-converting enzyme I have proved useful in the management of refractory heart failure.

- Angiotensin II, which functions via specific receptor subtypes, is responsible for stimulation of norepinephrine release and sympathetic activation.

Endothelin System
Endothelin is a 21-amino acid peptide that is produced by the endothelium. Much like angiotensin II, an endothelin-converting enzyme cleaves large endothelin into its biologically active form. Although its role in physiology continues to be elucidated, most likely, as with angiotensin II, it serves to maintain vascular tone and arterial blood pressure. In CHF, it functions as a compensatory mechanism to mediate vasoconstriction and possibly augment inotropic function.

Myocardial responsiveness to endothelin also may be preserved in late heart failure when the myocardium has become refractory to other endogenous agonists. As with angiotensin II, endothelin has growth-promoting and mitogenic potential and, therefore, may contribute to cardiac and vascular remodeling. Endothelin also serves to stimulate renin and aldosterone release and to augment activation of cardiac fibroblasts. Also, endothelin has potent renal vasoconstricting and sodium-retaining actions in CHF. Studies also have suggested that an increase in plasma endothelin may have prognostic implications in CHF. Preliminary studies suggest that specific endothelin receptor antagonists have beneficial hemodynamic effects in CHF. Hence, blockade of the endothelin system with receptor antagonists or endothelin-converting enzyme inhibitors may prove to be an important strategy in the management of CHF.

- An increase of plasma endothelin may have prognostic implications in CHF.
- Endothelin receptor blockade is emerging as a new strategy in the management of CHF.

Questions

Multiple Choice (choose the one best answer)

1. Arterial baroreflexes, which are located in the carotid sinus and aortic arch, respond to increases in arterial pressure and function to:
   a. Inhibit efferent sympathetic neural outflow to the heart and circulation
   b. Inhibit efferent parasympathetic neural outflow
   c. Increase the release of renin by the kidney
   d. Increase heart rate

2. In chronic congestive heart failure, despite the stimulus of increased cardiac filling pressures, cardiopulmonary baroreceptor reflexes are attenuated. This action results in which one of the following?
   a. Decreased adrenergic activity
   b. Increased adrenergic activity
   c. Systemic vasodilatation
   d. Suppression of the renin-angiotensin-aldosterone system

3. Atrial natriuretic peptide is of myocardial cell origin and is released in response to an increase in atrial stretch. Important biologic actions include which one of the following?
   a. Anti-natriuresis
   b. Activation of the renin-angiotensin-aldosterone system
   c. Mitogenic effect on vascular smooth muscle
   d. Vasodilatation

4. The development of neutral endopeptidase inhibitors is a new therapeutic strategy in congestive heart failure, designed to do which one of the following?
   a. Potentiate the natriuretic peptide system
   b. Inhibit the natriuretic peptide system
   c. Activate the renin-angiotensin-aldosterone system
   d. Stimulate the adrenergic nervous system

5. Nitric oxide is an endogenous endothelial cell-derived relaxing factor that functions via the second messenger, cyclic guanosine monophosphate. Which one of the following describes its action?
   a. Causes ventricular hypertrophy
   b. Contributes to essential hypertension
   c. Contributes to atherosclerosis
   d. Is an endogenous vasodilator

6. Angiotensin II mediates vasoconstriction via which of the following receptor subtypes?
   a. Endothelin-A receptor
   b. Angiotensin-II receptor
   c. Angiotensin-I receptor
   d. All of the above

7. Angiotensin-converting enzyme is responsible for which of the following?
   a. Degradation of angiotensin II
   b. Conversion of angiotensin I to angiotensin II
   c. Stimulation of norepinephrine
   d. All of the above

8. Inhibition of angiotensin-converting enzyme in chronic congestive heart failure:
   a. Increases the rate of hospitalization due to excessive hypotension
   b. Contributes to left ventricular hypertrophy and cardiac dilatation via increases in angiotensin II
   c. Increases mortality in congestive heart failure
   d. Inhibits aldosterone release via decreases in angiotensin II

9. Endothelin is:
   a. A potent endothelium cell-derived vasodilator
   b. A potent endothelium cell-derived vasoconstrictor
   c. An inhibitor of ventricular hypertrophy
   d. Decreased in congestive heart failure

10. Inhibition of endothelin in congestive heart failure may be accomplished by which of the following?
    a. Endothelin receptor antagonism
    b. Endothelin-converting enzyme inhibition
    c. Inhibition of angiotensin II
    d. All of the above

Answers

1. Answer a

Activation of arterial baroreflexes functions to inhibit sympathetic tone, slow heart rate, and inhibit activation of the renin-angiotensin system.

2. Answer b

In heart failure, attenuation of cardiopulmonary reflexes results in an impaired inhibition of the adrenergic nervous system, resulting in marked vasoconstriction with activation of the renin-angiotensin-aldosterone system.

3. Answer d

This peptide increases sodium excretion, inhibits the renin-angiotensin-aldosterone system, provides antimitogenic effects to vascular smooth muscle, and is vasodilatory.

4. Answer a

Neutral endopeptidase is an ectoenzyme that is co-localized with angiotensin-converting enzyme. This enzyme is responsible for the degradation of the natriuretic peptides and, therefore, inhibition of this ectoenzyme potentiates the biologic actions of the three natriuretic peptides (atrial natriuretic peptide, brain natriuretic peptide, and C-type natriuretic peptide).

5. Answer d

Nitric oxide is a potent vasodilating substance that also possesses growth-inhibiting actions.

6. Answer c

Angiotensin II mediates its vasoconstrictor action via the angiotensin-I receptor. It does not interact with the endothelin receptor nor mediate vasoconstriction via the angiotensin-II receptor subtype.

7. Answer b

Angiotensin-converting enzyme is an enzyme that converts angiotensin I to the active mature peptide angiotensin II, which has potent biologic actions.

8. Answer d

Inhibition of angiotensin-converting enzyme in heart failure decreases vasoconstriction, reduces ventricular hypertrophy and dilatation, reduces morbidity and mortality, and inhibits the release of aldosterone.

9. Answer b

Endothelin is a potent endothelium cell-derived vasoconstricting and growth-promoting peptide that is activated in congestive heart failure.

10. Answer d

Therapeutic strategies to oppose the endothelin system in heart failure may include selective and nonselective endothelin receptor antagonists to inhibit the endothelin A and B receptors, respectively. Also, because the increase in endothelin in congestive heart failure may involve processing of large endothelin to endothelin I, endothelin-converting enzyme inhibitors may play a role. Studies have suggested that endothelin activation may occur, in part, by stimulation by angiotensin II; therefore, inhibition of the renin-angiotensin-aldosterone system may inhibit activation of endothelin in congestive heart failure.

Chapter 3

Left Ventricular Systolic Function

John A. Rumberger, Ph.D., M.D.
Joseph G. Murphy, M.D.

> Candidates for the Cardiology Boards are expected to have an understanding of the fundamentals of left ventricular systolic function and its measurement.

Contraction of the left ventricle (LV) during systole is necessary for continuous perfusion of vital organs.

Cellular Aspects of LV Contraction

Microanatomy

Cardiac myocytes contain myofibrils that are composed of longitudinally repeating sarcomeres separated by Z bands (thickened and invaginated portions of the surface membrane, the sarcolemma). The sarcomeres occupy about 50% of the mass of cardiac cells. Thin filaments composed of actin are attached to each Z line and interdigitate with the thick filaments, composed of myosin molecules. The thick and thin myofilaments slide past one another in a "rowing-type" mechanism to generate force and shorten the myocyte. The myofilaments maintain a fixed length throughout contraction. Mitochondria compose about 20% of the cell volume and are the organelles in which adenosine triphosphate (ATP) is produced. They are situated in close apposition to the myofibrils, as well as just beneath the sarcolemma. Their platelike foldings, or cristae, contain the respiratory enzymes and project inward from the surface membrane (Fig. 1).

- Contractile sarcomeres occupy about 50% of the mass of cardiac cells.

Excitation and Contraction Coupling

The coupling of cardiac excitation (electrical event) and contraction (mechanical event) are fundamentally molecular events. The sarcolemma is a thin phospholipid layer and is the site of electrical polarization. The phospholipid bilayer acts as an ionic barrier and maintains high intracellular $[K^+]$ and low intracellular $[Na^+]$ and $[Ca^+]$ (Fig. 2).

Near the Z lines are wide invaginations of the sarcolemma, the T system, which branch through the cell. Closely coupled to but not continuous with the T system is the sarcoplasmic reticulum, a complex network of anastomosing, membrane-limited intracellular tubules that surround each myofibril and play a critical role in excitation of the muscle.

Troponin (which is composed of troponin C, I, and T) and tropomyosin are regulatory proteins found in the thin filaments. In the absence of troponin and tropomyosin, the contractile proteins actin and myosin are activated, requiring only the presence of Mg^{2+} and ATP. These regulatory proteins, when present, however, prevent cross-bridge formation between myosin and actin. When Ca^{2+} is bound to troponin C, the binding of troponin I to actin is inhibited, which in turn causes a conformational change in tropomyosin, so that the latter, instead of inhibiting, now enhances cross-bridge formation. Thus, Ca^{2+} blocks an inhibitor of the interaction between actin and myosin. The key element in the initiation of contraction is the release of

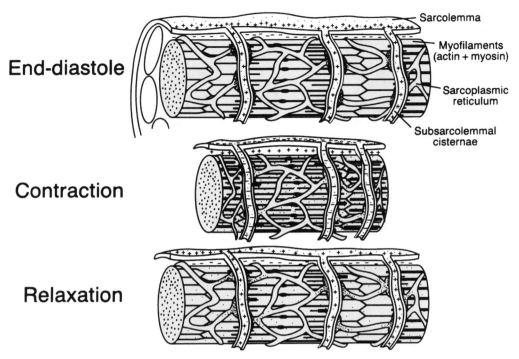

Fig. 1. The major shifts of calcium ions during myocyte excitation-contraction coupling and relaxation. The dots represent calcium ions, and the positive and negative signs indicate electrical charge across membrane partitions. (From Giuliani ER, Gersh BJ, McGoon MD, Hayes DL, Schaff HV [editors]: *Mayo Clinic Practice of Cardiology*. Third edition. Mosby, 1996, p 554. By permission of Mayo Foundation.)

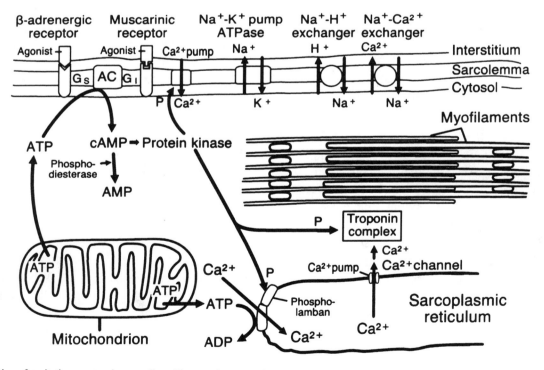

Fig. 2. The regulation of excitation-contraction coupling. The sarcolemma and sarcoplasmic reticulum modulate cytoplasmic calcium availability, and the troponin-tropomyosin complex regulates responsiveness to cytoplasmic calcium. AC, adenylate cyclase; ADP, adenosine phosphate; AMP, adenosine monophosphate; ATP, adenosine triphosphate; ATPase, adenosine triphosphatase; cAMP, cyclic adenosine monophosphate; Gi, guanine nucleotide-binding regulatory protein that inhibits adenylate cyclase; Gs, guanine nucleotide-binding regulatory protein that stimulates adenylate cyclase. (From Giuliani ER, Gersh BJ, McGoon MD, Hayes DL, Schaff HV [editors]: *Mayo Clinic Practice of Cardiology*. Third edition. Mosby, 1996, p 552. By permission of Mayo Foundation.)

sarcoplasmic [Ca^{2+}]. Depolarization of the sarcolemma caused by the upstroke of the action potential opens the ion channels that carry the inward Ca^{2+} current, which in turn triggers a release of the large stores of calcium in the sarcoplasmic reticulum. With cellular depolarization, the myoplasmic [Ca^{2+}] rises and is bound to troponin. Once each cross-bridge "stroke" is completed, the myosin head ejects its ATP breakdown products, binds another ATP molecule, and detaches from the actin site. The myosin head then returns to its original orientation and the cycle is repeated.

Relaxation is brought about by the active (ATP-requiring) reuptake of the calcium into the sarcoplasmic reticulum. Thus, calcium is essential to the excitation-contraction coupling, and when the calcium concentration decreases to a critical point, contraction ceases.

- Troponin and tropomyosin are regulatory proteins found in the thin filaments.
- The key element in the initiation of cardiac contraction is the release of sarcoplasmic [Ca^{2+}].
- The transmembrane calcium current does not directly cause cardiac contraction but secondarily releases sarcoplasmic calcium.

Mechanics of Contraction

The patterns of changes in the LV during contraction can be summarized in the mnemonic TARTT. During systole, the LV *T*ranslates (moves from side-to-side), *A*ccordions (moves with the base and apex attempting to approximate each other), *R*otates (about the LV "long axis"), *T*ilts (perpendicular to the long axis), and *T*hickens (Fig. 3).

Myocardial fibers are arranged in a spiral fashion around the central LV cavity. The subendocardial and subepicardial fibers run largely parallel to the long axis of the cavity, and the midwall fibers are mostly perpendicular to the long axis (that is, circumferential). During ventricular ejection, these fibers shorten and thicken, and as the LV cavity decreases circumferentially and longitudinally, the inner surface decreases more than the external surface, as dictated by geometry. Because muscle mass remains constant, an increase in wall thickness must occur.

During isovolumic LV contraction, the chordae tendineae become tense, the mitral valve closes, and the ellipsoid LV becomes more spherical. During LV ejection, the longitudinal axis shortens by only about 10%, whereas the short-axis diameter shortens by about 25%, thus accounting for 80% to 90% of the normal stroke volume.

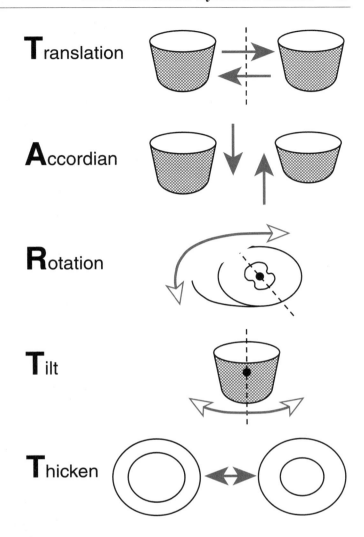

Fig. 3. Mechanisms of contraction and motion of the heart.

Isovolumic contraction refers to the interval (about 50 ms) between the onset of ventricular systole and the opening of the semilunar valves. The LV pressure must exceed that in the aorta during diastole. There is a small increase of pressure in the aorta just before the semilunar valves (aortic and pulmonary) open. Ventricular ejection is that phase of ventricular systole (about 350 to 400 ms in duration at a normal heart rate) in which blood is ejected through the aortic valve. The first phase (about 100 ms) is rapid, and then ejection slows toward the end of ventricular systole. The increase in ventricular pressure is more marked in the rapid phase.

- Myocardial fibers are arranged in a spiral fashion around the central LV cavity.

Determinants of Contraction of the Intact LV

The mechanical determinants of cardiac function are preload, afterload, contractility, and heart rate. When the intact heart is compared with isolated muscle, heart volume and pressure are analogous to muscle length and tension. *Starling's law of the heart* is a fundamental property of heart muscle in which the force of contraction at any given tension depends on the initial muscle fiber length. This, in turn, depends on the ultrastructural disposition of thick and thin myofilaments within the sarcomeres. It was in the classic isolated heart or muscle strip experiments that the concepts of preload, afterload, and contractility first became useful terms.

Alterations in preload, operating through changes in end-diastolic fiber length, are important determinants of the performance of the intact ventricle and provide the basis for the function curves of the intact ventricle. The ability to augment preload provides a functional reserve to the heart in situations of acute stress and exercise. Preload is thus an important factor in maintaining systolic LV performance in many disease states (Fig. 4).

Afterload

Afterload for the intact LV is the tension, force, or wall stress acting on the fibers of the LV after the onset of shortening. This is primarily the arterial pressure and is a major determinant of stroke volume. An abrupt increase in the impedance to LV ejection, when preload is constant, causes a decrease in fiber shortening and LV stroke volume. The LV becomes smaller during normal ejection and its walls thicken. Thus, despite an increase in aortic pressure during LV ejection, the afterload or wall stress decreases during ejection. Thus, in this situation, there is an inverse relationship between afterload (systolic pressure or wall stress) and stroke volume, extent of wall shortening, and velocity of shortening. In the normal individual, stroke volume can be maintained despite a modest increase in arterial pressure by augmenting LV end-diastolic pressure and volume; that is, the increment in afterload is met by an increase in preload. However, in the diseased heart with little preload reserve (such as heart failure), the LV stroke volume would decrease. Also, even in the normal heart, when there is relative hypovolemia (such as with sepsis or hemorrhage), the preload cannot increase sufficiently and an increase in afterload will reduce the stroke volume (Fig. 5). Table 1 shows LV loading in disease states.

Left Ventricular Preload:

- ¥ "Stretch" in isolated muscle preparations
- ¥ End-diastolic wall stress in intact heart
- ¥ Common to use LVEDV with substitution of LVEDP frequently in clinical situations

Contributing factors:

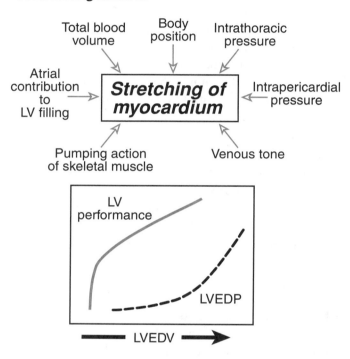

Fig. 4. Factors affecting myocardial stretch and left ventricular (LV) preload. LVEDP, left ventricular end-diastolic pressure; LVEDV, left ventricular end-diastolic volume.

Contractility

The term "contractility" has been used synonymously with "inotropic state." It is difficult to define in a quantitative sense because there is no clear-cut single measurement of contractility that provides a numeric value that can be assigned to a given heart. However, when loading (preload and afterload) conditions remain constant, an improvement in contractility augments cardiac performance, whereas a depression in contractility lowers cardiac performance. Inotropic influences generally act through altered Ca^{2+} availability to the myofilaments or through an alteration in myofilament Ca^{2+} sensitivity. Additional factors that directly or indirectly affect contractility are sympathetic nerve activity and circulating catecholamines (Fig. 6).

The LV pressure-volume relationship is a convenient

Table 1.—Left Ventricular Loading in Disease States

Condition	Preload	Afterload	Contractility	Therapy
Sepsis	↓	→↓	→↓	Fluids and antibiotics
Dehydration	↓	→	→	Fluids
Heart failure	↑	→	↓	Diuretics
Cardiogenic shock	↑	→	↓	Inotropes Intra-aortic balloon pump

RV infarct	↓	→	→	Increase intravenous fluids
				  to maintain high RV filling
				  pressure

Acute mitral regurgitation	↑	→	→	Intra-aortic balloon pump Surgery, if severe
Aortic stenosis	→	↑	→	Surgery, if severe
Systemic hypertension	→	↑	→	Antihypertensive medications

RV, right ventricular.

framework used to understand the responses of LV contraction to alterations in preload, afterload, and contractility.

● The ability to augment preload provides a functional reserve to the heart in situations of acute stress and exercise.

In its simplest sense, the average circumferential wall stress (σ, force per unit of cross-sectional area of wall) in the intact heart is the product of intraventricular pressure (P) and the internal radius of curvature of the chamber (a) divided by the thickness of the muscle walls (h x 2). Laplace's law for a spherical ventricle is

$$\sigma = Pa/2h$$

Preload
Defining preload for the intact LV as the ventricular end-diastolic wall stress provides a direct analogy to the preload of the isolated muscle strip, which determines the resting length of the sarcomeres. Increase in preload augments the stroke volume as well as the extent and velocity of wall shortening. At a constant preload, there is an inverse relation between systolic wall stress and stroke volume.

Heart Rate
Increasing the frequency of contraction does not produce a shift of the ventricular performance curve relating LV end-diastolic pressure and stroke work, but it does increase stroke power at any given level of filling pressure. Thus, increasing the heart rate will improve myocardial contractility,

because the systolic fraction of the cardiac cycle is increased. The positive inotropic effect resulting from an increase in heart rate is more prominent in the depressed heart than in the normal heart. In the normal heart, an artificial increase in heart rate (such as via a pacemaker) will not increase cardiac output, because venous return to the heart is reflexly and metabolically stabilized. However, if the diastolic volume of the LV is increased by increasing venous return, as during exercise, then tachycardia plays a major role in increasing cardiac output. This assumes, however, that not only the speed of contraction but also the speed of relaxation is increased, such that this effect requires preservation of both systolic and diastolic function. Of course, when the heart rate is too fast, the short duration of diastole can lead to interference with ventricular filling, and a decrease in cardiac output can be found, generally with rates of more than 180 beats/min (Table 2).

Myocardial Infarction
Myocardial infarction of approximately 30% or more of the LV mass results in a decrease in the LV ejection fraction. Initially, the cardiac output will be depressed and, in circumstances of considerable damage to the LV, function may deteriorate further, leading to death. However, in most circumstances, when adequate reserve is present, the cardiac stroke volume is augmented by increases in ventricular preload within hours of the infarction. This change is generally accomplished by an increase in left ventricular end-diastolic pressure and reflects a direct consequence to Starling's law of the heart. Increases in afterload may also accompany

Left Ventricular Afterload:

- ¥ Tension, force, or wall stress acting on the fibers of the LV **after** the onset of shortening
- ¥ Although LV systolic pressure and systemic vascular resistance can affect afterload, and thus cardiac output, neither is its equivalent

Contributing factors:

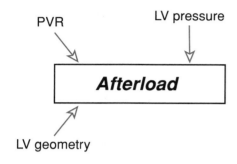

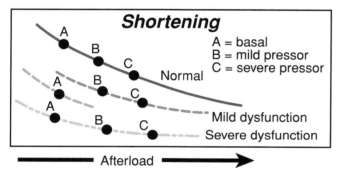

Fig. 5. Factors affecting left ventricular (LV) afterload. PVR, peripheral vascular resistance.

Left Ventricular Contractility:

- Synonymous with "inotropic state," but there is no single measurement of its value
- Generally mediated through altered Ca^{2+} availability or via alteration of myofilament Ca^{2+} sensitivity
- Contractility by definition is independent of loading conditions

Contributing factors:

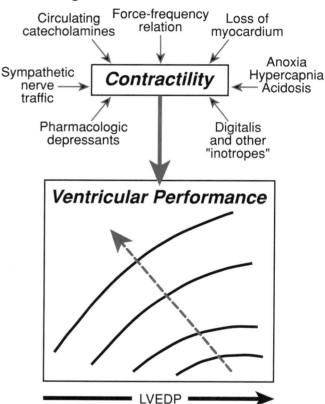

Fig. 6. Determinants of left ventricular contractility. LVEDP, left ventricular end-diastolic pressure.

these changes and thus may offset the increases in stroke volume brought about by increased preload. There are limits to preload reserve, and further increases in cardiac output must then be brought about by increased heart rate. This situation is also common in patients with a dilated cardiomyopathy and congestive heart failure. In such circumstances, use of agents to reduce afterload may be beneficial for augmenting LV stroke volume (Table 3).

- Myocardial infarction of approximately 30% or more of the LV mass results in a depression of the LV ejection fraction.

Left Ventricular Hypertrophy

Left ventricular hypertrophy can occur in conditions of pressure and volume overload. Acquired disorders associated with a pathologic increase in LV preload include chronic

aortic and mitral valvular regurgitation, idiopathic dilated cardiomyopathy, and, often, myocardial infarction. Disorders associated with a pathologic increase in LV afterload include severe aortic stenosis and chronic systemic hypertension. Although the changes in the sarcomeres are different for these two overload states, in both situations the overall mass of the LV is increased. Nevertheless, the hypertrophic response, which is an important adaptive process that enables the heart to compensate for overloading, is a complex process that is both beneficial and detrimental to LV performance. The hypertrophied cells are not necessarily normal, and abnormalities in inotropic response and vascular reactivity have been shown. LV hypertrophy increases myocardial

Table 2.—Effect of Heart Rate on Left Ventricular Systolic Function

Heart rate:
 Positive inotropic effect. Note there is little effect by ventricular pacing on stroke volume in normal patients because of reflex stabilization of venous return
 In the overloaded LV (e.g., CHF), increases in heart rate augment stroke volume (to a point)
 In exercise, with increased venous return, increases in heart rate are the major contributors to increased cardiac output; in normals, the speeds of LV contraction and relaxation are increased, facilitating accommodation of the increased venous return (up to 180-220 beats/min, but much lower rates in CHF)

CHF, congestive heart failure; LV, left ventricle.

oxygen demand and, along with changes in ventricular loading (primarily afterload) and heart rate, is a major contributor to increased myocardial oxygen consumption (Table 4).

Physiologic Measures of LV Systolic Function

Ejection Fraction

The most commonly available measure of systolic performance or contraction is the ejection fraction (EF). This is simply a ratio of the LV stroke volume (SV) to the LV end-diastolic volume. It can be determined with various imaging methods (Table 5). Many of these methods rely on an assumption that the LV shape can be approximated by an ellipsoid. However,

Table 3.—Effect of Loss of Myocardium on Left Ventricular Systolic Function

Loss of myocardium:
 Infarction (> 30% of LV mass), fibrosis, infiltration, "myopathies" all reduce LV systolic performance
 Generally, preload reserve (Starling's law) can assist in augmentation of stroke volume
 However, in some circumstances, reflex and intrinsic regulatory humoral factors may "pathologically" increase SVR (increase afterload); when preload reserve is exhausted, there is an afterload-preload "mismatch"

LV, left ventricle; SVR, systemic vascular resistance.

Table 4.—Effect of Left Ventricular Hypertrophy on Left Ventricular Systolic Function

Left ventricular hypertrophy:
 Common in both chronic "pressure" and "volume" overloading; also common in dilated cardiomyopathy and after myocardial infarction (if > 20% of LV)
 May assist in "normalizing" LV wall stress, but is a major component of myocardial oxygen demand and can be associated with reduced myocardial flow reserve (?mechanism of "angina" in aortic stenosis) and altered inotropic responsiveness

LV, left ventricle.

the geometry of the LV can be distorted by various diseases, and thus the accuracy of any individual measure of EF is dependent on the completeness of the measurements. For instance, use of simple formulas derived from two-dimensional echocardiographic measures of end-systolic and end-diastolic dimensions and estimates of LV long-axis length can be erroneous if there are regional abnormalities of contraction, such as after infarction. In such instances, accurate measures of EF can be derived with radionuclide ventriculography (which does not require assumptions of ventricular shape) or directly via quantitation of LV end-diastolic volume (EDV) and end-systolic volume (ESV) with magnetic resonance imaging or electron beam computed tomography. Thus:

$$\text{ejection (fraction EF)} = \frac{\text{EDV - ESV}}{\text{EDV}} = \frac{\text{SV}}{\text{EDV}}$$

Table 5.—Clinical Methods of Measuring Left Ventricular Systolic Function

1. Ejection fraction (EF) can be determined with available imaging tools; be cautious of methods that rely on assumptions of LV geometry; acute increase in preload or decrease in afterload will increase EF, and vice versa
2. The velocity of circumferential fractional shortening (VCF) is a better index of contractility than the actual amount of shortening; is relatively insensitive to acute changes in preload; difficult to calculate clinically
3. PER: peak LV systolic emptying rate; load-dependent index of systolic function; use angio, RNA, cine-CT

angio, angiography; cine-CT, cine-computed tomography; RNA, radionuclide angiography.

• The most commonly applied and clinically available measure of systolic performance or contraction is the ejection fraction.

Maximal Elastance

Another method for measurement of left ventricular contractility is the concept of Emax (maximal elastance). This is based on the observation that there is a linear relationship between pressure and volume at end-systole. Stated another way, all end-systolic pressure-volume points form a straight line on the pressure-volume curve for a given degree of contractility. The slope of this line is called the Emax. With an increase in contractility, there is an increase in the slope of the Emax; with a decrease in contractility, there is a decrease in the slope of the Emax. Calculation of Emax requires construction of pressure-volume curves and alteration of either preload or afterload (Fig. 7).

Myocardial Relaxation

Myocardial relaxation is the process by which the myocardium returns to its initial length and tension. Cardiac relaxation is an energy-dependent process that consumes high-energy phosphates. At the cellular level, abnormalities of calcium reuptake may account for LV diastolic abnormalities and failure of relaxation. Relaxation also depends on systolic and diastolic loads and the passive elastic characteristics of the ventricle.

Relaxation may be simplistically regarded as occurring during the isovolumic relaxation period and part of the rapid filling period. If the ventricle is able to fully and quickly complete relaxation, the ventricle will rapidly expand and a large portion of blood flows in from the left atrium to the LV after mitral valve opening. However, if there is a delay in the rate and duration of relaxation, the ventricle will continue to expand slowly even after mitral valve opening. There will thus be a decrease in the rate of early rapid filling.

Ventricular Compliance

In mid- and late diastole, pressure and volume increase, and the passive diastolic properties of the ventricle, namely, chamber stiffness (or its inverse, chamber compliance), can be assessed. LV compliance is the change in volume per unit pressure as the LV fills with blood from the left atrium. Thus, a decrease in compliance will result in less blood entering the LV for a given increase in pressure. Myocardial fibrosis from any cause can be expected to increase stiffness

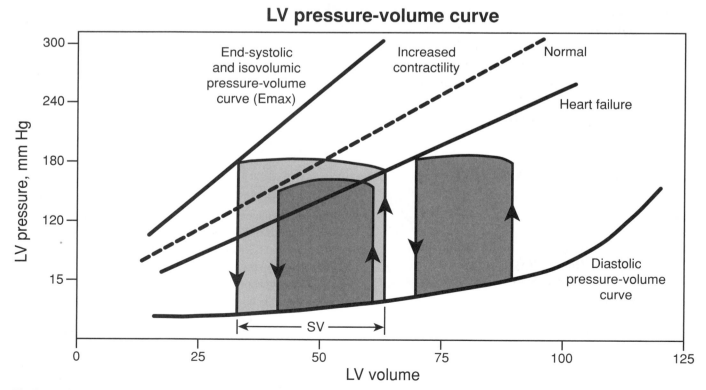

Fig. 7. Maximal elastance (Emax) is a sensitive measure of left ventricular (LV) function and is derived from LV pressure-volume loops.

because collagen fibers are very rigid, being virtually nondistensible at normal pressures.

The term "myocardial stiffness" is used to differentiate changes in the stiffness properties of each unit of muscle as opposed to overall chamber stiffness. Thickening of ventricular walls from any cause (for example, LV hypertrophy) tends to increase both myocardial and chamber stiffness. An increased volume/mass ratio is often associated with increased chamber stiffness, whereas in other cases, increased chamber stiffness may occur in the presence of a normal volume/mass ratio, implying increased myocardial stiffness.

Questions

Multiple Choice (choose the one best answer)

1. Arterial impedance is extremely difficult to treat mathematically for which of the following reasons?
   a. Blood is a non-newtonian fluid and therefore its apparent viscosity is dependent on flow rate and tube dimensions
   b. The arteries are viscoelastic
   c. The capacitance varies considerably with anatomical location
   d. The anatomical branching patterns are complex and therefore constitute an extremely irregular network of sites for producing reflected waves
   e. All of the above

2. The following can result in an increase in cardiac contractility *except*:
   a. Dobutamine infusion
   b. Premature ventricular contraction
   c. Increase in heart rate
   d. Angiotensin-converting enzyme inhibitor

3. The following statements about the heart are true *except*:
   a. The Frank-Starling principle relates initial myocardial fiber length to tension development by the ventricle
   b. The myocardium is very rich in mitochondria
   c. The center of the sarcomere is occupied by the dark A band and flanked by the Z bands
   d. The myocardium has about one capillary per fiber
   e. The T tubular system plays a role in excitation-contraction coupling

4. Which of the following is part of the left ventricular cardiac cycle?
   a. Isovolumic contraction
   b. Ventricular ejection
   c. Isovolumic relaxation
   d. Rapid filling phase
   e. All of the above

5.-9. Choose answer a or b for statements 5-9
   a. Isovolumic contraction
   b. Ejection

5. Distinguished by an increase in ventricular and aortic pressure and a greater aortic blood flow

6. Coincides with the peak of the R wave on electrocardiography

7. The earliest increase in ventricular pressure after atrial contraction

8. The interval between the start of ventricular systole and the opening of the semilunar valves

9. The sharp decrease in the left atrial pressure due to the descent of the base of the heart and stretch of the atria

10. The sarcotubular system is located within certain myocardial cells. It is composed of sarcoplasmic reticular and transverse tubules. Its purpose is:
    a. To enhance automaticity
    b. To facilitate electrical conduction and contraction
    c. To serve as an energy reserve for myocardial cell function
    d. To transport electrical impulses from the sinoatrial node to the atrioventricular node

11. The peak active tension (L_{max}) in the length-tension curve of a papillary muscle sarcomere occurs:
    a. At 2.0 µm
    b. At 2.2 µm
    c. At 3.0 µm
    d. At 3.65 µm
    e. Beyond 3.65 µm

12. Afterload steadily increases during systole:
    a. True
    b. False

13. The concept of "afterload/preload mismatch" is common in:
    a. Patients with congestive heart failure
    b. Patients with severe hemorrhage
    c. Patients with sepsis
    d. Patients with pulmonary embolism
    e. All of the above

14.-16. For statements 14-16, match the appropriate physiologic principle
    a. Bowditch ("treppe") effect
    b. Law of Laplace
    c. Anrep effect
    d. Woodworth phenomenon

14. The positive inotropic effect of an acute increase in afterload

15. The tension tending to expand the wall of a blood vessel is greater if the radius of the vessel is greater, or if the blood vessel wall is thinner

16. An increase in heart rate may in itself increase myocardial contractility

Answers

1. Answer e

The non-newtonian nature of blood makes the element of viscosity dependent on shear rate and thus does not lend itself to easy mathematical manipulation. The viscoelastic nature of the arteries alters not only the conductance but also the capacitance. The patterns of wave reflection (which account for the changes in the arterial pulse height and width as one proceeds distally from the central circulation) are complex and dependent on other factors, such as blood viscosity and the state of "stiffness" of the arteries and individual arterial segments.

2. Answer d

Dobutamine is a β-agonist and thus has a direct effect on ventricular contractility. Post-extrasystolic potentiation refers to the supernormal contraction that follows a premature ventricular depolarization. The more premature the extra beat, the more forceful the ventricular contraction following it. Increased availability of calcium ions at the contractile sites caused by the additional electrical activation is postulated as the major mechanism; however, the increased preload from the long filling period and decreased afterload from the ineffective contraction associated with the extra beat also play a role in augmenting cardiac performance. Increasing the frequency of contraction will improve myocardial contractility, because the systolic fraction of the cardiac cycle is increased (from the usual 30% to up to 50% of the cardiac cycle). The ventricle responds to repeated stimuli occurring at shorter intervals with increasing strength of contraction until a plateau is reached. The increase in force of contraction is attributed to an increase in intracellular calcium, because calcium enters the cell with every electrical action potential.

3. Answer c

The sarcomeres are flanked by the two (microscopically) lighter I, or isotropic, bands. The other statements are true.

4. Answer e

All are components of the ventricular cardiac cycle.

5. through 9. Answers are: 5. b; 6. a; 7. a; 8. a; 9. b.

10. Answer b

The sarcotubular system provides a mechanism for electromechanical coupling. It consists of a transverse tubular system, which facilitates electrical conduction, and the sarcoplasmic reticulum, which is stimulated to release large amounts of calcium for myocardial contraction. It does not have a part in "automaticity" or sinoatrial to atrioventricular node conduction. It does not function as a site for energy reserve.

11. Answer b

The length-tension studies done by Sonnenblick form the experimental validation of Starling's law. The maximal length of the sarcomere (after fixation) is around 2.2 μm, at which length the thin actin and thick myosin myofilaments are optimally overlapped to provide the greatest number of force-generating sites. At sarcomere lengths of less than 2.2 μm, the actin myofilaments first pass into the center of the sarcomere, and at 2.0 μm they bypass one another and developed tension decreases. At a length of 3.65 μm, the actin and myosin myofilaments are completely disengaged and the developed tension decreases by zero.

12. Answer b

In the simplest conceptualization of the law of Laplace for the heart, wall stress is directly proportional to arterial pressure and radius of curvature and inversely proportional to wall thickness. Although intracavitary pressure initially increases after commencement of mechanical systole, radius of curvature decreases and wall thickness increases. Thus, the combined effect is to actually decrease wall stress during systole from its value at end-diastole.

13. Answer e

Patients with congestive heart failure have the classic mismatch. They frequently are at the limit of their preload reserve because of ventricular dilatation and certain structural abnormalities that result in altered ventricular capacitance. When the preload reserve cannot be counted on to augment cardiac output, afterload reduction (to attempt a better matching of afterload with preload) is a common method of therapy. Both sepsis and hemorrhage act as situations of relative intravascular volume depletion or paralysis or inadequacy of venous constriction and thus result in lowering of preload pressures (volumes). Severe pulmonary embolism also can result in relative decreases in left atrial return and a subsequent reduction in left ventricular filling volumes and pressures.

14. through 16. Answers are: 14. c; 15. b; 16. a

The Bowditch effect (also called the "treppe" or staircase phenomenon) is a force-interval relationship in which an increase in pulse rate may also increase myocardial contractility. The law of Laplace reflects relationships between the distending pressure and tension in the wall of a blood vessel. The Anrep effect describes an additional influence in afterload changes whereby there is an increase in ventricular performance several beats after the aortic pressure is increased. This may be due to recovery from transient subendocardial ischemia caused by the sudden change in arterial impedance. The recuperative effect of a long pause on the strength of contraction is known as the Woodworth phenomenon.

Notes

Chapter 4

Left Ventricular Diastolic Function

Christopher P. Appleton, M.D.

Candidates for the Cardiology Boards are expected to know in outline the hemodynamic phases of diastole, the cellular events that occur in diastole, methods of measuring diastolic function of the left ventricle, and the effects of disease on ventricular diastolic function.

Left ventricular (LV) diastolic function can be defined as the ability of the ventricle to fill to a normal end-diastolic volume, during both rest and exercise, with a mean left atrial (LA) pressure that does not exceed 12 mm Hg. Abnormalities of LV diastolic function occur early in most cardiac diseases and increase in frequency with age, with up to 40% to 50% of patients older than 70 with symptoms of congestive heart failure having "LV diastolic dysfunction" as their primary cardiac problem. These patients either are unable to distend a slowly relaxing and stiffened left ventricle adequately or can do so only with increased filling pressures. As a result, symptoms due to pulmonary congestion and atrial arrhythmias are common, and a reduced exercise capacity often results. Although the mortality rate associated with "isolated" diastolic dysfunction appears to be only one-third of that associated with LV systolic dysfunction, the morbidity and functional disability may be severe. Recognition of patients whose main problem is diastolic dysfunction is important because therapy for these patients is usually different from that for patients with LV systolic dysfunction.

- In patients older than 60 years who have symptoms of heart failure, LV diastolic dysfunction should always be included in the differential diagnosis, especially if systolic function is normal.
- Although the mortality rate associated with "isolated" diastolic dysfunction is less than that associated with LV systolic dysfunction, the morbidity and functional disability may be severe.

Hemodynamic Phases of Diastole

Diastole is divided into four phases: 1) isovolumic relaxation, 2) early LV filling, 3) diastasis, and 4) filling at atrial contraction. As shown in Figure 1, the determinants of LV diastolic performance vary in their importance and interaction during these different phases. Isovolumic relaxation begins with aortic valve closure and continues until LV pressure decreases to less than LA pressure. Early diastolic LV filling begins with mitral valve opening and ends when the increasing ventricular pressure equals or exceeds the LA pressure. If the diastolic filling period is relatively long, a period of diastasis follows in which LA and LV pressures are nearly equal and little additional LV filling is occurring. Finally, atrial contraction reestablishes a transmitral pressure gradient, and a variable amount of blood is transferred from atrium to ventricle in late diastole.

- Diastole is divided into four phases: 1) isovolumic

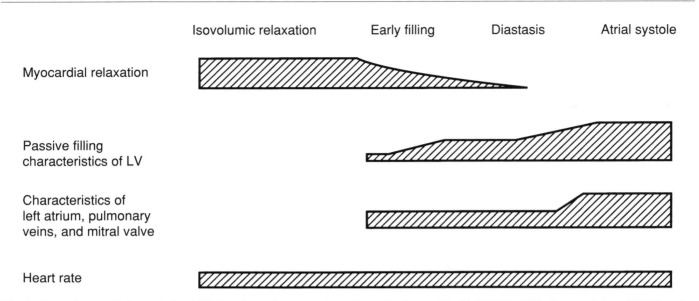

Fig. 1. Determinants of left ventricular (LV) diastolic performance. (From *Prog Cardiovasc Dis* 32:273-290, 1990. By permission of WB Saunders Company.)

relaxation, 2) early LV filling, 3) diastasis, and 4) filling at atrial contraction.

Although dividing diastole into phases aids description and quantitation of LV diastolic properties, in reality such a separation is artificial in that the factors that influence each phase usually influence all others, especially in disease states. This interaction of diastolic properties, the multiple other factors that influence these properties (such as systolic function, pericardial restraint, and coronary artery turgor), and the overlap of their effects on the different phases of diastole have contributed to the difficulty in understanding and studying LV diastolic function.

LV Diastolic Properties

LV Relaxation

The process of LV contraction and relaxation is dependent on myocardial cytosolic Ca^{2+} concentration. In mammalian hearts, contraction occurs after cellular depolarization results in the passive release of large stores of calcium from the sarcoplasmic tubular network or sarcoplasmic reticulum and subsequent activation of the Ca^{2+}-troponin-actin-myosin cascade. LV relaxation (actin-myosin crossbridge deactivation) occurs when cytosolic Ca^{2+} decreases, the result of an energy-dependent (adenosine triphosphate) reuptake of the calcium by a powerful sarcoplasmic reticulum Ca^{2+} pump. The faster the rate of Ca^{2+} reuptake, the faster the rate

of LV relaxation and decrease in LV pressure.

The cellular processes and molecular biology that influence myocyte Ca^{2+} handling and LV relaxation and the effect of cardiac diseases are becoming clearer (Fig. 2). The sarcoplasmic reticulum Ca^{2+} pump, which controls the rate of LV relaxation, has an endogenous regulator, phospholamban, which is stimulated by phosphorylation with a cyclic adenosine monophosphate-dependent protein kinase. LV contraction and relaxation also can be affected by various mechanisms that alter the availability of Ca^{2+} to the contractile proteins, or conversely the sensitivity of the proteins to Ca^{2+}. β_1-Adrenergic phosphorylation of phospholamban by drugs such as isoproterenol and mechanical stretch or load on the ventricle are posttranslational ways of modulating LV relaxation. Pretranslational changes in gene expression for the sarcoplasmic reticulum Ca^{2+} pump and phospholamban also appear to occur as a result of neurohumoral triggers, myocyte hypertrophy, or myocyte contractile dysfunction.

In contrast to LV contraction, in which Ca^{2+} is released "passively," LV relaxation is an energy-dependent process that requires the reuptake of Ca^{2+} into the sarcoplasmic reticulum. Thus, abnormalities of diastolic function occur earlier in disease states than abnormalities of systolic function.

- The sarcoplasmic reticulum Ca^{2+} pump, which controls the rate of LV relaxation, has an endogenous regulator, phospholamban.

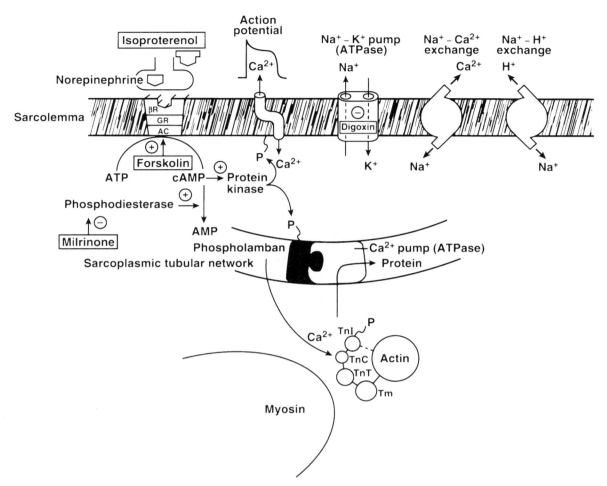

Fig. 2. Calcium use in excitation-contraction coupling in the mammalian heart. AC, adenylate cyclase; AMP, adenosine monophosphate; ATP, adenosine triphosphate; cAMP, cyclic AMP; βR, β-adrenergic receptor; GR, G protein-coupled receptor kinase; P, degree of phosphorylation; Tm, tropomyosin; TnC, troponin C; TnI, troponin I; TnT, troponin T. (From *Circulation* 87 Suppl 7:VII-31-VII-37, 1993. By permission of the American Heart Association.)

- LV contraction and relaxation also can be affected by various mechanisms that alter the availability of Ca^{2+} to the contractile proteins or, conversely, the sensitivity of the proteins to Ca^{2+}.

In the intact mammalian heart, both experimental and clinical studies suggest that the normal LV contracts to a volume below its equilibrium volume, compressing elastic cardiac elements, which creates early diastole-restoring forces that produce a "suction" effect that lowers LV minimal pressure and increases early LV filling. Rapid normal LV relaxation helps maximize the beneficial effect of these restoring forces, and together they result in a normal pattern of LV filling that occurs predominantly in early diastole. In contrast to the process of calcium release, the reuptake of cytosolic calcium into the sarcoplasmic reticulum is an active, energy-(adenosine triphosphate) and load-dependent process.

Deactivation of the contractile proteins can be delayed by several mechanisms, and this delay is a consistent finding that occurs early in the course of nearly all cardiac diseases. Ischemia, increased mechanical loading (hypertension, aortic stenosis), tachycardia, electrical dyssynchrony, and negative inotropic drugs are some of the posttranslational ways that LV relaxation is slowed or "impaired." Genetic alterations in the myocyte handling of calcium are induced by LV hypertrophy, thyroid hormones, and perhaps chronic catecholamine stimulation.

- In contrast to LV contraction, LV relaxation is an energy-dependent process and therefore more susceptible to disruption by disease states.

Slower LV relaxation antagonizes the "suction" effect of normal restoring forces on LV filling and results in a delayed mitral valve opening, lower early transmitral gradient, and a shift to an LV filling pattern that has reduced filling in early diastole and a greater proportion of filling at atrial contraction. This pattern is less favorable, especially during faster heart rates, because a shorter diastolic filling time may not allow the ventricle to relax and fill without increasing mean LA pressure and causing pulmonary congestion.

LV Passive Diastolic Properties

After LV relaxation is complete, the remainder of LV filling is influenced by more passive LV characteristics (Fig. 1). These are composed of inherent cardiac elements such as myocardial compliance, chamber compliance, and viscoelastic properties. They also are influenced by external constraints such as the pericardium and pulmonary airway pressure and volume. The sum effect of all components is described by the exponential diastolic LV pressure-volume relationship, which indicates the ability of a relaxed or passive LV to distend with increasing volume. A decrease in LV chamber compliance means that increased filling pressures will be required to maintain a normal cardiac filling volume and output.

Under normal circumstances, viscoelastic properties associated with LV filling are small and are usually ignored. Although an intact pericardium does contribute several millimeters of mercury to normal intracardiac pressures, the effect of pericardial restraint in limiting cardiac filling becomes clinically significant only during maximal exercise or when acute cardiac dilatation or pericardial disease is present. Similarly, only with a marked increase in pulmonary airway pressures, as in asthma or with positive-pressure ventilation, are intracardiac pressures affected sufficiently to inhibit LV filling or to decrease cardiac output.

- The effect of pericardial restraint in limiting cardiac filling becomes clinically significant only during maximal exercise or when acute cardiac dilatation or pericardial disease is present.

LV myocardial compliance is believed to be related mainly to the cardiac interstitial elements, the collagen-elastic struts and network that help connect and provide support for the cardiac myocytes. These elements are increased in the presence of pressure overload-induced LV hypertrophy. They also are increased in response to chronic LV ischemia and LV scarring, other conditions commonly associated with a decrease in LV compliance. LV chamber compliance decreases with increasing LV volume, in part due to the increased stretch on the elastic interstitial elements.

Measuring LV Diastolic Properties

LV Relaxation

The rate of LV relaxation can be measured from high-fidelity (micromanometer) pressure recordings taken during LV isovolumic relaxation (Fig. 3). A decrease in LV pressure is usually exponential between maximal -dP/dt (occurring approximately at aortic valve closure) and the time of mitral valve opening. The pressure decrease can be described by the relationship:

$$P(t) = P_o \cdot e^{-t/T}$$

where P_o is LV pressure at maximal -dP/dt (the point at which the rate of LV pressure decline is maximal), t is the time after onset of relaxation, and T is the time constant of isovolumic relaxation (τ). This time constant represents the time for the LV pressure to decrease to l/e of its initial value, τ typically being 30 to 40 ms in humans, with lower values of τ representing faster relaxation. Relaxation is believed to be "complete" after three time constants (90 to 120 ms in humans), which correspond in time to shortly after peak early diastolic filling in normals. In mammalian hearts, τ appears proportional to heart rate, being as short as 10 ms in rats, in which the normal resting heart rate is 350 beats/min.

- LV relaxation is quantitated by analyzing the exponential decrease in LV pressure during isovolumic relaxation.
- Tau (τ) is a quantitative measure of LV relaxation. Lower values represent faster relaxation of the LV.

Despite its usefulness, several limitations of quantitating LV relaxation with a simple exponential model are recognized. In patients with hypertrophic cardiomyopathy or markedly asynchronous relaxation, the decrease in LV pressure may significantly deviate from an exponential relationship. The simple model also assumes that LV pressure decays to zero pressure, which does not consider the effect of either LV restoring or external forces. Studies in normal animals suggest that if LV filling did not occur, LV minimal pressure would be negative. Although the addition of an intercept term to the original equation provides for a "floating" or non-zero LV asymptote pressure, the method to best quantify LV relaxation that is most appropriate under different circumstances remains controversial.

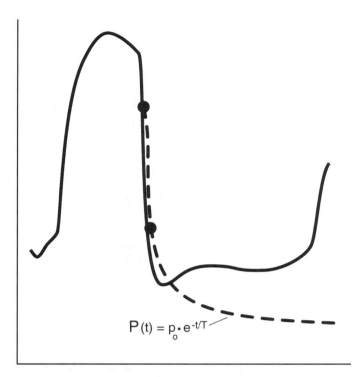

$$P(t) = p_o \cdot e^{-t/T}$$

Fig. 3. Calculation of time constant of myocardial relaxation (tau, τ). Pressure is plotted on y-axis, and time is plotted on x-axis. Pressure is measured by high-fidelity, manometer-tipped catheters. Pressure from time of aortic valve closure (upper dot) to mitral valve opening (lower dot) is fitted to a monoexponential equation. Time constant of relaxation (T) is obtained from equation, as shown. e, natural logarithm; p, pressure; t, time; T, τ. (From *Mayo Clin Proc* 64:71-81, 1989. By permission of Mayo Foundation for Medical Education and Research.)

LV Passive Properties

LV myocardial compliance, or the ability of the muscle to distend in response to a known stress, is quantitated by developing a stress-strain relationship. This requires deforming a known mass of myocardium with a given force while simultaneously measuring its deformation. Because of the many assumptions about LV geometry, and the inability to exclude the effects of external and "active" (relaxation, viscoelastic properties) LV forces, this has proved to be impractical in vivo. Therefore, the sum effect of myocardial compliance, chamber compliance, and external forces is studied by constructing LV pressure-volume (P-V) relationships obtained during diastasis (Fig. 4). Operating chamber compliance, or its reciprocal term "chamber stiffness," is defined as the slope of a tangent to this P-V relationship at a specified point. The steeper the slope, the less compliant or stiffer the ventricle (Fig. 4 *A*, in which point "b" is "stiffer" than "a"). Because chamber stiffness depends on which point of the P-V curve is used for assessment, several

methods have been proposed to normalize this value so that it can be compared after interventions, in serial studies, or between ventricles of different sizes. Although no consensus exists on this point, operating chamber compliance is most commonly measured at LV end-diastolic pressure.

- LV chamber compliance is evaluated by analyzing pressure-volume (P-V) relationships.

Shifts and shape changes in the LV P-V relationship have different implications. Because the P-V relationship is exponential, the same incremental increase in volume results in a greater pressure increase as the ventricle progressively distends (Fig. 4 *B*). If the shape of the P-V curve does not change, a shift leftward indicates decreased chamber compliance (same slope tangent at smaller LV volume), and a shift rightward indicates increased compliance. In reality, when measured in sequential studies, curve shifts to the right and left are usually accompanied by alterations in the shape of the P-V curve, and so the incremental change in pressure for a given volume is also changing (Fig. 4 *C*).

The requirements for accurate construction of LV P-V relationships are formidable. The points should be taken after LV relaxation is complete (during diastasis), so that only passive properties are in effect. High-fidelity LV pressure recordings should be used and transmural LV pressure (LV pressure-intrapleural pressure) should be calculated to avoid inaccuracies caused by respiratory-induced changes in intrapleural pressure. To characterize the P-V relationship over its entire clinical range, LV volume must be varied by rapid changes in preload and afterload without markedly affecting heart rate or LV contraction and relaxation. Accurate calculation of LV volume itself is difficult by current angiographic and echocardiographic methods. These requirements have proved impractical for most clinical studies. As a result, most research involving chamber compliance, or sequential changes in LV chamber compliance, has been performed in experimental studies only.

LV Diastolic Properties in Cardiac Disease States

The most common cardiac abnormality encountered in clinical practice is LV hypertrophy due to hypertension. Affected patients have impaired LV relaxation, and only a minority have evidence of reduced LV chamber compliance and increased LA pressures. Patients with ischemic

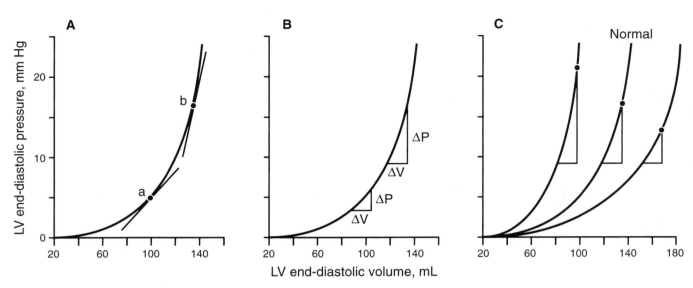

Fig. 4. Left ventricular (LV) pressure-volume relationships. P, pressure; V, volume.

heart disease are similar, with the great majority having mostly relaxation abnormalities and only about 10% having altered compliance that increases mean LA pressure to abnormal values. Patients with hypertrophic cardiomyopathy also have abnormal LV relaxation (sometimes severe), but a higher proportion of individuals also have a decrease in chamber compliance.

- The most common cause of isolated LV diastolic dysfunction is LV hypertrophy due to hypertensive heart disease.

Patients with dilated cardiomyopathies typically have both impaired LV relaxation and reduced chamber compliance. Interestingly, the LV P-V relationship is shifted right (more compliant) in most cases, but this is offset by the increase in LV volume, and therefore filling pressures are often increased. More rarely (< 10% of the time), operating chamber compliance and filling pressures remain normal.

- Shifting of the LV P-V relationship to the right indicates a more compliant ventricle and is common in patients with dilated cardiomyopathies, even though filling pressures are often increased.

In restrictive cardiomyopathy, LV relaxation is also usually impaired. However, the hallmark of this disorder is a severe decrease in LV chamber compliance at normal, or

near normal, LV volumes. This indicates a shift of the diastolic P-V relationship to the left. A similar leftward shift of the P-V relationship occurs in patients with constrictive pericarditis due to the thickened, noncompliant pericardium. Constrictive pericarditis is unusual in being one of the only cardiac disorders in which LV relaxation can be normal in the presence of severely altered chamber compliance.

- A leftward shift of the P-V relationship occurs in patients with restrictive cardiomyopathy as a result of increased muscle stiffness. A similar leftward shift is seen in constrictive pericarditis due to a thickened, noncompliant pericardium.

Patients with isolated mitral or aortic regurgitation often have little change in LV relaxation or chamber compliance. In patients with LV enlargement, this indicates a remodeling of the ventricle to an eccentric-type hypertrophy whose P-V relationship has shifted to the right, keeping filling pressures normal despite the increase in cardiac volume. A marked decrease in cardiac compliance usually indicates very severe regurgitation or additional cardiac abnormalities.

- Patients with isolated chronic mitral or aortic regurgitation often have little change in LV relaxation, and a shift of the P-V curve to the right helps keep filling pressures normal.

Relationship of LV Systolic and Diastolic Function

LV systolic and diastolic function are intimately related on a beat-to-beat basis. For example, through its effect on restoring forces, LV end-systolic volume affects the rate of LV relaxation, and thus patients with reduced LV ejection fractions are expected to have a prolonged τ. Conversely, by the Starling mechanism, LV end-diastolic pressure and stretch affect LV contractility. Loading conditions, inotropic stimulation, and neurohumoral factors likewise generally affect both systolic and diastolic function in parallel fashion.

- Loading conditions, inotropic stimulation, and neurohumoral factors generally affect both systolic and diastolic function in parallel fashion.

Despite this close interaction, a hysteresis of LV systolic and diastolic function does occur. This is common with LV hypertrophy, in which end-systolic volume and LV ejection fraction remain normal yet LV relaxation is impaired. As discussed previously, this dissociation occurs because changes in the rate of calcium reuptake, which controls the speed of LV relaxation, can occur without changes in LV ejection fraction or end-systolic volume. Hypertrophic and restrictive cardiomyopathies are diseases in which reduced chamber compliance, as well as prolonged relaxation, can occur with a normal LV ejection fraction. The reverse situation, abnormal LV systolic function with normal diastolic properties, is not observed, although shifts of the LV P-V relationship to the right frequently minimize the decrease in LV chamber compliance that could occur when ventricular volume is increased.

LV Diastolic Filling Pressures

Familiarity with different LV filling pressures and their pathophysiologic correlates aids understanding of LV diastolic function. The difference between LA and LV pressure (the transmitral pressure gradient) determines whether there is forward mitral blood flow and LV filling (Fig. 5). LV end-diastolic pressure, or the pressure immediately preceding systole, distends the myocardium and modulates stroke volume via the Frank-Starling mechanism. When increased LV end-diastolic pressure is needed to fill a noncompliant ventricle, two different mechanisms

may be present. In less advanced disease, a vigorous LA contraction confines the abnormal pressure increase to the short period in late diastole, so that mean LA pressure remains normal. In more advanced disease, LV compliance is reduced and mean LA pressure is increased, pulmonary congestion is often present, and pressure increases rapidly in early diastole and stays increased. In the patient with less severe disease, the loss of atrial contraction due

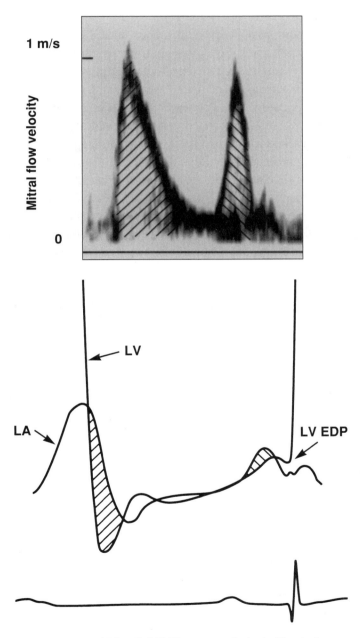

Fig. 5. *Upper Panel*, Diastolic LV filling pattern obtained with pulsed-wave Doppler technique. *Lower Panel*, Transmitral pressure gradient (hatched areas) that causes this filling. LA, left atrium; LV, left ventricle; LV EDP, left ventricular end-diastolic pressure.

to atrial fibrillation may precipitate pulmonary edema. Paradoxically, the same arrhythmia may have relatively less effect in the patient with reduced LV compliance because the atrium may already show signs of systolic decompensation and contribute relatively little to ventricular filling.

LV Filling Patterns

At Rest and With Exercise and Aging

Although many factors influence diastolic function, LV relaxation and LV chamber compliance (through its effect on LA pressure) are the chief determinants of the transmitral pressure gradient and LV filling. For a given LA pressure, slower LV relaxation results in later mitral valve opening, reduced early diastolic transmitral gradient and filling, and a compensatory increase in the proportion of filling at atrial contraction. Conversely, for the same rate of LV relaxation, higher LA pressure results in opposite effects. At normal heart rates and PR intervals, atrial contraction occurs after LV relaxation and early diastolic filling are complete. This separation of early and late diastolic filling optimizes mechanical efficiency and helps maintain normal LA filling pressures.

In young persons, LV relaxation is rapid, LV-restoring forces are prominent, and most LV filling (70%-90%) occurs in early diastole. With aging, LV relaxation slows in association with an increase in systolic blood pressure and LV mass, and the proportion of filling that occurs with atrial contraction increases, typically to 30% to 40% by age 65. During exercise, the rate of LV relaxation becomes faster and the PR interval shortens. These changes offset the reduction in diastolic filling time at faster heart rates and help maintain the separation between early and late diastolic filling. Despite increases in cardiac output of 3 to 5 times with exercise, LA pressure does not appreciably increase in normal subjects.

LV Filling Patterns in Disease States

Three basic abnormal LV filling patterns are recognized and are associated with changes in LV diastolic properties and filling pressures (Fig. 6). The most common and least abnormal pattern is reduced filling in early diastole due to "impaired" LV relaxation in the presence of normal LA pressure. Affected patients generally have minimal symptoms at rest, but they may show a limitation in exercise capacity. This may be due to an abnormal increase in LA

pressure or an inability to increase LV end-diastolic volume due to a premature "fusion" of early and late diastolic filling at faster heart rates.

A second abnormal LV filling pattern has been termed "pseudonormal," to indicate that although LV filling appears relatively normal, diastolic abnormalities are present. This seemingly paradoxical situation occurs when the effect of impaired LV relaxation on early diastolic filling is offset by a moderate decrease in LV compliance and increase in LA pressure. In contrast to a truly normal LV filling pattern, blood is forced, rather than sucked, into the LV in early diastole. Patients with this pattern have a moderate functional limitation that is between that of patients with impaired LV relaxation and those with restrictive-type physiology.

A third abnormal LV filling pattern is called "restrictive." Patients with this filling pattern also have impaired LV relaxation; however, a severe decrease in LV chamber compliance results in a markedly increased LA pressure, which forces blood into the ventricle in early diastole. This results in an increased proportion of filling in early diastole that has an abrupt, premature termination, with only minimal filling occurring at atrial contraction. A reduced atrial contribution indicates LA systolic failure is present as a result of chronic pressure overload. Patients with this pattern are severely symptomatic and have marked functional impairment.

- Three abnormal LV filling patterns are recognized. In order of increasing severity they are: "impaired" relaxation, "pseudonormal" filling, and "restrictive" filling.

Gradations in LV filling patterns among the three abnormalities are common. Unusual patterns also can occur in the presence of a prolonged PR interval or intraventricular conduction defects. However, the abnormal LV filling patterns remain specific to the alterations in LV relaxation and compliance rather than to the type of cardiac disease, and all three patterns (depending on disease stage) occur in disorders as diverse as restrictive and dilated cardiomyopathies. The progression of abnormalities in LV filling patterns with disease states (from impaired relaxation to pseudonormal to restrictive), together with changes in LV relaxation and compliance, has been documented in experimental models of congestive heart failure and clinically observed in patients with restrictive cardiomyopathies. When considered with the normal changes observed with aging, a "natural history" of LV filling patterns in health and disease can be constructed (Fig. 7).

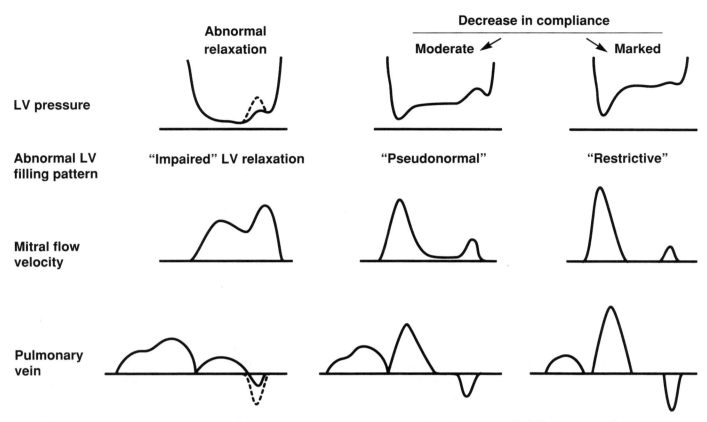

Fig. 6. The three basic abnormal left ventricular (LV) (mitral flow velocity) filling patterns together with representative LV pressure recordings and pulmonary venous flow velocity recordings.

Noninvasive Evaluation of LV Diastolic Function

Because of the impracticality of invasively measuring diastolic properties in most patients, noninvasive methods for indirectly evaluating LV diastolic function have been developed. These methods have focused on evaluating the LV filling pattern. The techniques have included digitized M-mode echocardiography, radionuclide ventriculography, pulsed-wave Doppler mitral flow velocity recordings, and, more recently, cine-computed tomography or magnetic resonance imaging angiography.

Radionuclide techniques that evaluate LV filling variables, such as peak filling rates and time to peak filling, have been studied in several disease states. Although sensitive for identifying impaired relaxation and restrictive-type filling abnormalities, a major limitation has been the inability of these variables to distinguish normal from pseudonormal filling patterns. Therefore, currently this technique is infrequently used to assess LV diastolic function.

Because of ease of performance, lack of ionizing radiation, and associated information about cardiac anatomy, valvular disease, and filling pressures, Doppler techniques have become the method most frequently used to assess LV filling and, indirectly, diastolic function. This analysis includes pulsed-wave Doppler recording of mitral, pulmonary venous, and right heart inflow velocities. Nomograms for normal age-related mitral and pulmonary venous flow velocities and related variables have been established. Although the differentiation of normal from pseudonormal LV filling from mitral inflow velocity alone can be challenging, ancillary data such as pulmonary venous flow velocities, LA size and function, response to the Valsalva maneuver, and rate of color M-mode mitral inflow propagation enable the distinction to be made in most cases. In addition, tissue Doppler imaging of mitral annular motion or myocardial velocities is a promising new technique that appears to help identify diastolic abnormalities.

As discussed previously, the three abnormal LV filling patterns have a general relationship to LV filling pressures. Several recent Doppler studies suggest that individual variables, such as atrial filling fraction, LA minimal volume,

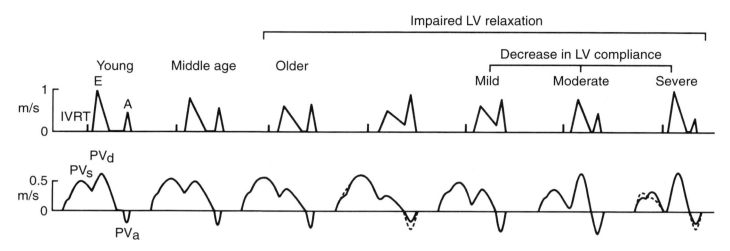

Fig. 7. Natural history of left ventricular (LV) filling patterns. A, mitral flow velocity at atrial contraction; E, mitral flow velocity in early diastole; IVRT, LV isovolumic relaxation time; PV_a, reverse pulmonary venous flow at atrial contraction; PV_d, pulmonary venous flow velocity in diastole; PV_s, pulmonary venous flow velocity in systole. (Modified from *Echocardiography* 9:437-457, 1992. By permission of Futura Publishing Company.)

the systolic fraction of pulmonary venous flow, or peak A-wave reversal in the pulmonary veins, also may be related to LV filling and end-diastolic pressures. Recent data show that regardless of age, when the extent of pulmonary venous flow at atrial contraction exceeds that of mitral flow velocity at atrial contraction by more than 30 ms, LV end-diastolic pressure and A-wave pressure are usually increased. The use of a combination of pulsed-wave and tissue Doppler variables is currently being explored as a possible way to help improve the estimate of mean LA pressure. However, differences in published results and a preponderance of older patients with coronary artery disease in all the studies suggest that further data will be necessary to determine the applicability of these methods to patients of all ages and with all types of cardiac disease.

- A pulsed-wave Doppler evaluation of mitral and pulmonary venous flow velocities is currently the most common method used for assessing LV diastolic function and filling pressures.
- Tissue Doppler imaging of mitral annular motion or myocardial velocities is a promising new technique that appears to help identify diastolic abnormalities.

The value of LV filling and mitral flow velocity patterns for predicting survival has been demonstrated in patients with dilated (Fig. 8) and restrictive cardiomyopathies. In some studies, the deceleration time of early mitral flow velocity was the strongest predictor of reduced survival and

was independent of LV systolic function. However, in other studies of dilated cardiomyopathy, LV systolic function was a more powerful predictor. Newer studies have shown that the response of the LV filling patterns to alterations in loading conditions also helps predict prognosis. Prospective studies are under way to compare the prognostic significance of LV systolic and diastolic indices in patients with heart failure.

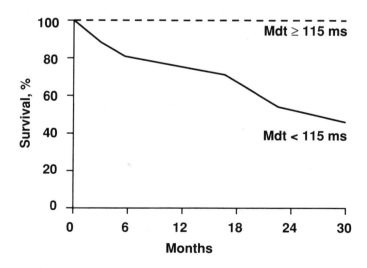

Fig. 8. Actuarial survival curves of patients with dilated cardiomyopathy, by Doppler pulsed-wave mitral deceleration time (Mdt). (From *J Am Coll Cardiol* 22:808-815, 1993. By permission of the American College of Cardiology.)

- The value of LV filling and mitral flow velocity patterns for predicting survival has been demonstrated in patients with dilated and restrictive cardiomyopathies.
- A restrictive LV filling pattern indicates a poor prognosis regardless of disease type or LV ejection fraction.
- The response of the LV filling patterns to alterations in loading conditions also helps predict prognosis in patients with reduced LV ejection fractions.

Although the evaluation of LV diastolic function by these Doppler techniques has become increasingly helpful, it should be remembered that the flow velocity patterns obtained represent the "net effect" of all the various factors that affect LV diastolic properties. Recently, Doppler methods have been described for more directly estimating the rate of LV relaxation in patients with aortic and mitral regurgitation. The deceleration time of early mitral flow velocity also has been demonstrated to be related to LV chamber compliance in experimental models of heart failure. Whether these methods will allow better direct quantification of LV diastolic properties, and under what circumstances, will require further study.

Therapy for LV Diastolic Dysfunction

Once diastolic dysfunction is identified, the immediate goals of therapy are to favorably improve cardiac loading conditions, heart rate, or atrioventricular coupling intervals and, simultaneously, treat the underlying cause of the diastolic dysfunction.

In patients with a marked reduction in LV ejection fraction and increased filling pressures, treatment with digitalis, diuretics, and reduction of afterload is appropriate. Patients with increased filling pressures and normal systolic function are also treated with diuretics to reduce pulmonary congestion, the exception being patients with thick-walled, restrictive-like cardiomyopathies when decreasing preload may result in a decrease in cardiac output and compensatory tachycardia.

In patients with an impaired relaxation-type LV filling pattern, therapy focuses more on reversing the underlying disease process that is contributing to the abnormally slow LV relaxation and altering diastolic filling mechanics in a way that offsets its effect and improves exercise tolerance. If normal or increased LV systolic function is present, Ca^{2+} channel or β-adrenergic blocking drugs may be beneficial by slowing the heart rate, which allows the ventricle to relax more completely and fill before atrial contraction. Over a long treatment period, the regression of hypertrophy with these agents alone or together with diuretics and angiotensin-converting enzyme inhibitors can lead to an improvement in relaxation and more normal LV filling. The potential beneficial effects of slowing the heart rate are most easily appreciated by examining a pulsed-wave Doppler mitral flow velocity pattern. Patients likely to have the most symptomatic benefit from lowering their heart rate are those with evidence of markedly delayed LV relaxation or near fusion of early and late LV diastolic filling with normal PR intervals. Patients with first-degree atrioventricular block respond less well, and the increase in PR interval with Ca^{2+} and β-blocking agents may actually result in an earlier atrial contraction, a more fused early and late diastolic LV filling pattern, and a reduced exercise tolerance. Dual-chamber cardiac pacing with a shortened PR interval, analogous to that used in patients with dilated cardiomyopathy, may be helpful for restoring a more normal filling profile if a pacemaker is present in patients with first-degree atrioventricular block and mitral E and A wave fusion.

- Therapy for diastolic dysfunction involves optimizing preload and afterload and treating the underlying abnormality that is causing the diastolic abnormality. Manipulating the heart rate (usually slower) or shortening the PR interval may also be helpful in some cases.

Suggested Review Reading

1. Appleton CP, Hatle LK: The natural history of left ventricular filling abnormalities: assessment by two-dimensional and Doppler echocardiography. *Echocardiography* 9:437-457, 1992.
This review article first proposed a "natural" history of LV filling patterns in health and disease. Its concepts helped explain how interaction of different rates of LV relaxation, LV compliance, and filling pressures could give similar-appearing LV filling patterns in normal subjects and patients with cardiac disease. These concepts were later validated in experimental models of heart failure.

2. Appleton CP, Hatle LK, Popp RL: Relation of transmitral flow velocity patterns to left ventricular diastolic function: new insights from a combined hemodynamic and Doppler echocardiographic study. *J Am Coll Cardiol* 12:426-440, 1988.
This is the original article describing the Doppler echocardiographic features of the three abnormal LV filling patterns (impaired relaxation, pseudonormal, and restrictive) and their hemodynamic and functional relations in patients with cardiac disease.

3. Bonow RO, Udelson JE: Left ventricular diastolic dysfunction as a cause of congestive heart failure. Mechanisms and management. *Ann Intern Med* 117:502-510, 1992.
The mechanisms by which LV diastolic dysfunction causes heart failure and potential treatments are described.

4. Brun P, Tribouilloy C, Duval AM, et al: Left ventricular flow propagation during early filling is related to wall relaxation: a color M-mode Doppler analysis. *J Am Coll Cardiol* 20:420-432, 1992.
This was the first study to use color M-mode Doppler technique for analysis of the rate of LV inflow propagation and how it is slowed in patients with impaired LV relaxation.

5. Cuocolo A, Sax FL, Brush JE, et al: Left ventricular hypertrophy and impaired diastolic filling in essential hypertension. Diastolic mechanisms for systolic dysfunction during exercise. *Circulation* 81:978-986, 1990.
This radionuclide study shows that a limitation to exercise in patients with LV hypertrophy and abnormal diastolic function is often the inability to fill to a normal LV end-diastolic volume, rather than any systolic abnormalities.

6. Garcia MJ, Ares MA, Asher C, et al: An index of early left ventricular filling that combined with pulsed Doppler peak E velocity may estimate capillary wedge pressure. *J Am Coll Cardiol* 29:448-454, 1997.
This article describes a promising new method of using a combination of pulsed-wave and color Doppler LV inflow propagation velocity to estimate LV filling pressures.

7. Isaaz K, Munoz del Romeral L, Lee E, et al: Quantitation of the motion of the cardiac base in normal subjects by Doppler echocardiography. *J Am Soc Echocardiogr* 6:166-176, 1993.
This study shows that normal LV diastolic function demonstrates more longitudinal shortening and lengthening of the heart near the base than the apex.

8. Kitzman DW, Higginbotham MB, Cobb FR, et al: Exercise intolerance in patients with heart failure and preserved left ventricular systolic function: failure of the Frank-Starling mechanism. *J Am Coll Cardiol* 17:1065-1072, 1991.
This Doppler exercise (bike) study shows a limitation to exercise in patients with LV hypertrophy and abnormal diastolic function is an abnormal increase in LV filling pressures in combination with an inability to fill to a normal LV end-diastolic volume.

9. Klein AL, Hatle LK, Taliercio CP, et al: Prognostic significance of Doppler measures of diastolic function in cardiac amyloidosis. A Doppler echocardiography study. *Circulation* 83:808-816, 1991.
In this landmark article, the Doppler technique was used to determine prognosis in the most common restrictive cardiomyopathy, amyloidosis. Prognosis was related to LV diastolic function and, specifically, chamber compliance.

10. Little WC, Downes TR: Clinical evaluation of left ventricular diastolic performance. *Prog Cardiovasc Dis* 32:273-290, 1990.
This is a review of techniques traditionally used at cardiac catheterization to quantitate LV diastolic properties.

11. Nishimura RA, Hayes DL, Holmes DR Jr, et al: Mechanism of hemodynamic improvement by dual-chamber pacing for severe left ventricular dysfunction: an acute Doppler and catheterization hemodynamic study. *J Am Coll Cardiol* 25:281-288, 1995.
This article underscores the importance of the cardiac

conduction system and proper timing of atrial contraction for normal LV systolic and diastolic function.

12. Nishimura RA, Housmans PR, Hatle LK, et al: Assessment of diastolic function of the heart: background and current applications of Doppler echocardiography. Part I. Physiologic and pathophysiologic features. *Mayo Clin Proc* 64:71-81, 1989.
This article reviews phases of diastole, factors affecting LV diastolic filling, and relation to Doppler echocardiographic techniques.

13. Nishimura RA, Tajik AJ: Quantitative hemodynamics by Doppler echocardiography: a noninvasive alternative to cardiac catheterization. *Prog Cardiovasc Dis* 36:309-342, 1994.
This article reviews how Doppler echocardiographic techniques can be used to estimate many hemodynamic and diastolic function variables that previously required cardiac catheterization.

14. Pozzoli M, Traversi E, Cioffi G, et al: Loading manipulations improve the prognostic value of Doppler evaluation of mitral flow in patients with chronic heart failure. *Circulation* 95:1222-1230, 1997.
Changes in LV filling patterns with alterations in loading conditions have prognostic ability in patients with systolic dysfunction and heart failure.

15. Takatsuji H, Mikami T, Urasawa K, et al: A new approach for evaluation of left ventricular diastolic function: spatial and temporal analysis of left ventricular filling flow propagation by color M-mode Doppler echocardiography. *J Am Coll Cardiol* 27:365-371, 1996.
In this article, delayed LV inflow propagation as assessed by color M-mode Doppler helped identify patients with pseudonormal LV filling patterns.

16. Vasan RS, Benjamin EJ, Levy D: Prevalence, clinical features and prognosis of diastolic heart failure: an epidemiologic perspective. *J Am Coll Cardiol* 26:1565-1574, 1995.
This is a review of previous studies of patients with diastolic heart failure. It summarizes data on the relation to specific disease, age-related prevalence of the problem, and estimated morbidity and mortality compared with LV systolic dysfunction.

17. Xie GY, Berk MR, Smith MD, et al: Prognostic value of Doppler transmitral flow patterns in patients with congestive heart failure. *J Am Coll Cardiol* 24:132-139, 1994.
This study of the Doppler technique showed that prognosis in dilated cardiomyopathy with LV systolic dysfunction is also directly related to LV diastolic function and, specifically, chamber compliance.

18. Nagueh SF, Middleton KJ, Kopelen HA, et al: Doppler tissue imaging: a noninvasive technique for evaluation of left ventricular relaxation and estimation of filling pressures. *J Am Coll Cardiol* 30:1527-1533, 1997.

19. Sohn DW, Chai IH, Lee DJ, et al: Assessment of mitral annulus velocity by Doppler tissue imaging in the evaluation of left ventricular diastolic function. *J Am Coll Cardiol* 30:474-480, 1997.
These two studies show that longitudinal shortening and lengthening of the heart near the base are reduced in patients with impaired LV relaxation and, when these factors are considered in association with Doppler mitral inflow patterns, can be used to identify pseudonormal LV filling patterns and to estimate LV filling pressures.

20. Nishimura RA, Tajik AJ: Evaluation of diastolic filling of left ventricle in health and disease: Doppler echocardiography is the clinician's Rosetta Stone. *J Am Coll Cardiol* 30:8-18, 1997.

21. Oh JK, Appleton CP, Hatle LK, et al: The noninvasive assessment of left ventricular diastolic function with two-dimensional and Doppler echocardiography. *J Am Soc Echocardiogr* 10:246-270, 1997.

22. Rakowski H, Appleton C, Chan KL, et al: Canadian consensus recommendations for the measurement and reporting of diastolic dysfunction by echocardiography: from the Investigators of Consensus on Diastolic Dysfunction by Echocardiography. *J Am Soc Echocardiogr* 9:736-760, 1996.
These three articles are reviews of current Doppler noninvasive evaluation of LV diastolic function.

Questions

Multiple Choice (choose the one best answer)

1. The most common symptom associated with abnormal left ventricular (LV) diastolic function is:
   a. Fatigue
   b. Exertional dyspnea
   c. Ventricular arrhythmias
   d. Exertional chest pain

2. During which phase of diastole is it most appropriate to measure the compliance characteristics of the LV?
   a. Early LV filling
   b. Isovolumic relaxation
   c. Filling at atrial contraction
   d. Mid-diastolic diastasis

3. The process of LV contraction and relaxation is dependent on myocardial cytosolic Ca^{2+} concentration. Which phase of Ca^{2+} cycling is energy-dependent and therefore affected early in cardiac disease states?
   a. LV contraction
   b. LV relaxation

4. LV pressure-volume (P-V) relations are used to define LV passive diastolic properties. A shift of the P-V curve to the left indicates which of the following?
   a. A decrease in LV operating chamber compliance
   b. An increase in LV operating chamber compliance
   c. No changes in operating chamber compliance
   d. Curves do not shift in most cardiac disease states

5. Familiarity with different LV filling pressures and their pathophysiologic correlates aids understanding of LV diastolic function and the clinical management of patients with cardiac disease. Increase of which pressure is most likely to be associated with pulmonary congestion?
   a. LV pressure minimum
   b. LV end-diastolic pressure
   c. Mean left atrial pressure
   d. Left atrial A-wave pressure

6. The most direct determinant of LV filling is:
   a. LV end-systolic volume
   b. Transmitral pressure gradient
   c. Rate of ventricular relaxation
   d. Mean left atrial pressure
   e. Viscoelastic properties of the LV

7. There are three basic abnormal LV filling patterns in disease states. Which pattern listed below is *not* one of these patterns?
   a. Restrictive filling pattern
   b. Impaired LV relaxation filling pattern
   c. Pseudonormal LV filling pattern
   d. Diastolic predominant filling pattern

8. Which LV filling pattern would be associated with the worst functional prognosis and the highest filling pressures?
   a. Pseudonormal filling pattern
   b. Impaired relaxation filling pattern
   c. Restrictive filling pattern

9. In a patient with LV hypertrophy, a normal ejection fraction, and impaired LV relaxation filling pattern, which of the following would *not* likely be helpful for improving symptoms related to diastolic dysfunction?
   a. Reducing blood pressure, if it were increased
   b. Slowing the heart rate with β-adrenergic blockers or calcium channel blockers
   c. Increasing the heart rate with peripheral vasodilators
   d. Adding angiotensin-converting enzyme inhibitors

10. A blunted cardiac output response in patients with impaired (slowed) LV relaxation has been shown to be due to which of the following?
    a. Pericardial restraint
    b. Failure to increase ejection fraction normally
    c. Inability to fill to a normal end-diastolic volume
    d. All of the above

11. The abnormal LV filling pattern that shows a reduced proportion of filling in early diastole and an increased proportion at atrial contraction is termed:
    a. Pseudonormal
    b. Impaired relaxation
    c. Restrictive
    d. None of the above

12. Patients with isolated chronic mitral or aortic regurgitation often have normal filling pressures despite significant LV enlargement. The mechanism by which this may happen is which of the following?
    a. A rightward shift in the LV pressure-volume relationship
    b. A leftward shift in the LV pressure-volume relationship

c. An increase in the speed of LV relaxation

d. Pericardial "stretch"

13. Currently, the most common method for assessing LV diastolic function and filling pressures is which of the following?
    a. Radionuclide techniques
    b. Echocardiographic Doppler techniques

c. Ultra-fast computed tomography angiography

d. Cardiac catheterization

14. Which abnormal LV filling pattern is least likely to benefit from therapies that decrease heart rate?
    a. Impaired relaxation
    b. Pseudonormal LV filling
    c. Restrictive LV filling

Answers

1. Answer b

LV diastolic dysfunction is defined as the inability of the ventricle to fill to a normal end-diastolic volume without causing increased filling pressures during either rest or exercise. The increase in filling pressures during exercise results in pulmonary congestion; dyspnea on exertion is thus the most common complaint. Fatigue is more likely in a patient with systolic dysfunction. Ventricular arrhythmias can be present in diastolic dysfunction but are uncommon and usually suggest other cardiac abnormality. Exertional chest pain is not typically associated with diastolic dysfunction unless large intracavitary gradients or coronary artery disease is present.

2. Answer d

The compliance characteristics of the LV are best measured after LV relaxation is complete and when there is no or very little cardiac filling. During the cardiac cycle, the only time that these criteria are met is between early diastolic filling and filling at atrial contraction, during the period known as mid-diastolic diastasis. In patients with fast heart rates or impaired relaxation, diastasis may not be present, which is one of the difficulties in measuring LV chamber compliance in vivo. Measuring compliance during isovolumic relaxation, early LV filling, or filling at atrial contraction is inappropriate because the ventricle is either relaxing or rapidly changing its volume or shape.

3. Answer b

LV contraction occurs after cellular depolarization results in the passive release of large stores of Ca^{2+} from the sarcoplasmic reticulum, which activates the contractile proteins.

Deactivation of the contractile elements occurs only when the cytosolic calcium decreases as a result of an energy-dependent (adenosine triphosphate) reuptake of calcium by a powerful sarcoplasmic reticulum Ca^{2+} pump. The impairment of this energy-dependent process and resultant slowing of the rate of calcium reuptake cause LV relaxation to be prolonged.

4. Answer a

The sum of all components contributing to passive LV characteristics after relaxation is finished is described by the exponential diastolic LV P-V relationship. The tangent to a line at a certain point, usually the end-diastolic pressure, describes the operating chamber compliance of the ventricle. A shift to the left indicates that for the same pressure, the ventricle holds less volume; therefore, such a shift would indicate a less compliant, or "stiffer," heart.

5. Answer c

In patients with slowly progressive cardiac disease, the first abnormality in pressure usually is confined to the pressure increase at atrial contraction (LV A-wave pressure), which increases LV end-diastolic pressure. With more severe disease, LV compliance decreases and mean left atrial pressure increases, and symptoms of pulmonary congestion result.

6. Answer b

Although many factors affect LV diastolic function and filling, they all exert their effect through the transmitral pressure gradient. Understanding the effects of various diastolic properties, such as LV relaxation and compliance, on this gradient is a key to understanding LV filling and diastolic function.

7. Answer d

Three basic abnormal LV filling patterns are recognized and associated with changes in LV diastolic properties and filling pressures. Most common is the impaired LV relaxation pattern, which shows reduced filling in early diastole and increased filling in atrial contraction. A more advanced pattern is called pseudonormal because filling resembles that in normal persons, although diastolic abnormalities are present. Patients with advanced disease have restrictive filling patterns, with vigorous filling in early diastole but little filling at atrial contraction as a result of atrial failure. A diastolic predominant pattern has little meaning because it is not specified when diastolic filling is occurring.

8. Answer c

Patients with restrictive filling patterns have both abnormally slow relaxation and a severe reduction in LV compliance with markedly increased mean left atrial pressure. These patients are usually in functional class III and IV and have symptoms of pulmonary congestion and a markedly reduced exercise tolerance.

9. Answer c

In patients with LV hypertrophy, an impaired relaxation-type filling pattern is common and often induced and aggravated by hypertension. If these patients have symptoms, they are typically exertional and due to a shortening of the diastolic filling time with inadequate time to fill the ventricle. Lowering blood pressure may improve LV relaxation and result in improvement in symptoms. Similarly, slowing the heart rate will allow a longer time for filling a ventricle, with prolonged relaxation. An increase in heart rate often makes symptoms worse, because it shortens the diastolic filling time, which for any given heart rate is already reduced compared with normal.

10. Answer c

Some patients with impaired LV relaxation have a reduced exercise tolerance as a result of a "blunted" cardiac output response. In both radionuclide and Doppler studies, this has been shown to be due to an inability of the ventricle to fill to a normal end-diastolic volume. Systolic function and end-systolic volume remain normal. The inability to fill to an increased end-diastolic volume is presumably due to the relaxation abnormality and the shortening of the diastolic filling time, which occur as the heart rate increases with exercise.

11. Answer b

The three basic abnormal LV filling patterns are impaired relaxation, pseudonormal filling, and restrictive filling. In patients with impaired LV relaxation, there is a reduced proportion of filling in early diastole, and slower relaxation reduces the early transmitral pressure gradient. As a compensatory mechanism, filling at atrial contraction is increased. This is the earliest diastolic abnormality in most cardiac disease states and the least abnormal of the three filling patterns.

12. Answer a

In patients with isolated cardiac volume overload, LV enlargement and eccentric LV hypertrophy develop. Under normal circumstances, the LV pressure-volume (P-V) relationship shifts to the right; thus, for an increased volume, there is no increase in filling pressures. A leftward shift of the P-V relationship is rare, except in restrictive or constrictive cardiomyopathies. In most cases of pure valvular heart disease, the speed of LV relaxation is not significantly altered. With chronic LV enlargement, the pericardium grows and there is no pericardial restraint or increase in pressures through "restraining" mechanisms.

13. Answer b

The current assessment of LV diastolic function focuses on analysis of LV filling patterns. Although all methods listed can be used to study LV filling, Doppler techniques are the most frequently used because of their ease of performance, lack of ionizing radiation, and associated information about cardiac anatomy, valvular disease, and filling pressures. Cardiac catheterization most accurately measures pressures, but special catheters and techniques are required to quantify LV diastolic properties.

14. Answer c

Patients with restrictive LV filling have a marked decrease in LV compliance and high LV filling pressures. LV filling in early diastole predominates and terminates abruptly as a result of the severe decrease in LV compliance. There is little filling in atrial contraction because of atrial systolic failure. A decrease in heart rate in these patients frequently results in a decrease in cardiac output and a worsening of symptoms. In contrast, patients whose predominant problem is impaired LV relaxation nearly always benefit from slowing of the heart rate (assuming the PR interval is not affected) because the slowly relaxing ventricle has more time to fill. Often, patients with pseudonormal LV filling also benefit from some heart rate slowing.

Chapter 5

Congestive Heart Failure: Diagnosis, Evaluation, and Surgical Therapy

Richard J. Rodeheffer, M.D.
Margaret M. Redfield, M.D.

Congestive Heart Failure

Chronic congestive heart failure is a clinical syndrome characterized by symptoms and signs of volume overload, with reduced exercise tolerance as a prominent feature. Classically, congestive heart failure has been defined as the pathophysiologic state in which an abnormality of cardiac function is responsible for failure of the heart to pump blood at a rate commensurate with the requirements of the metabolizing tissues, or to do so only when filling pressure is increased. Not all patients with systolic dysfunction have the clinical syndrome of congestive heart failure. Many patients with systolic dysfunction have compensated and asymptomatic ventricular dysfunction (Fig. 1). Likewise, not all patients with clinical congestive heart failure have systolic dysfunction. Patients with isolated diastolic dysfunction may have all the signs and symptoms of congestive heart failure.

Diastolic Heart Failure

Diastolic heart failure is a condition in which there is resistance to filling of one or both ventricles, leading to increased ventricular filling pressures and congestive symptoms in the presence of normal or near-normal systolic function. This entity is covered in more detail in the chapter "Diastolic Function and the Heart."

Asymptomatic Left Ventricular Dysfunction

Asymptomatic left ventricular dysfunction is defined as the presence of significant ventricular systolic dysfunction for prolonged periods in the absence of symptoms of or treatment for heart failure. A recent epidemiologic study conducted in Scotland reported that 2.9% of the population had systolic dysfunction and that 50% of patients with systolic dysfunction had no symptoms of heart failure (Fig. 2). In patients over 55 years, the prevalence of systolic dysfunction was 6%, again with nearly half of patients being asymptomatic. While several epidemiologic studies are under way worldwide to confirm this finding, it is clear that substantial numbers of patients have asymptomatic ventricular dysfunction.

The importance of recognizing and treating asymptomatic left ventricular dysfunction to prevent or to delay progression to the syndrome of congestive heart failure is increasingly recognized, as evidenced by recent trials targeted at patients with asymptomatic left ventricular dysfunction: Studies of Left Ventricular Dysfunction (SOLVD) and Survival and Ventricular Enlargement (SAVE) trials.

Patients with asymptomatic ventricular dysfunction progress to develop overt congestive heart failure and have excess mortality, as demonstrated in both the SAVE and the SOLVD trials (Fig. 3 and 4).

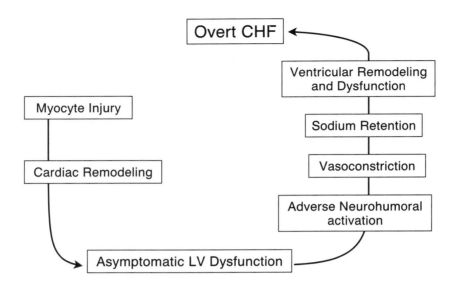

Fig. 1. Progression to heart failure. Myocardial damage leads to ventricular dilatation and hypertrophy (cardiac remodeling), but in the early stages a patient may be well compensated hemodynamically without fluid retention or symptoms or signs of congestive heart failure. Ultimately, adverse neurohumoral activation and progressive ventricular dysfunction lead to excessive vasoconstriction, sodium retention, and clinical congestive heart failure (CHF). LV, left ventricular.

Epidemiology of Heart Failure

More than 400,000 new cases of congestive heart failure are diagnosed each year in the United States, and 2 to 3 million Americans have congestive heart failure. The annual number of deaths approaches 200,000, and congestive heart failure is the leading diagnosis at hospital dismissal for patients older than 65 years. The annual health care cost of congestive heart failure exceeds $10 billion.

Congestive heart failure has been termed the "new epidemic of cardiovascular disease" in the next millenium. Although mortality rates from acute coronary syndromes have decreased with the widespread use of coronary care units, reperfusion therapy, aspirin, β-adrenergic blockers, and angiotensin-converting enzyme inhibitors, decreases in prevalence due to risk factor modification have not been great enough to counteract the increased prevalence of coronary disease related to reduced mortality. In combination with the aging of the population, the effect of decreasing mortality from coronary disease has been to increase the prevalence of congestive heart failure. This trend will continue. Mortality from hypertension-related cerebrovascular accidents has declined and thus more patients are surviving with chronic hypertensive heart disease and are at risk for congestive heart failure. Unfortunately, increases in awareness and control of hypertension have plateaued, and hypertensive heart disease continues to play a major role in the development of heart failure.

Causes of Systolic Ventricular Dysfunction

Systolic dysfunction and congestive heart failure are the common end points of a wide range of cardiovascular disease processes (Table 1). In the Framingham Heart Study, hypertension was the most common precursor of the development of congestive heart failure. Of patients with a clinical diagnosis of congestive heart failure, 75% had hypertension. Hypertension was the sole cause of heart failure in 25% of these patients. Hypertension or coronary artery disease (or both) is the major cause of heart failure in the United States. Many recent large trials in patients with heart failure indicate a much lower prevalence of hypertension and a higher proportion of patients with coronary artery disease as the presumed cause of their ventricular dysfunction.

The diagnosis of idiopathic dilated cardiomyopathy is increasing, and this may reflect a true increase in the incidence of this disease or an increased awareness of the entity and the increasing use of noninvasive assessment of systolic function, such as echocardiography.

Global ventricular dilatation and systolic dysfunction are often referred to as cardiomyopathy even when the underlying cause is well known (i.e., ischemic cardiomyopathy, alcoholic cardiomyopathy, hypertensive cardiomyopathy). A list of disease processes that produce cardiac dilatation and systolic dysfunction is provided in Table 2.

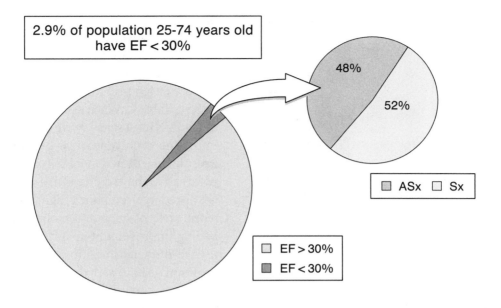

Fig. 2. Rates of symptomatic (Sx) and asymptomatic (ASx) ventricular dysfunction in North Glasgow, Scotland. Nearly 3% of the population had definite systolic dysfunction, and nearly 50% of these subjects had no symptoms of heart failure. EF, ejection fraction. (Data from *Lancet* 350:829-833, 1997.)

Two well-conducted studies demonstrated that idiopathic dilated cardiomyopathy is familial in 20% to 25% of cases. The affected genes and the affected gene product have not been completely identified.

Although conduction system disease due to Lyme disease is well established, it is unclear whether *Borrelia burgdorferi*, the causative agent of Lyme disease, is a significant cause of myocardial disease.

Increasingly, the cardiac manifestations of human immunodeficiency virus (HIV) infection are being described,

including pericarditis, myocarditis, and dilated cardiomyopathy.

Cardiac amyloidosis, an infiltrative cardiomyopathy that progresses from isolated diastolic dysfunction to systolic dysfunction in the advanced stages, is a rare cause of cardiomyopathy. The diastolic dysfunction associated with early amyloid cardiac disease progresses from abnormal relaxation associated with few symptoms to progressively more severe decreases in ventricular compliance with marked symptoms of heart failure in the setting of normal systolic function.

Early reports of small series of patients (mostly children or young adults) with incessant tachycardia and ventricular dysfunction that resolved with medical or surgical therapy demonstrated that chronic tachycardia in itself can produce ventricular dysfunction. It now is well recognized that in patients with atrial fibrillation, poorly controlled ventricular rates can result in a reversible dilated cardiomyopathy. These patients are often unaware of their tachycardia and may have reasonable resting heart rates, and exercise testing or Holter monitoring is needed to detect the poor rate control. Patients who do not respond to or are intolerant of negative chronotropic medications may require atrioventricular node ablation and pacemaker implantation or atrioventricular node modification.

Cocaine use is associated with a myocarditis with persistent ventricular dysfunction as well as microvascular

Table 1.—Causes of Ventricular Dysfunction in Recent Studies of Congestive Heart Failure

Study	History of hypertension, %	Ischemic, %	Nonischemic, %
CONSENSUS*	19	74	26
VHeFT I†	40	44	56
VHeFT II	50	54	46
SOLVD			
Treatment	42	72	28
SOLVD			
Prevention	37	83	17

*Cooperative North Scandinavian Enalapril Survival Study.
†Veterans Administration Cooperative Vasodilator-Heart Failure Trial.

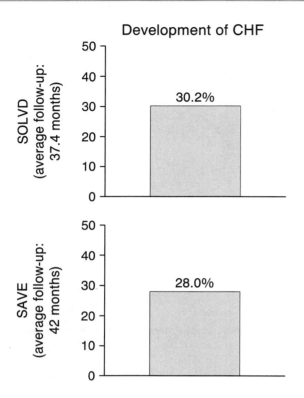

Fig. 3. Progression to overt congestive heart failure (CHF) in untreated patients with asymptomatic ventricular dysfunction in the SAVE (Survival and Ventricular Enlargement) and SOLVD (Studies of Left Ventricular Dysfunction) trials. (Data from *N Engl J Med* 327:669-677, 1992 and *N Engl J Med* 327:685-691, 1992.)

disease, coronary artery spasm, and myocardial infarction.

Reversible left ventricular dysfunction associated with severe sleep apnea has been described recently.

- Idiopathic dilated cardiomyopathy is familial in 20% to 25% of cases.
- In patients with atrial fibrillation, poorly controlled ventricular rates can result in a reversible dilated cardiomyopathy.

Natural History of Heart Failure

Accurate estimation of prognosis in patients with congestive heart failure is difficult because of the multiple causes that produce the syndrome, the large number of factors that influence prognosis, the different modes of death (ischemic events, progressive heart failure, and sudden death), and the variable and evolving treatment strategies. Observed mortality in patients enrolled in recent randomized trials of vasodilator therapy is shown in Figure 5. Rough estimates

of 2-year mortality based on recent randomized trials according to functional class in patients treated with adequate doses of angiotensin-converting enzyme inhibitors are provided in Table 3.

Poor prognostic factors in ventricular dysfunction are listed in Table 4. When ejection fraction and symptom class are similar, most studies have documented a poorer survival in patients with ventricular dysfunction due to coronary artery disease than in "nonischemic" ventricular dysfunction. Most studies have reported that in congestive heart failure, advanced age is a poor prognostic factor. Patients with recent onset of symptoms probably have a better chance of having improvement in systolic function (especially in myocarditis, peripartum cardiomyopathy, or alcoholic cardiomyopathy) and, thus, have a better prognosis. Left ventricular ejection fraction is a powerful independent prognostic factor in heart failure. Most patients with advanced heart failure have an ejection fraction less than 20%, and further decrements do not add significant prognostic value. Thus, in patients referred for cardiac transplantation, ejection fraction is not helpful in determining short-term prognosis and priority for early transplantation. Furthermore, among

Table 2.—Causes of Dilated Cardiomyopathy[*]

Idiopathic
Familial
Infectious agents: bacterial, viral (including **human immunodeficiency virus**), fungal, ***Borrelia burgdorferi* (Lyme disease)**
Acute rheumatic fever
Infiltrative disorders: **amyloid**, hemochromatosis, sarcoid
Toxic: heroin, **cocaine**, alcohol, amphetamines, doxorubicin (Adriamycin), cyclophosphamide, sulfonamides, lead, arsenic, cobalt, phosphorus, ethylene glycol, some antiviral agents
Nutritional deficiencies: protein, thiamine, selenium
Electrolyte disorders: hypocalcemia, hypophosphatemia, hyponatremia, hypokalemia
Collagen vascular disorders: lupus, rheumatoid arthritis, systemic sclerosis, polyarteritis nodosa, hypersensitivity vasculitis, Takayasu's syndrome, polymyositis, Reiter's syndrome
Endocrine and metabolic diseases: diabetes mellitus, thyroid disease, hypoparathyroidism with hypocalcemia, pheochromocytoma, acromegaly
Tachycardia-induced cardiomyopathy
Miscellaneous: peripartum cardiomyopathy, sleep apnea syndrome, Whipple's disease, L-carnitine deficiency

*Items in boldface type are the causes most often found in clinical practice.

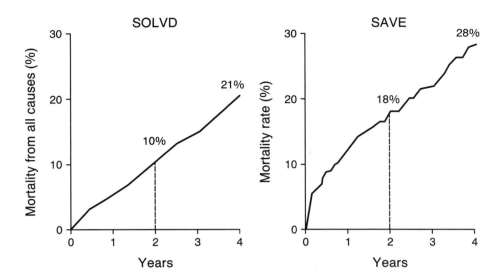

Fig. 4. Mortality among untreated patients with asymptomatic ventricular dysfunction in the SAVE and SOLVD trials. (Data from *N Engl J Med* 327:669-677, 1992 and *N Engl J Med* 327:685-691, 1992.)

patients with an ejection fraction less than 20%, symptoms and prognosis vary widely. Several small studies have suggested that symptoms and prognosis worsen markedly when *right* ventricular function deteriorates and that this may represent a useful prognostic factor in patients with very poor left ventricular function. Hemodynamic values measured after optimization of therapy have some value in predicting prognosis, especially pulmonary capillary wedge pressure and stroke work index. Likewise, several studies have demonstrated that abnormalities in diastolic function as determined with Doppler echocardiography have prognostic value. Specifically, a "restrictive" transmitral Doppler pattern (increased E/A, decreased deceleration time of E, short isovolumic relaxation time) was associated with a worse prognosis.

Table 3.—Approximate 2-Year Mortality of Patients With Left Ventricular Dysfunction Treated With Angiotensin-Converting Enzyme Inhibitors

New York Heart Association class	Mortality, %
I	10
II	20
III	30-40
IV	40-50

Clinical Presentation of Heart Failure

The symptoms of congestive heart failure are listed in Table 5. None of the symptoms are specific for systolic ventricular dysfunction. Dyspnea on exertion and fatigue are early but very nonspecific symptoms of congestive heart failure. Pulmonary disease, obesity, deconditioning, and advanced age also can produce these symptoms. Edema is also very nonspecific. Paroxysmal nocturnal dyspnea and true orthopnea are more specific for heart failure but are relatively insensitive symptoms.

The physical findings in congestive heart failure, listed in Table 6, are also not sensitive, and many are nonspecific. Patients with significant systolic dysfunction may not have any of these signs, and physical findings cannot be used to exclude the presence of systolic ventricular dysfunction.

Diagnostic criteria for heart failure were established before the widespread use of noninvasive assessments of systolic and diastolic function. Patients may have no signs or symptoms of heart failure despite a significant reduction of systolic function. Diagnostic criteria for diastolic heart failure have not been established. The Framingham criteria are listed in Table 7, but although they are accurate for identifying clinical heart failure, these criteria are neither sensitive nor specific for the detection of systolic ventricular dysfunction.

When heart failure is suspected, the physician should provide an estimation of the functional class of the patient based on an assessment of the patient's daily activity and

Table 4.—Poor Prognostic Factors in Ventricular Dysfunction

Ischemic cause*
Advanced age
Duration of symptoms
Ejection fraction
    Left ventricular < 25%*
    Right ventricular < 35%*
Hemodynamics
    Low cardiac index, stroke work index
    High pulmonary capillary wedge pressure, pulmonary
      artery systolic pressure
    "Restrictive" filling pattern on Doppler
      echocardiography
Functional
    NYHA functional class III or IV*
    Decreased exercise duration
    Peak oxygen consumption < 14 mL/kg per min*
    6-Minute walking distance < 350 m
Neurohumoral factors—increased levels of:
    Norepinephrine
    Plasma renin activity
    Aldosterone
    Angiotensin II
    Atrial or brain natriuretic factor
    Arginine vasopressin
    Endothelin
    Tumor necrosis factor
Arrhythmias
    Sudden death and symptomatic ventricular tachycardia*
    Asymptomatic premature ventricular contraction and
      nonsustained ventricular tachycardia

*Most useful clinically.
NYHA, New York Heart Association.

the limitations imposed by the patient's symptoms of heart failure. Although imperfect, the New York Heart Association classification has long been used to categorize patients with heart failure, and this classification provides important prognostic information (Table 8).

Exercise Testing in Heart Failure

Increasingly, more objective quantification of functional capacity is obtained with exercise testing with respiratory gas analysis for calculating oxygen consumption. The maximal oxygen consumption indexed to body surface area

Table 5.—Symptoms of Congestive Heart Failure

None
    Truly asymptomatic
    Asymptomatic because of sedentary lifestyle
Dyspnea on exertion
Decreased exercise tolerance
Orthopnea
Paroxysmal nocturnal dyspnea
Fatigue
Edema
Abdominal pain and distention
Palpitations
Syncope or presyncope
Embolic events (central nervous system, peripheral)

($\dot{V}O_2$ max) has prognostic value even in patients with severe systolic dysfunction and congestive heart disease who are being considered for transplantation. According to a study in patients with severe systolic dysfunction and advanced symptoms of congestive heart failure who were referred for cardiac transplantation, $\dot{V}O_2$ max less than 14 mL/kg per m^2 was predictive of a poorer 1-year survival with medical therapy than with cardiac transplantation, and $\dot{V}O_2$ max more than 14 mL/kg per m^2 was predictive of a 1-year survival at least equivalent to that afforded by transplantation. Thus, patients with preserved exercise tolerance can be followed closely on medical therapy until exercise capacity deteriorates. The prognostic value of $\dot{V}O_2$ max must be interpreted in view of the age, sex, and conditioning status of the person and should not be viewed as an inflexible guideline. In an active 60-year-old man, $\dot{V}O_2$ max of 14 mL/kg per m^2 represents 60% of the predicted maximal exercise capacity, whereas it is only 30% of predicted capacity in a 20-year-old man. Another recent study suggested using $\dot{V}O_2$ max less than 50% predicted a poor short-term prognosis and need for cardiac transplantation. A functional classification scheme based on respiratory gas exchange and $\dot{V}O_2$ max is presented in Table 9. Because $\dot{V}O_2$ max reflects the cardiac output during peak exercise, the corresponding levels of cardiac index are also presented.

- $\dot{V}O_2$ max less than 14 mL/kg per m^2 is predictive of a poorer 1-year survival with medical therapy than with cardiac transplantation.
- $\dot{V}O_2$ max more than 14 mL/kg per m^2 is predictive of a 1-year survival equivalent to that afforded by transplantation.

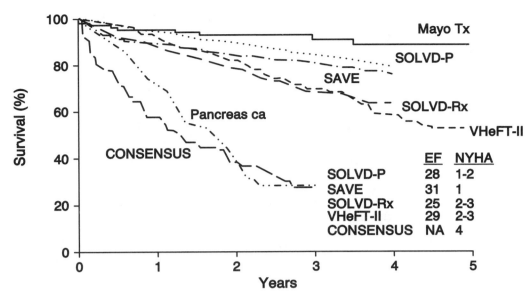

Fig. 5. Observed mortality in patients with systolic dysfunction and heart failure treated with angiotensin-converting enzyme inhibitors in recent clinical heart failure trials. EF, ejection fraction; NYHA, New York Heart Association.

Evaluation of Heart Failure

The goals of the evaluation in patients with chronic heart failure are 1) to determine the type of cardiac dysfunction (systolic vs. diastolic, right ventricular vs. left ventricular failure, valvular vs. myocardial), 2) to uncover correctable etiologic factors, 3) to determine prognosis, and 4) to guide therapy.

In addition to the history and physical examination, the routine laboratory evaluation for suspected heart failure or systolic dysfunction and the pertinent findings are listed in Table 10.

Who Needs Coronary Angiography?

Because most patients with systolic dysfunction have coronary artery disease, a major decision in the subsequent evaluation of a patient with documented systolic dysfunction is the need for coronary angiography and revascularization. Revascularization is considered to prevent further ischemic injury of the remaining functional myocardium and to restore function to "hibernating" myocardium. All major trials of coronary artery bypass grafting (CABG) versus medical therapy excluded patients with congestive heart failure or ejection fraction less than 35%. Several cohort studies in patients with systolic dysfunction and angina have demonstrated significant benefit of CABG over medical therapy. The role of CABG in patients without angina is less clear. The best study to predict "viability" of myocardium is con\phy (PET), thallium imaging, and dobutamine echocardiography suggests that

these methods can detect viability. In patients with severe systolic dysfunction who are candidates for revascularization, some assessment of viability with thallium imaging, PET scanning, or dobutamine echocardiography to document the extent of salvageable myocardium is reasonable.

Table 6.—Physical Findings in Congestive Heart Failure

Carotid	Normal or ↓ volume
Jugular venous pressure	Normal or ↑
Hepatojugular reflux	+ or -
Parasternal lift	+ or -
Apical impulse	Normal or diffuse in character, normal in position or laterally displaced
Palpable S_3, S_4, or P_2	+ or -
S_1	Normal or ↓ intensity
S_3, S_4	+ or -
MR or TR murmur	+ or -
Rales	+ or -
Pulsus alternans	+ or -
Edema	+ or -
Ascites	+ or -
Hepatomegaly	+ or -
Muscle wasting	+ or -
Blood pressure	Normal, ↑, orthostatic, or ↓

+ or -, Present or absent; MR, mitral regurgitation; TR, tricuspid regurgitation.

Table 7.—Framingham Criteria for the Diagnosis of Congestive Heart Failure

Major criteria
 Paroxysmal nocturnal dyspnea or orthopnea
 Neck vein distention
 Rales
 Cardiomegaly
 Acute pulmonary edema
 S_3 gallop
 Increased jugular venous pressure > 16 cm H_2O
 Circulation time > 25 s
 Hepatojugular reflux
Minor criteria
 Ankle edema
 Night cough
 Dyspnea on exertion
 Hepatomegaly
 Pleural effusion
 Vital capacity decreased 1/3 from maximum
 Tachycardia (heart rate > 120 beats/min)
Major or minor criterion
 Weight loss > 4.5 kg in 5 days in response to treatment

Definite congestive heart failure = 2 major criteria or 1 major and 2 minor criteria

Table 8.—New York Heart Association Functional Classification for Congestive Heart Failure

Class I	Patients with cardiac disease but without resulting limitations of physical activity. Ordinary physical activity does not cause undue fatigue, palpitation, dyspnea, or anginal pain
Class II	Patients with cardiac disease resulting in slight limitation of physical activity. They are comfortable at rest. Ordinary physical activity results in fatigue, palpitation, dyspnea, or anginal pain
Class III	Patients with cardiac disease resulting in marked limitation of physical activity. They are comfortable at rest. Less than ordinary physical activity causes fatigue, palpitation, dyspnea, or anginal pain
Class IV	Patients with cardiac disease resulting in inability to carry on any physical activity without discomfort. Symptoms of cardiac insufficiency or of anginal syndrome may be present even at rest. If any physical activity is undertaken, discomfort is increased

Endomyocardial biopsy for the detection of lymphocytic myocarditis is no longer routinely recommended because immunosuppression was not found to have an impact on survival in a multicenter trial of immunosuppressive therapy for myocarditis. A retrospective trial found that patients with biopsy-proven myocarditis had a prognosis similar to that of patients with idiopathic dilated cardiomyopathy. Endomyocardial biopsy is recommended if a systemic disease (amyloidosis or hemochromatosis) is strongly suggested by the clinical presentation. If giant cell myocarditis is suspected (acute onset, young patient, ventricular arrhythmias), preliminary studies suggest no prognostic importance to this finding.

Acute Decompensation of Chronic Heart Failure

The initial evaluation of patients with acute decompensation of chronic congestive heart failure includes clinical and hemodynamic stabilization. Look for and correct precipitating factors (Table 11). Optimize long-term therapy.

Acute Heart Failure

Acute heart failure may present as pulmonary edema ("backward failure") or cardiogenic shock ("forward failure"). The causes of acute heart failure include the following:
1. Coronary artery disease with ischemia, injury, or infarct
2. Mechanical complications of myocardial infarction (ventricular septal defect, acute mitral regurgitation, left ventricular rupture)
3. Arrhythmia (high-grade atrioventricular block or tachyarrhythmia)
4. Tamponade
5. Pulmonary embolus
6. Myocarditis
7. Valvular lesion (*a*, acute myocardial regurgitation due to papillary muscle or chordal rupture or endocarditis; *b*, acute aortic regurgitation due to dissection or endocarditis; *c*, prosthetic valve dysfunction due to acute thrombosis or dehiscence)
8. Hypertensive or ischemic heart disease, with an acute increase in hypertension or plasma volume
9. Acute renal failure or insufficiency leading to increased plasma volume, in association with underlying cardiac disease

Table 9.—Functional Classification for Congestive Heart Failure Based on $\dot{V}O_2$ max

Class	Severity	$\dot{V}O_2$ max, mL/kg per m^2	Maximal cardiac index, L/min per m^2
A	None	> 20	> 8
B	Mild	16-20	6-8
C	Moderate	10-15	4-6
D	Severe	6-9	2-4
E	Very severe	< 6	< 2

$\dot{V}O_2$ max, maximal oxygen consumption.

Initial Evaluation of Acute Pulmonary Edema

The initial evaluation of a patient presenting with pulmonary edema or cardiogenic shock includes the following:

1. A directed history and physical examination
2. 12-Lead electrocardiography (ECG) and continuous ECG monitoring
3. A hematologic examination—complete blood cell count, electrolytes, urea, creatinine, cardiac enzymes, and arterial blood gases
4. Chest radiography
5. Transthoracic echocardiography
6. Consider cardiac catheterization, transesophageal echocardiography, arterial catheter or pulmonary artery balloon catheter if needed

If there is no evidence of a specific cause that requires emergency intervention such as emergency percutaneous transluminal coronary angioplasty or cardiac surgery, stabilize the patient with oxygen, diuretic agents, afterload reduction, inotropic agents, and morphine sulfate. Perform further evaluation and treatment as needed.

Initial Evaluation of Cardiogenic Shock

Cardiogenic shock is associated with a high mortality rate if untreated (approximately 85%). Remember that 10% to 15% of patients presenting with cardiogenic shock have inadequate left ventricular filling pressures and need fluid. Consider right ventricular infarction, usually in the setting of an inferior infarct. The initial evaluation also should include determination of prothrombin time, activated partial thromboplastin time, serum glucose level, liver function, and lactate concentration. Focus on the following key steps:

1. Assess volume status—consider fluid challenge unless the signs of left-sided fluid overload are clear-cut

2. Assess left ventricular systolic function (transthoracic echocardiography or pulmonary artery catheter)
3. Rule out infarct or ischemia
4. Rule out correctable mechanical lesion (transthoracic echocardiography and perhaps transesophageal echocardiography)

If infarct or ischemia is suspected, catheterization with percutaneous transluminal coronary angioplasty, if available, is preferable to treatment with thrombolytic agents. Stabilize the patient with volume-expanding or diuretic agents, inotropic agents, and afterload reduction. Consider an intra-aortic balloon pump if the initial measures are inadequate, especially after revascularization. Intra-aortic balloon pump is most appropriate as a bridge to surgery (mitral regurgitation or ventricular septal defect) or transplantation. Exclude aortic regurgitation or dissection before placement. Continue evaluation for underlying cause.

Surgical Therapy

Conventional Surgery: Coronary Artery Bypass Graft, Valve Replacement and Repair, Congenital Heart Disease Repair

Large trials such as the Coronary Artery Surgery Study (CASS) established that patients with extensive coronary artery disease and systolic ventricular dysfunction have better survival after revascularization. Recent reports underscore the potential for improvement in ventricular systolic function after revascularization to viable but ischemic ventricular segments. Patients with coronary artery disease and ventricular dysfunction should be evaluated for the presence of "hibernating myocardium"; if present, revascularization should be considered.

When circulatory failure occurs in the setting of valve dysfunction or congenital heart disease, surgical correction may stabilize or improve ventricular function. Timing of surgery is essential to optimize the risk:benefit ratio for the procedure. Surgery should be performed before significant ventricular dysfunction develops.

Transplantation

Cardiac transplantation increased markedly in the 1980s, due in large part to better immunosuppression (cyclosporine) and improved survival. Currently, national databases indicate that a 1-year survival of approximately 85% can be anticipated; 5-year survival rates are 70% to 75%. Risk-adjusted program-specific survival rates are a matter of public record

Table 10.—Routine Laboratory Evaluation for Suspected Heart Failure or Systolic Dysfunction*

Class I—usually indicated, always acceptable

Chest radiography

    Cardiomegaly

    Pulmonary venous hypertension

    Edema

    Pleural effusions

Electrocardiogram

    Rhythm, Q waves, ST-T changes, left ventricular hypertrophy

Complete blood cell count

    Anemia as exacerbating condition

Urinalysis

    Nephrotic syndrome contributing to edema

Sodium, potassium, magnesium, calcium, BUN, creatinine, glucose

    Renal insufficiency

    Diabetes mellitus

    Electrolyte abnormality

Serum albumin

    Low, contributing to edema

T_4 and TSH or sensitive TSH

    If patient is > 65 years, in atrial fibrillation, or has symptoms suggestive of thyroid disease

Assessment of systolic, diastolic, valvular function

    Transthoracic echocardiography

Cardiac catheterization/coronary angiography—in patients:

    With angina

    With significant area of ischemia on noninvasive stress test

    At risk for coronary artery disease who are to undergo a corrective noncoronary cardiac surgical procedure

    With diastolic heart failure and angina or risk factors for coronary artery disease

Noninvasive stress testing—to detect ischemia in patients who are candidates for revascularization:

    Without angina but with a high probability of coronary artery disease

    Without angina but with previous myocardial infarction to detect viability and residual ischemia (thallium or

        dobutamine echocardiography probably is preferable to sestamibi to provide optimal information on viability)

Screening for other rare causes

    Only as suggested by history and physical examination findings

Exercise testing with respiratory gas analysis

    As needed for prognosis/timing of transplantation in transplantation candidates

Class II—acceptable but of uncertain efficacy and may be controversial

Serum iron and ferritin

    For patients without features to suggest hemochromatosis

Sensitive TSH

    In nonelderly patients in normal sinus rhythm with unexplained congestive heart failure

Noninvasive stress testing

    To detect ischemia in all patients with unexplained congestive heart failure who are candidates for revascularization

Coronary angiography

    In all patients with unexplained congestive heart failure who are candidates for revascularization

Table 10 (continued)

Endomyocardial biopsy—in patients:

    With recent onset of rapidly deteriorating cardiac function

    Receiving chemotherapy with doxorubicin

    With systemic disease and possible cardiac involvement (hemochromatosis, sarcoidosis, amyloidosis, Löffler's endocarditis, endomyocardial fibroelastosis); some argue that currently there is little to support its use to detect lymphocytic myocarditis because there is no proven benefit to standard immunosuppressive therapy and it has no prognostic value; exception for transplantation candidates

Exercise testing

    To determine functional limitation in patients for whom history is unclear

    To address specific clinical questions (rate control in patients with atrial fibrillation, chronotropic competence, exercise-induced arrhythmias, blood pressure control in those with congestive heart failure and hypertension, response to therapy)

Class III—generally not indicated

Endomyocardial biopsy

    Routine evaluation of patients with unexplained congestive heart failure

Screening for asymptomatic arrhythmias

    Patients who have symptoms suggestive of sustained arrhythmia or syncope should undergo electrophysiologic evaluation

Multiple echocardiographic or radionuclide studies

    For patients responding to therapy unless normalization of systolic function is suspected

Coronary angiography

    In patients who are not candidates for revascularization, valve surgery, or heart transplantation

---

*Based on guidelines of the American College of Cardiology and the American Heart Association.

BUN, blood urea nitrogen; T_4, thyroxine; TSH, thyroid-stimulating hormone.

and can be found on the Internet at *www.unos.org*.

Satisfactory transplant outcomes depend on careful selection of candidates and meticulous life-long posttransplantation follow-up. Currently, the number of patients on the waiting list is greater than the number of available donor hearts, and average waiting times have increased. Consequently, 25% to 30% of patients die while waiting for a donor. Patients selected for transplantation should have a good chance of achieving the expected 85% 1-year patient survival after transplantation.

Appropriate candidates are those with end-stage cardiac disease in whom conventional treatments have been exhausted and whose 1-year life expectancy without transplantation is thought to be poor. An upper age limit of 60 to 65 years is appropriate because long-term benefits are less impressive in the elderly. Patients should be free of other serious medical disease that might limit life expectancy or seriously compromise the effectiveness of the procedure. It is important that patients have good renal, liver, and pulmonary function. Although patients with diabetes mellitus may be appropriate candidates, they should be free of diabetes-related end-organ disease, and it should be recognized that the development of diabetic complications may have a negative impact on long-term transplant success. Persons who have had significant psychiatric disorders or unresolved substance abuse problems are frequently poor candidates. Finally, patients with fixed increased pulmonary vascular resistance (pulmonary vascular resistance index > 4 Wood units) are at increased risk for perioperative death.

Long-term follow-up involves frequent monitoring of immunosuppression. Conventional immunosuppression usually consists of corticosteroids, azathioprine, and cyclosporine. Newer agents such as mycophenolate mofetil and tacrolimus (FK506) also may be valuable in selected patients. Acute allograft rejection can occur at any time after transplantation and must be considered whenever there

Table 11.—Precipitating Factors for Acute Decompensation of Chronic Congestive Heart Failure

Noncompliance with diet or therapy
Arrhythmia
Systemic infection
Pulmonary embolism
High-output states—anemia, pregnancy, hyperthyroidism
Unrelated illness—renal, pulmonary, hypothyroidism, gastrointestinal
Ischemia
Hypertension
Toxins—alcohol, street drugs
Inappropriate drug therapy—negative inotrope, salt-retaining

is a significant change in clinical status. Endomyocardial biopsy remains the only reliable means of diagnosing rejection. Treatment of a high histologic grade of rejection requires acute augmentation of immunosuppression. If the rejection episode is not associated with hemodynamic compromise, a brief course of intravenous corticosteroids may be sufficient. If hemodynamic compromise is present, treatment with lymphocytolytic antibodies may be required. If repeated episodes of acute rejection occur, the level of chronic maintenance immunosuppression should be increased. During the periods of increased immunosuppression required to treat acute rejection, patients have an especially heightened risk of infection; cytomegalovirus infection often is reactivated in this context.

Hypertension develops in about 90% of patients who have had heart transplantation, and effective control may require more than one antihypertensive agent. Appropriate initial choices are an angiotensin-converting enzyme inhibitor and a diuretic. A long-acting calcium channel blocker and a diuretic also may be effective; calcium channel blockers interact with cyclosporine, causing increased cyclosporine levels and the need to readjust the dose of cyclosporine.

Hypercholesterolemia is also common after transplantation and needs both dietary and pharmacologic management. Pravastatin and simvastatin have been shown in controlled trials to reduce the development of the diffuse accelerated coronary atherosclerosis that tends to occur in the allograft heart. Pravastatin and simvastatin also have been shown to have an early salutary effect on mortality that is difficult to explain on the basis of their cholesterol-lowering properties alone (Fig. 6). Therefore, these drugs have been suggested to have immunosuppressive effects that contribute to their beneficial effect on mortality. Early and continuous treatment with 3-hydroxy-3-methylglutaryl coenzyme A (HMG-CoA) reductase inhibitors, therefore, is generally recommended for patients with cardiac transplants.

Immunosuppressed patients are at higher risk for the development of malignancy, and heightened tumor surveillance is indicated. There is a notable increase in the incidence of tumors associated with oncoviruses, such as

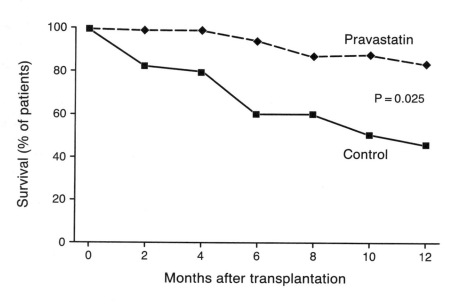

Fig. 6. Effect of pravastatin on survival during the first year after cardiac transplantation. (From *N Engl J Med* 333:621-627, 1995. By permission of Massachusetts Medical Society.)

squamous cell skin malignancies and non-Hodgkin lymphoma. The latter, known as posttransplant lymphoproliferative disease, is especially common in recipients without serologic evidence of past Epstein-Barr virus infection who receive a heart from a donor who has had previous Epstein-Barr viral infection.

Assessment of Donor Hearts

The standard approach includes assessment of the potential donor for cardiac dysfunction due to contusion, increased catecholamine levels (occasionally found in cases of cerebral trauma), or underlying coronary artery disease. Echocardiography is a standard form of assessment. Older donors with risk factors for coronary artery disease may need to undergo coronary angiography. In general, appropriate donor management requires maintaining adequate, but not excessive, filling pressures and sufficient cardiac output to ensure viability of the liver, kidneys, and other potential donor organs. If catecholamines are used to support the circulation, they should be used at the lowest possible dose.

Mechanical Ventricular Assist and Replacement Devices

The shortage of donor hearts has provided a continuing impetus for the development of mechanical devices to replace or to assist the heart. Initial attempts at total cardiac replacement in the 1980s were marked by unacceptable levels of infectious and embolic complications. Current efforts have been devoted to the development of implantable left ventricular assist devices that unload, rather than replace, the left ventricle. Single-chamber pumps that work in concert with the left ventricle (drawing in blood during ventricular systole and pumping blood into the aorta during ventricular diastole) are able to maintain excellent levels of systemic perfusion. These devices allow for free ambulation of the patient and can be worn for weeks or months. Currently, they are available as bridge-to-transplant devices, but they may eventually be used as permanent implants in lieu of transplantation. They are still associated with an increased incidence of emboli and infection.

Cardiac Myoplasty and Ventricular Resection

Skeletal muscle assist procedures have undergone a slow evolution during the past 15 years. Recent attention has focused on the "muscle wrap" procedure, in which the latissimus dorsi is maintained on its neurovascular pedicle and brought into the chest to be wrapped around the left and right ventricles. After the initial operation, the latissimus dorsi is "trained" by a pacemaker and assumes muscle energetics similar to those of cardiac muscle. The long-term safety and efficacy of this experimental surgery are unknown.

Resection of a portion of the left ventricular free wall, often in combination with mitral valve repair, has been proposed as a therapy for dilated cardiomyopathy (Batista operation). This "ventricular remodeling" procedure should still be considered experimental.

Suggested Review Reading

Practice Guidelines for the Evaluation of Suspected Heart Failure

1. Guidelines for the evaluation and management of heart failure. Report of the American College of Cardiology/American Heart Association Task Force on Practice Guidelines (Committee on Evaluation and Management of Heart Failure). *Circulation* 92:2764-2784, 1995.

2. Konstam MA, Dracup K, Baker DW, et al: *Heart Failure: Evaluation and Care of Patients With Left-Ventricular Systolic Dysfunction. Clinical Practice Guideline No. 11.* AHCPR Publication No. 94-0612. Rockville, Maryland: Agency for Health Care Policy and Research, Public Health Service, U.S. Department of Health and Human Services, June 1994.

These two references provide recommendations for the evaluation and management of patients with ventricular dysfunction and congestive heart failure. A comprehensive reference list is included in each as evidence supporting recommendations.

Epidemiology/Asymptomatic Left Ventricular Dysfunction

1. McDonagh TA, Morrison CE, Lawrence A, et al: Symptomatic and asymptomatic left-ventricular systolic dysfunction in an urban population. *Lancet* 350:829-833, 1997.

This study showed that systolic dysfunction was common in the general population and that 50% of patients with systolic dysfunction are asymptomatic.

2. Pfeffer MA, Braunwald E, Moye LA, et al: Effect of captopril on mortality and morbidity in patients with left ventricular dysfunction after myocardial infarction. Results of the Survival and Ventricular Enlargement trial. *N Engl J Med* 327:669-677, 1992.

3. The SOLVD Investigators: Effect of enalapril on mortality and the development of heart failure in asymptomatic patients with reduced left ventricular ejection fractions. *N Engl J Med* 327:685-691, 1992.

Two major trials, SAVE and SOLVD, demonstrated the natural history of asymptomatic ventricular dysfunction and the impact of angiotensin-converting enzyme inhibitor therapy on cardiovascular morbidity and mortality in patients with asymptomatic ventricular dysfunction.

Role of Metabolic Stress Testing in Determining Prognosis in Patients With Heart Failure

1. Mancini DM, Eisen H, Kussmaul W, et al: Value of peak exercise oxygen consumption for optimal timing of cardiac transplantation in ambulatory patients with heart failure. *Circulation* 83:778-786, 1991.

This study established the utility of metabolic stress testing in the assessment of short-term prognosis in patients with severe systolic dysfunction and heart failure, allowing risk stratification in patients suitable for cardiac transplantation.

Transplantation

1. Kobashigawa JA, Katznelson S, Laks H, et al: Effect of pravastatin on outcomes after cardiac transplantation. *N Engl J Med* 333:621-627, 1995.

This controlled trial showed that pravastatin reduced mortality in the first year after cardiac transplantation.

2. Rodeheffer RJ, Naftel DC, Stevenson LW, et al: Secular trends in cardiac transplant recipient and donor management in the United States, 1990 to 1994. A multi-institutional study. *Circulation* 94:2883-2889, 1996.

This multicenter database study describes current cardiac transplant waiting times and outcomes in the United States.

Questions

Multiple Choice (choose the one best answer)

1. Cardiac transplant rejection is most reliably detected by assessment of:
   a. Peripheral leukocyte count
   b. Echocardiographically determined systolic function
   c. Echocardiographically determined diastolic function
   d. Endomyocardial biopsy

2. Current center-specific cardiac transplant survival data:
   a. Show 1-year overall survival of about 75%
   b. Are available on the Internet
   c. Are generally uniform from center to center
   d. Are unrelated to the age of the recipient

3. Evaluation of a cardiac donor who is brain-dead includes all of the following *except*:
   a. Endomyocardial biopsy
   b. Echocardiography
   c. Electrocardiography
   d. Review of the hemodynamic stability of the donor before declaration of brain death

4. Evaluation of a potential cardiac transplant recipient includes all of the following *except*:
   a. Renal function assessment
   b. Measurement of pulmonary vascular resistance
   c. Measurement of plasma catecholamine values
   d. Measurement of left ventricular function

5. A 70-year-old man comes to the emergency department with a 1-week history of worsening dyspnea, abdominal fullness, and paroxysmal nocturnal dyspnea. He is known to have idiopathic dilated cardiomyopathy (ejection fraction, 20%) with stable class II to III congestive heart failure. Symptoms started shortly after he sustained an acute knee injury that was treated with rest, heat, compression wraps, and ibuprofen (Motrin). He denies chest pain.

Medical history:	Renal insufficiency with a creatinine value of about 1.7 mg/dL, chronically
Medications:	Digoxin, 0.125 mg/day
	Furosemide (Lasix), 80 mg/day
	Enalapril (Vasotec), 10 mg twice a day
	Ibuprofen (Motrin), 600 mg three times a day
	Warfarin (Coumadin), 5.0 mg/day
Physical examination:	Blood pressure, 120/60 mm Hg; heart rate, 96 beats/min, regular; respiratory rate, 28/min; afebrile
Lungs:	Rales, 2/3 of lung field
Heart:	Jugular venous pressure, 20 cm with a large "v" wave; left ventricle, dilated with the apex beat in the 6th space midaxillary line; gallop rhythm; 2/6 mitral regurgitation murmur
Extremities:	3+ edema to knee

   Laboratory findings:
   Chest radiography shows pulmonary edema and cardiomegaly
   Electrocardiography: normal sinus rhythm at 96 beats/min; typical left bundle branch block (also was present on electrocardiogram 1 year ago)
   Creatinine, 2.5 mg/dL; INR, 4.8; bilirubin, 2.3 mg/dL; creatine kinase, normal

   The next step should be:
   a. Administration of heparin and urgent ventilation-perfusion ($\dot{V}Q$) scanning
   b. Stop use of enalapril and warfarin, start diuresis with intravenous furosemide, start therapy with hydralazine and isosorbide dinitrate (Isordil)
   c. Emergency echocardiography to assess left ventricular function
   d. Oxygen, diuresis with intravenous furosemide, continue enalapril therapy, hold warfarin therapy for 2 days and then recheck INR, check digoxin level, stop use of ibuprofen

6. A 38-year-old man with a 5-year history of congestive heart failure due to idiopathic dilated cardiomyopathy presents with increasing dyspnea. Coronary angiography 4 years ago showed normal coronary arteries with an ejection fraction of 20% by ventriculography. Ejection fraction by multiple gated acquisition (MUGA) scanning 1 year ago was 15%. The patient is taking an angiotensin-converting enzyme inhibitor (enalapril, 10 mg twice a day), digoxin, furosemide (Lasix), warfarin (Coumadin), and metolazone (Zaroxolyn) as needed. He comes for routine follow-up. He is slightly more dyspneic and fatigued (has to pause for rest after

climbing 4 steps) and is requiring more frequent use of metolazone to control edema. Evaluation should include which of the following?

a. Repeat coronary angiography
b. MUGA to assess ejection fraction
c. Stress testing, with measurement of oxygen consumption
d. Holter monitoring

7. A 57-year-old obese woman presents with dyspnea on exertion, pedal edema, fatigue, and orthopnea. She has a long history of hypertension with suboptimal control. She does not have angina. She is a nonsmoker and has normal cholesterol levels.

Medications:	Atenolol, 50 mg/day
	Combination of triamterene and hydrochlorothiazide (Dyazide), 1 tablet/day
Physical examination:	Blood pressure, 170/90 mm Hg; heart rate, 64 beats/min; normal arterial waveform
Lungs:	Clear to auscultation
Heart:	Jugular venous pressure increased, left ventricular impulse prominent and sustained, heart sounds S_1 and S_2 normal and S_3 present; no murmurs
Abdomen:	Obese
Extremities:	2+ pedal edema

Laboratory findings:

Chest radiography shows cardiomegaly with pulmonary venous hypertension and Kerley B lines

Electrocardiography shows sinus rhythm, normal tracing

The next step should include which of the following?

a. Initiate therapy with digoxin, diuretics, and an angiotensin-converting enzyme inhibitor
b. Echocardiography
c. Treatment with verapamil for diastolic dysfunction
d. Coronary angiography

8. A 68-year-old woman presents with dyspnea on exertion and pedal edema that clears overnight. She has a long history of hypertension. She does not have angina. She is a nonsmoker and has normal cholesterol levels.

Medications:	Atenolol, 50 mg/day
	Combination of triamterene and hydrochlorothiazide (Dyazide), 1 tablet/day
Physical examination:	Blood pressure, 170/100 mm Hg; heart rate, 58 beats/min
Lungs:	Clear to auscultation
Heart:	Jugular venous pulse not well seen, left ventricular impulse was prominent, no murmurs, heart sound distant
Abdomen:	Obese
Extremities:	Mild pedal edema

Laboratory findings:

Chest radiography showed cardiomegaly and pulmonary venous hypertension

Electrocardiography showed normal sinus rhythm

Echocardiography: Normal left ventricular cavity size; ejection fraction, 70%; no regional wall motion abnormality

Left ventricular wall thickness, 16 mm; left ventricular mass index, 175 g/m^2

Left atrium enlarged

E:A wave ratio (E/A) of the mitral inflow Doppler velocity profile, 2.0; deceleration time, 140 ms; isovolumic relaxation time, 65 ms

Tricuspid regurgitation velocity, 3.2 m/s

On the basis of echocardiographic findings, one can conclude that:

a. This patient has isolated diastolic dysfunction causing heart failure
b. This patient has left ventricular hypertrophy
c. The left ventricular end-diastolic filling pressures are increased
d. All of the above

9. A 39-year-old man is referred for evaluation of atrial fibrillation and congestive heart failure. He was very active physically until 3 months ago, when he noted dyspnea on exertion when jogging. This progressed, and he saw his physician. He has no chest pain. Electrocardiography shows atrial fibrillation, with a resting heart rate of 140 beats/min. The patient is entirely unaware of his tachycardia. The physician begins treatment with digoxin and warfarin (Coumadin). Echocardiography shows a dilated left ventricle and an ejection fraction of 30%. An angiotensin-converting

enzyme inhibitor and a combination of triamterene and hydrochlorothiazide (Dyazide) are added to the treatment. Adequate anticoagulation has been used for 4 weeks. His symptoms are improved but he is still in New York Heart Association class II. The patient has no previous history of cardiac disease, no cardiac risk factors, no history of alcohol or drug use, and no family history of heart disease.

Physical examination: Blood pressure, 120/60 mm Hg; heart rate, 88 beats/min, irregular at rest and increasing to 140 after 1 minute of brisk stepping in place; afebrile; respiratory rate, 16/min

Lungs: Clear

Heart: Jugular venous pulse normal with hepatojugular reflux, left ventricle 1+ enlarged, no murmur

Extremities: No edema

Laboratory findings:

Electrocardiography shows atrial fibrillation with a ventricular rate of 88 beats/min; digoxin effect, otherwise normal

Chest radiography shows cardiomegaly

INR, 3.0; thyroid-stimulating hormone, normal; cholesterol, 158 mg/dL

The most appropriate next step in evaluation is:

a. Continue treatment with current medications, chemical or direct current cardioversion, and observation
b. Stress thallium test with reinjection at rest
c. Endomyocardial biopsy
d. Coronary angiography

10. A 53-year-old man with multiple cardiac risk factors presents with a 6-month history of dyspnea on exertion and exertional chest fullness. He has had orthopnea and an episode of paroxysmal nocturnal dyspnea.

Laboratory findings:

Electrocardiography shows nonspecific ST abnormalities

Echocardiography shows mildly dilated left ventricle; ejection fraction, 20%; global hypokinesis

The next step in diagnostic evaluation should be:

a. Exercise multiple gated acquisition (MUGA) scanning

b. Stress test with measurement of maximal oxygen consumption
c. Coronary angiography
d. Transplant consultation

11. A 58-year-old man with multiple cardiac risk factors presents with a 1-year history of dyspnea on exertion and exertional chest pressure. He has had orthopnea and an episode of paroxysmal nocturnal dyspnea.

Laboratory findings:

Electrocardiography shows nonspecific ST abnormalities

Echocardiography shows a mildly dilated left ventricle; ejection fraction, 20%; global hypokinesis

Coronary angiography shows an 80% stenosis of proximal left anterior descending artery, 85% proximal circumflex artery, 90% mid-right coronary artery; distal vessels are adequate in size

The appropriate next step includes:

a. Surgical consultation for coronary artery bypass grafting
b. Rest thallium test with delayed imaging
c. Initiation of therapy with an angiotensin-converting enzyme inhibitor
d. All of the above

12. A 56-year-old woman is active and completely asymptomatic. The results of her insurance physical examination were normal except for left bundle branch block detected on electrocardiography and cardiomegaly on chest radiography. Echocardiography was then performed and showed moderate left ventricular dilatation and ejection fraction of 33%.

Medical history: Postmenopausal and not taking estrogen

Normal lipid values

Family history:

Mother had sudden death at age 45 years

Maternal aunt and maternal grandmother died of heart failure

Sister was told she had an enlarged heart

Patient has 3 children of childbearing age

Laboratory findings:

Coronary angiography showed normal coronary arteries

$\dot{V}O_2$max, 75% of predicted

Further recommendations should include:

a. Digoxin, diuretic, angiotensin-converting enzyme inhibitor, genetic counseling

b. Angiotensin-converting enzyme inhibitor, genetic

counseling, and close follow-up

c. Genetic counseling, close follow-up, and initiation of therapy when symptoms of congestive heart failure develop

d. Transplant evaluation

Answers

1. Answer d

Endomyocardial biopsy remains the only reliable diagnostic method for detection of transplant rejection. Echocardiographic abnormalities may not occur until rejection is very advanced and potentially irreversible.

2. Answer b

Center-specific data are available on the Internet at *www.unos.org*. National average data show 1-year survival of about 85%, but results are variable in different centers. Long-term survival is less likely in patients older than 65 years.

3. Answer a

Endomyocardial biopsy is not indicated, but all of the other evaluations are important.

4. Answer c

Plasma catecholamine values correlate with survival in large groups of patients with heart failure but are not useful for making decisions about transplants in individual patients.

5. Answer d

This man presents with acute decompensation with a background of stable congestive heart failure. He has pulmonary edema with stable hemodynamic findings. He has known severe left ventricular dysfunction, and emergency echocardiography is not likely to be helpful because no new mechanical problem is suggested by examination findings and the ejection fraction is already severely reduced. Evaluation should focus on clinical stabilization (diuresis and oxygen) and identification of precipitating factors. The most likely scenario is sodium retention due to the ibuprofen. The patient has significant congestive heart failure and renal insufficiency at baseline and likely is very dependent on renal production of prostaglandins. Although pulmonary embolus is a concern, he is given anticoagulation therapy and has no other clinical features to suggest this diagnosis. The worsening renal insufficiency is probably due to ibuprofen; serum creatinine level was stable with angiotensin-converting enzyme inhibitors, and this therapy should be continued for now. A change to use of hydralazine and isosorbide dinitrate should be made only if the renal function does not respond to discontinuing treatment with ibuprofen.

6. Answer c

This man has progressive and severe congestive heart failure while receiving maximal standard therapy. The primary question is whether he needs a heart transplant. He is not at high risk for new coronary artery disease causing worsening congestive heart failure. He already has severe left ventricular dysfunction, and repeat MUGA will not likely provide much information to guide the decision. The most helpful prognostic information is his exercise capacity as assessed from his maximal oxygen uptake ($\dot{V}O_2$ max). If his $\dot{V}O_2$ max is less than 14 mL/kg per m^2 or less than 50% of predicted, transplant evaluation is appropriate. In the absence of symptoms of arrhythmias, screening with Holter monitoring is not warranted unless examination suggests extremely frequent ectopy with relative bradycardia and it is believed that ectopy is frequent enough to compromise cardiac output.

7. Answer b

On the basis of the symptoms, physical examination findings, and chest radiography, this woman has congestive heart failure, which could be due to systolic or isolated diastolic dysfunction. One needs to establish the type of cardiac dysfunction before selecting therapy, and echocardiography would be the best test to help make this distinction. Although coronary artery disease is possible, in the absence of angina a noninvasive screening test may be more appropriate than going directly to angiography. Empiric therapy for systolic or diastolic dysfunction is inappropriate, because studies have shown that physical examination and chest radiography are not able to differentiate systolic from diastolic dysfunction. The use of verapamil to treat diastolic dysfunction unrelated to hypertrophic cardiomyopathy is controversial.

8. Answer d

The echocardiographic findings are entirely consistent with hypertensive heart disease with advanced diastolic dysfunction and chronic increase of the left ventricular filling pressures. The patient has concentric left ventricular hypertrophy as evidenced by increased wall thickness and left ventricular mass index (< 125 g/m^2 is normal). The mitral inflow Doppler shows evidence of increased filling pressures, with increased E/A and short deceleration time. With left ventricular hypertrophy and normal atrial pressures, an abnormal relaxation pattern with decreased E/A and prolonged deceleration time are expected. The E/A of 2.0 and deceleration time are consistent with restrictive physiology and indicate reduced left ventricular compliance and increased filling pressures. The left atrial enlargement and mild pulmonary hypertension suggest that her filling pressures have been chronically increased. Despite the absence of regional wall motion abnormality, one could not assume an absence of epicardial coronary artery disease, and further evaluation of that would be appropriate.

9. Answer a

The most likely diagnosis in this patient is tachycardia-related cardiomyopathy. He could also have idiopathic dilated cardiomyopathy with provocation of symptoms with atrial fibrillation. He is at low risk for coronary artery disease, so neither thallium testing nor coronary angiography is needed. He has no features to suggest viral myocarditis, and, even if present, positive biopsy findings would not alter therapy because he is well compensated. Because he presented with atrial fibrillation, it was appropriate to evaluate the sensitive thyroid-stimulating hormone value. If the patient has tachycardia-related cardiomyopathy, his ejection fraction should improve within 3 to 12 months after cardioversion. If the patient has idiopathic dilated cardiomyopathy, he is stable in New York Heart Association class II with appropriate standard therapy, and transplant evaluation is not appropriate. Antiarrhythmic therapy is not appropriate before cardioversion.

10. Answer c

This patient is at high risk for coronary artery disease (risk factors and angina) and potentially is a candidate for revascularization. MUGA would only suggest the diagnosis of coronary artery disease, and even if the results were negative it would have a poor predictive value. MUGA would not provide information regarding viability. At this point, evaluation for a transplant and $\dot{V}O_2$ assessment are premature because this patient may be a candidate for a conventional bypass procedure.

11. Answer d

This patient has severe left ventricular dysfunction and congestive heart failure without clear evidence of transmural myocardial infarction on electrocardiography, and he has angina. He has severe three-vessel disease, which appears appropriate for bypass. Although the major surgical trials excluded patients with left ventricular dysfunction of this severity, many smaller studies have suggested that patients with severe left ventricular dysfunction and severe three-vessel disease do best with operation. Some suggest that the presence of angina improves the chance that there is significant viable hibernating myocardium, which will have improved function postoperatively. Most surgeons like some confirmation of the presence of a large amount of viable myocardium before deciding to operate in such a high-risk candidate. Thallium imaging, dobutamine echocardiography, or positron emission tomographic scanning, if available, is appropriate. Therapy with an angiotensin-converting enzyme inhibitor would be appropriate.

12. Answer b

This patient has asymptomatic left ventricular dysfunction, probably on the basis of familial dilated cardiomyopathy with high penetrance. Patients who are asymptomatic do not always have normal exercise capacity when tested objectively. This patient should be treated with angiotensin-converting enzyme inhibitors to help prevent the combined end point of death and progression to congestive heart failure on the basis of the SOLVD Prevention Trial. Because she is asymptomatic, digoxin and diuretics are probably not indicated. She should definitely see a geneticist, and she and her children should receive genetic counseling. Also, her children and siblings should probably be screened for cardiomyopathy. At this point, with an ejection fraction of 33% and only mild to moderate reduction in exercise capacity and lack of symptoms, transplant evaluation is premature.

Chapter 6

Medical Therapy of Systolic Ventricular Dysfunction and Heart Failure

Margaret M. Redfield, M.D.
Richard J. Rodeheffer, M.D.

Principles of Treatment

Concurrent with the evaluation of the underlying cause of systolic ventricular dysfunction, specific medical therapy should be commenced to reduce both morbidity and mortality. Aggressive treatment of the underlying cardiovascular disease, especially coronary artery disease, valvular heart disease, or hypertension, should be pursued if possible in all cases. Treatment strategies common to all patients with systolic dysfunction regardless of the underlying myocardial disorder are discussed below according to the level of symptoms of heart failure (Table 1). Therapies proven to reduce mortality and morbidity (angiotensin-converting enzyme [ACE] inhibitors) should be used in all patients with reduced systolic function. Therapies that control symptoms (digoxin, diuretics) but have not been proved to reduce mortality should be guided by symptoms. Nonpharmacologic measures appropriate for all patients with systolic dysfunction are outlined in Table 1.

- ACE inhibitors are indicated for all patients with systolic ventricular dysfunction regardless of symptoms.

ACE Inhibitors

Angiotensin II is an important regulator of blood pressure and has a large number of biologic actions (Fig. 1).

It is produced from the precursor angiotensin I peptide by an angiotensin-converting enzyme, and angiotensin I, in turn, is formed from cleavage of angiotensinogen by renin. This system is referred to as the "renin-angiotensin system" (RAS) or, because angiotensin II stimulates production of aldosterone, as the "renin-angiotensin-aldosterone system" (RAAS). Angiotensin may be produced by several tissues (including the heart and vasculature), and tissue RAS may be upregulated independently from circulating or systemic RAS. Circulating RAS is activated primarily in decompensated heart failure or in patients taking diuretics. Some studies have suggested that tissue RAS is activated in patients with systolic dysfunction without overt heart failure. On this basis, antagonism of the deleterious actions of angiotensin II should be beneficial in all patients with systolic dysfunction, regardless of the level of symptoms. This hypothesis is supported by the results of several large multicenter trials evaluating the impact of therapy with ACE inhibitors in patients with systolic dysfunction with or without overt heart failure (Table 2).

As summarized in Table 2, ACE inhibitor therapy reduces symptoms, retards progression of heart failure (including need for hospitalization), and reduces mortality among patients with systolic dysfunction regardless of functional class. Mortality reduction is most striking in the most symptomatic patients and in those with severe systolic dysfunction, especially post myocardial infarction.

Table 1.—General Approach to Medical Therapy for a Patient With Systolic Dysfunction

In all patients
    Assess and aggressively treat ischemia and cardiac risk factors
    Control hypertension
    Dietary counseling as needed
    Exercise program
    Maintain sinus rhythm if possible
    Monitor electrolytes
    Instruct in daily weights and adjustment of diuretics
    Referral to appropriate center if candidate for transplantation
NYHA class I before therapy (asymptomatic left ventricular dysfunction)
    ACE inhibitor*
    Consider warfarin
    Consider β-blocker
NYHA class II
    ACE inhibitor*
    Consider warfarin
    Consider β-blocker
    Loop diuretic if symptoms persist while taking ACE inhibitor
    Digoxin if symptoms persist while taking ACE inhibitor
NYHA class III
    Consider hospitalization for initiation of therapy
    ACE inhibitor*
    Loop diuretic
    Digoxin
    Consider warfarin
    Consider β-blocker
NYHA class IV
    Hospitalization
        Hemodynamic monitoring, inotropic support, and intravenous vasodilators to stabilize condition may be necessary, with gradual weaning and up-titration of oral regimen
    ACE inhibitor*
    Loop diuretic
    Digoxin
    Consider warfarin
    Consider additional vasodilator (hydralazine and isosorbide dinitrate or amlodipine)
    Consider combination diuretic therapy for diuretic resistance
    Consider amiodarone

ACE, angiotensin-converting enzyme; NYHA, New York Heart Association.
*Titrate to maximal recommended dose as tolerated; use hydralazine and isosorbide dinitrate or angiotensin II receptor blocker if patient cannot tolerate drug because of cough; use hydralazine and isosorbide dinitrate if patient cannot tolerate drug because of renal insufficiency.

Effects of ACE Inhibitors in Systolic Dysfunction

As combined arterial and venous vasodilators, ACE inhibitors have favorable hemodynamic effects in patients with systolic dysfunction. Reduction in afterload, preload, and wall stress are observed without an increase in heart rate.

ACE inhibitors augment renal blood flow and reduce production of aldosterone and antidiuretic hormone. Thus, they promote excretion of sodium and water.

ACE inhibitors have effects on cellular metabolism independent of their hemodynamic effects. Their potent anti-hypertrophic effects on ventricular and vascular cells may be at least partially independent of blood pressure reduction and contribute to their role in the prevention of ventricular remodeling. ACE inhibitors have been demonstrated to blunt progressive dilatation of the ventricle in patients with systolic dysfunction and are among the most potent agents against ventricular hypertrophy in patients with hypertension.

ACE inhibitors also have been demonstrated to reduce ischemic events in patients with systolic dysfunction due to myocardial ischemia. This has led to studies that have examined an expanded role for the use of ACE inhibitors in patients with acute myocardial infarction without definite systolic dysfunction (Table 2). Completed trials support the use of ACE inhibitors in patients with anterior or other large myocardial infarctions regardless of ejection fraction. Trials are under way to examine the effect of ACE inhibitors on ischemic events in unselected patients with coronary artery disease but no recent infarct.

Specific ACE Inhibitors

Specific ACE inhibitors differ in chemical structure, which imparts differences in potency, half-life, bioavailability, route of elimination, and affinity for tissue-bound ACE. The clinical relevance of these differences is unproven. The most widely prescribed ACE inhibitors (captopril, enalapril, lisinopril) are those used in the large clinical trials. ACE inhibitors with a sulfhydryl group (captopril) are more likely to produce rash, neutropenia, and nephrotic syndrome. These side effects are dose-related, and neutropenia is more likely to occur in patients with collagen vascular disease.

Special Considerations With ACE Inhibitors

Correct Dosage of ACE Inhibitors

Use of the optimal dose of ACE inhibitors is an important clinical issue. In clinical practice, ACE inhibitors commonly

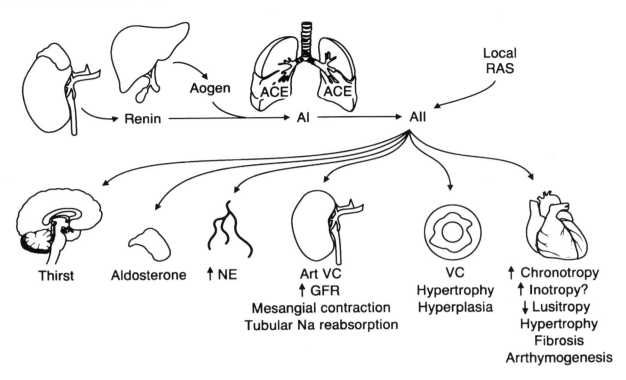

Fig. 1. Circulating and local renin-angiotensin system (RAS). Renin from kidney converts angiotensinogen (Aogen) to angiotensin I (AI), which is converted to angiotensin II (AII) by angiotensin-converting enzyme (ACE) in lungs. AII, either from this pathway or produced independently in tissues, exerts effects on brain, adrenals, sympathetic nervous system, kidney, vasculature, and heart. NE, norepinephrine; GFR, glomerular filtration rate; Na, sodium; VC, arterial vasoconstriction.

are prescribed at doses well below those demonstrated to be efficacious in clinical trials. Studies in animal models of heart failure and preliminary results from the ATLAS trial comparing high and low doses of lisinopril in patients with heart failure support the need for high doses of ACE inhibitors in patients with heart failure to achieve maximal symptomatic relief and survival benefit (Table 3). Careful monitoring of renal function, potassium, and blood pressure is required during the titration phase. Diuretic dosage may need to be decreased for systemic hypotension in the absence of pulmonary congestion. Avoid over-diuresis with diuretics before initiation and titration of ACE inhibitor dose. In the Evaluation of Losartan in the Elderly (ELITE) trial, more than 70% of elderly patients in the ACE inhibitor arm tolerated full doses of the drug and only about 10% of all patients developed a significant increase in creatinine levels.

ACE Inhibitors in Renal Dysfunction
Mild renal impairment and a mild increase in the serum level of creatinine during the up-titration of ACE inhibitors are not contraindications to initiation of goal doses of ACE inhibitors, although meticulous monitoring of electrolytes during up-titration is required. ACE inhibitors are contraindicated in the presence of significant renal artery stenosis.

Side Effects of ACE Inhibitors
In addition to renal insufficiency, hyperkalemia, and hypotension, other class-related side effects of ACE inhibitors include cough, angioedema, fetal anomalies, and dysgeusia (metallic taste). Cough is related to an increase in bradykinin and occurs in 5% to 10% of white persons but may be more common among Asians. Because of the teratogenicity of ACE inhibitors, they should not be used in the treatment of females of childbearing age who are not sterilized or using effective birth control.

Role of Bradykinin in Mediating Beneficial Effects of ACE Inhibitors
Because ACE inhibitors prevent the breakdown of bradykinin, the potentiation of bradykinin may mediate some of the beneficial effects of ACE inhibitors as well as some of the side effects mentioned above. Limited

Table 2.—Clinical Trials of ACE Inhibitors in Systolic Dysfunction

Study	Patient population	ACE inhibitor	Time of administration after MI	Treatment duration	Outcome
Studies in systolic dysfunction with heart failure					
CONSENSUS	NYHA IV ($n = 253$)	Enalapril vs placebo		1 day-20 mo	Decreased mortality; decreased CHF
SOLVD-Treatment	NYHA II and III ($n = 2,569$)	Enalapril vs placebo		22-55 mo	Decreased mortality; decreased CHF
V-HeFT II	NYHA II and III ($n = 804$)	Enalapril vs hydralazine isosorbide		0.5-5.7 yr	Enalapril decreased mortality compared with hydralazine and isosorbide
Studies in asymptomatic systolic dysfunction					
SOLVD-Prevention	Asymptomatic LV dysfunction ($n = 4,228$)	Enalapril vs placebo		14.6-62 mo	Decreased combined end point of mortality and CHF hospitalizations
SAVE	MI, decreased LV function ($n = 2,231$)	Captopril vs placebo	3-16 days	24-60 mo	Decreased mortality, progression to CHF and recurrent MI
Studies in systolic dysfunction/acute MI					
AIRE*	MI and CHF ($n = 2,006$)	Ramipril vs placebo	3-10 days	Minimum of 6 mo	Decreased mortality
TRACE*	MI, decreased LV function ($n = 1,749$)	Trandolapril vs placebo	3-7 days	24-50 mo	Decreased mortality
Studies in patients with acute MI					
CONSENSUS II	MI ($n = 6,090$)	Enalaprilat/enalapril vs placebo	24 hr	41-180 days	No change in survival; hypotension with enalaprilat
ISIS-4	MI ($n > 50,000$)	Captopril vs placebo	24 hr	28 days	Decreased mortality
GISSI-3	MI ($n = 19,394$)	Lisinopril vs control	24 hr	6 wk	Decreased mortality
SMILE	MI ($n = 1,556$)	Zofenopril vs placebo	24 hr	6 wk	Decreased mortality

ACE, angiotensin-converting enzyme; CHF, congestive heart failure; LV, left ventricular; MI, myocardial infarction; NYHA, New York Heart Association.
*Study involved patients with MI.

animal studies suggest that bradykinin is important in mediating the antihypertrophic, reverse remodeling, and vascular remodeling effects of ACE inhibitors. However, in the ELITE trial, the angiotensin II AT$_1$ receptor antagonist losartan had similar beneficial effects on symptoms and actually reduced mortality more than ACE inhibitors. Studies are under way to establish the clinical importance of potentiation of bradykinin by ACE inhibitors in patients with heart failure.

Other Vasodilators

Hydralazine and Isosorbide Dinitrate in Heart Failure

The combination of hydralazine and isosorbide dinitrate (Isordil) was shown in the VHeFT-I trial to reduce mortality and improve symptoms in patients with heart failure. In this trial, ACE inhibitors reduced mortality more than hydralazine and isosorbide dinitrate.

Table 3.—Recommended Dosage of Commonly Used
Angiotensin-Converting Enzyme Inhibitors
for Treatment of Systolic Dysfunction

Agent	Dose
Captopril	50 mg tid
Enalapril*	10 mg bid
Lisinopril*	20-40 mg qd

*Higher doses may be used if patients have persistent hypertension or symptoms.

- Although ACE inhibitors are considered first-line therapy and are superior to hydralazine and isosorbide dinitrate, hydralazine and isosorbide dinitrate are recommended for patients intolerant of ACE inhibitors, especially those who develop renal insufficiency with ACE inhibitors.
- Doses of hydralazine and isosorbide dinitrate recommended in heart failure are much higher than those used in hypertension or angina. Goal doses are 75 to 100 mg hydralazine 3 to 4 times daily in combination with 30 to 40 mg isosorbide dinitrate 3 or 4 times daily.

Angiotensin II Receptor Antagonists

These agents were developed as antagonists of the RAS that did not cause potentiation of bradykinin. The lack of bradykinin-related side effects may be beneficial; however, if bradykinin potentiation is important in the beneficial effects of ACE inhibitors, angiotensin II receptor antagonists theoretically may not be as effective as ACE inhibitors. The findings of the ELITE trial suggest that angiotensin II antagonists and ACE inhibitors have equivalent effects on symptoms, but the former agents potentially have a greater effect on survival. However, this trial was not powered to test mortality and was performed in elderly patients with milder heart failure. Thus, further studies are under way to determine if this class of agents has a role either as a substitute for or as *an addition to* ACE inhibitors in treating heart failure.

- Angiotensin II receptor antagonists do not have a lower incidence of renal insufficiency or hyperkalemia and thus are not an alternative to ACE inhibitors for patients intolerant of ACE inhibitors because of renal effects.
- Angiotensin II receptor antagonists do not cause cough.

Calcium Channel Blockers in Heart Failure

First-generation calcium channel blockers (verapamil, diltiazem, nifedipine) are contraindicated in the presence of heart failure because they reduce survival and exacerbate symptoms of heart failure.

Newer generation dihydropyridines have been tested recently in treating heart failure. These agents have higher vascular-to-myocardial specificity and fewer negative inotropic effects. The Prospective Randomized Amlodipine Survival Evaluation (PRAISE) trial tested amlodipine versus placebo (in addition to standard therapy, including ACE inhibitors) in patients with heart failure, and amlodipine had no effect on survival or hospitalization for major cardiovascular events. There was a suggestion of improved survival for patients with nonischemic cardiomyopathy. Currently, PRAISE-II is under way in patients with idiopathic dilated cardiomyopathy to determine whether amlodipine added to ACE inhibitors improves survival. The VHeFT-III trial examined felodipine, another dihydropyridine, in patients with heart failure. No beneficial (or detrimental) effect on survival or symptoms was demonstrated.

- Amlodipine may be an option for treating heart failure in patients who are still hypertensive while receiving maximal doses of standard therapy.

Digitalis Glycosides in Heart Failure

Although the consensus is that digitalis is of value in controlling ventricular rate in atrial fibrillation when this rhythm complicates congestive heart failure due to systolic ventricular dysfunction, its efficacy in ventricular dysfunction in patients in sinus rhythm has been questioned.

Observational studies have suggested that in many outpatients with the diagnosis of congestive heart failure, digitalis treatment could be discontinued without apparent symptomatic deterioration. Subsequent studies in patients with well-characterized cardiac dilatation and systolic dysfunction have shown that digitalis, compared with placebo, decreases pulmonary capillary wedge pressure, increases cardiac index, and improves symptoms and exercise tolerance.

In the RADIANCE trial, patients receiving digoxin treatment who were in sinus rhythm and had an ejection fraction of 35% or less and New York Heart Association class II or III symptoms were randomized to continuation of digoxin or substitution of digoxin by a placebo. All patients continued to take ACE inhibitors and diuretics. Those in whom digoxin treatment was discontinued had a 25% probability of clinical deterioration, in comparison with 5% of those who continued receiving digoxin (Fig. 2). The RADIANCE trial documented the benefit of digoxin in ventricular systolic dysfunction with sinus rhythm.

The Digoxin Mortality Study enrolled 6,800 patients with symptomatic congestive heart failure and sinus rhythm, with or without evidence of systolic dysfunction. There were few patients with class IV heart failure in this trial. Digoxin treatment did not alter overall mortality during an average follow-up of 3 years. Digoxin-treated patients had a reduced risk of hospitalization for worsening heart failure.

The dose of digoxin should be adjusted downward in patients with renal insufficiency and in those taking verapamil, amiodarone, quinidine, or propafenone. In the Digoxin Mortality Study, the incidence of hospitalization for suspected digoxin toxicity in actively treated patients was higher than for placebo, but still quite low.

- Digitalis provides symptomatic benefit but no documented mortality benefit in heart failure.

Diuretics in Heart Failure

Diuretics are required for patients with heart failure who remain symptomatic despite treatment with ACE inhibitors and digoxin. Patients who present with pulmonary edema need diuretics immediately, although the dose may be markedly reduced or eliminated when treatment with ACE inhibitors and digoxin has been started and up-titrated. Because diuretics are inexpensive and essential in the management of pulmonary edema, no trials have examined their effect on mortality in heart failure. Recent data from the Systolic Hypertension in the Elderly Program (SHEP) showed that diuretic-based therapy of hypertension reduced onset of heart failure, especially in patients with a history of myocardial infarction (80% decrease in initial episodes of heart failure).

The minimal dose of diuretics needed to control heart congestion should be used because over-diuresis further exacerbates the activation of the RAS that results from diuretic therapy and may result in hypotension, prerenal azotemia, hyponatremia, hypokalemia, and hypomagnesemia. Over-diuresis also results in excessive thirst, which reduces quality of life and may result in excessive fluid intake and "diuretic refractoriness."

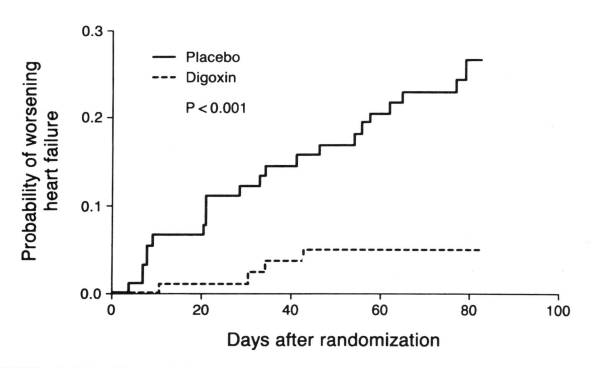

Fig. 2. RADIANCE study. Kaplan-Meier analysis of cumulative probability of worsening heart failure in patients continuing to receive digoxin ($n = 85$) and those with treatment switched to placebo ($n = 93$). Patients in the placebo group had a higher risk of worsening heart failure throughout the 12-week study (relative risk, 5.9; 95% confidence interval, 2.1 to 17.2; $P < 0.001$).

If congestive symptoms persist despite treatment with maximal doses of ACE inhibitors and digoxin, up-titration of diuretics may be needed. It is important to determine whether the current dose of diuretics produces a diuretic response. If not, the morning dose should be increased. In advanced heart failure, twice-daily dosing is often required. In the absence of renal failure, if there is need for doses greater than 120 mg furosemide twice daily, consideration should be given to combination therapy with a thiazide diuretic such as metolazone (Zaroxolyn). Metolazone potentiates the action of loop diuretics, because it blocks sodium reuptake further down the nephron. With chronic use of loop diuretics, there is hypertrophy and enhanced sodium retention by the distal nephron, blunting the response to loop diuretics. Blockade of the distal nephron by a thiazide prevents this augmented sodium reuptake. Such combination diuretic therapy often results in profound hypokalemia and volume depletion. Careful monitoring of electrolytes and blood pressure is required. Patients with refractory hypokalemia may benefit from a small dose of a potassium-sparing diuretic such as spironolactone (Aldactone). Careful monitoring of potassium levels is required, especially in patients taking ACE inhibitors.

- Diuretics are required for patients with heart failure who remain symptomatic despite treatment with ACE inhibitors and digoxin.
- The minimal dose of diuretics needed to control congestion should be used, because over-diuresis further exacerbates the activation of the RAS that results from diuretic therapy and may result in hypotension, prerenal azotemia, hyponatremia, hypokalemia, and hypomagnesemia.
- Metolazone potentiates the action of loop diuretics because it blocks sodium reuptake further down the nephron, but may result in profound hypokalemia and volume depletion.

β-Blockers in Heart Failure

The rationale for use of β-blockers in heart failure stems from sympathetic nervous system activation in asymptomatic left ventricular dysfunction. This activation increases linearly in relation to the severity of heart failure. Some experimental data suggest that chronic heightened sympathetic nervous system activation and increased plasma levels of norepinephrine may be directly toxic to myocytes. Up-regulation of β-receptors

was once believed to mediate improvement in clinical status and systolic function with β-blocker therapy; carvedilol does not up-regulate β_1 receptors. Thus, mechanisms other than β-receptor up-regulation may mediate the beneficial effects of this β-blocker.

- All patients with stable NYHA class II or III heart failure due to left ventricular systolic dysfunction should receive a β-blocker unless they have a contraindication or cannot tolerate the treatment; β-blockers are generally used with diuretics and ACE inhibitors
- Patients receiving a β-blocker should be advised that 1) side effects may occur early but do not generally prevent long-term use; 2) symptomatic improvement may not occur for 2-3 months; and 3) β-blockade may reduce the risk of disease progression even if symptoms have not responded favorably to treatment
- More data are needed on the effect of β-blockers in unstable patients and patients with current or recent class IV symptoms before they can be recommended for use in such patients
- β-Blockers are indicated for long-term management of chronic heart failure. They should not be used in acutely ill patients ("rescue" therapy), including those who are in the intensive care unit with refractory heart failure requiring intravenous support

Modified from Packer M, Cohn JN: Consensus recommendations for the management of chronic heart failure. *Am J Cardiol* 83 (no. 2A):1A-38A, 1999. By permission of Excerpta Medica.

Although acute administration of β-adrenergic blockade decreases contractility and heart rate in normal humans and animals or in those with heart failure, chronic administration improves contractility, according to several randomized and nonrandomized studies. This effect becomes apparent in 3 to 6 months, and, on average, patients receiving β-blockers have an increase of about 5% in ejection fraction. Improvement in diastolic function may also occur after treatment.

Some studies have shown improvement in functional class or quality of life with β-blockade in patients with heart failure. Fewer studies have shown improved exercise tolerance, as assessed by oxygen consumption tests or other objective exercise tests, perhaps because the chronotropic response to exercise is blunted by the β-blocker.

The effect of β-blockers on mortality of patients with heart failure is controversial. The largest studies with published mortality data are the Metoprolol in Dilated

Cardiomyopathy (MDC), the CIBIS, the Australia/New Zealand (ANZ), and the Carvedilol Study Group trials. The ANZ and the Carvedilol Study Group trials showed a statistically significant decrease in mortality. Meta-analysis of all the β-blocker trials suggests a beneficial effect. Large-scale mortality trials are under way and include the BEST trial (examining the effect of bucindolol), the CIBIS-II trial, and several trials with carvedilol. These larger trials, powered to detect mortality differences, are needed before firm recommendations can be made about the use of β-blockers in heart failure.

The β-blockers currently being investigated for treatment of heart failure include metoprolol (a selective β-blocker without any significant ancillary effects), carvedilol (a nonselective β-blocker with α-blocking and antioxidant activity), and bucindolol (a nonselective β-blocker with additional direct vasodilatory action). The vasodilatory properties of carvedilol and bucindolol are thought to make them better tolerated by patients with heart failure. It is unclear whether the other ancillary properties of these agents impart clinically significant differences in effects that may be the basis for recommending therapy with one β-blocker and not others. Until consensus is reached, pending results of ongoing trials and review by cardiology societies that recommend guidelines, the use of β-blockers in heart failure should be considered unproven, although certainly justifiable in patients with mild-to-moderate heart failure. Few studies have included a significant number of patients in class IV heart failure, and treatment with β-blockers in these patients is currently contraindicated.

Oral Inotropic Agents in Heart Failure

Phosphodiesterase inhibitors were developed as new inotropic agents for the treatment of heart failure. The first of these, amrinone, was shown to have effective inotropic and vasodilator properties when used for short-term, intravenous support of critically ill patients. A similar compound, milrinone, was developed for both short-term intravenous use and long-term oral administration.

These agents are hemodynamically effective and increase cardiac output, decrease pulmonary capillary wedge pressure, and improve exercise capacity. However, in a controlled clinical trial, when these agents were administered orally for long periods, their short-term efficacy was overshadowed by an increase in long-term mortality. The PROMISE trial, which compared oral milrinone with placebo, showed increased mortality in the milrinone group, with detrimental effects most prominent in patients

in New York Heart Association class IV heart failure. Because of the poor results of long-term oral administration, phosphodiesterase inhibitors currently are restricted to short-term use as intravenous inotropic support agents. They can be of value in the intensive care setting in stabilizing the condition of patients with heart failure who have hemodynamic decompensation.

Vesnarinone, a novel inotropic agent, was evaluated initially in a clinical trial that showed survival benefit. Subsequently, a larger trial revealed increased mortality in the vesnarinone-treated group. Final analyses of this trial are forthcoming and may shed light on the mechanisms of toxicity.

Two important lessons can be learned from these "failed drug" experiences:

- Short-term improvements in hemodynamic variables and exercise capacity do not necessarily imply a long-term mortality benefit in heart failure.
- Only adequately designed clinical trials with sufficient statistical power can assess the long-term safety and efficacy of drugs for heart failure.

Intermittent and Continuous Intravenous Inotropic Therapy

During the 1980s, a few small clinical studies suggested that the periodic use of short-term intravenous inotropic support provided long-lasting symptomatic benefit. It was hypothesized that short-term exposure to intravenous inotropic drugs resulted in "conditioning" of the myocardium, with subsequent sustained clinical improvement. Larger, more definitive clinical trials have not been performed, and the theoretical basis for this form of therapy is unproven.

Although continuous low-dose intravenous inotropic therapy administered on an outpatient basis has become popular in some medical centers, adequately controlled clinical trials have not been performed to demonstrate the safety and efficacy of this therapy. The potential for toxicity with home use of powerful inotropic drugs should be considered.

Anticoagulation in Heart Failure

The Stroke Prevention in Atrial Fibrillation (SPAF) trial and other atrial fibrillation trials have demonstrated that patients with decreased ejection fraction or clinical heart failure and atrial fibrillation are at high risk for cardioembolic events. The efficacy of warfarin (Coumadin) in reducing embolic events in these patients has also been well documented.

Similarly, patients with a recent anterior or large myocardial infarction are at markedly increased risk for cardioembolic events, and anticoagulation is recommended for at least the first 3 to 6 months after infarction. Patients with systolic dysfunction who have had a cardioembolic event are also at increased risk regardless of rhythm, and anticoagulation is recommended for them.

The value of chronic anticoagulation in patients with sinus rhythm and chronic ischemic or nonischemic dilated cardiomyopathy without a recent large myocardial infarction or previous cardioembolic event is a matter of controversy. The clinical practice guidelines of the National Health Care Policy and Research Agency for Heart Failure do not recommend anticoagulation for these patients. However, the American Heart Association/American College of Cardiology guidelines indicate that use of anticoagulation in patients with a very low ejection fraction (<25%) or an intracardiac thrombus is a "class II" therapeutic intervention, that is, "acceptable but of uncertain efficacy."

The rationale for anticoagulation is based largely on a retrospective study of patients with idiopathic dilated cardiomyopathy evaluated in the 1970s that demonstrated a high rate of cardioembolic events, which was lower in patients receiving warfarin. In an analysis of major heart failure studies, the incidence of arterial thromboembolism in the largest studies was 2.0% to 2.4% per 100 patient-years. A recent analysis of anticoagulation use in 6,513 patients enrolled in the SOLVD trials demonstrated that, after adjustment for baseline differences in other predictors of outcome in patients receiving warfarin and those not receiving it, warfarin treatment was associated with lower all-cause mortality and lower mortality due to cardiovascular disease. There was no decrease in deaths due to stroke, pulmonary embolism, or other vascular cause. After adjustment for baseline differences in other predictors of outcome in patients receiving warfarin and those not receiving it, warfarin treatment was also associated with lower rates of hospital admission for nonfatal myocardial infarction. The mortality benefit was evident in patients with ischemic or nonischemic cause of heart failure as well as in patients with or without atrial fibrillation and was independent of the treatment arm or symptom status of the patient. Because this was not a randomized trial, the mortality benefit may reflect other management factors not assessed in this observational study. Nonetheless, the findings can be used to justify anticoagulation treatment in patients with decreased systolic function. Until randomized trials are conducted, this issue remains a matter of debate.

- Chronic anticoagulation is indicated in patients with decreased ejection fraction and atrial fibrillation, previous cardioembolic event, or recent large myocardial infarction.
- Use of chronic anticoagulation in other patients with an ejection fraction <25% is a matter of controversy and is considered a "class II" therapy.

Other Therapeutic Issues

Atrial Fibrillation in Heart Failure
Atrial arrhythmias such as atrial fibrillation can aggravate congestive heart failure and increase the risk of stroke. Restoration of sinus rhythm may improve symptoms as well as left ventricular function itself. For most patients, an attempt to restore and to maintain sinus rhythm is warranted. If sinus rhythm cannot be restored, good rate control remains an important therapeutic goal.

The most appropriate antiarrhythmic agent for patients with heart failure and atrial fibrillation is quinidine or amiodarone, because other antiarrhythmic agents such as propafenone and sotalol may exacerbate heart failure and increase mortality in patients with ischemic heart disease as the basis of heart failure. Amiodarone does not increase mortality or symptoms in patients with heart failure and has been shown in some trials to decrease mortality. Also, amiodarone may improve symptoms in patients with heart failure. Thus, amiodarone is an attractive agent for patients with atrial fibrillation and heart failure.

- Excessive ventricular response rate in atrial fibrillation can in itself cause deterioration of left ventricular function. Restoration of normal sinus rhythm or at least good control of ventricular rate is an essential aspect of management.

Sudden Death and Sustained Ventricular Tachycardia in Heart Failure
Sudden death is common in congestive heart failure and accounts for approximately one-third of the deaths among these patients. Although sudden death was widely assumed to be a consequence of ventricular tachycardia or fibrillation, recent data suggest that bradyarrhythmias and electromechanical dissociation may account for a significant proportion of these cases of sudden death. Patients who survive an episode of cardiac arrest or who present with sustained ventricular tachycardia should be referred to an electrophysiologist for consideration of

electrophysiologically guided antiarrhythmic therapy or a defibrillator (or both).

Nonsustained Ventricular Arrhythmias

Although it has been suggested that antiarrhythmic agents would prevent sudden death in congestive heart failure, well-designed clinical trials are needed to demonstrate safety and efficacy, particularly with the potential for drug-related proarrhythmic side effects.

The two largest trials of amiodarone for the prevention of sudden death in heart failure were the Amiodarone in Patients with Congestive Heart Failure and Asymptomatic Ventricular Arrhythmia (CHF-STAT) and the Grupo de Estudio de la Sobrevida en la Insuficiencia Cardiaca en Argentina (GESICA) trials. The GESICA trial reported a 28% reduction in risk of death; however, the CHF-STAT trial did not demonstrate an overall statistical decrease in mortality, although there was a trend toward lower mortality in the patient subgroup with nonischemic cardiomyopathy. Neither trial showed any evidence of increased mortality. Currently, the Sudden Cardiac Death in Heart Failure Trial (SuCD-HeFT), which randomizes patients to standard therapy, amiodarone, or a defibrillator, is under way. Until completion of this trial, treatment of patients with heart failure and asymptomatic ventricular arrhythmias remains a "class III" unproven therapeutic intervention.

Exercise

Although exercise programs do not alter mortality in patients with congestive heart failure, physical conditioning improves exercise capacity and the sense of well-being. It is recommended that patients with chronic heart failure engage in regular exercise to maintain peripheral muscle tone. For many patients, a monitored exercise program is an important adjunctive therapy.

NEW TRIAL INFORMATION ADDED AT PROOF STAGE

Benefit of β-Blockers for Heart Failure

The benefit of β-blockers for treatment of chronic heart failure was confirmed in 1999 by two large studies: MERIT-HF and CIBIS-II.

MERIT-HF randomized 3,991 patients with heart failure (New York Heart Association functional class II to IV) and ejection fractions less than 40% to β-blocker therapy, in addition to standard therapy for congestive heart failure. Long-acting metoprolol reduced overall mortality by 34%, including both sudden deaths and deaths due to worsening heart failure.

CIBIS-II was a multicenter, double-blind, randomized trial of bisoprolol in 2,647 patients with chronic heart failure (New York Heart Association class III or IV, ejection fraction < 35%); in addition, the patients received ACE inhibitors and diuretics. CIBIS-II was stopped early because bisoprolol showed a significant mortality benefit. All-cause mortality was significantly lower with bisoprolol than placebo (11.8% versus 17.3%, $P < 0.0001$), and sudden deaths were also reduced significantly.

The effect of β-blockade on mortality is additive to that of ACE inhibition and is probably a class effect of β-blockade that has been proved thus far for carvedilol, bisoprolol, and metoprolol. The benefit of β-blocker therapy is independent of the severity or cause of heart failure.

Randomized Aldactone Evaluation Study (RALES)

RALES was a randomized trial of aldactone in 1,663 patients with severe heart failure and an ejection fraction less than 35% who were being treated with an ACE inhibitor, a loop diuretic, and, in some cases, digoxin. The trial was discontinued early after a mean follow-up period of 2 years because spironolactone decreased mortality (46% in the placebo group to 35% in the spironolactone group, $P < 0.001$). This 30% reduction in mortality among patients in the spironolactone group was due to a lower risk of both death from progressive heart failure and sudden death from cardiac causes. The frequency of hospitalization for worsening heart failure was 35% lower in the spironolactone group than in the placebo group. In addition, patients who received spironolactone had a significant improvement in the symptoms of heart failure, as assessed on the basis of the New York Heart Association functional class ($P < 0.001$). RALES concluded that blockade of aldosterone receptors by spironolactone, in addition to standard therapy, substantially reduces the risk of both morbidity and death among patients with severe heart failure.

Suggested Review Reading

Practice Guidelines for Treatment of Heart Failure

1. Committee on Evaluation and Management of Heart Failure: Guidelines for the evaluation and management of heart failure. Report of the American College of Cardiology/American Heart Association Task Force on Practice Guidelines. *Circulation* 92:2764-2784, 1995.

2. Konstam MA, Dracup K, Baker DW: *Heart Failure: Evaluation and Care of Patients With Left-Ventricular Systolic Dysfunction. Clinical Practice Guideline No. 11.* AHCPR Publication No. 94-0612. Rockville, Maryland: Agency for Health Care Policy and Research, Public Health Service, U.S. Department of Health and Human Services, June 1994.

Angiotensin-Converting Enzyme Inhibitors

1. Brown NJ, Vaughan DE: Angiotensin-converting enzyme inhibitors. *Circulation* 97:1411-1420, 1998.
Review of angiotensin-converting enzyme inhibitors and pertinent congestive heart failure trials.

2. Dzau VJ: Tissue renin-angiotensin system in myocardial hypertrophy and failure. *Arch Intern Med* 153:937-942, 1993.
Review of the role of the circulating and local renin-angiotensin system in the pathophysiology of heart failure.

3. Pitt B, Segal R, Martinez FA, et al: Randomised trial of losartan versus captopril in patients over 65 with heart failure. *Lancet* 349:747-752, 1997.
ELITE Trial results—Study comparing AII receptor blocker with angiotensin-converting enzyme inhibitors.

Calcium Channel Blockers in Congestive Heart Failure

1. Elkayam U, Shotan A, Mehra A, et al: Calcium channel blockers in heart failure. *J Am Coll Cardiol* 22(Suppl A):139A-144A, 1993.
Review of early use of traditional calcium channel blockers in congestive heart failure.

2. Packer M, O'Connor CM, Ghali JK, et al: Effect of amlodipine on morbidity and mortality in severe chronic heart failure. *N Engl J Med* 335:1107-1114, 1996.
Results of the PRAISE trial.

Digitalis and Inotropic Agents

1. Leier CV: Positive inotropic therapy: an update and new agents. *Curr Probl Cardiol* 21:521-581, 1996.
Review of digoxin and other inotropes.

β-Blockers

1. Packer M: Do beta-blockers prolong survival in chronic heart failure? A review of the experimental and clinical evidence. *Eur Heart J* 19(Suppl B):40B-46B, 1998.

Anticoagulation

1. Al-Khadra AS, Salem DN, Rand WM, et al: Warfarin anticoagulation and survival: a cohort analysis from the Studies of Left Ventricular Dysfunction. *J Am Coll Cardiol* 31:749-753, 1998.
Recent study of the effects of warfarin, also reviews available literature.

Questions

Multiple Choice (choose the one best answer)

1. A 53-year-old man was referred by his orthopedist after a routine preanesthetic electrocardiogram showed left bundle branch block. He has no history of cardiovascular disease. He is a physically active construction worker who denies angina, exertional dyspnea, edema, or palpitations. There is no family history of sudden death or heart disease. He has no specific cardiovascular risk factors and does not drink alcohol or take recreational drugs.

Physical examination findings:
   Blood pressure, 115/65 mm Hg
   Heart rate, 65 beats/min and regular

Lungs, clear to auscultation

Jugular venous pressure—normal in level and waveform, apical beat normal in location and character

S_1, S_2 paradoxically split

No S_3

S_4 present

Extremities, no edema

Laboratory findings:

Electrocardiogram—normal sinus rhythm, typical left bundle branch block

Chest radiograph—mild cardiomegaly

Echocardiogram—left ventricular end-diastolic dimension = 7.0 cm; ejection fraction = 30%; normal cardiac valves

Cholesterol = 185; high-density lipoprotein = 56

Adenosine thallium—no evidence of infarction or ischemia

Metabolic stress test—VO_2 max = 110% predicted

Creatinine, 1.0 mg/dL

Potassium, 4.2 mEq/L

The most appropriate therapy for this patient is:

a. Digoxin 0.25 mg, lisinopril titrated to 40 mg, furosemide 20 mg
b. Close follow-up
c. Hydralazine titrated to 75 mg four times daily and isosorbide dinitrate titrated to 40 mg three times daily
d. Enalapril titrated to 20 mg/day

2. A 76-year-old woman complains of mild exertional dyspnea, which she started to note on her previously well-tolerated morning walk. An echocardiogram performed elsewhere was reported as abnormal. She gets dyspneic with walking fast or on hills but still walks 1 mile/day and has no paroxysmal nocturnal dyspnea, orthopnea, or rest dyspnea. She has had mild edema in the evenings for several years. She has no angina, palpitations, or syncope. She is a nonsmoker. She has a long history of hypertension and takes two antihypertensive drugs. She has no other specific cardiac risk factors. She receives estrogen replacement therapy.

Medications:

Lisinopril 30 mg/day

Furosemide 80 mg/day

Potassium 20 mEq/day

Premarin/Provera

Physical examination findings:

Blood pressure, 178/95 mm Hg

Heart rate, 80 beats/min and regular

Lungs, clear to auscultation

Jugular venous pressure—normal in level and waveform

S_1, S_2 paradoxically split

No S_3

S_4 present

Extremities, trace of edema

Laboratory findings:

Electrocardiogram—normal sinus rhythm with left bundle branch block

Chest radiograph—cardiomegaly and pulmonary venous hypertension

Echocardiogram—left ventricular end-diastolic dimension = 6.5 cm; ejection fraction = 25%; normal valves

Cholesterol = 200; low-density lipoprotein = 107

Adenosine thallium—no evidence of ischemia or infarction

Creatinine, 2.0 mg/dL

Potassium, 4.5 mEq/L

The most appropriate additional therapy at this point is:

a. Hydralazine titrated to 75 mg four times daily and isosorbide dinitrate titrated to 40 mg three times daily
b. Digoxin 0.125 mg/day
c. Metolazone 2.5 mg/day 30 minutes before furosemide
d. Nifedipine (Procardia XL) 10 mg/day

3. A 70-year-old man was referred for a second opinion after a recent hospitalization in which he had a perioperative anterior myocardial infarction following radical prostate surgery. He did not receive thrombolysis or emergency percutaneous transluminal coronary angioplasty because of concern about postoperative bleeding. In the hospital, he had pulmonary edema, which responded to diuresis, digoxin, and initiation of enalapril, which was increased to 10 mg twice daily before dismissal. He tolerated initiation of a low dose of β-blockers. Exercise thallium testing performed before dismissal revealed a fixed anterior-septal-apical defect. On his return 1 week after dismissal, he reported being physically inactive but denied having angina, dyspnea, or palpitations.

Medications:

    Enalapril 10 mg twice daily

    Furosemide 40 mg/day

    Digoxin 0.25 mg/day

    Metoprolol 25 mg twice daily

    Aspirin 80 mg/day

Physical examination findings:

    Blood pressure, 110/50 mm Hg

    Heart rate, 60 beats/min and regular with normal arterial waveform

    Lungs, clear to auscultation

    Jugular venous pressure—normal in level and waveform

    S_1, S_2 normal

    No S_3

    S_4 present

    Extremities, no edema

Laboratory findings:

    Electrocardiogram—pathologic precordial leads, Q waves in V_1-V_4

    Chest radiograph—cardiomegaly with evidence of pulmonary edema

    Echocardiogram—dilated left ventricle with thinning and akinesis of the anterior wall and anterior septum, apex not well seen, ejection fraction estimated at 35%

    Creatinine, 1.7 mg/dL (previously 1.3 on admission and 1.8 on dismissal from hospital)

    Potassium, 4.9 mEq/L

The most appropriate therapeutic changes at this point include:

a. Discontinue treatment with enalapril; start treatment with hydralazine, isosorbide dinitrate, and warfarin

b. Add warfarin

c. Discontinue treatment with enalapril; start treatment with losartan and add warfarin

d. Discontinue treatment with enalapril and metoprolol; start treatment with warfarin, hydralazine, and isosorbide dinitrate

4. An 87-year-old woman was referred for a second opinion after 4 hospitalizations for heart failure in the last 6 months. She usually presented with progressive dyspnea over several days, which deteriorated to pulmonary edema that responded to aggressive diuresis in the hospital. She has a long history of hypertension. She denied having angina but refused to undergo stress imaging or angiography and wished to pursue a nonaggressive approach.

Medications:

    Lisinopril 5 mg/day

    Digoxin 0.125 mg/day

    Furosemide 20 mg/day

    Potassium 10 mEq/day

Physical examination findings:

    Blood pressure, 140/80 mm Hg

    Heart rate, 80 beats/min and regular rhythm

    Lungs, clear to auscultation

    Jugular venous pressure—elevated to 10 cm with a large v wave

    S_1, S_2 normal

    S_3 present

    Extremities, 2+ edema to knee

Laboratory findings:

    Electrocardiogram—normal sinus rhythm, left ventricular hypertrophy

    Chest radiograph—cardiomegaly and pulmonary venous hypertension

    Echocardiogram—left ventricular end-diastolic dimension = 6.0 cm, ejection fraction = 30%, global hypokinesis, left ventricular wall thickness = 1.3

    Creatinine, 1.2 mg/dL

    Potassium, 4.7 mEq/L

The most appropriate therapeutic change at this point is:

a. Add metolazone

b. Add amlodipine

c. Lisinopril titrated to 30-40 mg/day and furosemide increased to 40 mg/day

d. Urge the patient to have angiography

5. A 42-year-old man with well-documented idiopathic dilated cardiomyopathy for 7 years is on a transplant list in another state. While on vacation, he has acutely decompensated heart failure with dyspnea at rest, nightly paroxysmal nocturnal dyspnea, orthopnea, edema, and lightheadedness. His ejection fraction has been documented at 12%, and a recent metabolic stress test showed a peak oxygen consumption of 11 mL/kg per minute.

Medications:

    Lisinopril 20 mg/day

    Digoxin 0.25 mg/day

Furosemide 120 mg twice daily
Warfarin

Physical examination findings:

General—moderate respiratory distress at rest

Blood pressure, 80/60 mm Hg

Heart rate, 120 beats/min and normal arterial character

Lungs, rales halfway up posterior chest wall on auscultation

Jugular venous pressure—angle of jaw with large v waves; apex, dilated left ventricle with apex beat in the 6th space anterior axillary line

S_1, S_2, split paradoxically

S_3 present

II/VI holosystolic murmur at apex

Extremities, cool, grade 3+ edema

Laboratory findings:

Electrocardiogram—sinus tachycardia, left bundle branch block

Chest radiograph—cardiomegaly, pulmonary venous hypertension, interstitial and some alveolar edema

Creatinine, 2.5 mg/dL (previously, 1.3 mg/dL)

Potassium, 3.5 mEq/L

Sodium, 132 mEq/L

The most appropriate therapy at this point is:

a. Carefully add carvedilol

b. Titrate lisinopril up to 40 mg/day

c. Hemodynamic monitoring and intravenous inotropic and diuretic therapy and transfer to a cardiac transplant center as soon as possible

d. Add metolazone and titrate lisinopril up to 40 mg/day

6. A 67-year-old man with severe diffuse 3-vessel coronary artery disease presents for outpatient follow-up after a recent hospitalization. He has had recurrent episodes of heart failure. A typical episode starts with chest tightness and quickly progresses to pulmonary edema. The patient has recently had numerous surgical consultations and has not been offered surgery because of "nongraftable" distal vessels. Adenosine thallium testing has shown large areas of ischemia without fixed defects. His ejection fraction is 35%.

Past medical history:

Diabetes mellitus; he has taken an oral agent for

20 years

Hyperlipidemia, with low-density lipoprotein > 180

Hypertension

Strong family history of coronary artery disease

Medications:

Glyburide

Lisinopril 40 mg/day

Furosemide 80 mg twice daily

Digoxin 0.25 mg/day

Aspirin 325 mg/day

Isosorbide dinitrate 40 mg every 4 hr x 3 during the day

Atorvastatin 20 mg/day

Nifedipine (Procardia XL) 30 mg/day

Physical examination findings:

Blood pressure, 125/75 mm Hg

Heart rate, 90 beats/min and normal arterial waveform

Lungs, no rales on auscultation

Jugular venous pressure—12 cm; apex beat normal

S_1, S_2 normal

S_3 present

Extremities, no edema

Laboratory findings:

Electrocardiogram—sinus rhythm with nonspecific ST-T abnormalities

Chest radiograph—mild cardiomegaly

Creatinine, 1.3 mg/dL

Potassium, 4.7 mEq/L

The most appropriate therapy at this point is:

a. Add a low dose of β-blocker and titrate up as tolerated; discontinue treatment with nifedipine

b. Add hydralazine and titrate up to 100 mg four times daily

c. Change nifedipine to amlodipine

d. Refer for transmyocardial laser revascularization

7. You are asked to evaluate a 60-year-old woman who is hospitalized for treatment of cellulitis and is doing well, but nurses have been refusing to administer angiotensin-converting enzyme inhibitor because of hypotension. She has stable New York Heart Association functional class II heart failure symptoms. She denies any orthostatic lightheadedness, syncope, or presyncope. She insists that her blood pressure is always low. A review of her medical record shows blood pressure in the range of 70/50 mm Hg to 80/55 mm Hg. She has not received

captopril since admission. Her ejection fraction has been stable at 28%.

Medications:

  Captopril 50 mg three times daily

  Furosemide 40 mg/day

  Digoxin 0.25 mg/day

  Cephalosporin intravenously

Physical examination findings:

  Afebrile

  Blood pressure, 75/50 mm Hg supine, 72/55 mm Hg standing

  Heart rate, 78 beats/min and regular

  Lungs, clear to auscultation

  Jugular venous pressure—normal with positive hepatojugular reflex

  S_1, S_2 paradoxically split. Apex 5th space anterior axillary line

  No S_3

  S_4 present

  Extremities, trace edema, clearing cellulitis on foot

Laboratory findings:

  Electrocardiogram—normal sinus rhythm, left bundle branch block

  Chest radiograph—cardiomegaly

  Creatinine, 1.2 mg/dL

  Potassium, 4.2 mEq/L

The most appropriate therapy at this point is:

a. Discontinue captopril, start lisinopril at 5 mg/day

b. Resume captopril at previous dose

c. Discontinue furosemide

d. Discontinue captopril, start hydralazine and isosorbide dinitrate, and titrate up to goal doses as tolerated

8. A 59-year-old man is admitted to the hospital with refractory heart failure. He has a history of two subendocardial myocardial infarctions and had coronary artery bypass grafting 10 years ago complicated by a postpericardiotomy syndrome. Two years ago, his ejection fraction was 40%. Recent angiography showed patent grafts. He has ascites, severe edema, and dyspnea. He has no anginal symptoms.

Medications:

  Lisinopril 20 mg/day

  Furosemide 120 mg twice daily

  Metolazone 2.5 mg/day

  Digoxin 0.25 mg/day

  Potassium 40 mEq three times daily

Physical examination findings:

  Blood pressure, 90/50 mm Hg

  Heart rate, 98 beats/min and normal rhythm and arterial character

  Lungs, no rales on auscultation

  Jugular venous pressure—angle of jaw, no v waves, no inspiratory decrease

  S_1, S_2 normal

  Loud early filling sound audible at base and apex

  Extremities, pitting edema to the level of the umbilicus

  Abdomen, hepatomegaly (nonpulsatile), ascites

Laboratory findings:

  Electrocardiogram—sinus rhythm, ST-T abnormalities

  Chest radiograph—mild cardiomegaly, with a linear dense structure visible along the anterior and apical cardiac border

  Echocardiogram—normal right ventricular size and function; left ventricle is upper normal in size, with anterior and inferior hypokinesis; no areas of scar; ejection fraction = 40%; mild mitral regurgitation; "very abnormal septal motion." The inferior vena cava and hepatic veins were dilated

  Creatinine, 1.7 mg/dL

  Potassium, 3.9 mEq/L

  Urinalysis, no proteinuria

The most appropriate action at this point is:

a. Hemodynamic monitoring, inotropic therapy, and renal dose of dopamine (2 μg/kg per minute)

b. Increase lisinopril, furosemide, and metolazone

c. Add hydralazine and isosorbide dinitrate

d. Computed tomography of the chest and surgical consultation

9. A 68-year-old man with idiopathic dilated cardiomyopathy for 7 years has appeared for his regular physical examination. He has stable New York Heart Association functional class II-III symptoms and has noted no change in his exercise tolerance and no fluid retention. His ejection fraction has been 20%. He has no palpitations, syncope, or presyncope.

Past medical history:

  Gout—last episode 1 year ago

  Acute femoral arterial occlusion, treated with

embolectomy 3 years ago

Medications:

    Lisinopril 30 mg/day

    Furosemide 60 mg/day

    Digoxin 0.25 mg/day

    Potassium 20 mEq/day

    Warfarin 5 mg/day

    Allopurinol 200 mg/day

Physical examination findings:

    Blood pressure, 105/65 mm Hg

    Heart rate, 80 beats/min and normal arterial wave-form

    Lungs, clear to auscultation

    Jugular venous pressure—normal with positive hepatojugular reflex

    Apex beat in 6th midaxillary line

    S_1, S_2 normal

    No S_3

    S_4 present

    Extremities, 1+ edema, peripheral pulses strong without bruits

Laboratory findings:

    Electrocardiogram—sinus rhythm with 5-beat run nonsustained ventricular tachycardia

    Chest radiograph—cardiomegaly with pulmonary venous hypertension

    Creatinine, 1.2 mg/dL

    Potassium, 4.3 mEq/L

    INR, 2.3

The most appropriate action at this point is:

a. Invasive electrophysiologic testing

b. Empiric amiodarone treatment at 200 mg/day

c. Continue current therapy

d. Discontinue warfarin

10. A 76-year-old woman was admitted with pulmonary edema. She has a long history of coronary artery disease and has had two Q-wave myocardial infarctions but has not been evaluated by a physician in the last 2 years. Her only medications are aspirin, diltiazem, and isosorbide dinitrate. She was treated with furosemide intravenously and had a 9-kg weight loss in 2 days. Echocardiography revealed an ejection fraction of 15%, with a dyskinetic apex. Treatment was started with digoxin, and she receives 5 mg of enalapril. Her blood pressure has decreased from 100/50 mm Hg to 70/40 mm Hg, and she is lightheaded. You are asked to advise

on additional medical therapy.

Physical examination findings:

    Blood pressure, 90/50 mm Hg supine and 80/40 mm Hg standing

    Heart rate, 110 beats/min

    Lungs, clear to auscultation

    Jugular venous pressure—flat

    S_1, S_2 normal

    No S_3 or S_4

    Extremities, no edema, mucous membranes are dry

Laboratory findings:

    Electrocardiogram—sinus rhythm, Q waves in V_1-V_5

    Chest radiograph—cardiomegaly but no pulmonary edema

    Adenosine thallium—fixed anterior, septal, and apical perfusion defects

    Creatinine, 1.3 mg/dL on admission, 2.3 mg/dL 2 days later, before enalapril dose

    Potassium, 3.7 mEq/L

The most appropriate therapy at this point is:

a. Start treatment with hydralazine and isosorbide dinitrate and titrate up as tolerated

b. Hold diuretics for a few days and rechallenge with angiotensin-converting enzyme inhibitor

c. Start treatment with losartan and carefully titrate up

d. Hemodynamic monitoring and inotropic therapy

11. Drugs proven to improve survival in patients with reduced systolic function and congestive heart failure include:

a. Angiotensin-converting enzyme (ACE) inhibitors

b. Digoxin

c. Diuretics

d. All the above

12. Intravenous inotropic support is appropriate:

a. In acute hemodynamically unstable heart failure

b. In a patient awaiting transplantation who is hemodynamically unstable while receiving maximal oral therapy

c. As palliative therapy to allow dismissal of the patient with refractory heart failure receiving oral therapy who is not a candidate for transplantation or other surgical therapy

d. All the above

Answers

1. Answer d

This patient has asymptomatic left ventricular dysfunction. The SOLVD prevention trial would suggest that morbidity is decreased by therapy with angiotensin-converting enzyme (ACE) inhibitors, and there was a trend toward decreased mortality. V-HeFT II showed that in patients with symptomatic heart failure, ACE inhibitors are superior to hydralazine/isosorbide dinitrate. Digoxin and diuretics are indicated primarily only for symptoms—this patient is asymptomatic.

2. Answer a

This patient remains symptomatic with an effective dose of an angiotensin-converting enzyme (ACE) inhibitor and a diuretic. She also remains quite hypertensive. Although digoxin or more diuretic would be indicated for persistent symptoms while a patient takes an ACE inhibitor and a diuretic, additional vasodilator therapy is most appropriate at this time because of the persistent hypertension. Other options would be amlodipine, carvedilol, or an angiotensin II receptor antagonist. Nifedipine would be contraindicated because of its negative inotropic effects. Her dose of furosemide is not maximized and if additional diuretic were needed for her hypertension or dyspnea, furosemide should be increased before metolazone.

3. Answer b

This patient should be taking warfarin because of the large anterior myocardial infarction and akinetic wall. He does not need to discontinue taking the angiotensin-converting enzyme (ACE) inhibitor, with the relatively mild increase in creatinine, which is stable with an effective dose of ACE inhibitor. Because his heart failure is well controlled and he has had a recent myocardial infarction, treatment with the β-blocker should be continued. It is unclear whether this type of patient should be treated with carvedilol instead of metoprolol.

4. Answer c

Repeated hospitalizations are common in patients with heart failure, especially the elderly. Thus, it is crucial to ensure that the medical regimen is optimized. Despite the patient being elderly, she needs much higher doses of angiotensin-converting enzyme (ACE) inhibitor and diuretic. There is no apparent contraindication (hypotension, hyperkalemia, or renal insufficiency). If up-titration

of ACE inhibitor results in renal insufficiency, treatment could be switched to hydralazine and isosorbide dinitrate. Underdosage of ACE inhibitor and failure to titrate diuretics is one of the most common errors in the management of heart failure and may be responsible for repeated hospitalizations. Because the patient has marked fluid overload, simultaneous increase in diuretics is appropriate, although caution should be used while up-titrating the ACE inhibitor. Amlodipine is not indicated unless blood pressure is still elevated after up-titration of ACE inhibitor. Although she may have coronary artery disease, the absence of angina and her gradual deterioration rather than acute or "flash" pulmonary edema make it less crucial to rule out coronary artery disease to better manage her heart failure. Other important issues in this patient would be salt restriction and compliance with medication.

5. Answer c

This patient has end-stage dilated cardiomyopathy and acute pulmonary edema. If he were at a transplant center and his hemodynamic condition deteriorated after initiation of inotropic therapy, he should be considered for a left ventricular assist device. Approximately 30% of patients listed for transplantation die while on the waiting list. There is a clear indication for inotropic therapy in this patient. With his symptomatic hypotension, additional diuretic or angiotensin-converting enzyme inhibitor alone is unlikely to be tolerated or adequate to stabilize his condition. Management of transplant patients is increasingly done by the patient's primary cardiologist and mandates close communication with the patient's transplant physician in situations such as this. Carvedilol is not indicated for class IV heart failure and likely would not be tolerated at this time without (or even with) inotropic support.

6. Answer a

Although the use of β-blockers as standard therapy for heart failure is controversial, their use is clearly indicated in this patient, because he has 3-vessel disease, evidence of hibernating myocardium, and episodes of recurrent heart failure that likely are precipitated by ischemia. Currently, he is well compensated hemodynamically, so outpatient initiation of a low dose of carvedilol and careful up-titration would be reasonable, although hospital admission for initiation of β-blocker therapy would be advised by some physicians. Nifedipine (or any dihydropyridine) without added β-blockade is not an optimal antianginal choice, especially in the presence of heart failure, and is inappropriate in this patient. Although the addition of hydralazine is appropriate for a patient with persistent symptoms who is receiving effective doses of angiotensin-converting enzyme inhibitor, β-blockade is more appropriate with the scenario here. Transmyocardial laser revascularization is investigational but may be valuable in end-stage coronary artery disease.

7. Answer b

This patient has no symptoms of hypotension and no evidence of hypoperfusion. She has a history of tolerating angiotensin-converting enzyme (ACE) inhibitors despite low blood pressure. She does not appear dehydrated. The ACE inhibitor should be restarted at her usual dose. Asymptomatic hypotension is not an indication to reduce the dose of ACE inhibitor. The combination of hydralazine and isosorbide dinitrate offers no advantage here.

8. Answer d

"Refractory" heart failure while a patient is receiving effective doses of medications should always prompt careful evaluation and consideration of other factors contributing to the patient's symptoms, especially when the degree of heart failure is out of proportion to the degree of systolic dysfunction. The presence of significant residual myocardial ischemia has been addressed in this patient, and patent grafts were demonstrated on coronary angiography. Patients with constrictive pericarditis may have mild systolic dysfunction (as may patients with restrictive cardiomyopathy). This patient has pericardial calcification and evidence on physical examination of probable constriction (pericardial "knock," ascites, elevated jugular venous pressure), likely related to his previous cardiac surgery. Although additional diuresis will be needed preoperatively, the most appropriate intervention is pericardiectomy, following the demonstration of pericardial thickening on computed tomographic scanning of the heart.

9. Answer c

Asymptomatic nonsustained ventricular tachycardia is not an indication for antiarrhythmic therapy (although this is being tested in several clinical trials). In the absence of syncope or near syncope, invasive electrophysiology testing is not indicated. The patient has a strong indication for warfarin treatment (previous cardioembolic event and very low ejection fraction). His heart failure symptoms are stable. Treatment with carvedilol could be considered in such a patient, but it is not yet considered standard therapy.

10. Answer b

Over-diuresis before initiating treatment with angiotensin-converting enzyme (ACE) inhibitors can result in excessive activation of the renin-angiotensin system and hypotension. ACE inhibitors are more effective in terms of morbidity and mortality than hydralazine and isosorbide dinitrate and easier to take (less frequent dosing). It would be appropriate to try ACE inhibitors again after withholding diuretics for a few days and gentle rehydration. In the ELITE trial, losartan had a similar side-effect profile (except for cough), and it would not be expected to be better tolerated in this scenario. The patient is not in cardiogenic shock (clear lungs, no jugular venous pressure elevation). The physical examination findings and clinical scenario strongly suggest central volume depletion and dehydration; thus, hemodynamic monitoring is not appropriate at this time.

11. Answer a

Only angiotensin-converting enzyme inhibitors have consistently been proven to improve survival. Digoxin did not improve survival in patients with mild to moderate heart failure in the digoxin trial. The effect of diuretics on survival has never been tested. All these agents improve symptoms.

12. Answer d

Intravenous inotropic support has a limited (and understudied) role in the management of heart failure. All the above scenarios represent appropriate uses of inotropic therapy.

Chapter 7

Essentials of Cellular Heart Failure

Peter A. Brady, M.D.
Andre Terzic, M.D., Ph.D.

> The cellular mechanisms of heart failure are complex and incompletely understood. In Cardiology Examinations, emphasis is increasingly being placed on understanding molecular cardiology and the cellular pathophysiology of cardiac diseases. This chapter briefly outlines the cellular mechanisms underlying myocardial failure.

Congestive heart failure results from abnormalities both intrinsic and extrinsic to the heart (Fig. 1).

Cardiomyocyte Loss

A decrease in ejection fraction and heart failure may be due to a decrease in the number of viable cardiomyocytes due to either cellular necrosis (myocardial infarction) or apoptosis.

Cellular Necrosis
Cellular necrosis occurs after coronary artery occlusion, which, if the area of myocardium served is large, may result in ventricular dysfunction. Cardiomyocyte necrosis is characterized by depletion of adenosine triphosphate (ATP), damage to intracellular organelles, intracellular Ca^{2+} overload, cell swelling, and rupture of cell membranes, leading to myocyte death.

Apoptosis
Apoptosis, or "programmed cell death," has been described recently in end-stage heart failure. Apoptosis is an energy-requiring process that involves active intracellular signaling, loss of surface contact between cells, cell shrinkage, chromosomal DNA fragmentation, and phagocytosis.

- Apoptosis, or "programmed cell death," has been described recently in end-stage heart failure.

Structural Alteration of Cardiomyocytes

Structural alterations of cardiomyocytes in heart failure can be divided broadly into cellular hypertrophy and ultrastructural changes in the cardiomyocytes.

Cellular Hypertrophy
Cellular hypertrophy occurs in response to increased demand for cardiac work. In heart failure, this occurs principally as a compensatory mechanism for loss of viable cardiac muscle and to normalize abnormal ventricular wall stress, thereby improving contractile efficiency. Cellular hypertrophy involves an increase in length and/or width of cardiomyocytes, altered gene expression, changes in contractile protein content, and induction of embryonic markers (e.g., atrial natriuretic factor). In heart failure, both hemodynamic (pressure, volume) and nonhemodynamic signals stimulate the development of cellular hypertrophy.

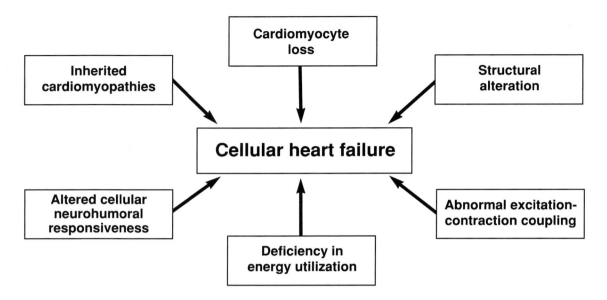

Fig. 1. Cellular mechanisms of heart failure. Many of the components of normal cardiomyocyte functioning may become abnormal in patients with heart failure. The contribution of specific cellular abnormalities to the pathogenesis of heart failure may vary from patient to patient and even in the same patient at different stages of disease.

Important mediators of the hypertrophic myocyte response include cellular stretch and release of growth factors (e.g., angiotensin II, endothelin, transforming growth factor-β, insulin-like growth factor). Hypertrophy results in more myofibrils that are available for cross-bridge cycling during contraction and an increase in the number of mitochondria that supply additional ATP to the cardiomyocyte. Hypertrophy serves as an important compensatory mechanism, but with increasing hypertrophy, energy consumption may outweigh energy production, leading to myocardial failure.

- Important mediators of the hypertrophic myocyte response include cellular stretch and release of growth factors.

Ultrastructural Changes

Ultrastructural changes associated with advanced heart failure include loss of myofibrils, proliferation of T-tubules, mitochondrial abnormalities, and increased amounts of cytoskeletal components such as tubulin (in microtubules), desmin, and vinculin (components of intermediate filaments). These abnormalities lead to heart failure by causing misalignment of contractile proteins and inefficient force transmission. Also, the extracellular matrix, an important element because it acts as the supporting structure surrounding the cell, may become abnormal with

progression of disease. The extracellular matrix maintains proper alignment of the cardiomyocytes during diastole and systole and ensures capillary patency during the cardiac cycle. An increase in fibronectin, laminin, and vimentin and increased deposition of collagen fibers I, III, IV, and VI have been found in hearts from patients with chronic heart failure. Collectively, these changes in the extracellular matrix lead to loss of myocyte attachment to the basement membrane and may result in impaired force transmission. In addition, changes in myocyte scaffolding and alignment may result in fiber slippage, fiber realignment, and thinning of the ventricular wall.

- Ultrastructural changes associated with advanced heart failure include loss of myofibrils, proliferation of T-tubules, mitochondrial abnormalities, and increased amounts of cytoskeletal components.

Abnormal Excitation-Contraction Coupling

Abnormalities in excitation-contraction coupling have also been described in failing myocardium and include altered membrane excitability, changes in Ca^{2+} handling, and myofilament abnormalities.

Altered Membrane Excitability

Altered membrane excitability is manifested as a prolongation of the duration of the action potential in ventricular cardiomyocytes (biopsy specimens) from patients with end-stage heart disease. This prolongation is believed to be due to abnormalities in K^+ channels responsible for the transient outward K^+ current (I_{To}) involved in early repolarization. Also, a partial depolarization of the cellular membrane in failing hearts is believed to be due to abnormalities in K^+ channels (I_{K1}) responsible for maintenance of the resting membrane potential. Because of the prolongation of the duration of the action potential in heart failure, the period during which Ca^{2+} influx can occur increases and could lead to intracellular Ca^{2+} loading, which may further impair cellular functioning.

Abnormalities in Ca²⁺ Handling

Abnormalities in Ca^{2+} handling may underlie systolic and diastolic dysfunction in heart failure. In comparison with normal cells, cardiomyopathic cells have higher diastolic levels of intracellular Ca^{2+} and exhibit slower decay in intracellular Ca^{2+} levels following systole. Such abnormalities may arise through decreased Ca^{2+} uptake in the sarcoplasmic reticulum or deficient Ca^{2+} storage in the failing heart. This may be associated with a decrease in the messenger RNA encoding for the Ca^{2+}-ATPase pump in the membrane of the sarcoplasmic reticulum and responsible for Ca^{2+} reuptake during diastole.

- Abnormalities in Ca^{2+} handling may underlie systolic and diastolic dysfunction in heart failure.

Myofilament Abnormalities

Myofilament abnormalities in patients with heart failure are manifested as a decrease in the number of myofibrils, changes in thin filament composition, and a decrease in total myosin content and myofibrillar Mg-ATPase activity. Changes include isoform switching of the contractile proteins, especially increased expression of the β-myosin heavy chain and actin, which correlates with alterations in cross-bridge cycling in the failing myocardium.

Deficit in Energy Utilization

No significant decreases in the steady-state levels of intracellular ATP have been found in heart failure, although the failing heart behaves in an energy-deficient manner. This suggests that a more subtle mechanism of bioenergetic deficit may be responsible for contractile dysfunction in heart failure. Markers of the cellular energetic state, such as the phosphocreatine-to-ATP ratio, have been identified as predictors of mortality in patients with dilated cardiomyopathy. Currently, it is believed that the failing myocardium has a decreased capacity to withstand metabolic stress, that is, failing myocardium has decreased myocardial bioenergetic reserve.

- Myofilament abnormalities in patients with heart failure are manifested as a decrease in the number of myofibrils, changes in thin filament composition, and a decrease in total myosin content and myofibrillar Mg-ATPase activity.
- No significant decreases in the steady-state levels of intracellular ATP have been found in heart failure, although the failing heart behaves in an energy-deficient manner.

Altered Cellular Neurohumoral Responsiveness

The best recognized alteration in cellular signaling during heart failure is the down-regulation of the β-adrenoceptor/adenylate cyclase signaling pathway. It is believed that such changes may contribute to decreased inotropic responsiveness to endogenous catecholamines. Recent research has indicated a potential role for gene therapy in the treatment of heart failure through overexpression of cardiac-specific β₂-adrenergic receptors, resulting in increased basal myocardial adenylate cyclase activity and enhanced contractility.

- The best recognized alteration in cellular signaling during heart failure is the down-regulation of the β-adrenoceptor/adenylate cyclase signaling pathway.

Inherited Forms of Cardiomyopathy

An increasing number of inheritable cardiomyopathies are being identified, including familial forms of hypertrophic and dilated cardiomyopathies.

Four major disease loci have been identified in familial hypertrophic cardiomyopathy. *CMH1* on chromosome 14 has been associated with mutations in the β-myosin heavy chain, a contractile protein of the thick filament of the sarcomere. *CMH2* on chromosome 1 has been associated with mutations in cardiac troponin T, a regulatory protein of the thin filament of the sarcomere. *CMH3* on chromosome 15 has been associated with mutations of α-tropomyosin, a contractile protein of the thin filament of the sarcomere. *CMH4* on chromosome 11 has been associated with mutations in cardiac myosin-binding protein C, a structural and regulatory protein of the sarcomere. Additional loci for familial hypertrophic cardiomyopathy have been discovered recently, including a locus for familial hypertrophic cardiomyopathy associated with Wolff-Parkinson-White syndrome mapped to chromosome 7. In addition to locus heterogeneity, a marked allelic heterogeneity also exists among the various forms of familial hypertrophic cardiomyopathy.

Genetic heterogeneity also exists among familial dilated cardiomyopathy. Missense mutations in the cardiac actin gene that cosegregate with hereditary idiopathic dilated cardiomyopathy have been identified recently in two unrelated families. Both mutations affect amino acids in domains of actin that attach to Z bands and intercalated disks, suggesting that defective force transmission in cardiac myocytes may be responsible for heart failure in these subsets of patients. In other affected families, disease genes have not been identified, but chromosomal locations of disease loci have been demonstrated and include the long and short arms of chromosome 1 and loci on chromosomes 3 and 9. In families with dilated cardiomyopathy, arrhythmia, and conduction defects, a candidate gene may be related to connexin 40, although this has not been confirmed. Additional candidate genes associated with dilated cardiomyopathy include the gene for tropomodulin and genes involved in the regulation of muscle growth.

- Four major disease loci have been identified in familial hypertrophic cardiomyopathy.
- Missense mutations in the cardiac actin gene that cosegregate with hereditary idiopathic dilated cardiomyopathy have been identified.

> To date, treatments for heart failure have been limited largely to alleviation of symptoms. With increased understanding of the cellular mechanisms of heart failure, future treatments will likely be aimed at molecular defects responsible for the pathogenesis of the disease.

Suggested Review Reading

1. Davies CH, Harding SE, Poole-Wilson PA: Cellular mechanisms of contractile dysfunction in human heart failure. *Eur Heart J* 17:189-198, 1996.

2. Niimura H, Bachinski LL, Sangwatanaroj S, et al: Mutations in the gene for cardiac myosin-binding protein C and late-onset familial hypertrophic cardiomyopathy. *N Engl J Med* 338:1248-1257, 1998.

3. Olivetti G, Abbi R, Quaini F, et al: Apoptosis in the failing human heart. *N Engl J Med* 336:1131-1141, 1997.

4. Olson TM, Michels VV, Thibodeau SN, et al: Actin mutations in dilated cardiomyopathy, a heritable form of heart failure. *Science* 280:750-752, 1998.

5. Schwartz K, Mercadier JJ: Molecular and cellular biology of heart failure. *Curr Opin Cardiol* 11:227-236, 1996.

6. Taylor DA, Atkins BZ, Hungspreugs P, et al: Regenerating functional myocardium: improved performance after skeletal myoblast transplantation. *Nat Med* 4:929-933, 1998.

Questions

Multiple Choice (choose the one best answer)

1. Cross-bridge cycling in the cardiac muscle refers to:
   a. Ca^{2+}-induced Ca^{2+} release that triggers systole
   b. Reuptake of Ca^{2+} by the sarcoplasmic reticulum that occurs in diastole
   c. Intercellular communication of two cardiomyocytes through connexin-40 junctions
   d. Interaction between actin and myosin and the sliding of these filaments across each other, leading to contraction

2. Phosphocreatine-to-ATP ratio:
   a. Does not predict mortality in patients with cardiomyopathy
   b. Is a predictor of mortality in patients with dilated cardiomyopathy
   c. Is not a marker of myocardial energy reserve
   d. Has not been tested in patients with cardiomyopathy

3. True statements about apoptosis include all the following *except*:
   a. It is also referred to as "programmed cell death"
   b. It has been described in humans with end-stage heart failure
   c. It is not an energy-requiring process
   d. It involves chromosomal DNA fragmentation

4. All the following statements are true for cardiomyocyte hypertrophy *except*:
   a. Is induced by cellular stretch
   b. Is induced by release of growth factors (e.g., angiotensin II, endothelin, transforming growth factor-β, and insulin-like growth factor)
   c. Occurs late in heart failure
   d. Is associated with altered genetic expression (e.g., induction of embryonic markers)

5. Beneficial effects on failing cardiomyocytes have been reported with the use of which of the following?
   a. Angiotensin-converting enzyme inhibitors
   b. Antagonists of the angiotensin II receptor
   c. Endothelin-1A receptor antagonists
   d. All the above
   e. None of the above

Answers

1. Answer d

Release and reuptake of Ca^{2+} by the sarcoplasmic reticulum are essential steps in the excitation-contraction-relaxation cycle. Although Ca^{2+} cycling governs the interaction between contractile proteins, cross-bridge cycling is defined specifically as the interaction between actin and myosin filaments. Connexin-40 are gap junction proteins.

2. Answer b

Phosphocreatine-to-ATP ratio has been used as a marker of the myocardial energetic status and recently has been shown to predict mortality in patients with dilated cardiomyopathy (*Circulation* 96:2190-2196, 1997).

3. Answer c

In contrast to necrosis, apoptosis, or "programmed cell death," is an energy-requiring process involving active intracellular signaling, loss of surface contact between cells, cell shrinkage, chromosomal DNA fragmentation, and, finally, extracellular degeneration and phagocytosis. It has been described recently in myocytes in end-stage heart failure (*N Engl J Med* 335:1182-1189, 1996, and 336:1131-1141, 1997).

4. Answer c

Cardiomyocyte hypertrophy occurs early in the progression of heart failure.

5. Answer d

Inhibitors of the angiotensin-converting enzyme or direct antagonists of the angiotensin II receptor may cause regression of cardiac hypertrophy, regardless of their effect on blood pressure. Another potent stimulus for myocardial cell growth and hypertrophy is endothelin. During development of ventricular hypertrophy, prepro endothelin-1 messenger RNA is increased, and overall production of endothelin-1 is markedly elevated in the failing myocardium. Therefore, endothelin-1A receptor antagonists, which abolish expression of genetic markers associated with cardiac hypertrophy, are being evaluated for their potential in improving long-term survival.

Chapter 8

The Endothelium

Amir Lerman, M.D.

The endothelium is more than a semipermeable barrier between the blood and the vascular smooth muscle. Indeed, the endothelial system must be regarded as a highly active endocrine organ. It contributes to local vascular regulation by releasing vasodilating substances (such as endothelium-derived relaxing factor) that have antiproliferative properties and vasoconstricting substances (such as endothelin) that have mitogenic properties. A critical balance between EDRF and endothelin may be the major determinant that regulates systemic and regional hemodynamic functions and cellular proliferation.

Pathogenesis of Atherosclerosis

Vascular endothelial injury is the critical first step in the pathogenesis of atherosclerosis. This leads to lipid accumulation and the adhesion of monocytes and platelets to the site of injury. These cells in concert with the endothelium release growth factors that cause migration and proliferation of smooth muscle cells. Oxidative stress and free radical production also have a role in the pathogenesis of atherosclerosis. Coronary artery disease risk factors such as hypercholesterolemia and hypertension may lead to the creation of free oxygen radicals that may mediate the vascular injury inflammatory response. Fuster proposed a classification that relates the extent of vascular injury with the progression of atherosclerosis and the acute coronary artery syndromes of myocardial infarction, unstable angina, and sudden cardiac death (Plate 1).

Type I vascular injury consists of a functional alteration of the vascular endothelium in the absence of morphologic change (Plate 2). This occurs with chronic injury to the endothelium from disturbances in blood flow, hypertension, hypercholesterolemia, cigarette smoking, and, in some persons, an increased level of homocysteine (Fig. 1). Although the macroscopic features characteristic of atherosclerosis are not present at this stage, evidence suggests that endothelial dysfunction is the earliest detectable event in the pathogenesis of atherosclerosis. Accumulation of lipids and monocytes/macrophages results from type I injury.

The release of various chemotactic factors by macrophages leads to the accumulation of platelets at the site of injury, with ensuing endothelial denudation and damage to the intima, which characterizes type II vascular injury (Plate 3). Inflammatory cells and platelets together with the endothelium stimulate the migration and proliferation of smooth muscle cells and may form either a fibrointimal lesion or an outer cap of a predominantly lipid-rich atherosclerotic lesion. A lipid-rich plaque surrounded by a thin cap can easily be disrupted to expose the underlying extremely thrombogenic matrix (Plates 4 and 5). This leads to type III vascular injury, which is manifested by endothelial denudation, with damage to both the intima and the media. During the evolution of atherosclerosis, growth factors, cytokines, and other molecules such as lipids and nitric oxide (NO) are involved in cell recruitment, migration, and

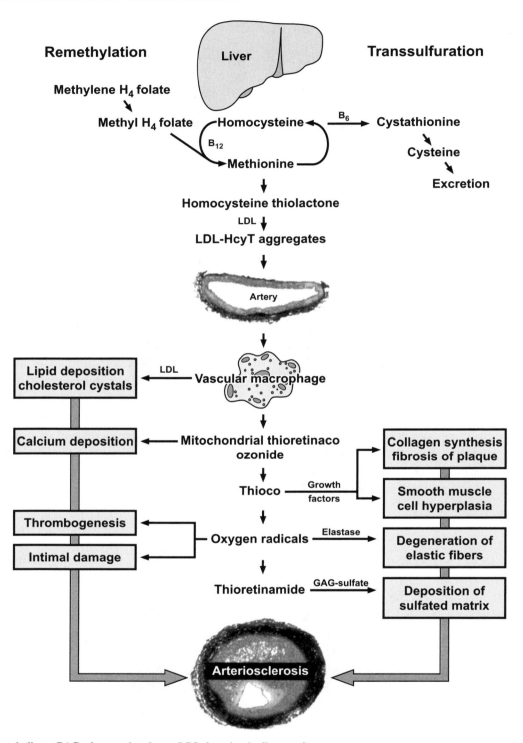

Fig. 1. Homocysteine metabolism. GAG, glycosaminoglycan; LDL, low-density lipoprotein.

proliferation as well as in lipid and protein synthesis (Plate 6). These molecules are also involved in vasomotor regulation, vascular remodeling, and the coagulation cascade.

• Type I vascular injury consists of a functional alteration

of the vascular endothelium in the absence of morphologic change.

• Endothelial denudation and damage to the intima characterize type II vascular injury.

• Type III vascular injury is manifested by endothelial

denudation, with damage to both the media and the intima.

- Endothelial dysfunction is the earliest detectable phase in the spectrum of atherosclerosis.

The pathogenesis of atherosclerosis can be regarded as a humoral-cellular activation that leads to an imbalance between vasoconstrictive factors with mitogenic properties and vasodilating factors with antimitogenic properties.

Many studies have documented that most acute coronary artery syndromes occur when the underlying coronary artery stenosis is not flow-limiting. Thus, the pathophysiology of acute myocardial ischemia is not necessarily dependent on the degree of coronary stenosis but rather on the characteristics of the underlying coronary atherosclerotic plaque. Moreover, evidence suggests that plaque rupture initiates the event of acute myocardial ischemic syndrome and is dependent on the tissue characterization of the plaque. A soft atherosclerotic plaque that is cellular and contains a lipid core has a greater tendency to rupture than fibrotic and calcified plaques. These observations have led to the hypothesis that to prevent the plaque from rupturing and to stabilize the plaque, an effort should be made to transfer the characteristics of the soft plaque to a more fibrotic plaque.

- Most acute coronary artery syndromes occur when the underlying coronary artery stenosis is not flow-limiting.
- The risk of plaque disruption/thrombosis depends more on plaque composition and vulnerability than on plaque size and stenosis severity seen angiographically.
- A soft atherosclerotic plaque has a greater tendency to rupture than fibrotic and calcified plaques do.

Role of Endothelium in Regulation of Vascular Tone

The first major insight into the importance of the endothelium as a modulator of vascular tone was the discovery that vascular rings of rabbit aorta contracted in response to norepinephrine and relaxed in response to acetylcholine. However, in the absence of a functional endothelium, no relaxation was observed in response to acetylcholine. This suggested the existence of a diffusible vasoactive substance, named "endothelium-derived relaxing factor" (EDRF).

To date, studies have supported the existence of EDRFs that are short-lived, diffuse into the vascular smooth muscle, and activate soluble guanylate cyclase, which mediates vasorelaxation (Fig. 2). EDRF is either NO or a closely related nitrosylated compound. An enzyme responsible for

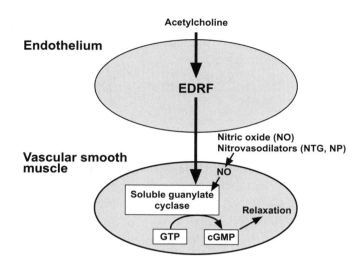

Fig. 2. Mechanism of action of acetylcholine on normal endothelium. cGMP, cyclic guanosine monophosphate; EDRF, endothelium-derived relaxing factor; GTP, guanosine triphosphate; NP, nitroprusside; NTG, nitroglycerin.

NO production by oxidation of the guanidino nitrogen of arginine, termed "nitric oxide synthase," has been identified in several mammalian tissues.

Our understanding of the role of EDRF/NO in the regulation of vascular tone has been advanced by the ability of the agent N^G-monomethyl-L-arginine (L-NMMA) to inhibit EDRF/NO production from L-arginine. Inhibition of EDRF/NO production by exogenous administration of L-NMMA results in a significant increase in systemic vascular resistance.

This observation was recently extended to the human coronary circulation, in which inhibition of EDRF/NO with increasing doses of L-NMMA induced an increase in basal epicardial coronary vascular resistance and attenuated flow-induced epicardial dilatation, supporting the view that EDRF/NO has a significant role in modulating basal vasomotion and endothelium-dependent dilatation. Moreover, the decrease in endogenous NO production in humans with endothelial dysfunction and cardiovascular disease risk factors results in attenuation of the decrease in coronary vascular resistance seen with exercise.

EDRF/NO is also a potent inhibitor of platelet adhesion and aggregation and has been shown in vitro to inhibit vascular smooth muscle and mesangial cell proliferation induced by serum- or platelet-derived growth factors (Plate 7). These studies support a significant role for EDRF/NO in the regulation of basal systemic and regional vascular tone and the control of vascular cell growth.

- EDRF is either NO or a related nitrosylated compound.
- NO activity is decreased in humans with coronary artery disease risk factors.

Endothelin

The endothelin family of peptides consists of three distinct 21-amino-acid chain peptides named "endothelin-1," "endothelin-2," and "endothelin-3." After binding to specific receptors, endothelin activates phospholipase and diacylglycerol, promoting the release of calcium ions (Ca^{2+}) from intracellular stores and the influx of Ca^{2+} through voltage-dependent Ca^{2+} channels.

Endothelin, the most potent vasoconstrictor known, produces contraction in isolated arteries and veins. The exogenous administration of pathophysiologic concentrations of endothelin in vivo results in increases in systemic, coronary, pulmonary, and renal vascular resistance. In addition to its vasoconstrictor properties, endothelin has mitogenic properties in vitro. It stimulates DNA synthesis in cultured vascular smooth muscle cells in a dose-dependent manner, which suggests that endothelin has a role as a growth factor. Increasing evidence indicates that in addition to its local vascular effect, endothelin is normally present in the plasma of humans and animals. The importance of its presence in the circulation is underscored by the finding of increased plasma concentrations of endothelin in cardiovascular, pulmonary, and renal disorders such as atherosclerosis, myocardial infarction, heart failure, and pulmonary hypertension. Moreover, plasma endothelin concentrations were found to be a prognostic marker after myocardial infarction.

An interaction between EDRF and endothelin is of potential importance in the pathophysiology of cardiovascular diseases. Several agonists such as thrombin stimulate the simultaneous release of EDRF and endothelin. Note that the thrombin-stimulated release of endothelin is inhibited by the inactivation of thrombin with hirudin, a specific thrombin inhibitor. Furthermore, the inhibition of EDRF synthesis in vitro in the presence of thrombin potentiates the release of endothelin, suggesting that EDRF in the presence of thrombin is an inhibitory stimulus for the synthesis or release (or both) of endothelin. These observations suggest that activation of the coagulation cascade under conditions of impaired EDRF formation such as atherosclerosis may induce the release of endothelin and contribute

to vasoconstriction. In human arteries, endothelin-induced vasoconstriction is inhibited by EDRF as well as by NO. Moreover, endothelin may release EDRF through activation of specific receptors on the endothelium.

- Endothelin, the most potent vasoconstrictor known, produces contraction in isolated arteries and veins.
- Plasma endothelin concentrations were found to be a prognostic marker after myocardial infarction.

In summary, significant evidence supports the hypothesis that the endogenous EDRF system serves as a functionally important modulator of the vasoconstrictor actions of endothelin. As demonstrated in vivo, the vasoconstrictor actions of endothelin are augmented by the inhibition of EDRF synthesis with L-NMMA. Thus, the delicate balance between endothelium-mediated vasodilatation and vasoconstriction is disrupted in disease states in which the endothelium is injured. This leads to the attenuated release of EDRF and the augmented release of endothelin, with subsequent vasoconstriction, thrombosis, and smooth muscle contraction.

- Endothelin releases intracellular Ca^{2+} to cause vasoconstriction in vascular smooth muscle cells.

Endothelial Dysfunction in Atherosclerotic Vascular Disease

A role for endothelial dysfunction in the pathophysiology of atherosclerosis continues to emerge. Increasingly, evidence suggests that hypercholesterolemia and atherosclerosis impair endothelium-dependent vasodilatation in humans, and several studies have demonstrated that the presence of early atherosclerosis and coronary risk factors is characterized by endothelial dysfunction in coronary epicardial and resistance vessels (Plate 8). Recent studies with sestamibi imaging have demonstrated that coronary endothelial dysfunction may result in myocardial perfusion defects indicating myocardial ischemia. Progressive impairment in endothelium-mediated modulation of coronary vasomotor tone in different stages of early atherosclerosis has been demonstrated (Plate 1).

Several researchers have suggested that the loss of endothelium-dependent vasodilatory response to acetylcholine, an endothelium-dependent vasorelaxing substance, may be an early marker of atherosclerosis in the absence of angiographically demonstrable lesions. An unexpected finding has been that coronary artery disease risk factors such as hypercholesterolemia, hypertension, and age older than 50 years can produce this "endothelial dysfunction" in microvessels, where overt atherosclerosis does not develop. Moreover, endothelium-dependent dilatation of the coronary arteries may be defective in patients with anginal-type chest pain and angiographically normal coronary arteries. As demonstrated recently, the impaired endothelium-dependent relaxation in atherosclerosis may be due to decreased activity of the enzyme responsible for the production of NO from arginine or to arginine deficiency, loss of incorporation of NO into a more potent compound, accelerated degradation of EDRF, or enhanced release of vasoconstrictors from the damaged endothelium. Indeed, this clinical situation is characterized by increased endothelin and decreased cyclic guanosine monophosphate (cGMP), the second messenger of EDRF, in coronary endothelial cells.

Recent investigations have focused on pharmacologic interventions to reverse and normalize endothelial dysfunction. These studies have demonstrated that lowering cholesterol levels, antioxidant therapy, angiotensin-converting enzyme inhibitors, and L-arginine (the precursor of NO) may improve peripheral and coronary endothelial function and may have a therapeutic role in the treatment of early atherosclerosis.

Consistent with this theory are the results of studies that investigated plasma and tissue endothelin in humans with symptomatic atherosclerotic disease that required arterial revascularization. The plasma concentrations of endothelin were increased in humans with advanced atherosclerosis and correlated with the extent of disease. Recent studies have demonstrated that early coronary atherosclerosis in humans is characterized by increased endothelin and decreased cGMP in coronary endothelial cells and is associated with coronary endothelial function.

Thus, it appears that in both early and advanced atherosclerosis, in which the endothelium is dysfunctional or injured, there is a state in which the balance between EDRF and endothelin is disrupted, leading to unopposed vasoconstriction and smooth muscle cell proliferation.

- The loss of endothelium-dependent vasodilatory response to acetylcholine, an endothelium-dependent vasorelaxing substance, may be an early marker of atherosclerosis.
- Coronary artery disease risk factors can produce "endothelial dysfunction" in microvessels, where overt atherosclerosis does not develop.

- Lowering cholesterol levels, antioxidant therapy, angiotensin-converting enzyme inhibitors, and L-arginine (the precursor of NO) may improve coronary endothelial function.

Endothelial Dysfunction in Acute Coronary Ischemic Syndromes

Flow-mediated arterial vasodilatation is important in the regulation of blood flow in an organ in response to physiologic demands. Normal arteries exhibit endothelium-dependent dilatation, whereas removal of the endothelium abolishes flow and acetylcholine-mediated dilatation. These physiologic responses are also lost in humans with advanced coronary artery disease and, in some patients, may be lost early in the course of atherosclerosis, preceding the appearance of stenosing and occlusive disease.

These concepts have been extended to ischemic syndromes because coronary artery dilatation during postocclusive hyperemia is an endothelium-dependent phenomenon involving EDRF/NO release. Hypoxia or anoxia inhibits the release of EDRF/NO, and ischemia and reperfusion induce impairment in endothelium-dependent relaxation to most EDRF/NO agonists. Studies also support that ischemic or reperfusion injury (or both) of the endothelium may be mediated by oxygen-derived free radicals that inactivate EDRF.

Although studies have emphasized alterations in EDRF/NO in ischemic syndromes, a role for endothelin has also been suggested. Ischemic syndromes are characterized by hypoxia and decreased blood flow and shear stress, which may induce endothelin gene expression and secretion. Increased circulating plasma concentrations of endothelin have also been observed in vivo in studies of arterial injury, with thrombus formation and coronary occlusion followed by reperfusion. The release of EDRF in the coronary artery is impaired early after global myocardial ischemia and reperfusion, and the ischemic event may also increase the production of an endothelium-derived *contracting* factor. These reports are supported by the recent demonstration of increased plasma concentrations of endothelin in the early hours of acute myocardial infarction, with a sustained increase in patients with continuing ischemia.

- Normal arteries exhibit endothelium-dependent dilatation, whereas removal of the endothelium abolishes flow and acetylcholine-mediated dilatation.
- Hypoxia or anoxia inhibits the release of EDRF/NO.

Thus, during coronary artery constriction and cardiac ischemia, endothelial damage and impaired EDRF release occur. The decreased release of EDRF may inhibit dilatation of the coronary arteries that supply the jeopardized myocardium and promote platelet adhesion and aggregation and platelet-induced constriction of the coronary arteries. Furthermore, vascular injury, decreased release of EDRF, ischemia, and decreased shear stress may all stimulate endothelin release, which, in turn, results in vasoconstriction leading to vasospasm and continuing ischemia and, thus, extension of the size of the myocardial infarct.

Coronary Artery Spasm

Although alterations in coronary vascular reactivity may be a hallmark of atherosclerotic coronary artery disease, spasm in angiographically normal coronary arteries most likely involves a local dysfunction of the vascular wall that could be related to hyperactivity of the vascular smooth muscle or to dysfunction of the endothelium. Coronary artery spasm may be provoked with various maneuvers, including immersion of the hand in ice water, and pharmacologic agents, such as ergonovine, acetylcholine, and serotonin, that produce vasospasm in patients with variant angina. Because increased levels of endothelin may be important in the vascular bed vasoconstrictor response, endothelin may be central to the pathogenesis of coronary artery spasm.

- Increased plasma concentrations of endothelin have been observed in vivo in studies of arterial injury, with thrombus formation and coronary occlusion followed by reperfusion.
- Coronary artery spasm may be provoked with various maneuvers, including immersion of the hand in ice water, and pharmacologic agents, such as ergonovine, acetylcholine, and serotonin.

Coronary Flow Reserve

Endothelium-Dependent Mechanisms of Coronary Vasodilatation

The normal physiologic response to increased myocardial demand, such as exercise or mental stress, is coronary vasodilatation to increase coronary blood flow. This process of coronary flow reserve to enhance myocardial flow is endothelium-dependent and mediated through the release of EDRF/NO. The functional integrity of the endothelium may be assessed by the administration of the endothelium-dependent vasodilator acetylcholine (Fig. 2). Acetylcholine causes the release of EDRF/NO from endothelial cells and the resultant vasodilatation by stimulation of muscarinic receptors on the cell membrane (Fig. 3). Stimulation of acetylcholine receptors produces a uniform endothelium-dependent dilatation of coronary vessels of all sizes. Several studies have demonstrated a correlation between the coronary vascular response to exercise and the response to intracoronary administration of acetylcholine.

Therefore, coronary endothelium-dependent vascular reactivity (epicardial and microvascular circulation) can be assessed by the intracoronary administration of acetylcholine in combination with coronary angiography and Doppler velocity analysis of coronary blood flow.

Normal coronary endothelial function is characterized by coronary vasodilatation and a three- to fourfold increase in coronary blood flow in response to acetylcholine. In the early stages of coronary atherosclerosis, endothelial dysfunction of the coronary microcirculation can be demonstrated. Although the results of coronary angiography are normal, the intracoronary administration of acetylcholine produces a significant attenuation of the increase in coronary blood flow or no change in coronary blood flow without epicardial vasoconstriction. At a later stage of the disease, coronary angiography may demonstrate mild atherosclerotic disease. The administration of acetylcholine at this stage shows microcirculatory as well as epicardial coronary vasoconstriction and a decrease in coronary blood flow. It may be that in the development of coronary artery disease, different stages of coronary endothelial dysfunction can be demonstrated.

- Normal coronary endothelial function is characterized by coronary vasodilatation and a three- to fourfold increase in coronary blood flow in response to acetylcholine.

Non-Endothelium-Dependent Mechanisms of Coronary Vasodilatation

Adenosine is formed in vivo by the action of nucleotidase enzymes on adenosine monophosphate (AMP). There are two subtypes of adenosine receptors: A_1 receptors on endothelial cells and A_2 receptors on coronary vascular smooth muscle cells. Adenosine is thought to act on the coronary vasculature via stimulation of A_2 receptors, which activates adenylate cyclase to produce cyclic adenosine monophosphate (cAMP) and smooth muscle relaxation. First, at pharmacologic doses (as given in a cardiac catheterization laboratory), adenosine can cross the endothelial barrier and directly stimulate the receptors on the smooth muscle

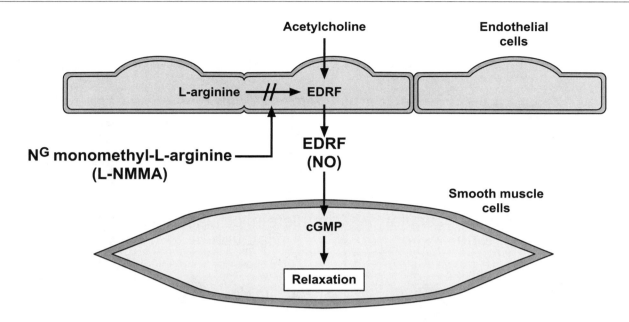

Fig. 3. Pathway of endothelial-derived relaxing factor (EDRF) synthesis and action. cGMP, cyclic guanosine monophosphate; NO, nitric oxide.

in an endothelium-independent mechanism. Second, adenosine acts predominantly on vessels smaller than 150 µm in diameter and, thus, mainly assesses changes in the coronary resistance vessels as reflected by changes in coronary blood flow. The administration of adenosine provides an endothelium-independent evaluation of the coronary microvasculature and may reveal abnormal coronary flow reserve in the presence of normal endothelial function. Furthermore, the measurement of coronary flow reserve in response to adenosine may provide important information about the functional significance of coronary artery disease and the need for revascularization procedures and their success.

● The two subtypes of adenosine receptors are A_1 receptors on endothelial cells and A_2 receptors on coronary vascular smooth muscle cells.

Nonendothelium-dependent vascular responses can be assessed in epicardial arteries with the administration of nitroglycerin. Nitroglycerin is a vasodilator that acts directly on vascular smooth muscle through a cGMP mechanism. Because the coronary microvessels lack the enzyme needed to convert nitroglycerin to its active form NO, nitroglycerin produces a dose-related dilatation of coronary vessels larger than 200 µm in diameter and has no effect on smaller coronary vessels.

Actual coronary blood flow can be measured by several methods, including coronary sinus thermodilution, gas clearance, contrast densitometric techniques, and intracoronary Doppler analysis. The availability of the intracoronary Doppler guidewire has facilitated the simple measurement of coronary blood flow in the cardiac catheterization laboratory, and the correlation between this measurement and those of more rigorous methods is good.

Coronary blood flow and flow reserve can be measured in response to arteriolar vasodilators to provide an assessment of the coronary microvasculature. The measurement of coronary flow can also provide important information about the physiologic significance of epicardial coronary artery disease.

The normal epicardial coronary arteries visible on coronary angiography provide minor resistance to coronary blood flow.

As stenosis develops in a coronary artery, blood pressure decreases across the lesion (Fig. 4). The microcirculation dilates to compensate for the decreased perfusion pressure, thus maintaining normal resting blood flow. During periods of increased myocardial demand, the capacity of the microcirculation to dilate further is limited, resulting in myocardial ischemia (Fig. 4). Thus, the physiologic severity of coronary stenosis may be assessed by determining the decrease in coronary flow reserve in response to hyperemia or by directly measuring the pressure gradient across the stenosis.

● The physiologic severity of coronary stenosis may be assessed by determining the decrease in coronary flow reserve in response to hyperemia.

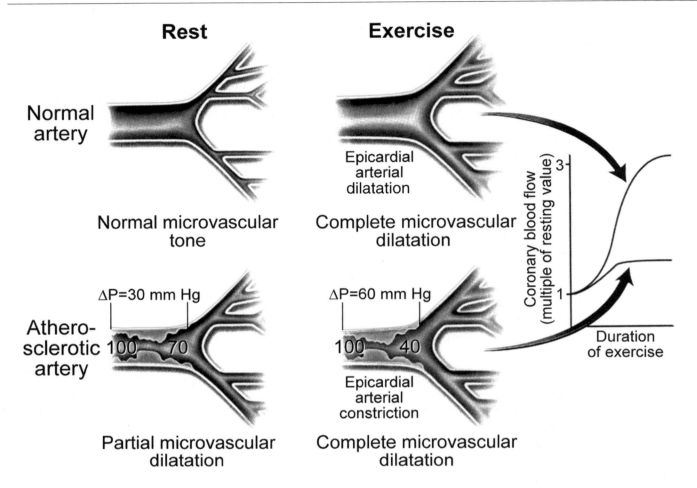

Fig. 4. Effect of epicardial stenoses and microvascular tone on coronary blood flow. (From *N Engl J Med* 334:1735-1737, 1996. By permission of the Massachusetts Medical Society.)

Questions

Multiple Choice (choose the one best answer)

1. The risk of plaque disruption depends primarily on all the following factors *except*:
   a. Severity of angiographic stenosis
   b. Plaque morphology
   c. Lipid content of the plaque
   d. Endothelial function

2. Plasma endothelin concentrations are increased in the following states:
   a. Heart failure
   b. Atherosclerosis
   c. Pulmonary hypertension
   d. All the above

3. Which of the following substances is *not* an endothelium-dependent dilator?
   a. Acetylcholine
   b. Substance P
   c. Bradykinin
   d. Nitroglycerin

4. Nitric oxide (endothelium-derived relaxing factor) mediates its vasorelaxation effect through:
   a. Specific receptors on the endothelium
   b. Specific receptors on smooth muscle cells
   c. Direct effect on smooth muscle cells
   d. Decrease in intracellular calcium

5. Endothelin exerts its vasoconstriction through:
   a. Activation of cGMP
   b. Direct effect on smooth muscle cells
   c. Injuring the endothelium
   d. Specific endothelin receptors

6. Endothelial dysfunction is characterized by:
   a. Vasoconstriction to endothelial-dependent vasodilator substances
   b. May occur without significant coronary artery disease
   c. May be causally linked to smoking
   d. All the above

7. Endothelial dysfunction may be reversed by
   a. Lowering cholesterol
   b. Stent implantation
   c. Thrombolytic therapy
   d. Nitroglycerin

Answers

1. Answer a
2. Answer d
3. Answer d
4. Answer c
5. Answer d
6. Answer d
7. Answer a

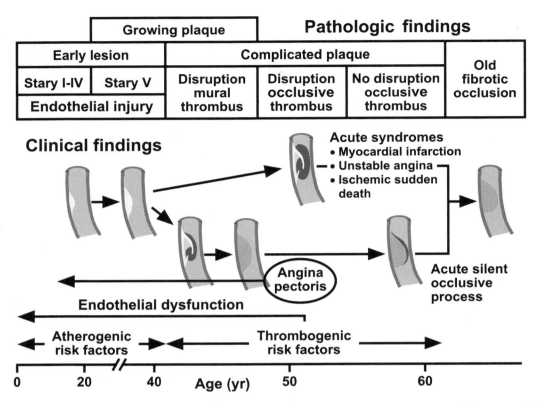

Pathologic findings					
	Growing plaque				
Early lesion		Complicated plaque			Old fibrotic occlusion
Stary I-IV	Stary V	Disruption mural thrombus	Disruption occlusive thrombus	No disruption occlusive thrombus	
Endothelial injury					

Plate 1. Evolution of atherosclerotic coronary artery disease. (From *N Engl J Med* 326:242-250; 310-318, 1992. By permission of the Massachusetts Medical Society.)

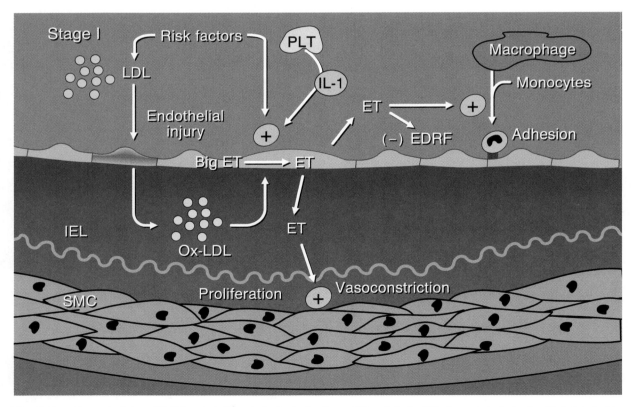

Plate 2. Stage I vascular injury. EDRF, endothelium-derived relaxing factor; ET, endothelin; IEL, internal elastic lamina; IL-1, interleukin 1; LDL, low-density lipoprotein particles; Ox-LDL, oxidized LDL particles; PLT, platelet; SMC, smooth muscle cell.

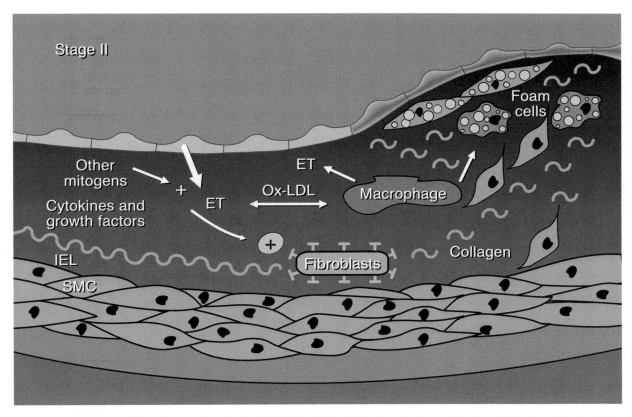

Plate 3. Stage II vascular injury. Interaction of endothelin (ET) and the atherosclerotic plaque. IEL, internal elastic lamina; Ox-LDL, oxidized low-density lipoprotein; SMC, smooth muscle cell. "+" indicates stimulation.

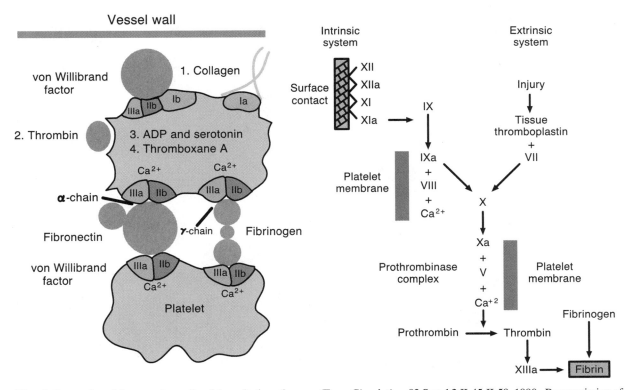

Plate 4. Interaction of the vascular wall and thrombotic pathways. (From *Circulation* 82 Suppl 2:II-45-II-59, 1990. By permission of the American Heart Association.)

Thrombosis

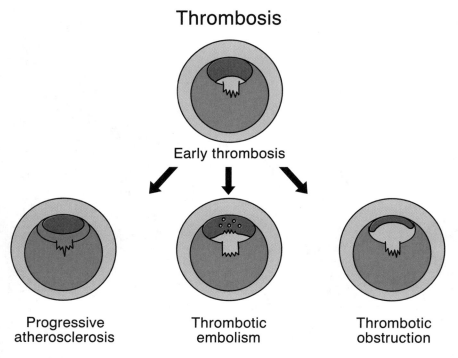

Plate 5. Sequelae of coronary artery thrombosis.

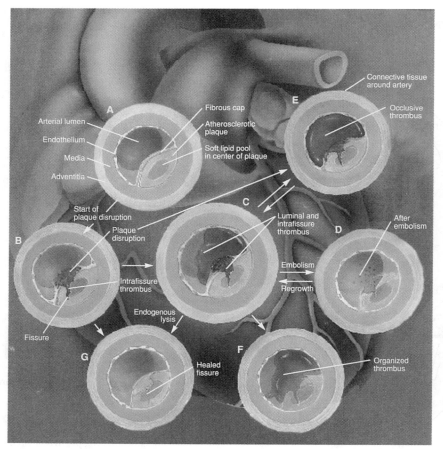

Plate 6. *A-G*, Progression of atherosclerosis.

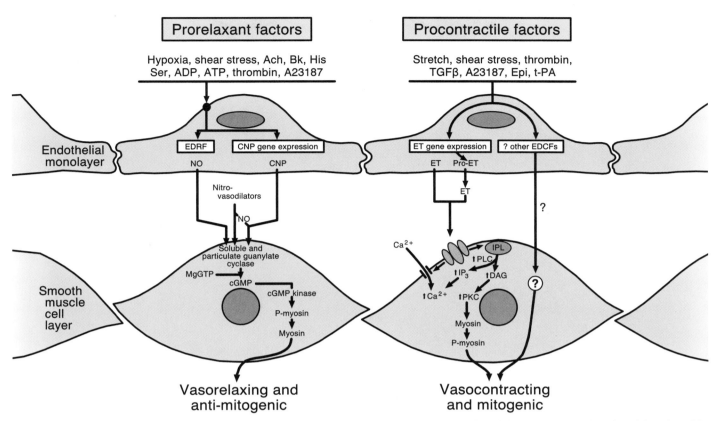

Plate 7. Prorelaxant and procontractile factors in the vascular wall. Ach, acetylcholine; ADP, adenosine diphosphate; ATP, adenosine triphosphate; Bk, bradykinin; C, cyclic; CNP, C-natriuretic peptide; DAG, diacylglycerol; EDRF, endothelium-derived relaxing factor; Epi, epinephrine; ET, endothelin; GMP, guanosine monophosphate; GTP, guanosine triphosphate; His, histamine; IP$_3$, inositol triphosphate; IPL, inositol phospholipids; PKC, protein kinase C; Ser, serotonin; TGFβ , transforming growth factor-beta; t-PA, tissue plasminogen activator.

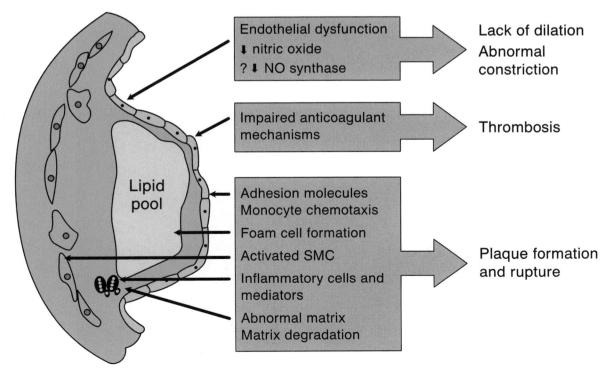

Plate 8. Consequences of endothelial dysfunction. NO, nitric oxide; SMC, smooth muscle cell.

Notes

Chapter 9

Pathogenesis of Atherosclerosis

Robert S. Schwartz, M.D.
Iftikhar J. Kullo, M.D.
William D. Edwards, M.D.

Prevalence of Coronary Artery Disease

Atherosclerotic disease of the cerebral, coronary, and peripheral arterial vasculature is the leading cause of morbidity, mortality, and health care expenditure in the U.S. and Western Europe (Table 1).

- More than 20 million North Americans have clinically significant coronary artery disease.
- Annually, nearly 300,000 North Americans die suddenly of undiagnosed coronary artery disease.
- There are 800,000 new myocardial infarctions annually in the United States.
- More than half a million patients are hospitalized in the United States annually with unstable angina.
- Currently, a typical North American has at least a 20% likelihood that clinical coronary artery disease will develop before age 60.
- Each year, 350,000 patients develop class III heart failure, principally as a consequence of coronary atherosclerosis.
- The cost of treating heart disease in the U.S. exceeds 50 billion dollars annually.

Arterial Wall Structure

Arteries are classified as either elastic (large vessels such as the aorta and carotid and iliac arteries) or muscular (medium-sized vessels such as the coronary, brachial, radial, and femoral arteries). All arteries have three distinct histologic layers: the intima (closest to the lumen), the media (consisting of smooth muscle cells and connective tissue), and the adventitia (tissue surrounding the artery). The arterial wall derives its blood supply from the vasa vasorum, which originates from the adventitial surface of the artery (Fig. 1).

- The aorta and the carotid and iliac arteries are elastic arteries.
- The coronary, brachial, radial, and femoral arteries are muscular arteries.

Elastic Arteries
The large peripheral arteries are conductance vessels, the media of which is mostly elastin folded into fenestrated layers. These vessels serve as the primary conduit leading from the heart. They expand in systole to convert the sudden systolic pressure impulse into potential energy. These vessels subsequently recoil elastically, converting the stored stretch potential energy into systemic blood flow and maintaining pressure throughout diastole. Unlike the muscular arteries, there is essentially no autoregulatory control of the diameter of conductance vessel by smooth muscle.

- The elastic arteries convert, in part, the systolic cardiac impulse into diastolic blood flow.

Table 1.—Cardiac Causes of Sudden Death

Coronary artery disease
  Atherosclerosis
  Infectious disease (syphilis)
  Inflammatory disorder (rheumatic vasculitis)
  Congenital anomaly
  Coronary artery embolism
  Coronary artery aneurysm
Valvular heart disease
  Mitral valve prolapse
  Aortic stenosis
Cardiomyopathy or myocarditis
  Idiopathic disorder
  Hypertrophic cardiomyopathy
  Infectious disease
  Sarcoidosis
  Amyloidosis
  Muscular dystrophy
  Arrhythmogenic ventricular dysplasia
Prolonged Q-T interval
  Idiopathic disorder
  Congenital anomaly
  Medication-related disorder
  Liquid protein diet
Metabolic abnormalities
  Hyperkalemia or hypokalemia
  Hypercalcemia or hypocalcemia
  Hypomagnesemia
  Increased levels of catecholamines
Congenital heart disease
  Primary pulmonary hypertension
  Tetralogy of Fallot
  Congenital heart block
  Ebstein anomaly of the heart
Medication
  Antiarrhythmic agents
  Antidepressant drugs
  Major tranquilizers
Intracardiac tumor
  Primary
  Metastatic
Cardiac ganglionitis
Wolff-Parkinson-White syndrome
No apparent underlying cardiac disease

From Giuliani ER, Gersh BJ, McGoon MD, Hayes DL, Schaff HV (editors): *Mayo Clinic Practice of Cardiology*. Third edition. Mosby, 1996, p 867. By permission of Mayo Foundation.

Muscular Arteries

The medium-sized muscular arteries contain substantially more smooth muscle than conductance vessels. The medial smooth muscle permits active changes in vessel diameter in response to end-organ need. Because atherosclerosis partly results from the migration and proliferation of smooth muscle cells, vessels that contain proportionally more smooth muscle might respond more vigorously to the inciting arterial injury that causes atherosclerosis.

- Muscular arteries can regulate blood flow in response to end-organ needs.

Endothelium

The endothelium, the single layer of cells in direct contact with the blood, lines the vascular system. Endothelial cells have several functions (Table 2).

- The endothelium is the largest endocrine organ in the body; it actively participates in the prevention of intravascular thrombosis and the regulation of vascular muscle tone.

Intima

The intima is between the endothelium and the internal elastic lamina. It is a highly fenestrated layer of elastin fibers that protects the media.

Media

The media consists almost entirely of smooth muscle cells. During growth and development, these cells have an extensive Golgi apparatus and endoplasmic reticulum, indicating active synthesis of proteins, collagen, elastin, and proteoglycans. In adults, the cells are comparatively quiet and contain little more than mitochondria and contractile filaments (actin and myosin). The outer third of the media is supplied by the vasa vasorum originating in the adventitia. Oxygen and nourishment reach the inner layer 1) from the vasa vasorum by diffusing through the outer layers and 2) from the blood in the lumen of the artery.

The primary function of the smooth muscle cells is to maintain vascular tone and to regulate local blood flow depending on metabolic requirements.

- Normally, smooth muscle cells of the media are synthetically quiescent, but they are capable of synthesizing collagen, elastin, and proteoglycans, which are inportant in the formation of complex atherosclerotic plaques and restenosis lesions that occur after percutaneous transluminal coronary angioplasty.

Adventitia

The adventitia is a loose connective tissue matrix that consists of collagen and proteoglycans intermixed with the

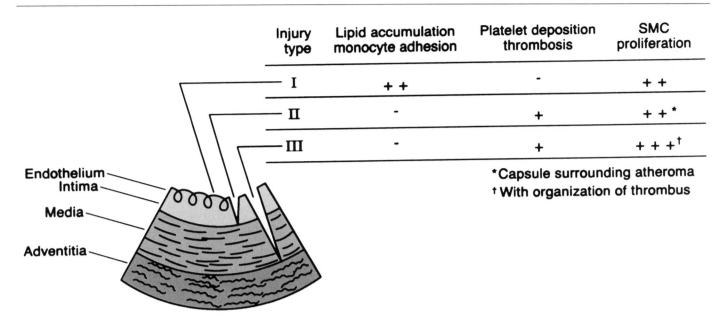

Injury type	Lipid accumulation monocyte adhesion	Platelet deposition thrombosis	SMC proliferation
I	+ +	-	+ +
II	-	+	+ + *
III	-	+	+ + + †

*Capsule surrounding atheroma
† With organization of thrombus

Endothelium
Intima
Media
Adventitia

Fig. 1. Classification of vascular injury or damage and vascular response. SMC, smooth muscle cell. (From Giuliani ER, Gersh BJ, McGoon MD, Hayes DL, Schaff HV [editors]: *Mayo Clinic Practice of Cardiology*. Third edition. Mosby, 1996, p 1058. By permission of Mayo Foundation.)

vasa vasorum and fat. The adventitia contains both fibroblasts and smooth muscle cells.

The Atherosclerotic Plaque

The atherosclerotic plaque typically is quite complex; however, atherosclerosis is fundamentally a disease of the arterial intima that, in its late stages, progresses to luminal narrowing (Plate 1).

Fatty Streak

The fatty streak consists predominantly of one cell type, the lipid-laden macrophage, which contains cholesteryl ester droplets and has the microscopic appearance of foam cells. Smooth muscle cells are interspersed among the macrophages, and as the fatty streak expands, smooth muscle cells accumulate at the site of the streak. The fatty streak also contains T lymphocytes (both CD8+ and CD4+).

The fatty streak was thought to be the precursor of atherosclerosis (Plate 2 A); however, its exact genesis is unclear. What is known is that macrophages phagocytose oxidized low-density lipoprotein (LDL), die, and contribute to the lipid of the fatty streak. In a typical cholesterol cleft, needle-shaped structures are filled with oxidized LDL (Plate 2 B). In a typical complex plaque, these regions of lipid deposition are

Table 2.—Functions of the Endothelium

Transport of low-density lipoproteins (LDL)—LDL bind to endothelial LDL receptors and are oxidized and transported across the endothelial cell to the intima
Prostacyclin production (PGI_2) to inhibit platelet deposition
Mitogen production (platelet-derived growth factor-like hormones)
Plasminogen secretion
Von Willebrand factor elaboration
Endothelin formation
Angiotensin-converting enzyme secretion
Endothelium-derived relaxing factor formation
Vascular adhesion molecule formation

walled off by the artery. Whether these structures promote inflammation and macrophage infiltration is uncertain, although it is clear that macrophages have a major role in the development of cholesterol clefts. It has been proposed that the fatty streak is one of the earliest lesions of atherosclerosis and that it progresses to a complex plaque. A major problem with this hypothesis is that fatty streaks found at autopsy occur at different locations and have a different distribution from that of mature, complex lesions. For example, complex lesions occur at bifurcations, and fatty streaks typically occur in straight arterial segments. Also, fatty streaks are common in the aortic arch of young persons, whereas advanced atherosclerosis occurs in the descending and abdominal aorta.

- The fatty streak is composed of lipid-laden macrophages and will regress with cholesterol lowering.

Fibrous Plaque

Collagen production is a principal feature of the atherosclerotic plaque, and hard fibrous plaques typically begin to develop in humans by age 25 years. Arterial remodeling, that is, the outward expansion of coronary arteries in response to increased plaque volume, also begins at this age. Arterial remodeling decreases the blood flow limitation of arterial stenosis because the outward arterial expansion accommodates increased plaque volume. The collagen deposition-remodeling process proceeds until the artery can no longer expand to accept additional growth of the plaque. This usually happens when the histopathologically measured arterial area stenosis is about 40%. Adventitial thickening resulting from collagen synthesis is thought to have a role in the limitation of arterial remodeling. The cells that populate these dense fibrous plaques are smooth muscle cells.

As a plaque ages, it develops an increasing amount of fibrous tissue and becomes a fibrous plaque. It usually is covered by a layer of connective tissue and populated by smooth muscle cells and fibrocytes (Table 3). This plaque may result from an inflammatory process induced by the lipid of the fatty streak. A fibrous cap occasionally forms across the top of a cholesterol-laden lipid reservoir. When this happens, the plaque is potentially "dangerous," because rupture of the fibrous layer can expose the underlying lipid to flowing blood, making a very thrombogenic surface. Coronary thrombosis is a frequent result; the thrombus is platelet rich. This thrombus can cause total or subtotal occlusion and result in an acute coronary syndrome such as sudden death, myocardial infarction, or unstable angina. Alternatively, this scenario can be played out as the plaque grows with time, with the accumulation of additional layers of cellular and fibrous tissue. The fibrous cap consists of smooth muscle cells, macrophages, and lymphocytes. It has been estimated that 30% to 50% of the cells are macrophages and 5% to 15% are T lymphocytes (Table 4).

- The fibrous cap of lipid-rich plaques may rupture and initiate an acute coronary syndrome.

Table 3.—Atherosclerosis: Extracellular Matrix

Collagens (I, III, IV, V, VI): structural
Elastin: structural
Proteoglycans: transport and regulation (cells, molecules)
Plasma components (low-density lipoprotein, fibrinogen, etc.)

Structure	Collagen type				
	I	III	IV	V	VI
Normal intima	-	-	+	-	-
Fibrous plaque	++	++	++	+	+
Atheromatous plaque, fibrous cap	+++	+++	+++	++	++

+, slight content; ++, significant content; +++, very significant content; -, no content.

From Giuliani ER, Gersh BJ, McGoon MD, Hayes DL, Schaff HV (editors): *Mayo Clinic Practice of Cardiology*. Third edition. Mosby, 1996, p 1067. By permission of Mayo Foundation.

Platelets

Platelets have an integral role in atherogenesis, especially in the elaboration of growth factors, including platelet-derived growth factor (PDGF) and transforming growth factors α and β (TGF-α and TGF-β). These potent mitogens are thought to be important in the migration and proliferation of smooth muscle cells in the wall of the artery. They also may be important in the organization of thrombus.

Macrophages

Several cell types are common in atherosclerotic plaques.

The monocyte is a blood-borne leukocyte that probes the endothelium and becomes localized just deep to this structure, in the intima along the basement membrane. On leaving the bloodstream, the monocyte becomes a macrophage and exits from the endothelial lining at the gap junctions. In animal models of lipid-induced atherosclerosis, endothelial cell dysfunction occurs after 3 or 4 months of a high fat diet. Specifically, there is substantial retraction of the endothelial cells—the cells actually separate, leaving the basement membrane completely uncovered. This phenomenon has also been demonstrated in humans. In patients with severe atherosclerosis, large areas of the arterial system have been found to be without any endothelial covering. This of course promotes platelet adhesion and aggregation, which in turn promote the release of growth factors for the influx of monocytes, macrophages, and subendothelial smooth muscle cells.

Table 4.—Atherogenesis: Influence of Risk Factors

Biology	Dyslipoproteinemia	Hypertension	Smoking	Genetics	Diabetes[*]
Endothelial injury (type I injury)	+	+	+	-	+
Lipoprotein—monocytes	++	-	-	++	++
Platelet deposition (over type II injury)	+	-	++	-	+
SMC—collagen	+	+	-	++	++
Plaque disruption (type III injury)	++	+	-	++	-
Thrombosis	+	-	++	+	++
Microvasculature	+	++	+	-	++[†]

SMC, smooth muscle cell; +, slight influence; ++, significant influence; -, no influence.

[*]Glycemia; advanced glycosylation end product (more so in insulin-dependent than in non-insulin-dependent diabetes mellitus).

[†]Insulin resistance (non-insulin-dependent diabetes mellitus); increased triglycerides, decreased high-density lipoprotein, hypertension.

From Giuliani ER, Gersh BJ, McGoon MD, Hayes DL, Schaff HV (editors): *Mayo Clinic Practice of Cardiology*. Third edition. Mosby, 1996, p 1058. By permission of Mayo Foundation.

Macrophages have a substantial role in atherogenesis. They secrete many growth factors, including PDGF, fibroblast growth factor (FGF), TGF-α, TGF-β, and interleukin-1. The monocyte must become activated after it becomes a macrophage and enters the tissue to begin synthesizing and secreting these factors.

Central to the current hypothesis of plaque growth is the role of growth factors (Table 5). These include three separate isoforms of PDGF (AA, AB, and BB). These isoforms are the principal mitogens for connective tissue-forming cells such as fibroblasts and smooth muscle cells. Acidic and basic FGF can also perform this function. However, unlike PDGF, FGF molecules are also mitogens for vascular smooth muscle cells and, thus, are powerful agents of neovascularization and angiogenesis. Most of the known mitogens appear to react specifically with the endothelium or mesodermal connective tissue such as smooth muscle cells and fibroblasts.

TGF-β appears to have primarily an inhibitory role in preventing cell growth, simultaneously inducing cellular differentiation. In the presence of other growth factors such as endothelial cell growth factor or PDGF, it facilitates fibrocyte growth in three dimensions. TGF-β has two effects on smooth muscle cells and fibroblasts, depending on concentration. At low doses, it stimulates smooth muscle cells and fibroblasts to upregulate PDGF-AA expression. At high doses of TGF-β, PDGF-AA continues to be secreted, but the PDGF-AA receptor is downregulated, inhibiting its autocrine response. Each growth factor binds specific cell surface receptors that stimulate eventual proliferation.

Table 5.—Regulatory Substances of Mitogenic and Other Cell Functions

Stimulators
  Platelet-derived growth factor
  Endothelial cell growth factor
  Fibroblast growth factor
  Smooth muscle cell-derived growth factor
  Interleukin-1
  Interleukin-6
  Transforming growth factor-β
  Low-density lipoproteins
  Vasoactive substances
    Angiotensin II
    Epinephrine
    Norepinephrine
    Serotonin
    Neuropeptide substances P and K
    Endothelin
  Thrombin
  Leukotrienes B_4, C_4, D_4
  Prostaglandin E_2, prostacyclin
Inhibitors
  Transforming growth factor-β
  Heparin-like factors
  Vasorelaxant substances
    Endothelium-derived relaxing factor
  Prostaglandin E, E_2; prostacyclin
  Interferon gamma

From Giuliani ER, Gersh BJ, McGoon MD, Hayes DL, Schaff HV (editors): *Mayo Clinic Practice of Cardiology*. Third edition. Mosby, 1996, p 1066. By permission of Mayo Foundation.

These cellular processes have been called the "response to injury" hypothesis for the genesis of atherosclerosis. According to this concept, endothelial injury, by chemical or other means, initiates a sequence of cellular events that results in a fibroproliferative lesion. The injury may be mild and/or chronic, as in hyperlipidemia. In these cases, the endothelial cells are phenotypically unchanged but demonstrate marked abnormalities of function. For example, patients with only minimal or mild luminal irregularities on coronary arteriography frequently demonstrate paradoxical responses to agents such as acetylcholine and other endothelium-dependent vasorelaxation drugs. The fatty streak is a major source of growth factors and, in conjunction with abnormal endothelial dysfunction, promotes formation of the fibroproliferative plaque.

The fatty streak is totally reversible in several animal models when normal cholesterol diets and metabolism are restored. Moreover, when studied with angiographic end points, the results of multiple regression trials suggest that the fibroproliferative plaques themselves can regress in patients. This suspicion has been confirmed in animal models in which fibrous plaque regression has been noted with cessation of high lipid diets.

Lymphocytes

T lymphocytes are often found in atherosclerotic lesions, but why they are there is not known. They may promote plaque growth. Several important cytokines such as interferon gamma and interleukin-1 are frequently associated with T lymphocytes. An important question is whether T lymphocytes occur in mature plaques or only in early lesions. Endothelial injury, platelet deposition and aggregation, plaque growth, and plaque rupture may be related directly to the presence of T cells and form a self-perpetuating cycle. If so, T lymphocytes may be an autoimmune component of atherosclerotic plaque growth.

The Intimal Cell Mass

An early histologic finding in atherosclerotic lesions is the intimal cell mass, which is composed of smooth muscle cells and associated connective tissue. The relationship of intimal cell masses to hypercholesterolemia is unknown. Lipid deposition and fatty streaks generally are not associated with intimal cell masses and can occur completely independently. In animal models, hypercholesterolemia from enhanced dietary fat intake promotes the development of intimal cell masses.

An example of a collection of intimal cells next to smooth muscle cells that have migrated toward the lumen and formed these intimal cell masses is shown in Plate 3. Proliferation is common in intimal cell masses, whereas there is little or no cell proliferation in regions of fatty streaks. The proliferation frequently referred to in atherosclerosis fundamentally occurs in intimal cell masses and can occur at any time in the life of the plaque.

Autopsy studies suggest that the intimal cell mass may be the beginning of an atherosclerotic plaque. These lesions are found in the arterial intima. In contrast to fatty streaks, which occur at sites different from those of mature lesions, many young people have intimal cell masses at arterial bifurcations, consistent with the location of mature lesions. Currently, it is thought that the intimal cell mass is more likely than the fatty streak to be the initiation of a true atherosclerotic plaque.

Some investigators suggest that the intimal cell mass may be part of a "normal" age-related thickening process. Indeed, older patients consistently have diffuse thickening of the arterial intima. Thus, an important question is whether there is a relationship between normal age-related intimal thickening and the progression of intimal cell masses into atherosclerotic plaques. Most experts believe that the two are separate processes despite the existence of proliferation in intimal cell masses.

Cellular Proliferation in Atherosclerosis

Because much of our knowledge about atherosclerosis comes from autopsy observations on mature and complex plaques, little is known about proliferation early in development. Proliferation is low or absent in late mature lesions. In malignant tumors, proliferation is frequently monoclonal. This means that all cells in the tumor, early and late, are from a common cell. This is true also for some nonmalignant tumors.

The monoclonality of arterial cells in arteriosclerotic plaques has been studied. With the use of marker enzymes, monoclonality was found in a large proportion of the atherosclerotic lesions examined, suggesting that each atherosclerotic plaque results from a single cell or, at most, a few cells. These monoclonality data are consistent with studies in pigs that also have shown intimal cell masses arising from monoclonal accumulation of intimal smooth muscle cells.

Hypotheses of Atherosclerosis

The three leading hypotheses of the pathogenesis of atherosclerosis are 1) the lipid, or insudation, hypothesis; 2) the platelet, or encrustation, hypothesis; and 3) the proliferative, or monoclonal, hypothesis. Importantly, these hypotheses are not mutually exclusive, and each one explains some of the pathologic observations made in atherosclerotic coronary artery disease.

The Lipid, or Insudation, Hypothesis

The insudation hypothesis suggests that the lipid component of the atherosclerotic plaque is derived from lipid-laden macrophages. This is supported by the well-proven relationship between increased plasma levels of lipoproteins and atherosclerosis. The insudation hypothesis is also substantiated by the finding that radioactively labeled lipid injected intravenously into patients accumulates in preexisting atherosclerotic plaques. Although the pathophysiology of initial lipid accumulation in the arterial wall is poorly understood, the deposition of lipid at sites of preexisting arterial damage is well proven.

However, there are problems with the insudation hypothesis. For example, no clinically significant atherosclerotic lesion is formed solely by lipids. Obstructive plaques have many other components, including loose and dense fibrous tissue, calcium, and smooth muscle cells. Another problem is that even if the atherosclerotic lesion begins as a fatty accumulation, how is the proliferation of smooth muscle cells, typical of complex atherosclerotic lesions, induced? Lipid concentrations that cause smooth muscle cell proliferation in vitro are considerably greater than those in the bloodstream. Thus, it appears that lipid accumulation itself is not sufficient to cause the proliferation of smooth muscle cells at lesion sites. Perhaps lipid deposition injures intimal cells that cause growth factor release and, thus, indirectly stimulates smooth muscle cell proliferation.

The Platelet, or Encrustation, Hypothesis

According to this hypothesis, platelets and thrombus from circulating blood drive atherosclerotic plaque formation. The accumulation of platelets initiates the process, and thrombus organization continues it. Atherosclerotic plaque contains recognizable platelet products. This is expected, because of the damage to the endothelium and the basement membrane and the exposure of highly thrombogenic subendothelial elements. Repeated thrombosis and plaque growth may occur, as shown in Plate 4.

In the encrustation hypothesis, the lipid in the plaque comes from the plasma, but its accumulation is passive and secondarily follows the thrombotic process, rather than being the primary instigator of the atherosclerotic plaque. Plaque expansion and volume growth result from repeated thrombotic episodes. Platelets are rich in growth factors, including PDGF and others, that promote smooth muscle cell growth and proliferation. Additional proliferation of smooth muscle cells depends on and is driven by the continuing deposition of platelets. The process can be self-sustaining, because thrombus is itself thrombogenic. Active thrombin is bound on the surface of the clot and perpetuates clot growth. Repeated episodes can cause the plaque to grow, producing severe luminal stenosis, or, alternatively, cause acute sudden arterial occlusion, precipitating an acute coronary syndrome.

The Proliferative, or Monoclonality, Hypothesis

According to this hypothesis, plaques begin as cell mutations or as an injury caused by a viral or other infectious event. A single isolated smooth muscle cell is the progenitor of a proliferative clone, which becomes the atherosclerotic cell mass. As atherosclerotic lesions mature, they become more definitively monoclonal than the initial fatty streak. This observation has been confirmed with DNA studies. This is to be expected because early lesions may be diluted by monocytes and other blood-borne elements.

Lipids and Atherosclerosis

The role of lipids in atherogenesis is supported by three major findings: the high lipid content of atherosclerotic plaques, induction of similar-appearing lesions in animals fed a high cholesterol diet, and strong clinical data supporting the relationship between serum levels of lipid and the epidemiology of coronary artery disease.

Lipids, especially cholesterol, are relatively insoluble in aqueous solutions such as blood and must be complexed with apolipoproteins to form lipoproteins to be transported within the vascular system. Lipid insolubility is the feature responsible for the ability of lipids to associate and form biologic structures such as cell membranes. Problems arise as lipid concentrations increase, likely because of their well-known detergent properties.

Lipoproteins are classified on the basis of density in ultracentrifugation: triglyceride-rich (chylomicra and remnants), very low-density lipoproteins (VLDL), intermediate-density lipoproteins (IDL), cholesterol-rich LDL, and protein-rich high-density lipoproteins (HDL). Recently, the apolipoproteins have been found to be essential in the determination of lipoprotein structure and the regulation of lipid transport. The major apolipoproteins are listed in Table 6. Apolipoproteins

A-I and A-II are the major components of HDL. One apolipoprotein (apo) B-100 molecule is contained in each VLDL particle in the liver and stays with that particle throughout its metabolism to IDL and LDL.

LDL

LDL is the best understood of the atherogenic proteins. Patients with increased ratios of plasma LDL apo-B to LDL cholesterol have a substantially increased risk of coronary atherosclerosis. This atherogenic risk occurs when LDL has an increased protein-to-cholesterol ratio and a large distribution of particle sizes. Typically, these are also hyper-triglyceridemic patients.

Lp(a) Lipoprotein

Lp(a) is an LDL particle that contains a large glycoprotein, apoprotein (a). Lp(a) has a higher density than LDL, but Lp(a) cholesterol is usually included in the LDL or VLDL cholesterol fraction. The role of Lp(a) is unknown, and its concentration usually is low (5 mg/dL). Genetically, some patients have increased Lp(a) levels that are highly correlated with coronary artery disease. On a per-particle basis, Lp(a) appears more atherogenic than LDL. Of interest, the genetic sequence for Lp(a) shares a high degree of homology with plasminogen, which suggests a link between Lp(a) and impaired fibrinolysis. The fibrinolytic pathways of patients may be inhibited by high concentrations of Lp(a).

HDL

HDL has an inverse relationship to coronary artery disease. In the Framingham study, low HDL cholesterol was a much stronger predictor of coronary risk than increased total LDL cholesterol in men and women 50 years and older. The major components of HDL are apo A-I and A-II. Tangier disease is characterized by hypercatabolism of apo A-I and apo A-II. HDL is essentially nonexistent in Tangier disease, and, in this disease, coronary artery disease generally occurs after age 40. An increased level of HDL has been described as a familial syndrome associated with lower overall rates of atherosclerosis. A key issue is whether HDL is truly antiatherogenic or whether there is only a statistical association between increased HDL and less disease.

In an atherosclerotic artery, cholesterol comes mainly from plasma lipoproteins, and the concentration of lipid in these atherosclerotic plaques is higher than in any other tissue of the body. In humans, LDL accumulates in the intima in preatherosclerotic states, as does Lp(a) (3 to 4

Table 6.—Apolipoproteins

Name	Distribution	Function
HDL A-I	Chylomicrons	Activates LCAT
HDL A-II	Chylomicrons	Unknown
B-100 LDL, VLDL	Chylomicrons	LDL receptor binding
HDL C-I, IDL, VLDL		Activates LCAT
E VLDL, chylo, HDL		Ligand for LDL receptor
Lp(a)	Chylomicrons	Unknown

HDL, high-density lipoprotein; IDL, intermediate-density lipoprotein; LCAT, lecithin-cholesterol acyltransferase; LDL, low-density lipoprotein; VLDL, very low-density lipoprotein; E VLDL, extremely VLDL.

times its concentration in the plasma). Concentrations of these lipids in the media are far less than in the intima. At about age 20, cholesteryl esters begin concentrating in the intima in normal arteries, and the concentration increases linearly. By age 60, cholesterol may be 2% to 3% of the total weight of a nonatherosclerotic coronary artery.

Other than the liver, most cells of the body derive the necessary cholesterol from plasma lipoproteins. Unesterified cholesterol in a cell is tightly regulated by three biochemical processes: inhibition of cholesterol synthesis by HMG-CoA reductase, activation of acyl-CoA:cholesterol acyltransferase, and downregulation of LDL receptors on the cell because of decreased mRNA for those receptors.

To summarize these concepts, a high serum cholesterol load is transmitted by the arterial intima in the form of LDL. Macrophages engulf this LDL, become foam cells, and die. Inflammatory responses ensue, generating a thrombus and involving the cellular organization of the thrombus. Healing occurs in the form of a fibrocalcific plaque that becomes a volume-occupying lesion. Typically, no capillaries are found in the arterial intima. Occasionally, neovascularization is seen in regions of plaque that likely were once thrombus, and these regions are typically associated with macrophages, foam cells, giant cells, and fibroblasts.

Homocysteine: A New Risk Factor for Coronary Atherosclerosis

The traditional risk factors for atherosclerosis are well known: smoking, diabetes mellitus, male sex, hypertension, and hyperlipidemia. Recently, increased plasma levels of homocysteine were shown to be an independent risk factor for coronary artery disease, stroke, and peripheral vascular disease and to promote arterial and venous thrombosis, although the exact mechanisms are uncertain. Renal disease, diabetes mellitus, and organ transplant dysfunction are also related to increased homocysteine levels. Homocysteine is toxic to endothelial cells and leads to their injury and dysfunction. The mechanisms are probably related to the generation of free radicals during homocysteine oxidation. Vascular smooth muscle cells proliferate on exposure to homocysteine, which also inhibits vascular endothelial cell growth. Homocysteine also is prothrombotic, because it increases thrombin generation at sites of vascular injury. Homocysteine may also lessen nitric oxide availability, increase collagen accumulation, and promote the adhesion of neutrophils and monocytes to the endothelium.

The odds ratio for coronary atherosclerosis is about 2.5 times that for fasting plasma homocysteine levels greater than the 95th percentile, which is similar in magnitude to conventional risk factors. Multivariate regression has shown that the interaction of hyperhomocysteinemia with hypertension and smoking is very strong, with the combined effects being greater than simply additive. Homocysteine and increased cholesterol levels are additive in cardiovascular risk.

The homocysteine concentration required for increased cardiovascular risk is unknown, as is the degree of homocysteine-lowering needed to prevent cardiovascular events. Because of these unknowns, it is not known in which populations homocysteine concentration should be evaluated. Folic acid and vitamins B_{12} and B_6 are beneficial in reducing plasma homocyteine levels. A randomized trial of folate supplementation has not been completed, and the potential benefits of prophylactic dietary folate on limiting atherosclerosis are unknown. Nevertheless, dietary folic acid supplementation is recommended for all patients with documented atherosclerosis. The enhanced folic acid diet suggested by the FDA uses enriched grain products and does not lower homocysteine levels in most patients. A typical multivitamin contains 400 µg of folic acid and should be considered for patients with coronary artery disease.

Regression of Coronary Atherosclerosis

As known for many years, hypercholesterolemia-induced experimental atherosclerosis in swine and monkeys regresses after the animal is returned to a nonatherogenic diet. This occurs with both the early fatty streak lesions and, to a lesser extent, the later fibrous plaques and smooth muscle proliferative lesions. Studies in humans with lipid-lowering drugs and dietary modification have conclusively demonstrated a reduction in the rate of cardiac events. Note that angiographic improvement in coronary stenoses is usually modest in coronary regression studies, suggesting that plaque stabilization due to a reduction in lipid content may be the main benefit of aggressive cholesterol lowering. The decrease in cardiac event rate correlates well with LDL cholesterol reduction. Noncoronary atherosclerosis may be affected less by aggressive cholesterol reduction than coronary atherosclerosis (Table 7).

Atherosclerosis: Possible Infectious Etiologies

The role of possible atherogenic bacterial and viral agents has not been defined, and it has not been proved that they are a cause of atherosclerosis. *Chlamydia pneumoniae* may be associated with both coronary and carotid atherosclerosis. *Chlamydia* is omnipresent and is known principally as a cause of acute respiratory disease. Serologic and epidemiologic data associate *C. pneumoniae* antibody with coronary artery disease, myocardial infarction, carotid artery disease, and cerebrovascular disease. This association is strengthened by finding the organism in atherosclerotic plaques in the arterial tree, including the aorta. Importantly, the organism is virtually absent from healthy arterial tissue. Data from animal experiments suggest the hematogenous dissemination of *Chlamydia* after pulmonary infection preferentially infects an atherosclerotic plaque. *Chlamydia* can infect and multiply in human vascular tissue and may elicit a release of cell-mediated cytokines with consequent local and systemic vascular effects.

The epidemiologic evidence is strong, even after adjusting for risk factors such as sex, age, hypertension, cigarette smoking, diabetes, and serum cholesterol. Calculation of odds ratios typically indicates a value of 2 times or greater, and several studies report that 20% to 25% of atherosclerotic specimens are positive for *Chlamydia*. An important question is whether chronic *Chlamydia* infection initiates or promotes disease progression or is a noncausal associate of atherosclerosis. To this end, several studies have recently shown that treatment of patients with macrolide antibiotics may decrease cardiovascular events and induce disease regression.

Table 7.—Progression and Regression of Coronary Atherosclerosis

Study	Progression (P) (control), %	Regression (R) (treated), %	Event reduction* (treated), %
NHLBI II	...	...	33
CLAS I II	...	...	34
POSCH	...	...	62
Lifestyle	3.4	2.2	...
FATS	2.1	0.8	75
UC-SCOR	0.8	1.5	...
STARS	5.8	1.5	79
SCRIP	...	...	50
CCAIT	...	...	47
Average	3.0(P)	1.4(R)	54

CCAIT, Canadian Coronary Atherosclerosis Intervention Trial; CLAS-I, -II, Cholesterol Lowering Atherosclerosis Study; FATS, Familial Atherosclerosis Treatment Study; NHLBI, National Heart, Lung, and Blood Institute; POSCH, Program on the Surgical Control of the Hyperlipidemias; SCRIP, Stanford Coronary Risk Intervention Project; STARS, St. Thomas' Atherosclerosis Regression Study; UC-SCOR, University of California-Stanford Coronary Regression Study .
*Death, myocardial infarction, unstable angina (revascularization).
From Giuliani ER, Gersh BJ, McGoon MD, Hayes DL, Schaff HV (editors): *Mayo Clinic Practice of Cardiology*. Third edition. Mosby, 1996, p 1080. By permission of Mayo Foundation.

Helicobacter pylori has also been implicated in atherosclerosis. *H. pylori* is a well-documented cause of chronic gastric infection. As a cause of atherosclerosis, *Helicobacter* has recently become controversial, with several studies reporting negative results. A possible mechanism by which *Helicobacter* causes atherosclerosis is through the generation of an adverse lipid profile, despite corrections for smoking, age, body mass index (BMI), and social class.

Infectious agents may also cause mutagenesis. Portions of the herpes genome have been found by in situ hybridization in atherosclerotic plaques. Cytomegalovirus antigen has also been found within plaque smooth muscle cells. Cytomegalovirus is at the forefront of investigations into the association of viruses and atherosclerosis, and strong seroepidemiologic evidence connects the cellular evidence with the clinical syndrome.

There are also problems with the concept of a viral cause of atherosclerosis. If atherosclerosis is caused by a virus, the hypothesis must fulfill the Koch postulates. Latent infection by cytomegalovirus is quite common in adult humans, and its prevalence increases with age. Indeed, the majority of Americans have been infected at one time or another during their adult years with cytomegalovirus. Because cytomegalovirus is found in atherosclerotic plaques does not indicate causality. Other interesting seroepidemiologic connections have been found, although they are tenuous. For example, coxsackie B4 antigen has been found in atherosclerotic plaques. Herpesvirus types 1 and 2 are common in aortic smooth muscle cells in adult humans and produce important cellular changes consistent with early aortic atherosclerosis. Thus, a series of viruses (herpes, coxsackie, and cytomegalovirus) have been identified that may have a mutational role that gives rise to the monoclonal cellular proliferation in atherosclerosis.

Many infections, both viral and bacterial, can clinically mimic vasculitic syndromes. Sometimes these vasculitides can be treated successfully with antibiotics. An example is Wegener granulomatosis. Hepatitis viruses (especially hepatitis C) are another potential cause.

Although direct infection of the vessel wall may be a cause of atherosclerosis, it is also possible that a humoral response to the infection can accentuate the problem of T-cell activation and other inflammation (Plate 5*A* and *B*). The inflammatory component of plaque rupture and consequent acute coronary syndromes may result from the infection. Consequently, chronic infection may have a role in the initiation, progression, or destabilization of atherosclerotic plaques.

In summary, a unified hypothesis has been proposed for the pathogenesis of atherosclerosis. The principal features, as summarized by Dr. Stephen Schwartz, are as follow:

1. All clinically significant atherosclerotic plaque involves smooth muscle cells. An important question is whether smooth muscle cell replication is a cause or an effect of the atherosclerotic lesion.

2. Focal smooth muscle cell masses occur in the intima at birth. The sites of these lesions with cellular collections correlate with the locations of atherosclerotic lesions later in life. This suggests that the intimal cell mass increasingly is a likely candidate for an early lesion that develops into an atheromatous plaque.

3. Fatty arterial lesions also are found at birth. These locations do *not* correlate well with the locations of plaques later in life.

4. Atherosclerotic plaques typically occur only in the intima. This may imply special characteristics of the smooth muscle cells trapped in the intima. For example, can these cells be transformed by infectious viral or bacterial vectors or by other physicochemical mutagenic agents?

5. The monoclonal hypothesis suggests that the smooth muscle cell component of plaque arises from one or, at most, a few cells. The mechanism for the initiation of proliferation is unknown.

6. Atherosclerosis is accelerated by hyperlipidemia. It is unclear whether there is a direct causal relationship between atherosclerosis and hyperlipidemia. Lipid accumulation may be a strong feature of plaque progression. Cholesterol lowering mediated by HMG CoA reductase inhibitors can cause disease regression and lower the incidence of adverse events mediated by vasculopathy. This suggests the contribution of hyperlipidemia to progression; it does not address the issue of plaque initiation.

7. Growth factors are present in atherosclerotic vascular lesions. It is unclear whether these are derived from exogenous or endogenous sources. Many potential sources exist for these growth factors and include exogenous blood-borne sources and endogenous cells such as smooth muscle cells, T lymphocytes, and macrophages. Each of these cells is very common in plaques.

8. The response to injury may precede plaque growth, as in other nonarterial lesions. However, the monoclonal hypothesis suggests that atherosclerotic lesions may not arise according to the "response-to-injury" concept.

9. PDGF likely has a role in propagating the atherosclerotic lesion. Although there are difficulties with the response-to-injury hypothesis, continued injury very likely has a role in plaque progression.

10. Cellular proliferation and growth control is critical; it is a complex balance of forces. Whatever the initiating factor may be, more important is what strategy or strategies might be used to slow or to stop plaque progression.

11. The cycle of denudation, thrombosis, and growth factor effects is likely mediated through macrophages and smooth muscle cells. These cells may initiate and stimulate the process in a complex, but poorly understood, chronic process.

Acute Coronary Syndromes

Acute coronary syndromes of unstable angina, non-ST-segment elevation (non-Q-wave) myocardial infarction, ST-segment elevation (Q-wave) myocardial infarction, and sudden cardiac death have a similar pathophysiologic mechanism, with atherosclerotic plaque fissuring, plaque rupture, and thrombus formation. Which acute coronary syndrome a patient has is determined by 1) the rapidity of vessel occlusion, 2) whether the obstruction is total or subtotal, 3) the ability of the infarct-related artery to recruit distal collaterals, and 4) whether the occlusion is transient, with recurrent cycles of thrombosis and spontaneous lysis that may allow time for myocardial conditioning and development of collateral vessels.

Vulnerable Plaque: Causes of Acute Coronary Syndrome

Certain types of atherosclerotic plaque may undergo sudden changes that may result in catastrophic consequences when thrombus forms on these plaques. An example of a ruptured plaque is shown in Plate 6, and examples of completely occluded atherosclerotic plaques are shown in Plate 7. Such plaques are termed "vulnerable." They rupture, causing acute coronary syndrome. The study of such plaques is beginning only now, but many important findings have emerged. Plaques may rupture from "intrinsic vulnerability" or mechanical stresses or they may be subjected to extrinsic "triggers," all of which are important in the pathogenesis of acute coronary syndrome.

Intrinsic plaque vulnerability includes important structural, cellular, and molecular characteristics. Large lipid cores covered by thin fibrous caps give rise to plaque vulnerability. Although stenotic coronary plaques are predominantly fibrous, a large lipid core is usually present in culprit lesions that are responsible for acute coronary syndromes. The lipid composition is much higher in vulnerable than in stable plaques, and the risk of rupture in aortic plaques is related to the size of the lipid core. The lipid type in a plaque is also a factor, because cholesteryl esters soften plaque and cholesterol in crystalline form likely hardens it. Cap thinning with reduced collagen also leads to plaque vulnerability. Of interest, the fibrous cap covering a mild stenosis is more likely to rupture than a stenotic plaque, because of more tension in the former and differential hydrodynamic shear forces in accord with the law of Laplace and the Bernoulli principle. As the heart beats, repetitive stretching, compression, bending, flexion shear, and pressure fluctuations "fatigue" and weaken a fibrous cap, leading to spontaneous rupture.

A hallmark of plaque vulnerability is inflammatory cell infiltrates. This strongly suggests an immune component to plaque vulnerability. The immune system has been strongly implicated in the coronary artery changes that promote thrombosis at a site of plaque rupture. Recent studies have suggested there is increased production of interferon gamma in patients with unstable angina. This molecule, in turn, can cause the release of many other growth factors, including cytokine interleukin-6 (IL-6), which promotes an acute phase response. A rare lymphocyte (CD4+CD28^{null}) is associated with substantial infiltrative characteristics, and it has been suggested recently that such cells may be responsible for converting a stable plaque to an unstable one. Only now, the potential immune features of atherosclerosis are being investigated.

The site of intimal rupture or erosion of thrombosed coronary atherosclerotic plaques may have inflammatory infiltrates regardless of plaque morphology. Several stimuli have been proposed to incite a chronic inflammatory reaction in atherosclerotic plaques, including lipoproteins (oxidized lipoproteins), the infectious vectors noted above, and an immune response to autoantigens such as heat shock proteins. These stimuli can activate macrophages and T lymphocytes in the plaque or attract such cells to the plaque. After the inflammatory reaction has begun, cytokines and matrix-degrading proteins weaken the connective tissue framework of the plaque and promote vulnerability. Smooth muscle cells may protect against plaque rupture by producing matrix, collagen, and inhibitors of matrix-degrading enzymes, the so-called matrix metalloproteinases.

The cytokines and matrix metalloproteinases are important molecular factors in causing plaque vulnerability. Matrix metalloproteinases are proteolytic enzymes that degrade various components of the extracellular matrix. In the atherosclerotic plaque, foam cell macrophages, activated T cells, and smooth muscle cells secrete these enzymes upon stimulation by various cytokines such as interferon gamma, tumor necrosis factor, interleukin-1, and macrophage colony-stimulating factor.

Blood pressure on the vessel wall exerts circumferential stress on a plaque. Regions of high stress correspond to sites of rupture found in autopsy specimens and have a characteristic angiographic appearance (Plate 8). Thinner fibrous caps are less capable of withstanding wall stress. The stresses in ruptured plaques are highest at the point where such caps attach to the arterial wall. Plaque rupture may occur spontaneously or it can be triggered under special circumstances. More than half of all patients with myocardial infarction report having a triggering event that is either emotional stress or physical exertion. These events cause rapid, strong sympathetic activity and they increase blood pressure, heart rate, the force of cardiac contraction, and coronary blood flow. Another trigger of plaque rupture is coronary vasospasm, which compresses the atheromatous

core. It can cause what has been described as "volcano-like eruption" of lipid into the lumen. Hypercoagulability and impaired fibrinolytic activity may also promote occlusive thrombus formation and an acute coronary syndrome.

Plaques can be stabilized. Several classes of drugs may stabilize rupture-prone plaques, including statins, antioxidants, angiotensin-converting enzyme inhibitors, and β-blockers. Lipid-lowering trials with statins have shown that lowering plasma LDL levels reduces the risk of acute ischemic events and death. Yet, these drugs are associated with only modest changes in stenosis. The two mechanisms most commonly proposed for positive results of statins on sudden vascular-mediated events are plaque stabilization and improved endothelial function, likely through endothelial-derived relaxing factor (or nitric oxide) activity. A favorable effect on thrombosis and fibrinolysis may also have a role. Enhanced endothelial function and blood coagulation-fibrinolysis have a beneficial effect on plaques in early developmental stages. Older and more mature plaques may benefit from reduction in lipid composition and size.

> Acute coronary syndromes are a large segment of the practice of clinical cardiology and questions are asked about them in detail on the Cardiology Boards. This section briefly outlines the pathologic mechanisms underlying these syndromes.

Unstable Angina

Unstable angina is a sudden acceleration in the severity of previously stable angina, rest angina, or post-myocardial infarction angina. Pathologically, unstable angina is characterized by incomplete or transient coronary artery occlusion, usually in association with rupture of the ulcer or fibrous cap of a lipid-rich atherosclerotic plaque. Usually, the initial thrombus is platelet-derived and may be associated with a variable vasoconstrictor response secondary to overpowering of the normal vasodilator functions of the endothelium. Platelet activation may be induced by the binding of thrombin, epinephrine, collagen, or serotonin to specific platelet-surface receptors. Platelet activation leads, in turn, to the release of adenosine-5-diphosphate (ADP) and phospholipase A_2 that mediate the hydrolysis of arachidonic acid, leading to the release of thromboxane A_2. Further activation of platelets is stimulated by phospholipase A_2 and thromboxane A_2. Platelet aggregation occurs by the binding of fibrinogen, vitronectin, fibronectin, and von Willebrand factor to specific platelet receptors, the glycoprotein integrin receptor, GPIIb/IIIa receptor. The clinical importance of the GPIIb/IIIa receptor is that antibody (abciximab) and nonantibody (tirofiban) receptor blockers are available to block platelet aggregation. Unstable angina is not associated with significant amounts of fibrin-rich thrombus, and controlled clinical trials have not documented a significant benefit of thrombolytic agents in unstable angina or ST-segment elevation (non-Q-wave) myocardial infarcts (TIMI-III trial). Inhibition of platelet aggregation by abciximab, a monoclonal antibody fragment that binds to the GPIIb/IIIa platelet receptor, decreases the number of episodes of ischemia in patients with unstable angina, in comparison with placebo.

Non-ST-Segment Elevation (Non-Q-Wave) Myocardial Infarction

Non-ST-segment elevation myocardial infarction is myocardial cell necrosis as evidenced by an increase in creatine kinase (muscle and brain subunits) in the absence of ST-segment elevation on the electrocardiogram. ST-segment elevation (Q-wave) and non-ST-segment elevation (non-Q-wave) myocardial infarction have replaced—but are not synonymous with—the earlier terms "transmural" and "non-transmural" myocardial infarction. In a non-ST-segment elevation infarction, myocardial damage is limited by one of several mechanisms: 1) spontaneous thrombolysis of the occluded coronary artery, 2) relief of coronary spasm, or 3) recruitment of distal collateral flow or the correction of a factor that adversely shifted the myocardial oxygen supply/demand ratio, such as heavy exertion or ischemia in a watershed territory secondary to systemic hypotension. Non-Q-wave myocardial infarction is usually associated with a complex disrupted atherosclerotic plaque in the infarct-related artery, with subtotal occlusive thrombus in most patients. Approximately one-fourth of the patients with non-Q-wave myocardial infarction have a total coronary artery occlusion.

ST-Segment Elevation Myocardial Infarction

ST-segment elevation infarction is usually caused by the occlusion of an epicardial coronary artery by a fibrin-rich thrombus. Most patients have a disrupted atherosclerotic plaque, but in a few, only the endothelium and intima of the coronary artery are injured. In the absence of good collateral circulation, persistent occlusion of a major coronary artery results in ST-segment elevation myocardial infarction, which is different from non-ST-segment elevation myocardial infarction in several important ways.

1. ST-segment elevation myocardial infarction is associated with more myocardial damage and has a worse in-hospital prognosis than non-ST-segment elevation myocardial infarction.
2. ST-segment elevation myocardial infarction is associated with fibrin-rich thrombus (red thrombus on angioscopy), whereas non-ST-segment elevation myocardial infarction is associated with platelet thrombi (gray-white appearance).
3. ST-segment elevation myocardial infarcts, being fibrin-rich, frequently lyse with thrombolysis, but non-ST-segment elevation myocardial infarcts do not benefit with thrombolysis.
4. Emergency angiography in a patient with non-ST-segment elevation myocardial infarction usually demonstrates patent coronary vessels but in ST-segment elevation myocardial infarction shows vessels occluded by thrombus.
5. Patients with ST-segment elevation myocardial infarction frequently have only single-vessel coronary artery disease and the underlying atherosclerotic plaque that triggered the acute thrombus may be less than 50% in many cases. Patients with non-ST-segment elevation infarction generally have more extensive coronary artery disease and, frequently, a more developed distal collateral network.

Although platelet thrombus is not the dominant thrombus type in ST-segment elevation myocardial infarction, platelet aggregation appears to be important in the instigation of ST-segment elevation myocardial infarction, as evidenced by the preventive benefit aspirin has on ST-segment elevation myocardial infarction.

Sudden Cardiac Death

Sudden cardiac death occurs either in the presence of myocardial infarction when the sudden cessation of coronary blood flow precipitates a malignant cardiac arrhythmia or in the absence of myocardial infarction in patients who have an arrhythmogenic substrate, usually in association with previous ventricular scarring or left ventricular dysfunction. Sudden cardiac death in patients who recently had a myocardial infarction may also be due to mechanical complications such as ventricular or papillary muscle rupture. Patients with left ventricular dysfunction, three-vessel coronary artery disease, or previous myocardial infarction are more likely to have a primary arrhythmogenic death and less likely to have an acute coronary thrombus with a secondary fatal arrhythmia than patients without a previous history of myocardial infarction, single-vessel coronary artery disease, and previously normal left ventricular function. Excluding patients with nonischemic heart disease, angiography in survivors of sudden cardiac death shows significant coronary artery disease in at least one vessel in almost all cases. In patients who subsequently had inducible ventricular tachycardia at electrophysiologic study suggesting an arrhythmogenic substrate, less than one-fourth had unstable complex atherosclerotic plaques, whereas most patients who were not inducible at electrophysiologic study had a complex unstable atherosclerotic plaque.

● Sudden cardiac death may occur in the absence of myocardial infarction in patients with scarred, poorly functioning left ventricles in whom an underlying arrhythmogenic substrate is present.

Questions

Multiple Choice (choose the one best answer)
Note: The following questions may have *more than* one correct answer.

1. In vivo, the subendothelium contains many types of collagen. All the following are types of subendothelial collagen *except*:
   a. Collagen II
   b. Collagen III
   c. Collagen IV
   d. Collagen V
   e. Collagen VI

2. Endothelium secretes all the following substances in large amounts *except*:
   a. Collagen
   b. Elastin
   c. Glycosaminoglycans
   d. Fibronectin
   e. Mucopolysaccharides

3. Which substance(s) is (are) secreted by the endothelium?
   a. Procoagulants
   b. Anticoagulants
   c. Vasoconstriction
   d. Vasorelaxation
   e. Proliferative

4. Which of the following is/are not true about platelets?
   a. Platelet activation can occur through many biochemical pathways and receptors
   b. Platelet aggregation occurs through many different surface receptors

c. Platelet adhesion occurs principally through subendothelial von Willebrand factor

d. Platelet-activating factor (PAF) also activates monocytes and polymorphonuclear leukocytes

e. Removal of the endothelium exposes subendothelium and creates intense platelet adhesion

5. Atherosclerosis principally affects which of the following component(s) of the vessel wall?
   a. Intima
   b. Adventitia
   c. Media
   d. Endothelium

6. The major cell type of the normal coronary artery intima is the:
   a. Macrophage
   b. Smooth muscle cell
   c. Lymphocyte
   d. Endothelial cell
   e. Foam cell

7. The foam cell is a lipid-laden cell derived from:
   a. Macrophage
   b. Smooth muscle cell
   c. Endothelial cell
   d. Lymphocyte
   e. Polymorphonuclear leukocyte

8. Which of the following is/are true about atherosclerotic plaques?
   a. Studies in arteries of patients with atherosclerosis show high rates of proliferation
   b. Intimal cell masses found in normal young patients suggest that proliferation may have an early role in the development of the atherosclerotic lesion
   c. Cells normally accumulate in the coronary arterial intima with aging
   d. Evidence suggests that the fatty streak may not be an early lesion of coronary atherosclerotic plaque
   e. The cells of atherosclerotic plaques are polyclonal in origin, that is, originating from many cells

9. In the "insudation hypothesis" of atherosclerosis, which of the following is/are true?
   a. Lipid accumulation in the atherosclerotic plaque comes from circulating lipid

b. Smooth muscle cell proliferation is induced by lipid accumulation at physiologic lipid concentration

c. Fatty deposition is required for plaque growth

d. Lipids in foam cells come from synthesis by local cellular activity

10. Which of the following is/are true of the fatty streak?
    a. It is found frequently in young children and infants
    b. It is found at the same anatomical sites in young persons and adults
    c. T lymphocytes may be found in many fatty streaks
    d. The principal lipid of the fatty streak is unoxidized cholesteryl esters
    e. The fatty streak is found principally in males at older ages

11. Which of the following is/are true of the "vulnerable" plaque?
    a. The vulnerable plaque typically has a fibrous cap covering a lipid-rich layer
    b. These plaques typically rupture at the central portion of the fibrous layer, where hydrodynamic forces are greatest
    c. Evidence suggests that vulnerable plaques may come from hemorrhage into the coronary artery vessel wall at certain locations
    d. The vulnerable plaque is typically associated with a severe angiographic stenosis
    e. There is evidence suggesting that more than 90% of myocardial infarctions causing death are associated with plaque rupture or ulceration

12. Which of the following is/are true of calcification of coronary artery plaque?
    a. Coronary calcification may proceed in a biochemical fashion similar to that in bone
    b. The principal component of plaque calcification is calcium carbonate and, thus, is related to vitamin D intake
    c. The degree of calcification is related to the overall volume of atherosclerotic plaque in coronary arteries
    d. Calcific medial sclerosis as a cause of coronary arterial calcification is associated with increased probability of an acute coronary syndrome
    e. The coronary artery develops calcification late in plaque development and nearly always is associated with large plaque burden

Answers

1. Answer a

2. Answer e

3. Answers a, b, c, d, and e

4. Answers b and e

5. Answers a and c

6. Answer b

7. Answers a and b

8. Answers b, c, and d

9. Answer a

10. Answers a, b, and c

11. Answers a, c, d, and e

12. Answers a and c

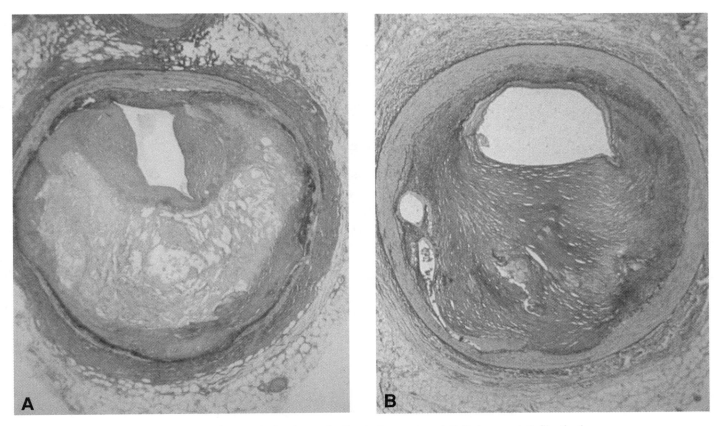

Plate 1. Histologic sections of advanced atherosclerosis showing marked luminal narrowing. *A*, Soft plaque and, *B*, fibrotic plaque.

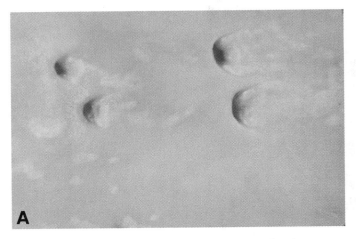
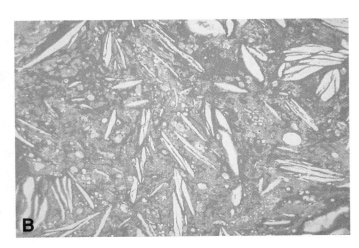

Plate 2. *A*, Fatty streaks. *B*, Cholesterol clefts in atherosclerosis.

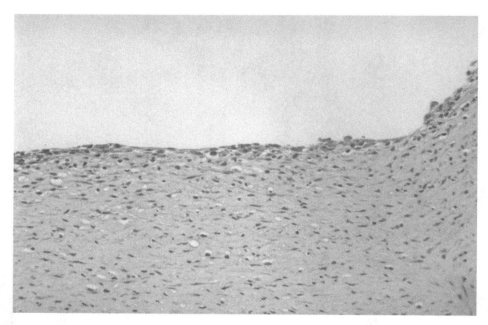

Plate 3. Intimal cells in proximity to smooth muscle cells.

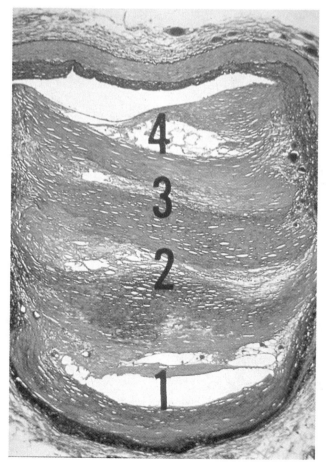

Plate 4. Histologic section showing that plaque progression occurs
in several distinct laminations (1-4).

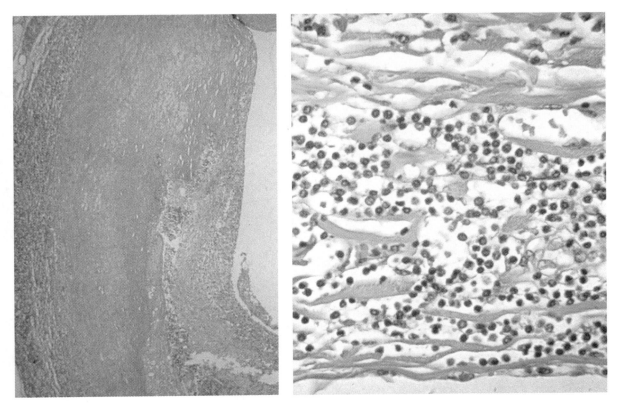

Plate 5. Foam cells in atherosclerosis.

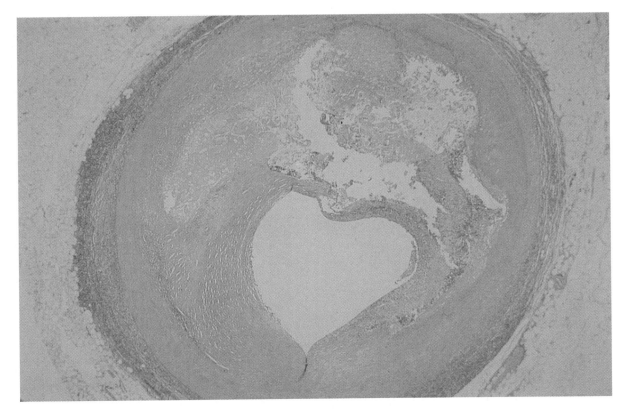

Plate 6. Acute rupture of plaque.

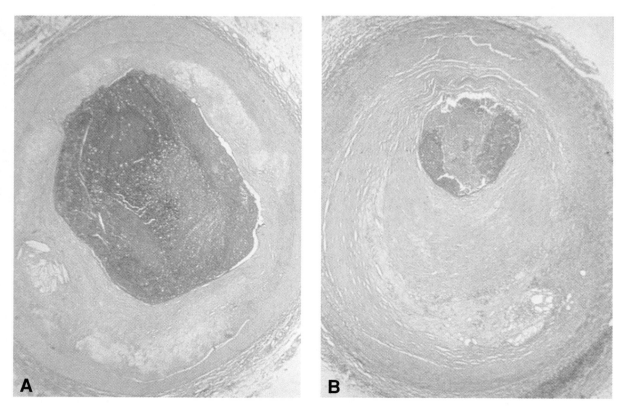

Plate 7. Histologic section showing occlusive coronary thrombosis in underlying, *A*, mild and, *B*, severe atherosclerotic luminal narrowing.

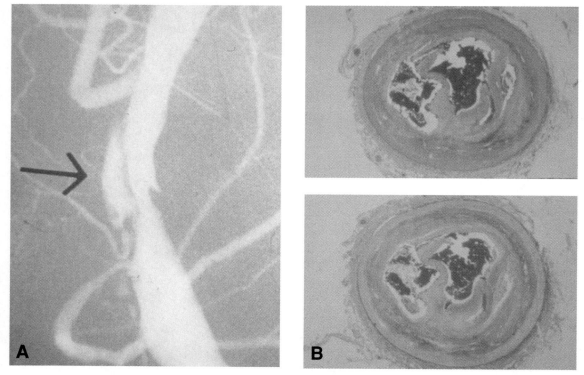

Plate 8. *A*, angiographic and, *B*, histologic correlation of plaque rupture and ulceration (*arrow* in *A*) of the right proximal coronary artery, with the appearance of pseudodissection.

Chapter 10

Hyperlipidemia and Other Risk Factors for Atherosclerosis

R. Scott Wright, M.D.
Thomas E. Kottke, M.D.
Gerald T. Gau, M.D.

Epidemiology

Increases in total and low-density lipoprotein (LDL) serum cholesterol values are associated with an increased risk of coronary artery disease, as demonstrated by the Framingham longitudinal study. Multiple epidemiologic studies that compared the incidence of coronary artery disease in different countries showed a direct correlation between the mean population total cholesterol and LDL cholesterol levels and the incidence of coronary artery disease. In contrast, there was an inverse correlation between the incidence of coronary artery disease and the mean serum high-density lipoprotein (HDL) level (Table 1).

- Epidemiologic studies have shown a direct correlation between mortality from coronary artery disease and total serum cholesterol and LDL cholesterol levels and an inverse correlation with serum HDL levels.

Country-specific age-adjusted death rates from coronary artery disease differ markedly. Rates of death from coronary artery disease for middle-aged men (45-64 years) in Scotland during the early 1980s were in excess of 540 per 100,000, which is more than 13 times that of Japanese men of the same age (about 40 per 100,000). What is less well realized is that the same 13-fold difference in the rate of death from coronary artery disease was also present in women; the rate was 170 per 100,000 in Scotland and 14 per 100,000 for middle-aged Japanese women of the same age.

- Mortality from coronary artery disease was 13 times higher in both middle-aged men and women in Scotland than in age-matched Japanese in the early 1980s.

LDL Subtypes and Coronary Artery Disease

The epidemiologic link between LDL cholesterol and the development of coronary artery disease is well established, and multiple randomized trials have conclusively demonstrated that treatment with a statin agent significantly reduces future cardiovascular events and mortality from all causes across all patient subgroups with hypercholesterolemia (Plate 1).

LDL cholesterol is a heterogeneous collection of lipoproteins; there are at least 15 distinct subspecies of LDL cholesterol. LDL cholesterol can be broadly classified into three classes: large, light LDL; intermediate LDL; and small, dense LDL. The major differences among these classes is the ratio of cholesterol molecules to apolipoprotein B. The large, light LDL cholesterol has the greatest cholesterol:apolipoprotein B ratio, and the small, dense LDL cholesterol has the lowest cholesterol:apolipoprotein B ratio.

- LDL cholesterol is a heterogeneous collection of lipoproteins.
- There are at least 15 distinct subspecies of LDL cholesterol.

Table 1.—Factors Influencing Levels of High-Density Lipoprotein

Relatively high levels	Relatively low levels
Females	Males
Blacks in United States	Whites in United States
Exercise	Diabetes
Estrogen	Hypertriglyceridemia
Alcohol	High-carbohydrate diet
Weight reduction	Obesity
Nicotinic acid	Smoking
Fibric acid derivatives	Progesterone
Chlorinated hydrocarbons	Antihypertensive drugs
Familial hyperalphalipo-proteinemia	Sedentary lifestyle
Insulin	

From Giuliani ER, Gersh BJ, McGoon MD, Hayes DL, Schaff HV (editors): *Mayo Clinic Practice of Cardiology*. Third edition. Mosby, 1996, p 492. By permission of Mayo Foundation.

Small, Dense LDL Cholesterol

The intermediate LDL particles predominate in middle-aged, normolipemic persons, and the small, dense LDL particles seem to predominate in persons with coronary artery disease, non–insulin-dependent diabetes mellitus, hypertriglyceridemia, and familial hyperlipidemia. The small, dense LDL particles have the poorest affinity of all LDL subparticles for the LDL receptor, and hence they are cleared least from plasma by hepatic uptake. The small, dense LDL particle seems very atherogenic because of its relative ease at penetrating the arterial intima, its great affinity for the arterial wall matrix through binding of chondroitin sulfate proteoglycans, and its tendency to be efficiently taken up by human macrophages. The small, dense LDL particles have the least inherent resistance to oxidative modification, and thus they become very atherogenic when incorporated into the lipid-rich atherosclerotic plaque. Figure 1 depicts the proposed pathophysiologic process of small, dense LDL particles.

- The small, dense LDL particles have the poorest affinity of all LDL subparticles for the LDL receptor, are cleared least from plasma by hepatic uptake, have the least inherent resistance to oxidative modification, and are probably the most atherogenic type of LDL.

Currently, no strong epidemiologic data independently establish an association of increased small, dense LDL to an increased risk of development of coronary artery disease. However, there is indirect evidence that links the small, dense LDL particle to an increased risk of development of coronary artery disease in that multiple studies demonstrate an association between hypertriglyceridemia and the development of coronary artery disease. The small, dense LDL particle is a major fraction of LDL cholesterol in persons with concurrent hypertriglyceridemia.

Treatment of small, dense LDL cholesterol remains controversial. It is unclear whether statin therapy has a significant beneficial effect on small, dense LDL cholesterol. Fibrates may play a role in the treatment of small, dense LDL cholesterol. A recent study with fenofibrate (200 mg/day) demonstrated a 50% reduction in the concentration of small, dense LDL particles and a significant increase in intermediate LDL particles. The conversion of LDL then facilitates clearance by the LDL receptor. Treatment of small, dense LDL will depend on the results of epidemiologic studies that establish its association with the development of coronary artery disease. Future treatment strategies may combine fenofibrate with a statin to facilitate conversion of the small, dense LDL particle to an intermediate-density LDL particle, which is then more easily cleared by the LDL receptor.

- The small, dense LDL particle is frequently a major fraction of LDL cholesterol in patients with concurrent hypertriglyceridemia.
- Fenofibrate may alter cholesterol metabolism away from dense LDL particle production to intermediate LDL particles, which are more easily removed by the LDL receptor.
- Fenofibrate is probably the agent of choice to reduce an increased concentration of small, dense LDL particles.

Lipoprotein (a)

Lipoprotein (a) is a complex of apolipoprotein (a) bound to LDL cholesterol by a disulfide bond. Several epidemiologic studies have linked increased lipoprotein (a), Lp(a), to the development of coronary artery disease. Lp(a) has structural similarity to plasminogen, and the two molecules are coded by closely associated genes on chromosome 6.

Lp(a) has multiple pathophysiologic effects, including the following:

1. Inhibition of fibrinolysis through direct competition with plasminogen for tissue binding sites
2. Binding to fibrin, tissue factor inhibitor, endothelial cells, monocytes, and thrombospondin

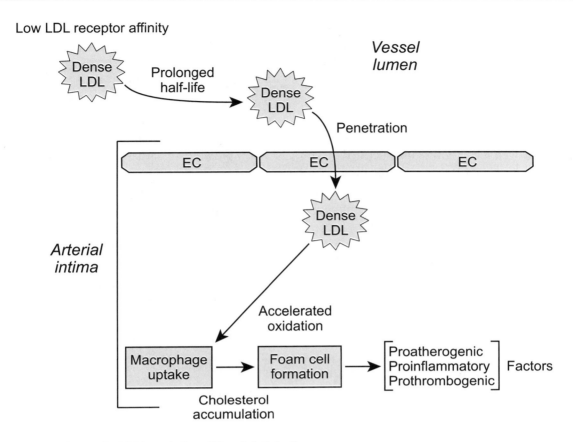

Fig. 1. Dense low-density lipoprotein (LDL) metabolism. EC, endothelial cell.

3. Competition with tissue plasminogen activator for binding sites and stimulation of synthesis of tissue plasminogen activator inhibitor
4. Facilitation of oxidation of LDL cholesterol and induction of formation of oxygen-free radicals in human monocytes
5. Inhibition of endothelial cell-independent vasorelaxation and, perhaps, promotion of smooth muscle proliferation

Lp(a) can be measured in plasma by an enzyme-linked immunosorbent assay method, but reference levels vary by race and perhaps by sex. Levels of Lp(a) are increased severalfold during an acute myocardial infarction, in response to pregnancy, in advanced malignancy, and in end-stage renal disease.

Multiple studies have shown a strong epidemiologic link between Lp(a) and the development of coronary artery disease. Data from the Framingham study suggest that the relative risk of development of coronary artery disease from Lp(a) is comparable to the relative risk of development of coronary artery disease from an increased LDL cholesterol level or a low HDL cholesterol level, but it is less than that observed for smoking and diabetes mellitus. The prevalence of an Lp(a) increase was lower than the prevalence of an increased total cholesterol or a low HDL cholesterol level in the Framingham data set (Plate 2).

In addition to epidemiologic data, Lp(a) appears mechanistically linked to the development of and progression of coronary artery disease. Lp(a) has been demonstrated in the arterial intima of native coronary arteries with atherosclerotic plaque and in saphenous vein grafts with atherosclerotic plaque. Increased Lp(a) has been associated with an increased risk of restenosis after percutaneous transluminal coronary angioplasty and with development of allograft vasculopathy in recipients of orthotopic heart transplants.

- Levels of Lp(a) are increased severalfold during an acute myocardial infarction, in response to pregnancy, in advanced malignancy, and in end-stage renal disease.

Despite the strong epidemiologic links between an increased Lp(a) concentration and the development of coronary artery disease, no study to date has demonstrated a reduction in future cardiac events by treatment of an increased

Lp(a) level. Several pharmacologic agents are effective for reducing Lp(a) concentrations. Nicotinic acid (niacin) can reduce Lp(a) concentrations up to 38%. Estrogen replacement can reduce Lp(a) concentrations by as much as 50% in postmenopausal women. The effect of estrogen is reduced when progesterone therapy is added in combination. No peer-reviewed published data exist with regard to the effect of the selective estrogen receptor modulators (SERMs) on Lp(a) concentrations. Fenofibrate and benzafibrate both reduce Lp(a) concentrations by as much as 30% to 40%, but gemfibrozil does not seem to affect Lp(a) concentrations. Statin drugs and cholestyramine do not affect Lp(a) concentrations. LDL apheresis can reduce Lp(a) concentrations, but LDL apheresis is not approved by the Food and Drug Administration for the treatment of an increased Lp(a) level. Finally, angiotensin-converting enzyme inhibitors, neomycin, and N-acetylcysteine lower Lp(a) concentrations in certain patient populations.

- Nicotinic acid, estrogens, fenofibrate, and benzafibrate reduce Lp(a), whereas statins and cholestyramine do not affect Lp(a) concentrations.

There is no consensus as to which populations are best served by screening for increased Lp(a) concentrations. Screening of low-risk patients for Lp(a) increase is not warranted, but Lp(a) should always be measured in patients with atherosclerosis who are nonsmokers, do not have diabetes, and have apparently normal LDL cholesterol levels while not taking lipid-lowering medication. Additionally, it is important to screen for increased Lp(a) in patients in whom statin treatment does not lower the LDL cholesterol to the desired target level, because Lp(a) can inhibit LDL clearance. Finally, it is appropriate to perform screening tests for increased Lp(a) and homocysteine levels in patients with a strong family history of premature coronary artery disease.

- It is important to screen for increased Lp(a) when statin treatment does not lower the LDL cholesterol level.

Fibrinogen and C-Reactive Protein

Increased fibrinogen and C-reactive protein levels are now recognized risk factors for the development of coronary artery disease. Several studies have demonstrated an epidemiologic link between increased fibrinogen and C-reactive protein levels and an increased risk of development of an acute

myocardial infarction. Data from the European Concerted Action on Thrombosis and Disabilities Angina Pectoris Study (ECAT) are shown in Plate 3. The data show an important interaction between fibrinogen, C-reactive protein, and increased serum cholesterol concentrations with regard to the risk of development of an acute coronary syndrome. One study found that an increased C-reactive protein value portends a poor prognosis in unstable angina.

It is unclear whether increased C-reactive protein and fibrinogen levels play direct mechanistic roles in the pathophysiology of the acute coronary syndrome or simply serve as markers of an inflammatory response process that is modulating the acute coronary syndrome. Several treatment options are available for patients with increased fibrinogen values. Smoking cessation and exercise are the best first-line therapies for reducing the fibrinogen level. Pravastatin and fenofibrate reduce fibrinogen concentrations. There are no outcome data on the effect of treatment for increased fibrinogen on the likelihood of future cardiac events.

- Smoking cessation, exercise, pravastatin, and fenofibrate reduce serum fibrinogen levels.

Homocysteine and Cardiovascular Disease

Several epidemiologic studies have linked hyperhomocysteinemia with an increased risk for coronary artery, cerebrovascular, and peripheral vascular disease. The exact mechanism(s) that explains the association between hyperhomocysteinemia and vascular disease remains unknown, but some investigators have postulated that hyperhomocysteinemia results in direct endothelial injury and a predisposition to a prothrombotic state.

One recent study underscored the potential importance of hyperhomocysteinemia to the risk of disease development. The relative risk for developing coronary artery disease was calculated at 1.9, whereas the relative risk for development of vascular disease was 3.3. This observed degree of magnitude is comparable to that of increased total cholesterol and low HDL cholesterol levels.

The treatment of hyperhomocysteinemia is relatively straightforward. The mainstay of therapy is folic acid supplementation (1 mg of folic acid supplementation daily). Many patients with hyperhomocysteinemia and atherosclerotic vascular disease are also deficient in vitamin B_6 or B_{12}, and we recommend that supplemental vitamin B_6 and B_{12} be given to all patients receiving folic acid for treatment of hyperhomocysteinemia. There are no outcome data on the impact of treatment of hyperhomocysteinemia on the development of future cardiovascular events. However, given the strong association between hyperhomocysteinemia and premature coronary artery and peripheral vascular disease, it seems prudent to treat all persons who have hyperhomocysteinemia.

- Treatment of hyperhomocysteinemia should be with supplementation with folic acid (1 mg/day), daily vitamin B_6, and monthly vitamin B_{12}.

Chlamydia pneumoniae Infection and Coronary Artery Disease

Several reports have identified staining antibodies for *Chlamydia pneumoniae* in the atherosclerotic plaque of patients with coronary artery disease. Several studies have linked an acute increase in IgG antibodies to *Chlamydia pneumoniae* during the course of an acute coronary syndrome. No studies have elucidated the mechanistic link between *Chlamydia pneumoniae* and the development of the acute coronary syndrome. Some authors have postulated that chronic or subacute infection with *Chlamydia pneumoniae* can serve to destabilize a previously stable atherosclerotic plaque and thus trigger the development of an acute coronary syndrome. Two small trials have empirically treated patients with increased IgG antibodies to *Chlamydia pneumoniae* with macrolide antibiotics. Several major trials are currently under way to test the efficacy of macrolide antibiotics in acute coronary syndromes, and it would be premature to recommend any course of treatment until the results are available.

- Two small trials have empirically treated patients with increased IgG antibodies to *Chlamydia pneumoniae* with macrolide antibiotics, but no specific recommendations for general therapy can be given at this stage.

Possible Risk Factors for Coronary Artery Disease

Several prospective additional risk factors also may have a mechanistic role in the development of atherosclerosis. Preliminary data have demonstrated an association between the angiotensin-converting enzyme gene and coronary artery disease. The D/D genotype occurs more frequently in persons with acute myocardial infarction than the I/D or I/I genotypes. These genotypes can be identified as circulating in plasma and may become important markers for identifying persons at high risk for development of coronary artery disease. At least two studies have examined the association between the expression of vascular disease in adults and the expression of the D/D and I/D genotypes in the grandchildren of adults with vascular disease. Both genotypes were increased in expression among second-degree relatives of patients with vascular disease.

- The D/D angiotensin-converting enzyme genotype occurs more frequently in persons with acute myocardial infarction than the I/D or I/I genotypes.

A recent report described a polymorphism in the glycoprotein IIb/IIIa receptor that may identify persons at highest risk for development of acute coronary syndromes. A single point mutation explains this polymorphism. Preliminary analysis of the Cholesterol and Recurrent Events (CARE) trial suggests that this polymorphism may have affected a significant percentage of patients in whom events occurred during follow-up. There may be an interaction between pravastatin and this polymorphism, which may explain some of the event reduction observed in the CARE trial.

Treatment Strategies and Goals for Therapy in Hyperlipidemia

Hyperlipidemia is appropriately identified and aggressively managed in less than 25% of all patients. The standard of care for patients with hyperlipidemia focuses on guidelines published by the National Cholesterol Education Program (NCEP) in 1993, outlining the nonpharmacologic and pharmacologic treatment of hyperlipidemia (Tables 2 through 7). The major target of therapy has been the LDL cholesterol, although recommendations regarding HDL cholesterol have been incorporated in the guidelines (Table 4). At least two ongoing randomized statin studies (atorvastatin, Lipitor; simvastatin, Zocor) are evaluating the effect of reducing the LDL value to targets that are lower than those advocated by the NCEP in the treatment of hyperlipidemia.

- The current standard of care for patients with hyperlipidemia centers on the guidelines published by the National Cholesterol Education Program (NCEP) in 1993.

Table 2.—National Cholesterol Education Program Recommendations for Dietary Treatment of Hyperlipidemia

	Initiating level	Minimal goal
Without CAD or two other risk factors	≥ 160 mg/dL (4.14 mmol/L)	< 160 mg/dL (4.14 mmol/L)
Without CAD and ≥ two other risk factors	≥ 130 mg/dL (3.36 mmol/L)	< 130 mg/dL (3.36 mmol/L)
With CAD	> 100 mg/dL (2.59 mmol/L)	≤ 100 mg/dL (2.59 mmol/L)

CAD, coronary artery disease.

Table 3.—National Cholesterol Education Program Recommendations for Drug Treatment of Hyperlipidemia

	Initiating level	Minimal goal
Without CAD or two other risk factors	≥ 190 mg/dL (4.91 mmol/L)	< 160 mg/dL (4.14 mmol/L)
Without CAD and ≥ two other risk factors	≥ 160 mg/dL (4.14 mmol/L)	< 130 mg/dL (3.36 mmol/L)
With CAD	> 130 mg/dL (3.36 mmol/L)	≤ 100 mg/dL (2.59 mmol/L)

CAD, coronary artery disease.

Table 4.—Treatment Strategies for Hyperlipidemia

Patient characteristics	LDL goal	HDL goal	Treatment strategies
Asymptomatic patient with no or one CAD risk factor	< 160 mg/dL or 4.1 mmol/L	> 35 mg/dL or 0.9 mmol/L	Diet, exercise, smoking cessation, weight loss, control of diabetes, consider statin agent, niacin, BAS
Asymptomatic patient with 2 or more CAD risk factors and normal triglycerides	< 130 mg/dL or 3.4 mmol/L	> 35 mg/dL or 0.9 mmol/L	Statin BAS Niacin Statin + BAS Statin + niacin
Asymptomatic patient with 2 or more CAD risk factors and elevated triglycerides (> 200 mg/dL)	< 130 mg/dL or 3.4 mmol/L	> 35 mg/dL or 0.9 mmol/L	Niacin Statin Gemfibrozil Statin + gemfibrozil Statin + niacin
Patient with known CAD and normal triglycerides	< 100 mg/dL or 2.6 mmol/L	> 35 mg/dL or 0.9 mmol/L	Statin BAS Niacin Statin + BAS Statin + niacin
Patient with known CAD and elevated triglycerides (> 200 mg/dL)	< 100 mg/dL or 2.6 mmol/L	> 35 mg/dL or 0.9 mmol/L	Niacin Statin Gemfibrozil Statin + gemfibrozil Statin + niacin

BAS, bile acid sequestrants; CAD, coronary artery disease; HDL, high-density lipoprotein; LDL, low-density lipoprotein.

Table 5.—Practical Treatment Strategy

Lipid profile	Diet	Drug
↑ LDL cholesterol (type II-A) ↑ Cholesterol Triglycerides normal	Low fat Low cholesterol	Statin BAS Niacin Statin + BAS Statin + niacin
↑ VLDL (type IV and V) ↑ Cholesterol ↑ Triglycerides (1/5 x TG)	↓ Wt ↓ Sugar ↓ Alcohol Low fat Low cholesterol	Niacin Gemfibrozil
↑ LDL and ↑ VLDL (type II-B) ↑ Cholesterol ↑ Triglycerides	↓ Wt ↓ Sugar ↓ Alcohol Low fat Low cholesterol	Statin Niacin Gemfibrozil Statin + niacin Statin + gemfibrozil

BAS, bile acid sequestrants; LDL, low-density lipoprotein; TG, triglycerides; VLDL, very low-density lipoprotein; wt, weight.

Table 6.—Risk Factors for Coronary Artery Disease

Positive risk factors
    Age, years
        Male ≥ 45
        Female ≥ 55
    Family history of premature CAD (≤ 55 years of age in
      father or first-degree male relative, ≤ 65 years of age in
      mother or first-degree female relative)
    Cigarette smoking (current or quit < 2 years ago)
    Hypertension (BP ≥ 140/90 mm Hg) or on treatment for
      hypertension
    Increased LDL cholesterol (LDL cholesterol > 130
      mg/dL)
    Low HDL cholesterol (HDL cholesterol < 35 mg/dL)
    Diabetes mellitus (treated or not)
Negative risk factors
    High HDL cholesterol (HDL cholesterol > 60 mg/dL)[*]

BP, blood pressure; CAD, coronary artery disease; HDL, high-density lipoprotein; LDL, low-density lipoprotein.
[*]Subtract one from the number of positive risk factors if high HDL cholesterol is present.

Approach to the Patient with Hyperlipidemia

All patients with hyperlipidemia, irrespective of their use of lipid-lowering drugs, should be managed with a low-fat, low-cholesterol diet with less than 30% of calories derived from total fat (less than 40 grams of fat per day), less than 300 mg of cholesterol a day, and enough calories to maintain a desirable weight. They should also initiate a regular aerobic exercise program. Patients who smoke also should be counseled to quit smoking immediately. Concurrent illnesses that have an impact on serum lipids (diabetes mellitus, hypothyroidism, nephrotic syndrome, chronic renal failure, excess alcohol consumption) should be managed as appropriate.

In clinical practice, less than 20% of patients with coronary disease will attain the NCEP guidelines without medication. Strict low-fat diets, including the Ornish diet and vegetarian diets, are effective for lowering lipid values for the committed patient. It is important to achieve the target LDL cholesterol value established by the NCEP guidelines within a short time for persons with documented coronary artery disease or diabetes mellitus. The overwhelming benefit (secondary prevention) achieved through lowering of the cholesterol value appears to begin early after the initiation of therapy. Because most patients cannot achieve the desired target LDL cholesterol value by nonpharmacologic

intervention alone, it is very reasonable to initiate the combined approach of pharmacologic and nonpharmacologic treatment of hyperlipidemia as soon as possible for persons with known coronary artery disease or diabetes. We recommend that the combined approach of pharmacologic and nonpharmacologic treatment of hyperlipidemia begin during the hospitalization period for persons hospitalized for unstable angina or myocardial infarction. Data will

Table 7.—Causes of Secondary Hyperlipidemia

Hypertriglyceridemia	Hypercholesterolemia
Excessive alcohol or simple sugars	Excessive dietary cholesterol or saturated fats (or both)
Contraceptives, estrogen, pregnancy	Hypothyroidism
Obesity	Obstructive liver disease
Diabetes mellitus	Nephrotic syndrome
Chronic renal failure	Multiple myeloma or dysglobulinemia
Cushing's disease, corticosteroid therapy	Progestational agents and anabolic steroids

From *Mayo Clin Proc* 63:605-621, 1988. By permission of Mayo Foundation for Medical Education and Research.

soon be published demonstrating enhanced 1-year compliance with treatment of hyperlipidemia when it is initiated during hospitalization.   No patient with coronary artery disease or diabetes mellitus should try nonpharmacologic therapy for any longer than 6 weeks before a decision is made regarding initiation of treatment with a lipid-lowering agent. Equally, if a patient can achieve the NCEP guidelines without medication, this is an acceptable approach. For patients without diabetes who have moderate hyperlipidemia, but without documented coronary artery disease,

a trial of nonpharmacologic therapy for up to several months may be reasonable.

- All patients with hyperlipidemia, irrespective of their use of lipid-lowering drugs, should follow a low-fat, low-cholesterol diet.
- Pharmacologic *and* nonpharmacologic management of hyperlipidemia are often necessary for persons with known coronary artery disease or diabetes mellitus, and they *can be initiated together during the hospitalization.*

Suggested Review Reading

1. The Agency for Health Care Policy and Research Smoking Cessation Clinical Practice Guideline. *JAMA* 275:1270-1280, 1996.

2. Consensus Conference: Lowering blood cholesterol to prevent heart disease. *JAMA* 253:2080-2086, 1985.

3. Gordon DJ: Cholesterol-lowering and total mortality. In *Lowering Cholesterol in High-Risk Individuals and Populations.* Edited by BM Rifkind. New York, Marcel Dekker, 1995, p 33.

4. Holme I: Cholesterol reduction and its impact on coronary artery disease and total mortality. *Am J Cardiol* 76:10C-17C, 1995.

5. Kannel WB: Range of serum cholesterol values in the population developing coronary artery disease. *Am J Cardiol* 76:69C-77C, 1995.

6. Neaton JD, Blackburn H, Jacobs D, et al: Serum cholesterol level and mortality findings for men screened in the Multiple Risk Factor Intervention Trial. *Arch Intern Med* 152:1490-1500, 1992.

7. O'Connor GT, Buring JE, Yusuf S, et al: An overview of randomized trials of rehabilitation with exercise after myocardial infarction. *Circulation* 80:234-244, 1989.

8. Oldridge NB, Guyatt GH, Fischer ME, et al: Cardiac rehabilitation after myocardial infarction. Combined experience of randomized clinical trials. *JAMA* 260:945-950, 1988.

9. Rossouw JE, Rifkind BM: Lowering cholesterol concentrations and mortality (III). *BMJ* 301:814-815, 1990.

10. Rubins HB, Robins SJ, Collins D, et al: Distribution of lipids in 8,500 men with coronary artery disease. *Am J Cardiol* 75:1196-1201, 1995.

11. Summary of the second report of the National Cholesterol Education Program (NCEP) Expert Panel on Detection, Evaluation, and Treatment of High Blood Cholesterol in Adults. *JAMA* 269:3015-3023, 1993.

12. Thom TJ, Epstein FH, Feldman JJ, et al: Total mortality and mortality from heart disease, cancer, and stroke from 1950 to 1987 in 27 countries. (NIH Publication No. 92-3088.) Bethesda, Maryland, National Institutes of Health, 1992, pp 159; 166.

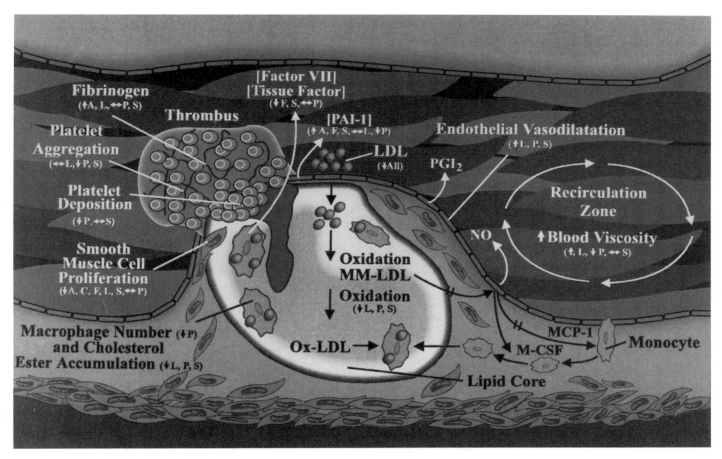

Plate 1. Coronary plaque disruption and major pathophysiologic pathways as influenced by various statin therapies. The diagram depicts an acute plaque disruption and resultant thrombus formation. Recirculation zones increase blood viscosity, which foster rapid plaque formation. NO, nitric oxide; PAI-1, plasminogen activator inhibitor 1; PGI$_2$, prostacyclin; MCP-1, monocyte chemotactic protein 1; M-CSF, monocyte colony-stimulating factor; LDL, low-density lipoprotein; Ox-LDL, oxidized low-density lipoprotein; MM-LDL, minimally modified low-density lipoprotein; A, atorvastatin; C, cerivastatin; F, fluvastatin; L, lovastatin; P, pravastatin; S, simvastatin. ↑, increase; ↓, decrease; ↔, no effect. (From *JAMA* 279:1643-1650, 1998. By permission of the American Medical Association.)

Factor	Relative risk	95% CI	Prevalence
Lp (a)	1.9	1.2-2.9	11.3
TC ≥ 240	1.8	1.2-2.7	14.3
HDL ≤ 35	1.8	1.2-2.6	19.2
Smoking	3.6	2.2-5.5	46.7
Glucose ≥ 120	2.7	1.4-5.3	2.6
Hypertension	1.2	0.8-1.8	26.3

Plate 2. Impact of risk factors for coronary artery disease. HDL, high-density lipoprotein; Lp(a), lipoprotein (a); TC, triglycerides. (Modified from *JAMA* 276:544-548, 1996. By permission of the American Medical Association.)

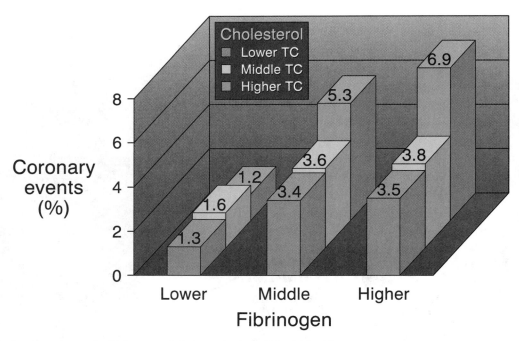

Plate 3. Risk of coronary events, by fibrinogen and cholesterol values. TC, triglycerides.

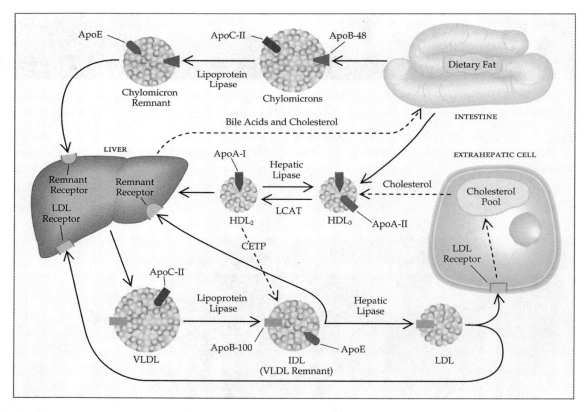

Plate 4. Metabolism of the major lipoproteins within the plasma. The intestine absorbs dietary fat into chylomicrons that contain apoB-48. Lipoprotein lipase and its cofactor, apoC-II, hydrolyze chylomicrons to remnants that are taken up by the liver by the binding of apoE. The liver secretes lipids as very low-density lipoprotein (VLDL) with apoB-100. VLDL is hydrolyzed to IDL, some of which is taken up by the liver. IDL is further hydrolyzed by hepatic lipase to become low-density lipoprotein (LDL). Hepatic and extrahepatic cells remove LDL from the circulation when apoB-100 binds to the LDL receptor. High-density lipoprotein (HDL) is thought to remove excess cholesterol from cells and target it to the liver for excretion in the bile. The metabolism of lipoproteins is shown by *solid arrows*, and the transport of cholesterol, when not contained within lipoproteins, is indicated by *broken arrows*. CETP, cholesterol ester transfer protein; LCAT, lecithin: cholesterol acyltransferase. (From Haber E: *Molecular Cardiovascular Medicine.* Scientific American, 1995, p 98. By permission of the publisher.)

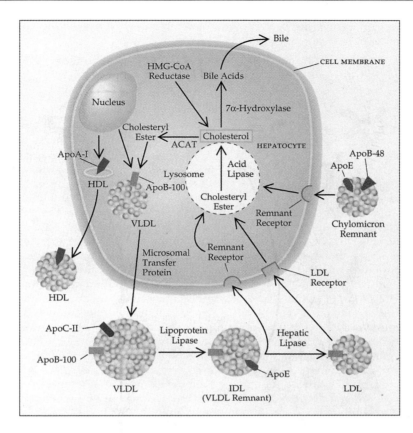

Plate 5. Metabolism of cholesterol and lipoproteins by the hepatocyte. Intracellular cholesterol is derived from new synthesis via HMG-CoA reductase or from hydrolysis by acid lipase of cholesteryl esters derived from uptake of lipoprotein. Cholesterol can be converted to bile acids, excreted directly into the bile, or esterified to cholesteryl ester by acyl-cholesterol acyltransferase for secretion in very low-density lipoprotein (VLDL). HDL, high-density lipoprotein; LDL, low-density lipoprotein. (From Haber E: *Molecular Cardiovascular Medicine*. Scientific American, 1995, p 105. By permission of the publisher.)

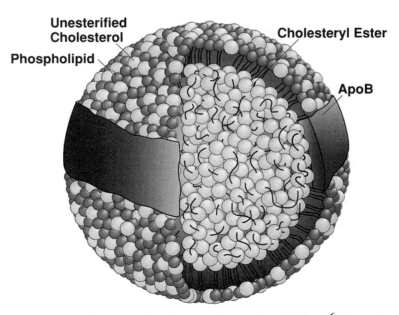

Plate 6. Low-density lipoprotein is a complex spherical particle with a mass of approximately 2.5×10^6 daltons. It consists of a hydrophobic core containing approximately 1,500 cholesteryl ester molecules and an amphipathic lipid monolayer shell of unesterified cholesterol and phospholipid in which the protein apolipoprotein B-100 (approximately 513 kilodaltons) is embedded. Apolipoprotein B-100 is responsible for binding native LDL to LDL receptors and for binding chemically modified LDL to macrophage scavenger receptors. (From Haber E: *Molecular Cardiovascular Medicine*. Scientific American, 1995, p 33, as modified from *Scientific Am* 251: 58-66, 1984. By permission of Ikuyo Tagawa Garber.)

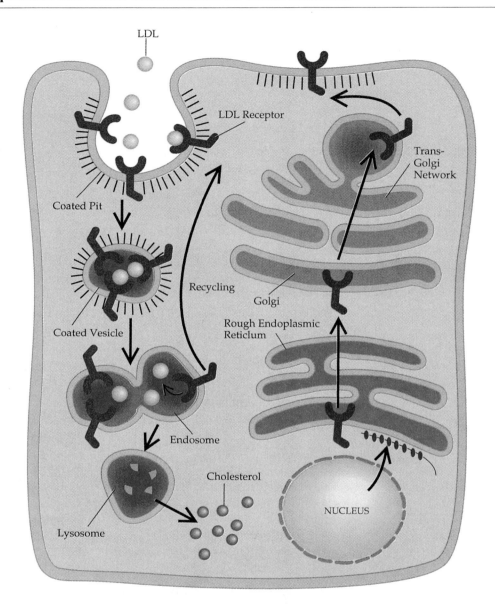

Plate 7. Low-density lipoprotein (LDL) receptors are synthesized as integral membrane proteins in the rough endoplasmic reticulum, where they are covalently modified by asparagine-linked and serine/threonine-linked glycosylation. The receptors are transported to the Golgi apparatus and the trans-Golgi network for additional processing of their polysaccharide chains and sorting to the cell surface. Receptor-mediated endocytosis of LDL occurs via a coated pit–coated vesicle-mediated pathway. In brief, after high-affinity binding of ligands to the receptor, invagination of cell surface coated pits that contain the receptor-ligand complex results in the formation of coated endocytic vesicles. These are converted to endosomes. The low pH in the lumen of the endosome induces receptor-ligand dissociation, after which the receptors recycle to the cell surface and the LDL is delivered to lysosomes for enzymatic digestion. This digestion leads to the release of cholesterol from the LDL (see Plate 6) and its subsequent entry into the metabolic pool of the cell. As a consequence, LDL receptor and cholesterol synthesis is suppressed and cholesterol storage as cholesteryl esters is stimulated. (From Haber E: *Molecular Cardiovascular Medicine*. Scientific American, 1995, p 35. By permission of the publisher.)

Chapter 11

Percutaneous Transluminal Coronary Angioplasty and Bypass Surgery in Coronary Artery Disease

Charanjit S. Rihal, M.D.
Hugh C. Smith, M.D.

There are three broad indications for myocardial revascularization in coronary artery disease:

1. To treat the symptoms of angina pectoris
2. To improve long-term survival
3. To prevent nonfatal events such as nonfatal myocardial infarction, congestive heart failure, or serious ventricular arrhythmias.

Trials of Coronary Artery Bypass Grafting Versus Medical Therapy

Seven prospective randomized trials, performed mainly in the 1970s, directly compared coronary artery bypass grafting (CABG) with medical therapy for chronic coronary artery disease. The three largest trials were the Veterans Administration Cooperative Study (VAC), the European Coronary Surgery Study (ECSS), and the Coronary Artery Surgery Study (CASS). Although a relatively small number of patients (2,649) were enrolled in these randomized trials, the data constitute the bulk of the evidence on which current myocardial revascularization strategies are based. In these trials, 20% of the patients had an ejection fraction less than 50%, and the majority of patients had either three-vessel (51%) or left main coronary artery (7%) disease. Almost all patients were men 40 to 60 years old, and only

3% were taking antiplatelet drugs upon enrollment. These trials were performed before the widespread use of effective lipid-lowering agents. A systematic overview (meta-analysis) of these trials was published by Yusuf et al. (*Lancet*, 1994).

Long-term follow-up of the patients over 12 years revealed a significant survival benefit of CABG, although there was an initial risk at the time of the procedure (Fig. 1). At 5 and 10 years, 10% and 26% of patients, respectively, initially treated with CABG had died, compared with 16% and 31% of those who received medical treatment. These values correspond to significant risk reductions (relative risk, 0.61 and 0.83). The significant risk reductions occurred even though a 40% "crossover" to CABG occurred by 10 years among patients in the medical treatment group.

Subgroup analysis identified particular subsets of patients in whom a greater benefit was found. The survival benefit of CABG compared with medical therapy is proportional to the baseline cardiac risk, as assessed by the number of diseased coronary arteries, the degree of left ventricular dysfunction, and the extent of myocardial ischemia. Patients with greater abnormalities of these characteristics derive the greatest benefit. At long-term follow-up, the relative risk of dying with CABG (compared with medical therapy) was 0.58 for three-vessel disease and 0.32 for left main coronary artery disease. In particular, a survival benefit was

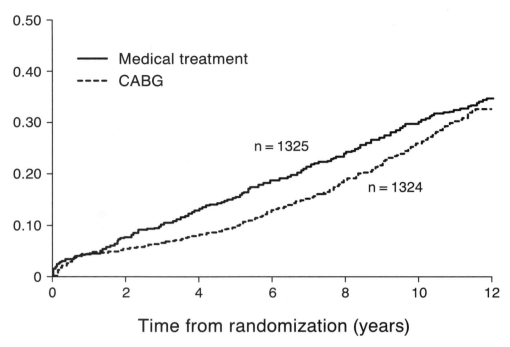

Fig. 1. Overall survival after random allocation to medical treatment of coronary artery bypass graft (CABG). (From *Lancet* 344:563-570, 1994. By permission of The Lancet.)

found if the left anterior descending artery was involved with disease (relative risk of 0.58 even in one- or two-vessel disease). Although the relative benefit was similar whether or not left ventricular dysfunction was present, the *absolute* benefit was greater among patients with low ejection fractions, because this group has a much higher absolute risk with medical treatment (Table 1).

- The survival benefit of CABG compared with medical therapy is proportional to the baseline cardiac risk, as assessed by the number of diseased coronary arteries, the degree of left ventricular dysfunction, and the extent of myocardial ischemia.

No benefit in reducing myocardial infarction could be demonstrated. This was due primarily to the risk of perioperative death or myocardial infarction (10% at 30 days). Overall, the 5-year incidence of death or myocardial infarction was 24% for the CABG group and 31% for the medical group.

In summary, the prospective randomized trials of CABG versus medical therapy indicate that CABG can reduce the risk of mortality by about 40% compared with medical therapy. The benefits of bypass surgery are maximized among the highest risk patients, specifically those with left main coronary artery disease, three-vessel disease, involvement of the

proximal left anterior descending artery, left ventricular dysfunction, and severe myocardial ischemia. No net benefit in terms of reducing myocardial infarction has been demonstrated. These trials are significantly limited by their age, the overwhelming predominance of male subjects, and the relatively low use of antiplatelet agents and effective lipid-lowering drugs. Also, the proportion of patients older than 60 years or with low ejection fraction was small (Table 2).

Percutaneous Transluminal Coronary Angioplasty for Single-Vessel Disease

To date, few prospective randomized studies have directly compared percutaneous transluminal coronary angioplasty (PTCA) with medical therapy among patients with single-vessel disease. The Angioplasty Compared to Medicine (ACME) study, a comparison of angioplasty with medical therapy, enrolled 212 patients with stable single-vessel disease and a positive stress test. Patients were randomly assigned to either angioplasty or medical therapy and were followed prospectively for 6 months. No patient in the PTCA arm died, but one patient in the medical arm died after a nonprotocol PTCA. The proportion of patients completely free of angina was greater in the PTCA arm, and the number of anginal episodes among the rest of them was

Table 1.—Outcomes of Various Subgroups in Medical Therapy Versus CABG Trials at 5 Years

Subgroup	Overall numbers		Medical treatment mortality rate, %	Odds ratio (95% CI)	P for CABG vs medical treatment	P for inter-action
	Deaths	Patients				
Vessel disease						0.19
One vessel	21	271	9.9	0.54 (0.22-1.33)	0.18	
Two vessels	92	859	11.7	0.84 (0.54-1.32)	0.45	
Three vessels	189	1,341	17.6	0.58 (0.42-0.80)	< 0.001	
Left main artery	39	150	36.5	0.32 (0.15-0.70)	0.004	
No LAD disease						0.06
One or two vessels	50	606	8.3	1.05 (0.58-1.90)	0.88	
Three vessels	46	410	14.5	0.47 (0.25-0.89)	0.02	
Left main artery	16	51	45.8	0.27 (0.08-0.90)	0.03	
Overall	112	1,067	12.3	0.66 (0.44-1.00)	0.05	
LAD disease present						0.44
One or two vessels	63	524	14.6	0.58 (0.34-1.01)	0.05	
Three vessels	143	929	19.1	0.61 (0.42-0.88)	0.009	
Left main artery	22	96	32.7	0.30 (0.11-0.84)	0.02	
Overall	228	1,549	18.3	0.58 (0.43-0.77)	0.001	
LV function						0.90
Normal	228	2,095	13.3	0.61 (0.46-0.81)	< 0.001	
Abnormal	115	549	25.2	0.59 (0.39-0.91)	0.02	
Exercise test status						0.37
Missing	102	664	17.4	0.69 (0.45-1.07)	0.10	
Normal	60	585	11.6	0.78 (0.45-1.35)	0.38	
Abnormal	183	1,400	16.8	0.52 (0.37-0.72)	< 0.001	
Severity of angina						0.69
Class 0, I, II	178	1,716	12.5	0.63 (0.46-0.87)	0.005	
Class III, IV	167	924	22.4	0.57 (0.40-0.81)	0.001	

CABG, coronary artery bypass graft; CI, confidence interval; LAD, left anterior descending; LV, left ventricle.
From *Lancet* 344:563-570, 1994. By permission of The Lancet.

decreased by angioplasty. Medication use was reduced among angioplasty patients, but it was not eliminated. An objective, modest increase in treadmill exercise test duration was demonstrated among the PTCA arm, even though all antianginal medications being taken were withheld.

Two emergency bypass operations and four myocardial infarctions occurred in the PTCA group, and by 6 months, 7 patients had undergone bypass surgery and 16 required nonprotocol angioplasty. In the medical arm, 11 patients required nonprotocol PTCA for increasing symptoms, but none required CABG. No difference in the rates of myocardial infarction was found (five in the PTCA arm versus three in the medical arm).

The Randomized Intervention Treatment of Angina (RITA)-2 trial was a prospective randomized trial of 1,018 patients with stable coronary artery disease conducted at 20 sites in the UK and Ireland. It tested the hypothesis that elective PTCA would decrease the combined frequency of all-cause death and nonfatal myocardial infarction. Patients with recent unstable symptoms were excluded and 80% of patients had class 0 to 2 angina. Also, 78% of patients were taking one or two antianginal drugs at enrollment, 60% had single-vessel coronary artery disease, 33% had two-vessel disease, and 7% had three-vessel disease. Only 6% of the patients had significant left ventricular dysfunction. Results over a median follow-up of 2.7 years are shown in Figure 2. Eighteen patients died, and the primary end point of death or myocardial infarction occurred in 6.3% of the PTCA group and in 3.3% of the medical therapy group (absolute difference, 3.0%; 95% confidence interval, 0.4%-5.7%; P = 0.02). The difference was

Table 2.—Clinical and Angiographic Characteristics of Patients Enrolled in Randomized Trials of CABG Versus Medical Therapy

Characteristic	% of patients
Age distribution, yr	
< 40	8.5
41-50	38.2
51-60	46.0
> 60	7.3
Ejection fraction ($n = 2,474$)	
< 40	7.2
40-49	12.5
50-59	28.0
≥ 60	52.3
Male	96.8
Severity of angina	
None	11.2
Class I or II	53.8
Class III or IV	35.0
History	
Myocardial infarction	59.6
Hypertension	26.0
Heart failure	4.0
Diabetes mellitus	9.6
Smoking ($n = 1,949$)	83.5
Current smokers ($n = 2,298$)	45.5
ST-segment depression > 1 mm	
Resting ($n = 2,423$)	9.9
Exercise ($n = 1,985$)	70.5
Drugs at baseline	
β-Blockers ($n = 2,308$)	47.4
Antiplatelet agents ($n = 1,195$)	3.2
Digitalis ($n = 2,319$)	12.9
Diuretics ($n = 1,940$)	12.6
No. of vessels diseased	
Left main artery	6.6
One vessel*	10.2
Two vessels*	32.4
Three vessels*	50.6
Location of disease	
Proximal left anterior descending	59.4
Left anterior descending diagonal	60.4
Circumflex	73.8
Right coronary	81.6

Data on some characteristics are not available for all patients: for data available for less than 90% of patients, numbers of patients with available data are shown in parentheses.
CABG, coronary artery bypass graft.
*Without left main coronary artery.
From *Lancet* 344:563-570, 1994. By permission of The Lancet.

attributable mainly to one death and seven infarctions among patients who had PTCA. The combined rates of death, myocardial infarction, and nonprotocol revascularization were about 25% in both groups by 3 years of follow-up, primarily due to worsening of symptoms of those in the medical group. Angina pectoris and treadmill exercise time improved significantly in both groups, but especially in the PTCA group (absolute 16.5% excess of class 2 or worse angina in the medical group at 3 months). In both groups, as patients with severe symptoms underwent nonprotocol revascularization over 3 years of follow-up, the difference in reported angina decreased (absolute 7.6% difference in class 2 angina or worse). Patients with class 2 or worse angina appeared to benefit from PTCA, with a 20% lower incidence of angina and 1-minute longer treadmill exercise time, whereas patients with mild symptoms at enrollment derived no significant improvement in symptoms.

The results of these randomized trials, which enrolled relatively low-risk patients (average mortality, 0.7%/year in RITA-2) with coronary artery disease, indicate that PTCA (plus needed antianginal medications) can improve symptoms compared with medical treatment alone. However, there is no apparent reduction in need for subsequent PTCA or CABG and little apparent impact on myocardial infarction or risk of death (and, in fact, an increase, because of periprocedural complications). These data suggest that for low-risk patients, PTCA is indicated only if the desired level of anginal relief cannot be achieved with medical therapy. On the basis of these data, "prophylactic" PTCA for mild symptoms or symptoms controlled by medical therapy cannot be recommended. Because the total number of patients enrolled in these trials was relatively small, the possibility of missing clinically important differences (type II errors) cannot be excluded. It cannot be determined from these data whether newer interventional and medical therapies, in particular stents (used in only 8% of patients in RITA-2), HMG-CoA reductase, and the newer more powerful antiplatelet agents, may significantly mitigate the observed risks and benefits.

Comparison of PTCA and CABG for Single-Vessel Disease

In general, medical therapy is indicated for single-vessel coronary artery disease, and no significant improvement in long-term survival can be expected following revascularization. Revascularization may be indicated for symptom relief, and three prospective randomized trials have compared

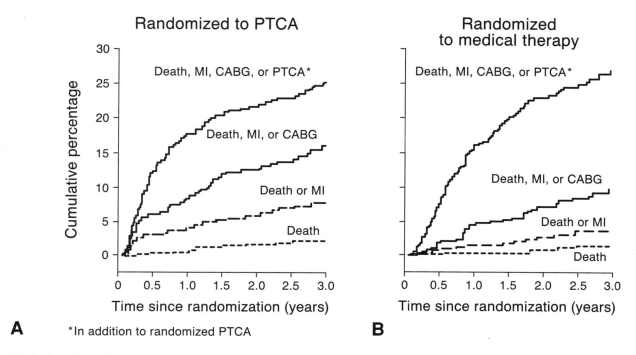

Fig. 2. Cumulative risk of percutaneous transluminal coronary angioplasty (PTCA), coronary artery bypass graft (CABG), myocardial infarction (MI), or death. *A*, Randomized to PTCA; *B*, randomized to medical therapy. (From *Lancet* 350:461-468, 1997. By permission of The Lancet.)

PTCA with CABG in this population. These have included the European Laussane, the British RITA, and the South American (Medicine, Angioplasty, or Surgery Study [MASS]) studies. The largest of these was the RITA study, which included 456 patients with single-vessel disease. The observed results were consistent across the three studies and indicated relief of angina in a high proportion of patients, whether treated with PTCA or CABG, but no significant differences in death plus myocardial infarction. Patients randomly assigned to angioplasty required a greater number of repeat interventions for the treatment of restenosis. These studies confirmed that both PTCA and CABG are highly effective in improving symptoms among patients with single-vessel disease when the disease becomes refractory to medical therapy. Neither of the revascularization modalities was associated with a clear decrease in either mortality or subsequent myocardial infarction. Because of the unsolved problem of restenosis, patients undergoing angioplasty require more repeat procedures.

Multivessel Disease

Historically, CABG has been the mainstay of therapy for patients with multivessel coronary artery disease, especially in the presence of left ventricular dysfunction. Nine recent prospective randomized studies have compared PTCA with CABG for the treatment of patients with multivessel disease (Table 3). Because of the relatively small size of each trial, none was adequately powered statistically to detect or to exclude differences in mortality, and various composite clinical end points were used. A systematic overview of eight of these trials was published by Pocock et al. (*Lancet*, 1995). When pooled, 3,371 patients were included, with 1,661 randomly assigned to CABG and 1,710 to PTCA. Mean follow-up was 2.7 years. Overall mortality was relatively low: 4.4% of patients in the CABG group and 4.6% of those in the PTCA group died (P = NS). The composite end point of death or myocardial infarction occurred in 7.6% of the CABG group and 7.9% of the PTCA group (P = NS) (Fig. 3). As expected, repeat revascularization within 1 year was required more often in the PTCA group, specifically in 33.7% (including 18% who crossed over to bypass surgery) but in only 3.3% of those assigned to bypass surgery. The prevalence of angina pectoris class II or greater was higher in the PTCA group at 1 year, but this difference was minimal by 3 years of follow-up (Fig. 4).

The Bypass Angioplasty Revascularization Investigation (BARI) trial was published in early 1996 in the *New England Journal of Medicine* and represents the single largest recent

Table 3.—Main Characteristics of Nine Prospective, Randomized Trials of Percutaneous Transluminal Coronary Angioplasty Versus Coronary Artery Bypass Grafting*

	BARI	CABRI	EAST	ERACI	GABI	MASS	RITA	Swiss	Toulouse
Location	North America, multicenter	Europe multi-center	Emory University (Atlanta, GA), single-center	Argentina, single-center	Germany, multi-center	SA, single-center	Britain, multi-center	Switzerland, single-center	France, single-center
No. of patients screened	25,200	?	5,118	1,409	8,981	?	17,237	?	?
Randomized (%)	1,829 (7.3)	1,054	392 (7.7)	127 (9.0)	359 (4.0)	214	1,011 (4.8)	142	152
Equivalent revascularization required	No	No	No	No	Yes	Yes	Yes	Yes	Yes
Follow-up duration planned (yr)	10	5-10	3	3	1	3.5	5	2.5	3
Completed	No	No	Yes	Yes	Yes	Yes	No	Yes	Yes
Primary end point	Mortality, MI	Mortality, nonfatal MI, angina, functional capacity	Combined death, MI, and large thallium defect	Combined death, MI, and angina	Freedom from angina at 1 year (> CCS 2)	Combined cardiac death, MI, refractory angina	Combined death and MI	Death, MI, repeat revascularisation	?

CCS, Canadian Cardiovascular Society class; MI, myocardial infarction; SA, South America.

*Names of trials: BARI, Bypass Angioplasty Revascularization Investigation; CABRI, Coronary Angioplasty Versus Bypass Revascularization Investigation; EAST, Emory Angioplasty Versus Surgery Trial; ERACI, Argentine Randomized Trial of Percutaneous Transluminal Coronary Angioplasty Versus Coronary Artery Bypass Surgery in Multivessel Disease; GABI, German Angioplasty Bypass Surgery Investigation; MASS, Medicine, Angioplasty, or Surgery Study; RITA, Randomized Intervention Treatment of Angina.

From Kusof S, Cairns JA, Fallen E, et al (editors): *Evidence Based Cardiology.* BMJ Publishing Group, 1998. By permission of the publisher.

PTCA versus CABG trial. It enrolled 1,829 patients who were prospectively followed for 5 years. Five-year Kaplan-Meier mortality was 11% among the CABG group and 14% among those assigned to PTCA. The incidence of death or Q-wave myocardial infarction at 5 years was 19% and 21% for the CABG and PTCA groups, respectively. Of the PTCA group, 54% required additional procedures, compared with 8% of the CABG group. In most cases, this was due to restenosis and was effectively treated by repeat angioplasty, with the result that 69% of the patients initially assigned to PTCA did not require subsequent CABG surgery. The overall 3% mortality difference did not reach statistical significance except for one subgroup, treated diabetics. Among diabetics requiring medical treatment, 5-year mortality was 19% in the CABG group and 35% in the PTCA group ($P = 0.003$). The authors concluded that PTCA does not compromise 5-year survival, with the exception of treated diabetics, and that repeat procedures are required more frequently among patients undergoing multivessel angioplasty.

Several secondary substudies have demonstrated that both PTCA and CABG produce similar benefits in quality of life measures and return to employment and are nearly equivalent in cost after 3 to 5 years of follow-up, although a slight advantage toward PTCA persists. In total, these

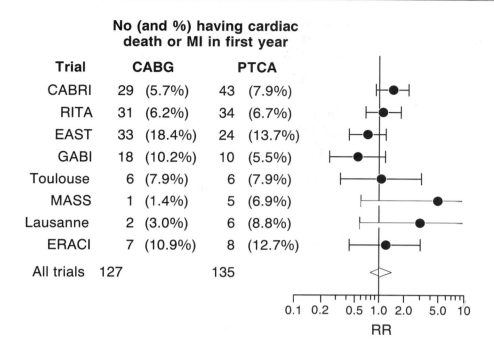

No (and %) having cardiac death or MI in first year

Trial	CABG		PTCA	
CABRI	29	(5.7%)	43	(7.9%)
RITA	31	(6.2%)	34	(6.7%)
EAST	33	(18.4%)	24	(13.7%)
GABI	18	(10.2%)	10	(5.5%)
Toulouse	6	(7.9%)	6	(7.9%)
MASS	1	(1.4%)	5	(6.9%)
Lausanne	2	(3.0%)	6	(8.8%)
ERACI	7	(10.9%)	8	(12.7%)
All trials	127		135	

Fig. 3. Cardiac death or myocardial infarction (MI) for percutaneous transluminal coronary angioplasty (PTCA) group compared with coronary artery bypass graft (CABG) group in the first year after randomization. For full names of trials, see Table 3. (From *Lancet* 346:1184-1189, 1995. By permission of The Lancet.)

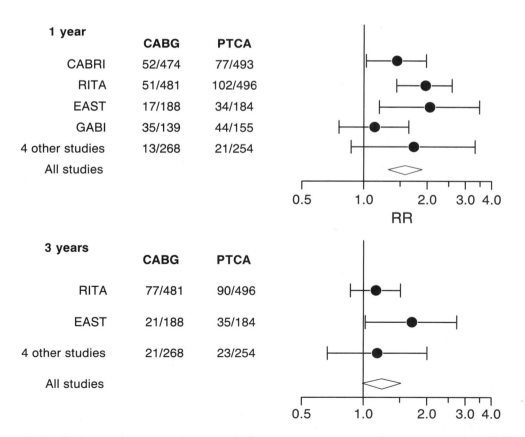

1 year

	CABG	PTCA
CABRI	52/474	77/493
RITA	51/481	102/496
EAST	17/188	34/184
GABI	35/139	44/155
4 other studies	13/268	21/254
All studies		

3 years

	CABG	PTCA
RITA	77/481	90/496
EAST	21/188	35/184
4 other studies	21/268	23/254
All studies		

Fig. 4. Prevalence of ≥ class 2 angina pectoris after random allocation to percutaneous transluminal coronary angioplasty (PTCA) or to coronary artery bypass graft (CABG). For full names of trials, see Table 3. (From *Lancet* 346:1184-1189, 1995. By permission of The Lancet.)

nine studies have randomly assigned 5,200 patients with multivessel coronary artery disease to either PTCA or CABG. Updated meta-analyses for mortality, myocardial infarction, and nonprotocol revascularization are shown in Tables 4 to 6. No clear advantage of one procedure has been demonstrated conclusively for any group of patients, except possibly for treated diabetics. Both procedures provide good symptom relief, and by 3 years, overall angina relief is nearly equivalent. Restenosis remains the major limitation of PTCA, but this can be managed with repeat PTCA, and bypass surgery can be avoided in most patients. Of note, even though CABG generally provides more complete revascularization, this has not translated into major survival benefit with CABG .

Limitations of Current Data

From a clinical standpoint, the important question when confronted with a patient is whether it is safe to assume PTCA and CABG are equivalent for multivessel disease. Although no statistical benefit has been demonstrated

Table 4.—All-Cause Mortality After Randomized Assignment to Percutaneous Transluminal Coronary Angioplasty (PTCA) or Coronary Artery Bypass Grafting (CABG)

Trial*	PTCA, Obs/Tot	CABG, Obs/Tot	Odds ratio	95% CI
BARI	125/915	111/914	1.14	0.87-1.50
CABRI	21/541	14/513	1.43	0.73-2.81
EAST	14/198	12/194	1.15	0.52-2.55
ERACI	3/63	3/64	1.02	0.20-5.20
GABI	4/182	9/177	0.44	0.15-1.32
MASS	1/72	1/70	0.97	0.06-15.70
RITA	16/510	18/501	0.87	0.44-1.72
Swiss	3/68	1/66	2.70	0.37-19.60
Toulouse	5/76	7/76	0.70	0.22-2.26
Total	192/2,625	176/2,575	1.09	0.88-1.35

CI, confidence interval; Obs, observed; Tot, total.
Between-trial test for heterogeneity, χ^2 (df = 8) = 5.17.
Fixed effects model.
*For full names of trials, see Table 3.
From Kusof S, Cairns JA, Fallen E, et al (editors): *Evidence Based Cardiology*. BMJ Publishing Group, 1998. By permission of the publisher.

Table 5.—Death or Myocardial Infarction After Random Assignment to Percutaneous Transluminal Coronary Angioplasty (PTCA) or Coronary Artery Bypass Grafting (CABG)

Trial*	PTCA, Obs/Tot	CABG, Obs/Tot	Odds ratio	95% CI
BARI	195/915	179/914	1.11	0.89-1.40
CABRI	35/541	32/513	1.04	0.63-1.71
EAST	43/198	50/194	0.80	0.50-1.27
ERACI	9/63	8/64	1.17	0.42-3.22
GABI	11/182	22/177	0.47	0.23-0.95
MASS	3/72	2/70	1.47	0.25-8.68
RITA	50/510	43/501	1.16	0.76-1.77
Swiss	11/68	3/66	3.43	1.14-10.35
Toulouse	6/76	6/76	1.00	0.31-3.24
Total	363/2,625	345/2,575	1.05	0.89-1.23

CI, confidence interval; Obs, observed; Tot, total.
Between-trial test for heterogeneity, χ^2 (df = 8) = 11.33.
Fixed effects model.
*For full names of trials, see Table 3.
From Kusof S, Cairns JA, Fallen E, et al (editors): *Evidence Based Cardiology*. BMJ Publishing Group, 1998. By permission of the publisher.

conclusively, it may be premature to conclude that the two procedures are, in fact, equivalent. In the recent trials, the enrolled patients were relatively low risk, in contrast to the previous CABG versus medical therapy trials. Less than 20% of patients in the PTCA versus CABG trials had left ventricular dysfunction and almost 70% had one- or two-vessel disease. Therefore, these trials enrolled a greater proportion of low- and moderate-risk patients, and their results may not be appropriately extrapolated to high-risk patients, such as those with severe three-vessel disease or left ventricular dysfunction (or both). Because these patients are relatively lower risk, a much larger number of patients would be required to demonstrate a clinically important difference in the 20% to 30% range. It is safe to conclude, however, that large mortality differences such as 40% to 50% can be ruled out.

To date, the major limitation of all trials and studies has been the rapid evolution that has occurred in the treatment of coronary artery disease. All three major therapeutic modalities—medical therapy, PTCA, and CABG—have

Table 6.—Nonprotocol Revascularization After Randomized Assignment to Percutaneous Transluminal Coronary Angioplasty (PTCA) or Coronary Artery Bypass Grafting (CABG)

Trial*	PTCA, Obs/Tot	CABG, Obs/Tot	Odds ratio	95% CI
BARI	494/915	73/914	8.58	7.04-10.46
CABRI	163/541	18/513	6.49	4.71-8.93
EAST	107/198	25/194	6.28	4.13-9.55
ERACI	20/63	2/64	7.26	2.91-18.14
GABI	91/182	9/177	9.29	5.86-14.73
MASS	29/72	0/70	11.72	5.20-26.42
RITA	189/510	20/501	7.50	5.53-10.16
Swiss	29/68	2/66	9.13	4.10-20.32
Total	1,122/2,549	149/2,499	7.87	6.92-8.95

CI, confidence interval; Obs, observed; Tot, total.
Between-trial test for heterogeneity, χ^2 (df = 7) = 4.92.
Fixed effects model.
*For full names of trials, see Table 3.
From Kusof S, Cairns JA, Fallen E, et al (editors): *Evidence Based Cardiology*. BMJ Publishing Group, 1998. By permission of the publisher.

experienced major advances and developments during the last decade. The importance of antiplatelet and lipid-lowering agents for secondary prevention has been demonstrated conclusively. Not only can cardiovascular death be reduced by these agents, medical therapy remains the only modality that has been demonstrated to reduce the incidence of nonfatal myocardial infarction. The development of new interventional devices has had a major effect on coronary angioplasty and has allowed ever widening application of these techniques. The development of intracoronary stents in particular has reduced the risks of perioperative death, myocardial infarction, and emergency bypass surgery and has had a modest salutary effect on restenosis. The widespread use of internal thoracic arterial conduits for bypass surgery has led to improved long-term outcomes. New, less invasive surgical approaches are being investigated, but their ultimate role is unclear.

Current Recommendations for Myocardial Revascularization

CABG Versus Medical Therapy

The current data indicate that among patients with refractory angina pectoris, revascularization is indicated for the relief of symptoms. Among certain high-risk subsets (such as left main coronary artery disease and three-vessel disease), CABG is indicated for prolongation of life. In addition, CABG may be indicated for prolongation of life if there is involvement of the proximal left anterior descending artery.

Single-Vessel Disease

Generally, for single-vessel disease, medical therapy should be considered the initial treatment of choice. PTCA is indicated if symptoms are refractory to medical therapy. If PTCA is technically not feasible, bypass surgery is indicated. Currently, no randomized evidence supports a strategy of "prophylactic" PTCA if symptoms are adequately controlled medically.

PTCA Versus CABG for Multivessel Disease

For treated diabetics, current evidence supports CABG as the treatment of choice, unless other mitigating factors are present. For nondiabetics, both multivessel PTCA and CABG are acceptable, bearing in mind the following caveats:
1) Large differences in mortality can be excluded, but smaller differences, 20% or less, cannot be ruled out yet.
2) CABG is associated with more complete revascularization and better early relief of angina; however, these differences are minimized after 3 to 5 years.
3) Repeat revascularization procedures are required more often after PTCA because of restenosis.
4) Initial cost, quality of life, and return to work are more favorable with PTCA but roughly equalize over 3 to 5 years of follow-up. No significant differences in rates of myocardial infarction have been demonstrated.

Suggested Review Reading

Original Descriptions of CABG and PTCA

1. Favaloro RG: Saphenous vein autograft replacement of severe segmental coronary artery occlusion: operative technique. *Ann Thorac Surg* 5:334-339, 1968.

2. Gruntzig AR, Senning A, Siegenthaler WE: Nonoperative dilatation of coronary-artery stenosis: percutaneous transluminal coronary angioplasty. *N Engl J Med* 301:61-68, 1979.

CABG Versus Medical Therapy Trials: Primary Sources

1. Alderman EL, Bourassa MG, Cohen LS, et al: Ten-year follow-up of survival and myocardial infarction in the randomized Coronary Artery Surgery Study. *Circulation* 82:1629-1646, 1990.

2. Davies RF, Goldberg AD, Forman S, et al: Asymptomatic Cardiac Ischemia Pilot (ACIP) study two-year follow-up: outcomes of patients randomized to initial strategies of medical therapy versus revascularization. *Circulation* 95:2037-2043, 1997.

3. European Coronary Surgery Study Group: Long-term results of prospective randomised study of coronary artery bypass surgery in stable angina pectoris. *Lancet* 2:1173-1180, 1982.

4. Prospective randomised study of coronary artery bypass surgery in stable angina pectoris. Second interim report by the European Coronary Surgery Study Group. *Lancet* 2:491-495, 1980.

5. The VA Coronary Artery Bypass Surgery Cooperative Study Group: Eighteen-year follow-up in the Veterans Affairs Cooperative Study of Coronary Artery Bypass Surgery for stable angina. *Circulation* 86:121-130, 1992.

CABG Versus Medical Therapy: Key Subgroup Papers

1. Caracciolo EA, Davis KB, Sopko G, et al: Comparison of surgical and medical group survival in patients with left main coronary artery disease. Long-term CASS experience. *Circulation* 91:2325-2334, 1995.

2. Caracciolo EA, Davis KB, Sopko G, et al: Comparison of surgical and medical group survival in patients with left main equivalent coronary artery disease. Long-term CASS experience. *Circulation* 91:2335-2344, 1995.

3. Myers WO, Schaff HV, Fisher LD, et al: Time to first new myocardial infarction in patients with severe angina and three-vessel disease comparing medical and early surgical therapy: a CASS registry study of survival. *J Thorac Cardiovasc Surg* 95:382-389, 1988.

4. Passamani E, Davis KB, Gillespie MJ, et al: A randomized trial of coronary artery bypass surgery. Survival of patients with a low ejection fraction. *N Engl J Med* 312:1665-1671, 1985.

CABG Versus Medical Therapy: Systematic and Qualitative Overviews

1. Gersh BJ, Califf RM, Loop FD, et al: Coronary bypass surgery in chronic stable angina. *Circulation* 79 (Suppl 1):I-46-I-59, 1989.

2. Yusuf S, Zucker D, Peduzzi P, et al: Effect of coronary artery bypass graft surgery on survival: overview of 10-year results from randomised trials by the Coronary Artery Bypass Graft Surgery Trialists Collaboration. *Lancet* 344:563-570, 1994.

PTCA Versus Medical Therapy

1. Parisi AF, Folland ED, Hartigan P: A comparison of angioplasty with medical therapy in the treatment of single-vessel coronary artery disease. *N Engl J Med* 326:10-16, 1992.

2. RITA-2 Trial Participants: Coronary angioplasty versus medical therapy for angina: the second Randomised Intervention Treatment of Angina (RITA-2) trial. *Lancet* 350:461-468, 1997.

3. Sievers B, Hamm CW, Herzner A, et al: Medical therapy versus PTCA: a prospective, randomized trial in patients with asymptomatic coronary single vessel disease (abstract). *Circulation* 88 (Suppl 1):I-297, 1993.

PTCA Versus CABG Trials: Primary Sources

1. The Bypass Angioplasty Revascularization Investigation (BARI) Investigators: Comparison of coronary bypass surgery with angioplasty in patients with multivessel disease. *N Engl J Med* 335:217-225, 1996.

2. CABRI Trial Participants: First-year results of CABRI (Coronary Angioplasty versus Bypass Revascularisation Investigation). *Lancet* 346:1179-1184, 1995.

3. Coronary angioplasty versus coronary artery bypass surgery: the Randomized Intervention Treatment of Angina (RITA) trial. *Lancet* 341:573-580, 1993.

4. Goy JJ, Eeckhout E, Burnand B, et al: Coronary angioplasty versus left internal mammary artery grafting for isolated proximal left anterior descending artery stenosis. *Lancet* 343:1449-1453, 1994.

5. Hamm CW, Reimers J, Ischinger T, et al: A randomized study of coronary angioplasty compared with bypass surgery in patients with symptomatic multivessel coronary disease. *N Engl J Med* 331:1037-1043, 1994.

6. Hueb WA, Bellotti G, de Oliveira SA, et al: The Medicine, Angioplasty or Surgery Study (MASS): a prospective, randomized trial of medical therapy, balloon angioplasty or bypass surgery for single proximal left anterior descending artery stenoses. *J Am Coll Cardiol* 26:1600-1605, 1995.

7. King SB III, Lembo NJ, Weintraub WS, et al: A randomized trial comparing coronary angioplasty with coronary bypass surgery. *N Engl J Med* 331:1044-1050, 1994.

8. Puel J, Karouny E, Marco F, et al: Angioplasty versus surgery in multivessel disease: immediate results and in-hospital outcome in a randomized prospective study (abstract). *Circulation* 86 (Suppl 1):I-372, 1992.

9. Rodriguez A, Boullon F, Perez-Balino N, et al: Argentine randomized trial of percutaneous transluminal coronary angioplasty versus coronary artery bypass surgery in multivessel disease (ERACI): in-hospital results and 1-year follow-up. *J Am Coll Cardiol* 22:1060-1067, 1993.

10. Williams DO, Baim DS, Bates E, et al: Coronary anatomic and procedural characteristics of patients randomized to coronary angioplasty in the Bypass Angioplasty Revascularization Investigation (BARI). *Am J Cardiol* 75:27C-33C, 1995.

PTCA Versus CABG: Systematic Overview

1. Pocock SJ, Henderson RA, Rickards AF, et al: Meta-analysis of randomised trials comparing coronary angioplasty with bypass surgery. *Lancet* 346:1184-1189, 1995.

Revascularization Overviews

1. Jones RH, Kesler K, Phillips HR III, et al: Long-term survival benefits of coronary artery bypass grafting and percutaneous transluminal angioplasty in patients with coronary artery disease. *J Thorac Cardiovasc Surg* 111:1013-1025, 1996.

2. Mark DB, Nelson CL, Califf RM, et al: Continuing evolution of therapy for coronary artery disease. Initial results from the era of coronary angioplasty. *Circulation* 89:2015-2025, 1994.

3. Rihal CS, Gersh BJ, Yusuf S: Chronic coronary artery disease: coronary artery bypass surgery vs percutaneous transluminal coronary angioplasty vs medical therapy. In *Evidence Based Cardiology*. Edited by S Yusuf, JA Cairns, E Fallen. BMJ Publishing Group, 1998, pp 368-392.

Questions

The following questions pertain to *chronic* coronary artery disease only:

Note: The following questions may have *more than one* correct answer.

1. Which of the following indications for coronary artery bypass grafting have been objectively proven?
   a. Prolongation of life
   b. Relief of severe angina pectoris
   c. Prevention of acute myocardial infarction
   d. Preservation of hibernating myocardium and prevention of congestive heart failure

2. Which of the following possible indications for percutaneous transluminal coronary angioplasty have been objectively proven?
   a. Prolongation of life
   b. Relief of severe angina pectoris
   c. Prevention of acute myocardial infarction
   d. Preservation of hibernating myocardium and prevention of congestive heart failure

3. In patients with stable coronary artery disease, coronary artery bypass grafting has been shown to improve survival in which of the following anatomical subgroups?
   a. Left main artery disease
   b. Three-vessel disease
   c. Two-vessel disease with normal left ventricular function
   d. One-vessel disease, except for left main coronary artery or proximal left anterior descending coronary artery
   e. One- or two-vessel disease with involvement of left anterior descending coronary artery

4. In the coronary artery bypass graft (CABG) pooling project, the odds ratio for death over long-term follow-up (CABG vs. medical treatment) was almost identical for patients who had normal and abnormal left ventricular function; however, CABG is thought to have greater benefit in patients with left ventricular dysfunction. Possible reasons for this include:
   a. The higher absolute risk of death while receiving medical treatment

   b. Because of small sample sizes, improvement in mortality with CABG could not be detected among patients with normal left ventricular function in individual trials
   c. In the Coronary Artery Surgery Study (CASS), CABG was initially shown to have a survival advantage for patients with three-vessel disease and left ventricular dysfunction
   d. All survival curves converge with time

5. Of the three major coronary artery bypass grafting (CABG) vs. medical therapy trials, which of the following showed an *overall* survival benefit for CABG?
   a. Coronary Artery Surgery Study (CASS)
   b. European Cooperative Surgery Study (ECSS)
   c. Veterans Administration Cooperative Study (VAC)

6. At the time of the coronary artery bypass grafting vs. medical therapy randomized trials, which of the following medical therapies were widely used for coronary artery disease?
   a. Aspirin
   b. β-Blockers
   c. HMG-CoA reductase inhibitors
   d. Calcium channel blockers
   e. Nitrates

7. In the coronary artery bypass grafting vs. medical therapy trials, which of the following subgroups were well represented?
   a. Females
   b. Patients older than 65 years
   c. Patients with an ejection fraction less than 35%
   d. Asymptomatic patients
   e. Patients with a previous infarction
   f. Smokers
   g. Patients with hypertension

8. Because numerous technological advances in coronary artery bypass grafting (CABG) have occurred since these randomized trials, which of the following statements can be expected to be true?
   a. CABG would be even more efficacious if trials were repeated today
   b. CABG in fact would be less efficacious because medical therapy has improved as well
   c. Because medical therapy has improved markedly, a much larger number of patients would be

necessary to show a survival benefit, if any, for CABG

9. Among patients with mild (class 0-2) angina with stable one- or two-vessel disease, percutaneous transluminal coronary angioplasty is indicated for which of the following?
   a. Prevention of death
   b. Prevention of myocardial infarction
   c. Prevention of severe angina pectoris
   d. To alleviate asymptomatic ischemia

10. Which of the following statements are true for percutaneous transluminal coronary angioplasty (PTCA) vs. coronary artery bypass grafting (CABG) trials (BARI, RITA etc.) for multivessel disease?
   a. In comparison with the older CABG vs. medical therapy trials, patients of equivalent risk were enrolled
   b. These trials showed that overall survival was better after CABG
   c. In these trials, survival was better after CABG only in the diabetic subgroup
   d. Repeat procedures were necessary more often after PTCA
   e. Although relief of angina was initially superior after CABG, the differences diminish with time
   f. Because of the risk of perioperative infarction, PTCA was superior to CABG in preventing myocardial infarction

11. Which of the following new treatments have been shown to improve procedural outcomes (and possibly tilt the balance in favor of that procedure)?
   a. Directional coronary atherectomy
   b. Intracoronary stent deployments
   c. Intravenous abciximab as adjuvant therapy for coronary angioplasty
   d. Oral glycoprotein IIb/IIIa receptor antagonist
   e. Minimally invasive coronary artery bypass grafting
   f. Use of radial artery grafts for coronary artery bypass grafting
   g. Hirudin

Answers

1. Answers a and b

2. Answer b

3. Answers a, b, and c

4. Answers a, b, c, and d

5. Answer b

6. Answers b and e

7. Answers e, f, and g

8. Answer c

9. Answer d

10. Answers c, d, and e

11. Answers b and c

Chapter 12

Unstable Angina

Stephen L. Kopecky, M.D.

Pathophysiology

Unstable angina usually is caused by plaque rupture and thrombus formation in the coronary artery, which, in turn, cause a sudden decrease in myocardial blood flow. This results in myocardial ischemia and either rest pain or an acceleration in previously stable angina. Unstable angina may also be manifested as new angina or post-myocardial infarct angina. Rarely, unstable angina can be caused by coronary artery spasm, which produces a decrease in myocardial blood flow, or by diseases that increase myocardial oxygen demand (hypermetabolic states such as hyperthyroidism, fever, anemia, pheochromocytoma, arteriovenous fistula, aortic valve disease, hypertrophic cardiomyopathy, and severe hypertension).

The initial therapy for unstable angina should be directed at treating the intracoronary thrombus with antiplatelet and anticoagulant agents in combination with drugs that reduce myocardial oxygen demand.

- Unstable angina is usually caused by coronary artery plaque rupture with thrombus formation.
- Rare causes of unstable angina include hyperthyroidism, hypertrophic cardiomyopathy, and severe hypertension (the "3 Hs").

Natural History

The natural history of unstable angina has improved markedly in the last three decades. In the late 1950s and early 1960s, before the widespread use of antiplatelet (aspirin) and anticoagulant (heparin) agents, progression to myocardial infarction occurred in 40% to 50% of patients, with mortality of 20% to 30%. Currently, with the use of antiplatelet and anticoagulant agents in combination with medications to decrease myocardial oxygen demand (i.e., β-blockers), the myocardial infarction rate has decreased to about 10% and mortality to approximately 5%. This decrease occurred even before the widespread use of percutaneous revascularization techniques in the late 1970s and early 1980s.

- Unstable angina progresses to myocardial infarction in about 10% of patients and to death in 5%.

Definition

By definition, unstable angina has three possible presentations: 1) symptoms of angina at rest (usually prolonged for more than 20 minutes), 2) new onset of exertional angina in the preceding 2 months (of at least Canadian Cardiovascular Society Class III [CCSC III]), or 3) acceleration of preexisting angina of the preceding 2 months to at least CCSC III (Tables 1 and 2). Variant angina, angina more than 24 hours after myocardial infarction, and non-Q-wave myocardial infarction are also considered part of the unstable angina syndrome.

Table 1.—Definition and Diagnosis of Unstable Angina*

Definition

    Symptoms of angina at rest (> 20 min)

    New onset (< 2 months) exertional angina of at least Canadian Cardiovascular Society class III

    Recent acceleration of angina to at least Canadian Cardiovascular Society class III

Diagnosis

    Symptoms--definitely, probably, probably not, definitely not

    History of symptoms of coronary artery disease

    Sex, age, and number of major risk factors (congestive heart failure)

    Physical examination--transient S_3, S_4, mitral regurgitation murmur, or left ventricular lift

    Electrocardiogram-- > 1 mm ST-segment depression or elevation, multiple T-wave inversions (*any* other transient ST-T-wave changes indicate intermediate probability of severe coronary artery disease)

*Includes variant angina, non-Q-wave myocardial infarction, angina more than 24 hours after myocardial infarction.

Evaluation

The risk of death or complications from myocardial ischemia in patients with unstable angina is higher than for patients with stable angina but lower than for those with acute myocardial infarction. The prognosis for a patient with symptoms suggestive of unstable angina depends on the likelihood of significant coronary artery disease being present (Table 3). A "high likelihood" is a greater than 85% chance of significant flow-limiting coronary artery disease being present, an "intermediate likelihood" is a 15% to 85% chance, and a "low likelihood" is a less than 15% chance. The prognosis also depends on the type of symptoms and the patient's comorbid conditions. Important points in the patient's history are the severity of angina, the frequency of angina, and the change in frequency in the preceding 2 months. Prolonged episodes of chest pain (longer than 20 minutes) in conjunction with rest pain or the presence of worsening mitral regurgitation or pulmonary edema or new electrocardiographic (ECG) changes with chest pain are important markers of high-risk patients (Table 4).

- "High likelihood" is a > 85% chance of severe coronary artery disease.

Table 2.—Canadian Cardiovascular Society Classification of Angina

Class	Activity provoking angina	Limits to normal activity
I	Prolonged exertion	None
II	Walking > 2 blocks	Slight
III	Walking < 2 blocks	Marked
IV	Minimal or rest	Severe

- "Low likelihood" is a < 15% chance of severe coronary artery disease.
- Chest pain > 20 minutes, ECG changes, significant mitral regurgitation, and pulmonary edema are poor risk factors.

Physical Examination

Physical examination of patients with unstable angina during an episode of pain is very useful. The presence of a new mitral regurgitation murmur or increased intensity of a preexisting murmur indicates a papillary muscle or mitral apparatus dysfunction due to ischemia. Note that a small amount of ischemic myocardium can cause ischemic mitral regurgitation. A large amount of myocardial ischemia can cause a third or fourth heart sound, left ventricular lift, or systemic hypotension, all of which adversely affect prognosis.

The ECG During Unstable Angina

A normal ECG is seen in approximately 5% of patients with unstable angina. More common are baseline nonspecific ST-T-wave changes that have no significant prognostic implications. Deep symmetrical precordial T-wave inversions (leads V_1-V_4) suggest acute ischemia in the distribution of the left anterior descending coronary artery. Transient ST- or T-wave changes that are present during pain but disappear with the resolution of symptoms strongly suggest unstable angina with a high likelihood of significant underlying coronary artery stenosis. Comparison with previous ECGs is helpful in adding to the prognostic power of ECG during pain. New ST-segment elevation of more than 1 mm in two or more contiguous leads that is prolonged for more than 30 minutes is diagnostic of an acute myocardial infarction. New ST-segment depression of 1 mm or more suggests a high-risk patient with either acute myocardial ischemia or non-Q-wave myocardial infarction. In general, ST-segment depression infarcts or unstable angina has not been shown to respond favorably to thrombolytic therapy. The only subgroup with ST-segment depression that has benefited from thrombolytic therapy is the subgroup with acute posterior infarction manifested by ST-segment depression in leads V_1-V_3.

- Deep symmetrical T-wave inversion in V_1-V_4 suggests left anterior descending coronary artery disease.
- Transient ST-segment changes with chest pain suggest significant coronary artery disease.

Initial Risk Stratification

When evaluating a patient with unstable angina for hospitalization and treatment, is it important to begin the evaluation within 20 minutes after the patient's arrival in the emergency department. The initial risk stratification depends on the likelihood of the patient having coronary artery disease (Table 3). The prognostic factors for death or nonfatal myocardial infarction are listed in Table 4. Patients with a high likelihood of coronary artery disease (high-risk patients) should be hospitalized on a monitored bed for intensive medical management. Patients with an intermediate likelihood of coronary artery disease (intermediate-risk patients) should be hospitalized for nonintensive inpatient management. Patients with a low likelihood of coronary artery disease (low-risk patients) can be treated as outpatients (Fig. 1).

Initial Laboratory Testing

In all patients in whom unstable angina is highly suspected clinically and who are hospitalized, the total creatine kinase (CK) and creatine kinase-muscle and brain subunits (CK-MB) should be measured at admission and every 8 hours for the first 24 hours after admission. Measuring troponin I or T may be useful in detecting myocardial damage in patients who are evaluated between 24 and 72 hours after the onset of pain and in whom serial measurements of CK and CK-MB are normal. An ECG should be performed at admission and 24 hours after admission if clinically indicated. Also, an ECG should be considered if the patient has recurrent pain while in the hospital or a significant change in clinical status (e.g., new pulmonary edema). A chest radiograph is useful in patients with evidence of hemodynamic instability or pulmonary edema. Serum lipids should be measured within 24 hours after the onset of chest pain because measurements made after that time may give falsely low readings of serum cholesterol.

Initial Medical Treatment

According to the *Unstable Angina Guidelines* recommended by the Agency for Health Care Policy and Research, treatment should be initiated within 1 hour after the patient arrives in the emergency department. Initial treatment should be centered on correcting the causes of myocardial ischemia (Table 5). Specifically, causes of increased myocardial oxygen demand should be assessed and addressed (i.e., tachycardia, hypertension, and hypoxia). Aspirin should be given to all patients, and the first dose (324 mg) should be chewed by the patient. This ensures rapid absorption because the amount of oral absorption is increased and interference with

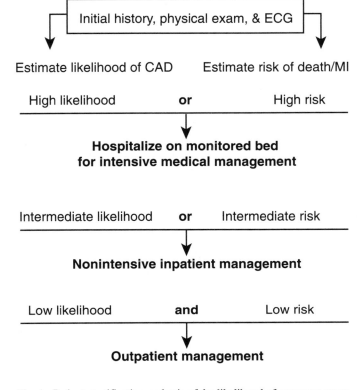

Fig. 1. Patient stratification on basis of the likelihood of coronary artery disease (CAD) and initial risk assessment. ECG, electrocardiogram; MI, myocardial infarction.

Table 3.—Likelihood of Significant CAD in Unstable Angina

High likelihood	Intermediate likelihood	Low likelihood
History of CAD	Definite angina	Chest pain, probably not angina
Definite angina	Males < 60 yr	One risk factor but not in diabetic patients
Males ≥ 60 yr	Females < 70 yr	T wave flat or inverted < 1 mm in leads
Females ≥ 70 yr	Probable angina	with dominant R waves
Hemodynamic changes or ECG changes	Males > 60 yr	Normal ECG
with pain	Females > 70 yr	
Variant angina	Probably not angina in DM or non-DM	
ST-segment elevation or depression	patients with ≥ 2 other risk factors	
≥ 1 mm from baseline	Vascular disease	
Marked symmetrical T-wave inversion	ST-segment depression of 0.05-1 mm	
in multiple chest leads	T-wave inversion ≥ 1 mm in leads	
	with dominant R waves	

CAD, coronary artery disease; DM, diabetes mellitus; ECG, electrocardiogram.

Table 4.—Factors Increasing Short-Term Risk of Death or Nonfatal MI in Unstable Angina

High risk	Intermediate risk	Low risk
Prolonged pain (> 20 min)	Rest angina resolved but	Increased angina frequency, severity, or
Pulmonary edema	increased chance of CAD	duration
Angina with new or worsening MR	Rest angina (> 20 min or	Angina provoked at lower threshold
Rest angina with dynamic ST changes	relieved with NTG)	New onset angina (2 weeks-2 months)
≥ 1 mm	Angina with T-wave changes	Normal or unchanged ECG
Angina with S_3 or rales	Nocturnal angina	
Angina with hypotension	New onset CCSC III or IV in	
	preceding 2 weeks but increased	
	chance of CAD	
	Age > 65 yr	
	Q waves or ST-segment depression	
	> 1 mm in multiple leads	

CAD, coronary artery disease; CCSC, Canadian Cardiovascular Society Classification; ECG, electrocardiogram; MI, myocardial infarction; MR, mitral regurgitation; NTG, nitroglycerin.

absorption by stomach contents is avoided. Heparin should be given to all patients with unstable angina who are in the high-risk or intermediate-risk category.

Therapy

Low-Molecular-Weight Heparin

Two large multicenter randomized trials have been completed on the use of low-molecular-weight heparin, specifically

enoxaparin, in the unstable angina/non-Q-wave myocardial infarction population. The first is the Efficacy and Safety of Subcutaneous Enoxaparin in Non-Q-Wave Coronary Events (ESSENCE) study. In this study, patients with the recent onset of rest angina who had their last pain within 24 hours of presentation and definite evidence of underlying coronary artery disease were randomly assigned to either unfractionated heparin or subcutaneous enoxaparin (1 mg/kg every 12 hours). The primary end point of death, myocardial infarction, or recurrent angina at 14 and 30 days was significantly

Table 5.—Treatment of Unstable Angina*

Drug	Clinical condition	Dose
ASA	Unstable angina	324 mg/day (160-324 mg/day)

Heparin	Unstable angina in high- and intermediate-risk populations	Low-molecular-weight heparin:
		    Enoxaparin 1 mg/kg s.c. every 12 hours for ≥ 48 hours *or*
		    dalteparin 120 IU/kg s.c. twice a day for 5 days *or*
		Unfractionated heparin:
		    70 U/kg (i.v. bolus), then 15 U/kg per hour (aPTT, 1.5-2.5)

Nitrates	Ongoing pain	1-3 tablets sublingual followed by 5-100 µg/min i.v.

β-Blockers	Any unstable angina	Low- and intermediate-risk groups:
		    Oral preparation
		High-risk group:
		    Metoprolol--1-5 mg i.v. every 5 min to 15 mg *or*
		    Propranolol--0.5-1.0 mg i.v. *or*
		    Atenolol--5 mg i.v. every 5 min to 10 mg *or*
		    Esmolol--i.v. drip, 50 µg/kg per min and titrate up

Narcotics	Persistent pain after treatment with nitroglycerin and β-blockers	Morphine--2-5 mg i.v.

aPTT, activated partial thromboplastin time; ASA, acetylsalicylic acid; i.v., intravenous; s.c., subcutaneously.
*Use calcium channel blockers only after treatment with nitrates and β-blockers and if systolic blood pressure is > 150 mm Hg and refractory ischemia is present; use also for vasospastic angina.

reduced by 16% and 15%, respectively, in the enoxaparin group. The Thrombolysis in Myocardial Infarction (TIMI)-XIB study showed similar benefit. Early in their course, patients with unstable angina are indistinguishable from those with non-Q-wave myocardial infarction, and it is reasonable to treat these patients with low-molecular-weight heparin, specifically enoxaparin, in the first 2 or 3 days of hospitalization. Studies have shown efficacy of other low-molecular-weight heparins, but not superiority, in comparison with unfractionated heparin. The primary difficulty with low-molecular-weight heparin use is the transition of patients to the cardiac catheterization laboratory where the exact dose regimen has not been determined for angioplasty patients.

Nitrates

Nitrates are given to patients with ongoing chest pain. Treatment with sublingual nitroglycerin tablets should be started provided that the patient is not hypotensive (systolic blood pressure < 90 mm Hg). If this is inadequate for controlling pain, nitroglycerin should be given intravenously.

β-Blockers

β-Blockers are a mainstay of therapy and should be given to all patients with unstable angina unless contraindicated (e.g., heart block, heart failure, asthma, severe peripheral vascular disease). The low-risk or intermediate-risk group can be given oral drugs, but it is recommended that the high-risk group initially be given β-blockers intravenously if pain

persists after the above treatment or if hypertension or tachycardia is present. Of the intravenous β-blockers, propranolol, metoprolol, atenolol, or esmolol can be given. Narcotics are administered to help decrease anxiety and to relieve pain if the above treatment is not effective. Calcium channel blockers may be used only after treatment with nitrates and β-blockers has been initiated and when patients have systolic blood pressure greater than 150 mm Hg or refractory ischemic symptoms. Calcium channel blockers are also indicated for vasospastic angina. Certain clinical conditions are relative contraindications for the use of the above-mentioned drugs in patients with unstable angina. Each patient must be evaluated independently, and the risks versus benefits of a drug must be assessed (Table 6).

Thrombolytics

Thrombolytic therapy has not been shown to clinically benefit patients with unstable angina. The TIMI-IIIA and IIIB studies showed no benefit of thrombolytic therapy versus standard therapy in this group of patients. In fact, thrombolytic agents increase the risk of myocardial infarction in this group of patients, possibly because of a procoagulant effect due to platelet activation.

- Aspirin, heparin, nitrates, and β-blockers are the mainstay of medical treatment of unstable angina.
- Thrombolytic therapy has *no* documented benefit in unstable angina.

Table 6.—Compatibility and Use of Unstable Angina Treatment With Other Clinical Conditions

	Clinical condition									
Drug	Allergy	Bleeding	Recent stroke	↓BP	Confusion	Heart block	CHF	Asthma	COPD	Renal failure
ASA	No	No	Ok	Ok	Ok	Ok	Ok	Ok	Ok	Ok
Heparin	No	No	No	Ok	No	Ok	Ok	Ok	Ok	Caution with LMWH
Nitrates	No	Ok	Ok	No	Ok	Ok	Ok	Ok	Ok	Ok
β-Blocker	No	Ok	Ok	No	Ok	No	No*	No*	Ok	Ok
Narcotics	No	Ok	No	No	No	Ok	Ok	Ok	Ok	Ok

ASA, acetylsalicylic acid; BP, blood pressure; CHF, congestive heart failure; COPD, chronic obstructive pulmonary disease; i.v., intravenous; LMWH, low-molecular-weight heparin.
*Possibly esmolol given intravenously.

IIb/IIIa Platelet Inhibitors

Currently, three drugs have been approved in the U.S. for treatment of patients with unstable angina with or without angioplasty: abciximab, eptifibatide, and tirofiban. Studies of these agents in patients with unstable angina included a large number of patients who also had angioplasty. Therefore, it is difficult to differentiate the benefits of angioplasty from those of the IIb/IIIa platelet inhibitors. It is believed that these drugs should be reserved first for high-risk patients with unstable angina refractory to the standard medications as listed above. The second group of patients that may benefit from IIb/IIIa inhibitors are those with unstable angina who are scheduled to have an interventional coronary procedure, in which case the decision to treat with a IIb/IIIa inhibitor should be made by the interventional cardiologist. There is good evidence that recurrent event rates are reduced after angioplasty in patients receiving glycoprotein IIb/IIIa platelet inhibitors. The role of these agents before angioplasty has not been determined, and it is reasonable to withhold these agents until a patient is en route to cardiac catheterization if early intervention is planned. However, if the patient is being treated at a hospital that does not have interventional capabilities or if the intention is to avoid intervention if possible, the early use of these agents is suggested. Additional studies are needed to determine the exact timing of the use of these drugs.

Intra-Aortic Balloon Pump

Intra-aortic balloon pumping should be considered in patients with unstable angina refractory to the aggressive medical management outlined above. Contraindications to intra-aortic balloon pumping are 1) severe peripheral vascular disease, 2) significant aortic insufficiency, and 3) severe aortoiliac disease, including aortic aneurysm. If patients have persistent chest discomfort for more than 1 hour after aggressive medical therapy, emergency cardiac catheterization should be considered.

Risk Stratification in Patients With Unstable Angina

After a patient's condition has been stabilized in the inpatient setting, the patient should be considered for further risk stratification, with either noninvasive stress testing or coronary angiography. Both inpatients and outpatients whose condition is stable should begin receiving medical therapy before being considered for risk stratification. Exercise or pharmacologic stress testing is an important part of the outpatient evaluation of those with unstable angina. In most cases, testing may be done within 72 hours after presentation. The choice of the type of the initial stress test depends on the patient's rest ECG, the ability to perform exercise, and the available methods and expertise.

Exercise treadmill testing is the standard mode of stress testing in patients with a normal ECG who are able to exercise. Concomitant conditions that preclude adequate interpretation of the stress ECG include digoxin therapy, widespread resting ST-segment depression (≥ 1 mm), left ventricular hypertrophy, left bundle branch block, significant interventricular conduction delay, and preexcitation syndrome. Patients who have these conditions should be considered for an imaging modality such as radionuclide agent (thallium, sestamibi, exercise multiple-gated acquisition [MUGA] scanning, or exercise echocardiography if available) (Tables 7 and 8).

Patients who are unable to exercise because of general debility, chronic obstructive pulmonary disease, peripheral vascular disease, or orthopedic limitations should undergo pharmacologic stress testing with an imaging modality. Available pharmacologic agents include adenosine, dobutamine, and dipyridamole. However, local expertise and patient factors are important in choosing the modality. Patients who are able to exercise to a high workload (i.e., ≥ 5 metabolic equivalents [METs]) without ischemia have a good prognosis and may be managed medically. However, patients who have evidence of ischemia, on the basis of symptoms, ECG, or imaging modality, at a low workload

Table 7.—Guidelines for Stress and Imaging Method in Coronary Artery Disease Patients

Choosing an Exercise Method Based on Patient Factors
If a patient has normal ECG and can walk, use exercise treadmill
If possible, exercise the patient (to ≥ 5 METs or to chest discomfort)

If:	Then do the following exercise (potential imaging)
Patient can walk or if goal is to prescribe an exercise regimen	ETT with imaging by thallium, sestamibi, echocardiography if increased sensitivity or specificity is needed
Can ride cycle (no knee arthritis)	Upright cycle exercise
Cannot walk or cycle	Arm exercise or pharmacologic stress test
To test for pulmonary vs. cardiac etiology of dyspnea	Cardiopulmonary ETT protocol with metabolic oxygen study

Deciding Which <u>Stress</u> Method to Use
If patient has normal ECG and can walk, use exercise treadmill
If possible, exercise the patient (to ≥ 5 METs or to chest discomfort)

Patient factors	Exercise (treadmill, cycle, arm)	Dipyridamole* (thallium, sestamibi)	Adenosine* (thallium, sestamibi)	Dobutamine (thallium, sestamibi, RNA, echocardiography)
Carotid bruits				
Without symptoms	Yes	Yes	Yes	Yes
With recent symptoms	Yes	No[†]	Yes[‡]	No[†]
Lung disease				
Mild/moderate COPD	Yes	Yes	Yes	Yes
Severe COPD/asthma	Yes	No	No	Yes
Theophylline medication	Yes	No	No	Yes
LBBB	No	Yes	Yes	No
β-Blocker medication	Yes	Yes	Yes	No
Dipyridamole medication	Yes	Yes	No	Yes
Fixed heart rate (PPM)	No	Yes	Yes	No
Poorly controlled hypertension	No	Yes	Yes	No
Significant ventricular ectopy	Yes	Yes	Yes	No

COPD, chronic obstructive pulmonary disease; ECG, electrocardiogram; ETT, exercise treadmill test; LBBB, left bundle branch block; MET, metabolic equivalent; PPM, non-rate-responsive permanent pacemaker; RNA, radionuclide angiography.
*For dipyridamole and adenosine, withhold caffeine for 12 hours.
[†]Because of possible high/low blood pressure response.
[‡]Graduated infusion with blood pressure monitoring suggested.

Table 8.—Deciding Which Imaging Modality to Use*

	Treadmill only	Echo	Thallium	Sestamibi	RNA
Goal of test					
Ventricular function (EF)	No	Yes	No	Yes (ask for 1st pass EF)	Yes
Screening test	Yes	Yes	Yes	Yes	Yes
Low cost desired	Yes	No	No	No	No
Post MI viability	No	Yes	Yes	Yes	Yes
Patient factors					
Large chest	Yes	No	Yes	Yes	Yes
Weight (females > 80 kg, males > 100 kg)	Yes	Yes	No	Yes	Yes
COPD	Yes	No	Yes	Yes	Yes
ECG factors					
LBBB	No	No	Yes	Yes	No
Nonspecific ST-T wave changes due to digoxin, WPW, MVP	No	Yes	Yes	Yes	Yes
LVH, PPM	No	No	Yes	Yes	No
Irregular rhythm (Afib, frequent PVCs)	No	Yes	Yes	Yes	No
Cannot exercise (see Table 7)	No	Yes	Yes	Yes	No

Afib, atrial fibrillation; COPD, chronic obstructive pulmonary disease; EF, ejection fraction; LBBB, left bundle branch block; LVH, left ventricular hypertrophy; MI, myocardial infarction; MVP, mitral valve prolapse; PPM, non-rate-responsive permanent pacemaker; PVC, premature ventricular contraction; WPW, Wolff-Parkinson-White syndrome.

*Local expertise/availability is extremely important in choosing imaging modality.

Bruce predicted time (male) = 16 - (0.11 x age)

(female) = 13.3 - (0.1 x age)

~1 Minute Bruce exercise time = 1 MET

(< 5 METs) may be considered for coronary angiography. Patients who can exercise only to a low workload without ischemia or those who have ischemia at a high workload are at intermediate risk, and their ongoing treatment should be individualized depending on many factors, including patient preference, physician preference, adequacy of follow-up, and tolerance of medical therapy. Patients with a low risk of significant coronary artery disease on the basis of exercise testing have a predicted average cardiac mortality of less than 1% per year, compared with 4% or greater for those with a high risk. Intermediate-risk patients may be considered for medical therapy, additional testing with an imaging agent, or cardiac catheterization. However, patients in the intermediate-risk category who have left ventricular dysfunction should be considered for cardiac angiography, because in many studies of patients with unstable angina, left ventricular ejection fraction is one of the most important factors for long-term outcome.

It should be remembered that all forms of exercise testing have been shown to be less accurate in women than in men. This is due partly to the lower pretest likelihood of coronary artery disease in women than in men. However, it is still reasonable to use noninvasive testing for risk stratification in women.

Exercise testing should be performed within the first few days after medical stabilization of the patient, because more than one-half of the subsequent cardiac ischemic events that will occur in the first year occur in the first month after the patient's initial presentation.

- An exercise capacity ≥ 5 METs without ischemia indicates

a good prognosis.

- Low-risk patients have < 1% annual cardiac mortality.
- High-risk patients have ≥ 4% annual cardiac mortality.

Cardiac Catheterization and Myocardial Revascularization

Patients whose clinical condition fails to stabilize with medical therapy or those in the high-risk category because of clinical findings or noninvasive test results should be considered for coronary angiography. Also, patients with congestive heart failure, severe left ventricular dysfunction, previous angioplasty, previous coronary bypass surgery, or myocardial infarction are in the high-risk category and should be considered for early cardiac catheterization. Patients also may have a preference for an early invasive strategy. The TIMI-IIIB study randomly assigned patients to either an "early invasive" or an "early conservative" strategy. The difference in the outcomes between these groups with regard to cardiovascular events was not significant. Cardiac catheterization should be performed only in patients who are potential candidates for revascularization (coronary artery bypass grafting [CABG] or percutaneous transluminal coronary angioplasty [PTCA]). Currently, either the early conservative or early invasive strategy is acceptable.

Overall, high-risk patients such as those who previously have had revascularization or patients with associated congestive heart failure, depressed left ventricular function, ventricular arrhythmia, or recurrent pain/ischemia or patients at high risk on the basis of a functional study should be considered for coronary angiography. However, diagnostic cardiac catheterization should not be performed in patients with extensive comorbid conditions and for whom the risk of revascularization outweighs the benefits. Also, for patients with a significantly decreased life span because of a comorbid condition such as malignancy, the decision whether to have cardiac catheterization should be individualized.

Among patients with unstable angina who undergo coronary angiography, 10% to 20% have normal coronary arteries or insignificant coronary artery disease, 5% to 10% have significant left main coronary artery disease, 20% to 25% have three-vessel disease, 25% to 30% have two-vessel disease, and 30% to 35% have single-vessel disease. Patients who are found to have significant coronary artery stenosis (i.e., > 70% stenosis of the left anterior descending, circumflex, or right coronary artery or more than 50% stenosis of the left main coronary artery) may be considered for revascularization. If catheterization shows left main coronary artery disease or three-vessel disease with depressed left ventricular function, the patient should be referred for CABG. Those with two-vessel disease with a proximal severe stenosis of the left anterior descending coronary artery and depressed left ventricular function should also be considered for CABG. In general, CABG has been shown to result in a better long-term outcome than medical management. Patients with the following conditions should be considered for PTCA or CABG: medical therapy that fails to stabilize their condition, recurrent angina/ischemia that occurs at rest or with a low level of exercise, ischemia that occurs with congestive heart failure symptoms, an S_3 gallop mitral regurgitation that is detected on physical examination, or significant ST-segment depression that occurs during pain.

- Coronary arteries are normal or minimally diseased in 10% to 20% of patients with unstable angina.
- Significant left main coronary artery disease is present in 5% to 10% of patients with unstable angina.
- Early conservative or invasive approaches to cardiac catheterization in patients with unstable angina are acceptable.

Patient Risk Factor Modification

All patients with unstable angina should have a complete risk factor assessment for hyperlipidemia, hypertension, family history, tobacco use, and diabetes mellitus. Patients with hyperlipidemia should be counseled in proper dietary therapy, and if this fails, they should be treated aggressively with medication according to the National Cholesterol Education Program guidelines (see chapter "Hyperlipidemia"). Hypertension should also be treated aggressively. All patients who use tobacco should be counseled to stop. Patients with a high-stress lifestyle that results in conflict and frustration may be at high risk for the development of coronary artery disease and may benefit from relaxation and stress-reduction therapy. Also, a regular exercise program has been shown to decrease stress levels, to help patients lose weight, and to lower their blood pressure and lipid levels.

Suggested Review Reading

1. Cohen M, Demers C, Gurfinkel EP, et al: A comparison of low-molecular-weight heparin with unfractionated heparin for unstable coronary artery disease. *N Engl J Med* 337:447-452, 1997.

2. The EPIC Investigation: Use of a monoclonal antibody directed against the platelet glycoprotein IIb/IIIa receptor in high-risk coronary angioplasty. *N Engl J Med* 330:956-961, 1994.

3. Klein W, Buchwald A, Hillis SE, et al: Comparison of low-molecular-weight heparin with unfractionated heparin acutely and with placebo for 6 weeks in the management of unstable coronary artery disease. Fragmin in unstable coronary artery disease study. *Circulation* 96:61-68, 1997.

4. The PURSUIT Trial Investigators: Inhibition of platelet glycoprotein IIb/IIIa with eptifibatide in patients with acute coronary syndromes. *N Engl J Med* 339:436-443, 1998.

Questions

Multiple Choice (choose the one best answer)

1. In patients with unstable angina who undergo coronary angiography, what percentage have normal coronary arteries or insignificant coronary artery disease?
   a. < 10%
   b. 10%–20%
   c. 40%–50%
   d. 60%–70%
   e. > 80%

2. The current *Unstable Angina Guidelines* from the Agency for Health Care Policy and Research recommend the following time schedule for patients with unstable angina presenting to the emergency department.
   a. Begin evaluation within 20 minutes and initiate medical therapy within another 20 minutes
   b. Begin evaluation within 20 minutes and initiate medical therapy within another hour
   c. Begin evaluation within 1 hour and initiate medical therapy within another hour

3. Which of the following is not a contraindication to intra-aortic balloon pump use in patients with unstable angina?
   a. Severe peripheral vascular disease
   b. Severe aortic stenosis
   c. Severe aortic insufficiency
   d. Severe aortoiliac disease

4. Which of the following is least likely to be a cause of unstable angina?
   a. Anemia
   b. Fever
   c. Hypothyroidism
   d. Severe aortic stenosis
   e. Severe hypertension

5. Which of the following drugs has been shown to decrease cardiovascular events in patients with unstable angina who are unable to take aspirin?
   a. Ticlopidine
   b. Sulfinpyrazone
   c. Dipyridamole
   d. All the above
   e. None of the above

6. Which patients with unstable angina who have the following ECG subsets have been shown to benefit from acute intravenous thrombolytic therapy?
   a. ST-segment depression > 1 mm in leads V_5-V_6
   b. T-wave inversion > 2 mm in leads V_1-V_4

c. Peaked T waves > 2 mm in leads V_1-V_4
d. All the above
e. None of the above

7. Which of the following diagnoses should be considered in the differential diagnosis of unstable angina?
   a. Aortic dissection
   b. Pericarditis
   c. Pneumothorax
   d. Pulmonary embolus
   e. None of the above
   f. All the above

8. Which of the following historic features indicates the lowest risk of death or nonfatal myocardial infarction in patients with unstable angina?

a. Rest pain > 20 minutes
b. Pulmonary edema associated with ischemia
c. Angina associated with ST-segment depression ≥ 1 mm
d. Angina with new mitral regurgitation murmur
e. Angina provoked at a workload lower than normal

9. Which of the following is indicated for the use of calcium channel blockers in patients with unstable angina?
   a. Vasospastic angina
   b. Ischemic symptoms refractory to nitrates and β-blockers
   c. Systolic blood pressure > 150 mm Hg refractory to nitrates and β-blockers
   d. All the above
   e. None of the above

Answers

1. Answer b

Normal or minimally diseased epicardial coronary arteries are found in 10% to 20% of patients with unstable angina.

2. Answer b

Ideally, patients with unstable angina should be evaluated and treated as soon as possible. Evaluation within 20 minutes and treatment within 60 minutes are considered the standard of care.

3. Answer b

Aortic incompetence—but not aortic stenosis—is a contraindication to intra-aortic balloon pump implantation.

4. Answer c

Hyperthyroidism—but not hypothyroidism—may precipitate unstable angina.

5. Answer a

Ticlopidine—but not sulfinpyrazone or dipyridamole—decreases cardiac events in unstable angina.

6. Answer e

Thrombolytic agents have no documented benefit in the absence of acute ST-segment elevation myocardial infarct, with the exception of patients with left bundle branch block in whom a new myocardial infarct is masked or in patients with a posterior infarct and ST-segment depression in leads V_1-V_3.

7. Answer f

The differential diagnosis of unstable angina includes all the above.

8. Answer e

Unstable angina associated with any of the following is associated with a worse prognosis: rest pain, ST-segment depression ≥ 1 mm, a new mitral regurgitation murmur, or pulmonary edema.

9. Answer d

Aspirin, heparin, β-blockers, and nitrates have been shown to be beneficial in unstable angina. Calcium channel blockers are indicated in subsets of patients with vasospastic angina or increased systolic blood pressure or in those refractory to conventional treatment.

Notes

Chapter 13

Diagnosis of Acute Myocardial Infarction

R. Scott Wright, M.D.
Paula J. Santrach, M.D.
Stephen L. Kopecky, M.D.

The diagnosis of acute myocardial infarction (MI) is based on a classic triad of chest pain persisting longer than 30 minutes, ST-segment elevation in two or more concurrent leads on electrocardiography (ECG), and an increase in serum markers of myocardial necrosis. Less than half of patients presenting to emergency rooms with an acute MI have this classic triad, which allows prompt and early diagnosis of infarction (Table 1).

Chest Pain in MI

MI is associated with the classic symptoms of severe retrosternal pressure in about 25% of patients, whereas 25% of patients have chest discomfort that closely mimics reflux esophagitis. A further 25% of patients have infarctions that are clinically silent, and the remaining patients complain of aching or stabbing chest pain; jaw, neck, and left arm discomfort; or, more rarely, back pain.

Typically, MI pain is prolonged beyond 30 minutes and is associated with diaphoresis, olyspnea, and anxiety. Inferior wall MI may be associated with epigastric discomfort, nausea, and vomiting that closely simulate cholelithiasis or peptic ulcer disease.

MI pain may respond to sublingual nitroglycerin, but so also may esophageal pain due to smooth muscle spasm. Infarction pain is rarely pleuritic, positional, or reproduced by chest wall pressure or inspiration.

The occurrence of infarction pain decreases with advancing age (older than 75 years), when syncope and confusional states increase in frequency as the presenting symptoms of MI.

In patients with diabetes and patients who have had a heart transplantation, MI is frequently clinically silent because of pain fiber denervation..

ECG in Acute MI

The development of modern reperfusion therapy has added urgency to the correct diagnosis of MI. All patients presenting to an emergency room with chest pain should have ECG

Table 1.—World Health Organization Criteria for Diagnosis of Acute Myocardial Infarction (MI)

ST-elevation MI	Non–ST-Elevation MI
Chest pain or classic symptoms ≥ 30 minutes	Chest pain or classic symptoms ≥ 30 minutes
ST-segment elevation of at least 1 mV in 2 contiguous leads, or new LBBB left bundle branch block	ST-segment depression or T-wave inversion persisting for 24 hours
Increase of cardiac enzyme levels	Increase of cardiac enzyme levels

within 10 minutes of arrival and thrombolysis started within 30 minutes or they should be transferred to a cardiac catheterization laboratory if ST-segment elevation MI is present.

A finding of new ST-segment elevation in two contiguous ECG leads of 0.1 mV or more in height has a sensitivity of about 50% but a specificity of 90% for the diagnosis of acute MI. About 20% of patients with enzyme-proven MI will have ECG criteria for infarction.

Infarctions should be classified as ST-segment elevation or non–ST-segment elevation infarction rather than the older terms of Q-wave and non–Q-wave or transmural and non-transmural infarction.

The ECG diagnostic criteria for acute MI in the Multicenter Investigation of the Limitation of Infarct Size (MILIS) study were as follows:

1. New Q waves (> 30 ms wide and 0.2 mV deep) in two contiguous leads)

2. New ST-segment elevation or depression of 0.1 mV or more measured 20 ms after the J point in two contiguous leads

3. New left bundle branch block in the appropriate clinical setting

The ECG criteria for the different anatomical locations are given in the ECG chapter of the book.

Inferior lead ST-segment depression in association with acute anterior wall MI may represent electrical reciprocal phenomena or true inferior wall ischemia due to obstruction of a "wrap-around"-type left anterior descending coronary artery distribution.

Anterior lead ST-segment depression in association with acute inferior wall infarction suggests a large inferior wall infarct and a high-risk patient cohort.

Markers of Myocardial Necrosis

The ideal marker of myocardial necrosis does not as yet exist. An ideal marker of acute myocardial necrosis would be present solely in the myocardium, become increased in the plasma only after acute myocardial necrosis, and would otherwise circulate at very low concentrations. It would appear quickly in the plasma after the onset of necrosis, yet be cleared by the body in such a way that detection would be possible for at least 24 hours after an episode of necrosis, and then would return to normal plasma levels.

Creatine Kinase

An increase in the level of creatine kinase (CK) and its myocardial isoform (MB) is the standard by which acute MI is diagnosed. Unfortunately, it typically takes 6 to 12 hours from symptom onset to accurately diagnose acute MI with standard serum enzyme determination. Consequently, new markers of acute myocardial necrosis are being tested to determine whether the diagnosis of acute MI can be made both more accurately and more timely.

CK is an enzyme that catalyzes the transfer of high-energy phosphates from ATP to creatine and is located within the mitochondria and the cytosol of both cardiac and noncardiac muscle cells. The MB isoform is highly expressed in cardiac myocytes, where it accounts for up to 20% of the total CK level. It is also present in low concentration in the smooth muscle of the gastrointestinal and genitourinary tracts. The CK level becomes increased in plasma when only 1 or 2 g of myocardial necrosis has occurred. The plasma CK level begins to increase 6 to 10 hours after the onset of myocardial necrosis, and it peaks at about 24 hours. The plasma CK level may peak earlier in non–Q-wave MI than in Q-wave MI. The plasma CK value returns to baseline by 48 to 72 hours after the onset of necrosis. The sensitivity of plasma CK and CK-MB values is excellent when serial measurements are made over 24 to 48 hours. However, the emphasis now is on the early diagnosis of acute MI, such that thrombolysis or angioplasty can be instituted before the onset of large-scale myocardial necrosis.

Several studies have analyzed the sensitivity and specificity of the plasma CK-MB value during the initial hours of an acute MI. The Biochemical Markers for Acute Myocardial Ischemia (BAMI) study demonstrated that although the specificity of the CK-MB value for the diagnosis of MI is almost 100%, its sensitivity at less than 3 hours after the onset of chest pain is only 30%, increasing to 70% between 6 and 9 hours and more than 97% at 9 to 12 hours.

Although the CK-MB value is an excellent marker for the retrospective diagnosis of acute MI, it is short of being ideal in the patient population with nondiagnostic ECG findings and chest pain onset within 4 to 6 hours of presentation to the emergency room. Several plasma markers recently have been tested to determine their value in identifying acute MI within the 4- to 6-hour window when reperfusion therapy is beneficial.

CK-MB Mass Measurements

Conventional measurement of the plasma CK-MB level is based on migration of the CK isoenzymes on agarose gel electrophoresis. Recently developed fluorometric enzyme immunoassays utilizing monoclonal antibodies allow direct measurement and quantification of the CK-MB isoform.

Measurement of CK-MB mass is faster than traditional gel agarose electrophoresis and may soon be available as a "point of service" test—one that can be easily performed in the emergency department or at the patient's bedside in the cardiac care unit.

Multiple studies have examined the sensitivity and specificity of CK-MB mass measurements early in the course of evolving MI (Table 2). All have found CK-MB mass to have higher sensitivity than that reported with conventional CK-MB by agarose gel electrophoresis.

The data suggest that CK-MB mass may be a good marker for the early diagnosis of acute MI. Frequent plasma sampling for CK-MB mass during the first 6 hours after onset of chest pain symptoms may result in an earlier diagnosis of acute MI.

CK-MB Isoform Analysis

The CK-MB molecule exists as a dimer and undergoes cleavage by serum carboxypeptidases upon release into plasma. This conversion is rapid and provides for at least two forms of circulating CK-MB: $CK-MB_1$ and $CK-MB_2$. Both isoforms can be measured and quantified. Several investigators have analyzed the efficacy of the $CK-MB_2 / CK-MB_1$ ratio with regard to early diagnosis of acute MI. Two studies by Puleo et al. utilized an absolute cutoff of $CK-MB_2$ of 1.0 U/L or more and a $CK-MB_2/CK-MB_1$ ratio of 1.5 or more as positive for MI. A third study by Laurino used an absolute $CK-MB_2$ value of 3 µg/L or more or a $CK-MB_2/CK-MB_1$ ratio or 2.3 or more as positive for MI. Their results are summarized in Table 3.

CK-MB isoforms, specifically $CK-MB_2$, appear promising as "early" markers of evolving MI.

Myoglobin

Myoglobin is a low-molecular-weight protein released by necrotic myocardium within 1 to 3 hours after the onset of necrosis. It is also released after injury to skeletal muscle, and thus skeletal muscle injury cannot be distinguished from cardiac muscle injury with this enzyme.

Kontos et al. and Laurino et al. both examined the diagnostic accuracy of the plasma myoglobin level in patients presenting with chest pain to emergency departments. The myoglobin level was most accurate within the first 12 hours after the onset of chest pain (Table 4).

Troponin Complexes

The troponin complex is the main regulatory protein of the thin filament of the cardiac myofibril and regulates calcium-dependent ATP hydrolysis and the actin-myosin interaction

Table 2.—Use of Creatine Kinase-MB Value in Evolving Myocardial Infarction

Study	Sensitivity/ specificity at < 2 hours, %*	Sensitivity/ specificity at 2-4 hours, %*
Kontos et al. ($n = 20$)	30/100	90/100
Young et al. ($n = 1,042$)	57/97	88/96
Brogan et al. ($n = 136$)	29/97	43/100

*After onset of chest pain.

Table 3.—Use of Creatine Kinase Isoform in Evolving Myocardial Infarction

Time from onset of chest pain, hours	Study, sensitivity/specificity, %		
	Laurino ($n = 100$)	Puleo ($n = 1,110$)	Puleo ($n = 49$)
0-2	20/100	8/93	13/NA
2-4	32/97	...	59/NA
4-6	85/95	56/93	92/NA
6-8	95/90	96/94	100/NA
8-10	100/86	...	100/NA
10-12	100/85	...	100/NA

that causes cardiac contraction. There are three subunits within the troponin complex: troponin I (TnI), which inhibits actin-myosin interaction; troponin T (TnT), which binds to tropomyosin; and troponin C (TnC), which binds calcium.

Cardiac Troponin T (cTnT)

Cardiac troponin T (cTnT) is a cardiac-specific contractile protein and is not found elsewhere in the body. The release of cTnT from necrotic myocardium starts 4 to 8 hours after the onset of infarction and peaks at 24 to 48 hours, similar to CK and CK-MB enzymes. It remains increased up to 10 days after infarction and is not a useful marker of reinfarction (Table 5).

The strengths of cTnT as a marker of MI are its cardiac specificity and persistent increase for several days after symptom onset. It will likely replace lactate dehydrogenase as the serum enzyme for retrospective diagnosis of late MI (> 24 hours old).

Cardiac Troponin I (cTnI)

Cardiac troponin I (cTnI) is a cardiac-specific contractile

Table 4.—Sensitivity and Specificity of Myoglobin in the Diagnosis of Acute Infarction

		Time after onset of chest pain, hours					
	Study	< 2	2-4	4-6	6-8	8-10	10-12
Sensitivity, %	Kontos	70	...	85	...	...	...
	Laurino	22	27	81	95	98	98
Specificity, %	Kontos	81	...	81	...	...	...
	Laurino	92	80	70	63	61	59

Table 5.—Sensitivity and Specificity of Troponin T for the Diagnosis of Myocardial Infarction

		Sensitivity, %		Specificity, %	
Study	Cutoff, µg/L	0-4 Hours	4-8 Hours	0-4 Hours	4-8 Hours
Burlina (n = 262)	0.2	57	87	N/A	N/A
Antman (n = 26)	0.2	50	75	100	100
Bakker (n = 322)	0.1	54	74	N/A	N/A
Bakker (n = 143)	0.1	51	65	74	88

N/A, not available.
Modified from *J Emerg Med* 16:67-78, 1998. By permission of Elsevier Science.

protein and an excellent marker of acute MI. The release of cTnI from necrotic myocardium starts 3 to 6 hours after the onset of acute MI, and it peaks at 24 to 48 hours. It remains increased for up to 10 days after the onset of acute MI. It is an excellent and specific "late" marker of acute MI, but, like troponin T, it is not a useful marker for infarct extension. It is not increased in acute skeletal muscle injury or renal failure, and thus it is useful for distinguishing acute MI from skeletal muscle injury. Although cTnT has been reported to be increased in a small number of patients with acute muscle injury or patients with chronic renal failure insufficiency, to date no reports exist of such increases for cTnI.

Brogan et al., in the BAMI study, compared the sensitivity of cTnI with that of CK-MB for the diagnosis of acute MI.

The sensitivity of cTnI is almost 100% at 9 to 12 hours after onset of infarction, and its sensitivity early in acute MI (30% at < 3 hours, 42% at 3-6 hours, and 70% at 6-9 hours) is reduced because of its large molecular size and relative "slowness" at migrating across the myocyte membrane to enter plasma. It remains increased for several days after an acute MI and so cannot be used to distinguish reinfarction from the initial MI.

Lactate Dehydrogenase (LDH)
LDH is the late enzyme of acute MI and is increased between 24 and 48 hours after infarction. It returns to normal 10 days after infarction. Cardiac troponins have replaced LDH for the late diagnosis of MI.

Early Diagnosis of MI—Which Marker to Use?
There is no consensus about which marker is "best" for early diagnosis of acute MI. No single current marker is "adequate" in itself. The practice at our institution is to obtain an initial ECG, plasma CK-MB mass measurement, and troponin I value for all patients with chest pain. Serial samples are measured every 2 to 3 hours for 4 samples after onset of chest pain. Postoperatively, only serial cTnI measurements are made. Other conditions also can lead to increases of cardiac markers of acute MI (Table 6).

Table 6.—Conditions Associated With Increases of Serum Cardiac Enzyme Markers

Plasma creatine kinase-MB	Troponin T
Acute muscle injury	Skeletal muscle injury
Postoperative patients	Chronic renal failure
Chronic renal failure	Marathon running
Dialysis	
Chronic muscle conditions	
Marathon running	

Chapter 14

Thrombolytic Trials for Acute Myocardial Infarction

Sze-Man J. Wong, M.D.
Joseph G. Murphy, M.D.

The Role of Thrombosis in Acute Myocardial Infarction

The cause of myocardial infarction in the great majority of patients is rupture of an atheromatous plaque that leads to occlusive intracoronary thrombus formation. In animal models of myocardial infarction, ischemic myocardial necrosis proceeds in a "wavefront" manner, spreading from subendocardium to epicardium. This process begins 20 minutes after acute coronary occlusion and involves most of the myocardial wall within 6 hours. In humans, the time to complete myocardial infarction is variably affected by the presence or absence of collateral vessels to the ischemic territory, ischemic preconditioning of the myocardium, and the occurrence of brief intervening periods of spontaneous reperfusion.

Fibrinolysis

The endogenous fibrinolytic system can spontaneously lyse the intracoronary thrombus and lead to a patency rate at 90 minutes of about 20%. Therapeutic administration of thrombolytic agents results in significantly higher patency rates. Thrombolytic agents differ in their efficiency of thrombolysis, fibrin selectivity, and ability to activate thrombosis and platelet aggregation (Table 1). Even for the same thrombolytic agent, different doses, different administration regimens, and concomitant use of adjunctive agents modify patency rates significantly.

Principles of Thrombolysis

Thrombolytic agents were first used for the treatment of acute myocardial infarction in 1958 and gained wide acceptance in the 1980s after several prospective, randomized, controlled trials showed a clear mortality benefit. The single most important predictor of benefit in all thrombolytic trials is the time from vessel occlusion to the restoration of TIMI-3 (normal) coronary flow. The benefit of thrombolytic therapy is age- and sex-independent. Patients who benefit the most are those treated early, the elderly, and those with anterior myocardial infarction. Intracoronary administration of thrombolytic agent was initially thought to be superior to systemic administration, but systemic administration is now considered the method of choice.

All patients with acute ST-segment elevation myocardial infarction presenting within 12 hours of the onset of chest pain should be considered for thrombolysis or the alternative, primary percutaneous transluminal coronary angioplasty (PTCA) (if cardiac catherization facilities and trained interventional staff are available within 60 to 90 minutes).

TIMI Classification of Coronary Flow
- TIMI-0 No antegrade flow
- TIMI-1 Partial penetration of contrast past the point of occlusion
- TIMI-2 Opacification but delayed filling of the distal vessel
- TIMI-3 Normal flow

Table 1.—Summary of Thrombolytic Agents in Clinical Practice or Clinical Trials

Agents	Comments
First-generation	
Streptokinase	Plasma half-life 18-25 min; patency at 90 min is 40%, and 32% achieve TIMI-3 flow; incidence of intracerebral hemorrhage about 0.3%; antigenic and therefore not used within 5 days to 2 years after prior administration; about 25 lives saved per 1,000 treated. Dose 1.5 million units over 1 hour intravenously
Urokinase	Plasma half-life 15 min; not considered antigenic; administered as 1.5 million units intravenous bolus, followed by 1.5 million units over 90 minutes
Anisoylated plasminogen streptokinase activator complex	Plasma half-life 100 minutes; patency at 90 minutes is 63%, and 43% achieve TIMI-3 flow; incidence of intracerebral hemorrhage is 0.6%; antigenic; about 25 lives saved per 1,000 treated; dose: 30 mg over 5 minutes intravenously
Second-generation	
Tissue-type plasminogen activator	
rt-PA (one chain)	Plasma half-life 5 minutes
t-PA (two chain), alteplase (by recombinant technology)	Plasma half-life 5 minutes; no antigenicity and causes moderate systemic fibrinogen depletion; about 35 lives saved per 1,000 treated; dose: 1) accelerated t-PA: administered as 15-mg bolus intravenously, then 50 mg over 30 minutes, and 35 minutes over the next 60 minutes; 2) 100 mg over 90 minutes intravenously
Single-chain urokinase-type plasminogen activator (r-scu-PA, Saraplase, Prourokinase)	Plasma half-life 5 minutes; effect requires concomitant use of heparin and even enhanced with preliminary bolus of heparin; reported to have higher rate of intracranial hemorrhage; dose: 20 mg intravenous bolus
Staphylokinase	Plasma half-life 1-2 minutes; high fibrin selectivity; limited systemic plasminogen activation; associated with high incidence of antibody formation; dose: 10 mg intravenously over 30 minutes
Third-generation	
Mutant	
TNK-tPA	Reduced plasma clearance with prolonged plasma half-life; can be administered as single intravenous bolus; 14 times more fibrin selective than t-PA; 80 times more resistant to PAI-1; intrinsically less thrombogenic and causes less platelet aggregation; dose: 30-40 mg intravenous bolus
r-PA	Deletion mutant of t-PA; preferential binding of fibrin-bound plasminogen; plasma half-life 18 minutes; does not require body weight adjustment
n-PA	Plasma half-life 37 minutes; improved lytic activity relative to t-PA; reduced fibrin affinity
Vampire bat plasminogen activator	Long plasma half-life, 2.8 hours; can be produced by recombinant technology; highly fibrin selective; can induce antibody formation

Mortality Trials of Thrombolytics in Acute Myocardial Infarction

Several landmark studies (GISSI-1 and ISIS-2) showed the convincing beneficial effect of thrombolytic therapy in patients with acute myocardial infarction. The beneficial effect also was found in elderly patients, patients with diabetes, and patients with previous myocardial infarction, despite previous reports that had suggested a possible increased complication risk associated with thrombolytic agents in these patients.

Thrombolytic trials designed to optimize therapy can be classified into mortality, patency, and recanalization studies. Various factors studied in these trials include different thrombolytic agents, timing of administration, and conjunctive and adjunctive therapies. Patients with new ST-elevation myocardial infarction and new-onset left bundle branch block benefit the most from thrombolysis. Patients with non–ST-elevation myocardial infarction and unstable angina do not benefit from thrombolysis. Patients with cardiogenic shock respond poorly to thrombolysis, probably because of poor penetration of the thrombolytic agent into the occlusive thrombus and the lack of adequate coronary perfusion pressure in the setting of severe hypotension, which is necessary to maintain vessel patency. Cardiogenic shock is an indication for primary PTCA.

There are many thrombolytic trials. From a learning perspective, it is important to know the key conclusions of the major trials. Each trial generally has one or two key conclusions, and these are summarized below. Thrombolytic trials are frequently classified by sponsoring organizations (as in GISSI, ISIS, TIMI, ECSG, TAMI, GUSTO, and MITI, discussed in detail in the following pages).

GISSI (Gruppo Italiano per lo Studio della Streptochinasi nell'Infarto Miocardico)

The GISSI Trial (also called the GISSI-1 trial) was a landmark study that first reported the benefit of intravenous streptokinase in a very large cohort of patients with infarction. Mortality benefits at 21 days and at 1 year were the primary end points. A total of 11,816 patients were enrolled. All patients had chest pain accompanied by ST-segment elevation or depression of 1 mm or more in any limb leads or of 2 mm or more in one or more of the precordial leads. All patients were treated within 12 hours of symptom onset. Streptokinase (1.5 million units) administered intravenously over 1 hour was compared with no thrombolysis.

The GISSI trial reported a reduction in mortality of 17% at 21 days and at 1 year in patients with ST-elevation myocardial infarction treated within 6 hours of infarction. Early administration resulted in better outcome (Table 2). The 21-day mortality was 10.7% in the treated group and 13% in the placebo group ($P < 0.001$). The 1-year mortality was 17.2% in the treated group and 19.0% in the placebo group ($P < 0.01$). Follow-up study showed that the mortality benefit lasted 10 years.

There was no significant mortality benefit in patients with ST-segment depression infarction or in those treated later than 6 hours.

GISSI-2 Trial

The GISSI-2 trial was one of the great head-to-head trials of streptokinase and tissue plasminogen activator (t-PA). It compared intravenous streptokinase (1.5 million units over 1.5

Table 2.—Mortality Reduction in Myocardial Infarction, by Time of Administration of Streptokinase: GISSI-1

Time after therapy	Reduction in mortality, %*		
	0-1 hours[†]	1-3 hours[†]	3-6 hours[†]
21 days	47	23	17
1 year	64	15	17

*All the values are statistically significant when compared with the group that did not have thrombolysis; thrombolysis given beyond 6 hours of the onset of pain showed no mortality benefit.
[†]From onset of chest pain to administration of streptokinase.

hours) with t-PA (100 mg over 3 hours) with or without heparin in 12,490 patients admitted within 6 hours after the onset of chest pain. There were no significant differences in mortality rate, rate of reinfarction, stroke rate, or the incidence of postinfarction angina. The GISSI-2 trial concluded that streptokinase and t-PA were equally effective in the treatment of ST-elevation myocardial infarction when administered within 6 hours of the onset of symptoms. Subcutaneous heparin had no added benefit on mortality, incidence of heart failure, or occurrence of severe ventricular dysfunction (Table 3) but did increase bleeding complications.

GISSI-3

The GISSI-3 trial evaluated adjunctive therapy to thrombolysis in patients with infarction. Specifically, GISSI-3 evaluated the effect of an angiotensin-converting enzyme (ACE) inhibitor (lisinopril), transdermal nitrate, or a combination on survival and left ventricular function in more than 18,000 patients after myocardial infarction. The ACE inhibitor reduced mortality (6.3% versus 7.1% for the control group [no ACE inhibitor or nitrate], $P = 0.03$) at 6 weeks

Table 3.—Comparison of Streptokinase and Tissue Plasminogen Activator (t-PA): GISSI-2

Factor	% of patients		P value
	t-PA	Streptokinase	
Mortality	9.0	8.6	NS
Heart failure	7.7	8.1	NS
Severe ventricular dysfunction	2.5	2.2	NS

NS, not significant.

and reduced the combined end point of death or severe ventricular dysfunction at 6 months (18.1% versus 19.3% in the control group, $P = 0.03$). The benefit was even larger in diabetic patients. Nitrates were of no statistical benefit for reduction in death or severe left ventricular dysfunction.

ISIS-1 (International Study of Infarct Survival)
This was a trial of β-adrenergic blocker without thrombolysis in just more than 16,000 patients. Mortality decreased with atenolol in patients with suspected myocardial infarction who were treated within 12 hours of presentation.

ISIS-2
The ISIS-2 trial is the famous aspirin and streptokinase (2 x 2) trial. It tested four regimens (streptokinase 1.5 million units over 1 hour, aspirin 162.5 mg daily for 1 month, combination, or placebo), more than 17,000 patients, within 24 hours of the onset of infarction. The key conclusion of this study was that aspirin and streptokinase both independently reduced mortality and had a synergistic benefit when used together without increasing the stroke risk. The benefit was still present at late follow-up more than 1 year later. The combination of streptokinase and aspirin reduced mortality by 53% when administered within 4 hours of symptoms and by 38% when administered within 12 to 24 hours of infarction (Table 4).

ISIS-3 Trial
ISIS-3 was a head-to-head comparison of streptokinase, anisoylated plasminogen streptokinase activator complex (APSAC), and duteplase (a nearly pure two-chain form of recombinant t-PA, rt-PA) in 41,299 patients; the median time from symptom onset to treatment was 4 hours. There was no difference in the 35-day and 6-month mortality rates for the different thrombolytic agents. The frequencies of reinfarction were comparable in the streptokinase and APSAC groups, but lower in patients receiving t-PA (Table 5). Allergic reactions were most frequent with APSAC and least with t-PA. Concurrent administration of subcutaneous heparin had no effect on mortality at 35 days or at 6 months.

ISIS-4
The ISIS-4 trial compared an adjuvant ACE inhibitor (captopril), oral mononitrate, and intravenous magnesium in 58,050 patients with myocardial infarction who presented within 24 hours of symptom onset. Magnesium and oral nitrates had no mortality benefit, but captopril reduced 5-week mortality by 7% ($P = 0.02$).

TIMI (Thrombolysis in Myocardial Infarction) Trials
The TIMI trials were 14 trials (at least 4 more are planned) on the efficacy of t-PA (TIMI 1-4), hirudin (TIMI 5-9B), TNK (a mutant form of rt-PA with higher fibrin specificity, slower plasma clearance, more resistance to plasma proteinase inhibitors, and greater enzymatic activity against fibrin compared with native rt-PA) (TIMI 10A-10B), enoxaparin (11A-11B), and gycoprotein IIb/IIIa inhibitors (TIMI-12, 14, 15, 16, 18). TIMI-13 was never planned because of the fate of Apollo XIII (Conti CR: Summary of the TIMI Trials. *Clin Cardiol* 21: 459-461, 1998).

TIMI-1
rt-PA resulted in more rapid myocardial reperfusion than streptokinase when assessed angiographically. There was no added mortality or ejection fraction benefit with rt-PA than with streptokinase, and bleeding complications were similar in both groups.

At 90 minutes after thrombolysis, TIMI-2 or 3 coronary flow reperfusion rates were 60% with rt-PA and 35% with streptokinase ($P < 0.001$). At 21 days, mortality was 4% with rt-PA and 5% with streptokinase (not a significant difference).

Table 4.—Overall Cardiovascular Mortality at 5 Weeks: ISIS-2

Treatment	Mortality, %
Streptokinase	9.2
Aspirin	9.4
Aspirin + streptokinase	8.0
Placebo	13.2

Table 5.—Comparison of Thrombolytic Agents for Myocardial Infarction: ISIS-3

Factor	Treatment		
	Streptokinase	APSAC	t-PA
35-Day mortality, %	10.6	10.5	10.6
Frequency of reinfarction, %	3.5	3.6	3.0

APSAC, anisoylated plasminogen streptokinase activator complex; t-PA, tissue plasminogen activator.

TIMI-2

In patients who received rt-PA, heparin, and aspirin for acute myocardial infarction, an invasive strategy of PTCA within 18 to 48 hours of infarction was of no added benefit over a conservative strategy of PTCA only in patients with spontaneous or exercise-induced myocardial ischemia. There was no difference at 6 weeks or 1 year in mortality or reinfarction rates. Death and nonfatal reinfarction at 1 year were 14.7% and 15.2%, respectively, in the invasive and conservative treatment groups (not a significant difference).

TIMI-2A

This study differed from the TIMI-2 trial by the addition of an immediate PTCA group (< 2 hours of rt-PA administration). This approach was compared with a delayed invasive strategy of PTCA within 18 to 48 hours of rt-PA administration and a conservative arm of PTCA for spontaneous or exercise-induced myocardial ischemia. Again, the conservative strategy was equally effective with the invasive arms when judged according to predismissal vessel patency and ejection fraction and 1-year mortality and reinfarction rates.

TIMI-2B

This study evaluated the effect of a β-adrenergic blocker (metoprolol) given immediately after rt-PA administration versus delayed administration 6 days after rt-PA administration in patients with ST-elevation myocardial infarction. Early reinfarction at 6 weeks was less in the immediate treatment group, but 1-year mortality rates, reinfarction rates, and ventricular function were similar in both groups.

TIMI-4

This study compared the efficacy of three thrombolytic regimens: anistreplase (APSAC), front-loaded rt-PA, or both agents in combination. Front-loaded rt-PA was superior for early vessel patency and close to statistical significance for a lower 6-week mortality rate and improved clinical outcome.

At 90 minutes, TIMI grade 3 blood flow patency was 60% with rt-PA ($P < 0.05$ compared with both other groups), 43% with APSAC, and 45% with rt-PA plus APSAC. The 6-week mortality rates among the treatment groups were 2.2% with rt-PA ($P = 0.06$ compared with both other groups), 8.8% with APSAC, and 7.2% with rt-PA plus APSAC.

TIMI Hirudin Studies (TIMI-5, 6, 7, 8, 9A, 9B)

The TIMI-5 trial evaluated the benefit of hirudin compared with heparin as an adjunct to front-loaded rt-PA in the treatment of ST-elevation myocardial infarction.. Hirudin was associated with a higher 18- to 36-hour vessel patency and a lower in-hospital reinfarction and death rate, but at the price of more major hemorrhagic complications. The TIMI-9 study showed that hirudin had no benefit over heparin in patients with acute myocardial infarction treated with thrombolysis.

European Cooperative Study Group (ECSG) Trials

The European Cooperative Study Group (ECSG) trials 1-6 analyzed infarct artery patency with t-PA and various conjunctive therapies, including PTCA and heparin. The overall conclusion of these studies was that infarct patency with t-PA was superior to that with streptokinase (ECSG-1), heparin improved patency (ECSG-6), but routine PTCA was detrimental (ECSG-4)

TAMI (Thrombolysis and Angioplasty in Myocardial Infarction)

The TAMI trials consisted of 10 studies (TAMI 1-9 and TAMI-UK), with more planned, on the efficacy of t-PA, urokinase, and adjuvant therapies (including fluosol, prostacyclin, and glycoprotein IIb/IIIa inhibitors) in acute myocardial infarction. The TAMI-1 trial evaluated the role of immediate PTCA in addition to t-PA in acute infarction and reported no advantage over delayed PTCA. Prostacyclin (TAMI-4) and fluosol (TAMI-9) had no benefit when added to t-PA for acute infarction.

GUSTO-1 (Global Utilization of Streptokinase and Tissue Plasminogen Activator for Occluded Coronary Arteries)

The GUSTO-1 trial randomized 41,021 patients to different thrombolysis regimens to test the hypothesis that early and sustained patency of the infarct-related vessel would improve survival in patients with evolving infarction. This study reported that rapid restoration of coronary flow with t-PA was associated with improved survival and a 14% reduction in mortality at 30 days when compared with streptokinase and intravenous or subcutaneous heparin. Accelerated t-PA also was associated with a significantly higher incidence of hemorrhagic stroke when compared with streptokinase. For overall benefit, as assessed from the combined end point of total mortality and disabling stroke, t-PA was significantly better than streptokinase (Table 6). The higher-risk patients had the greatest benefit.

In summary, the GUSTO-1 trial found that accelerated

t-PA and intravenous heparin resulted in a lower mortality than streptokinase combined with either subcutaneous or intravenous heparin. A secondary finding was that patients with cardiogenic shock benefited from emergency PTCA. The angiographic substudy of GUSTO-1 showed that the 1-year mortality rates remained in favor of t-PA (9.1%, versus 10.1% for streptokinase) combined with either intravenous or subcutaneous heparin ($P \leq 0.01$).

GUSTO-2A

The GUSTO-2A trial was a hirudin study that was stopped prematurely because of excessive bleeding. It found a small benefit for hirudin over heparin in patients with infarction.

GUSTO-2B Angiographic Substudy Trial

The GUSTO-2B Angiographic Substudy Trial was a head-to-head comparison of primary PTCA and thrombolysis. Primary PTCA was found to be an excellent alternative to thrombolysis in skilled hands and had a small short-term advantage over thrombolysis with t-PA.

GUSTO-3

The GUSTO-3 trial was a head-to-head trial of two forms of recombinant t-PA: alteplase and reteplase (a longer-acting mutant variety of alteplase). The study included more than 15,000 patients with ST-segment elevation or new left bundle branch block myocardial infarction who presented within 6 hours of symptom onset. The results with both agents were almost identical.

Mortality at 30 days was 7.22% with alteplase and 7.43% with reteplase (not a significant difference), and the incidence of hemorrhagic stroke was 0.88% and 0.91%, respectively (not significant).

INJECT (International Joint Efficacy Comparison of Thrombolytics)

In this study, 6,010 patients were randomized to receive either 1.5 million units of streptokinase or two bolus doses of 10 units of reteplase (r-PA) 30 minutes apart. Aspirin (93%) and intravenous heparin (99%) also were given. Mortality was assessed at 35 days and at 6 months. The 35-day mortality rates were 9.0% for r-PA and 9.5% for streptokinase (not significant). Mortality at 6 months was 11.% and 12.5%, respectively (not significant). Hypotension and allergic reactions were more common in the streptokinase group, and there was a small, nonstatistically significant excess in nonfatal in-hospital strokes in the r-PA group.

RAPID (Reteplase Angiographic Patency International Dose-Ranging) Study

The study was designed to determine the best regimen for administering r-PA (bolus versus infusion). The three intravenous r-PA regimens were: 1) a single bolus of 15 units, 2) two boluses of 10 units given 30 minutes apart followed by 5 units, and 3) three boluses of 10 units each given 30 minutes apart. Standard t-PA was used as a control. Patency of the infarct-related artery was evaluated angiographically at 30, 60, and 90 minutes after initiation of therapy and again at hospital dismissal (5 to 14 days later). r-PA given in a double bolus of 10 units plus 10 units 30 minutes apart resulted in better patency rate and improvement in left ventricular ejection fraction and regional wall motion abnormalities. The complication rates were comparable in all groups.

RAPID-2

The RAPID-2 trial compared double-bolus reteplase with front-loaded accelerated alteplase for achieving infarct-related artery patency and TIMI-3 flow at 90 minutes. A

Table 6.—Results of Thrombolysis: GUSTO-1

	Treatment				
Factor	SK and SC heparin	SK and iv heparin	t-PA and iv heparin	SK, t-PA, iv heparin	P value, t-PA vs. both SK groups
No. of patients	9,796	10,377	10,344	10,328	
24-hour mortality, %	2.8	2.9	2.3	2.5	0.005
30-day mortality, %	7.2	7.4	6.3	7.0	0.001
Or nonfatal stroke, %	7.9	8.2	7.2	7.9	0.006
Nonfatal hemorrhage stroke, %	7.4	7.6	6.6	7.4	0.004
Or nonfatal disabling stroke, %	7.7	7.9	6.9	7.6	0.006

SC, subcutaneous; SK, streptokinase; iv, intravenous.

total of 324 patients were recruited. Aspirin and heparin were given as adjunctive therapy to both treatment groups. The rate of patent infarct-related arteries with TIMI-2 or -3 flow was higher with reteplase (83.4%) than alteplase (73.3%, $P = 0.03$). TIMI-3 flow rates were 60% and 45%, respectively ($P = 0.01$). In addition, the reteplase group required fewer additional interventions (13.6%) in the subsequent 6 hours than the alteplase group (26.5%, $P = 0.004$). The 35-day mortality was 4.1% and 8.4%, respectively (not significant). The differences in the late patency rate and TIMI-3 coronary blood flow rate were not statistically significant. Other factors compared, including rate of stroke and adverse outcomes at 35 days (death, reinfarction, congestive heart failure and shock, or an ejection fraction < 40%), also showed no statistically significant difference.

PARADIGM (Platelet Aggregation Receptor Antagonist Dose Investigation and Reperfusion Gain in Myocardial Infarction)

This three-part clinical trial examined the effect of thrombolysis in combination with the platelet glycoprotein IIb/IIIa inhibitor lamifiban. Patients with ST elevations presenting within 12 hours of symptom onset treated with t-PA or streptokinase were enrolled. The primary efficacy end point was a composite of angiographic, continuous electrocardiographic, and clinical markers of reperfusion. Rate of bleeding was the primary safety end point. The mean time to reperfusion, defined electrocardiographically as more than 50% recovery of the ST-segment elevation,was significantly reduced in patients receiving lamifiban. At 90 minutes, more patients in the lamifiban group achieved reperfusion (80.1% vs. 62.5%, $P = 0.001$). The use of lamifiban resulted in more rapid reperfusion but a higher incidence of bleeding (16.1% in the lamifiban group and 10.3% with placebo).

MITI-1 and -2 (Myocardial Infarction Triage and Intervention)

The MITI trials evaluated the benefit of prehospital administration of thrombolyis. The trials concluded that although there was no demonstrable benefit to prehospital administration of thrombolysis, treatment within 70 minutes of symptom onset was extremely beneficial compared with treatment given 70 minutes or later from symptom onset (Table 7).

GREAT Trial

This trial was conducted in rural Britain and reported a reduction of more than 50% in 1-year mortality (10.5% versus 21.5%, $P \leq 0.01$) and a time saving of about 2 hours when at-home thrombolysis was compared with in-hospital thrombolysis. This trial is particularly relevant to patients with projected prolonged transport times to a hospital.

European Myocardial Infarct Trial

This was a large randomized trial of nearly 5,500 patients in which prehospital treatment with anistreplase was compared with in-hospital thrombolysis. Cardiovascular mortality at 30 day follow-up decreased from 9.7% to 8.3% ($P = 0.05$) with prehospital thrombolysis, and the time saving was about 1 hour for drug administration.

- Give thrombolysis in the emergency room if the transport time to a cardiac catheterization facility with available staff is more than 90 minutes.
- Give prehospital thrombolysis if the transport time to an emergency room is more than 60 minutes.

Conjunctive Therapy With Thrombolytic Agents

Aspirin

In acute ST-elevation myocardial infarction, aspirin reduces mortality by 23% and reocclusion rate by 50%.

Glycoprotein IIb/IIIa Receptor Antagonists

These drugs bind to platelet glycoprotein IIb/IIIa receptor site and prevent platelet aggregation. Two agents (abciximab and eptifibatide) are approved by the Food and Drug Administration for conjunctive use with intracoronary stents. Tirofiban and eptifibatide are approved for use in unstable angina and non–Q-wave myocardial infarction. Clinical trials (Table 8) of combinations of thrombolytic agents with glycoprotein IIb/IIIa receptor antagonists have shown improved patency rates of the infarct-related artery.

Table 7.—Results of Prehospital Thrombolysis: MITI Trials

	Time to treatment, minutes		
	< 70	≥ 70	P value
Mortality, %	1.2	8.7	< 0.05
Infarct size, %	4.9	11.2	< 0.05
Ejection fraction, %	53	49	< 0.05

Thienopyridines (Ticlopidine and Clopidogrel)

These are relatively weak antiplatelet agents that inhibit adenosine diphosphate-induced platelet aggregation, thus prolonging bleeding time and reducing blood viscosity. Currently, there are no studies of their conjunctive use in acute myocardial infarction.

Heparin

In GUSTO-1, the patency of the infarct-related artery was significantly higher at 5 to 7 days in patients receiving intravenous heparin (84% vs. 72%, $P = 0.04$) after initial t-PA, even though there was no difference in the patency rate at 90 minutes and 24 hours. The finding suggests that heparin can prevent reocclusion of the infarct-related artery in acute ST-elevation myocardial infarction. The benefit for heparin with streptokinase is less clear. Mortality in the t-PA groups with and without heparin showed no statistically significant difference.

Low-Molecular-Weight Heparin

Low-molecular-weight heparin is a class of depolymerized, fractionated heparinoid compounds with molecular weights ranging from 4,000 to 6,000 daltons. They have anti-thrombotic and anti-Xa activities. Different preparations differ in their anti-IIa to anti-Xa activities (e.g., 1:2 for dalteparin and 1:3 for enoxaparin and nadroparin). There is greater release of tissue factor pathway inhibitor that is not inhibited by platelet factor 4. The bioavailability is much higher for this class of compounds, with significantly less variability in activity. The incidence of heparin-associated thrombocytopenia and bleeding complications is much less for these agents than heparin. In clinical trials comparing intravenous heparin and enoxaparin (initially intravenous followed by subcutaneous), the cardiac event rates (death, recurrent myocardial infarction, and readmission for acute coronary syndrome) at 3 months are 36.4% and 25.5%, respectively ($P = 0.04$). The rate of reinfarction from day 4 to day 6 was 6.6% for heparin and 2.2% for enoxaparin ($P = 0.05$).

Direct Thrombin Inhibitor

Hirudin is a direct thrombin inhibitor that is available as an extract from medicinal leeches or produced by recombination technology. The rate of reinfarction is reduced, and there is a trend toward a lower rate of reocclusion. However, in a randomized trial (TIMI-7), there was no improvement in the primary end point, including death, ventricular function, or severe congestive heart failure.

Adjunctive Therapy With Thrombolytic Agents

Adjunctive therapy with thrombolytic agents in acute myocardial infarction includes β-adrenergic blockers, angiotensin-converting enzyme (ACE) inhibitors, nitrates, and, in hypomagnesemic patients, magnesium. β-Blockers and ACE inhibitors have been shown to reduce infarct size and improve mortality. Nitrates are clinically helpful in relieving symptoms, but do not improve survival.

β-Blockers

The effect of β-blockers in conjunction with thrombolytics was studied in TIMI-2B. The 1,431 patients were randomly assigned to immediate metoprolol (intravenous followed by oral) or oral metoprolol at day 6 after infarction. There

Table 8.—Trials of Thrombolytics With Glycoprotein IIb/IIIa Receptor Antagonists

Trial	Agent	Outcome
TAMI-8	Murine 7E3 with t-PA	Dose-dependent relationship of antiplatelet action, improved vessel patency at day 5, less recurrent ischemia
IMPACT-AMI	Accelerated t-PA, aspirin, and heparin together with eptifibatide	Highest tolerable eptifibatide is associated with higher TIMI-3 flow rate (66% vs. 39%, $P = 0.006$)
PARADIGM	Lamifiban in conjunction with t-PA or streptokinase in ST-elevation myocardial infarction	Lamifiban induced more rapid reperfusion, as evidenced by continuous electrocardiography factors; however, there was more bleeding in lamifiban-treated patients

IMPACT-AMI, Integrilin to Manage Platelet Aggregation to Prevent Coronary Thrombosis in Acute Myocardial Infarction; PARADIGM, Platelet Aggregation Receptor Antagonist Dose Investigation and Reperfusion Gain in Myocardial Infarction; TAMI-8, Thrombolysis and Angioplasty in Acute Myocardial Infarction.

was no difference in overall mortality and resting ejection fraction at dismissal. The incidence of reinfarction and recurrence of chest pain at day 6 were lower in the immediate metoprolol group than the later group (reinfarction: 2.7% vs. 5.1%, $P = 0.02$; recurrent chest pain: 18.8% vs. 24.1%, $P < 0.02$), and there was a trend toward lower intracerebral hemorrhage in the immediate metoprolol group. In patients receiving rt-PA within 2 hours of onset of symptoms, the immediate β-blocker group had a lower mortality rate at 6 weeks, but the mortality benefit was not found at 1 year. β-blocker trials in acute myocardial infarction in the prethrombolytic era showed benefit, with about a 15% reduction in the incidence of ventricular fibrillation, 15% to 30% reduction in infarct size, and 18% reduction in reinfarction and recurrence of myocardial ischemia during hospitalization.

ACE Inhibitors

ACE inhibitors are well studied in several large, randomized, controlled trials involving patients with overt signs of heart failure (Survival and Ventricular Enlargement, SAVE; Acute Infarction Ramipril Efficacy, AIRE; Survival of Myocardial Infarction Long-Term Evaluation, SMILE; Trandolapril Cardiac Evaluation, TRACE) and asymptomatic patients (Cooperative New Scandinavian Enalapril Survival Study II, CONSENSUS II; GISSI-3, ISIS-4, Chinese Captopril Trial). There is a significant reduction in mortality rate regardless of time of administration after acute myocardial infarction. The mechanism of action of ACE inhibitors is inhibition of postinfarct remodeling and thus preservation of left ventricular function, resulting in improved survival.

Nitrates

No studies have shown a survival benefit associated with routine use of nitrates in acute myocardial infarction (GISSI-3, ISIS-4). Nevertheless, nitrates are helpful for managing ongoing ischemic pain, congestive heart failure, pulmonary edema, hypertension, and significant mitral regurgitation.

Magnesium

The use of magnesium in acute myocardial infarction remains controversial. In the prethrombolytic era, the Leicester Intravenous Magnesium Intervention II Trial (LIMIT-2) showed a lower mortality rate in patients randomized to receive 2 g of magnesium followed by 15 g continuous infusion over 24 hours compared with controls (7.8% vs.10.3%, $P = 0.02$). However, ISIS-4 failed to show a mortality benefit with magnesium in 23,000 patients randomized within 6 hours after the onset of symptoms (7.9% in magnesium group vs. 7.6% in control, not significant). ISIS-4 also showed an increased incidence of hypotension (1.1%) requiring termination of use of the study drug, bradycardia (0.3%), and cutaneous flushing and burning (0.3%). The current recommendation for patients with acute myocardial infarction receiving thrombolytics is to check the serum magnesium level and maintain it at more than 2 mEq/L.

Complications of Thrombolytic Therapy and Conjunctive Therapy

Bleeding

Intracerebral hemorrhage is the most serious complication that occurs in patients receiving thrombolytics (0.5%), usually within the first 2 days of hospitalization; the incidence with t-PA (0.7%) is higher than with streptokinase (0.4%). The mortality and permanent neurologic damage rate remains high (about two-thirds of patients) despite early detection and aggressive treatment, and this rate is even higher in patients older than 75 years.

The most common bleeding site is the site of vascular access, which can usually be managed by local pressure for 30 minutes. Other bleeding sites include gastrointestinal, genitourinary, and, rarely, retroperitoneal.

In case of uncontrolled, life-threatening bleeding, the thrombolytic and heparin therapy should be discontinued. In addition to blood transfusion, appropriate antidotes should be administered. For bleeding due to thrombolytics, cryoprecipitate (10 units) and fresh frozen plasma may be needed to correct a hypofibrinogenemic state. ε-Aminocaproic acid is an antifibrinolytic agent that competes with plasminogen for lysine binding site on the fibrin. It is used as a last resort because it may cause thrombosis. It is administered at a loading dose of 5 g, followed by continuous infusion of 0.5 to 1.0 g/hour until bleeding stops. Heparin can be neutralized by protamine administration intravenously (1 mg of protamine neutralizes 100 U of heparin). Platelet transfusion is required for bleeding due to glycoprotein IIb/IIIa antagonists. Hemorrhage due to hirudin requires administration of prothrombin complex and not fresh frozen plasma because it merely corrects the laboratory abnormality and does not stop the bleeding.

Allergic Reactions

A common nonhemorrhagic complication is allergic reaction. Both streptokinase and APSAC (both are derived from group C streptococci) can cause hypotension, flushing, chills, fever, vasculitis, interstitial nephritis, and life-threatening anaphylaxis. Streptokinase and APSAC are not recommended if prior use occurred within 2 years because of the presence of neutralizing antibodies in more than 50% of such patients. Reteplase, t-PA, and urokinase do not usually cause such reactions and can be safely used in patients with prior streptokinase or APSAC exposure.

Clinical Detection of Reperfusion

It is important to know how effective the thrombolytic therapy is for achieving rapid reperfusion after administration. Resolution of chest pain, resolution of ST-segment elevation, and presence of "reperfusion arrhythmia" have limitations as markers for reperfusion. Chest pain may resolve with narcotics or myocardial denervation due to myocardial ischemia or necrosis. The ST-segment elevation may return to pre-infarct level as a result of natural post-infarction evolution or the dynamic blood flow pattern so characteristic of the first 12 hours after infarction. Ventricular tachycardia after infarction occurs more often in patients who do not receive reperfusion therapy or patients who do not achieve successful reperfusion. Findings that are reasonably specific for successful reperfusion are the sudden relief of chest pain with full resolution of electrocardiographic abnormalities and the occurrence of accelerated idioventricular rhythm.

Thus, there are no useful clinical reperfusion indicators. Continuous 12-lead electrocardiographic monitoring or serial assessment of 12-lead electrocardiography may be more useful for assessing completeness of reperfusion than other variables. There is not a complete correlation between the extent of ST-segment resolution and the completeness of coronary flow. Biochemical markers of infarction have not proved to be clinically useful to judge reperfusion in a timely manner. Other noninvasive tests such as echocardiography, high-frequency QRS monitoring, continuous vector electrocardiography, and cine magnetic resonance angiography are investigational tools for this purpose.

Chapter 15

Management of Acute Myocardial Infarction

Joseph G. Murphy, M.D.
R. Scott Wright, M.D.
Stephen L. Kopecky, M.D.
Guy S. Reeder, M.D.

This chapter reviews the management of acute myocardial infarction (MI) based on the American College of Cardiology/American Heart Association (ACC/AHA) recommendations published in the *Journal of the American College of Cardiology* (1). The ACC/AHA classification system of diagnostic or therapeutic benefit is as follows:

Class I: Conditions for which there is evidence for and/or general agreement that a given procedure or treatment is beneficial, useful, and effective.

Class II: Conditions for which there is conflicting evidence and/or divergence of opinion about the usefulness/efficacy of a procedure or treatment.

Class IIa: Weight of evidence/opinion is in favor of usefulness/efficacy.

Class IIb: Usefulness/efficacy is less well established by evidence/opinion.

Class III: Conditions for which there is evidence and/or general agreement that a procedure/treatment is not useful/effective and in some cases may be harmful.

Management of Myocardial Infarction

Out-of-Hospital Management of Acute Myocardial Infarction

The out-of-hospital management of suspected MI should include the early recognition of patients with possible infarction, including those with typical chest pain as well as those with atypical chest pain, jaw pain, back or abdominal pain, unexplained dyspnea, or syncope or near-syncope. Out-of-hospital bystander cardiopulmonary resuscitation (CPR) and/or defibrillation by trained paramedics or untrained personnel using the automatic defibrillator may be lifesaving for ventricular fibrillation. Aspirin (325 mg) should be administered to all patients with suspected MI.

The ACC recognizes that "the single most effective therapy for myocardial infarction is early TIMI [Thrombolysis in Myocardial Infarction] grade 3 reperfusion of the infarct-related artery by either thrombolysis or PTCA [percutaneous transluminal coronary angioplasty]" (1); thus, rapid emergency transport to a hospital emergency room is of paramount importance. Prehospitalization thrombolysis has a class IIb ACC/AHA indication when hospital transport time is projected to be longer than 90 minutes, but out-of-hospital thrombolysis is more widely used in European centers.

Emergency Room Management of Suspected Myocardial Infarction

"The underlying principle of the early in-hospital evaluation of patients with suspected myocardial infarction is that the loss of time equals the loss of myocardial cells" (1). Mortality, infarct size, and loss of ventricular function are directly dependent on the time from vessel occlusion to restoration of TIMI grade 3 blood flow irrespective of the mode of reperfusion (PTCA or thrombolysis) or the thrombolytic agent used. The ACC/AHA suggested that the standard of care should be initial evaluation of the patient within 15 minutes after arrival in the emergency room and thrombolysis or emergency PTCA initiation within 30 minutes.

All patients with suspected MI should receive 1) oxygen, 2) sublingual nitroglycerin (unless contraindicated by hypotension), 3) adequate opiate analgesia, 4) aspirin (if not give earlier), and 5) a 12-lead electrocardiogram (ECG).

The generally accepted criteria for thrombolysis is a new ST-segment elevation MI (> 0.1 mV elevation in 2 or more contiguous leads) presenting within 6 hours after the onset of chest pain in the absence of contraindications to thrombolysis. A longer time period may be considered on an individual basis in patients with continuing chest pain, a stuttering clinical course, or a nonevolving ECG pattern (persistent ST-segment elevation without the development of Q waves). Symptoms of acute MI in patients with left bundle branch block (LBBB) should be managed like those of an ST-segment elevation MI. Patients with non-ST-segment elevation infarcts (non-Q-wave MI) or unstable angina should not receive thrombolytic therapy. Although complications of thrombolysis are increased in the elderly (older than 75 years), MIs in the elderly carry a high mortality, which is decreased by thrombolysis.

Contraindications to Thrombolysis

The physician should balance the potential benefits of thrombolysis against the risks of thrombolysis-induced bleeding in each patient and whether alternative options (PTCA) are available. Thus, every effort should be made to give thrombolysis to a patient having a large anterior wall infarct who presents within 6 hours even if some contraindications are present; however, the same calculated risk may not be justified in a patient presenting late with a small inferior infarct.

The only absolute contraindications to thrombolysis are active internal bleeding, a previous cerebrovascular event (stroke or transient ischemic attack), and the patient's request not to have thrombolysis. The major and minor relative contraindications are outlined in Table 1.

Rapid primary PTCA in experienced hands is an excellent alternative to thrombolysis for most MI patients and is superior to thrombolysis in patients with cardiogenic shock or contraindications to thrombolysis and in those not eligible for thrombolysis with non-ST-segment elevation MI in which circumflex artery occlusion is suspected (lateral wall ECG or echocardiographic changes).

Hospital Management of Patients With Myocardial Infarction

1. All patients with acute MI who are candidates for CPR and defibrillation should have continuous ECG monitoring in a coronary care unit for at least the first 24 hours. MI

Table 1.—Major and Minor Relative Contraindications to Thrombolysis

Major relative contraindications:
1. High risk of internal bleeding because of recent internal surgery (< 10 days)
2. Severe recent gastrointestinal tract bleeding (< 3 mo)
3. Prolonged cardiopulmonary resuscitation (> 15 min)
4. Recent severe trauma, particularly head injury
5. Severe uncontrolled hypertension (> 175 mm Hg systolic)

Minor relative contraindications:
1. Recent minor trauma
2. Endocarditis
3. Known intracavitary left heart thrombus (atrium or ventricle)
4. Pregnancy
5. Coagulation disorder
6. Proliferative diabetic retinopathy
7. Concomitant warfarin therapy (mechanical heart valves, atrial fibrillation, etc.)

Modified from Click R and the Mayo Clinic Coronary Care Unit Staff: Thrombolytic therapy in acute myocardial infarction.

should be confirmed by serial ECGs and cardiac enzyme studies. Prophylactic treatment with lidocaine for ventricular arrhythmias is not recommended.

2. In the absence of any contraindication (hypotension, bradycardia, or excessive tachycardia), nitroglycerin should be administered intravenously for 24 to 48 hours after acute infarction. Nitrates are unique in that they do not rely on an intact endothelium for their vasodilator properties. Oral nitrates are less useful in an acute setting because the dose cannot be finely titrated to the hemodynamic condition of the patient.

3. β-Blockers should be administered to MI patients who are without contraindications to these agents, regardless of whether reperfusion therapy was administered.

4. Calcium channel blockers generally are not indicated for patients with acute MI (exceptions include severe coronary vasospasm not responsive to nitrates or rate control of supraventricular arrhythmias in patients with contraindication to β-blockers).

5. All patients with an acute ST-segment elevation MI, LBBB, or ventricular dysfunction should receive an angiotensin-converting enzyme (ACE) inhibitor within hours after hospitalization unless contraindicated for other reasons (e.g., hypotension or renal artery stenosis). This

agent should be continued for 6 weeks in all patients and indefinitely in those with left ventricular systolic dysfunction (ejection fraction < 40%) or clinical heart failure.

6. All MI patients should receive aspirin, 160 to 325 mg/day, indefinitely.

7. Magnesium sulfate should be given to correct diuretic-induced magnesium deficits.

Preventive Cardiology

After MI, all patients should have a low-density lipoprotein level (LDL) less than 100 mg/dL, preferably by diet but, if not, by lipid-lowering medication. An ideal body weight, a high-density lipoprotein (HDL) level greater than 40 mg/dL, and a triglyceride level less than 120 mg/dL are also highly desirable. Smoking cessation and a structured exercise program are also important.

Summary of Medications in Acute Myocardial Infarction

Intravenous Nitroglycerin

Class I Indications

1. For the first 24 to 48 hours in patients with acute MI and heart failure, large anterior infarction, persistent ischemia, or hypertension

2. Continued use (beyond 48 hours) in patients with recurrent angina or persistent pulmonary congestion

Class IIb Indications

1. For the first 24 to 48 hours in all patients with acute MI who do not have hypotension, bradycardia, or tachycardia

2. Continued use (beyond 48 hours) in patients with a large or complicated infarction (long-acting oral or transdermal patches may be substituted)

Oral Aspirin

Long-term daily aspirin (160 to 325 mg) is an ACC/AHA Class I indication for all MI patients unless the patient has true aspirin allergy, in which case other antiplatelet agents should be substituted.

Intravenous Atropine

Class I Indications

1. Sinus bradycardia with evidence of low cardiac output and peripheral hypoperfusion or frequent premature ventricular

complexes at onset of symptoms of acute MI

2. Acute inferior infarction with type I second- or third-degree atrioventricular (AV) block associated with symptoms of hypotension, ischemic discomfort, or ventricular arrhythmias

3. Sustained bradycardia and hypotension after administration of nitroglycerin

4. For nausea and vomiting associated with administration of morphine

5. Ventricular asystole

Class IIa Indication

1. Symptomatic patients with inferior infarction and type I second- or third-degree heart block at the level of the AV node (i.e., with narrow QRS complex or with known existing bundle branch block)

Class IIb Indications

1. Administration concomitant with (before or after) administration of morphine in the presence of sinus bradycardia

2. Asymptomatic patients with inferior infarction and type I second-degree heart block or third-degree heart block at the level of the AV node

3. Second- or third-degree AV block of uncertain mechanism when pacing is not available

Atropine is not indicated for either mild sinus bradycardia (> 40 beats/min without signs or symptoms of hypoperfusion or frequent premature ventricular contractions) or advanced heart block (type II AV block and third-degree AV block and third-degree AV block with new wide QRS complex) when a temporary pacemaker is indicated.

Intravenous Heparin

Class I Indication

All patients undergoing percutaneous or surgical revascularization

Class IIa Indications

1. Intravenously in patients undergoing reperfusion therapy with alteplase

2. Intravenously or subcutaneously in all patients not treated with thrombolysis who do not have a contraindication to heparin. For patients who are at high risk for systemic emboli (large or anterior MI, atrial fibrillation, previous embolus, or known left ventricular thrombus), intravenous heparin is preferred

3. Intravenously in patients treated with nonselective

thrombolytic agents (streptokinase, anistreplase, urokinase) who are at high risk for systemic emboli (large or anterior MI, atrial fibrillation, previous embolus, or known left ventricular thrombus)

Class IIb Indication

1. Patients treated with nonselective thrombolytic agents, not at high risk for systemic embolism, subcutaneous heparin, 7,500 U to 12,500 U twice daily until completely ambulatory

Routine intravenous heparin is not required within 6 hours for patients receiving a nonselective fibrinolytic agent (streptokinase, anistreplase, urokinase) who are not at high risk for systemic embolism.

β-Blocking Agents

β-Blockers are indicated for almost all patients after MI who do not have contraindications to β-blocker therapy. β-Blockers are particularly useful in patients with continuing or recurrent ischemic pain and in those with tachyarrhythmias, such as atrial fibrillation with a rapid ventricular response.

Angiotensin-Converting Enzyme Inhibitors

Class I Indications

1. Patients within the first 24 hours after suspected acute anterior wall MI or clinical heart failure in the absence of significant hypotension or known contraindications to ACE inhibitor treatment.

2. Patients with MI and left ventricular ejection fraction less than 40% or those with clinical heart failure on the basis of systolic pump dysfunction during and after convalescence from acute MI

Class IIa Indications

1. All other patients within the first 24 hours after suspected or established acute MI, provided significant hypotension or other clear-cut contraindications are absent

2. Asymptomatic patients with mildly impaired left ventricular function (ejection fraction of 40% to 50%) and a history of old MI

Class IIb Indication

1. Patients who have recently recovered from MI but have normal or mildly abnormal global left ventricular function

Calcium Channel Blockers

There are no class I indications for the use of calcium channel blockers in acute MI.

Class IIa Indications

Verapamil or diltiazem may be given to patients for whom β-blockers are ineffective or contraindicated (i.e., bronchospastic disease) for relief of ongoing ischemia or control of a rapid ventricular response with atrial fibrillation after acute MI in the absence of clinical heart failure, left ventricular dysfunction, or AV block.

Short-acting nifedipine is contraindicated in the routine treatment of acute MI because of its negative inotropic effects and the reflex sympathetic activation, tachycardia, and hypotension associated with its use.

Diltiazem and verapamil are contraindicated in patients with acute MI and associated left ventricular dysfunction or heart failure.

ACC/AHA Indications for Nonmedical Treatment in Myocardial Infarction

Indications for Primary PTCA

Class I Indication

1. As an alternative to thrombolytic therapy if performed in a timely fashion by a skilled operator at a high-volume PTCA center

Class IIa Indications

1. As a reperfusion strategy in patients who are candidates for reperfusion but in whom thrombolytic therapy is contraindicated because of a risk of bleeding

2. Patients in cardiogenic shock

Class IIb Indications

1. As a reperfusion strategy in patients who do not qualify for thrombolytic therapy for some reason other than risk of bleeding

2. Patients with evolving large or anterior infarcts treated with thrombolytic agents in whom the artery is believed not to be patent

Indications for Emergency Coronary Artery Bypass Graft Surgery

Class I Indications

1. Failed angioplasty with persistent ischemia or hemodynamic instability in patients with coronary anatomy suitable for surgery

2. Acute MI with persistent or recurrent ischemia

refractory to medical therapy in patients with coronary anatomy suitable for surgery who are not candidates for catheter intervention

3. At the time of surgical repair of postinfarction ventricular septal defect or mitral valve insufficiency

Class IIa Indication

1. Cardiogenic shock with coronary anatomy suitable for surgery

Indications for Early Coronary Angiography and/or Interventional Therapy in Non-ST-Segment Elevation Myocardial Infarction

Class I Indication

1. Patients with recurrent (stuttering) episodes of spontaneous or induced ischemia or evidence of shock, pulmonary congestion, or left ventricular dysfunction

Class IIa Indications

1. Patients with persistent ischemic-type discomfort despite medical therapy and an abnormal ECG or two or more risk factors for coronary artery disease

2. Patients with chest discomfort, hemodynamic instability, and an abnormal ECG

Class IIb Indications

1. Patients with chest discomfort and an unchanged ECG

2. Patients with ischemic-type chest discomfort and a normal ECG and more than two risk factors for coronary artery disease

Indications for Hemodynamic Monitoring

Hemodynamic monitoring consists of intracardiac placement of a balloon-tipped flotation catheter for monitoring pulmonary artery capillary wedge pressure, pulmonary artery pressure, cardiac output, and pulmonary arteriolar resistance and for measuring systemic intra-arterial blood pressure.

Class I Indications for Pulmonary Artery Hemodynamic Monitoring

1. Severe or progressive clinical heart failure or pulmonary edema

2. Cardiogenic shock or progressive hypotension

3. Suspected mechanical complications of acute infarction (i.e., ventricular septal defect, papillary muscle rupture, or pericardial tamponade)

Class IIa Indication

1. Hypotension that does not respond promptly to fluid administration in a patient without pulmonary congestion

Class I Indications for Invasive Systemic Arterial Pressure Monitoring

1. Patients with severe hypotension (systolic arterial pressure < 80 mm Hg) and/or cardiogenic shock

2. Patients receiving vasopressor agents

Class IIa Indication

1. Patients receiving intravenous sodium nitroprusside or other potent vasodilators

Class IIb Indications

1. Hemodynamically stable patients receiving nitroglycerin intravenously for myocardial ischemia

2. Patients receiving inotropic agents intravenously

Routine hemodynamic monitoring in patients with acute infarction without evidence of cardiac or pulmonary complications is not indicated.

Indications for Intra-Aortic Balloon Counterpulsation

Intra-aortic balloon counterpulsation (IABP) increases diastolic blood pressure and coronary perfusion and is valuable to "buy time" in hemodynamically unstable patients pending definitive treatment.

Class I Indications

1. Cardiogenic shock not quickly reversed with pharmacologic therapy as a stabilizing measure before angiography and prompt revascularization

2. Acute mitral regurgitation or ventricular septal defect complicating MI as a stabilizing therapy for angiography and repair/revascularization

3. Recurrent intractable ventricular arrhythmias with hemodynamic instability

4. Refractory post-MI angina as a bridge to angiography and revascularization

Class IIa Indication

1. Signs of hemodynamic instability, poor left ventricular function, or persistent ischemia in patients with large areas of myocardium at risk

Class IIb Indications
1. In patients with successful PTCA after failed thrombolysis or those with three-vessel coronary artery disease, to prevent reocclusion
2. In patients known to have large areas of myocardium at risk, with or without active ischemia

Indications for Emergency Surgical Repair of Mechanical Defects Complicating Acute Myocardial Infarction

Class I Indications
1. Papillary muscle rupture with severe acute mitral insufficiency
2. Postinfarction ventricular septal defect or free wall rupture and pulmonary edema or cardiogenic shock (emergency or urgent)
3. Postinfarction ventricular aneurysm associated with intractable ventricular tachyarrhythmias and/or pump failure (urgent)

Indications for Risk Stratification after Myocardial Infarction

Treadmill Exercise Test (TMET)

Class I Indications
1. Before dismissal for prognostic assessment or functional capacity (submaximal at 4 to 6 days or symptom-limited at 10 to 14 days)
2. Early after dismissal for prognostic assessment and functional capacity (14 to 21 days)
3. Late after dismissal (3 to 6 weeks) for functional capacity and prognosis if early stress was submaximal

Exercise or pharmacologic stress nuclear or echocardiographic imaging is indicated when baseline ECG abnormalities are present.

TMET or pharmacologic stress test is not indicated within the first 48 hours after MI or in patients with unstable symptoms (angina, heart failure, or arrhythmia).

Indications for Coronary Angiography after Myocardial Infarction

Class I Indications
1. Patients with spontaneous episodes of myocardial ischemia or episodes of myocardial ischemia provoked by minimal exertion during recovery from infarction

2. Before definitive therapy of a mechanical complication of infarction, such as acute mitral regurgitation, ventricular septal defect, pseudoaneurysm, or left ventricular aneurysm
3. Patients with persistent hemodynamic instability

Class IIa Indications
1. When MI is suspected to have occurred by a mechanism other than thrombotic occlusion at an atherosclerotic plaque; this would include coronary embolism, certain metabolic or hematologic diseases, coronary artery spasm
2. Survivors of acute MI with depressed left ventricular systolic function (ejection fraction $\leq 40\%$), heart failure, previous revascularization, or malignant ventricular arrhythmias
3. Survivors of acute MI who had clinical heart failure during the acute episode but subsequently demonstrated well-preserved left ventricular function

Class IIb Indications
1. Coronary angiography performed in all patients after infarction to find persistently occluded infarct-related arteries in an attempt to revascularize the artery or to identify patients with three-vessel disease
2. All patients after a non-Q-wave MI
3. Recurrent ventricular tachycardia or ventricular fibrillation or both, despite antiarrhythmic therapy, in patients without evidence of ongoing myocardial ischemia

Routine coronary angiography and PTCA after successful thrombolytic therapy are not indicated in the absence of spontaneous or exercise-induced myocardial ischemia.

ACC/AHA Recommendations for Long-Term Treatment

Indications for Long-Term β-Blocker Therapy in Survivors of Myocardial Infarction
β-Blocker therapy is an ACC/AHA Class I indication in survivors of MI in all but very low-risk patients without a clear contraindication to β-blocker therapy, whereas β-blocker therapy is a class IIa indication in low-risk patients without a clear contraindication to β-blocker therapy.

Indications for Long-Term Anticoagulation After Acute Myocardial Infarction

Class I Indications
1. Secondary prevention of MI in post-MI patients unable to take daily aspirin

2. Post-MI patients in persistent atrial fibrillation
3. Patients with LV thrombus

Class IIa Indications
1. Post-MI patients with extensive wall motion abnormalities

2. Patients with paroxysmal atrial fibrillation

Class IIb Indication
1. Post-MI patients with severe left ventricular systolic dysfunction, with or without clinical heart failure

Suggested Review Reading

1. Ryan TJ, Anderson JL, Antman EM, et al: ACC/AHA guidelines for the management of patients with acute myocardial infarction. A report of the American College of Cardiology/American Heart Association Task Force on Practice Guidelines (Committee on Management of Acute Myocardial Infarction). *J Am Coll Cardiol* 28:1328-1428, 1996.

Notes

Chapter 16

Coronary Angioplasty in Myocardial Infarction

Joseph G. Murphy, M.D.

Acute myocardial infarction results from thrombotic occlusion of a coronary artery, which almost always is triggered by rupture of a lipid-rich atherosclerotic plaque due to a combination of mechanical, inflammatory, and biochemical forces.

Emergency treatment of myocardial infarction aims to restore TIMI grade 3 blood flow to the ischemic myocardium as rapidly and reliably as possible. Lesser degrees of restoration of coronary flow are associated with a significantly poorer prognosis, not dissimilar to that of an occluded vessel. In patients with myocardial infarction, primary percutaneous transluminal coronary angioplasty (PTCA) restores TIMI-3 flow in 90%, compared with about 60% in those treated with thrombolysis.

Limitations of Thrombolysis in Acute Myocardial Infarction

Although thrombolysis is the treatment of choice for acute ST-segment elevation myocardial infarction in patients remote from a cardiac catheterization laboratory, current generation thrombolytic agents have significant limitations in the treatment of myocardial infarction, including the following:

1. Limitation of efficacy
   Restoration of TIMI-3 flow in approximately 50% of patients
   Restoration of TIMI-2 flow in an additional 20% of patients
2. Hemorrhagic complications
   Intracranial bleeding in about 1% of patients (frequently fatal)
   Gastrointestinal tract bleeding
   Genitourinary tract bleeding
   Bleeding at venous or arterial access sites
3. Many patients, especially the elderly (up to 40%), have contraindications to thrombolysis
4. Early hazard effect
   This is the unexpected paradoxical increase in mortality seen in the first 24 hours among patients receiving thrombolysis, in comparison with controls, and documented in the GISSI-1 Trial and all other major randomized trials. It possibly is related to myocardial reperfusion injury. After the first 24 hours, thrombolytic deaths are fewer than those among controls.
5. Thrombolysis does not treat the unstable plaque that triggers the thrombotic episode, and, in some cases, a high-grade residual stenosis that will cause spontaneous or exercise-induced ischemia remains.
6. Thrombolysis is of poor efficacy in cardiogenic shock.

An atlas illustrating pathologic conditions associated with coronary angioplasty in myocardial infarction is found at the end of the chapter (Plates 1-9).

Coronary angioplasty may be performed as a primary emergency treatment for myocardial infarction, as a rescue procedure after failed thrombolysis, electively after thrombolytic therapy for spontaneously occurring or exercise-induced myocardial ischemia, or in special situations such as cardiogenic shock.

TIMI (Thrombolysis in Myocardial Infarction) Classification of Coronary Flow

- TIMI-0   No antegrade flow
- TIMI-1   Partial penetration of contrast past the point of occlusion
- TIMI-2   Opacification but delayed filling of the distal vessel
- TIMI-3   Normal flow

Primary Angioplasty

Advantages

Primary angioplasty is the performance of emergency angioplasty in the setting of acute myocardial infarction without the previous use of thrombolytic agents. The potential advantages of primary angioplasty over thrombolytic therapy in the treatment of acute myocardial infarction are listed in Table 1. The principal advantages of primary PTCA are the higher number of patients who attain TIMI-3 flow in the occluded vessel, the lower risk of intracerebral hemorrhage in comparison with thrombolysis, and the absence of contraindications to cardiac catheterization in most patients. Also, PTCA may be associated with a lower incidence of hemorrhagic myocardial infarction, but the validity and clinical benefit of this have not been proved.

Disadvantages

The disadvantages of primary PTCA as a treatment for myocardial infarction are primarily logistic and related to the availability of resources required to maintain on-call cardiac catheterization facilities and the time delay that accrues to the patient by transfer to an appropriately equipped hospital. The results of primary PTCA are highly operator dependent and may not be equally efficacious in both community and academic environments. PTCA also requires the placement of an arterial access sheath, with the attendant risk of vascular complications. PTCA in the presence of thrombus is associated with a higher reocclusion rate and restenosis rate than elective PTCA.

Table 1.—Potential Benefits of PTCA Over Thrombolysis for Acute Myocardial Infarction

Very low rates of intracerebral hemorrhage or stroke

Rapid, accurate confirmation of vessel occlusion in patients with nondiagnostic ECGs

Full anatomical evaluation of the entire epicardial coronary circulation and determination of the extent and severity of both infarct and noninfarct vessel disease

Reperfusion rates > 95%

TIMI-3 flow rates > 90%

Assessment of left ventricular function

Rapid evaluation of high-risk coronary anatomy (left main disease or severe 3-vessel disease with decreased left ventricular function) or mechanical complications of myocardial infarction requiring emergency cardiac surgery (acute mitral regurgitation, ventricular septal defect, or myocardial rupture)

Confirmation of reperfusion and vessel patency after therapy

Vascular access for temporary pacemaker or intra-aortic balloon pump placement

Treatment of underlying coronary stenosis

Fewer contraindications and greater applicability than thrombolysis

ECG, electrocardiogram; PTCA, percutaneous transluminal coronary angioplasty; TIMI, Thrombolysis in Myocardial Infarction.

Management of Patients With Suspected Acute Myocardial Infarction Based on Angiographic Findings

The approach to patients with suspected acute myocardial infarction referred to the cardiac catheterization laboratory should be individualized on the basis of angiographic findings.

Possible Findings at Coronary Angiography

1. Normal left ventricular function, normal coronary flow, and no critical coronary artery stenosis or normal angiographic vessels—consider a noncardiac cause of chest pain or transient intracoronary event (spasm, embolus, or thrombus with spontaneous thrombolysis). Conservative strategy.

2. Significant regional wall motion abnormality (RWMA) on left ventriculography consistent with acute infarct, no critical (> 70%) coronary artery stenosis, and TIMI-3 flow in all vessels. Conservative strategy.

3. No or small RWMA on left ventriculography, occluded small coronary vessel 2 mm or less in diameter. Probably conservative strategy if the risk of PTCA exceeds the benefit.

4. Consider conservative strategy if culprit vessel cannot be identified on angiography.

5. Consider PTCA or a stent (or both) for coronary stenosis of 70% or greater in the probable culprit vessel (identified by left ventriculography or electrocardiography [ECG] by ST-segment elevation) if TIMI blood flow is grade 2 or less and the anatomy is favorable for intervention. If TIMI blood flow is grade 3, weigh the option for immediate intervention versus delayed intervention (allows plaque to heal but increases the risk of reocclusion).

6. Consider emergency coronary artery bypass graft (CABG) if there is a critical stenosis of 60% or greater of the unprotected left main coronary artery or severe three-vessel coronary artery disease. Culprit-vessel PTCA later followed by CABG may be appropriate for some patients.

7. Saphenous vein graft thrombosis. Consider option of subselective thrombolytic infusion, thrombectomy, or PTCA. The results are poorer than for native arteries.

Advantages and Disadvantages of Thrombolysis in Myocardial Infarction

Thrombolysis is an effective treatment for myocardial infarction and has been studied from a scientific perspective in a greater number of patients in randomized controlled trials than primary PTCA. Thrombolysis is not operator-specific and generally can be administered earlier than primary PTCA, frequently in a community setting. Thrombolysis does not require access to cardiac catheterization facilities and has greater applicability in populations without emergency access to cardiac catheterization laboratories.

Although thrombolysis is targeted directly at dissolving the occluding coronary thrombus, reperfusion rates, especially TIMI-3 flow (approximately 60%), are generally less than those achieved with primary PTCA (approximately 90%). Thrombolysis is frequently contraindicated because of hypertension or cerebrovascular disease, and even when not contraindicated, it often is not administered in a timely manner. Thrombolysis is ineffective in patients in cardiogenic shock. Two other disadvantages of thrombolytic therapy are the difficulty in reliably assessing myocardial reperfusion and, in many cases, the frequent need for subsequent PTCA to treat the underlying stenosis.

Contraindications to Primary PTCA

Contraindications to primary PTCA in myocardial infarction are rare and include a contraindication to heparin usage (e.g., recent [< 48 hours] intracranial neurosurgical procedure or active significant gastrointestinal tract bleeding), a history of severe angiographic contrast anaphylaxis, or severe upper and lower limb vascular disease that would preclude vascular access. Patients with unprotected left main coronary artery stenoses (without a patent bypass graft to either the left anterior descending or left circumflex coronary arteries) generally require emergency CABG and are not appropriate candidates for PTCA. Thrombolysis should not be administered if primary PTCA is planned, because this increases the risk of vascular complications, increases length of hospital stay and costs, and does not improve final left ventricular function or vessel patency.

Primary PTCA may be difficult in patients with excess thrombus burden, especially in occluded saphenous vein grafts, and may lead to a recurrent cycle of no reflow or reclosure. Technical problems with primary PTCA include the inability to steer the guidewire across the lesion, subintimal dissection by the guidewire, and reflex hypotension and bradycardia following reperfusion of the right coronary artery or dominant left circumflex coronary artery.

- Contraindications to primary PTCA in myocardial infarction are rare and include severe contrast allergy, absence of vascular access, and inability to use heparin.
- Primary PTCA allows the rapid assessment of coronary anatomy and ventricular function.
- Primary PTCA is associated with a very low rate of stroke.
- Reflex hypotension following primary PTCA may require low doses of intravenous boluses of epinephrine (25-50 µg).

> The Cardiology Boards will present several scenarios of chest pain and myocardial infarction. It is important to know which patients would be better candidates for PTCA or thrombolytic agents or whether either strategy would be equally acceptable.

Primary Angioplasty Trials

Primary angioplasty has been compared with thrombolysis in 10 randomized trials: 4 trials using streptokinase, 3 using standard regimen tissue plasminogen activator (rt-PA), and

3 using accelerated regimen rt-PA. The major problem with these trials was that they lacked statistical power and none demonstrated a statistically significant mortality benefit for one treatment modality over the other.

Four of these trials (PAMI, Netherlands, Mayo Clinic, and GUSTO-IIb) were prospective controlled trials.

PAMI (Primary Angioplasty in Myocardial Infarction) Trial

This trial tested the hypothesis that PTCA is superior to t-PA (100 mg infused over 3 hours) in the prevention of the combined end point of in-hospital death and nonfatal reinfarction. The study randomly assigned 395 patients at 10 centers (195 were assigned to PTCA, of whom 175 [90%] received PTCA, and 200 to t-PA). The technical results of PTCA were excellent (patency, 99%; good angiographic result without hemodynamically significant stenosis, 97%, and TIMI-3 flow, 94%). The clinical end points were all better in the PTCA arm but did not reach conventional statistical significance (death rate was 2.6% and 6.5% in the PTCA and t-PA arms, respectively [$P = 0.06$]; reinfarction rate was also 2.6% and 6.5% [$P = 0.06$]). No strokes or intracerebral hemorrhages occurred in the PTCA arm; the t-PA arm had a high incidence (28%) of ischemia and nonprotocol coronary angiography and angioplasty before hospital dismissal. The disappointing finding in the study was that 6 weeks after myocardial infarction the rest or exercise ejection fraction was not different between the PTCA and t-PA groups. In high-risk patients (anterior infarct, age older than 70 years, or tachycardia at admission), PTCA had a mortality benefit (2% for PTCA vs. 10% for t-PA [$P = 0.01$]); however, it had no such benefit in low-risk patients (3% for PTCA vs. 2% for t-PA).

Mayo Clinic Study

This was the smallest of the four randomized studies, but it used a novel approach to estimate myocardial salvage by comparing rest nuclear sestamibi scans before and after reperfusion. Anterior infarcts threatened a mean of 48% of the left ventricular mass, of which PTCA salvaged a mean of 31% and t-PA 27% ($P = 0.06$). For inferior infarcts, 18% of the myocardium was threatened, and PTCA salvaged 5% and t-PA 7% ($P = 0.47$). The PTCA group showed a beneficial trend but no statistical benefit in the ejection fraction at hospital dismissal and 6 weeks after infarction. Similar to the PAMI Trial, the t-PA group had more recurrent ischemic events and nonprotocol coronary angiography and angioplasty. No mortality benefit was found, and mortality

was low in both the PTCA (4.3%) and t-PA (3.5%) groups. No strokes occurred in either group.

Netherlands (Zwolle) Trial

In this trial, 301 patients were randomly assigned to streptokinase (149 patients) or PTCA (152 patients). Mortality was lower in the PTCA (2%) than in the streptokinase (7.4%) group ($P = 0.02$), as was reinfarction (1.3% vs. 10%; $P < 0.001$). One patient in the PTCA (0.7%) and three in the streptokinase (2%) group had a stroke ($P = NS$). Similar to the PAMI Trial and Mayo Clinic Study, recurrent ischemia, unscheduled coronary angiography, and angioplasty were higher in the thrombolytic group.

GUSTO-IIb (Global Utilization of Streptokinase and Tissue Plasminogen Activator for Occluded Coronary Arteries) Angioplasty Study

This is the largest of the PTCA vs. t-PA trials, and, unlike the other major trials, it used front-loaded t-PA. Patients were randomly assigned to either PTCA (565 patients) or t-PA (573 patients). No significant difference occurred in the individual end points of death, reinfarction, or disabling stroke. However, when the end points were combined, the PTCA group had a significant (33%) decrease in the event end point, compared with 13.7% for accelerated t-PA ($P = 0.033$). Recurrent ischemia and intracranial hemorrhage were also significantly higher in the t-PA group.

Conclusions of the PTCA vs. thrombolysis trials—Meta-analysis of the four major trials would indicate that PTCA has a clear benefit compared with t-PA in respect to the following:

1. Mortality—4.4% vs. 6.7% ($P = 0.02$)
2. Reinfarction—3.5% vs. 6.9% ($P = 0.007$)
3. Recurrent ischemia—7.1% vs. 18.1% ($P < 0.001$)
4. Stroke—0.8% vs. 2.3% ($P = 0.008$)

The benefit was projected to be higher if the TIMI-3 flow rate had been greater than the 90% expected in the GUSTO-IIb study.

PAMI-II Trial

The PAMI-II trial, conducted in both academic and community settings, tested three separate hypotheses in 1,100 patients with acute myocardial infarction. This trial considered important management issues in acute infarction.

1. Can primary angioplasty be performed safely in nonacademic settings? The answer was "yes." PTCA was successful in 96% of patients (TIMI-3 flow in

93%). Overall mortality among the 1,100 patients was 2.9%. Of the patients, 982 (89%) had PTCA, and 5% required CABG because of unfavorable anatomy for PTCA; 6% of the patients received medical therapy.

2. Will routine prophylactic use of the intra-aortic balloon pump for 36 to 48 hours improve the prognosis for high-risk but hemodynamically stable patients (age older than 70 years, three-vessel disease, ejection fraction of 45% or less, saphenous vein graft occlusion, poor or suboptimal PTCA result, malignant ventricular arrhythmias) by augmenting coronary blood flow? In these patients, including 45% of all those who had PTCA, intra-aortic balloon pump had no significant benefit on mortality, reinfarction, stroke, heart failure, infarct vessel reocclusion, or ejection fraction at dismissal or 6 weeks after dismissal. However, PAMI-II included only patients with a hemodynamically stable condition, and no conclusion should be drawn from this study about the use of intra-aortic balloon pump in those with unstable hemodynamics—where it is strongly advised.

3. Can low-risk patients (55% of those receiving primary PTCA in the PAMI study) be safely dismissed early (day 3 after admission) or is observation in a cardiac care unit needed, with dismissal on day 5 to 7 after admission? The study concluded that low-risk patients may be managed safely in a step-down unit rather than in a cardiac care unit and can receive an abbreviated heparin regimen. Also, they do not need predismissal exercise testing.

All studies reported a longer time to treatment in the PTCA arm than in the thrombolytic arm. This is probably less critical than it initially appears, because the time from vessel occlusion to arterial patency ("pain-to-balloon" time) is the key interval, which could not be reported with any degree of accuracy for the thrombolytic study arms. Major bleeding requiring blood transfusion was a problem for both treatment strategies. It should be noted that all these studies had fewer patients than the thrombolytic trials. Significant improvements in PTCA treatment have occurred since the publication of these trials, including the use of intracoronary stents and the use of GP IIb/IIIa inhibitors.

Stents and Acute Myocardial Infarction

Balloon angioplasty alone in acute myocardial infarction is associated with a high rate of vessel restenosis (40% in one series), probably associated with the presence of significant residual intracoronary thrombus. In the GUSTO IIb and MITI Trials, the acute benefit of primary PTCA seen at 1 month was lost at 6 months, with a higher requirement for further revascularization in PTCA patients than in patients treated with thrombolysis at 12-month follow-up.

Meanwhile, the development of potent GP IIb/IIIa receptor inhibitors has reduced the occurrence of acute stent thrombosis in the setting of acute myocardial infarction to less than 2%.

The combination of the above has led to the evaluation of stenting in acute myocardial infarction.

Three major trials (Stent-PAMI, ADMIRAL, and FRESCO trials) and several small studies have evaluated stents in acute myocardial infarction.

ADMIRAL Study (Abciximab With PTCA and Stent in Acute Myocardial Infarction)

This study evaluated the role of abciximab in acute myocardial infarction. Patients were randomly assigned to either abciximab or placebo before undergoing PTCA or stent implantation. The study included 300 patients with acute myocardial infarction, but more patients in the abciximab than in the placebo group had a history of myocardial infarction (14.8% vs. 8%). The primary study end point was the combined incidence of death, recurrent myocardial infarction, and urgent target vessel revascularization at 30 days. The principal findings of the study were the following:

1. At 24 hours, the TIMI-3 flow rates were 86% in the abciximab group and 78% in the placebo group ($P < 0.05$).

2. Left ventricular function was greater in the abciximab group than in the placebo group at 24 hours (55% vs. 51%; $P < 0.05$).

3. The primary end point of the trial—the combined incidence of death, recurrent myocardial infarction, and urgent target vessel revascularization at 30 days—was decreased by nearly half from 20% in the placebo group compared with 10.7% in the abciximab group ($P < 0.03$).

4. Also, all the individual components of the end point favored abciximab: death was reduced from 4.7% to 3.3%, recurrent myocardial infarction from 4.7% to 2%, and urgent target vessel revascularization from 14% to 6% ($P = 0.03$).

5. The rate of major bleeding at 30 days was not significantly higher in the abciximab group (4% vs. 2.6%), but a significant increase in minor bleeding was observed (6.7% vs. 1.3%, $P = 0.02$).

These data support the benefit of combining abciximab with PTCA or stent in the treatment of acute myocardial infarction. The improved TIMI-3 flow at 24 hours with abciximab translated to improved left ventricular function at 24 hours in the abciximab group. The use of abciximab ensured better short-term vascular wall stability (30-day incidence of death, recurrent myocardial infarction, and urgent target vessel revascularization was decreased). Abciximab did not cause excess hemorrhagic complications.

Stent-PAMI (Stent-Primary Angioplasty in Myocardial Infarction) Trial

The Stent-PAMI Trial was designed to test the safety, efficacy, and short-term and long-term outcomes of stenting as a primary strategy in anterior myocardial infarction. The trial enrolled 1,458 patients with myocardial infarction at 62 centers in 12 countries within 12 hours after symptom onset. Patients who were either ineligible for stenting (considered to be best managed either medically or surgically) or in whom the operator thought stent placement was mandatory were excluded from randomization and enrolled in a registry ($n = 558$). All other patients were randomly assigned to receive a Palmaz-Schatz heparin-coated stent ($n = 452$) or no further coronary intervention after primary angioplasty ($n = 448$).

Almost all (98%) the patients assigned to stent placement received a stent. For the patients who did not, the stent either could not be deployed or a proper stent size was not available. Of the PTCA-only group, 67 patients (15%) ultimately had stenting; thus, 85% of this group had PTCA alone. For both groups, procedural success was greater than 99%.

Acute angiographic results showed significantly greater residual stenosis in the primary PTCA group than in the primary stent group (24.8% vs. 11%, $P = 0.0001$). This difference remained at 6 months of follow-up, with 20% of the stent group showing greater than 50% stenosis compared with 32% of the primary PTCA group. Both acute and 6-month angiographic data showed that the minimal luminal diameter was larger in the stent group.

Target vessel revascularization at 6 months was more likely in the PTCA group (21.4% vs. 12.8%, $P < 0.001$). Patients in the primary stent group also showed significantly reduced postprocedural anticoagulant use as well as decreased angiographic restenosis and reocclusion.

Overall, stenting was associated with a decrease in the combined end point of death, recurrent myocardial infarction, disabling stroke, and ischemia-driven target vessel revascularization at 6 months (12.4% vs. 20.1%, $P < 0.01$). This difference appeared to be related almost entirely to a decrease in ischemia-driven target vessel revascularization.

FRESCO (Florence Randomized Elective Stenting in Acute Coronary Occlusions) Trial

This study aimed to compare stenting of the primary infarct-related artery with optimal primary PTCA with respect to clinical and angiographic outcomes of patients with an acute myocardial infarction. The trial randomly assigned patients treated for acute infarction in whom primary angioplasty had already achieved an excellent result (defined as residual stenosis < 30% and TIMI-3 flow) to either adjunctive stenting or no stenting. After successful primary PTCA, 150 patients were randomly assigned to elective stenting or no further intervention. The primary end point of the trial was a composite end point defined as death, reinfarction, or repeat target vessel revascularization as a consequence of recurrent ischemia within 6 months after randomization. The secondary end point was angiographic evidence of restenosis or reocclusion at 6 months afer randomization. Rates of recurrent ischemia, restenosis, and reocclusion were significantly improved in the stented patients. This improvement was maintained at 6 months.

Stenting of the infarct-related artery was successful in all patients assigned to stent treatment. At 6 months, the incidence of the primary end point was 9% in the stent group and 28% in the PTCA group ($P = 0.003$), and the incidence of restenosis or reocclusion was 17% and 43% ($P = 0.001$).

The conclusion of the study was that primary stenting of the infarct-related artery, compared with optimal primary angioplasty, has a lower rate of major adverse events related to recurrent ischemia and a lower rate of angiographically detected restenosis or reocclusion of the artery. The benefit of coronary stenting in decreasing the incidence of restenosis or reocclusion was evident both early (within the first 30 days) and late (from 1 to 6 months) after the procedure.

The authors suggested that in the acute phase, coronary stenting prevented vessel wall recoil and reocclusion because of latent intimal wall dissection. The latter mechanism, they suggested, was relevant because in nearly all patients in the PTCA group with in-hospital recurrent ischemia, emergency coronary angiography revealed occlusive or subocclusive dissection. The larger postprocedural luminal diameter provided by stenting and the beneficial effect of stenting on vascular remodeling may explain the better long-term results of stenting in decreasing the rates of late restenosis and reocclusion.

The ESCOBAR trial randomly assigned 204 patients with acute myocardial infarction to either PTCA or stent. The success rates were 96% and 98%, respectively. The difference in the frequency of subacute closure and recurrent myocardial infarction was significant, with the stent group having improved outcome. Recurrent myocardial infarction occurred in 2% in the stent group and in 7% in the PTCA group.

Two other small trials of stenting in acute MI have been reported: PASTA (Primary Angioplasty Versus Stent Implantation in Acute Myocardial Infarction) and GRAMI (GRII Stent in Acute Myocardial Infarction). Both have reported a higher primary success rate, a lower target vessel in-hospital revascularization rate, and a lower in-hospital death rate with stenting than with PTCA alone in acute myocardial infarction.

Management of Specific Myocardial Infarction Scenarios

The management of specific myocardial infarction scenarios is frequently a subject on the Cardiology Boards and is outlined below.

Distant or Remote Geographic Location

If the transportation time for a patient is more than 90 minutes to a hospital with an available primary PTCA service, thrombolysis is advised, in the absence of contraindications. Any potential gain from PTCA in this setting would be nullified by the delay in reperfusion caused by the transportation time. For patients within 90 minutes' transportation time to a primary PTCA center, other factors should be considered, including relative contraindications to thrombolysis and patient and physician preference.

- Myocardial infarction in patients more than 90 minutes from a primary PTCA center should be treated with thrombolytic agents unless contraindicated.

Hypertension

In patients with a sustained systolic pressure greater than 180 mm Hg or a diastolic pressure greater than 110 mm Hg, thrombolytic agents should be avoided because of the increased risk of intracranial hemorrhage, and PTCA should be recommended. If the hypertension is transient and easily controlled, thrombolytic agents may be acceptable, but PTCA would be the optimal approach. If thrombolytic agents are used, streptokinase may be the better agent because it has a lower risk of intracranial bleeding than t-PA.

- Primary PTCA is the treatment of choice in patients at increased risk for stroke because of uncontrolled hypertension.

Previous CABG

Myocardial infarction in patients with previous bypass surgery has several special features and may be due to native artery occlusion distal to the graft insertion, occlusion of a native nongrafted vessel, saphenous vein graft occlusion, or, more rarely, internal mammary artery graft occlusion.

Overall, thrombolysis has a lower success rate (about 50%) in patients who previously had CABG. Thrombolytic agents are less effective for vein graft occlusion than for native artery occlusion, probably because of the increased thrombus burden in the occluded saphenous vein grafts in comparison with that of native vessels. ECG findings may be subtle and nondiagnostic of myocardial infarction (< 2 mm ST-segment elevation in about 50% of patients) in patients with occlusion of a saphenous vein graft.

Coronary angiography is useful in this setting to define the occlusion of a culprit vessel. PTCA of occluded vein grafts has a significantly lower success rate (about 70%) than PTCA for native vessel occlusions (about 90%). PTCA may be more effective if the occlusion is in the distal native vessel or an ungrafted native vessel. Administration of thrombolytic agents without the benefit of previous angiography in patients who have had CABG and acute myocardial infarction is acceptable if a cardiac catheterization laboratory is not available, but it has a lower success rate overall than in patients who have not had CABG.

- Overall, thrombolysis has a success rate of approximately 50% in patients with previous CABG.
- ECG findings may be subtle and nondiagnostic of myocardial infarction in about 50% of patients with myocardial infarction and previous CABG.
- PTCA of occluded saphenous vein grafts has a lower success rate (about 70%) than PTCA for native vessel occlusions (about 90%).

ST-Segment Depression Myocardial Infarction

Patients with ST-segment depression myocardial infarction have poorer left ventricular function and more multivessel disease than those with ST-segment elevation myocardial infarction. Thrombolytic therapy has not been shown to be beneficial in this setting, and a nonstatistical trend toward increased mortality with thrombolytic agents was noted in one trial. Patients with ST-segment depression myocardial infarction overall have a mortality rate of about 15%, and PTCA is advised if possible.

Some patients with ST-segment depression myocardial infarction will have left circumflex coronary occlusion, which is electrically silent without ST-segment elevation.

- Thrombolytic therapy is not beneficial in patients with ST-segment depression myocardial infarction.

Left Bundle Branch Block

Patients with myocardial infarction complicated by new left bundle branch block usually have large infarcts and high mortality rates if coronary perfusion is not restored. Primary PTCA and thrombolytic therapy are both effective in reducing mortality and improving left ventricular function. Left bundle branch block makes the diagnosis of myocardial infarction difficult, especially if it antedates myocardial infarction.

Stroke

Thrombolysis is contraindicated in patients with a recent history of stroke or transient ischemic attacks, because of the risk of intracranial hemorrhage or secondary hemorrhage into the infarcted zone. PTCA is the preferred strategy in patients presenting with myocardial infarction in whom there is a recent history of cerebrovascular disease.

Elderly Patients

Elderly patients (older than 70 years) have a higher in-hospital mortality (approximately 25%) from myocardial infarction than younger patients and benefit significantly from either thrombolytic agents or primary PTCA. Elderly patients have higher complication rates with both primary PTCA and thrombolytic therapy than younger patients. The decision to proceed with either revascularization strategy is reasonable in elderly patients, although primary PTCA has the benefit of a lower stroke rate in a population at higher risk for stroke with thrombolytic agents.

Coronary Angioplasty in Cardiogenic Shock

Cardiogenic shock develops in about 8% of patients with acute myocardial infarction, of whom approximately 70% to 80% will die with conservative management. Thrombolytic agents are ineffective in reversing cardiogenic shock, probably because the low coronary perfusion pressure makes penetration of the thrombus by the thrombolytic agent ineffective and any coronary thrombolysis that does occur is rapidly followed by vessel reocclusion. The only thrombolytic studies to include cardiogenic shock patients were the Gruppo Italiano per lo Studio della Streptochinase Nell'Infarcto Miocardico (GISSI)-1 and 2 and GUSTO studies, in which the mortality was 70%, 78%, and 56%, respectively. Multiple nonrandomized series have reported a beneficial effect of PTCA in cardiogenic shock, with a survival of approximately 70% in patients in whom reperfusion is accomplished. Mortality without reperfusion was about 20%. Predictors of mortality in cardiogenic shock include poor left ventricular function, triple-vessel disease, delayed presentation, and failure to reperfuse with PTCA. In the GUSTO study, mortality from cardiogenic shock was lower in the U.S. than in other countries, probably because of greater use of PTCA in the U.S.

Technical Aspects of Primary PTCA in Acute Myocardial Infarction

In the absence of severe hemodynamic instability or renal failure, left ventriculography should always be performed in the setting of suspected myocardial infarction. This allows the assessment of overall left ventricular function, RWMAs, mechanical complications of myocardial infarction (severe mitral regurgitation, ventricular septal defect, and myocardial rupture) and may help with identification of the infarct-related artery. Next, a diagnostic coronary catheter should be inserted into the non-infarct-related artery to look for the presence of collateral filling of the infarct-related artery. The infarct-related artery should then be visualized.

The most common angiographic finding is total coronary occlusion by thrombus. In the presence of hemodynamic instability, an intra-aortic balloon pump should be placed via the contralateral femoral artery. Aspirin and clopidogrel should be administered orally together with abciximab intravenously if there is significant intracoronary thrombus and no major bleeding contraindication to therapy. A soft guidewire should be chosen initially to cross the occluded coronary vessel, and the initial dilation should be performed at low pressure with an appropriate but not oversized PTCA balloon. After flow has been restored to the occluded vessel, further dilation or stent placement can be performed.

Complications of Primary PTCA

Malignant Arrhythmias

Malignant ventricular arrhythmias (ventricular tachycardia, ventricular fibrillation) occur most frequently at the time of reperfusion, because of the sudden release of the products of ischemia, including potassium ions. These arrhythmias are usually transient but may require defibrillation. Ventricular fibrillation in the setting of severe multivessel disease or severe ventricular dysfunction may be refractory to defibrillation.

No-Reflow or Slow-Reflow Phenomenon

No-reflow or slow-coronary reflow is the restoration of less than TIMI-3 coronary flow in the presence of an apparently successful PTCA. It is due to a combination of factors, including distal embolization of thrombus, microvascular endothelial injury, tissue edema, and reperfusion injury. Strategies to treat this condition include intracoronary administration of adenosine, nitroglycerin, or verapamil and intra-aortic balloon pump placement to augment diastolic coronary blood flow.

Distal Embolization

Mechanical disruption of an occlusive intracoronary thrombus by primary PTCA may lead to embolism of thrombus either distally into the coronary bed or, more rarely, proximally out of the coronary circulation into the systemic arterial vasculature.

Intimal Dissection

Initial poor vessel visualization increases the risk of intimal dissection, which may be difficult to distinguish from intracoronary thrombus. Intimal dissection is best treated with stent placement.

Incessant Thrombus

A frustrating problem is the generation of new intracoronary thrombus at the time of primary PTCA. Physiologically, there is a balance between the procoagulant and anticoagulant properties of the coagulation cascade. The strategy behind primary PTCA is to restore coronary flow in the infarct-related artery and shift the coagulation balance in favor of the anticoagulant factors. In some primary PTCA patients, procoagulant factors still dominate, even with the use of adjuvant aspirin, clopidogrel, heparin, and abciximab. In the past, conventional therapy for this complication was to infuse intracoronary thrombolytic agents. Paradoxically, this may exacerbate new thrombus formation by activating platelets and exposing additional clot-bound thrombin.

RESCUE Angioplasty

Rescue angioplasty is emergency PTCA performed following failed thrombolysis. Failure to reperfuse after thrombolysis occurs in about 20%-30% of patients and is associated with a high mortality (approximately 10%). The cause of thrombolysis failure is likely multifactorial:

1. A higher proportion of platelet-rich (gray-white in appearance) and thrombolysis-insensitive thrombi
2. Acute or chronic thrombus formation with layering of new thrombus on existing layers of partially organized thrombus that is thrombolysis-insensitive
3. Subintimal and subfibrous cap thrombus inaccessible to thrombolyis
4. Active inhibitors of thrombolysis such as plasminogen activator inhibitor (PAI)-1 present in activated platelets and shown to occur in animal models of resistant thrombi
5. Predominant nonthrombotic mechanism of coronary occlusion such as vessel spasm or hemorrhage into an atherosclerotic plaque
6. Failure to achieve adequate lytic levels at the thrombus site

Although newer thrombolytic agents or dosing regimens such as front-loaded rt-PA may improve vessel patency, a significant number of patients likely still will not achieve vessel patency with lytic agents; their best chance of myocardial salvage will be emergent PTCA.

Two studies (RESCUE and CORAMI) evaluated the results of PTCA after failed thrombolysis.

1. The RESCUE Trial (Randomized Comparison of Rescue Angioplasty With Conservative Management of Patients With Early Failure of Thrombolysis for Acute Anterior Myocardial Infarction)—This trial compared 151 patients with failed thrombolysis for first anterior wall myocardial infarction with documented occluded arteries within 8 hours after symptom onset. The PTCA patency rate was 92%, and PTCA decreased the occurrence of the combined end point of death and severe heart failure at 30 days after infarction (6% for PTCA vs. 17% for conservative management [$P = 0.055$]). The PTCA mortality was 5%, compared with 10% in the non-PTCA group ($P = NS$). PTCA significantly improved exercise ejection fraction but not rest ejection fraction or mortality.

2. The CORAMI Study (Cohort of Reserve Angioplasty in Myocardial Infarction)—This study included 72 patients and had a procedural success rate of 90%, with three in-hospital deaths (4%) and an actuarial survival of 92% among patients dismissed from the hospital.

The published Mayo experience of 34 patients with rescue angioplasty has also been favorable, with a 4-year survival of 89% even though the average predismissal ejection fraction was 36%, suggesting that a patent infarct-related artery may be beneficial even in the absence of ventricular salvage.

The benefits of rescue angioplasty may be enhanced in the future as better methods are developed to diagnose failed thrombolysis in a timely manner without the need for angiography and the newer GP IIb/IIIa inhibitors that block platelet aggregation gain widespread use as an adjunct to rescue angioplasty. Pooled data suggest that rescue PTCA following rt-PA has a lower success rate and a higher reocclusion rate than PTCA following streptokinase or urokinase.

The experience with nonrandomized rescue PTCA from the TIMI and TAMI trial databases has been reported. In-hospital mortality was 6% (TAMI) and 10% (TIMI) with successful rescue PTCA. Unsuccessful PTCA has a very high mortality, 39% (TAMI) and 33% (TIMI), much higher overall than for patients with unsuccessful thrombolysis but in whom rescue PTCA was not attempted (about 8%). The excess mortality seen with unsuccessful rescue PTCA may be due partly to selection bias of very ill patients in whom thrombolysis failed and for whom rescue PTCA was the last option for survival.

- Rescue angioplasty for failed thrombolysis may be beneficial if performed within 12 hours after the onset of chest pain.
- Rescue PTCA following rt-PA may have a lower success rate and a higher reocclusion rate than PTCA following streptokinase or urokinase.

Elective Angioplasty Following Thrombolytic Therapy for Myocardial Infarction

Three trials have been performed to evaluate immediate routine PTCA following thrombolytic administration (TIMI-2A, TAMI, ECSG). No benefit and possibly a slight detriment to routine immediate PTCA following thrombolysis were shown by all these studies. Two trials have evaluated delayed routine PTCA (SWIFT [Should We Intervene Following Thrombolysis], TIMI-2B) after the administration of thrombolytic agents, whereas DANAMI evaluated myocardial revascularization as a long-term strategy after myocardial infarction. These studies demonstrated no benefit to the patient either at the time of dismissal or at 1 year with delayed routine PTCA following thrombolytic administration (Tables 2 and 3).

In summary, PTCA for myocardial infarction is indicated as an alternative to thrombolysis as the primary mode of reperfusion, as a rescue procedure following failed thrombolysis, in cardiogenic shock when thrombolysis is ineffective, or as an elective procedure in the presence of spontaneous or exercise-induced myocardial ischemia after myocardial infarction. PTCA is not indicated as a routine procedure after successful thrombolysis in the absence of ongoing or exercise-induced myocardial ischemia.

DANAMI Trial (Danish Trial in Acute Myocardial Infarction)

The DANAMI Trial was a randomized trial that evaluated myocardial revascularization by either PTCA or CABG compared with conservative medical management in patients with either spontaneous or inducible myocardial ischemia at the time of predischarge stress testing following thrombolysis for a first myocardial infarction in 1,008 patients younger than 70 years.

At the 30-month follow-up point, there was no significant mortality benefit to myocardial revascularization but recurrent myocardial infarction was decreased by almost half (5.6% vs. 10.5%, $P < 0.005$) in the invasive strategy group, as were hospital admissions for unstable angina (18% vs. 30%, $P < 0.00001$).

Table 2.—PTCA Following Thrombolysis

Study	Patients	Strategy following thrombolysis trials
TIMI-2A	389	Immediate PTCA vs. PTCA at 18-48 hr after rt-PA
TAMI	386	Immediate PTCA vs. PTCA at 7 days after rt-PA infusion
ECSG	387	Immediate PTCA vs. no PTCA following rt-PA infusion
TIMI-2B	3,262	PTCA 18-48 hr after rt-PA or PTCA for recurrent ischemia
SWIFT	800	PTCA < 48 hr after APSAC or no catheterization or PTCA

APSAC, anisoylated plasminogen streptokinase activator complex; ECSG, European Cooperative Study Group; PTCA, percutaneous transluminal coronary angioplasty; rt-PA, tissue plasminogen activator; SWIFT, Should We Intervene Following Thrombolysis; TAMI, Thrombolysis and Angioplasty in Myocardial Infarction; TIMI, Thrombolysis in Myocardial Infarction.

Table 3.—PTCA Following Thrombolysis*

Study	Early mortality, %	Left ventricular ejection fraction, %
TIMI-2A		
Immediate PTCA	7.2	50
18-48-hour PTCA	5.7	49
TAMI		
Immediate PTCA	4.0	53
7-day PTCA	1.0	56
ECSG		
Immediate PTCA	7.0	51
No PTCA	3.0	51
TIMI-2B		
Conservative	5.2	50
Invasive	4.6	50
SWIFT		
Conservative	2.7	52
Invasive	3.3	51

ECSG, European Cooperative Study Group; SWIFT, Should We Intervene Following Thrombolysis; TAMI, Thrombolysis and Angioplasty in Myocardial Infarction; TIMI, Thrombolysis in Myocardial Infarction.
*Comparison of early and late PTCA and of PTCA and conservative management had no statistical benefit for mortality or ventricular function in the trials.

Suggested Review Readings

1. Gibbons RJ, Holmes DR, Reeder GS, et al: Immediate angioplasty compared with the administration of a thrombolytic agent followed by conservative treatment for myocardial infarction. *N Engl J Med* 328:685-691, 1993.

In patients with acute myocardial infarction, immediate angioplasty does not appear to result in greater myocardial salvage than the administration of a thrombolytic agent followed by conservative treatment, although a small difference between these two therapeutic approaches cannot be excluded.

2. Grines CL, Browne KF, Marco J, et al: A comparison of immediate angioplasty with thrombolytic therapy for acute myocardial infarction. *N Engl J Med* 328:673-679, 1993.

In comparison with t-PA therapy for acute myocardial infarction, immediate PTCA decreased the combined occurrence of nonfatal reinfarction or death, was associated with a lower rate of intracranial hemorrhage, and resulted in similar left ventricular systolic function.

3. The Global Use of Strategies to Open Occluded Coronary Arteries in Acute Coronary Syndromes (GUSTO IIb) Angioplasty Substudy Investigators: A clinical trial comparing primary coronary angioplasty with tissue plasminogen activator for acute myocardial infarction. *N Engl J Med* 336:1621-1628, 1997.

The results of this trial suggest that angioplasty provides a small-to-moderate short-term clinical advantage over thrombolytic therapy with t-PA. Primary angioplasty, when it can be accomplished promptly at experienced centers, should be considered an excellent alternative method for myocardial infarction.

4. de Boer MJ, Hoorntje JC, Ottervanger JP, et al: Immediate coronary angioplasty versus intravenous streptokinase in acute myocardial infarction: left ventricular ejection fraction, hospital mortality and reinfarction. *J Am Coll Cardiol* 23:1004-1008, 1994.

This study found that immediate coronary angioplasty without antecedent thrombolytic therapy results in better left ventricular function and lower risk of death and recurrent myocardial infarction than treatment with streptokinase given intravenously.

5. Zijlstra F, de Boer MJ, Hoorntje JCA, et al: A comparison of immediate coronary angioplasty with intravenous streptokinase in acute myocardial infarction. *N Engl J Med* 328:680-684, 1993.

Immediate angioplasty after acute myocardial infarction was associated with a higher rate of patency of the infarct-related artery, a less severe residual stenotic lesion, better left ventricular function, and less recurrent myocardial ischemia and infarction than streptokinase given intravenously.

6. Boden WE, O'Rourke RA, Crawford MH, et al: Outcomes in patients with acute non-Q-wave myocardial infarction randomly assigned to an invasive as compared with a conservative management strategy. *N Engl J Med* 338:1785-1792, 1998.

Most patients with non-Q-wave myocardial infarction do not benefit from routine, early invasive management consisting of coronary angiography and revascularization. A conservative, ischemia-guided initial approach is both safe and effective.

7. Every NR, Parsons LS, Hlatky M, et al: A comparison of the thrombolytic therapy with primary coronary angioplasty for acute myocardial infarction. *N Engl J Med* 335:1253-1260, 1996.

In a community setting, no benefit was observed in terms of either mortality or the use of resources with a strategy of primary angioplasty rather than thrombolytic therapy in a large cohort of patients with acute myocardial infarction.

8. Malacrida R, Genoni M, Maggioni AP, et al: A comparison of early outcome of acute myocardial infarction in women and men. *N Engl J Med* 338:8-14, 1998.

The gender effect on the outcome of myocardial infarction is small and, at most, consists of only a small independent association between female sex and early mortality and morbidity after suspected acute myocardial infarction.

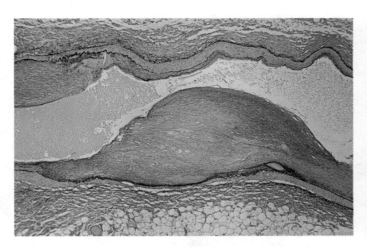

Plate 1. Right coronary artery plaque (longitudinal section, similar to angiographic view).

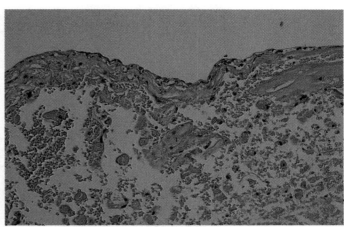

Plate 2. Grade 4 right coronary artery atherosclerosis with thin cap and plaque hemorrhage. (x50.)

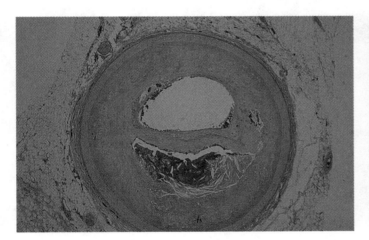

Plate 3. Plaque hemorrhage in right coronary artery.

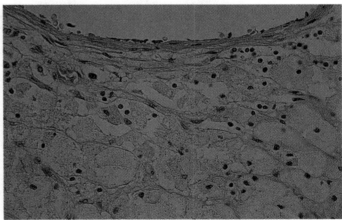

Plate 4. Collection of foam cells beneath thin cap of right coronary artery plaque. (x100.)

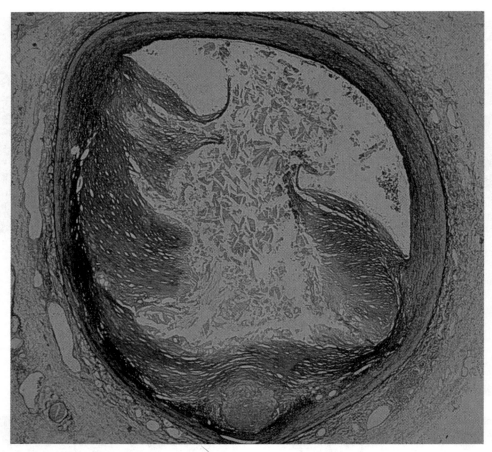

Plate 5. Acute plaque rupture with apparent atheroembolism.

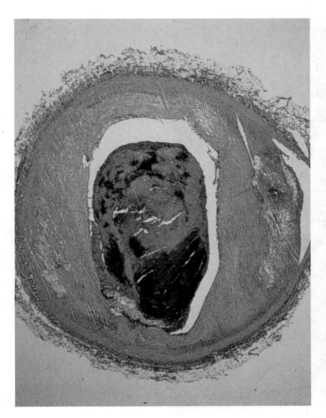
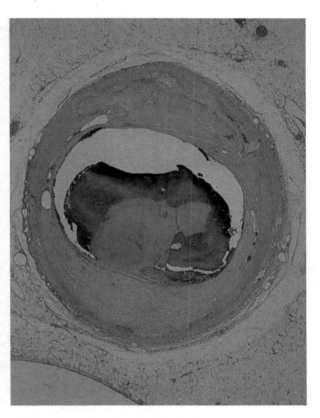

Plate 6. Thrombosis and grade 2 atherosclerotic plaques. Note that the underlying plaque is not flow-limiting in either artery.

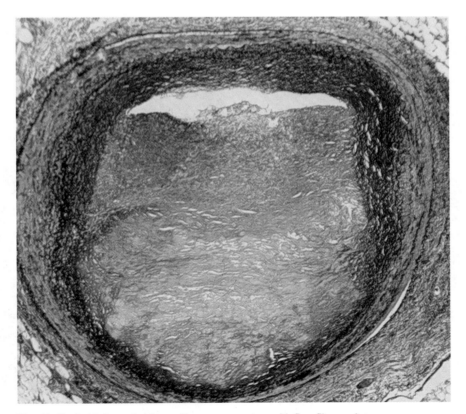

Plate 7. Grade 4 left anterior descending coronary artery with firm fibrous plaque.

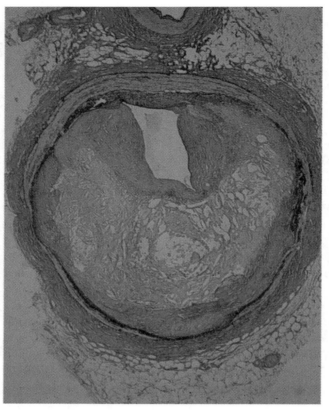

Plate 8. Grade 4 right coronary artery with eccentric soft plaque.

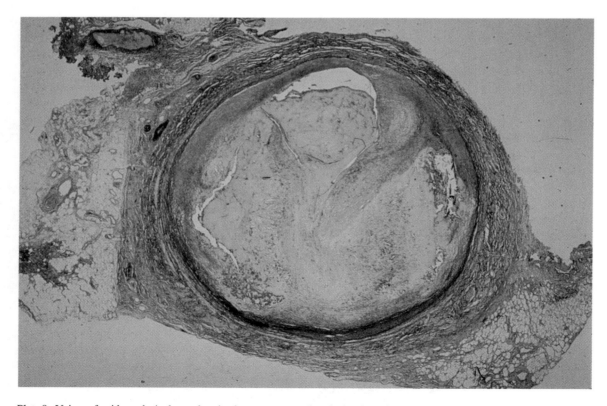

Plate 9. Vein graft with grade 4 atherosclerotic plaque rupture and occlusive thrombus.

Chapter 17

Essentials of Interventional Cardiology

Joseph G. Murphy, M.D

> The general Cardiology Boards require that candidates be familiar with the principles of interventional cardiology, including indications and complications of percutaneous transluminal coronary angioplasty (PTCA), risk stratification of coronary lesions for interventional procedures, the results of major interventional trials, and indications for the newer interventional devices, including atherectomy, stents, laser, and intravascular ultrasound. Less emphasis is placed on knowledge of the procedural techniques involved.

Randomized trials comparing PTCA and coronary artery bypass grafting (CABG) are discussed in Chapter 11 and those comparing primary PTCA and thrombolysis for acute myocardial infarction, in Chapter 16. Thrombolytic trials are reviewed in Chapter 14 and GPIIb/IIIa inhibitors in Chapter 81.

Mechanism of Coronary Angioplasty (PTCA)

The mechanism by which PTCA improves coronary blood flow is complex and includes two primary pathophysiologic mechanisms, namely fracture of the atheromatous plaque with creation of a localized intramural vessel wall dissection and stretching of the non-atheromatous elements of the arterial wall. Other mechanisms of PTCA considered less important include plaque compression and stretching without fracture of the underlying atheromatous plaque. The indications and contraindications for PTCA are summarized in Tables 1 and 2, respectively.

Complications of Coronary Angioplasty

Abrupt vessel closure after PTCA due to vessel wall dissection, in situ thrombus formation, no reflow or slow reflow phenomenon or distal embolism (especially in saphenous vein grafts), and late vessel restenosis due to smooth muscle proliferation are numerically the most important complications of PTCA and other interventional coronary procedures.

Abrupt Vessel Closure
Abrupt vessel closure is defined as the precipitate closure of the dilated lesion during or shortly after an interventional cardiology procedure. The incidence of abrupt vessel closure is about 7% (5% in the cardiac laboratory and 2% after the procedure). Before stenting, abrupt closure was the major cause of death, myocardial infarction, and the need for emergency CABG after PTCA.

An atlas of percutaneous transluminal coronary angiographic (PTCA) images is found at the end of the chapter (Plates 1-9).

Table 1.—Selection Criteria for PTCA

Myocardial ischemia (angina or ischemia demonstrated on
   functional testing)
Revascularization necessary (or preferable to medical
   treatment)
Lesions approachable with PTCA
High likelihood of success
Absence of factors in favor of surgery: left main artery
   disease, old bypass graft, diffuse disease, chronic total
   occlusion, high-risk anatomy, heavy vessel and lesion
   calcification

Additional indications
   Cardiogenic shock
   Rescue PTCA following failed thrombolysis
   Primary PTCA in acute myocardial infarction

PTCA, percutaneous transluminal coronary angioplasty.
Modified from Giuliani ER, Gersh BJ, McGoon MD, Hayes DL, Schaff
   HV (editors): *Mayo Clinic Practice of Cardiology*. Third edition. Mosby,
   1996, p 369. By permission of Mayo Foundation.

Table 2.—Contraindications to PTCA

Unprotected left main stenosis—unless the patient is not a
   candidate for CABG
Likely nondilatable lesion with large area of ischemia (may
   be a candidate for Rotablator or CABG)
Revascularization unnecessary or no inducible myocardial
   ischemia present
Diffuse disease or many lesions (surgery preferable)
Low anticipated success rate
Stenosis (< 60%) of indeterminate effect on coronary blood
   flow
Variant angina with mild fixed stenoses
Other coexistent cardiac disease requiring cardiac surgery
   (valve disease)
Chronic total occlusion if CABG is a better option

CABG, coronary artery bypass graft; PTCA, percutaneous transluminal
   coronary angioplasty.
Modified from Giuliani ER, Gersh BJ, McGoon MD, Hayes DL, Schaff
   HV (editors): *Mayo Clinic Practice of Cardiology*. Third edition. Mosby,
   1996, p 370. By permission of Mayo Foundation.

Preprocedural predictors of death following abrupt vessel closure complicating PTCA are poor ventricular function, a history of heart failure or unstable angina, advanced age, and a large area of myocardium at risk, including a large amount of myocardium collateralized from the target vessel to another coronary territory. The leading causes of abrupt closure are arterial wall dissection, in situ arterial thrombosis, and vessel spasm (especially after laser angioplasty) and distal embolism in degenerated saphenous vein grafts and microembolism after Rotablator use.

- Abrupt vessel closure is the major cause of acute complications following PTCA and other interventional coronary procedures.

The predictors of abrupt vessel closure include the following:
(1) Patient characteristics—multivessel disease, unstable angina, and female sex
(2) Preprocedural angiographic characteristics—vessel angulation and tortuosity, total occlusion, long lesion, calcification, ostial location, major side branches at risk, preexisting thrombus, bifurcation lesions, and vein graft lesions
(3) Postprocedural angiographic characteristics—arterial wall dissection
Abrupt closure is reduced by periprocedural platelet

inhibition (aspirin, ticlopidine, clopidogrel, abciximab) and heparin anticoagulation.

EPIC Trial
The EPIC (Evaluation of 7E3 for the Prevention of Ischemic Complications) trial demonstrated that abciximab (ReoPro), a human-murine chimeric monoclonal antibody Fab fragment against the platelet glycoprotein IIb/IIIa fibrinogen receptor reduced the abrupt closure rate, mortality, myocardial infarct rate, and need for emergency CABG by about 35% in high-risk PTCA patients.

- The EPIC trial demonstrated that abciximab reduced the risk of abrupt vessel closure in high-risk PTCA patients.

EPILOGUE Trial
A subsequent trial by the EPILOGUE (Evaluation in PTCA to Improve Long-Term Outcome With Abciximab GP IIb/IIIa Blockade) study group demonstrated that abciximab, when combined with lower-dose, weight-adjusted heparin (70 units/kg bolus), reduced the risk of acute ischemic complications in patients undergoing percutaneous coronary revascularization without increasing the risk of hemorrhage compared with abciximab combined with standard heparin therapy (100 units/kg bolus plus added heparin to maintain the activated clotting time > 300 seconds).

The American College of Cardiology and the American Heart Association have classified coronary artery stenoses on the basis of expected success rates and complication rates (Table 3).

Restenosis Following PTCA

Restenosis develops after interventional coronary procedures in about 20% to 40% of patients. Several unique features distinguish coronary restenosis from progression of native coronary disease. These include the time course for clinical restenosis (recurrent ischemic symptoms within 6 months after the original procedure), the rare occurrence of myocardial infarction due to restenosis lesions, and the lack of a strong association between restenosis and many of the established risk factors for atherosclerosis (for example, increased serum levels of low-density lipoprotein [LDL] cholesterol). Restenosis following unprotected left main PTCA or stent may, however, present with sudden death.

Mechanism of Post-PTCA Restenosis

Restenosis is a complex process associated with elastic recoil of the vessel wall, remodeling of the arterial wall, proliferation of fibrous tissue and smooth muscle cells of the intima, excess formation of extracellular matrix, residual plaque within the artery, and thrombus formation. Histologic examination of directional atherectomy specimens from restenotic lesions has found proliferation of smooth muscle cells in more than 90% of samples. Several studies using different interventional devices have documented that the greater the initial luminal gain, the greater the stimulus to late neointimal proliferation.

Predictors of Restenosis

Clinical predictors of restenosis following PTCA include diabetes mellitus and unstable angina, and angiographic predictors include intraluminal thrombus, saphenous vein graft lesions, proximal left anterior descending coronary artery anatomical location, a nonoptimal angiographic result after PTCA, long stenotic lesions, chronic total occlusions, ostial stenosis, and heavily calcified lesions. Intravascular ultrasonography was predictive of a higher restenosis rate following PTCA if a concentric ring of plaque without dissection or rupture remained after the procedure. Stents are the only FDA-approved device to decrease the restenosis rate, although in the CAVEAT-1 trial directional coronary atherectomy was shown to modestly reduce restenosis rates.

At least 20 drugs (aspirin, ticlopidine, angiopeptin, seratonin antagonists, antiproliferative agents, fish oils, trapadil,

---

Table 3.—American College of Cardiology and American Heart Association Angioplasty Guidelines: Lesion-Specific Characteristics of Type A, B, and C Lesions

Type A lesions (high success, > 85%; low risk)
- Discrete (< 10 mm long)
- Concentric
- Readily accessible
- Nonangulated segment, < 45°
- Smooth contour

- Little or no calcification
- Less than totally occluded
- Not ostial in location
- No major branch involvement
- Absence of thrombus

Type B lesions (moderate success, 60% to 85%; moderate risk)
- Tubular (10 to 20 mm long)
- Eccentric
- Moderate tortuosity of proximal segment
- Moderately angulated segment, > 45°, < 90°
- Irregular contour

- Moderate to heavy calcification
- Total occlusions < 3 months old
- Ostial in location
- Bifurcation lesions requiring double guidewires
- Some thrombus present

Type C lesions (low success, < 60%; high risk)
- Diffuse (> 2 cm long)
- Excessive tortuosity of proximal segment
- Extremely angulated segments, > 90°

- Total occlusions > 3 months old
- Inability to protect major side branches
- Degenerated vein grafts with friable lesions

From *J Am Coll Cardiol* 12:529-545, 1988. By permission of the American College of Cardiology.

steroids, angiotensin-converting enzyme inhibitors, calcium antagonists, prostacyclin analogues, thromboxane A_2 inhibitors, antioxidants) have been tested in angiographic restenosis trials, but all have been negative to date.

According to some studies, catheter-based radiotherapy with iridium-192 following PTCA and coronary stent implant significantly decreases the risk of further angiographic restenosis (defined as stenosis > 50% at follow-up) in patients with previous coronary restenosis after an interventional coronary procedure. In one study, the restenosis rate was 17% for radiotherapy versus 54% for placebo.

Different interventional devices achieve a luminal enlarging effect in different ways and, thus, may provoke the restenotic response to greater or lesser degrees. Although devices such as atherectomy debulk the atherosclerotic lesion and achieve an excellent initial angiographic result, they are associated with more arterial wall injury and exposure of intramural tissue than nondebulking techniques such as PTCA.

Intravascular ultrasonographic studies have documented that plaque compression/fracture is responsible for about 95% of the luminal gain after PTCA and only about 50% of the gain after atherectomy (Table 4).

Experimental animal data have documented the strong linear correlation between the degree of arterial wall injury and the thickness of subsequent neointimal formation.

Stenting, which is associated with a lower restenosis rate, probably achieves this result through a combination of reduction in arterial wall elastic recoil, better apposition of the arterial wound edges (leading to better wound healing), a more circular arterial lumen, and better vessel blood flow characteristics because of the "tacking-up" of small nonobstructive intimal dissections. Several angiographic studies have documented a loss of luminal area up to 50% because of elastic recoil of the vessel wall after PTCA, compared with approximately 5% after stent implant.

- Clinical predictors of restenosis include diabetes mellitus and unstable angina.

Internal Mammary Artery Interventions

Internal mammary arteries have a very low incidence of atherosclerosis even in patients with advanced coronary artery and peripheral disease. Patients with diabetes mellitus and previous mediastinal irradiation are at higher risk of internal mammary artery disease. Internal mammary graft stenoses are usually at the distal anastomotic site and may be dilated, with a procedural success rate of more than 90%.

Table 4.—Comparison of DCA and PTCA in Enlarging the Vessel Lumen

	DCA	PTCA
Plaque fracture/compression	50%	95%
Plaque removal	40%	0%
Vessel expansion	10%	5%

DCA, directional coronary atherectomy; PTCA, percutaneous transluminal coronary angioplasty.

New Interventional Devices

An increasing number of interventional devices are availables that optimize the results of PTCA (primarily stents), treat the complications of PTCA (stents), or allow an interventional approach to lesions not considered optimal for PTCA (Rotablator, excimer laser, directional atherectomy). Atherectomy, laser angioplasty, and stents are discussed below, and intravascular ultrasonography and intravascular Doppler studies are discussed in Chapter 54.

Atherectomy

Atherectomy is a catheter-based technique in which the atheromatous plaque is removed with interventional cutting devices. Three atherectomy devices are in clinical use.

Directional Coronary Atherectomy

Directional coronary atherectomy (DCA) was the first new interventional device approved by the FDA after PTCA. It has been studied in several large randomized trials (CAVEAT-1, CAVEAT-2, CCAT, and BOAT).

CAVEAT-1

CAVEAT-1 (Coronary Angioplasty Versus Excisional Angioplasty Trial-1) compared DCA with PTCA in de novo native coronary stenoses. DCA was associated with a higher initial angiographic success rate and a smaller postprocedure residual stenosis rate but was associated with an approximate doubling of the procedural complication rate (5% to 11% for death, myocardial infarction, CABG) compared with PTCA. The excess mortality associated with DCA was maintained at 6 months and 1 year follow-up. There was a trend toward a lower restenosis rate in the DCA group.

CAVEAT-2

CAVEAT-2 (Coronary Angioplasty Versus Excisional Angioplasty Trial-2) compared DCA and PTCA for saphenous vein graft stenosis and found no significant benefit for DCA compared with PTCA.

CCAT

CCAT (Canadian Coronary Atherectomy Trial) evaluated DCA and PTCA for proximal left anterior descending artery stenoses, and although the angiographic result was initially better with DCA, at late follow-up there was no significant benefit to DCA.

BOAT

BOAT (Balloon Versus Optimal Atherectomy Trial) was a randomized trial in which 989 patients were assigned to either PTCA or DCA. The major complication rate was low in the DCA arm (no deaths, 2% Q-wave myocardial infarction, 1% emergency CABG, and 1.4% perforation). The angiographic restenosis rate was 31% in the DCA arm and 40% in the PTCA-only arm at 7 months after the procedure. The non–Q-wave myocardial infarction rate was 16% in the DCA arm and 6% in the PTCA arm. Many patients in the DCA group required adjunctive PTCA or stenting.

At 1 year, there was no statistically significant difference in the incidence of major clinical events (death, Q-wave myocardial infarction, or the requirement for further target-vessel revascularization) between the DCA and PTCA study arms.

OARS

OARS (Optimal Atherectomy Restenosis Study) was a nonrandomized study of directional coronary atherectomy in 199 patients at four experienced centers. The angiographic success rate was high (97.5%), with a low rate of major complications (no deaths, 1.5% Q-wave myocardial infarction, 1% emergency CABG, and 1% perforation). The 6-month restenosis rate was 29%. The negative aspect of OARS was the 14% incidence of non-Q-wave myocardial infarction (defined as a creatine kinase increase more than three times normal) and the requirement for adjuvant PTCA or stent in 87% of patients.

START

START (Stent Versus Directional Atherectomy Randomized Trial), from Japan, is the only randomized trial to compare DCA guided by intravascular ultrasonography (IVUS) with Palmaz-Schatz stent implantation.

The acute angiographic results were comparable for the two treatment groups. Post-procedure plaque volume as assessed by IVUS was significantly less with DCA than with stent. At 3-month follow-up, the angiographic restenosis rate was 8.5% in the DCA group and 23% in the stent group. Follow-up is continuing.

In summary, the DCA versus PTCA randomized trials documented no statistically significant sustained benefit for DCA in either native vessel or saphenous vein graft disease. Currently, directional atherectomy is used less frequently than before because of the availability of stents and Rotablator. DCA is now reserved for large vessels (≥ 3.0 mm) with severely eccentric atheromatous plaques or ostial lesions in native vessels and saphenous vein grafts.

Transluminal Extraction Atherectomy

The transluminal extraction atherectomy (TEC) device is a percutaneous over-the-wire hollow catheter system with two angulated stainless steel cutting blades in its arrow-shaped, motor-driven rotating head. TEC has the advantage of debulking atheromatous or thrombotic lesions using the conical cutting head and continuous removal of debris through the hollow catheter lumen. TEC is used primarily for treating stenoses in degenerated vein grafts, where its debulking ability may reduce the risk of distal embolization compared with PTCA, and in nondegenerated, thrombus-containing occluded saphenous grafts where the thrombus burden is generally excessive for lysis by thrombolytic agents or reperfusion by PTCA. TEC may also be useful in acute myocardial infarction because of its ability to remove fresh thrombus.

The largest experience with TEC has been that of the U.S. TEC Multicenter Registry, which reported a procedural success rate of about 90% in both native coronary arteries and degenerated saphenous vein grafts (mean bypass graft age, 8 years). The major procedural complication rate was about 6% for native coronary vessels and 4% for saphenous vein grafts. The angiographic restenosis rate was about 50% for native vessels and 60% for degenerated saphenous vein grafts.

TEC is contraindicated in very angulated lesions ($> 45°$) and markedly eccentric lesions, because of the risk of vessel perforation. Bifurcation lesions should be avoided because of the risk of side branch occlusion. If TEC is used as a rescue procedure after PTCA dissection, it may extend an existing intimal dissection. Heavily calcified lesions or ulcerated lesions without significant thrombus are also poor targets for TEC intervention. TEC does not decrease the coronary restenosis rate and is not useful as a treatment for the complications of PTCA. TEC generally requires adjunctive PTCA and stenting to achieve an optimal result.

Rotablator (Rotational Atherectomy)

Rotablator uses a diamond-studded burr that spins at a very high speed (160,000-180,000 revolutions/min) to selectively abrade the atheromatous plaque. It is effective in opening many arterial lesions not amenable to conventional PTCA techniques, such as heavily calcified lesions. Rotablator functions by selectively abrading the relatively more rigid tissues within the arterial wall (calcium and atheromatous plaque), with relative sparing of the normal elastic arterial wall constituents (differential cutting phenomenon). In theory, the abraded arterial wall elements are pulverized to particles smaller than 10 µm in diameter that should pass through the microcirculation unhindered. In practice, microembolization leading to no reflow with myocardial infarction or slow reflow (TIMI grade 2 flow) with regional wall hypokinesia may occur.

Rotablator use is contraindicated in the presence of intraluminal thrombus or in lesions likely to contain thrombus, for example, ulcerated lesions associated with unstable angina. However, it is frequently used in situations in which PTCA has failed to open the coronary stenosis because of an inability to cross or dilate the lesions with the PTCA balloon. In this situation, it is important that the Rotablator not be used if there is evidence of angiographic dissection from previous PTCA attempts to dilate the lesion. Eccentric lesions can be treated with Rotablator, provided great care is used to ensure that the guidewire is coaxial with the vessel lumen (minimize guidewire bias), thus minimizing the risk of vessel perforation. Guidewire protection of a major vessel sidebranch is not possible with Rotablator. Rotablator may be used for bifurcated lesions with the above proviso. The luminal area produced by Rotablator is usually greater than the bur size used. Rotablator is followed by adjunctive low-pressure PTCA in almost all patients and frequently by stent implant. Rotablator does not decrease coronary restenosis rates but may be valuable as a treatment for densely fibrotic restenotic lesions or calcified lesions because of its debulking effect.

Rotablator is generally contraindicated in degenerated or thrombus-containing saphenous vein grafts because of the risk of distal embolization; an exception is a distal graft anastomotic site, where Rotablator is very effective. Long lesions, calcified lesions, and restenotic lesions are all suitable for Rotablator.

Rotablator is associated with specific complications, including slow coronary flow and no coronary reflow phenomenon, arterial wall dissection and perforation, and guidewire fracture.

- Rotablator is the interventional cardiology technique of choice for heavily calcified lesions.
- Regional wall hypokinesia after Rotablator use may be due to the slow reflow phenomenon due to microemboli.

ERBAC Trial

The ERBAC (Excimer Laser, Rotational Atherectomy and Balloon Angioplasty Comparison) trial was a randomized trial in which a head-to-head comparison was made at a single center of PTCA, excimer laser coronary angioplasty (ELCA), and Rotablator in 685 patients with complex coronary lesions. The procedural success rates were 80% for PTCA, 77% for ELCA, and 90% for Rotablator, which represented a statistically significant improvement ($P < 0.002$) for Rotablator compared with ELCA and PTCA. The incidence of major procedural adverse events (death, Q-wave myocardial infarction, and emergency CABG) was not statistically different among the treatment groups. The angiographic restenosis rate was high for all treatment groups, as might be expected with complex coronary artery lesions: PTCA, 47%; ELCA, 59%; and Rotablator, 57%.

The conclusion of the ERBAC trial was that Rotablator allowed procedural success in an added 10% of complex coronary lesions than either PTCA or ELCA allowed, but this early benefit was lost by the time of late follow-up, with no overall benefit in the requirement for target-vessel revascularization compared with PTCA or laser.

STRATAS Trial

The STRATAS (Study to Determine Rotablator System and Transluminal Angioplasty Strategy) trial was performed to determine the optimal Rotablator debulking strategy (aggressive debulking of the coronary lesion with a bur-to-artery ratio of 0.7 to 0.9, followed by no PTCA or low-pressure PTCA at < 1 atm, compared with moderate debulking with bur-to-artery ratio of < 0.7, followed by PTCA at > 4 atm). There was no significant difference in the incidence of major procedural complications (death, Q-wave myocardial infarction, or emergency CABG). There was a trend toward a higher requirement for target-vessel revascularization in the aggressive treatment group, 35% versus 27% for the conservative group ($P = 0.08$) at the time of late follow-up, but no difference in restenosis rate (54% versus 50%).

DART

DART (Dilatation Versus Ablation Revascularization Trial) was a comparison of Rotablator and PTCA in noncomplex coronary stenosis (A and B$_1$ lesions). The procedural success rate was greater than 99% in both groups, but bailout stenting and emergency CABG were required in more PTCA patients and the no-reflow phenomenon was seen in 8% of Rotablator patients, compared with 0.5% of PTCA patients ($P = 0.01$).

ELCA

ELCA (excimer laser coronary angioplasty) is a niche device that, despite initial enthusiasm when it was first introduced, is rarely used in most interventional laboratories. It is used predominantly in the treatment of in-stent restenosis, aorto-ostial disease (frequently using an eccentric laser fiber), and noncalcified diffuse lesions as an alternative to Rotablator. Potentially, ELCA may be useful for revascularization of chronic total occlusions. The AMRO trial, performed in Holland, compared the immediate and long-term results of ELCA with PTCA in 308 patients with stable angina and long, diffuse coronary lesions. In this study, there was no significant difference in early or late results using ELCA or conventional PTCA. The angiographic success rate was 80% in the ELCA arm, similar to that with PTCA (79%). The difference in the major acute complication rate between ELCA and PTCA was not significant. In the ELCA arm, there were no deaths, the Q-wave myocardial infarction rate was 2.6%, non-Q-wave myocardial infarction rate was 2%, and emergency CABG rate was 4.5%. The 6-month restenosis rate for ELCA was 52%, compared with 41% for PTCA ($P = $ NS).

ELCA has also been associated with coronary perforation and dissections that may occur unpredictably. In animal experiments, expanding water vapor bubbles with a maximum diameter of three times that of the laser catheter caused microsecond arterial dilatation and may explain some of the vascular complications.

ELCA is contraindicated in acute myocardial infarction and lesions with ongoing thrombus formation. It is also contraindicated in very tortuous coronary vessels and angulated lesions ($> 45°$), in the presence of a previous PTCA-induced coronary dissection, in severely calcified lesions, and in bifurcation lesions.

Intracoronary Stents

Intracoronary stents have revolutionized the practice of interventional cardiology. Before the advent of stenting, PTCA had about reached the limit of its technology, with a restenosis rate of about 30%, a suboptimal dilatation rate of about 15%, and an abrupt closure rate of about 5%.

Intracoronary stents were initially introduced as bailout devices to treat obstructive coronary dissections and abrupt closure after PTCA. Their use has now expanded to optimization of post-PTCA angiographic results and reduction in coronary restenosis rate and primary stent placement for many lesions. The mechanisms by which stents are beneficial are complex and multifactorial, including scaffolding of coronary artery dissections, better endothelial wound apposition after PTCA with a reduction in the exposure of thrombogenic subintimal arterial wall elements to blood, and an improvement in blood flow characteristics because of a more regular intraluminal surface.

Currently, more than 50 stent designs are being investigated or used clinically. Stents are classified by

1. The nature of the stent delivery system (self-expanding [wallstent, RADIUS, Magic Wallstent, Cardiocoil] and balloon expandable [Palmaz-Schatz, Gianturco-Rubin I, II, Wiktor, ACS multi-link, Crown, AVE, NIR])
2. The cell pattern of the predeployed stent (slotted tube [Palmaz-Schatz, Crown], coil [AVE, Wiktor, Gianturco-Rubin I, II], mesh [ACS, NIR, RADIUS, wallstent])
3. The metal used (tantalum, which is more radiopaque [Tensum, Wiktor], stainless steel, which is less radiopaque [most stents], cobalt alloy [Wallstent], nitinol [RADIUS, PARAGON, Cardiocoil])

Major Randomized Stent Studies

STRESS

STRESS (Stent Restenosis Study) randomly assigned 407 patients to a Palmaz-Schatz stent or PTCA for de novo native coronary stenoses. The stent group had a greater primary success rate (96% vs. 90%), fewer dissections (7% vs. 34%), less angiographic restenosis (32% vs. 42%, $P = 0.05$), and a trend toward better event-free survival at follow-up (80% vs. 74%, $P = $ NS).

BENESTENT Study

BENESTENT (Belgium and Netherlands Stent) study randomly assigned 516 patients to a Palmaz-Schatz stent or PTCA for de novo native coronary stenoses. The stent group had a lower restenosis rate (22% vs. 32%, $P = 0.02$) and a lower repeat PTCA rate (10% vs. 21%, $P = 0.001$) at late follow-up. Vascular and bleeding complications were more common in the stent patients.

SAVED Trial

The SAVED (Saphenous Vein De Novo) trial evaluated the role of stenting in the treatment of coronary bypass graft disease. The trial randomly assigned 270 patients with saphenous vein graft disease to either PTCA or Palmaz-Schatz stent implant. There was a higher initial procedural success rate and a better gain in luminal diameter in the stent group. The restenosis rate was similar in the stent (37%) and PTCA (46%) groups (P = NS). The stent group had fewer clinical cardiovascular events (27%) than the PTCA group (42%) at 6-month follow-up (P < 0.05).

SICCO Trial

The SICCO (Stenting in Chronic Coronary Occlusion) trial evaluated the role of stenting in chronic coronary occlusion. The study randomly assigned 117 patients who had successful PTCA of a chronically occluded coronary artery to either no further intervention or to a Palmaz-Schatz stent implant. The results at 1 year were much better in the stent group than in the PTCA-alone group. The restenosis rate was 32% in the stent group and 74% in the PTCA group (P < 0.001), and for reocclusion, the rates were 12% and 26% (P = 0.058), respectively.

BENESTENT II Trial

The BENESTENT II trial included a much broader patient population than BENESTENT I and was more representative of an unselected cardiology patient population. BENESTENT II compared heparin-coated Palmaz-Schatz stent implantation with PTCA. Bailout stenting was needed in 13% of PTCA patients. Procedural success was higher in the stent group (97%) than in the PTCA group (86%). The restenosis rate in the stent group was 16%, compared with 30% in the PTCA group (P = 0.001). Major adverse coronary events (death, myocardial infarction [Q-wave or non-Q-wave], CABG, repeat PTCA) at 7-month follow-up were 13% for the stent group and 19% for the PTCA group (P = 0.03).

Optimal PTCA Versus Primary Stenting

Several trials (OPUS, DESTINI, UPSIZE, EPISTENT, ERACI II) have examined methods of improving PTCA results and whether a stent-like angiographic result with PTCA combined with a strategy of provisional stenting in patients with a suboptimal PTCA result would yield long-term results comparable to those of primary stent implantation.

OPUS Trial

The OPUS (Optimal Angioplasty Versus Primary Stenting) trial randomly assigned 479 patients to PTCA alone (with provisional stenting if a suboptimal result was obtained with PTCA) or to primary stenting. In the PTCA arm, 37% of patients had stenting. At 6 months, the results in the stent arm were superior to those in the PTCA arm, and slightly less expensive. Target-vessel revascularization was 10% in the PTCA arm and 4% in the stent arm. The rate of death, myocardial infarction, or target-vessel revascularization was 15% in the PTCA arm and 6% in the stent arm (P = 0.003).

UPSIZE Pilot Study (Balloon Dilatation Guided by Intravascular Ultrasonography)

This pilot study assessed the role of IVUS-guided PTCA in optimizing angioplasty results. The study enrolled 252 patients, of whom 58% had type B2 coronary stenosis. IVUS detected calcification in 59% of patients. This study was nonrandomized, but several important findings came from the study.

- Vessel diameter measured with IVUS is larger than that measured by quantitative coronary angiography (QCA).
- IVUS-guided PTCA resulted in optimization of PTCA results.
- IVUS-guided PTCA had an angiographic restenosis rate of 19% (angiographic follow-up in 71% of patients).
- IVUS detected dissection in 70% of patients, compared with 58% by QCA.

DESTINI

DESTINI (Doppler and QCA-Guided Aggressive PTCA Trial) randomly assigned 779 patients to either PTCA with guidance by Doppler and quantitative angiography to obtain an optimal PTCA result compared with patients who had primary lesion stenting.

An optimal PTCA result was obtained in only 43% of selected patients, with a cross-over of the remaining 57% of PTCA patients to stenting. Six-month follow-up of both groups showed no difference in the incidence of major cardiovascular events or target-vessel revascularization. The conclusion of the study was that if an excellent PTCA result is obtained (residual coronary stenosis < 35%, coronary flow reserve > 2.0, and no arterial dissection of grade C or higher), then the 6-month results can be expected to be similar to stenting, and this excellent PTCA result is attainable in less than 50% of PTCA patients.

EPISTENT Trial
The EPISTENT trial (Randomized Trial of Primary Versus Provisional Coronary Stenting in Patients With Platelet Glycoprotein IIb/IIIa Blockade) enrolled 1,590 patients, 61% of whom had type B2 or C coronary lesions and 20% of whom were diabetic. All patients received abciximab, heparin, aspirin, and ticlopidine. The study compared primary stenting with PTCA with provisional stenting if abrupt or threatened target-vessel closure occurred or if the residual stenosis after PTCA was greater than 50%. At 6-month follow-up, the results of primary stenting were superior to those of provisional stenting. The death rate among the primary stent group was 0.4% and 1.8% for the PTCA with provisional stenting ($P < 0.02$). The rate of target-vessel revascularization was 8.7% in the primary stent group and 15.4% in the PTCA with provisional stenting group ($P < 0.001$).

DEBATE I
DEBATE I (Doppler End-Point Angioplasty Trial of Europe), among others, established that a coronary flow reserve greater than 2.5 and a residual stenosis less than 35% were good predictors of a favorable prognosis with respect to future cardiovascular events and angiographic restenosis. In DEBATE I, 45 of 48 patients achieved these criteria after stenting, whereas only 19 of 48 patients met these criteria after PTCA.

Stents and Anticoagulation
When stents were initially introduced, patients received aggressive anticoagulation (combinations of warfarin, heparin, dextran, and aspirin) because of concerns about stent thrombosis. This led to a high rate of bleeding and vascular complications. Intravascular ultrasonography documented that the main reason for stent thrombosis was probably inadequate stent expansion and poor apposition of the stent to the arterial vessel wall.

Stent thrombosis has been reduced from about 20% in the early days of coronary stenting to about 1% currently because of the realization of the importance of correct stent-to-artery sizing and the need for adequate stent expansion by high-pressure balloon dilatation and the use of potent antiplatelet agents.

Aggressive anticoagulation regimens are not required for optimally deployed stents. A combination of aspirin and platelet inhibitors (aspirin, clopidogrel, or ticlopidine and a IIB/IIIa receptor blocker) is effective in preventing acute closure due to stent thrombosis by minimizing platelet deposition.

Future stent designs probably will incorporate coatings to minimize platelet and fibrin deposition, as in the BENESTENT II with heparin-coated Palmaz-Schatz stents. The pharmacology of platelet inhibitors is discussed in Chapter 81.

Ticlopidine and Clopidogrel
Ticlopidine and clopidrogel are both potent inhibitors of ADP-induced platelet aggregation and act synergistically with aspirin, which itself prevents platelet aggregation by thromboxane A_2.

Intracoronary Stenting and Antithrombotic Regimen (ISAR) Trial
This trial compared two antithrombotic regimens in 517 patients following Palmaz-Schatz coronary artery stenting: ticlopidine (for 4 weeks), aspirin (indefinitely), and heparin (for 12 hours after the procedure) were compared with phenprocoumon, a warfarin derivative (for 4 weeks), aspirin (indefinitely), and heparin (for 5 to 10 days after the procedure). The antiplatelet group did better in all clinical end points than the anticoagulation group: stent occlusion, 0.8% versus 5.4% ($P < 0.005$); major bleeding complications, 0% versus 6.5% ($P < 0.001$). There was an approximately 80% reduction in the occurrence of acute myocardial infarction (0.8% vs. 4.2%, $P = 0.02$) and the need for repeat coronary intervention (1.2% vs. 5.4%, $P = 0.01$) in the antiplatelet group. At 6 months, there was no difference in angiographic restenosis rates (27% for the antiplatelet group and 29% for the anticoagulation group, $P = NS$).

STARS Trial
The STARS (Stent Antithrombotic Regimen Study) trial compared aspirin alone, aspirin and coumadin, or aspirin and ticlopidine in 1,650 patients after Palmaz–Schatz stent implantation. Similar to the ISAR trial, the combination of aspirin and ticlopidine was associated with the lowest stent thrombosis rate (0.6% in the STARS trial).

Ticlopidine has been associated with life-threatening neutropenia and has largely been supplanted at many interventional cardiology centers by clopidogrel, a drug chemically related to ticlopidine. Clopidogrel has the same specific mechanism of action as ticlopidine against the ADP-activated pathway of platelet aggregation, but it has a more rapid onset of antiplatelet action, its antiplatelet effect is severalfold more powerful, and it is associated with a lower incidence of neutropenia (0.1%) than ticlopidine (2.4%).

- Stent deployment may be optimized by using intravascular ultrasonographic imaging or high-pressure PTCA balloon inflation.
- Aggressive anticoagulation regimens using warfarin are not required for optimally deployed stents and are associated with an increased risk of bleeding and vascular complications.

Angiojet Trial and VEGAS-2 Trial

The angiojet is a new interventional device that infuses saline at high pressure that is directed backward into the infusion catheter. This removes intravascular thrombus by a Venturi or suction effect.

The VEGAS-2 study compared the angiojet with a prolonged infusion of urokinase thrombolysis in vein graft or coronary artery lesions with clear angiographic thrombus. In-hospital mortality was less in the angiojet group (1.7%) than in the urokinase group (3.0%), as was periprocedural myocardial infarction, 14% versus 31%, and procedural cost.

Suggested Review Reading

1. The Bypass Angioplasty Revascularization Investigation (BARI) Investigators: Comparison of coronary bypass surgery with angioplasty in patients with multivessel disease. *N Engl J Med* 335:217-225, 1996.
Compared with CABG, an initial strategy of PTCA did not significantly compromise 5-year survival in patients with multivessel disease, although subsequent revascularization was required more often with this strategy. For treated diabetics, 5-year survival was significantly better after CABG than after PTCA.

2. The EPIC Investigators: Use of a monoclonal antibody directed against the platelet glycoprotein IIb/IIIa receptor in high-risk coronary angioplasty. *N Engl J Med* 330:956-961, 1994.
Ischemic complications of coronary angioplasty and atherectomy were reduced with a monoclonal antibody directed against the platelet IIb/IIIa glycoprotein receptor, although the risk of bleeding was increased.

3. The EPILOG Investigators: Platelet glycoprotein IIb/IIIa receptor blockade and low-dose heparin during percutaneous coronary revascularization. *N Engl J Med* 336:1689-1696, 1997.
Inhibition of the platelet glycoprotein IIb/IIIa receptor with abciximab, together with low-dose, weight-adjusted heparin, markedly reduces the risk of acute ischemic complications in patients undergoing percutaneous coronary revascularization, without increasing the risk of hemorrhage.

4. The EPISTENT Investigators: Randomised placebo-controlled and balloon-angioplasty-controlled trial to assess safety of coronary stenting with use of platelet glycoprotein-IIb/IIIa blockade. *Lancet* 352:87-92, 1998.
Platelet glycoprotein IIb/IIIa blockade with abciximab substantially improves the safety of coronary-stenting procedures. Balloon angioplasty with abciximab is safer than stenting without abciximab.

5. Erbel R, Haude M, Hopp HW, et al: Coronary-artery stenting compared with balloon angioplasty for restenosis after initial balloon angioplasty. *N Engl J Med* 339:1672-1678, 1998.
Elective coronary stenting was effective in the treatment of

restenosis after balloon angioplasty. Stenting resulted in a lower rate of recurrent stenosis despite a higher incidence of subacute thrombosis.

6. Fischman DL, Leon MB, Baim DS, et al. A randomized comparison of coronary-stent placement and balloon angioplasty in the treatment of coronary artery disease. *N Engl J Med* 331:496-501, 1994.
In selected patients, placement of an intracoronary stent, compared with balloon angioplasty, results in an improved rate of procedural success, a lower rate of angiographically detected restenosis, a similar rate of clinical events after 6 months, and a less frequent need for revascularization of the original coronary lesion.

7. Leon MB, Baim DS, Popma JJ, et al: A clinical trial comparing three antithrombotic-drug regimens after coronary-artery stenting. *N Engl J Med* 339:1665-1671, 1998.
Compared with aspirin alone and a combination of aspirin and warfarin, treatment with aspirin and ticlopidine resulted in a lower rate of stent thrombosis, although there were more hemorrhagic complications than with aspirin alone. After coronary stenting, aspirin and ticlopidine should be considered for the prevention of the serious complication of stent thrombosis.

8. Pitt B, Waters D, Brown WV, et al: Aggressive Lipid-Lowering Therapy Compared with Angioplasty in Stable Coronary Artery Disease. *N Engl J Med* 341:70-76, 1999.
In low-risk patients with stable coronary artery disease, aggressive lipid-lowering therapy is important to reduce the incidence of ischemic events. The PTCA-treated patients were not treated according to the NCEP lipid guideline. Unfortunately, the combined effect of PTCA and aggressive lipid lowering on ischemic events was not studied in this trial.

9. Savage MP, Douglas JS Jr, Fischman DL, et al: Stent placement compared with balloon angioplasty for obstructed coronary bypass grafts. *N Engl J Med* 337:740-747, 1997
Compared with balloon angioplasty, stenting of selected venous bypass-graft lesions resulted in superior procedural outcomes, a larger gain in luminal diameter, and a reduction in major cardiac events. There was no significant reduction in the rate of angiographic restenosis, which was the primary end point of the study.

10. Schomig A, Neumann F-J, Kastrati A, et al: A randomized comparison of antiplatelet and anticoagulant therapy after the placement of coronary-artery stents. *N Engl J Med* 334:1084-1089, 1996.
Compared with conventional anticoagulation, combined antiplatelet therapy with ticlopidine and aspirin after the placement of coronary artery stents reduces the incidence of both cardiac events and hemorrhagic and vascular complications.

11. Serruys PW, de Jaegere P, Kiemeneij F, et al: A comparison of balloon-expandable-stent implantation with balloon angioplasty in patients with coronary artery disease. *N Engl J Med* 331:489-495, 1994.
In more than 7 months of follow-up, the clinical and angiographic outcomes were better in patients who received a stent than in those who received standard coronary angioplasty. However, this benefit was achieved at the cost of a significantly higher risk of vascular complications at the access site and a longer hospital stay.

12. Serruys PW, van Hout B, Bonnier H, et al: Randomised comparison of implantation of heparin-coated stents with balloon angioplasty in selected patients with coronary artery disease (BENESTENT II). *Lancet* 352:673-681, 1998.
Over 12 months of follow-up, a strategy of elective stenting with heparin-coated stents is more effective but also more costly than balloon angioplasty.

13. Teirstein PS, Massullo V, Jani S, et al: Catheter-based radiotherapy to inhibit restenosis after coronary stenting. *N Engl J Med* 336:1697-1703, 1997.
In this preliminary, short-term study of patients with previous coronary restenosis, coronary stenting followed by catheter-based intracoronary radiotherapy substantially decreased the rate of subsequent restenosis.

14. Versaci F, Gaspardone A, Tomai F, et al: A comparison of coronary-artery stenting with angioplasty for isolated stenosis of the proximal left anterior descending coronary artery. *N Engl J Med* 336:817-822, 1997.
In patients with symptomatic isolated stenosis of the proximal left anterior descending coronary artery, stenting is better than standard coronary angioplasty, with a lower rate of restenosis and a better clinical outcome.

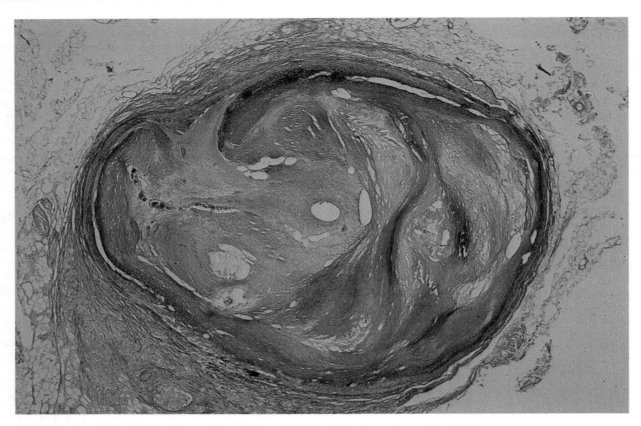

Plate 1. Restenosis after PTCA, with complete occlusion of the left anterior descending coronary artery.

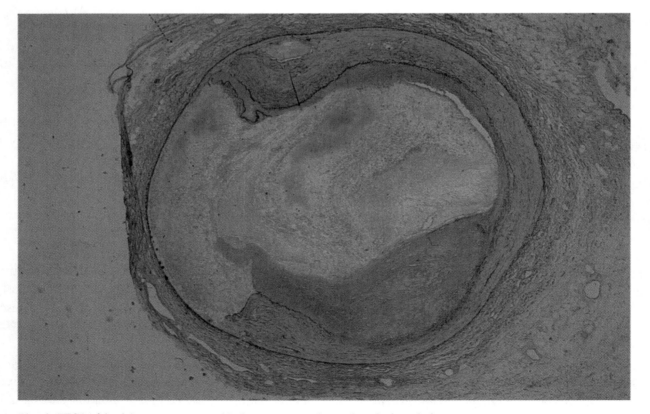

Plate 2. PTCA of the right coronary artery with plaque rupture and acute thrombotic occlusion.

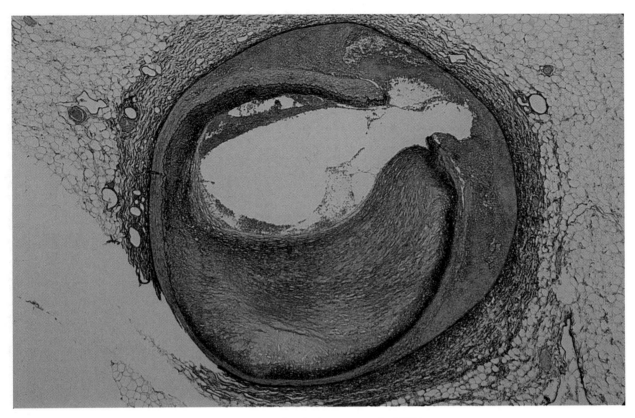

Plate 3. Tear and dissection of the mid-left anterior descending coronary artery after PTCA.

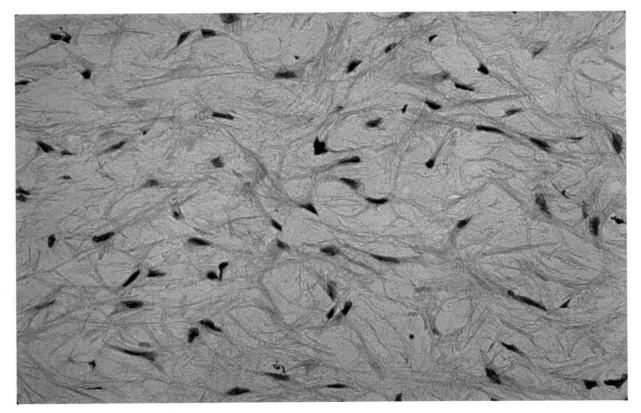

Plate 4. Restenosis after PTCA (x100.)

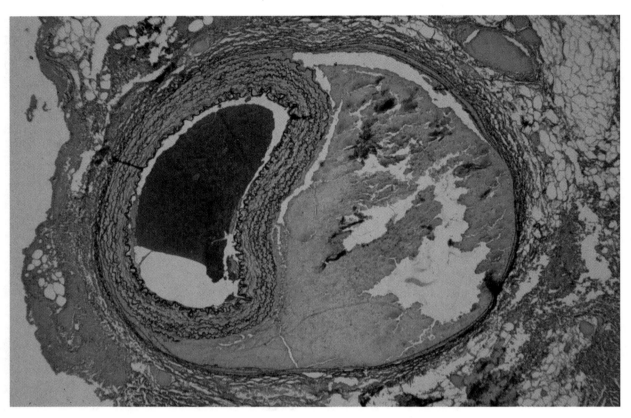

Plate 5. Left internal mammary artery graft with an acute dissection and obstruction.

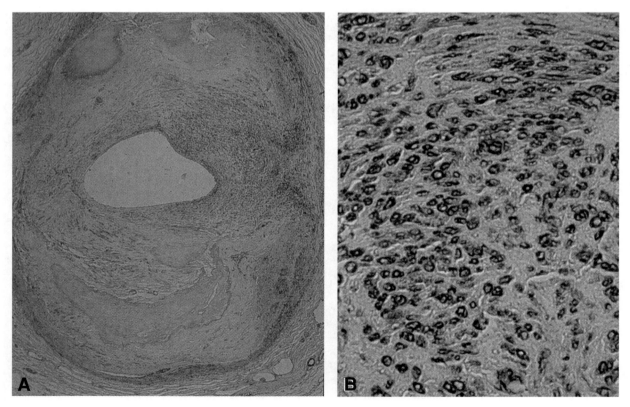

Plate 6. *A*, PTCA of the left circumflex coronary artery. *B*, Smooth muscle cells in restenosis tissue (actin stain).

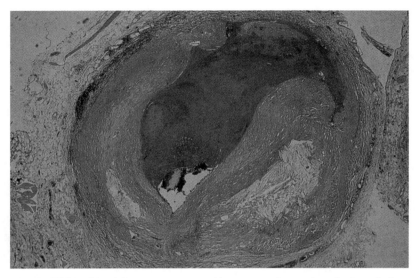

Plate 7. PTCA of the right coronary artery with rupture and acute thrombotic occlusion.

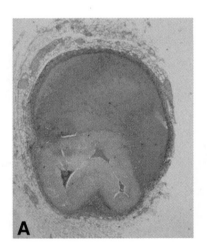

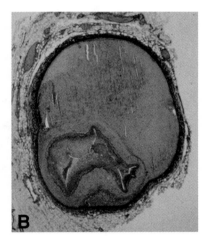

Plate 8. Right coronary artery showing acute dissection with luminal compression. (*A*, Hematoxylin and eosin; *B*, Verhoeff-van Gieson.)

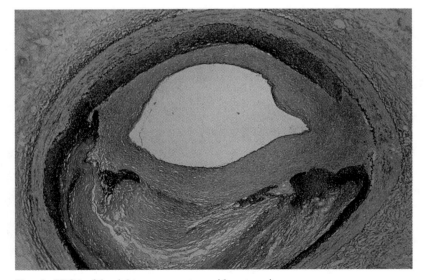

Plate 9. PTCA of the right coronary artery with restenosis.

Notes

Chapter 18

Arrhythmias Complicating Acute Myocardial Infarction

Margaret A. Lloyd, M.D.

At least 75% of patients with acute myocardial infarction (MI) have an arrhythmia during the peri-infarct period.

Supraventricular Arrhythmias

Sinus Bradycardia

Sinus bradycardia is the most common arrhythmia occurring during the early hours after MI and may occur in up to 40% of inferior and posterior infarctions. Bradycardia may be related to autonomic imbalance or to atrial and sinus node ischemia (or to both). Profound bradycardia may predispose the patient to ventricular ectopy. This arrhythmia usually resolves spontaneously, and treatment is reserved for hemodynamically symptomatic arrhythmias and those accompanied by bradycardia-dependent ventricular arrhythmias. Atropine is often successful in treating symptomatic bradycardia, but it may cause transient rebound tachycardia. Temporary pacing is rarely required (Table 1).

Sinus Tachycardia

Sinus tachycardia may occur in up to one-third of patients in the peri-infarct period, especially those with anterior MI. The ischemic left ventricle may have a relatively fixed stroke volume; thus, augmentation of cardiac output is primarily dependent on an increase in heart rate. Sinus tachycardia may also occur as a result of sympathetic stimulation from locally released and circulating catecholamines, concurrent anemia, hypo- or hypervolemia,

Table 1.—Indications for Temporary Pacing in the Peri-Infarct Period

Sinus bradycardia with hypotension, bradycardia-dependent ventricular arrhythmias, angina, syncope/presyncope, or congestive heart failure and refractory to atropine

Accelerated idioventricular rhythm with symptomatic rate < 40 beats/min

Prolonged (> 3 s) sinus pauses

Atrial fibrillation with inadequate ventricular rate

Asystole

Mobitz II second-degree block

Third-degree (complete heart) block

New or progressive bifascicular block

hypoxia, pericarditis, inotropic drugs, pain, or fear. Treatment includes optimizing hemodynamics and oxygenation, correction of anemia and electrolyte and acid-base abnormalities, pain control, and anxiolytic agents. β-Blockers are indicated for patients without evidence of significant left ventricular dysfunction or hypovolemia. Persistent sinus tachycardia as an early manifestation of heart failure is an indicator of poor prognosis.

Premature Atrial Contractions

Premature atrial contractions may be present in up to one-half of patients with MI. Their occurrence may be due to atrial or sinus node ischemia, atrial infarction, pericarditis, anxiety, or pain. The combination of atrial asystole and rapid ventricular rate markedly decreases cardiac output and increases myocardial oxygen demands. Attempts should be made to restore sinus rhythm; if not successful, rate control should be pursued aggressively to minimize myocardial oxygen demand. Premature atrial contractions have no prognostic significance after MI.

Atrial Fibrillation

New atrial fibrillation occurs in association with 10% to 20% of cases of MI and is usually transient. It may be due to atrial or sinus node ischemia, associated right ventricular infarction, pericarditis, heart failure, or increased atrial pressures. It usually occurs in older patients with a history of hypertension, mitral regurgitation, and larger left atria. New atrial fibrillation in the peri-infarct period is associated with a higher infarct mortality.

Atrial systole may contribute up to one-third of the cardiac output in patients with an ischemic left ventricle. Patients with persistent or refractory atrial fibrillation in the peri-infarct period have higher pulmonary capillary wedge pressures and lower ejection fractions and are in a poorer Killip class overall compared with patients who maintain sinus rhythm.

Atrioventricular Block

First-Degree Block

Approximately 5% to 10% of patients with MI have first-degree block at some point during the peri-infarct period. Almost all have supra-Hisian conduction abnormalities. Rare cases of infranodal block are seen in patients with anterior MI and associated fascicular block; these patients are at risk for progressive block, including third-degree block with ventricular asystole. First-degree block may be associated with drugs that prolong atrioventricular conduction.

Second-Degree, Mobitz Type I Block (Wenckebach)

Wenckebach may be seen with up to 10% of cases of MI, typically inferior infarcts, and is due to increased vagal tone and ischemia. The conduction defect is usually in the atrioventricular node; when seen early in the course of an MI, it usually responds to atropine. Resolution usually occurs after 48 to 72 hours. Treatment is initially with atropine and, rarely, temporary pacing for symptomatic bradycardia. Late-occurring Wenckebach is less sensitive to atropine and may be due to recurrent ischemia. Very rarely, Wenckebach will progress to higher grades of block that require permanent

pacing. Wenckebach rhythm in the peri-infarct period has no impact on long-term prognosis.

Second-Degree, Mobitz Type II Block

Mobitz type II block occurs in 1% of cases of MI and is more common after anterior MI. There is a high risk of progression to higher degrees of block, including sudden complete heart block with ventricular asystole. Patients should have a temporary pacing wire placed prophylactically at the first sign of Mobitz type II block in the peri-infarct period. The conduction defect is more likely to be infranodal than Mobitz type I block, and most patients should be treated with permanent pacing. If it is uncertain whether permanent pacing is indicated, electrophysiologic evaluation should be performed before hospital dismissal to assess the integrity of the infranodal conduction system. Long-term prognosis is related primarily to the size of the infarct rather than to the conduction abnormality.

Third-Degree (Complete) Block

Complete heart block may occur with either an anterior or inferior MI. With inferior infarcts, the conduction defect is likely to be in the atrioventricular node, with escape rhythms exceeding 40 beats/min and exhibiting a narrow QRS complex. With an anterior MI, the conduction defect is infranodal and the escape rhythm (if present) is usually less than 40 beats/min with a wide QRS complex. Typically, complete heart block seen with anterior MI is preceded by progressive fascicular, bundle, or Mobitz type II block.

Temporary pacing may be required for complete heart block in association with inferior MI if the patient is hemodynamically unstable. Temporary pacing should always be used in patients with anterior infarcts if progressive or complete block is present. Permanent pacing is almost always required for high-grade block in the setting of anterior MI; the prognosis is poor for these patients because of the large amount of myocardium involved. Electrophysiologic evaluation before hospital dismissal should be considered for patients with anterior MI and transient complete heart block to assess the integrity of the infranodal conduction system. Transient complete heart block in the setting of inferior MI rarely requires permanent pacing and usually resolves spontaneously.

Bundle Branch Block

New bundle branch block (BBB) has been reported in about 15% of cases of MI and is associated with an increased risk of complete heart block, congestive heart failure, cardiogenic shock, ventricular arrhythmias, and sudden death. Most commonly seen is right BBB, with left BBB and alternating BBB being less common. This may be related to the discrete anatomical size of the right bundle compared with the broad, fan shape of the left bundle. The correlation between the infarct-related artery and the presence of BBB is strong, with the highest incidence (more than half) of all BBBs occurring in infarcts involving the left anterior descending coronary artery. Progressive infra-Hisian block indicates a significant risk of sudden complete heart block and asystole, and patients demonstrating progression should have temporary pacing wires placed. Persistent BBB confers a significantly higher mortality, because of the large amount of myocardium that must be involved in the infarct to include the bundle branches. Thrombolytic therapy and catheter-based early reperfusion appear to decrease the incidence of BBB in the peri-infarct period.

Intraventricular Block

New isolated left anterior hemiblock occurs in 3% to 5% of patients with MI; new isolated left posterior hemiblock occurs in 1% to 2% of patients with acute MI. Anatomically, left posterior hemiblock is larger; hence, a larger infarct is required to produce block. Mortality is greater among these patients. Left anterior hemiblock in combination with new right BBB is also indicative of a larger infarct and higher subsequent mortality.

Ventricular Arrhythmias

Ventricular Fibrillation

Many studies have reported that the incidence of primary ventricular fibrillation (VF) in MI is about 5% in patients in whom a documented rhythm is obtained and occurs without antecedent warning arrhythmias in over half. The true incidence of primary VF is probably much higher, because it has been estimated that one-half of all patients with coronary artery disease die of sudden cardiac death, presumably VF. Factors associated with an increased incidence of VF include current smoking, left BBB, and hypokalemia. Patients with anterior MI and VF have a worse long-term prognosis than those with VF associated with inferior MI. VF may occur with reperfusion after thrombolytic therapy or catheter-based therapy. Treatment consists of prompt defibrillation. β-Blockers appear to decrease the incidence of lethal ventricular arrhythmias, including VF, in the peri-infarct period.

Ventricular Tachycardia

Ventricular tachycardia (VT) occurs in 10% to 40% of cases of MI. Early VT (during the first 24 hours) is usually transient and benign. Late-occurring VT is associated with transmural infarction, left ventricular dysfunction, hemodynamic deterioration, and a markedly higher mortality, both in-hospital and long-term. Treatment of sustained VT consists of cardioversion; if the rate is slow and hemodynamically tolerated, cardioversion may be attempted with drugs. Rapid VT (> 150 beats/min) or VT associated with hemodynamic deterioration should be treated with prompt DC cardioversion.

Accelerated Idioventricular Rhythm

Accelerated idioventricular rhythm (AIVR) is an ectopic ventricular rhythm consisting of three or more consecutive ventricular beats with a rate faster than the normal ventricular escape rate of 30 to 40 beats/min, but slower than VT. Onset and offset usually are gradual, and isorhythmic dissociation is often present. AIVR has been reported in 10% to 40% of cases of MI, especially (but not necessarily) with early reperfusion. The incidence is equal in inferior and anterior infarcts and is not related to infarct size. The presence of AIVR during the peri-infarct period is not correlated with increased mortality or incidence of VF. AIVR may also be seen with digitalis toxicity, myocarditis, and cocaine use. Symptoms may be related to loss of atrioventricular synchrony or slow ventricular rates (or both).

Premature Ventricular Complexes

PVCs occur frequently during MI. Their significance in predicting ventricular tachycardia and fibrillation is unclear. Treatment of PVCs in the peri-infarct period has not been shown conclusively to decrease the incidence of malignant ventricular arrhythmias or to improve mortality; in fact, pooled results of randomized trials in which PVCs were treated prophylactically in the peri-infarct period with lidocaine demonstrated an increased mortality. β-Blockers may be the best option for treating PVCs and preventing malignant ventricular arrhythmias.

Miscellaneous Considerations

Reperfusion Arrhythmias

Typically, AIVR has been credited with being a marker for reperfusion. However, any arrhythmia (or no arrhythmia) may be seen with reperfusion; conversely, AIVR may occur without reperfusion. Other clinical factors should be considered when deciding whether reperfusion has occurred, such as resolution of chest pain, improved hemodynamics, and normalization of electrocardiographic (ECG) changes. The appearance of reperfusion arrhythmias is related to size of infarct, length and severity of ischemia, rate of reperfusion, heart rate, extracellular potassium concentration, and the presence of congestive heart failure or left ventricular hypertrophy (or both).

Asystole and Electromechanical Dissociation

Asystole and electromechanical dissociation occur in a small fraction of patients with MI and are usually associated with large infarcts. The prognosis is extremely poor even with aggressive therapy. Defibrillation should be attempted in patients with apparent asystole, because the rhythm may actually be fine VF.

T-Wave Alternans

This is a transient ECG finding usually seen with ischemia and most pronounced in leads overlying the affected myocardium.

Other ECG Findings

Regional pericarditis sometimes seen after Q-wave infarctions may present with PR depression, but more commonly with atypical ST-segment and T-wave changes. These changes typically consist of gradual premature reversal of initially inverted T waves or persistent/recurrent ST-segment elevation (or both). Persistent ST-segment elevation after infarct may be due to continuing ischemia or aneurysm formation or may herald free wall rupture.

Left ventricular free wall rupture occurs in approximately 10% of cases of fatal transmural MI. ECG findings include failure of the characteristic evolution of the ST segment, T wave, or both. Persistent, progressive, or recurrent ST-segment elevation in the absence of recurrent ischemia may be seen. Failure of the T wave to invert or initial inversion followed by reversion to the upright may also be seen. Abrupt bradycardia responsive to atropine may occur and is believed to mark the time of rupture.

Other ECG findings may include U waves with hypokalemia and tall peaked T waves with hyperkalemia.

Suggested Review Reading

1. Birnbaum Y, Sclarovsky S, Herz I, et al: Admission clinical and electrocardiographic characteristics predicting in-hospital development of high-degree atrioventricular block in inferior wall acute myocardial infarction. *Am J Cardiol* 80:1134-1138, 1997.

2. Hindman MC, Wagner GS, JaRo M, et al: The clinical significance of bundle branch block complicating acute myocardial infarction. 1. Clinical characteristics, hospital mortality, and one-year follow-up. *Circulation* 58:679-688, 1978.

3. Jensen GV, Torp-Pedersen C, Kober L, et al: Prognosis of late versus early ventricular fibrillation in acute myocardial infarction. *Am J Cardiol* 66:10-15, 1990.

4. Ryden L, Ariniego R, Arnman K, et al: A double-blind trial of metoprolol in acute myocardial infarction. Effects on ventricular tachyarrhythmias. *N Engl J Med* 308:614-618, 1983.

Questions

Multiple Choice (choose the one best answer)

1. The appearance of reperfusion arrhythmias is related to all except which of the following?
   a. Duration of ischemia
   b. Left ventricular hypertrophy
   c. Serum concentration of sodium
   d. Myocardial extracellular potassium concentration

2. Electrocardiographic findings in patients with acute myocardial infarction associated with left ventricular free wall rupture include all the following *except*:
   a. Evidence of regional pericarditis
   b. Left posterior hemiblock
   c. Recurrent ST-segment elevation
   d. Lack of T-wave inversion

3. Which of the following is true about accelerated idioventricular rhythm?
   a. More common in inferior acute myocardial infarctions
   b. More common in large infarctions
   c. Pacing is never indicated
   d. Does not portend increased mortality

4. Prophylactic temporary pacing should be urgently considered in all the following arrhythmic complications of acute anterior myocardial infarction *except*:
   a. Sinus bradycardia during the first hour after acute myocardial infarction
   b. New right bundle branch block and new left anterior hemiblock
   c. New left bundle branch block and new first-degree atrioventricular block
   d. New right bundle branch block and new first-degree atrioventricular block
   e. All the above

5. Which of the following is *false* regarding the occurrence of complete (third-degree) heart block in inferior acute myocardial infarction?
   a. It may take 5 to 7 days to resolve
   b. The rate is usually greater than 40 beats/min
   c. The QRS is usually wide
   d. Pacing may be required if the patient is hemodynamically unstable

6. Which of the following is *true* about second-degree atrioventricular (AV) block?
   a. Type I second-degree AV block almost always requires permanent pacing
   b. Type II second-degree AV block is never seen with intraventricular block
   c. Type I second-degree AV block is never seen with intraventricular block
   d. Type I second-degree AV block may require temporary pacing
   e. All the above

7. Which of the following is *false* regarding new atrial fibrillation in the peri-infarct period?
   a. Restoration of sinus rhythm may improve hemodynamics
   b. There is no effect on subsequent mortality
   c. Rate control may improve hemodynamics
   d. Concurrent complete heart block may be present
   e. All the above

8. Autonomic imbalance in the early hours after acute myocardial infarction contributes to the occurrence of all *except*:
   a. Mobitz type II block
   b. Sinus bradycardia
   c. Sinus tachycardia
   d. Mobitz type I block

9. The only drugs demonstrated to reduce ventricular ectopy and to improve mortality in acute myocardial infarction are:
   a. Class I antiarrhythmic agents
   b. β-Blockers without intrinsic sympathomimetic activity
   c. Intravenous amiodarone
   d. Lidocaine
   e. All the above

10. In a patient with acute anterior myocardial infarction and third-degree heart block complicated by congestive heart failure requiring temporary ventricular pacing, all the following may improve hemodynamics *except*:
    a. Reperfusion of the culprit artery
    b. Increasing the pacing rate
    c. Atrial-based pacing
    d. Intra-aortic balloon pump
    e. All the above

Answers

1. Answer c

Serum concentration of sodium has no correlation with the presence or absence of reperfusion arrhythmias. The appearance of reperfusion arrhythmias correlates with all the other choices.

2. Answer b

Left posterior hemiblock is not associated with myocardial rupture. All the others may be seen in association with free wall rupture in acute myocardial infarction.

3. Answer d

The presence of accelerated idioventricular rhythm in the peri-infarct period has no effect on subsequent mortality. The rest of the choices are false.

4. Answer a

Sinus bradycardia may be seen in the early hours after both anterior and inferior myocardial infarction and does not warrant pacing unless symptomatic and refractory to atropine. The other choices may all involve infranodal conduction disturbance, and pacing should be considered.

5. Answer c

The QRS is usually narrow, because the conduction disturbance most often is intranodal.

6. Answer d

Type I second-degree AV block may require temporary pacing if the ventricular rate is too slow to maintain satisfactory hemodynamics.

7. Answer b

All other things being equal, patients with acute myocardial infarction complicated by new atrial fibrillation have a higher subsequent mortality than those who do not.

8. Answer a

Mobitz type II block usually results from infarction of infranodal conduction tissue; all other choices may be modulated by autonomic instability.

9. Answer b

All other choices either have no effect on or worsen mortality.

10. Answer e

All the listed choices may improve hemodynamic status in this situation.

Chapter 19

Mechanical Complications of Myocardial Infarction

Joseph G. Murphy, M.D.
Guy S. Reeder, M.D.
John F. Bresnahan, M.D.

> Questions about the diagnosis and management of the complications of myocardial infarction are frequent in both Internal Medicine and Cardiology Boards.

Mechanical complications after myocardial infarction are common and frequently result in death.

Patients with acute myocardial infarction can be divided into four hemodynamic subsets on the basis of the cardiac examination (Killip class, Table 1) or invasive monitoring (Forrester classification, Table 2). Although there is overlap between the two classifications, they are not interchangeable in terms of either prognosis or management. Table 3 provides data regarding hemodynamic patterns in cardiovascular disease.

Cardiogenic Shock

Cardiogenic shock is persistent hypotension (systolic pressure < 80 mm Hg) for more than 30 minutes in the absence of hypovolemia (an adequate left ventricular filling pressure measured as pulmonary capillary wedge pressure > 18 mm Hg). It frequently is associated with anuria, acidosis, peripheral hypoperfusion, and cerebral hypoxia. The cardiac index in cardiogenic shock is usually less than 2.0 L/min per m^2.

The causes of cardiogenic shock include 1) large left ventricular infarct (usually > 40% of left ventricle) in 80% of shock patients, 2) right ventricular infarct in 10% of shock patients, and 3) mechanical complications (ventricular septal defect, acute mitral regurgitation, tamponade) in 10% of shock patients. Cardiogenic shock develops in most patients several hours after the initial insult.

The incidence of cardiogenic shock is about 10% of all patients with acute infarction, and mortality is about 80% with conservative management. Thrombolytics are generally ineffective once hypotension has become established in cardiogenic shock. Primary percutaneous transluminal coronary angioplasty is the treatment of choice for cardiogenic shock, with added inotropic support, including an intra-aortic balloon pump and positive inotropic drugs, as described in Chapter 77.

Table 1.—Killip Class: Clinical Examination

Class	Finding
I	No S$_3$ or rales
II	Rales in less than half of lung field
III	Rales in more than half of lung field
IV	Cardiogenic shock

S$_3$, left ventricular third heart sound.

An atlas illustrating the pathologic conditions associated with myocardial infarction is at the end of the chapter (Plates 1-13).

Table 2.—Forrester Classification: Invasive Monitoring

Class	Finding	PCWP, mm Hg	CI, L/min per m^2
I	Normal hemodynamics	≤18	2.2
II	Good cardiac output, pulmonary congestion	> 18	≥ 2.2
III	Low cardiac output, no pulmonary congestion	≤ 18	< 2.2
IV	Low cardiac output, pulmonary congestion	> 18	< 2.2

CI, cardiac index; PCWP, pulmonary capillary wedge pressure.

Percutaneous transluminal coronary angioplasty reduces the mortality in cardiogenic shock by about 35% in absolute numbers if reperfusion is established in a timely manner. However, overall mortality in cardiogenic shock is still about 45% with angioplasty.

Hemodynamic Monitoring in Acute Myocardial Infarction

The indications for invasive pulmonary artery pressure monitoring in acute myocardial infarction are as follows:
1. Cardiogenic shock
2. Right ventricular infarction
3. Hypotension unrelated to bradycardia and unresponsive to fluids
4. Combined hypotension and heart failure
5. Suspected or actual mechanical complications of acute myocardial infarction
6. To guide use of inotropic drugs in patients with poor hemodynamics after infarction

Intra-aortic Balloon Counterpulsation

Hemodynamic Effects
1. Increased diastolic arterial blood pressure with augmented coronary diastolic blood flow and cardiac output
2. Increased or decreased systolic arterial blood pressure and reduction in left ventricular afterload with lower impedance to left ventricular ejection
3. The above results in a reduction in myocardial oxygen consumption, diminished heart rate, and increased urinary output

Table 3.—Typical Hemodynamic Patterns in Cardiovascular Disease*

	Pressure				Pulmonary arteriolar resistance index
	RA	PA	PCW	CI	
Normal	< 6	< 28/12	< 18	> 2.4	< 2
Tamponade	High	Variable	Low	Low	Normal
Right ventricular infarction	High	Low-normal	Low	Low	Normal
Acute pulmonary embolus	High	Normal-high	Low	Low	Normal-high
Left ventricular failure	Normal	Normal-high	High	Low-normal	Normal
High-output heart failure	High	Normal-high	High	High	Normal
Right ventricular failure	High	Variable	Low-normal	Low-normal	Normal
Cardiogenic shock	High	Normal-high	High	Low	Normal
Septicemia	Low	Low-normal	Low	High	Low
Chronic pulmonary hypertension	High	High	Normal	Low-normal	High
Hypovolemia	Low	Low-normal	Low	Low	Low

*The values and descriptions given reflect typical clinical scenarios, but there is significant patient-to-patient variation. RA, PA, and PCW pressures are in mm Hg. CI is in L/min per m^2. Pulmonary arteriolar resistance is in Wood units (multiply by 80 to convert Wood units to dynes · s · cm^5).
CI, cardiac index; PA, pulmonary artery; PCW, pulmonary capillary wedge; RA, right atrial.

Indications

1. Cardiogenic shock
2. Refractory myocardial ischemia
3. To stabilize the patient in association with a myocardial revascularization procedure (coronary artery bypass or angioplasty)
4. Mechanical complications of infarction

Complications

1. Vascular complications (insertion site, aortic wall, damage from repeated balloon inflations)
2. Hematologic problems (hemolysis, systemic emboli)
3. Balloon dependence (unable to wean from support)
4. Vascular complications are increased in elderly female patients of small stature and in patients with diabetes mellitus or peripheral vascular disease

Contraindications

1. Patient not a candidate for aggressive revascularization
2. Aortic incompetence
3. Severe peripheral vascular disease
4. Aortic aneurysm (thoracic or descending aorta)
5. Aortic dissection

Right Ventricular Infarction

Suspect significant right ventricular infarction in any patient with an inferior myocardial infarction complicated by hypotension. Other hemodynamic features of right ventricular infarction include an increased right atrial pressure (> 12 mm Hg) in the presence of normal or decreased right ventricular and pulmonary artery systolic pressures and an increased ratio of right ventricular to left ventricular filling pressures. In general, the central venous pressure, right atrial pressure, and right ventricular diastolic pressure are all increased and right ventricular systolic pressure and cardiac output are decreased. A hemodynamic pattern that suggests pericardial disease (steep right atrial Y descent and square root sign) may occur. With significant right ventricular infarction, the right ventricle dilates acutely, with resultant pericardial constriction-type pathophysiology and an increased jugular venous pressure and, more rarely, a positive Kussmaul sign. A clear lung field on chest radiography in a hypotensive patient is a hallmark of right ventricular infarction.

- Significant right ventricular infarction is associated with hypotension, an increased jugular venous pressure, and clear lung fields.
- Significant right ventricular infarction rarely occurs in the absence of evidence of an inferior wall infarction.

Diagnosis

Right ventricular infarction is diagnosed on the basis of classic clinical features, ST-segment elevation on right-sided chest leads (V_3R/V_4R), and right ventricular dilatation and hypokinesia on imaging studies. Echocardiography is the single best diagnostic imaging method and will show an increase in right ventricular dimensions, a depressed right ventricular function, and tricuspid regurgitation. The hemodynamic findings are low cardiac output, low pulmonary wedge pressure, and increased right atrial pressure (> 12 mm Hg). Other findings may include significant tricuspid regurgitation due to dilatation of the right ventricle and a significant right-to-left intracardiac shunt through a patent foramen ovale as a result of increased right atrial pressure. Patients with prior right ventricular hypertrophy due to congenital heart disease or advanced pulmonary disease may have significant hemodynamic problems even with a moderate-sized right ventricular infarction.

> Always consider either a pulmonary embolus or a new right-to-left shunt across a patent foramen ovale in a patient with marked arterial desaturation complicating an inferior wall infarction.

- The hemodynamic findings associated with right ventricular infarction are low cardiac output, low pulmonary wedge pressure, and increased right atrial pressure.
- Right ventricular infarction may be complicated by tricuspid regurgitation due to tricuspid annular dilatation.
- The differential diagnosis of right ventricular infarction is pulmonary embolus, constrictive pericarditis, pericardial tamponade, and cardiogenic shock due to any cause.

Management

Thrombolytics or primary percutaneous transluminal coronary angioplasty may be beneficial when administered early in the course of inferior or true posterior infarction complicated by right ventricular infarction even in the absence of ST-segment elevation in the right-sided chest leads. This is currently the only non-ST–elevation myocardial infarction for which thrombolytics should be administered. Patients with hypotension or decreased urinary output due to right ventricular infarction should have volume loading to achieve a pulmonary wedge pressure of 18 mm Hg or more. Inotropic support with dopamine also may be beneficial. Many patients with right ventricular infarction in the presence of normal or mildly depressed left ventricular function have a good prognosis, but 72 hours may pass before right ventricular function starts to improve. Overall, right ventricular infarction increases mortality significantly.

- True posterior infarction complicated by right ventricular infarction is the only non-ST–elevation myocardial infarction for which thrombolytics should be administered.
- Patients with hypotension or decreased urinary output due to right ventricular infarction should have volume loading to achieve a pulmonary wedge pressure of 18 mm Hg or more.

> A common examination question addresses the diagnosis and management of patients with a myocardial infarction complicated by a new systolic murmur. Possible diagnoses include papillary muscle dysfunction or rupture, interventricular septal rupture, and tricuspid regurgitation due to right ventricular infarction or pulmonary embolus.

Rupture of the Ventricular Free Wall

Rupture of the ventricular free wall usually presents catastrophically with either sudden death, usually due to electromechanical dissociation, or tamponade with cardiogenic shock. Rarely, patients present with subacute ventricular rupture manifested by pericardial pain, electrocardiographic evidence of pericarditis, and a pericardial rub. Rupture typically occurs within 4 days after infarction. Significant predisposing factors for ventricular rupture in the TIMI 9B trial were elderly age (> 70 years; odds ratio, 5.0) and female sex (odds ratio, 3.6). Possible risk factors also include the use of steroids, anticoagulation, or late thrombolysis.

Myocardial ruptures are of three types:

1. A slit-like tear that occurs early after infarction and is associated with single-vessel disease without any thinning of the left ventricular wall and good left ventricular function (most common type of rupture).
2. Rupture that results from a subacute process with localized necrosis of myocardium.

3. Rupture that is preceded by the development of myocardial thinning, with rupture in the center of the thinned area.

Late ruptures are associated with multivessel disease and occur days to weeks after infarction. Rupture usually occurs in the left ventricle (8 times more than in the right ventricle), in the terminal distribution of the left anterior descending coronary artery (anterior wall rupture), or in diagonal branches (lateral wall rupture) at the junction of normal and infarcted myocardium.

The treatment of rupture of the ventricular free wall is emergency cardiac operation. Rarely, the rupture may be walled off to produce a left ventricular false aneurysm or pseudoaneurysm. Echocardiography is the diagnostic imaging method of choice, and cardiac operation is almost always required because of the tendency for false aneurysms to rupture without warning. Pseudoaneurysms are also associated with heart failure caused by loss of myocardial power and systemic thromboembolism.

- Predisposing factors for ventricular rupture are elderly age (> 70 years) and female sex.
- Elderly women are also at higher risk for rupture of the ventricular free wall.

Rupture of the Ventricular Septum

Rupture of the ventricular septum is similar in many ways to rupture of the ventricular free wall in that it almost always occurs within days of acute infarction, is frequently a serpiginous tract rather than a discrete hole, is associated with transmural infarction, and probably also is associated with hypertension. Ventricular septal rupture usually presents abruptly with hypotension, acute right ventricular failure, and a new pansystolic murmur frequently associated with a systolic thrill. Echocardiography is the diagnostic imaging method of choice. Inferior infarctions cause septal rupture in the basal inferior septum, whereas anterior infarctions cause rupture in the apical septum.

Treatment of rupture of the ventricular septum is emergency cardiac surgery.

- Ventricular septal rupture presents with hypotension, acute right ventricular failure, and a new pansystolic murmur frequently associated with a systolic thrill.
- Patients with acute ventricular septal defect can lie supine, but patients with mitral rupture develop pulmonary edema rapidly and cannot lie flat.

Acute Mitral Regurgitation

Acute mitral regurgitation after myocardial infarction can be due to papillary muscle dysfunction caused by fibrosis or ischemia, papillary muscle rupture (either partial or complete), or mitral annular dilatation associated with left ventricular failure. The blood supply to the posteromedial papillary muscle (derived only from the posterior descending artery) is more tenuous than that to the anterolateral papillary muscle (derived from both the left anterior descending and the left circumflex arteries). Consequently, 90% of papillary muscle ruptures involve the posteromedial papillary muscle. This is fortuitous because the posteromedial papillary muscle usually has multiple heads (in contrast to the single head of the antero-lateral papillary muscle), and rupture of an individual head is frequently survivable, at least in the short term. Infarctions associated with papillary muscle rupture are usually small, and frequently there is only single-vessel coronary disease. Patients with papillary muscle rupture usually present up to 1 week after myocardial infarction with acute pulmonary edema. The loudness of the mitral regurgitation murmur is variable and may not correlate with the degree of mitral regurgitation. The murmur may be completely absent in some patients with severe mitral regurgitation. A thrill is rarely present in acute mitral regurgitation. Large V waves are present in the pulmonary wedge tracing, and, more rarely, the regurgitant jet may be transmitted through the pulmonary vasculature to lead to increased oxygen saturation in the pulmonary artery; this may suggest an erroneous diagnosis of ventricular septal rupture. Echocardiography is the diagnostic imaging method of choice, and urgent cardiac operation is generally indicated (Fig. 1).

- In 90% of papillary muscle ruptures, the posteromedial papillary muscle ruptures.
- A thrill is rarely present in acute mitral regurgitation.
- A murmur may not be audible.
- Heart block complicating inferior infarction increases mortality significantly.

Heart Block

The principles of the treatment of heart block complicating myocardial infarction are as follows:

1. Anterior infarctions cause heart block because of septal injury that leads to necrosis of the infra-atrioventricular nodal conduction system, including the His bundle and

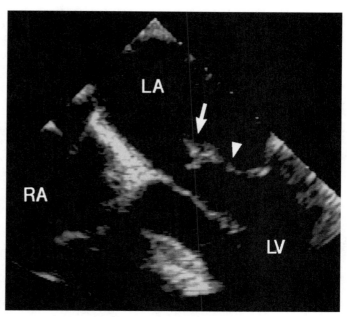

Fig. 1. Papillary muscle rupture complicating acute inferior myocardial infarction; magnified transverse four-chamber view. The ruptured head of the posteromedial papillary muscle (*arrow*) prolapses freely into the left atrium; the posterior mitral valve leaflet (*arrowhead*) is flail. (From Freeman WK, Seward JB, Khandheria BK, Tajik AJ: *Transesophageal Echocardiography.* Little, Brown and Company, 1994, p 554. By permission of Mayo Foundation.)

bundle branches. Inferior infarctions usually cause heart block because of activation of abnormal cardiovascular reflexes or transient ischemic injury of the atrioventricular node. Necrosis of the atrioventricular node is rare in inferior infarction because of the presence of collateral vessels from the left anterior descending vessel in addition to the normal blood supply from the atrioventricular nodal artery (supplied by the right coronary artery in 85% of cases and the left circumflex artery in the remaining 15% of patients with a left dominant coronary circulation).

2. First-degree heart block and second-degree heart block type I (Wenckebach) are usually atrioventricular nodal in location and frequently are transient, whereas second-degree heart block type II and complete heart block are usually due to injury to the infranodal conduction system and may be permanent.

3. Patients with second-degree atrioventricular block and anterior infarction can progress to high-grade atrioventricular heart block very rapidly and should be paced at an early stage, whereas inferior infarctions usually progress in a stepwise fashion and can be observed without temporary pacing for a longer time if clinically stable.

4. Inferior infarctions usually are paced for symptoms of hypoperfusion, whereas anterior infarctions are paced early on the basis of electrocardiographic criteria alone, frequently without symptoms of hypoperfusion.

NEW TRIAL INFORMATION ADDED AT PROOF STAGE

The SHOCK Trial (Should We Emergently Revascularize Occluded Coronaries for Cardiogenic Shock)

SHOCK was a randomized trial of emergency percutaneous transluminal coronary angioplasty (PTCA) and coronary artery bypass grafting (CABG) versus initial medical stabilization in patients with acute myocardial infarction complicated by cardiogenic shock. All patients were eligible to receive intra-aortic balloon pump support or inotropic medication. Patients in the revascularization group were treated with thrombolysis if clinically indicated and then underwent emergency PTCA or CABG within 6 hours. The medically treated patients were required to receive thrombolytic therapy, unless there was an absolute contraindication. Exclusion criteria included acute mechanical shock and isolated right ventricular infarction. Importantly, of all patients screened, only 26% (302) patients with acute myocardial infarction and shock were successfully randomized.

At 30 days, the all-cause mortality rate was 46% for the revascularization group and 56% for the medical group; the absolute risk reduction was 9.3%, and the relative risk reduction was 17% ($P = 0.11$). At 30 days the mortality rate was 38% in patients with successful PTCA and 78% in patients with unsuccessful PTCA. The mortality rate in the CABG group was 42%.

At 60 days, the mortality rate was lower in the revascularization group (54%) than in the medical group (68%; $P = 0.04$). Adverse events, including stroke, peripheral vascular occlusion, persistent angina, sepsis, hemorrhage, and refractory shock, were similar in both groups, except that acute renal failure occurred more frequently in the medical group. In subgroup analysis, age was significantly associated with outcome: younger patients (< 75 years) had a greater benefit from revascularization than older patients (≥ 75 years), who had a greater benefit from medical therapy. At 6 months, younger patients in the revascularization group had a lower mortality rate (48%) than those in the medical group (69%, $P < 0.01$), suggesting a lesser effect of revascularization with increasing age. Prior myocardial infarction had a significant interaction with outcome at 30 days but not at 6 months.

The conclusion of the study was that early revascularization was better than initial medical management but that all patients with cardiogenic shock still have a high mortality, in excess of 50%, despite advances in emergency care.

Suggested Review Reading

1. Killip T III, Kimball JT: Treatment of myocardial infarction in a coronary care unit. A two year experience with 250 patients. *Am J Cardiol* 20:457-464, 1967.
   This classic article describes the Killip classes for myocardial infarction.

2. Forrester JS, Diamond G, Chatterjee K, et al: Medical therapy of acute myocardial infarction by application of hemodynamic subsets (part 1). *N Engl J Med* 295:1356-1362, 1976.
   This classic article describes the Forrester classification for myocardial infarction.

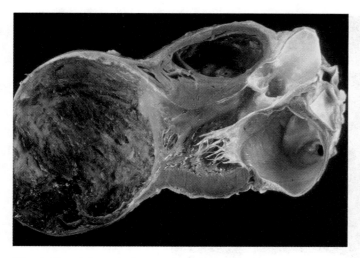

Plate 1. Huge left ventricular aneurysm with shallow mural thrombus, after myocardial infarction.

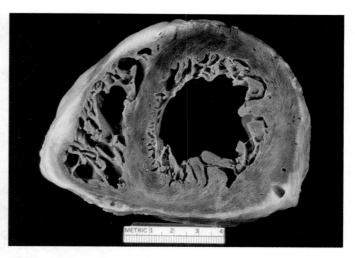

Plate 2. Cardiogenic shock with large acute myocardial infarction.

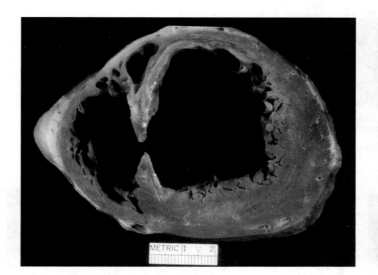

Plate 3. Ventricular septum rupture, after myocardial infarction.

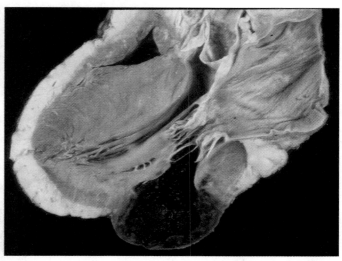

Plate 4. False aneurysm (contained left ventricle rupture), after myocardial infarction.

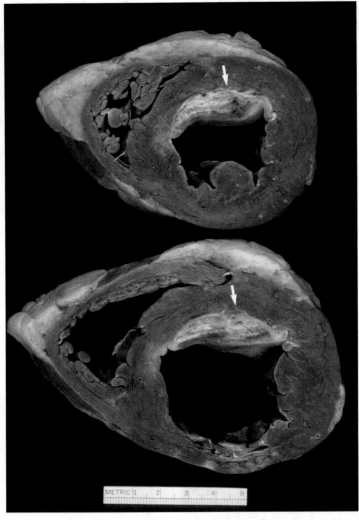

Plate 5. Old mural thrombus (*arrows*), after myocardial infarction.

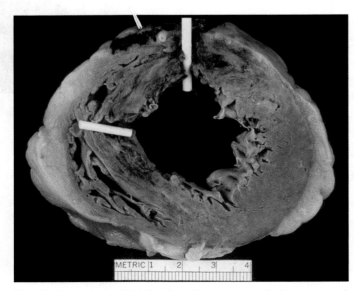

Plate 6. Acute myocardial infarction with two ruptures in the septum and ventricular free wall.

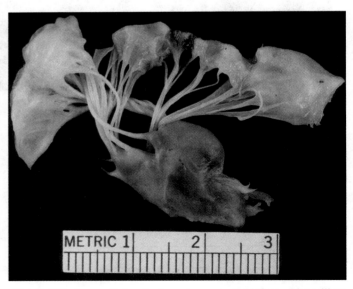

Plate 7. Mitral regurgitation due to acute myocardial infarct with papillary muscle rupture.

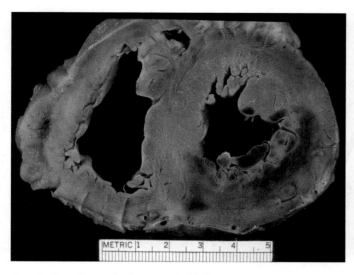

Plate 8. Acute hemorrhagic myocardial infarct.

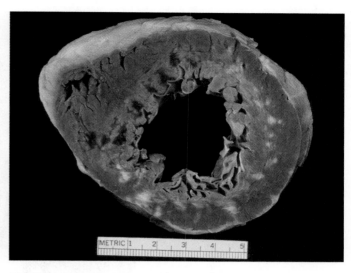

Plate 9. Multiple old infarcts and an acute subendocardial myocardial infarct.

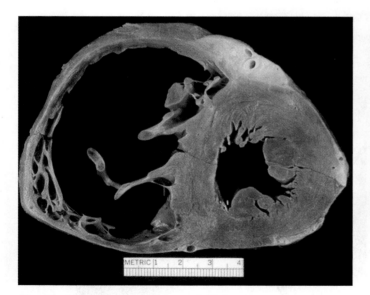

Plate 10. Acute right ventricle myocardial infarct.

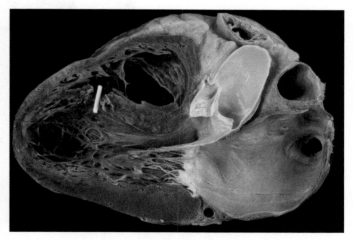

Plate 11. Ventricular septal defect, after myocardial infarction.

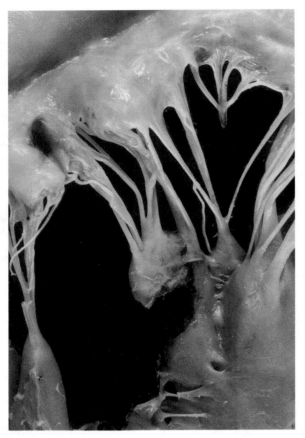

Plate 12. Partial mitral valve papillary muscle rupture.

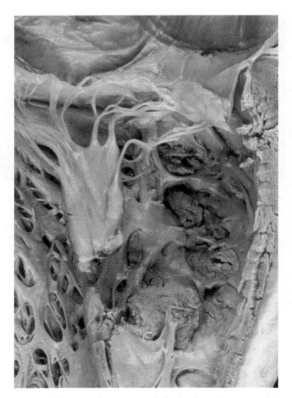

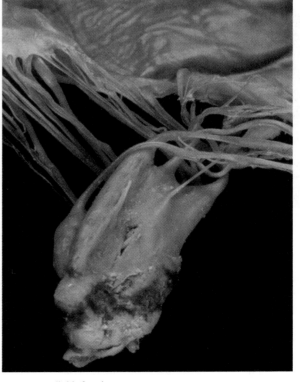

Plate 13. Ruptured posteromedial mitral papillary muscle in acute myocardial infarction.

Chapter 20

Cardiac Rehabilitation

Joseph G. Murphy, M.D.
Gerald T. Gau, M.D.

Cardiac rehabilitation is an area frequently overlooked by examination candidates. Candidates for the Cardiology Boards should know the phases of cardiac rehabilitation, the physiologic benefits of exercise, and the contraindications to enrollment of patients in a rehabilitation program.

Cardiac rehabilitation is the restoration of physical, psychological, and social well-being in patients who have had a cardiac event or in patients with chronic cardiac disease. It includes the prevention of sudden death, relief of cardiac symptoms, decrease in cardiac morbidity, and stabilization or reversal of the disease process. Cardiac rehabilitation combines exercise training with modification of coronary risk factors in patients with documented cardiac disease.

Basic Physiology of Exercise

Isometric exercise (weight lifting) predominantly increases blood pressure and involves an abrupt increase in cardiac work and a modest increase in cardiac output. It is contraindicated in patients with poor left ventricular function. Apart from peripheral muscle toning, it is of little cardiovascular benefit.

Dynamic exercise (walking, cycling, swimming) increases cardiac output with a decrease in total peripheral resistance but local vasoconstriction of the splanchnic and renal arterioles, thus shunting blood to the working muscle beds. Systolic blood pressure increases and diastolic blood pressure decreases or remains constant.

Heart rate increases as a result of decreased vagal nerve activity and increased sympathetic discharge. Myocardial oxygen demand ($M\dot{V}o_2$) during exercise is determined by heart rate, ventricular contractility, and ventricular wall tension. $M\dot{V}o_2$ is approximated by the rate-pressure product (heart rate x peak systolic blood pressure).

Training Effect (Response to Chronic Exercise)

Population-based studies have shown that regular physical activity levels from 500 kcal/week to 3,500 kcal/week energy expended have an incremental beneficial effect on lowering the risk of cardiac death when all other risk factors are controlled.

Training increases maximal oxygen uptake ($\dot{V}o_2$ max) in both healthy persons and those with ischemic heart disease. Resting heart rate decreases, as do $M\dot{V}o_2$, heart rate, and systolic blood pressure, for any given exercise level, unlike in deconditioned persons. Collateral blood flow to ischemic myocardium is augmented by exercise training. Skeletal muscle alters its biochemical profile after chronic exercise with an increased number of mitochondria, an increased myoglobin content, and an increased myocardial capillary/myocyte ratio. Exercise increases the use of fatty acids but has little effect on carbohydrate metabolism (Tables 1 and 2).

Cardiac rehabilitation is usually divided into four phases (Table 3). Phase I is the hospitalization phase, in which the goal is primarily education and prevention of deconditioning. Phase II is the supervised convalescent phase after hospital dismissal. Phase III is the unsupervised at-home recovery phase, which merges into phase IV, the maintenance of health stage.

The indications for cardiac rehabilitation include 1) myocardial infarction, 2) coronary artery bypass surgery, 3) percutaneous transluminal coronary angioplasty or other interventional coronary procedures, 4) stable angina, 5) class II or III heart failure, 6) heart transplantation, 7) valvular heart surgery, and 8) surgery for congenital heart disease.

Rehabilitation After Myocardial Infarction

Cardiac rehabilitation after myocardial infarction decreases cardiac death by 20%-25%, but no change occurs in the incidence of nonfatal reinfarction. Phase I is the inpatient portion, which lasts 4 to 6 days, during which much of the hospitalization time is taken up by interventions. Most patient education has been shifted to the immediate out-of-hospital phase II program. Phase II lasts from 1 week up to 3 months; patient risk stratification depends on the degree of cardiac dysfunction and comorbid conditions. Phase III is the late recovery program, in which patients continue to be medically supervised for a minimum of 6 months. Phase IV is nonmedically supervised; the patient exercises on his or her own, usually with a group of other patients who have also been part of the same program.

Patients in the 1990s have smaller myocardial infarctions, are left with better left ventricular function, have shorter

Table 1.—Benefits Resulting From Long-Term Outpatient Cardiac Rehabilitation

Physiologic
- ↑ $\dot{V}o_2max$
- ↓ $M\dot{V}o_2$ for given workload
- ↑ Muscle strength and endurance
- ↑ Blood fibrinolytic activity
- ↓ Platelet aggregation
- ↓ Catecholamines

Improved left ventricular function[*]

Increased resistance to ventricular fibrillation[*]

Symptomatic
- ↓ Angina pectoris
- ↓ Dyspnea
- ↓ Claudication
- ↓ Fatigue

Anatomical
- ↓ Progression of disease[*]
- ↑ Regression of disease[*]
- ↑ Improved myocardial perfusion[*]

Psychologic
- ↓ Anxiety and depression
- ↑ Confidence and self-esteem
- ↑ Knowledge

Epidemiologic
- ↓ Morbidity[*]
- ↓ Mortality[*]

Risk factors
- ↓ Smoking
- ↓ Total cholesterol and triglycerides
- ↑ High-density lipoprotein cholesterol
- ↓ Obesity
- ↓ Hypertension
- ↑ Carbohydrate metabolism

Economic
- ↑ Patient productivity[*]
- ↓ Disability cases[*]
- ↓ Physician office visits[*]
- ↓ Medications

$\dot{V}o_2max$, maximal oxygen uptake; $M\dot{V}o_2$, myocardial oxygen demand.

*Potential benefits.

From Giuliani ER, Gersh BJ, McGoon MD, Hayes DL, Schaff HV (editors): *Mayo Clinic Practice of Cardiology*. Third edition. Mosby, 1996, p 540. By permission of Mayo Foundation.

Table 2.—Adaptations to Exercise Training in Cardiac Patients

1. ↑ $\dot{V}o_2$ max resulting from:
   a. Skeletal muscle adaptation (↑ $c(a - \bar{v})O_2$)
   b. Improvement in left ventricular function in selected patients (↑ maximal cardiac output)
2. ↓ HR and SBP for a given submaximal exercise intensity resulting from:
   a. ↑ $c(a - \bar{v})O_2$
   b. ↓ Submaximal cardiac output
3. As a result, symptoms of angina pectoris, fatigue, and dyspnea improve

$\dot{V}o_2$ max, maximal oxygen uptake; $c(a - \bar{v})O_2$, difference in oxygen content between the arterial and mixed venous blood; HR, heart rate; SBP, systolic blood pressure.
From Giuliani ER, Gersh BJ, McGoon MD, Hayes DL, Schaff HV (editors): *Mayo Clinic Practice of Cardiology*. Third edition. Mosby, 1996, p 540. By permission of Mayo Foundation.

hospital stays, have lower morbidity and mortality, and return to work earlier than patients who had infarctions before this decade. Risk factor modification is the main focus of phase II rehabilitation, in addition to addressing quality of life issues and early return to work.

Cardiac rehabilitation programs include not only patients who have had myocardial infarction but also patients who have had interventional cardiac procedures, coronary artery bypass, and cardiac transplantation and those with chronic heart failure and high cardiovascular risk.

Risk Stratification After Myocardial Infarction

Before hospital dismissal, patients are given an exercise test to stratify them into a low-, intermediate-, or high-risk group (Table 4). If the result of the exercise test is normal and the patient is defined as low risk, the patient can enter the exercise program and be prescribed an individualized program that is either a supervised or nonsupervised program, depending on the degree of cardiac abnormality. Usually, patients are monitored electrocardiographically for a short time and then are quickly weaned from monitoring to prevent any psychological dependence.

Patients are defined as high risk if they 1) have reduced left ventricular function, exercise tolerance of less than 5 METs on the predismissal treadmill test, a history of complex

Table 3.—Phases of Cardiac Rehabilitation

Phase	Type of program	Duration
I	Inpatient	Days
II	Outpatient, immediate post-hospitalization	1-12 wk
III	Late recovery period	Minimum of 6 mo beyond phase II
IV	Maintenance program	Indefinite

From Giuliani ER, Gersh BJ, McGoon MD, Hayes DL, Schaff HV (editors): *Mayo Clinic Practice of Cardiology*. Third edition. Mosby, 1996, p 530. By permission of Mayo Foundation.

ventricular arrhythmias, angina with activity, exercise hypotension, or abnormal electrocardiographic changes on a good pharmacologic program or 2) are survivors of sudden out-of-hospital cardiac arrest. Patients with compensated congestive heart failure are all considered high risk. All high-risk patients need supervised, electrocardiography-monitored, and individualized programs (Table 5).

One of the most important aspects of cardiac rehabilitation

Table 4.—Risk Stratification After a Cardiac Event

High risk
    1. Low functional capacity (< 5 METs) or unable to exercise for any reason
    2. Severe left ventricular dysfunction (EF < 30%)
    3. Severe residual myocardial ischemia
    4. Complex ventricular ectopy
    5. Complicated hospital course (heart failure, arrhythmia, ischemia)
    6. Post-cardiac arrest
Intermediate risk
    1. Functional capacity 5-6 METs
    2. Moderate left ventricular dysfunction (EF 30%-50%)
    3. Moderate residual myocardial ischemia
    4. Noncomplex ventricular ectopy
Low risk
    1. Functional capacity > 6 METs
    2. Normal left ventricular function (EF > 50%)
    3. No residual myocardial ischemia
    4. No significant ventricular ectopy
    5. Uncomplicated hospital course

EF, ejection fraction; MET, unit of energy required for basal metabolism.

Table 5.—Absolute Contraindications to Exercise Training

Unstable angina pectoris	Thrombophlebitis
Dangerous arrhythmias	Recent systemic or pulmo-
Overt cardiac failure	nary embolus
Severe left ventricular outflow tract obstruction	Severe hypertension (> 200 mm Hg resting systolic or
Hypertrophic cardiomyopathy or aortic stenosis	> 110 mm Hg resting diastolic blood pressure)
Dissecting aneurysm	Overt psychoneurotic distur-
Serious systemic disease	bances
Myocarditis (acute)	Uncontrolled diabetes mellitus
Large pericardial effusion	Severe orthopedic limitation
Pulmonary hypertension (> 60 mm Hg at rest)	Intraventricular thrombus
Significant inflammatory or infectious disease	Third-degree heart block without pacemaker

Modified from Giuliani ER, Gersh BJ, McGoon MD, Hayes DL, Schaff HV (editors): *Mayo Clinic Practice of Cardiology*. Third edition. Mosby, 1996, p 530. By permission of Mayo Foundation.

is the awareness that low-intensity exercise, usually 40% to 70% of exercise capacity, exerts a positive training effect that can be done with increasing safety and leads to much better compliance with the program.

Exercise and cardiac rehabilitation programs are very safe—the cardiac death rate is about 1 patient per million patient-hours. The higher the degree of exercise training, the lower the incidence of cardiac arrest induced by intense activity.

The exercise prescription in cardiac rehabilitation is generally 40% to 70% of the aerobic capacity. Patients may start with just 3 to 5 minutes of exercise and gradually increase the time until able to do 20 to 60 minutes of continuous aerobic activity, usually 3 to 7 days a week. Activity should be aerobic, either treadmill or bike-type activities (Table 6).

Exercise Training and Heart Failure

Patients with chronic heart failure benefit significantly from exercise training. Results include a decrease in myocardial oxygen demand, an increased functional capacity, an increased cardiac output at peak exercise due to reduced vascular resistance, and decreased sympathetic activity. Peak oxygen uptake increases up to 25%, and exercise duration increases up to 33%. There is a poor correlation between resting ejection fraction and exercise time on an exercise symptom-limited protocol.

In one study of patients with chronic heart failure, forearm blood flow-dependent vasodilatation that was abnormal before training was restored toward normal with exercise training in association with enhanced endothelial release of nitric oxide and improved endothelial function. Mild exercise training at low levels in obese males without any change in weight is associated with decreased insulin levels, decreased resting blood pressure, and decreased levels of low-density lipoprotein; these results emphasize some of the biochemical and hemodynamic changes that occur in response to low-level exercise training.

Table 6.—Aerobic Exercise Prescription for Cardiac Rehabilitation

Phase	Intensity	Duration, min	Frequency	Mode
I	RHR + 20	5-20	2-3 times/day	Slow walk, or cycle or arm ergometry[*]
II	RHR + 20 40%-70% of functional capacity; perceived exertion 11 to 14	10-45	5-6 times/wk	Walk, cycle or arm ergometry, rowing, stair climbing, cross-country skiing simulator, walk-jog, low-level games
III	50%-75% of functional capacity; perceived exertion 12 to 14	20-45	3-6 times/wk	Walk, walk-jog, jog, cycle or arm ergometry or other aerobic equipment, outdoor cycle, games, swimming
IV	50%-80% of functional capacity; perceived exertion 12 to 15	20-45	3-6 times/wk	Same as above (III)

RHR, resting heart rate.
[*]Arm ergometry during phase I is limited to nonambulatory patients.
From Giuliani ER, Gersh BJ, McGoon MD, Hayes DL, Schaff HV (editors): *Mayo Clinic Practice of Cardiology*. Third edition. Mosby, 1996, p 539. By permission of Mayo Foundation.

Risks Associated With Cardiac Rehabilitation

Risk of cardiac arrest during supervised exercise:
    about 1 in 110,000 person-hours
Risk of death during supervised exercise:
    1 in 750,000 person-hours
Risk of death with uncontrolled vigorous exercise (such as jogging):
    1 in 60,000 person-hours
Risk of death with uncontrolled vigorous exercise in the normal healthy population:
    1 in 550,000 person-hours

METs (Metabolic Equivalent System)

One MET is the unit of energy that is required for basal metabolism (that is, in a person at rest in the postabsorptive state). It approximates 3.5 mL O_2/kg per minute. Table 7 lists the number of METs associated with various activities.

Table 7.—METs Required for Various Activities

No. of METs	Activity
2-3	Walking at 2 mph
	Clerical work
	Playing billiards
	Driving a car
4-5	Walking at 4 mph
	Light assembly work
	Doubles tennis
	Painting
6-7	Walking at 5 mph
	Construction
	Singles tennis
	Yard work
8-9	Jogging at 5 mph
	Digging trenches
	Touch football
	Sawing wood
10-11	Running at 6 mph
	Lumberjack work
	Squash

MET, unit of energy required for basal metabolism.

Notes

Chapter 21

Risk Stratification After Myocardial Infarction

Guy S. Reeder, M.D.

Clinicians are adept at recognizing patients at high risk for mortality or morbidity after myocardial infarction. Thus, patients with congestive heart failure, recurrent ischemia, diabetes mellitus, resting ejection fraction less than 40%, nonsustained ventricular tachycardia, and other high-risk clinical characteristics are appropriately selected for coronary angiography and revascularization. Clinicians search less diligently for patients who are at low risk for future adverse events after myocardial infarction; such patients are candidates for early dismissal and might logically avoid unnecessary and possibly harmful laboratory investigation and revascularization procedures.

- Patients at high risk for mortality or morbidity after myocardial infarction are those with congestive heart failure, recurrent ischemia, diabetes mellitus, resting ejection fraction less than 40%, and nonsustained ventricular tachycardia.

Why Identify a Low-Risk Group of Patients?

In the United States, patients surviving myocardial infarction often undergo many noninvasive and invasive tests and subsequent revascularization procedures. In the Global Utilization of Streptokinase and t-PA for Occluded Coronary Arteries (GUSTO-1) trial, elective angiography was performed in 70%, angioplasty in 30%, and bypass grafting in 13% of patients during their initial hospitalization for myocardial infarction. In one analysis of this trial, the use of angiography and angioplasty was compared in the United States and Canada. Despite an approximately threefold higher rate of angiography and angioplasty and fourfold higher rate of bypass grafting in the United States than in Canada, survival at 1 year differed by only four-tenths of 1% (Table 1). A similar comparison of post-thrombolytic procedures and 30-day survival between U.S. and non-U.S. patients in this trial demonstrated no difference in death or nonfatal stroke at 1-year follow-up, despite a threefold to fourfold higher rate of revascularization procedures within the United States. The Survival and Ventricular Enlargement (SAVE) study also found an almost threefold difference in revascularization between U.S. and Canadian patients and no significant difference in mortality or reinfarction at 1 year (Table 2). Examination of regional variation within the United States in the utilization of procedures after myocardial infarction demonstrates no relationship between procedure rates and subsequent death or reinfarction. In fact, GUSTO-1, and other studies, demonstrated that the performance of angiography after infarction is most closely correlated with its availability at the particular hospital studied (Fig. 1). Such marked variability in utilization of resources after infarction suggests the unnecessary use of such procedures in some patients—most likely those who are already at low risk of adverse events.

- The performance of angiography after infarction is most closely correlated with its availability at the particular hospital studied.

Table 1.—U.S.-Canadian Comparison of Procedures After Myocardial Infarction: GUSTO-1

Variable	U.S.	Canada
No. of patients	23,105	2,898
Angiography, %*	72	25
PTCA, %*	29	11
Bypass, %*	14	3
Total revascularization (1 yr), %	53	24
Survival, %		
24 hr	97.3	96.8
30 days†	93.2	92.4
1 yr	90.7	90.3

GUSTO-1, Global Utilization of Streptokinase and t-PA for Occluded Coronary Arteries trial; PTCA, percutaneous transluminal coronary angioplasty.
*In-hospital.
†$P = 0.02$
Data from *N Engl J Med* 331:1130-1135, 1994.

What Constitutes "Low Risk" After Myocardial Infarction?

An idealistic definition of "low risk" is the absence of any adverse event after infarction; obviously, this is an unachievable goal. What then is a practical benchmark with which to establish low risk? One approach is to consider only the two *irreversible* adverse events after myocardial infarction:

Table 2.—U.S.-Canadian Comparison of Procedures After Myocardial Infarction: SAVE

Variable	U.S.	Canada
All revascularization, %	31	12
Morbidity, 1 yr, %	11	11
Reinfarction, 1 yr, %	8	9

SAVE, Survival and Ventricular Enlargement Study.
Data from *N Engl J Med* 328:779-784, 1993.

death and nonfatal reinfarction. All other events are treatable as they occur and, therefore, assume much less importance in prevention. A practical definition of "low risk" might be constructed, then, as follows: a population of patients with an incidence of adverse irreversible events so low that prophylactic intervention would be unlikely to alter it. Such patients, by definition, would not require extensive postinfarction testing, because their event rates would be so low as to negate any value of subsequent intervention. The most recent benchmark results of intervention (angioplasty or bypass) in patients with single- and multiple-vessel coronary artery disease have been established by the multiple randomized trials comparing these methods. In these trials, the average 1-year mortality for patients undergoing angioplasty was approximately 3%. Given that such trials tended to exclude patients with advanced disease, recent infarction, and poor ventricular function, their

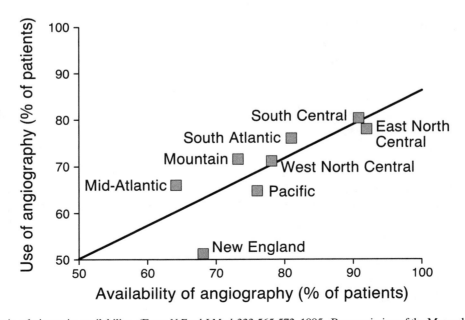

Fig. 1. Use of angiography in relation to its availability. (From *N Engl J Med* 333:565-572, 1995. By permission of the Massachusetts Medical Society.)

results may reflect an overly optimistic goal when compared with an average population of patients after myocardial infarction. Nonetheless, there can be little disagreement that if a population of patients who have had infarction could be found who had a similar 1-year mortality risk of about 3%, they could certainly be described as low-risk. Parenthetically, one might observe that searching for such a patient population would be most worthwhile if it constituted a significant proportion of patients seen after infarction.

- Average 1-year mortality for patients undergoing angioplasty was approximately 3%.

How to Detect Low-Risk and High-Risk Patients

In the prethrombolytic era, an uncomplicated clinical course and negative treadmill test predicted a low risk of death after infarction. Treadmill testing has been of little predictive value, however, in patients undergoing thrombolysis, primarily because of very low event rates after dismissal. In the thrombolytic era, three trials (TIMI-II, GISSI-2, GUSTO-1) prospectively examined clinical and noninvasive laboratory data to predict patients at low and high risk of death or reinfarction. The Thrombolysis in Myocardial Infarction (TIMI-II) trial was a randomized comparison of aggressive and conservative intervention after thrombolytic therapy in 3,339 patients with acute myocardial infarction. The average 6-week mortality rate was 4.8%, and the subsequent mortality rate during the year after hospital dismissal ranged from 2.0% to 3.3%. In that trial, eight "not low-risk" factors were prospectively tested with the end point of 6-week mortality (Table 3). Patients with none or only one of these risk factors constituted a relatively low-risk group with a mortality rate of 1.5% to 2.3% cumulative at 6 weeks, respectively (Fig. 2). In those with two or more risk factors, mortality ranged from 13% to 17%. These risk factors can be used clinically for patients receiving thrombolytic therapy.

Gruppo Italiano per lo Studio della Sopravvivenza nell'Infarto Miocardico 2 (GISSI-2) was a thrombolytic comparison trial in which 12,381 patients with acute myocardial infarction were prospectively randomized to streptokinase or tissue-plasminogen activator. In-hospital mortality was 9.4%, and the 6-month all-cause mortality rate was 3.5%. Cox regression modeling was used to analyze prespecified demographic and clinical variables and the presence

Table 3.—"Not Low-Risk" Factors: TIMI-II

Risk factor	Patients with risk factor, %	Deaths in 6 wk, %
Age ≥ 70 yr	11.5	11.2
Previous infarction	13.7	7.9
Anterior infarction	51.5	5.6
Atrial fibrillation	2.0	10.6
Rales in more than one-third of lung field	3.2	12.4
Hypotension and sinus tachycardia	4.8	10.1
Female sex	17.7	7.1
Diabetes mellitus	13.0	8.5

From *J Am Coll Cardiol* 16:313-315, 1990. By permission of the American College of Cardiology.

of recovery-phase left ventricular dysfunction, defined as an echocardiographic left ventricular ejection fraction of less than 40%, or a percentage of akinetic or dyskinetic myocardial segments of 36% or more. The five most important independent predictors of mortality included ineligibility for exercise testing, left ventricular failure, echocardiographic left ventricular dysfunction, electrical instability, and age older than 70 years (Table 4). A positive exercise test did not assume independent predictive ability. The strong relationship between resting echocardiographic ejection fraction and 6-month mortality is shown in Figure 3. For patients with an ejection fraction more than 40%, 6-month mortality was only 2.2%. Additionally, two "low-risk" subsets were identified by multivariate analysis. These "low-risk" subsets are described in Table 5. (These were not tested prospectively in a validation data set.) In patients younger than 70 years with an ejection fraction more than 40% by echocardiographic testing (prevalence, 62.5% of the population), the additional 6-month mortality was only 1.2%. For patients of any age with an echocardiographic ejection fraction more than 40% who were eligible for exercise testing (prevalence, 53% of population), the additional 6-month mortality was only 0.86%. Was in-hospital revascularization responsible for the low 6-month mortality in these subgroups? This explanation is extremely unlikely because cumulative 6-month revascularization (percutaneous transluminal coronary angioplasty and bypass) was only 7% and predominantly confined to unstable or high-risk patients (Table 6). Thus, GISSI-2 (unlike many contemporary trials because of its low rate of subsequent revascularization) offers

Table 4.—Independent Predictors of 6-Month Mortality: GISSI-2

Variable	Relative risk	95% confidence interval
Factors predictive		
Ineligibility for exercise test		
Cardiac reason	3.31	2.31-4.76
Noncardiac reason	2.89	1.93-4.34
Early LV failure	2.51	1.89-3.33
Echocardiographic LV dysfunction	2.51	1.93-3.27
Electrical instability	1.63	1.24-2.13
Age > 70 yr	1.56	1.19-2.04
Late LV failure	1.41	1.03-1.93
History of treated hypertension	1.39	1.08-1.79
Factors not predictive		
Female sex	0.83	0.62-1.11
Previous myocardial infarction	1.21	0.90-1.63
History of angina	1.07	0.81-1.41
History of insulin-dependent diabetes	1.30	0.72-2.34
Postinfarction angina	1.12	0.80-1.57
Anterior (Q-wave) site	1.06	0.82-1.37
QRS score > 10	0.97	0.71-1.31
Positive exercise test	1.51	0.94-2.43

LV, left ventricular.
From *Circulation* 88:416-429, 1993. By permission of the American Heart Association.

a unique perspective of the "natural history" of patients after thrombolysis, almost free from possible confounding influences of revascularization procedures.

Six-month reinfarction rate in GISSI-2 was 2.5%. A similar multivariate analysis identified risk factors for nonfatal infarction, including ineligibility for exercise testing, previous infarction, and postdismissal angina (Table 7). However, prediction of recurrent infarction remained poor, because 50% of reinfarction occurred in patients without any identified risk factors. A positive exercise test was not predictive of reinfarction in GISSI-2.

The GUSTO-1 trial was a thrombolytic comparison trial involving 41,021 patients. The primary trial end point of 30-day mortality occurred in 7.0% of patients, and 1-year mortality was 3.5%. With multivariate analysis, the five most important clinical predictors of 30-day mortality in the GUSTO-1 trial were age, systolic blood pressure, Killip

Table 5.—Low-Risk Subsets: GISSI-2

Subset 1
    Age < 70 yr
    Ejection fraction > 40% by echocardiography
    Prevalence 62.5% of population
    Additional mortality at 6 mo = 1.2%
Subset 2
    Any age
    Ejection fraction > 40% by echocardiography
    Eligible for exercise test
    Prevalence 53% of population
    Additional 6 mo mortality = 0.86%

Data from *Circulation* 88:416-429, 1993.

class, heart rate, and infarct location (Fig. 4). An a priori definition of "uncomplicated infarction" included the absence of death, reinfarction, ischemia, stroke, shock, heart failure, bypass surgery, balloon pumping, emergency catheterization, cardioversion, or defibrillation *in the first four hospital days*. On prospective application of this definition, 57% of surviving patients were without these events on day 4. These patients subsequently had a 30-day mortality of 1%, reinfarction 1.7%, heart failure 2.6%, and recurrent ischemia 6.7%. The 1-year mortality was 2.6% in this group and 4.5% in the "complicated" group.

- In the thrombolytic era, three trials (TIMI-II, GISSI-2, GUSTO-1) prospectively examined clinical and noninvasive laboratory data to predict patients at low and high risk of death or reinfarction.
- The five most important independent predictors of mortality in GISSI-2 included ineligibility for exercise testing, left ventricular failure, echocardiographic left ventricular dysfunction, electrical instability, and age older than 70 years.
- A positive exercise test was not predictive of reinfarction in GISSI-2.
- The five most important clinical predictors of 30-day mortality in the GUSTO-1 trial were age, systolic blood pressure, Killip class, heart rate, and infarct location.

Role of Exercise Testing

Exercise testing has failed to predict death or nonfatal myocardial infarction in patients treated with thrombolysis. As demonstrated in the GISSI-2 database, the highest late

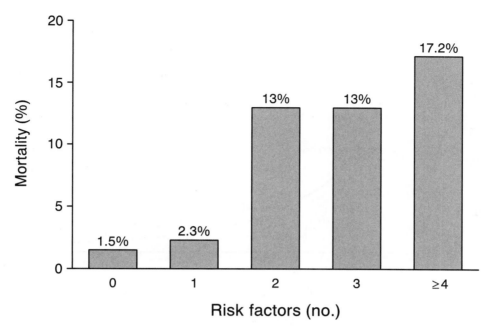

Fig. 2. Mortality at 6 weeks relative to the number of "not low-risk" factors, TIMI-II trial.

mortality occurred in patients who were not candidates for an exercise test because of cardiac or noncardiac causes (7.1% 6-month mortality). The 6-month mortality was 1.7% in patients with a positive exercise test and 0.9% in those with a negative test. Thus, although a negative test is reassuring, patients with a positive exercise test still had a 98.3% chance of not having myocardial infarction during the ensuing 6 months. Although the addition of echocardiographic or nuclear imaging techniques increases the sensitivity of functional testing, the very low event rates preclude a useful predictive accuracy for such tests because many false-positive results (evidence of ischemia without infarction) will occur.

Table 6.—Six-Month Revascularization: GISSI-2*

	In-hospital		Cumulative 6 mo	
	PTCA, %	CABG, %	PTCA, %	CABG, %
Entire cohort	0.6	0.4	2.5	4.5
Post MI angina	2.6	1.8	20.1	14.7
+ETT	1.3	0.7	5.8	8.9

CABG, coronary artery bypass grafting; +ETT, positive exercise treadmill test; MI, myocardial infarction; PTCA, percutaneous transluminal coronary angioplasty.
*N = 12,381.

- Exercise testing has failed to predict death or nonfatal myocardial infarction in patients treated with thrombolysis.

Role of Angiography

Coronary angiography is frequently performed in patients hospitalized for myocardial infarction and is clearly justified in patients at high risk, especially those with low ejection fraction or clinical manifestations of left ventricular failure or unstable angina. No data exist, however, to support performing angiography in *all* patients after infarction, especially those assessed to be at low risk. Coronary angiography and left ventriculography can clearly identify patients with reduced left ventricular function and multivessel coronary artery disease. However, such patients constitute a minority of those undergoing thrombolytic therapy, and these patients often can be identified by clinical characteristics. In addition, angiography cannot predict which patients will have occlusion after thrombolysis. Furthermore, because no study has ever shown a benefit of revascularization after thrombolysis in patients who have no manifestations of ischemia, the widespread application of routine angiography in low-risk patients cannot be scientifically justified. Nonetheless, it is widely performed.

- Angiography cannot predict which patients will have occlusion after thrombolysis.

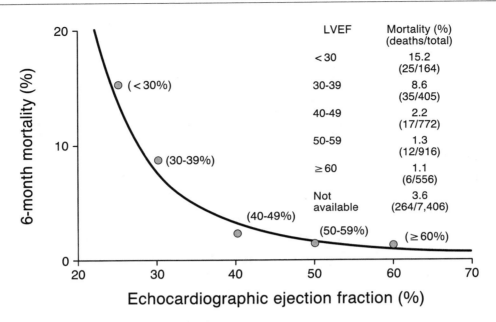

Fig. 3. Six-month mortality versus ejection fraction in GISSI-2. LVEF, left ventricular ejection fraction. (From *Circulation* 88:416-429, 1993. By permission of the American Heart Association.)

Primary Angioplasty

Primary angioplasty yields results comparable to or better than those with thrombolysis when performed by experienced operators with minimal delay. Fewer long-term data exist regarding mortality after primary angioplasty than after thrombolysis. In patients meeting usual inclusion criteria for thrombolytic therapy, the outcome after primary angioplasty is very good. In the Primary Angioplasty in Myocardial Infarction (PAMI) trial, the 6-month subsequent mortality was only 1%. To a substantial extent, such good results are likely due to selection effects, as alluded to for thrombolytic therapy. For patients judged not to be candidates for thrombolysis who undergo primary angioplasty, fewer good long-term results are likely. A large observational study including nonthrombolysis candidates compared 1,050 patients who had primary angioplasty with 2,095 patients receiving thrombolysis. A 5.5% hospital mortality and approximately 5% subsequent 1-year mortality were observed, and there were no differences between primary percutaneous transluminal coronary angioplasty and thrombolysis.

- Primary angioplasty yields results comparable to or better than those with thrombolysis when performed by experienced operators with minimal delay.

Summary

1. Patients at low risk after myocardial infarction can be identified from simple clinical characteristics (Fig. 5), including treatment with thrombolysis (or primary angioplasty in a patient without thrombolytic exclusions), a stable postreperfusion clinical course with no evidence of heart failure or recurrent ischemia, preserved left ventricular function (ejection fraction > 40%), and no clinical contraindications to post-infarction treadmill exercise testing.
2. Low-risk patients can be expected to have a 6-month to 1-year mortality of less than 4% and may constitute upwards of half of patients treated with thrombolysis. It is highly

Table 7.—Independent Predictors of Nonfatal Reinfarction: GISSI-2

Variable	Relative risk	95% confidence interval
Ineligibility (cardiac) for exercise test*	2.32	1.41-3.82
Previous MI	1.78	1.20-2.64
History of angina pre-MI	1.58	1.10-2.25
Angina at follow-up	1.47	1.01-2.15

MI, myocardial infarction.
*A negative exercise text was the reference category.
From *J Am Coll Cardiol* 24:608-615, 1994. By permission of the American College of Cardiology.

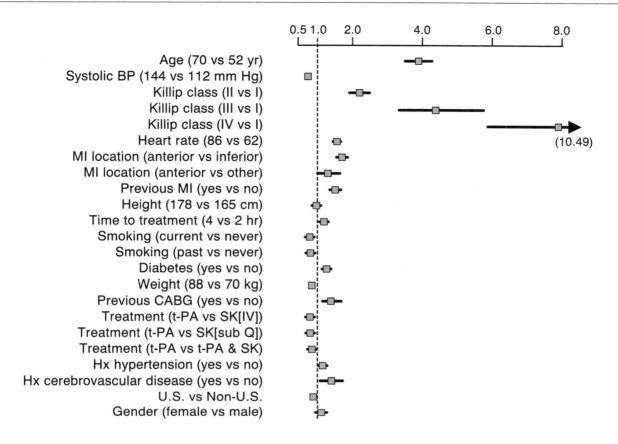

Fig. 4. Independent predictors of 30-day mortality in GUSTO-1. BP, blood pressure; CABG, coronary artery bypass grafting; MI, myocardial infarction; SK (IV, sub Q), streptokinase (intravenous, subcutaneous); t-PA, tissue-plasminogen activator. (From *Circulation* 91:1659-1668, 1995. By permission of the American Heart Association.)

unlikely that aggressive testing and intervention would have any measurable beneficial effect on such a good outcome.

3. There is no current evidence that death or reinfarction can be reliably predicted by functional testing or angiographic features of the infarct-related artery, and *routine* angiography and revascularization in patients with acute infarction after thrombolysis should not be advocated for this purpose. For patients judged not to be at low risk (i.e., all others), more aggressive investigation and intervention are clearly warranted. This latter group includes all patients who did not receive early reperfusion therapy and patients with a complicated hospital course after thrombolysis.

Unstable Coronary Syndromes: Strategy for Cardiology Examinations

Management of unstable coronary syndromes is important for cardiology examinations and, more importantly, for clinical practice. Multiple clinical situations will likely be presented, including the ones described here.

Unstable Angina

Initial management includes medical therapy with aspirin, heparin, a β-adrenergic blocker, and nitroglycerin (intravenously), unless there is a definite contraindication (such as heart block or hypotension). Never use a first-generation dihydropyridine calcium blocker as first-line or sole therapy. Proceed to coronary angiography in patients with continued symptoms, positive exercise treadmill test while receiving adequate medications, ejection fraction less than 40%, diabetes, heart failure, ventricular tachycardia, or ventricular fibrillation.

Non–Q-Wave Myocardial Infarction

Try medical therapy first, and consider catheterization and revascularization for patients with continued symptoms or ischemia on functional testing. No trial has shown a bene-

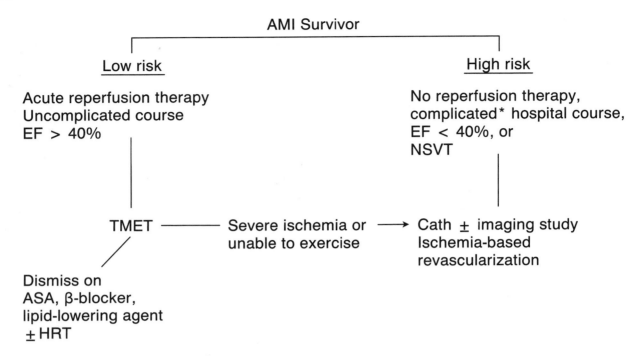

Fig. 5. Strategy for risk stratification after acute myocardial infarction (AMI). ASA, acetylsalicylic acid; Cath, catheterization; EF, ejection fraction; HRT, hormone replacement therapy; NSVT, nonsustained ventricular tachycardia; TMET, treadmill exercise test. *Complications include recurrent pain, congestive heart failure, diabetes mellitus, mechanical complication, and multiple high-risk clinical variables.

fit of aggressive early intervention in stable (pain-free) patients. Avoid calcium channel blockers in patients with pulmonary congestion.

Q-Wave Myocardial Infarction

Remember to give ancillary therapy with aspirin, β-blockers, angiotensin-converting enzyme inhibitors (for ejection fraction of 45% or more), and, later, lipid-lowering therapy and hormone replacement.

Primary percutaneous transluminal coronary angioplasty (PTCA) is effective treatment, but make sure, as guidelines state, it "is performed by experienced operators in a timely fashion." "Timely" usually means within an hour of presentation. If you are given the option of thrombolysis or delayed primary PTCA (more than 1 hour from "door to balloon time"), lysis is probably the better choice if there are no contraindications.

Primary PTCA is the best choice for patients at high risk of stroke (age > 75 years, history of cerebrovascular accident or transient ischemic attacks, hypertension), with cardiogenic shock, and, of course, with other lytic contraindications.

Strong indications for catheterization after myocardial

infarction include recurrent pain, left ventricular dysfunction (ejection fraction ≤ 40%), diabetes, heart failure, or substantial ischemia on functional testing. In fact, it is probably acceptable to perform angiography on most patients, but be careful not to recommend revascularization in patients without high-risk anatomy (left main, three-vessel, or proximal left anterior descending coronary artery disease) or demonstrable ischemia.

Search for ischemia as the first step in evaluation of late (> 48 hours) nonsustained ventricular tachycardia.

Do *not* advise:

- PTCA as routine with lysis or afterward
- PTCA without ischemia after Q-wave myocardial infarction
- PTCA in general without considering medical therapy
- Calcium channel blockers as first-line therapy after myocardial infarction
- Empiric antiarrhythmic therapy for asymptomatic nonsustained ventricular tachycardia or premature ventricular complexes
- Prophylactic lidocaine after myocardial infarction
- Thrombolysis for non–ST-elevation myocardial infarction

Suggested Review Reading

1. Epstein SE, Palmeri ST, Patterson RE: Current concepts: evaluation of patients after acute myocardial infarction: indications for cardiac catheterization and surgical intervention. *N Engl J Med* 307:1487-1492, 1982.
This is a classic article about risk stratification after infarction using treadmill testing for patients with uncomplicated infarction in the prethrombolytic era. In this setting, a positive treadmill test was associated with an increased incidence of adverse outcomes and was clinically useful.

2. The GUSTO Investigators: An international randomized trial comparing four thrombolytic strategies for acute myocardial infarction. *N Engl J Med* 329:673-682, 1993.
This is the most recent landmark trial of thrombolytic therapy comparing four different strategies, including the most clinically effective one—accelerated tissue-plasminogen activator.

3. Hillis LD, Forman S, Braunwald E: Risk stratification before thrombolytic therapy in patients with acute myocardial infarction. *J Am Coll Cardiol* 16:313-315, 1990.
Clinical risk stratification using simple variables in patients receiving thrombolytic therapy is useful for predicting high- and low-risk groups.

4. Kalynych AM, King SB: PTCA versus CABG for angina pectoris: a look at the randomized trials. *Coron Artery Dis* 6:788-796, 1995.
An overview of the randomized trials of angioplasty compared with bypass grafting for treatment of patients with multivessel coronary artery disease showed that mortality was similar between the two treatment groups, but patients receiving angioplasty required more repeat revascularization, especially in the first year after entry into the study.

5. Lee KL, Woodlief LH, Topol EJ, et al: Predictors of 30-day mortality in the era of reperfusion for acute myocardial infarction. Results from an international trial of 41,021 patients. *Circulation* 91:1659-1668, 1995.
This multivariate analysis of the GUSTO trial showed the importance of advanced age and features of left ventricular dysfunction as clinical predictors of poor outcome after infarction.

6. Newby LK, Califf RM, Guerci A, et al: Early discharge in the thrombolytic era: an analysis of criteria for uncomplicated infarction from the Global Utilization of Streptokinase and t-PA for Occluded Coronary Arteries (GUSTO) trial. *J Am Coll Cardiol* 27:625-632, 1996.
This important article evaluates the outcomes of patients with uncomplicated infarction in the GUSTO trial. Patients who were clinically stable and had not had complications by day 4 had a generally good outcome and low event rate after dismissal.

7. Pilote L, Califf RM, Sapp S, et al: Regional variation across the United States in the management of acute myocardial infarction. *N Engl J Med* 333:565-572, 1995.
One of the main correlates of angiography after infarction is the availability of angioplasty in the hospital in which the patient is being treated.

8. Reeder GS, Gibbons RJ: Acute myocardial infarction: risk stratification in the thrombolytic era. *Mayo Clin Proc* 70:87-94, 1995.
This article is an overview of risk stratification principles in the thrombolytic era. Treadmill testing and all forms of noninvasive testing are less useful in patients who have had thrombolysis because the outlook in these patients is generally good and the incidence of repeat infarction or death during the ensuing year is sufficiently low that the predictive accuracy of a positive functional test is diminished.

9. Reiner JS, Lundergan CF, van den Brand M, et al: Early angiography cannot predict postthrombolytic coronary reocclusion: observations from the GUSTO angiographic study. Global Utilization of Streptokinase and t-PA for Occluded Coronary Arteries. *J Am Coll Cardiol* 24:1439-1444, 1994.
Angiography after thrombolysis for acute infarction is not useful for predicting which patients will have reocclusion of the infarct-related artery.

10. Rouleau JL, Moye LA, Pfeffer MA, et al: A comparison of management patterns after acute myocardial infarction in Canada and the United States. *N Engl J Med* 328:779-784, 1993.
Even though patients in the United States are much more aggressively managed in terms of procedures and interventions after infarction, early-term and 1-year outcome are virtually identical in Canadian patients in terms of mortality and reinfarction.

11. Van de Werf F, Topol EJ, Lee KL, et al: Variations in patient management and outcomes for acute myocardial infarction in the United States and other countries. Results from the GUSTO trial. Global Utilization of Streptokinase and Tissue Plasminogen Activator for Occluded Coronary Arteries. *JAMA* 273:1586-1591, 1995.

Aggressive patient management after infarction in the United States, compared with non-U.S. centers in the GUSTO trial, failed to affect mortality during follow-up.

12. Villella A, Maggioni AP, Villella M, et al: Prognostic significance of maximal exercise testing after myocardial infarction treated with thrombolytic agents: the GISSI-2 data-base. *Lancet* 346:523-529, 1995.

Maximal exercise testing after myocardial infarction treated with thrombolysis in the GISSI-2 database failed to identify patients who were at risk for reinfarction or death during follow-up.

13. Volpi A, De Vita C, Franzosi MG, et al: Determinants of 6-month mortality in survivors of myocardial infarction after thrombolysis. Results of the GISSI-2 data base. *Circulation* 88:416-429, 1993.

The GISSI-2 trial was the single best "natural history" trial of patients undergoing thrombolytic therapy, because the rate of intervention during the first year in this trial was only 7% (angioplasty plus bypass grafting). The low late mortality and the usefulness of clinical predictors and left ventricular ejection fraction at rest are highlighted. Inability to exercise was an important predictor of adverse outcomes; a positive exercise test after thrombolytic therapy did not predict a poor outcome.

14. Volpi A, de Vita C, Franzosi MG, et al: Predictors of nonfatal reinfarction in survivors of myocardial infarction after thrombolysis. Results of the Gruppo Italiano per lo Studio della Sopravvivenza nell'Infarto Miocardico (GISSI-2) Data Base. *J Am Coll Cardiol* 24:608-615, 1994.

No clinical or laboratory tests predicted nonfatal reinfarction in patients treated with thrombolysis for acute myocardial infarction in the GISSI-I trial. Recurrent infarction is not related to exercise-induced ischemia but to plaque instability and associated thrombus, which often persist in the first weeks to month after thrombolytic therapy.

15. Boden WE, O'Rourke RA, Crawford MH, et al: Outcomes in patients with acute non–Q-wave myocardial infarction randomly assigned to an invasive as compared with a conservative management strategy. *N Engl J Med* 338:1785-1792, 1998.

16. Lange RA, Hillis LD: Use and overuse of angiography and revascularization for acute coronary syndromes. *N Engl J Med* 338:1838-1839, 1998.

The trial and the accompanying editorial emphasize that in this group of patients with non–Q-wave myocardial infarction randomized to an invasive or a conservative management strategy, there were no significant differences in the primary end point of death or nonfatal myocardial infarction at follow-up. In fact, mortality was slightly higher in the invasive strategy group. This trial and three others published in the literature examining urgent angiography and aggressive revascularization with medical therapy and ischemia-based revascularization all fail to identify any substantial benefit for an aggressive approach. Critics of these trials point out that intervention was relatively late and that very unstable patients were excluded, and these points are certainly true. For patients not able to be stabilized medically, urgent catheterization with plans for revascularization is mandatory. However, on the basis of these trials, stable patients after non–Q-wave infarction are probably best managed with an initial conservative approach and revascularization based on subsequent demonstration of ischemia, either spontaneously or with functional testing.

Questions

Multiple Choice (choose the one best answer)

1. Angiography after myocardial infarction:
   a. Predicts who will have reinfarction
   b. Predicts mortality
   c. Often leads to revascularization
   d. Is a cost-effective risk-stratification strategy
   e. Is necessary in all patients after infarction

2. Treadmill testing after myocardial infarction in patients who have had thrombolysis:
   a. Predicts reinfarction
   b. Predicts mortality
   c. Is vastly inferior to nuclear or exercise echocardiography
   d. Is useful for exercise prescription and reassurance of the patient
   e. Is mandatory in all patients after myocardial infarction

3. Clinical risk factors for a poor outcome after myocardial infarction include all *except*:
   a. Shock
   b. Pulmonary congestion
   c. Age older than 70 years
   d. Current cigarette smoker
   e. Recurrent rest angina

4. The average 1-year post-dismissal mortality rate for patients receiving thrombolytic therapy in a clinical trial is:
   a. 1%
   b. 2% to 4%
   c. 8%
   d. More than 15%
   e. More than 40%

5. The average 1-year post-dismissal mortality rate in a large observational registry of patients after reperfusion (primary percutaneous transluminal coronary angioplasty or thrombolysis) was:
   a. 1%
   b. 3%
   c. 5% to 6%
   d. 10% to 15%
   e. More than 20%

6. In GISSI-2:
   a. There was a high (> 50%) rate of angiography after myocardial infarction
   b. There was considerable (> 40%) revascularization after myocardial infarction
   c. Treadmill testing gave incremental prognostic information over clinical assessment
   d. A resting ejection fraction less than 40% was associated with a 6-month mortality rate of more than 8%
   e. Female patients had a higher mortality rate than male patients

7. All of the following are true about the GUSTO-1 trial *except*:
   a. 20% of patients had an uncomplicated myocardial infarction
   b. The 30-day mortality rate was 1%, and the 1-year additional mortality rate was 3.5%
   c. Patients with uncomplicated infarction by day 4 had 1% 30-day and 2.6% additional 1-year mortality rates
   d. Age, hypotension, Killip class II or higher, increased heart rate, and location of infarct were the five most important clinical predictors of mortality at 30 days

8. For patients with non–ST-segment elevation myocardial infarction:
   a. Urgent angiography and aggressive intervention are indicated
   b. Thrombolytic therapy reduces mortality
   c. Initial medical therapy is indicated, and nonresponders are selected for angiography and revascularization
   d. Patients with noncritical single-vessel disease and well-preserved ejection fraction are prime candidates for subsequent revascularization

9. Ancillary therapy for ST–segment elevation myocardial infarction involves:
   a. Aspirin
   b. β-Adrenergic blockers
   c. Angiotensin-converting enzyme inhibitors for ejection fraction less than 45%
   d. Lipid-lowering therapy for low-density lipoprotein cholesterol value less than 100 mg/dL
   e. All of the above

10. Nonsustained ventricular tachycardia after myocardial infarction:
    a. Is a risk factor for sudden death
    b. Should prompt a search for ischemia
    c. Should not be treated with empiric antiarrhythmic agents
    d. When associated with an ejection fraction < 40%, consider electrophysiologic study
    e. All of the above

11. For patients not receiving thrombolysis or primary percutaneous transluminal coronary angioplasty:
    a. Mortality is lower than in candidates for thrombolysis
    b. Angiography and stress testing are useful to select patients for revascularization vs. medical therapy
    c. Ancillary therapy (aspirin, β-adrenergic blockers, angiotensin-converting enzyme inhibitors) is unimportant
    d. Revascularization prolongs survival in asymptomatic patients with well-preserved ejection fraction and single-vessel (not left main coronary artery) disease

12. Which patient is at the highest risk after myocardial infarction?
    a. Received thrombolysis as part of a trial
    b. Received primary percutaneous transluminal coronary angioplasty as part of a trial
    c. Received thrombolysis or angioplasty in a nontrial setting within 1 hour of presentation
    d. Received thrombolysis, is in Killip class II with an ejection fraction of 36%
    e. Received thrombolysis, had an uncomplicated hospital course, has asymptomatic 1-mm ST depression on rehabilitation treadmill exercise test at 6 METs

Answers

1. Answer c

Angiography after myocardial infarction frequently leads to revascularization, including angioplasty, stent placement, or coronary artery bypass grafting. It is not a good predictor of mortality and does not predict reinfarction with any degree of accuracy. Angiography is not necessary in low-risk patients and is not a cost-effective risk-stratification method if applied to all patients. Angiography is best applied to high-risk patients, including those with ongoing ischemia, congestive heart failure, significant ventricular arrhythmias beyond the immediate post-infarction period, and evidence of ischemia on stress testing.

2. Answer d

Treadmill testing after myocardial infarction in patients who have received thrombolysis differs significantly from that in patients treated in the pre-thrombolytic era or in those who have not received thrombolytic therapy. Treadmill testing does not accurately predict either mortality or reinfarction. It is, however, useful for exercise prescription and reassurance of the patient. Although stress testing in combination with either nuclear or exercise imaging has improved diagnostic accuracy, in general, compared with treadmill testing alone, the incremental prognostic value after thrombolysis is not large. Treadmill testing is not mandatory in all patients after myocardial infarction.

3. Answer d

Risk factors associated with a poor outcome after myocardial infarction include shock or advanced Killip class on presentation; the presence of congestive heart failure, including pulmonary congestion; advanced age, especially older than 70 years; or recurrent ischemia or rest angina. Paradoxically, cigarette smokers have an improved survival compared with those who do not smoke, provided the patients cease smoking.

4. Answer b

The average 1-year post-dismissal mortality rate for a patient receiving thrombolytic therapy in a clinical trial is 2% to 4%.

5. Answer c

The average 1-year post-dismissal mortality rate in a large observational registry after reperfusion with either thrombolysis or percutaneous transluminal coronary angioplasty was 5% to 6%, which is significantly higher than that for patients in clinical trials referred to in the previous question, which was 2% to 4%. Selection bias for patients included in clinical trials is thought to explain the difference.

6. Answer d

In the GISSI-2 trial, an ejection fraction less than 40% was associated with a mortality rate of more than 8% 6 months after infarction. Female patients did not have a higher mortality rate than male patients. Exercise testing did not give any incremental prognostic information over good clinical assessment. The GISSI-2 trial was notable in that there was a relatively low rate of angiography after infarction in comparison with present-day practice in the United States.

7. Answer a

In the GUSTO-1 trial, the 30-day mortality rate was approximately 1% and the additional 1-year mortality rate was 3.5%. Patients with uncomplicated infarction by day 4 had a 1% 30-day mortality rate and 2.6% additional 1-year mortality rate. Older age, hypotension, Killip class II or higher, increased heart rate, and location of infarct were the strongest clinical predictors of mortality at 30 days. In comparison, the uncomplicated infarction rate was 57% higher in the GISSI study.

8. Answer c

For patients with non–ST-segment elevation myocardial infarction, medical management is the initial treatment of choice, whereas patients with evidence of ongoing ischemia or continuing pain should have angiography and revascularization, if appropriate. There is no demonstrated survival benefit to urgent angiography and aggressive intervention. Thrombolytic therapy has never been shown to reduce mortality in patients with non–ST-segment elevation. Patients with noncritical single-vessel disease and a good ejection fraction do not seem to benefit significantly from emergency revascularization.

9. Answer e

Important ancillary therapy for ST-segment elevation myocardial infarction includes aspirin and β-adrenergic blockers in patients without contraindications. Also, angiotensin-converting enzyme inhibitors are used if the ejection fraction is less than 45%, and aggressive lipid-lowering therapy is used to achieve a low-density lipoprotein cholesterol value of less than 100 mg/dL.

10. Answer e

Nonsustained ventricular tachycardia after myocardial infarction has been demonstrated in numerous studies to be a risk factor for sudden death, but in the Coronary Artery Surgery Study (CASS), suppression of nonsustained ventricular tachycardia with encainide, flecainide, or moricizine led to an increased mortality rate. The presence of nonsustained ventricular tachycardia should prompt an aggressive search for the presence of ongoing myocardial ischemia in patients with reduced ejection fraction, and an electrophysiologic study should be considered once the ischemia has been corrected.

11. Answer b

For patients not receiving thrombolysis or primary percutaneous transluminal coronary angioplasty, the mortality is generally higher than in those receiving thrombolysis or considered candidates for thrombolysis. Angiography and stress testing are useful to select patients for revascularization therapy or those who may be safely managed with medical therapy. In patients who do not receive thrombolysis, the importance of ancillary therapy (including aspirin, β-adrenergic blockers, and angiotensin-converting enzyme inhibitors) is comparable to that in patients receiving thrombolysis. There is no evidence that revascularization prolongs survival in patients who are asymptomatic with good ventricular function and have single-vessel coronary artery disease, excluding flow-limiting left main coronary artery disease or probable proximal left anterior descending coronary artery disease.

12. Answer d

The highest risk of death after myocardial infarction occurs in patients presenting in Killip class II or higher with significantly decreased left ventricular function. Patients considered to be at relatively low risk are those who received thrombolysis or primary percutaneous transluminal coronary angioplasty as part of a trial, because trials generally seem to select patients at lower risk than those excluded from participation. Patients who are not part of a clinical trial but who present early are also in a favorable prognostic category. Patients with uncomplicated myocardial infarction after thrombolysis also have a favorable prognosis, even with the presence of 1 mm of asymptomatic depression on rehabilitation treadmill at 6 METs.

Chapter 22

Physical Examination

Clarence Shub, M.D.

General Appearance

Important clues to a cardiac diagnosis can be obtained from inspection of the patient (Table 1).

Blood Pressure

Blood pressure should always be determined in both arms and in the legs if there is any suspicion of coarctation of the aorta. Differences in blood pressure between both arms of more than 10 mm Hg systolic or 5 mm Hg diastolic are abnormal (Table 2).

Palpation of Precordium

The patient should be examined in both the supine and the left lateral decubitus position. Examining the apical impulse by the posterior approach with the patient in the sitting position may at times be the best method to appreciate subtle abnormalities of precordial motion. The normal apical impulse occurs during early systole with an outward motion imparted to the chest wall. During mid- and late systole, the left ventricle (LV) is diminishing in volume and the apical impulse moves away from the chest wall. Thus, outward precordial apical motion occurring in late systole is abnormal. Remember that the point of maximal impulse is not synonymous with the apical impulse.

Abnormalities on Apex Palpation

Constrictive pericarditis or tricuspid regurgitation produces a subtle systolic precordial retraction.

The apical impulse of LV enlargement is usually widened or diffuse (> 3 cm in diameter), can be palpated in two interspaces, and is displaced leftward. A subtle presystolic ventricular filling wave (A wave)—frequently associated with LV hypertrophy—may be better visualized than palpated by observing the motion of the stethoscope applied lightly on the chest wall, with appropriate timing during simultaneous auscultation. The apical impulse of LV hypertrophy without dilatation is sustained but should not be displaced.

Causes of a palpable A wave (presystolic impulse) include the following:

> aortic stenosis
> hypertrophic obstructive cardiomyopathy
> acute mitral regurgitation
> systemic hypertension

- The apical impulse of LV hypertrophy without dilatation is sustained and localized. It should not be displaced but may be accompanied by a palpable presystolic outward movement, the A wave.
- Outward precordial apical motion occurring in late systole is abnormal.
- Multiple abnormal outward precordial movements may occur: presystolic, systolic, late systolic rebound, and a rapid filling wave in early diastole.

Table 1.—Clinical Clues to Specific Cardiac Abnormalities Detectable From the General Examination

Condition	Appearance	Associated cardiac abnormalities
Marfan syndrome	Tall	Aortic root dilatation
	Long extremities	Mitral valve prolapse
Acromegaly	Large stature	Cardiac hypertrophy
	Coarse facial features	
	"Spade" hands	
Turner syndrome	Web neck	Aortic coarctation
	Hypertelorism	Pulmonary stenosis
	Short stature	
Pickwickian syndrome	Severe obesity	Pulmonary hypertension
	Somnolence	
Friedreich ataxia	Lurching gait	Hypertrophic cardiomyopathy
	Hammertoe	
	Pes cavus	
Duchenne-type muscular dystrophy	Pseudohypertrophy of calves	Cardiomyopathy
Ankylosing spondylitis	Straight back syndrome	Aortic regurgitation
	Stiff ("poker") spine	Heart block (rare)
Jaundice	Yellow skin or sclera	Right-sided congestive heart failure
		Prosthetic valve dysfunction (hemolysis)
Sickle cell anemia	Cutaneous ulcers	Pulmonary hypertension
	Painful "crises"	Secondary cardiomyopathy
Lentigines (LEOPARD syndrome*)	Brown skin macules that do not increase with sunlight	Hypertrophic obstructive cardiomyopathy
		Pulmonary stenosis
Hereditary hemorrhagic telangiectasia (Osler-Weber-Rendu disease)	Small capillary hemangiomas— on face or mouth, with or without cyanosis	Pulmonary arteriovenous fistula
Pheochromocytoma	Pale, diaphoretic skin	Catecholamine-induced secondary dilated cardiomyopathy
	Neurofibromatosis—café-au-lait spots	
Lupus	Butterfly rash on face	Verrucous endocarditis
	Raynaud phenomenon—hands	Myocarditis
	Livedo reticularis	Pericarditis
Sarcoidosis	Cutaneous nodules	Secondary cardiomyopathy
	Erythema nodosum	Heart block
Tuberous sclerosis	Angiofibromas (face; adenoma sebaceum)	Rhabdomyoma
Myxedema	Coarse, dry skin	Pericardial effusion
	Thinning of lateral eyebrows	Left ventricular dysfunction
	Hoarseness of voice	
Right-to-left intracardiac shunt	Cyanosis and clubbing of distal extremities	Any of the lesions that cause Eisenmenger syndrome
	Differential cyanosis and clubbing	Reversed shunt through patent ductus arteriosus
Holt-Oram syndrome	Rudimentary or absent thumb	Atrial septal defect
Down syndrome	Mental retardation	Endocardial cushion defect
	Simian crease of palm	
	Characteristic facies	

Table 1 (continued)

Condition	Appearance	Associated cardiac abnormalities
Scleroderma	Tight, shiny skin of fingers with contraction	Pulmonary hypertension
		Myocardial, pericardial, or endocardial disease
	Characteristic taut mouth and facies	
Rheumatoid arthritis	Typical hand deformity	Pericardial, endocardial, or myocardial disease
	Subcutaneous nodules	(often subclinical)
Thoracic bony abnormality	Pectus excavatum	Pseudocardiomegaly
	Straight back syndrome	Mitral valve prolapse
Carcinoid syndrome	Reddish cyanosis of face	Right-sided cardiac valve stenosis or regurgitation
	Periodic flushing	

*LEOPARD syndrome: *l*entigines, *e*lectrocardiographic changes, *o*cular hypertelorism, *p*ulmonary stenosis, *a*bnormal genitalia, *r*etardation of growth, *d*eafness.
Data from Abrams J: *Essentials of Cardiac Physical Diagnosis.* Lea & Febiger, 1987.

Abnormalities on Palpation of Lower Sternum

Precordial motion in the lower sternal area usually reflects right ventricular (RV) motion. RV hypertrophy due to systolic overload (such as in pulmonary stenosis) causes a sustained outward lift. Diastolic overload (such as in atrial septal defect [ASD]) causes a vigorous nonsustained motion. In severe mitral regurgitation, the left atrium expands in systole but is limited in its posterior motion by the spine. The RV may then be pushed forward, and the parasternal region is "lifted" indirectly.

Significant *overlap* of sites of maximal pulsation occurs in LV and RV overload states. For example, in RV overload, the abnormal impulse can overlap with the LV in the apical sternal region (between the apex and the left lower sternal border). An LV apical aneurysm may produce a delayed outward motion and cause a "rocking" motion.

Table 2.—Causes of Blood Pressure Discrepancy Between Arms or Between Arms and Legs

Arterial occlusion or stenosis of any cause
Dissecting aortic aneurysm
Coarctation of the aorta
Patent ductus arteriosus
Supravalvular aortic stenosis
Thoracic outlet syndrome

Abnormalities on Palpation of Left Upper Sternum

Abnormal pulsations at the left upper sternal border (pulmonic area) can be due to a dilated pulmonary artery (for example, poststenotic dilatation in pulmonary valve stenosis, idiopathic dilatation of the pulmonary artery, or increased pulmonary flow related to ASD or pulmonary hypertension). Pulsations of increased blood flow are dynamic and quick, whereas pulsations due to pressure overload cause a sustained impulse.

> If the apical impulse is not palpable and the patient is hemodynamically unstable, consider cardiac tamponade as the first diagnosis.

Abnormalities on Palpation of Right Upper Sternum

Abnormal pulsations at the right upper sternal border (aortic area) should suggest an aortic aneurysm. An enlarged left lobe of the liver associated with severe tricuspid regurgitation may be appreciated in the epigastrium, and the epigastric site may be the location of the maximal cardiac impulse in patients with emphysema or an enlarged RV.

- RV hypertrophy due to systolic overload causes a sustained outward lift. Diastolic overload (as in ASD) causes a vigorous nonsustained motion.

- In severe mitral regurgitation, the left atrium expands in systole but is limited in its posterior motion by the spine. The RV may then be pushed forward, and the parasternal region is "lifted" indirectly.
- Significant *overlap* of sites of maximal pulsation occurs in LV and RV overload states.
- Pulsations of increased blood flow are dynamic and quick, whereas pulsations due to pressure overload cause a sustained impulse.

Jugular Veins

Abnormal waveforms in the jugular veins reflect abnormal hemodynamics of the right side of the heart. In the presence of normal sinus rhythm, there are two visible positive or outward moving waves (A and V) and two visible negative or inward moving waves (X and Y). The X descent is sometimes referred to as the "systolic collapse." Ordinarily, the C wave is not readily visible. The A wave can be identified by simultaneous auscultation of the heart and inspection of the jugular veins. The A wave occurs at about the time of S_1. The X descent follows. The V wave, a slower, more undulating wave, occurs near S_2. The Y descent follows. The A wave is normally larger than the V wave, and the X descent is more marked than the Y descent (Tables 3 through 5).

Normal jugular venous pressure decreases with inspiration and increases with expiration. Veins that fill, however, with inspiration (Kussmaul sign) are a clue to constrictive pericarditis, pulmonary embolism, or RV infarction (Table 5).

- Jugular veins that fill with inspiration (Kussmaul sign) are a clue to constrictive pericarditis, pulmonary embolism, or RV infarction.

Hepatojugular (Abdominojugular) Reflux Sign

The neck veins distend with steady (> 10 seconds) upper abdominal compression while the patient continues to breathe normally without straining. Straining may cause a false-positive hepatojugular reflux sign. The neck veins may collapse or remain distended. Jugular venous pressure that remains increased and then falls abruptly (≥ 4 cm H_2O) indicates an abnormal response. It may occur in LV failure with secondary pulmonary hypertension. In patients with chronic congestive heart failure, a positive hepatojugular reflux sign (with or without increased jugular venous pressure), a third heart sound, and radiographic pulmonary vascular redistribution are independent predictors of increased pulmonary capillary wedge pressure. The hepatojugular maneuver can also be useful for eliciting venous pulsations if they are difficult to visualize.

- A positive hepatojugular (abdominojugular) reflux sign may be found in LV failure with secondary pulmonary hypertension.

> If the jugular veins are engorged but not pulsatile, consider superior vena caval obstruction.

Table 3.—Timing of Jugular Vein Pulse Waves

A wave precedes the carotid arterial pulse and is
  simultaneous with the S_4 just before S_1
X descent is between S_1 and S_2
V wave is just after S_2
Y descent is after the V wave in early diastole

Table 4.—Abnormal Jugular Vein Pulse Waves

Increased A wave
  1. Tricuspid stenosis
  2. Decreased right ventricular compliance due to right ventricular hypertrophy in severe pulmonary hypertension
      Pulmonary stenosis
      Pulmonary hypertension
  3. Severe left ventricular hypertrophy due to pressure by the hypertrophied septum on right ventricular filling (Bernheim effect)
      Hypertrophic obstructive cardiomyopathy
      Severe aortic stenosis (uncommon)
      Severe systemic hypertension (uncommon)
  4. Lutembacher syndrome

Rapid X descent
  Cardiac tamponade
Increased V wave
  Tricuspid regurgitation
  Atrial septal defect
Rapid Y descent (Friedreich sign)
  Constrictive pericarditis

Table 5.—Differentiation of Internal Jugular Vein Pulse and Carotid Pulse

Jugular vein pulse	Carotid pulse
Double peak when in sinus rhythm	Single peak
Obliterated by gentle pressure	Unaffected by gentle pressure
Changes with position and inspiration	Unaffected by position or inspiration

Arterial Pulse

Abnormalities of the Carotid Pulse

Hyperdynamic Carotid Pulse

A vigorous, hyperdynamic carotid pulse is consistent with aortic regurgitation. It may also occur in other states of high cardiac output or be caused by the wide pulse pressure associated with atherosclerosis, especially in the elderly.

Dicrotic and Bisferiens Pulse

A dicrotic pulse occurs in myocardial failure, especially in association with hypotension, decreased cardiac output, and increased peripheral resistance. Dicrotic and bisferious are the Greek and Latin terms, respectively, for "twice beating," but in cardiology they are not equivalent. The second impulse occurs in early diastole with the dicrotic pulse and in late systole with the bisferiens pulse. The bisferiens pulse usually occurs in combined aortic regurgitation and aortic stenosis, but occasionally in pure aortic regurgitation.

Aortic Stenosis

Pulsus parvus (soft or weak) classically occurs in aortic stenosis but can also result from severe stenosis of any cardiac valve or can occur with low cardiac output of any cause. Severe aortic stenosis also produces a slowly increasing delayed pulse (pulsus tardus). Because of the effects of aging on the carotid arteries, the typical findings of pulsus parvus and tardus may be less apparent or absent in the elderly, even with severe degrees of aortic stenosis.

Hypertrophic Obstructive Cardiomyopathy

In hypertrophic obstructive cardiomyopathy, the ventricular obstruction begins in mid-systole, increases as contraction proceeds, and decreases in late systole. The initial carotid impulse is brisk. The pulse may be bifid (bisferious) as well (Table 6).

Inequality of the carotid pulses can be due to carotid atherosclerosis, especially in elderly patients. In a young patient, consider supravalvular aortic stenosis. (The right side then should have the stronger pulse.) Aortic dissection and thoracic outlet syndrome may also produce inequality of arterial pulses. A pulsating cervical mass, usually on the right, may be caused by atherosclerotic "buckling" of the right common carotid artery and give the false impression of a carotid aneurysm.

Transmitted Murmurs

Transmitted murmurs of aortic origin, most often due to aortic stenosis (less often due to coarctation, patent ductus arteriosus, pulmonary stenosis, and ventricular septal defect), decrease in intensity as they ascend the neck, whereas a carotid bruit is usually louder higher in the neck and decreases in intensity as the stethoscope is inched proximally toward the chest. Both conditions may coexist, especially in elderly patients. An abrupt change in the acoustic characteristics (pitch) of the bruit as the stethoscope is inched upward may be a clue to the presence of combined lesions.

Pulsus Paradoxus

Paradoxical pulse is an exaggeration of the normal (up to 10 mm) inspiratory decline in arterial pressure and occurs classically in cardiac tamponade, but occasionally with other cardiac abnormalities such as severe congestive heart failure, pulmonary embolism, or chronic obstructive pulmonary disease (Table 7).

Table 6.—Causes of a Double-Impulse Arterial Pulse

Dicrotic pulse (systolic + diastolic impulse)
    Cardiomyopathy
    Left ventricular failure
Bisferiens pulse (two systolic impulses)
    Aortic regurgitation
    Combined aortic valve stenosis and regurgitation
    (dominant regurgitation)
Bifid pulse (two systolic impulses with intervening pulse collapse)
    Hypertrophic cardiomyopathy

Pulsus Alternans

Pulsus alternans (alternation of stronger and weaker beats) rarely occurs in normal subjects, and when it does it is transient after a premature ventricular contraction. It usually is associated with severe myocardial failure and is frequently accompanied by a third heart sound, both of which impart an ominous prognosis. Pulsus alternans may be affected by alterations in venous return and may disappear as congestive heart failure progresses. Electrical alternans (alternating variation in the height of the QRS complex) is unrelated to pulsus alternans (Table 8).

- A dicrotic pulse occurs in myocardial failure, often in association with hypotension, decreased cardiac output, and increased peripheral resistance.
- Pulsus parvus (soft or weak) classically occurs in aortic stenosis but can also result from severe stenosis of any cardiac valve or can occur with severe low cardiac output of any cause.
- Because of the effects of aging on the carotid arteries, the typical findings of pulsus parvus and tardus may be less apparent or absent in the elderly, even with severe degrees of aortic stenosis.
- Inequality of the carotid pulses can be due to carotid atherosclerosis, especially in elderly patients. In a young patient, consider supravalvular aortic stenosis. (The right side then should have the stronger pulse.)
- Transmitted murmurs of aortic origin, most often due to aortic stenosis (less often due to coarctation, patent ductus arteriosus, pulmonary stenosis, or ventricular septal defect) decrease in intensity as they ascend the neck, whereas a carotid bruit is usually louder higher in the neck and decreases in intensity as the stethoscope is inched proximally toward the chest.
- Paradoxical pulse occurs classically in cardiac tamponade, but occasionally with other cardiac abnormalities such as severe congestive heart failure, pulmonary

Table 7.—Causes of Pulsus Paradoxus

Constrictive pericarditis
Pericardial tamponade
Severe emphysema
Severe asthma
Severe heart failure
Pulmonary embolism
Morbid obesity

Table 8.—Pulsus and Electrical Alternans

Pulsus alternans
    Severe heart failure
Electrical alternans
    Pericardial tamponade
    Large pericardial effusions

embolism, or chronic obstructive pulmonary disease.
- Pulsus alternans usually is associated with severe myocardial failure and is frequently accompanied by a third heart sound, both of which impart an ominous prognosis.

Abnormalities of the Femoral Pulse

In hypertension, simultaneous palpation of radial and femoral pulses may reveal a delay or relative weakening of the latter pulses, suggesting aortic coarctation. Finding a femoral (or carotid) bruit in an adult may suggest diffuse atherosclerosis.

Heart Sounds

First Heart Sound (S_1)

Only the mitral (M_1) and tricuspid (T_1) components of S_1 are normally audible. M_1 occurs before T_1 and is the loudest component. Wide splitting of S_1 occurs with right bundle branch block and Ebstein anomaly.

Factors Influencing the Intensity of S_1

PR Interval

The PR interval varies inversely with the loudness of S_1—with a long PR interval, the S_1 is soft; conversely, with a short PR interval, the S_1 is loud.

Mitral Valve Disease

Mitral stenosis produces a loud S_1 if the valve is pliable. When the valve becomes calcified and immobile, the intensity of S_1 decreases. The S_1 may also be soft in severe aortic regurgitation (related to early closure of the mitral valve) caused by rapidly filling LV diastolic pressure.

The Rate of Increase of Systolic Pressure Within the LV

A loud S_1 can be produced by hypercontractile states, such as fever, exercise, thyrotoxicosis, and pheochromocytoma. Conversely, a soft S_1 can occur in LV failure.

If S_1 seems to be louder at the lower left sternal border than at the apex (implying a loud T_1), suspect ASD or tricuspid stenosis. Atrial fibrillation produces a variable S_1 intensity. (The intensity is inversely related to the previous RR cycle length; a longer cycle length produces a softer S_1.) Mitral stenosis, because of the immobility of the valve, is an exception to this general rule. A variable S_1 intensity during a wide complex regular tachycardia suggests atrioventricular dissociation and ventricular tachycardia. The marked delay of T_1 in Ebstein's anomaly is related to the late billowing effect of the deformed (sail-like) anterior leaflet of the tricuspid valve as it closes in systole. Table 9 lists causes of an abnormal S_1.

- If S_1 seems to be louder at the base than at the apex, suspect an ejection sound masquerading as S_1. If the S_1 is louder at the lower left sternal border than at the apex (implying a loud T_1), suspect ASD or tricuspid stenosis.
- A variable S_1 intensity during a wide complex regular tachycardia suggests atrioventricular dissociation and ventricular tachycardia.
- The marked delay of T_1 in Ebstein's anomaly is related to the late billowing effect of the deformed (sail-like) anterior leaflet of the tricuspid valve as it closes in systole.

Systolic Ejection Clicks or Sounds

The ejection click follows S_1 closely and can be confused with a widely split S_1 or, occasionally, with an early non-ejection click. Clicks can originate from the left or right side of the heart.

The three possible mechanisms for production of the clicks are as follows:

1) Intrinsic abnormality of the aortic or pulmonary valve, such as congenital bicuspid aortic valve
2) Pulsatile distention of a dilated great artery, as occurs in increased flow states such as truncus arteriosus (aortic click) or ASD (pulmonary click) or in idiopathic dilatation of the pulmonary artery
3) Increased pressure in the great vessel, such as in aortic or pulmonary hypertension. Because aortic click is not usually heard with uncomplicated coarctation, its presence should suggest associated bicuspid aortic valve. In the latter condition, the click diminishes in intensity, becomes "buried" in the systolic murmur, and ultimately disappears as the valve becomes heavily calcified and immobile later in the course of the disease. Although a click implies cusp mobility, its presence does not necessarily exclude severe stenosis.

Table 9.—Abnormalities of S_1 and Their Causes

Loud S_1
    Short PR interval
    Mitral stenosis
    Left atrial myxoma
    Hypercontractile states
Soft S_1
    Long PR interval
    Depressed left ventricular function
    Early closure of mitral valve in acute severe aortic incompetence
    Left bundle branch block

A click would be expected to be absent in subvalvular stenosis. The timing of the pulmonary click in relationship to S_1 (reflecting the isovolumic contraction period of the RV) is associated with hemodynamic severity in valvular pulmonary stenosis. With higher systolic gradient and lower pulmonary artery systolic pressure, the isovolumic contraction period shortens, and thus the earlier the click occurs in relationship to S_1. A pulmonary click can occur in idiopathic dilatation of the pulmonary artery, and this condition may be a masquerader of ASD, especially in young adults. The pulmonary click due to valvular pulmonary stenosis is the only right-sided heart sound that *decreases* with inspiration. Most other right-sided auscultatory events either increase in intensity with inspiration (most commonly) or show minimal change. The pulmonary click is best heard along the upper left sternal border, but if it is loud enough or if the RV is markedly dilated, it may be heard throughout the precordium. The aortic click radiates to the aortic area and the apex and does not change with respiration.

- The presence, absence, or loudness of the ejection click does not necessarily correlate with the degree of valve stenosis.
- An aortic click is not heard with uncomplicated coarctation; its presence should suggest associated bicuspid aortic valve.
- An ejection click is absent in subvalvular or supravalvular aortic stenosis or hypertrophic obstructive cardiomyopathy.
- A pulmonary click can occur in idiopathic dilatation of the pulmonary artery, a condition that may mimic ASD, especially in young adults.

- The pulmonary click is best heard along the upper left sternal border. The aortic click radiates to the aortic area and the apex and does not change with respiration. The causes of ejection clicks are listed in Table 10.

Mid-Late Nonejection Clicks

Nonejection systolic clicks are most commonly due to mitral valve prolapse. Rarely, nonejection clicks can be caused by papillary muscle dysfunction, rheumatic mitral valve disease, or hypertrophic obstructive cardiomyopathy. Other rare causes of nonejection clicks (that can masquerade as mitral prolapse) include ventricular or atrial septal aneurysms, ventricular free wall aneurysms, and ventricular and atrial mobile tumors, such as myxoma. A nonejection click not due to mitral valve prolapse does not have the typical responses to bedside maneuvers found with mitral valve prolapse, as outlined below.

Mitral Valve Prolapse

Maneuvers that decrease LV volume, such as standing or the Valsalva maneuver, move the click earlier in the cardiac cycle. Conversely, maneuvers that increase LV volume, such as assuming the supine position and elevating the legs, move the click later in the cardiac cycle. With a decrease in LV volume, a systolic murmur, if present, would become longer. Interventions that increase systemic blood pressure make the murmur louder.

- Miscellaneous causes of nonejection clicks (that can masquerade as mitral prolapse) include ventricular or atrial septal aneurysms, ventricular free wall aneurysms, and

Table 10.—Causes of Ejection Clicks

Aortic
    Congenital valvular aortic stenosis
    Congenital bicuspid aortic valve
    Truncus arteriosus
    Aortic incompetence
    Aortic root dilatation or aneurysm
Pulmonary
    Pulmonary valve stenosis
    Atrial septal defect
    Chronic pulmonary hypertension
    Tetralogy of Fallot with pulmonary valve stenosis
      (absent if there is only infundibular stenosis)
    Idiopathic dilation of the pulmonary artery

ventricular and atrial mobile tumors, such as myxoma.
- Maneuvers that decrease LV volume, such as standing or the Valsalva maneuver, move the click earlier in the cardiac cycle. Conversely, maneuvers that increase LV volume, such as assuming the supine position and elevating the legs, move the click later in the cardiac cycle.

Second Heart Sound (S_2)

S_2 is often best heard along the upper and middle left sternal border and not necessarily in the classic "pulmonary" area. Splitting of S_2 is best heard during normal breathing with the subject in the sitting position.

Determinants of S_2 include the following:
1) Ventricular activation (bundle branch block delays closure of the ventricle's respective semilunar valve)
2) Ejection time
3) Valve gradient (increased gradient with low pressure in the great vessel delays closure)
4) Elastic recoil of the great artery (decreased elastic recoil delays closure, such as in idiopathic dilatation of the pulmonary artery)

Splitting of S_2

Wide but physiologic splitting of S_2 may be due to the following:
1) Delayed electrical activation of the RV, such as in right bundle branch block or premature ventricular contraction originating in the LV (which conducts with a right bundle branch block pattern)
2) Delay of RV contraction, such as in increased RV stroke volume and RV failure
3) Pulmonary stenosis (prolonged ejection time)

In ASD, there is only minimal respiratory variation in S_2 splitting. This is referred to as "fixed" splitting. Fixed splitting should be verified with the patient in the sitting or standing position because normal subjects occasionally appear to have fixed splitting in the supine position. When the degree of splitting is unusually wide, especially when the pulmonary component of the second heart sound (P_2) is diminished, suspect concomitant pulmonary stenosis. Indeed, this condition is the cause of the most widely split S_2 that can be recorded.

Wide, fixed splitting, although considered typical of ASD, occurs in only 70% of patients with ASD. However, persistent expiratory splitting is audible in most. Normal respiratory variation of the S_2 occurs in up to 8% of patients with ASD. With Eisenmenger physiology, the left-to-right shunting decreases and the degree of splitting narrows.

A pulmonary systolic ejection murmur (due to increased flow) is common in patients with ASD, and with significant left-to-right shunt, a diastolic tricuspid flow murmur can be heard as well. Similar to aortic stenosis, as pulmonary stenosis increases in severity, P_2 decreases in intensity, and ultimately S_2 becomes single.

The wide splitting of S_2 in mitral regurgitation and ventricular septal defect is related to early aortic valve closure (in ventricular septal defect, P_2 is delayed as well), which, in turn, is due to decreased LV ejection time, but the loud pansystolic regurgitant murmur often obscures the wide splitting of S_2 and then the S_2 appears to be "single."

Partial anomalous pulmonary venous connection may occur alone or in combination with ASD (most often of the sinus venosus type). Wide splitting of S_2 occurs in both conditions, but it usually shows normal respiratory variation in isolated partial anomalous pulmonary venous connection.

Pulmonary hypertension may cause wide splitting of S_2, although the intensity of P_2 is usually increased and widely transmitted throughout the precordium.

- Fixed splitting should be verified with the patient in the sitting or standing position because normal subjects occasionally appear to have fixed splitting in the supine position.
- Wide, fixed splitting, although considered typical of ASD, occurs in only 70% of patients with ASD.
- Wide splitting of S_2 occurs in both partial anomalous pulmonary venous connection and ASD, but it usually shows normal respiratory variation in isolated partial anomalous pulmonary venous connection.
- Pulmonary hypertension may or may not cause wide splitting of S_2, although the intensity of P_2 is usually increased and widely transmitted throughout the precordium.

Paradoxic (Reversed) Splitting of S_2

This is usually caused by conditions that delay aortic closure. Examples include the following:
1) Electrical delay of LV contraction, such as left bundle branch block (most commonly)
2) Mechanical delay of LV ejection, such as aortic stenosis and hypertrophic obstructive cardiomyopathy
3) Severe LV systolic failure of any cause
4) Patent ductus arteriosus, aortic regurgitation, and systemic hypertension are other rare causes of paradoxic splitting

Paradoxic splitting of S_2 (in the absence of left bundle branch block) may be an important bedside clue to significant LV dysfunction. In severe aortic stenosis, the paradoxic splitting is only rarely recognized because the late systolic ejection murmur obscures S_2. However, when paradoxic splitting of S_2 is found in association with aortic stenosis, usually in young adults (assuming left bundle branch block is absent), severe aortic obstruction is suggested. Similarly, paradoxic splitting in hypertrophic obstructive cardiomyopathy implies significant resting LV outflow tract gradient. Transient paradoxic splitting of S_2 can occur with myocardial ischemia, such as during an episode of angina, either alone or in combination with an apical systolic murmur of mitral regurgitation (papillary muscle dysfunction) or prominent fourth heart sound (S_4).

- When paradoxic splitting of S_2 is found in association with aortic stenosis, usually in young adults (assuming left bundle branch block is absent), severe aortic obstruction is suggested. Similarly, paradoxic splitting in hypertrophic obstructive cardiomyopathy implies significant resting LV outflow tract gradient.
- Transient paradoxic splitting of S_2 can occur with myocardial ischemia, such as during an episode of angina, either alone or in combination with an apical systolic murmur of mitral regurgitation (papillary muscle dysfunction) or a prominent S_4.

Intensity of S_2

Loud S_2
Ordinarily, the intensity of the aortic component of the second heart sound (A_2) exceeds that of the pulmonic component (P_2). In adults, a P_2 that is louder than A_2, especially if P_2 is transmitted to the apex, implies either pulmonary hypertension or marked RV dilatation, such that the RV now occupies the apical zone. The latter may occur in ASD (approximately 50% of patients). Hearing two components of the S_2 at the apex is abnormal in adults, because ordinarily only A_2 is heard at the apex. Thus, when both components of S_2 are heard at the apex in adults, suspect ASD or pulmonary hypertension.

Soft S_2
Decreased intensity of A_2 or P_2, which may cause a single S_2, reflects stiffening and decreased mobility of the aortic or pulmonary valve (aortic stenosis or pulmonary stenosis, respectively). A single S_2 may also be heard in older patients and the following cases:
1) With only one functioning semilunar valve, such as

in persistent truncus arteriosus, pulmonary atresia, or tetralogy of Fallot

2) When one component of S_2 is enveloped in a long systolic murmur, such as in ventricular septal defect

3) With abnormal relationships of great vessels, such as in transposition of the great arteries

● When both components of S_2 are heard at the apex in adults, implying an increased pulmonary component of S_2, suspect ASD or pulmonary hypertension.

Opening Snap (OS)

A high-pitched snapping sound related to mitral or tricuspid valve opening, when present, is abnormal and is referred to as an OS. This may arise from either a doming stenotic mitral valve or tricuspid valve, most commonly the former. The intensity of an OS correlates with valve mobility. Rarely, an OS can occur in the absence of atrioventricular valve stenosis in conditions associated with increased flow through the valve, such as significant mitral regurgitation.

In mitral stenosis, the presence of an OS, often accompanied by a loud S_1, implies a pliable mitral valve. The OS is often well transmitted to the left sternal border and even to the aortic area. In mitral stenosis, the absence of an OS implies the following:

1) Severe valve immobility and calcification (note that an OS can still be heard in some of these cases)

2) Mitral regurgitation is the predominant lesion

3) Mitral stenosis is very mild

● Significant mitral stenosis may be present in the absence of an OS if the mitral valve leaflets are fixed and immobile.

S_2-OS Interval

The S_2-mitral OS interval reflects the isovolumic relaxation period of the LV. With increased severity of mitral stenosis and greater increase in left atrial pressures, the S_2-OS interval becomes shorter and may be confused with a split S_2. The S_2-OS interval should not vary with respiration. The S_2-OS interval widens on standing, whereas the split S_2 does not change or narrows. Mild mitral stenosis is associated with an S_2-OS interval of more than 90 ms, and severe mitral stenosis with an interval of less than 70 ms. However, the S_2-OS interval is an unreliable predictor of the severity of mitral stenosis. Other factors that increase left atrial pressures, such as mitral regurgitation or LV failure, can also affect this interval. When the S_2-OS interval is more than 110 to 120 ms, the OS may be confused with

an LV third heart sound (S_3). In comparison, the LV S_3 is usually low-pitched and is localized to the apex.

Tricuspid valve OS can be recognized by its location along the left sternal border and its increase with inspiration.

An S_3, which implies that rapid LV filling can occur, is rare in pure mitral stenosis. Also, an RV S_3 can occur in mitral stenosis with severe secondary pulmonary hypertension and RV failure. An RV S_3 is found along the left sternal border and increases with inspiration. A tumor "plop" due to an atrial myxoma has the same early diastolic timing as an OS and can be confused with it.

● In mitral stenosis, the presence of an OS, often accompanied by a loud S_1, implies a pliable mitral valve that is not heavily calcified. (In such cases, the patient may be a candidate for mitral commissurotomy or balloon valvuloplasty rather than mitral valve replacement.)

● In general, mild mitral stenosis is associated with an S_2-OS interval of more than 90 ms, and severe mitral stenosis with an interval of less than 70 ms.

● A tumor "plop" due to atrial myxoma has the same early diastolic timing as an OS and can be confused with it.

Third Heart Sound (S_3)

The exact mechanism of S_3 production remains controversial, but its timing relates to the peak of rapid ventricular filling with rapid flow deceleration. Factors related to S_3 intensity include the following:

1) Volume and velocity of blood flow across the atrioventricular valve

2) Ventricular relaxation and compliance

Although a physiologic S_3 can be heard in young normal subjects, it should not be audible after age 40. Both LV and RV S_3, but especially the latter, may be augmented with inspiration. The physiologic S_3 may disappear in the standing position; the pathologic S_3 persists. An S_3 in a patient with mitral or aortic regurgitation implies severe regurgitation or a failing LV or both. The presence of a diastolic flow rumble ("relative" mitral stenosis) after the S_3 suggests severe mitral regurgitation. An S_3 is less common in conditions that cause thick, poorly compliant ventricles, for example, LV hypertrophy that occurs with pressure overload states (such as aortic stenosis or hypertension), until late in the disease. An S_3 may occur in hypertrophic obstructive cardiomyopathy with normal systolic function.

The pericardial knock of constrictive pericarditis is similar to an S_3 and is associated with sudden arrest of ventricular expansion in early diastole. The pericardial knock is of higher frequency than S_3, occurs slightly earlier in diastole, may vary with respiration, and is more widely transmitted. The causes of S_3 are listed in Table 11.

- An S_3 in a patient with mitral or aortic regurgitation implies severe regurgitation or a failing LV or both.
- An S_3 is less common in conditions that cause thick, poorly compliant ventricles, for example, LV hypertrophy that occurs with pressure overload states.
- The pericardial knock is of higher frequency than S_3, occurs slightly earlier in diastole, may vary with respiration, and is more widely transmitted.

Fourth Heart Sound (S_4)

The S_4 is thought to originate within the ventricular cavity and results from a forceful atrial contraction into a ventricle having limited distensibility, such as in hypertrophy or fibrosis. It is not heard in healthy young persons. Common pathologic states in which an S_4 is often present include the following:

1) Aortic stenosis
2) Hypertension
3) Hypertrophic obstructive cardiomyopathy
4) Pulmonary stenosis
5) Ischemic heart disease

As the S_4 becomes closer to S_1, the intensity of the latter increases. Sitting or standing may attenuate the S_4. A loud S_4 can be heard in acute mitral regurgitation (for example, with ruptured chordae) or regurgitation of recent onset (the left atrium has not yet significantly dilated). With chronic mitral regurgitation due to rheumatic disease, the left atrium dilates, becomes more distensible, and generates a less forceful contraction. Under these circumstances, an S_4 is usually absent. An S_4 can still be heard in some patients with LV hypertrophy or ischemic heart disease, despite enlargement of the left atrium.

Although an S_4 can be heard in otherwise normal elderly patients, a palpable S_4 ("a" wave) should not be present unless the LV is abnormal. An S_4 can originate from the RV. A right-sided S_4 is increased in intensity with inspiration, is often associated with large jugular venous "a" waves, and is best heard along the left sternal border rather than at the apex (this is the usual site of an LV S_4).

In patients with aortic stenosis who are younger than 40 years, the presence of an S_4 usually indicates significant obstruction. Similarly, the presence of right-sided S_4, in association with pulmonary stenosis, indicates severe pulmonary

Table 11.—Causes of S_3

Physiologic in young adults and children
Severe left ventricular dysfunction of any cause
Left ventricular dilatation without failure due to:
Mitral regurgitation
Ventricular septal defect
Patent ductus arteriosus
Aortic regurgitation
Right ventricular S_3 in right ventricular failure and severe volume overload
S_3 is augmented in intensity with an increase in venous return due to leg elevation, exercise, or the release phase of Valsalva
Increased systemic peripheral resistance due to sustained handgrip will also augment S_3

valve obstruction. An S_4 is present in most patients with hypertrophic obstructive cardiomyopathy and in patients with acute myocardial infarction and is often found in patients with systemic hypertension.

- A loud S_4 can be found in acute mitral regurgitation (for example, with ruptured chordae) and can be a clue that the regurgitation is of recent onset.
- Although an S_4 can be heard in otherwise normal elderly patients, a palpable S_4 ("a" wave) should not be present unless the LV is abnormal.
- An S_4 is present in most patients with hypertrophic obstructive cardiomyopathy and in patients with acute myocardial infarction and is often found in patients with systemic hypertension.

Cardiac Murmurs

Systolic Murmurs

Systolic murmurs may be divided into two categories:

1) Ejection types, such as aortic or pulmonary stenosis
2) Pansystolic or regurgitant types, such as mitral regurgitation, tricuspid regurgitation, or ventricular septal defect

Most, but not all, systolic murmurs fit into this simple classification scheme. Factors that differentiate the various causes of LV outflow tract obstruction are shown in Table 12.

Table 12.--Factors That Differentiate the Various Causes of Left Ventricular Outflow Tract Obstruction

	Valvular	Supravalvular	Discrete subvalvular	HOCM
Valve calcification	Common after age 40	0	0	0
Dilated ascending aorta	Common	Rare	Rare	Rare
PP after VPB	Increased	Increased	Increased	Decreased
Valsalva effect on SM	Decreased	Decreased	Decreased	Increased
Murmur of AR	Common	Rare	Sometimes	0
Fourth heart sound (S_4)	If severe	Uncommon	Uncommon	Common
Paradoxic splitting	Sometimes[*]	0	0	Rather common[*]
Ejection click	Most (unless valve calcified)	0	0	Uncommon or 0
Maximal thrill & murmur	2nd RIS	1st RIS	2nd RIS	4th LIS
Carotid pulse	Normal to anacrotic[*] (parvus et tardus)	Unequal	Normal to anacrotic	Brisk, jerky; systolic rebound

AR, aortic regurgitation; HOCM, hypertrophic obstructive cardiomyopathy; LIS, left intercostal space; PP, pulse pressure; RIS, right intercostal space; SM, systolic murmur; VPB, ventricular premature beat.

[*]Depends on severity.

From Marriott HJL: *Bedside Cardiac Diagnosis*. JB Lippincott Company, 1993, p 116. By permission of the publisher.

Aortic and Pulmonary Stenosis

Stenosis of the aortic or pulmonary valves causes a delay in the peak intensity of the systolic murmur related to prolongation of ejection. The magnitude of the delay is proportional to the severity of obstruction. The intensity (loudness) of an ejection systolic murmur may not reflect the severity of obstruction. Thus, for example, a patient with mild aortic stenosis or a normal mechanical aortic prosthesis and increased cardiac output may have a loud murmur (grade 3 or 4). Conversely, a patient with severe aortic stenosis and low cardiac output may have only a grade 1 or 2 murmur. However, the timing of peak intensity may still be delayed. For valvular pulmonary stenosis, early timing of the ejection click, a widely split S_2, and delayed peak intensity of systolic murmur suggest severe stenosis.

Hypertrophic Obstructive Cardiomyopathy

Patients with hypertrophic obstructive cardiomyopathy can have three different types and locations of systolic murmurs:

1) Mid- (and lower) left sternal border (left ventricular outflow tract obstruction)
2) Apex (associated mitral regurgitation)
3) Upper left sternal border (right ventricular outflow tract obstruction)—uncommon (a bedside clue is a prominent jugular venous "a" wave)

Frequently, the louder systolic murmur at the mid-left sternal border, which can be widely transmitted, may mask the others.

Aortic Stenosis Versus Aortic Sclerosis

A frequent clinical problem is the differentiation of aortic stenosis from benign aortic sclerosis. With aortic sclerosis, there should be no other clinical, electrocardiographic, or roentgenographic evidence of heart disease. The systolic murmur is generally of grade 1 or 2 intensity and peaks early. The carotid upstroke should be normal. A normal S_2 (that is, A_2 preserved) supports a benign process, but remember that S_2 can appear single in normal elderly subjects. The systolic murmur of aortic stenosis, in contrast, is delayed (peaking late in systole) and is usually louder, and the carotid pulse is weakened and delayed (parvus et tardus) (remember the exception of the elderly, who may have normal carotid pulses despite having significant aortic stenosis). The apical impulse in aortic stenosis is frequently abnormal also (see Palpation of Precordium).

Supravalvular Aortic Stenosis

The systolic murmur of supravalvular aortic stenosis is maximal in the first or second right intercostal space, and a carotid pulse inequality may be present (see Abnormalities of the Carotid Pulse). Patients are usually young. (The differential diagnosis of left ventricular outflow tract obstruction is shown in Table 12.)

Mitral Regurgitation

Although mitral regurgitation is usually pansystolic, at times it can be late systolic in timing (in this case, suspect mitral prolapse, papillary muscle dysfunction, and, less commonly, rheumatic disease). The systolic murmur of mitral regurgitation can also be early systolic in timing; this can be heard in cases of acute, severe mitral regurgitation with markedly increased left atrial pressures, reducing the late systolic LV-left atrial gradient. In such cases, the patients are usually hemodynamically unstable and have evidence of significant pulmonary congestion. The systolic murmur of severe chronic mitral regurgitation is usually loud (grade 3-4 or louder). The systolic murmur of severe acute mitral regurgitation can be variable, especially in the presence of low cardiac output states or shock (such as acute myocardial infarction with left ventricular dysfunction and papillary muscle dysfunction). Under these circumstances, the systolic murmur may be unimpressive or even absent. The systolic murmur of "posterior mitral leaflet syndrome" can be well transmitted to the aortic area and be confused with aortic stenosis. Except in the elderly, palpation of the carotid pulse helps differentiate these two conditions. In about 15% of cases, pure aortic stenosis can cause a localized apical systolic murmur. Auscultation during inhalation of amyl nitrite can help differentiate this murmur from mitral regurgitation (Tables 13 and 15). The systolic murmur of "anterior mitral leaflet syndrome" is transmitted posteriorly and can be heard along the thoracic spine and even at the base of the skull.

Tricuspid Regurgitation

The systolic murmur of tricuspid regurgitation is usually best heard at the lower left sternal border or over the xyphisternum, but it may also be heard to the right of the sternum, over the apicosternal area, or over the apex (if the RV is sufficiently dilated and occupies the position usually taken by the LV). The systolic murmur of significant tricuspid regurgitation may be subtle or even inaudible clinically, but large "v" waves can almost always be seen in the jugular venous pulse. Inspiration may accentuate the murmur of tricuspid regurgitation, but not consistently so, and the absence of inspiratory augmentation does not exclude tricuspid regurgitation (with severe tricuspid regurgitation, the X descent becomes obliterated).

Ventricular Septal Defect

Depending on the size of the defect and the pressure gradient between the LV and the RV, the systolic murmur of ventricular septal defect is typically pansystolic and associated with a thrill along the left sternal border, but the murmur can be variable in contour and the thrill absent. The murmur parallels the pressure difference between the two ventricles (in turn related to pulmonary and systemic vascular resistances). With significant pulmonary hypertension, the murmur duration shortens and may resemble an early systolic ejection-type murmur. If the maximal intensity of the systolic murmur is in the first and second left intercostal spaces with radiation to the left clavicle, suspect supracristal ventricular septal defect or patent ductus arteriosus. The systolic murmur of multiple ventricular septal defects is indistinguishable from that of single defects. The same is true for LV-right atrial shunts. The loud pansystolic murmur of ventricular septal defect may mask associated defects, such as patent ductus arteriosus. A wide pulse pressure suggests the latter or associated aortic regurgitation. The combination of ventricular septal defect and aortic regurgitation may suggest patent ductus arteriosus, but the systolic murmur in patent ductus arteriosus peaks at S_2 and it does not in the combination of ventricular septal defect and aortic regurgitation. A systolic murmur in the posterior thorax may be caused by the following:

1) Coarctation
2) Aortic dissection
3) "Anterior mitral leaflet syndrome" (with posteriorly directed jet of mitral regurgitation)
4) Peripheral pulmonary artery stenosis
5) Pulmonary arteriovenous fistula

- Stenosis of a semilunar valve causes a delay in the peak intensity of the systolic murmur related to prolongation of ejection. The magnitude of the delay is proportional to the severity of obstruction.
- For valvular pulmonary stenosis, early timing of the ejection click, a widely split S_2, and delayed peak intensity of systolic murmur suggest severe stenosis.
- The systolic murmur of supravalvular aortic stenosis is maximal in the first or second right intercostal space, and a carotid pulse inequality may be present.
- Although mitral regurgitation is usually pansystolic, at

times it can be late systolic in timing (in this case, suspect mitral prolapse, papillary muscle dysfunction, and, less commonly, rheumatic disease).

- Mitral regurgitation that is early systolic in timing can be heard in acute, severe cases with markedly increased left atrial pressures, reducing the late systolic LV-left atrial gradient.

- The systolic murmur of "posterior mitral leaflet syndrome" can be transmitted to the aortic area and be confused with aortic stenosis.

- The systolic murmur of "anterior mitral leaflet syndrome" is transmitted posteriorly and can be heard along the thoracic spine and even at the base of the skull.

- Inspiration may accentuate the murmur of tricuspid regurgitation, but not consistently so, and the absence of inspiratory augmentation does not exclude tricuspid regurgitation.

- The systolic murmur of ventricular septal defect is typically pansystolic and associated with a thrill along the left sternal border, but the murmur can be variable in contour.

- If the maximal intensity of a systolic murmur is in the first and second left intercostal spaces with radiation to the left clavicle, suspect supracristal ventricular septal defect or patent ductus arteriosus.

- A loud pansystolic murmur of ventricular septal defect may mask associated defects, such as patent ductus arteriosus. A wide pulse pressure suggests the latter or associated aortic regurgitation.

- The combination of ventricular septal defect and aortic regurgitation may suggest patent ductus arteriosus, but the murmur in the latter peaks at S_2, and it does not in the combination of ventricular septal defect and aortic regurgitation.

Innocent Systolic Murmurs

Innocent systolic murmurs are generally related to increased blood flow or turbulence across a semilunar valve, especially the aortic valve. These murmurs are common at all ages. In young patients, they are apt to be heard over the pulmonary area. Innocent systolic murmurs usually are soft (grade 2 or less), are short (never pansystolic), and have no associated abnormal clinical findings (e.g., S_2 is normal, there are no clicks). In older patients, they generally emanate from a sclerotic aortic valve or dilated aortic root. Such murmurs can be heard at the aortic area, left sternal border, or apex. If heard at the apex, they may be confused with the murmur of mitral regurgitation. In younger patients, an innocent systolic murmur may originate from

the RV outflow tract or pulmonary artery. Remember that a patent ductus arteriosus or ventricular septal defect also can masquerade as an "innocent" murmur.

An innocent systolic murmur heard at the lower left sternal border should be differentiated from the systolic murmur of ventricular septal defect, tricuspid regurgitation, infundibular pulmonary stenosis, or hypertrophic obstructive cardiomyopathy. When uncertain about the cause of a systolic murmur, a Valsalva maneuver should be performed (Table 13). The findings of a pathologic systolic murmur are listed in Table 14.

- Innocent systolic murmurs usually are soft (grade 2 or less), are short, and have no associated abnormal clinical findings.

- In younger patients, an innocent systolic murmur often originates from the RV outflow tract or pulmonary artery.

- Remember that a patent ductus arteriosus or ventricular septal defect can masquerade as an "innocent" murmur.

Diastolic Murmurs

In general, the loudness of a diastolic murmur correlates with the severity of the underlying abnormality.

Aortic Regurgitation (AR)

The murmur of mild AR may be difficult to hear and may be clinically "silent." A grade 1 chronic AR murmur is rarely, if ever, severe. This murmur is best heard with the patient in the sitting position, leaning forward, in held expiration. Consider AR when there is a wide arterial pulse pressure, especially in young or middle-aged patients (older patients may have generalized atherosclerosis causing wide pulse pressure). The murmur of AR is typically early diastolic (immediately after S_2) and decrescendo in timing, but occasionally it appears later in diastole or has varying configurations. In the presence of mitral stenosis, an early diastolic murmur may be caused by AR or pulmonary regurgitation (Graham Steell murmur), more often the former. Severe AR, especially if acute, may be associated with markedly increased LV end-diastolic pressures. These pressures will decrease the gradient between the aorta and LV in diastole, and the murmur will taper rapidly. Thus, a short, early diastolic murmur does not exclude significant acute AR, especially if the patient has evidence of acute heart failure. A patient with severe AR due to infective endocarditis may present in this way. In mild AR, the LV end-diastolic pressure remains normal, the gradient persists throughout most of diastole, and the

Table 13.--Effect of Selected Physiologic Changes and Physical or Pharmacologic Maneuvers on Common Cardiac Murmurs

	Effect on murmur		
	Augmented	Little or no change	Decreased
Amyl nitrite	HOCM AS; PS Innocent SM MS TS		MR VSD] SM AR Austin Flint] DM
Hand grip	AR MR VSD MS*	AS, TR PR TS	HOCM
Long cardiac cycle length (e.g., atrial fibrillation or with premature ventricular contraction)	AS PS HOCM	MR AR	
Valsalva maneuver	HOCM MV prolapse†		AS PS
Posture			
Standing	HOCM MV prolapse†		AS PS
Squatting	AR, MR, VSD		HOCM MV prolapse‡

AR, aortic regurgitation; AS, aortic stenosis; DM, diastolic murmur; HOCM, hypertrophic obstructive cardiomyopathy; MR, mitral regurgitation; MS, mitral stenosis; MV, mitral valve; PR, pulmonary regurgitation; PS, pulmonary stenosis; SM, systolic murmur; TR, tricuspid regurgitation; TS, tricuspid stenosis; VSD, ventricular septal defect.

*Related to increased cardiac output.

†Duration of systolic murmur increased (earlier onset), variable augmentation effect.

‡Duration of systolic murmur decreased (later onset), variable intensity effect.

murmur may persist longer into diastole. With severe chronic AR, there is often a wide pulse pressure (with hyperdynamic pulses), a systolic ejection murmur that usually peaks early (related to increased aortic flow), reduced diastolic blood pressure, and LV enlargement by palpation.

Remember that the anatomical location of the aortic valve is not under the second right intercostal space (the "aortic area") but is situated lower in the thorax under the mid-upper sternum. AR is often best heard along the left sternal border. AR can be primarily transmitted down the right sternal border. If so, one should suspect diseases of the aortic root, such as aortic aneurysm or dissection. The combination of hypertension, chest pain, and right sternal border transmission of AR should suggest proximal aortic dissection. When the AR is of valvular origin, it can be heard at the aortic area, but it is also transmitted along the left sternal border and to the apex.

Table 14.—Findings That Suggest a Systolic Murmur Is Pathologic

Loud (grade 3 or more) in intensity

Long in duration

Increased jugular venous pressure

Abnormal carotid pulse

Abnormal S_2

Associated with ejection or nonejection click

Presence of an opening snap

Presence of left or right ventricular hypertrophy or heave

Fixed or expiratory splitting of S_2

- Consider AR when there is a wide arterial pulse pressure, especially in young or middle-aged patients.
- In the presence of mitral stenosis, an associated early diastolic murmur may be due to AR or pulmonary regurgitation (Graham Steell murmur), more often the former.
- A short, early diastolic murmur does not exclude significant acute AR, especially if the patient has evidence of acute heart failure.
- AR, although often heard at the left sternal border, can be primarily transmitted down the right sternal border. If so, one should suspect diseases of the aortic root, such as aortic aneurysm or dissection.
- The combination of hypertension, chest pain, and right sternal border transmission of AR should suggest proximal aortic dissection.

Austin Flint Murmur

An Austin Flint murmur is related to mitral inflow turbulence caused by the AR jet and implies a significant AR leak. Because this may produce an apical diastolic rumble that is mid-diastolic in timing with presystolic accentuation, it may be confused with mitral stenosis. The presence of radiographic left atrial enlargement or atrial fibrillation favors mitral stenosis rather than isolated AR. Administration of amyl nitrite can help differentiate these murmurs (Table 13): the Austin Flint murmur decreases (as the LV afterload decreases), whereas the mitral stenosis murmur increases (as do all valvular stenotic murmurs in response to amyl nitrite). Also, there should be no OS or other features of mitral valve disease. Obviously, a patient with rheumatic heart disease can have both AR and mitral stenosis. When AR has a "honking" or "cooing" quality, consider a perforated, everted, or ruptured aortic cusp, such as with infective endocarditis.

- With administration of amyl nitrite, the Austin Flint murmur decreases (as the LV afterload decreases), whereas the murmur of mitral stenosis increases (as do all valvular stenotic murmurs in response to amyl nitrite).
- When AR has a "honking" or "cooing" quality, consider a perforated, everted, or ruptured aortic cusp, such as with infective endocarditis.

Pulmonary Regurgitation

Although pulmonary regurgitation may sound similar to the murmur of AR, it is usually localized to the pulmonary area and, like most right-sided events, gets louder with inspiration. The murmur characteristics depend on the cause.

Pulmonary regurgitation due to pulmonary hypertension begins in early diastole (immediately after P_2) and is long and high-pitched. In comparison, the murmur of pulmonary regurgitation due to organic pulmonary valve disease is lower pitched, harsher, and rumbling, beginning slightly later in diastole and often ending in mid-diastole. Pulmonary regurgitation, especially when mild or even moderate, is frequently inaudible. In the presence of mitral stenosis, an early diastolic murmur heard at the left sternal border is more likely to be AR than pulmonary regurgitation.

- Pulmonary regurgitation due to pulmonary hypertension begins in early diastole and is long and high-pitched. In comparison, the murmur of pulmonary regurgitation due to organic pulmonary valve disease is lower pitched, harsher, and rumbling, begins slightly later in diastole, and often ends in mid-diastole.

Mitral Stenosis

The diastolic murmur of mitral stenosis is very localized (to the apex), is low-pitched, and begins at the time of mitral valve opening. The presence of a loud S_1 or an OS should prompt a careful search for this easily overlooked diastolic murmur. With the patient in the left lateral decubitus position, the stethoscope may have to be inched around the apical region to find the highly localized, subtle, flow rumble of mitral stenosis. If it is not audible, exercise, such as sit-ups, may augment mitral flow and bring out the murmur. Other provocative maneuvers that increase flow across the mitral valve, such as administration of amyl nitrite, also augment the murmur of mitral stenosis (Table 13). The duration of the diastolic murmur is related to the severity of mitral stenosis, persisting as long as there is a significant pressure gradient across the mitral valve. Therefore, a pandiastolic murmur implies severe mitral stenosis. The murmur may crescendo in late diastole (presystolic accentuation), even in atrial fibrillation, suggesting that atrial contraction is not required for this phenomenon.

Rarely in mitral stenosis, the diastolic murmur is not heard (so-called silent mitral stenosis). The usual reasons for silent mitral stenosis are as follows:

1) Improper auscultation (most commonly)
2) Very mild mitral stenosis
3) A decrease in flow rates across the mitral valve, such as in severe congestive heart failure or concomitant aortic or tricuspid stenosis
4) Abnormal chest wall configuration limiting auscultation, such as in obesity or severe chronic obstructive

pulmonary disease, in which case all sounds should be indistinct or distant

Consider mitral stenosis and focus the cardiac examination accordingly with new onset of atrial fibrillation or when atrial fibrillation is found in association with any of the following clinical scenarios:

1) Stroke or other systemic or peripheral embolus (an atrial myxoma may also present in this way)
2) "Unexplained" pulmonary hypertension
3) "Unexplained" congestive heart failure
4) "Unexplained" recurrent pleural effusions

- The duration of the diastolic murmur is related to the severity of mitral stenosis, persisting as long as there is a significant pressure gradient across the mitral valve.
- Even in the apparent absence of a murmur, important auscultatory clues to the presence of mitral stenosis include a loud S_1 and an OS.
- Consider mitral stenosis when atrial fibrillation is found in association with any of the following clinical scenarios: 1) stroke or other systemic or peripheral embolus, 2) "unexplained" pulmonary hypertension, 3) "unexplained" congestive heart failure, and 4) "unexplained" recurrent pleural effusions.

Tricuspid Stenosis

The bedside differentiation of tricuspid and mitral stenosis includes the following:

1) Response to inspiration (murmur of tricuspid stenosis increases)
2) Location: the diastolic murmur of tricuspid stenosis is best heard at the left sternal border, whereas the murmur of mitral stenosis is localized to the apex. The associated OS, if present, augments with inspiration
3) Frequency: tricuspid stenosis is higher in frequency and begins earlier in diastole than mitral stenosis (these differences may be difficult to appreciate at the bedside)
4) A large jugular venous A wave with a slow Y descent should suggest tricuspid stenosis. (Other causes of large A waves, including pulmonary stenosis or pulmonary hypertension, should not interfere with RV filling and therefore are not associated with a slow Y descent.) Rarely, there may be a diastolic thrill palpable along lower left sternal border and hepatic (presystolic) pulsation. Other causes of RV inflow obstruction, such as thrombus

or extrinsic RV compression, can masquerade as tricuspid stenosis

Note that tricuspid stenosis usually occurs in patients with rheumatic heart disease (although there are other, rarer causes, such as carcinoid). In patients with rheumatic heart disease, especially females, concomitant mitral valve disease is almost always present. The clinical findings of the left-sided valve lesions often overshadow the tricuspid involvement, and the murmur of tricuspid stenosis may be mistaken for aortic or pulmonary regurgitation.

- A large jugular venous A wave with a slow Y descent should suggest tricuspid stenosis.
- The clinical findings of the left-sided valve lesions often overshadow the tricuspid involvement, and the murmur of tricuspid stenosis may be mistaken for aortic or pulmonary regurgitation.

Mid-Diastolic Flow Murmurs

Almost any condition that increases flow across atrioventricular valves (such as mitral regurgitation, patent ductus arteriosus, intracardiac shunts, or complete heart block) can also cause a short mid-diastolic flow rumble (functional diastolic murmur) in the absence of organic atrioventricular valve stenosis. (Actually, the rumble begins in early rather than mid-diastole, but it is delayed in comparison with the early diastolic murmur of semilunar valve regurgitation.) The murmur may begin after a prominent S_3 and does not show presystolic accentuation.

- Almost any condition that increases flow across atrioventricular valves (such as mitral regurgitation, patent ductus arteriosus, intracardiac shunts, or complete heart block) can also cause a short mid-diastolic flow rumble (functional diastolic murmur) in the absence of organic atrioventricular valve stenosis.

Continuous Murmurs

Continuous murmurs should be differentiated from to-and-fro murmurs (such as occur in combined aortic stenosis and regurgitation). In aortic regurgitation, the systolic component decreases before S_2, whereas the continuous murmur of patent ductus arteriosus, for example, typically peaks at S_2. Murmurs caused by coronary arteriovenous fistula, venous hum, and ruptured sinus of Valsalva aneurysm peak later in diastole. When the murmur is due to dilated bronchial vessels, such as in pulmonary atresia, it can be heard anywhere in the chest, axillae, or back. When a continuous murmur is loudest in the posterior thorax, consider the following:

1) Coarctation
2) Pulmonary arteriovenous fistula
3) Peripheral pulmonary stenosis

● Continuous murmurs should be differentiated from to-and-fro murmurs (such as occur in combined aortic stenosis and regurgitation). In aortic regurgitation, the systolic component decreases before S_2, whereas the continuous murmur of patent ductus arteriosus typically peaks at S_2.

Bedside Physiologic Maneuvers to Differentiate Different Types of Murmurs (Table 13)

Valsalva

The Valsalva maneuver is useful for differentiating right-sided from left-sided murmurs. During the active strain phase, with decreased venous return, most murmurs decrease in intensity. There are two important exceptions to this rule:

1) The murmur of hypertrophic obstructive cardiomyopathy typically gets louder
2) The murmur of mitral valve prolapse may get longer (and possibly louder)

After the release of the strain phase of the Valsalva maneuver, with a sudden increase in venous return, right-sided murmurs return immediately (within one or two cardiac cycles), whereas left-sided murmurs gradually return after several cardiac cycles. Thus, differentiation between aortic and pulmonary stenosis and between aortic and pulmonary regurgitation is possible.

Respiration

The effect of normal respiration is also useful for distinguishing right-sided and left-sided murmurs. In general, right-sided murmurs are augmented with inspiration (frequent exceptions occur with tricuspid regurgitation). In cases of severe RV failure, the RV may be unable to augment its output with inspiration, and pulmonary or tricuspid murmurs may fail to become louder with inspiration.

R-R Cycle Length

Varying R-R cycle length (such as in atrial fibrillation or with frequent premature ventricular contractions) affects murmurs in specific ways that can be of diagnostic value at the bedside. In general, systolic ejection murmurs (such as aortic or pulmonary stenosis) increase after a long cycle length, whereas regurgitant murmurs (such as mitral or

tricuspid regurgitation) do not. The systolic murmur of hypertrophic obstructive cardiomyopathy is augmented with the increased contractility of a post-premature ventricular contraction beat, but the peripheral arterial pulse volume decreases because left ventricular outflow tract obstruction worsens.

Handgrip

Isometric exercise (such as handgrip), by increasing systemic blood pressure (afterload), augments the murmurs of mitral or aortic regurgitation or ventricular septal defect but does not significantly alter the murmur of aortic stenosis and tends to decrease the murmur of hypertrophic obstructive cardiomyopathy.

Squatting

Prompt squatting causes a rapid transient increase in venous return and a sustained increase in peripheral resistance. The latter may augment the murmurs of mitral and aortic regurgitation. Because LV volume and peripheral resistance increase, the murmur of hypertrophic obstructive cardiomyopathy becomes softer. Then, after the upright position is assumed, with decreased LV volume and peripheral resistance, the murmur of hypertrophic obstructive cardiomyopathy becomes louder.

Amyl Nitrite

Administration of amyl nitrite is simple, inexpensive, and, in most patients, safe (exceptions are in acute myocardial infarction or critical carotid artery stenosis, in which even transient hypotension should be avoided if possible). Amyl nitrite causes acute systemic vasodilation, resulting in a transient (30 to 45 seconds) decline in systemic blood pressure, followed by reflex tachycardia and an increase in venous return and cardiac output. All stenotic murmurs, including hypertrophic obstructive cardiomyopathy, become louder. The murmur of mitral regurgitation usually decreases because of the decrease in LV afterload (during the vasodilation phase). The diastolic murmur of aortic regurgitation diminishes, whereas the murmur of mitral stenosis becomes louder because of the increased flow across the mitral valve, especially during the tachycardia phase. The systolic murmur of mitral prolapse may become longer (as LV volume decreases initially) but not necessarily louder, because LV pressures also are decreased. The major usefulness of amyl nitrite is to differentiate (Tables 13 and 15) the following:

1) A small ventricular septal defect (murmur decreases)

from pulmonary stenosis (murmur increases)

2) Aortic stenosis (increase) from mitral regurgitation (decrease)
3) Aortic regurgitation (decrease) from mitral stenosis (increase)
4) Aortic regurgitation (decrease) from pulmonary regurgitation (increase)
5) Mitral regurgitation (decrease) from tricuspid regurgitation (increase)

- After release of the Valsalva maneuver, with a sudden increase in venous return, right-sided murmurs return immediately (within one or two cardiac cycles), whereas left-sided murmurs gradually return after several cardiac cycles.
- Systolic ejection murmurs (such as aortic or pulmonary stenosis) increase after a long cycle length, whereas regurgitant murmurs (such as mitral or tricuspid regurgitation) do not.

- Amyl nitrite causes all stenotic murmurs, including hypertrophic obstructive cardiomyopathy, to become louder.

Miscellaneous

The mammary soufflé can be continuous and can mimic patent ductus arteriosus. It can be obliterated by pressure with the examining finger next to the stethoscope. Innocent venous hums are loudest in the neck but can be transmitted to the precordium and be mistaken for patent ductus arteriosus or atrioventricular fistula. The venous hum is loudest in the sitting or standing position. Motion of the neck or jugular vein compression affects the intensity of the murmur.

- The innocent venous hum is loudest in the neck but can be transmitted to the precordium and be mistaken for patent ductus arteriosus or atrioventricular fistula.
- The venous hum is of variable quality, is loudest in the sitting or standing position, and decreases in the supine position.

Table 15.--Effect of Amyl Nitrite and Vasopressors on Various Murmurs

Diagnosis	Amyl nitrite	Phenylephrine
	Systolic murmurs	
Mitral insufficiency	Decrease	Increase
Ventricular septal defect	Decrease	Increase
Patent ductus arteriosus	Decrease	Increase
Tetralogy of Fallot	Decrease	Increase
Atrial septal defect	Increase	Increase or no change
Idiopathic hypertrophic subaortic stenosis	Increase	Decrease
Aortic stenosis (valvular)	Increase	No change
Pulmonary stenosis (valvular and muscular)	Increase	No change
Tricuspid insufficiency	Increase	No change
Systolic ejection murmur (innocent)	Increase	Decrease
	Diastolic murmurs	
Aortic insufficiency	Decrease	Increase
Austin Flint murmur	Decrease	Increase
Mitral stenosis	Increase	Decrease
Pulmonary insufficiency	Increase	No change
Pulmonary insufficiency due to Eisenmenger syndrome	Decrease	Increase
Tricuspid stenosis	Increase	No change

From Tavel ME: *Clinical Phonocardiography and External Pulse Recordings.* Fourth edition. Year Book Medical Publishers, 1985, p 198. By permission of Mosby.

Questions

Multiple Choice (choose the one best answer)

1. The carotid pulse in isolated, severe aortic stenosis may show each of the following characteristics *except*:
   a. Bisferiens pulse
   b. Slowed upstroke
   c. Delayed peak
   d. Reduced volume
   e. Palpable vibrations ("shudder")

2. All the following findings in aortic stenosis suggest severe aortic obstruction or left ventricular decompensation *except*:
   a. Paradoxic splitting of S_2
   b. An S_3 in an adult
   c. An S_4 in an adolescent
   d. Prolonged, late-peaking systolic ejection murmur
   e. Ejection sound

3. All the following are typical diagnostic features of hypertrophic obstructive cardiomyopathy *except*:
   a. An S_4 is common
   b. An aortic ejection sound is heard
   c. An S_3 may be present even in the absence of ventricular systolic dysfunction
   d. The carotid pulse may have a bifid, "jerky" quality
   e. The apical impulse may be "trifid" with three outward (positive) waves

4. A 42-year-old woman complains of palpitations and progressive dyspnea over a 2-week period. Physical examination reveals a normal body habitus, a blood pressure of 130/80 mm Hg, and an irregular pulse of 140 beats/min. Auscultation of the posterior thorax reveals bibasilar crackles. The jugular venous pressure is increased (approximately 17 cm) with an absent A wave, a prominent V wave, and a slow Y descent. The carotid pulse (although of variable intensity) is brisk. On precordial palpation, a left parasternal lift and an enlarged, inferolaterally displaced apical impulse are present. S_1 is of variable intensity, and both components of S_2 are audible. S_2 is narrowly split in inspiration and becomes single in expiration. A high-pitched early diastolic sound is audible at the base, left sternal border, and apex and does not vary appreciably with respiration. The following murmurs are audible: a grade 2/4 holosystolic murmur at the lower and mid-left sternal border which augments with inspiration; a grade 2/4 mid-diastolic murmur at the lower left sternal border which augments with inspiration; a grade 2/6 apical holosystolic, blowing murmur that radiates to the axilla; and a grade 1/6 mid-diastolic rumbling murmur localized to the apex. The most likely cardiac diagnosis on the basis of these findings is multivalvular heart disease with:
   a. Combined aortic stenosis and aortic regurgitation, tricuspid regurgitation, mitral stenosis, and mitral regurgitation
   b. Combined aortic regurgitation (with an Austin Flint murmur at the apex), tricuspid regurgitation, and mitral regurgitation
   c. Combined tricuspid regurgitation and tricuspid stenosis, mitral regurgitation, and mitral stenosis
   d. Combined pulmonic regurgitation and stenosis with tricuspid regurgitation and tricuspid stenosis

5. In regard to the clinical scenario described in question 4, all the following statements are correct *except*:
   a. Atrial fibrillation is common in this clinical setting
   b. The enlarged, displaced apical impulse suggests left ventricular enlargement
   c. The apical systolic murmur would be expected to become louder after a long cardiac cycle length
   d. The valve abnormalities present are most likely "postinflammatory" (rheumatic) in cause
   e. The variable intensity of S_1 is consistent with atrial fibrillation

6. An 18-year-old female patient has had a heart murmur since birth and has exertional dyspnea. Examination reveals no clubbing or cyanosis. Vital signs are normal. The chest is clear to auscultation. The apical impulse is diffuse with a thrill palpable at the mid-left sternal border. The carotid and jugular venous pulses are normal. S_1 is normal. S_2 is normal. A grade 4/6 harsh, long systolic murmur beginning immediately after S_1 is audible and is loudest at the lower left sternal border but heard throughout the precordium. An S_3 is present at the apex, followed by a short diastolic rumble. In this clinical scenario, the most likely diagnosis is:
   a. Ventricular septal defect
   b. Ostium secundum atrial septal defect
   c. Sinus venosus atrial septal defect

d. Patent ductus arteriosus

e. Pulmonary stenosis

7. All the following clinical findings are typical for uncomplicated atrial septal defect *except*:
   a. Pulmonic component of S_2 is audible at the apex
   b. Pulmonary ejection sound
   c. Large A waves are present in jugular venous pulse contour
   d. Systolic ejection murmur is audible over the pulmonary area
   e. Wide, persistent splitting of S_2

8. An asymptomatic 21-year-old college student is referred for evaluation of a cardiac murmur. On examination, the patient is anxious. The blood pressure is 160/110 mm Hg in both arms, and the pulse is 90 beats/min and regular. The chest is clear to auscultation. The jugular venous pressure and carotid pulses are normal. The apical impulse, although not displaced, demonstrates a palpable presystolic (A) wave. There is no palpable thrill. S_1 and S_2 are normal. An ejection sound is audible at the upper right sternal border and apex. A grade 3/6 systolic ejection-type murmur is audible at the left upper chest and left infraclavicular area. A grade 1/6 early diastolic decrescendo murmur is audible at the upper right sternal border and left lower sternal border. The constellation of findings in this clinical scenario suggests which of the following as the diagnosis?
   a. Patent ductus arteriosus
   b. Coarctation of the aorta
   c. Atrial septal defect
   d. Pulmonary stenosis
   e. Ventricular septal defect

9. A 46-year-old man has a 6-month history of vague right upper quadrant abdominal discomfort with gradually progressive dyspnea and bilateral leg edema. On cardiac examination, the blood pressure is 130/84 mm Hg and the pulse is 88 beats/min and regular. No crackles or wheezes are heard on auscultation of the chest. The carotid pulse is normal. The jugular venous pressure is increased (to approximately 20 cm H_2O) with a small X descent and a prominent, rapid Y descent. The apical impulse is indistinct, and there is no parasternal lift. S_1 is normal. S_2 is prominently split but narrows normally with expiration. S_2P is normal. A prominent third heart sound is audible along the left lower sternal border and apex. No significant murmurs are audible. There is hepatic enlargement and tenderness with 2+ bilateral pretibial pitting edema noted. There is no clubbing or cyanosis. The constellation of findings in this clinical scenario suggests which of the following diagnoses?
   a. Dilated cardiomyopathy with biventricular failure
   b. "Silent" mitral stenosis with secondary pulmonary hypertension
   c. Pericardial tamponade
   d. Constrictive pericarditis
   e. Atrial septal defect with severe pulmonary hypertension

10. A 28-year-old woman is being evaluated for exertional dizziness and chest pain. Clinical examination reveals normal vital signs. The chest is clear to auscultation. The carotid pulse is bifid with a rapid upstroke. The jugular venous pressure is normal. The apical impulse is bifid and sustained. There is no parasternal lift. S_1 is normal. S_2 is paradoxically split. An S_4 is audible at the apex. A harsh grade 3/6 mid-peaking systolic ejection murmur is audible at the mid-left sternal border and apex. No diastolic murmur and no edema, cyanosis, or clubbing are present. The constellation of findings in this clinical scenario is most consistent with which of the following diagnoses?
    a. Hypertrophic obstructive cardiomyopathy
    b. Severe pulmonic stenosis
    c. Severe aortic stenosis
    d. Combined aortic stenosis and tricuspid stenosis
    e. Atrial septal defect

11. All the following maneuvers or interventions or physiologic events would be expected to increase the intensity of the systolic murmur of hypertrophic obstructive cardiomyopathy *except*:
    a. Valsalva maneuver
    b. Prompt squatting
    c. Arising to the upright position after squatting
    d. Amyl nitrite administration
    e. Post-premature ventricular contraction beat

12. A 50-year-old woman has a 1-week history of intermittent fever, chills, night sweats, and progressive dyspnea. A heart murmur has been present since childhood. Examination reveals a blood pressure of 140/85 mm Hg, a pulse of 90 beats/min and regular, and a

temperature of 38°C. Jugular venous pressure is 10 cm H_2O with a predominant V wave. The carotid pulses are bounding. There are bibasilar crackles in the posterior lung fields. The apical impulse is dynamic with a palpable thrill. There is a left parasternal lift. S_1 is normal. S_2 is prominently split but varies normally with respiration. S_2P is increased. A grade 4/6 harsh pansystolic murmur is audible at the apex and left sternal border but is also well heard at the base. An S_4 and S_3 are audible at the apex with a grade 2/6 mid-diastolic rumble following the S_3. There is 1+ bilateral pretibial pitting edema. The abdomen is normal,

and there is no clubbing, cyanosis, or petechiae of the extremities. The most likely diagnosis in this clinical scenario is infective endocarditis associated with:

a. Complicating ostium secundum atrial septal defect with chronic pulmonary hypertension
b. Complicating pulmonary stenosis and regurgitation
c. Severe mitral regurgitation, mitral prolapse, ruptured chord, and "posterior leaflet syndrome"
d. Severe mitral regurgitation, mitral prolapse, ruptured chord, and "anterior leaflet syndrome"
e. A congenitally bicuspid aortic valve with aortic stenosis and regurgitation

Answers

1. Answer a

A bisferiens pulse, which has a rapid initial upstroke and an interruption at peak followed by a second outward impulse (giving the pulse a bifid character), occurs in selected cases of aortic regurgitation and especially with combined aortic regurgitation and aortic stenosis. It is not found in isolated, severe aortic stenosis. The other choices, including a slowed carotid upstroke, delayed peak, and reduced pulse volume, are classic for severe aortic stenosis. A palpable "shudder" is found in some cases of severe aortic stenosis.

2. Answer e

An ejection sound, typically heard in the presence of a bicuspid aortic valve, usually disappears as the aortic valve becomes calcified and immobile. The presence of an ejection sound provides a clue to the cause (i.e., bicuspid aortic valve) but not the severity. Paradoxic splitting of S_2 can be heard, especially in younger patients, and is a manifestation of significant aortic obstruction when it is found. In older patients, as the aortic valve becomes calcified and restricted in its motion, the aortic component becomes inaudible and S_2 is single. An S_3 in an adult patient with aortic stenosis implies cardiac decompensation. An S_4 in an adolescent is a manifestation of left ventricular hypertrophy and also implies significant aortic stenosis in this age group. A prolonged, late-peaking systolic ejection murmur is typical for severe aortic stenosis.

3. Answer b

The aortic ejection sound implies valvular abnormality (e.g., bicuspid aortic valve) but can also be heard in some patients with systemic hypertension. It is not typical of hypertrophic obstructive cardiomyopathy. A mid to late (nonejection) sound can be heard in some patients. The other findings, although not necessarily present in every patient, are nonetheless typical diagnostic features, including an S4, a carotid pulse with a bifid, "jerky" quality, and the apical impulse having three outward (positive) waves (also referred to as the "triple ripple"). An S_3 is present in some patients with hypertrophic obstructive cardiomyopathy who are "rapid fillers" (with normal left ventricular systolic function) and can also be heard when left ventricular systolic decompensation is present.

4. Answer c

This is a complex and challenging case from the standpoint of the examination and requires synthesis of all of the clinical findings. You are told that multivalvular disease is present. The presence of a normal second heart sound, in which case both components of S_2 are audible (including the aortic component by definition), and the variable but brisk upstroke of the carotid pulse and the characteristics of the systolic murmur (holosystolic rather than ejection type) are not consistent with aortic stenosis. A mid-diastolic rumbling murmur at the apex may be due to either mitral stenosis or an "Austin Flint" murmur. In this case it represents mitral stenosis. The high-pitched early diastolic sound is an opening snap of the mitral valve and is often widely transmitted throughout the precordium, as opposed to the diastolic murmur, which is very localized to the apex in mitral stenosis. The slow Y descent of the jugular venous waveform and a mid-diastolic murmur at the left sternal border which augments with inspiration are important clues to the presence of tricuspid stenosis. The characteristics of the systolic murmurs are not typical of either aortic or pulmonary stenosis (which are ejection in quality). The holosystolic murmur at the lower and mid-sternal border which augments with inspiration represents tricuspid regurgitation.

5. Answer c

Augmentation after a long cycle length does not typically happen with mitral regurgitation (which this apical systolic murmur represents). The increase in murmur intensity following a long cardiac cycle length (such as with atrial fibrillation) typically occurs with stenotic lesions, rather than regurgitant ones. The presence of atrial fibrillation should suggest the presence of mitral valve disease in this clinical setting. The enlarged, displaced apical impulse is consistent with left ventricular enlargement. Although there are other rare causes of multivalvular heart disease in a female of this age, it is most likely "post-inflammatory" (rheumatic) in cause.

6. Answer a

Atrial septal defect by itself (either ostium secundum or sinus venosus type) is not typically associated with a palpable thrill, nor is patent ductus arteriosus. Although pulmonary stenosis can produce a thrill, especially when it is severe, it is typically located at the upper left sternal border, it is ejection in type, and S_2 is not normal. (S_2 is either widely split or single as the pulmonary component diminishes.) The presence of a short diastolic (in this case, flow) rumble at the apex is related to the left-to-right shunt (volume effect) that is present and is not typically seen with pulmonary stenosis. The murmur of patent ductus arteriosus is typically audible at the upper left sternal border or infraclavicular area and peaks at the time of S_2.

7. Answer c

The predominant jugular venous waveform in atrial septal defect is a V wave. The pulmonary component of S_2 that is audible at the apex is typical for atrial septal defect. A pulmonary ejection sound related to increased flow and expansion of the pulmonary artery (due to the left-to-right shunt) is also typical, as is the systolic ejection (flow) murmur over the pulmonary area. Wide, persistent splitting of S_2 is classic for atrial septal defect.

8. Answer b

The presence of systemic hypertension in a patient of this age should raise the possibility of secondary causes of hypertension, including coarctation of the aorta. Missing from the clinical description is the notation of palpation of the femoral pulses, which are typically either diminished in amplitude or delayed (in comparison with simultaneous palpation of the radial artery). The palpable A wave of the apical impulse reflects the presence of left ventricular hypertrophy. An ejection sound at the upper right sternal border (although possibly related to the hypertension itself) should raise the possibility of a concomitant bicuspid aortic valve (which should be suspected in patients with coarctation even if this sign is absent). Likewise, the early decrescendo diastolic murmur at the upper right sternal border and left sternal edge is related to aortic regurgitation due to the same abnormality, possible aggravated by the systemic hypertension. The murmur of patent ductus arteriosus peaks at the time of the second heart sound and usually has a diastolic component. The systolic murmur of coarctation can sometimes be heard in the posterior thorax. The presence of a normal second heart sound and the other clinical findings are against the diagnosis of atrial septal defect. The second heart sound is typically abnormal (widely split or single, from loss of the pulmonary component with pulmonary stenosis). Likewise, the associated murmur of pulmonic regurgitation, if present, is more likely to be heard along the upper left sternal border. (Refer to question 6 for the findings of ventricular septal defect.)

9. Answer d

The history and clinical findings are consistent with systemic venous congestion. The jugular venous pressure is increased with a rapid Y descent. The third heart sound along the left sternal border and apex, which is typically high-pitched and may vary with respiration, is consistent with a "pericardial knock." The hepatic enlargement and edema are consistent with systemic venous congestion. With dilated cardiomyopathy and biventricular failure, the jugular venous pressure would demonstrate prominent A and V waves (assuming normal sinus rhythm is present). The apical impulse, although possibly hypokinetic, should still be visibly or palpably enlarged. Likewise, parasternal lift representing right ventricular overload also may be present.

One would expect murmurs of mitral or tricuspid regurgitation related to atrioventricular annular dilation in dilated cardiomyopathy. The appearance of the jugular venous waveform is not compatible with pulmonary hypertension (which causes prominent A waves), and the pulmonary component of S_2 is normal, also arguing against the presence of severe pulmonary hypertension. A normal S_2P does not exclude milder degrees of pulmonary hypertension. Pericardial tamponade may also produce a "quiet heart" on palpation, but the typical jugular venous waveform shows a prominent X descent more frequently than a prominent Y descent. With tamponade, there should not be a third heart sound present unless there is combined effusive-constrictive pericarditis or another cause of S_3. The jugular venous waveform is not consistent with atrial septal defect, which is associated with a predominant V wave. Likewise, the normal physiologic response of S_2 (even though S_2 is prominently split) is not consistent with atrial septal defect.

10. Answer a

Think of this diagnosis in a patient who has any combination of angina pectoris, dyspnea, or exertional dizziness or syncope (the "triad" of left ventricular outflow tract obstruction). The bifid carotid pulse is typical of hypertrophic cardiomyopathy with obstruction, as is the bifid sustained apical impulse. A third impulse may be found in some cases (sometimes referred to as the "triple ripple," trifid). The paradoxic split S_2 (in the absence of left bundle branch block) is an important physical sign that, in this setting, suggests significant left ventricular outflow tract obstruction. Paradoxic splitting of S_2 should not be present in pulmonary stenosis. It could be heard in severe aortic stenosis, especially in young patients, but the bifid carotid pulse with the rapid upstroke is not consistent with this diagnosis. Likewise, the data do not support combined aortic stenosis and tricuspid stenosis. Atrial septal defect does not cause paradoxic splitting of the second heart sound, nor the palpable abnormalities of the carotid pulse and apical impulse as described in this case. Bedside physiologic maneuvers should be considered when a systolic murmur is audible in a patient with this history or when the cause of a systolic murmur is unclear (see question 11).

11. Answer b

Prompt squatting would be expected to decrease the systolic murmur of hypertrophic cardiomyopathy by the combination of increased venous return and increased systemic vascular resistance. All the other maneuvers listed would be expected to augment the intensity of the systolic murmur, including the Valsalva maneuver, arising to the upright position after squatting (reduced ventricular volume), amyl nitrite administration, and the augmentation after a premature ventricular contraction (post-ectopic potentiation).

12. Answer c

The clinical history should obviously alert the examiner to the possibility of an infection. A heart murmur since childhood, although possibly related to rheumatic heart disease, in this case reflects long-standing mitral valve prolapse. The transmission of the murmur to the left sternal border and the base of the heart is related to the anterior direction of the mitral regurgitant jet, in turn related to a ruptured chord subserving the posterior mitral valve leaflet. The murmur is directed anteriorly and is heard in the upper chest region (at the base). Although there is a predominant V wave in the jugular venous waveform and S_2 is prominently split, it does vary normally with respiration, arguing against atrial septal defect. The pulmonic component of S_2 would not be expected to be increased in pulmonary stenosis, and the quality (pansystolic as opposed to ejection type) and location of the murmur are not typical of pulmonary stenosis. (In severe pulmonary stenosis, the murmur may be widely transmitted, however.) The "anterior mitral valve leaflet syndrome" would be expected to direct the mitral regurgitant jet posteriorly, which then can be heard in the axilla and over the posterior thorax, including the thoracic spine, and even at the base of the skull posteriorly. The physical findings (e.g., the hyperdynamic carotid pulse) are not compatible with a congenital bicuspid aortic valve with aortic stenosis and regurgitation (although it would be compatible with severe, *isolated* aortic regurgitation, in which case the pulse pressure also would be expected to be wide). The harsh pansystolic (as opposed to ejection type) murmur at the apex and left sternal border is unusual for aortic stenosis, especially in this age group. On occasion, the systolic murmur of aortic stenosis can be heard loudest or even localized to the apex, especially in the elderly. The diastolic rumble following S_3 is related to increased forward flow across the mitral valve and should be differentiated from the diastolic murmur of aortic regurgitation, which immediately follows S_2, a subtle but important bedside clinical feature. At 50 years old, a patient with a congenital bicuspid aortic valve frequently would have an ejection sound also (although this is not a consistent feature).

Chapter 23

Valvular Stenosis

Rick A. Nishimura, M.D.

Aortic Stenosis

Definition and Causes

Aortic stenosis is a disease in which there is progressive obstruction to left ventricular outflow which results in the following: 1) pressure hypertrophy of the left ventricle; 2) symptoms of angina, dyspnea, and syncope; and 3) if untreated, death. The presentation, diagnosis, and eventual treatment of aortic stenosis depend on the cause and severity of the outflow obstruction. The causes can be divided into supravalvular aortic stenosis, fixed subvalvular aortic stenosis, and valvular aortic stenosis (Table 1). Valvular aortic stenosis has many causes, including congenital, unicuspid, or bicuspid aortic valves, rheumatic heart disease, and senile degenerative disease. Two-dimensional/Doppler echocardiography can be used to determine reliably the level of obstruction and to assess the severity of obstruction.

Supravalvular Aortic Stenosis

Supravalvular aortic stenosis is a congenital abnormality in which the ascending aorta superior to the aortic valve is narrowed. This is the rarest site of aortic stenosis. The stenosis is seen as either a single discrete constriction or a long tubular narrowing. Important associations with supravalvular aortic stenosis include elfin facies, hypercalcemia, and peripheral pulmonic stenosis. The diagnosis of supravalvular aortic stenosis should be suspected in a young patient who has a left ventricular outflow murmur. Typically,

a thrill is felt on palpation of the right carotid artery but not of the left one, because the obstructive jet is directed toward the innominate artery. The diagnosis can be made on the basis of two-dimensional echocardiography (visualization of the narrowed ascending aorta) and Doppler echocardiography (provides information about the magnitude of the obstruction). Aortic root angiography or transesophageal echocardiography may be required to show the extent of narrowing of the ascending aorta if surgical intervention is contemplated.

Subvalvular Aortic Stenosis

Discrete subvalvular stenosis is seen in approximately 10% of all patients with aortic stenosis. It can be secondary to a subvalvular ridge that extends into the left ventricular

Table 1.—Causes of Aortic Stenosis

Supravalvular
Subvalvular
Discrete
Tunnel
Valvular
Congenital (1 to 30 years old)
Bicuspid (40 to 60 years old)
Rheumatic (40 to 60 years old)
Senile degenerative (> 70 years old)

outflow tract or to a tunnel-like narrowing of the outflow tract. The obstruction is frequently accompanied by aortic regurgitation due to malformation of the aortic valve from the high-velocity jet emanating from the subvalvular obstruction. The diagnosis can be made at the time of echocardiography by visualization of a narrowing or discrete subvalvular ridge extending into the left ventricular outflow tract and a high-velocity turbulence on continuous-wave Doppler echocardiography. A discrete ridge may be difficult to visualize directly in older patients, but it should be suspected when there is high-velocity flow across the outflow tract in the presence of a structurally normal aortic valve with early systolic closure. If the site of obstruction is not visualized on the initial echocardiogram, transesophageal echocardiography should be performed to confirm the diagnosis.

The diagnosis of subvalvular aortic stenosis needs to be differentiated from the dynamic outflow obstruction of hypertrophic obstructive cardiomyopathy, because their treatment differs. Many cardiologists recommend resection of the discrete subvalvular stenosis in all patients who are candidates for operation, both to relieve the degree of left ventricular outflow obstruction and to prevent progressive aortic regurgitation. The treatment of patients with hypertrophic obstructive cardiomyopathy is discussed in the chapter on cardiomyopathy.

- Supravalvular aortic stenosis is associated with elfin facies, hypercalcemia, and peripheral pulmonic stenosis.
- Supravalvular aortic stenosis should be suspected when there is a palpable thrill in the right carotid artery.
- Discrete subvalvular aortic stenosis presents with a high Doppler velocity across the aortic outflow tract and a structurally normal aortic valve on two-dimensional echocardiography.

> Be alert for supravalvular or subvalvular aortic stenosis in a young person presenting with signs and symptoms of aortic stenosis but with a normal aortic valve on echocardiography.

Valvular Aortic Stenosis

Obstruction at the valvular level accounts for most cases of aortic stenosis. The cause depends on the age at presentation. In patients who have symptomatic aortic stenosis in their teens and early twenties, the cause is usually a congenitally unicuspid or fused bicuspid aortic valve. Patients in their forties to sixties who have symptoms usually have a calcified bicuspid aortic valve or the stenosis may be the end result of rheumatic heart disease. In the 1990s, the most common presentation is an elderly patient who has senile degeneration of the valve, with calcific deposits at the base of the cusps in the absence of commissural fusion.

- The most common cause of aortic stenosis in the 1990s is senile degenerative changes.
- In patients with aortic stenosis due to rheumatic disease, "silent" mitral stenosis should be ruled out.
- A bicuspid or rheumatic cause should be suspected in a patient with aortic stenosis who presents in the sixth decade of life.

Pathophysiology

Progressive left ventricular outflow obstruction results in concentric pressure hypertrophy of the left ventricle caused by an increase in left ventricular wall thickness. The increase in wall thickness is a compensatory mechanism to "normalize" wall stress. In most patients, the size of the left ventricular cavity remains normal and systolic function is usually well preserved. When the left ventricle fails to compensate for the long-standing pressure overload, ventricular dilatation and progressive decrease in systolic function occur.

The pathophysiology of aortic stenosis is due to the following: 1) increase in afterload, 2) decrease in systemic and coronary flow from obstruction, and 3) progressive hypertrophy. These mechanisms result in the classic symptom triad of dyspnea, angina, and syncope. Exertional dyspnea is common, even in the presence of normal systolic function. Abnormalities of diastolic function are common in patients with aortic stenosis and result in increased left ventricular filling pressures that are reflected onto the pulmonary circulation. Diastolic dysfunction occurs from prolonged ventricular relaxation and decreased compliance and is caused by myocardial ischemia, a thick noncompliant left ventricle, and increased afterload. Symptoms of exertional angina may be present in the absence of epicardial coronary artery obstruction. Myocardial ischemia results from myocardial oxygen supply/demand mismatch due to high diastolic pressure, decreased myocardial perfusion gradient, and increased myocardial mass. The cause of exertional syncope is multifactorial and may include ventricular arrhythmias, a sudden decrease in systemic flow caused by the obstruction, or abnormal vasodepressor reflexes caused by the high left ventricular intracavitary pressure. As progressive, long-standing pressure overload is placed upon the left ventricle, systolic decompensation may occur from the afterload mismatch and lead to symptoms of both left-sided and right-sided heart failure.

A "death spiral" may occur in patients with critical aortic stenosis. With the onset of systemic hypotension (due to either drugs or a vasovagal reaction), perfusion of the coronary arteries may decrease. This increases the myocardial oxygen demand/supply mismatch and results in myocardial ischemia. The myocardial ischemia, in turn, reduces forward cardiac output, and aortic diastolic pressure decreases, further decreasing coronary perfusion pressure. Unless immediate steps are taken to increase perfusion pressure, progressive hemodynamic deterioration and death may occur.

- Diastolic dysfunction is due to abnormalities of relaxation and compliance and is one of the primary pathophysiologic processes present in patients with aortic stenosis.
- Myocardial ischemia occurs in patients with aortic stenosis despite normal epicardial coronary arteries, because of myocardial oxygen demand/supply mismatch.
- The most common cause of syncope in patients with aortic stenosis is vasodepressor syncope.

> Suspect critical aortic stenosis in a patient with syncope and an aortic murmur.

Clinical Presentation

The clinical presentation of aortic stenosis varies. Patients may be completely asymptomatic and have a heart murmur detected on physical examination. Others have one or more of the classic triad of symptoms of exertional dyspnea, angina, and syncope. Uncommonly, patients with end-stage aortic stenosis and concomitant left ventricular dysfunction present with anasarca and cardiac cachexia. Albeit rare, sudden death may be the initial manifestation of aortic stenosis.

Physical examination of a patient with aortic stenosis reveals classic characteristic findings. Severe aortic stenosis is diagnosed on the basis of a dampened upstroke of the carotid artery, a sustained bifid left ventricular impulse, an absent A_2, and a late-peaking systolic ejection murmur. A concomitant systolic thrill indicates the presence of aortic stenosis (mean gradient, > 50 mm Hg). In some patients, the systolic ejection murmur may be heard with equal intensity at the apex and the base. It is not necessarily the intensity of the murmur that corresponds to the severity of aortic stenosis but

rather the timing of the peak and duration of the murmur. The murmur of aortic stenosis must be differentiated from that of hypertrophic obstructive cardiomyopathy or mitral regurgitation due to a flail posterior leaflet.

> Know how to distinguish between hypertrophic cardiomyopathy and aortic stenosis on the basis of physical examination findings.

Laboratory Tests

Electrocardiography and Radiography
Electrocardiography usually shows normal sinus rhythm with left ventricular hypertrophy. If atrial fibrillation is present, concomitant mitral valve disease or thyroid disease must be suspected. Chest radiography shows left ventricular predominance, with dilatation of the ascending aorta. Aortic calcification is frequently seen on lateral chest radiographs.

Echocardiography
Two-dimensional/Doppler echocardiography is the imaging modality of choice for diagnosing aortic stenosis and estimating its severity. The location of the obstruction (supravalvular, valvular, or subvalvular) can be identified with two-dimensional echocardiography. In patients with valvular aortic stenosis, the cause (bicuspid versus rheumatic versus senile degenerative) may be assessed from the parasternal short-axis view. Although the presence or absence of aortic stenosis is readily diagnosed on two-dimensional echocardiography, the severity of the stenosis cannot be judged on the basis of the two-dimensional echocardiographic image alone.

Doppler echocardiography is an excellent modality for assessing the severity of aortic stenosis. By using the modified Bernoulli equation ($\Delta P = 4v^2$), a maximal instantaneous and mean aortic valve gradient can usually be derived from the continuous-wave Doppler velocity across the aortic valve. However, accurate measurement of the aortic valve gradient requires a detailed, meticulous study using multiple sites of interrogation to ensure that the Doppler beam is parallel to the stenotic jet. In laboratories with experienced echocardiographers, the Doppler-derived aortic valve gradients are accurate and reproducible and correlate well with those obtained with cardiac catheterization. The mean gradient from the integral of the aortic valve velocity curve should be used to determine the severity of aortic stenosis. If the mean gradient is greater than 50 mm Hg, severe aortic stenosis can be diagnosed with certainty. In a patient with clinical findings of severe aortic stenosis and a Doppler-derived mean gradient greater than 50 mm Hg, no other hemodynamic information is needed to assess the severity of stenosis.

Aortic valve gradients depend not only on the severity of obstruction but also on flow. In patients with low cardiac output, the stenosis may still be severe, with mean gradients less than 50 mm Hg. To overcome these problems, an aortic valve area has been derived using the hydraulic equation of Gorlin and Gorlin. In the cardiac catheterization laboratory, the aortic valve area (AVA) is calculated from the pressure gradient and an independent measure of cardiac output.

$$AVA = \frac{1,000 \times CO}{44 \times SEP \times HR \times \sqrt{\Delta P}}$$

where CO = cardiac output, HR = heart rate, and SEP = systolic ejection period.

Two-dimensional/Doppler echocardiography can also provide reliable estimations of aortic valve area by the continuity equation:

$$AVA = \frac{LVOT_{area} \times LVOT_{TVI}}{AV_{TVI}}$$

where AV = aortic valve flow velocity, LVOT = left ventricular outflow tract, and TVI = time velocity integral.

Severe aortic stenosis should be considered if a patient has clinical findings consistent with severe aortic stenosis, a mean gradient greater than 50 mm Hg, and a valve area less than 1.0 cm^2 (Table 2).

There are limitations to using Doppler echocardiography in estimating the severity of aortic stenosis. The major problem occurs when the Doppler beam is not parallel to the aortic stenosis velocity jet, because the mean gradient will be underestimated. Thus, in a patient with the clinical features of severe aortic stenosis but echocardiographic/Doppler findings of mild-to-moderate stenosis, further evaluation with either repeat Doppler echocardiography or cardiac catheterization is required. Doppler echocardiography will not overestimate the mean gradient, except in rare instances of severe anemia (hemoglobin < 8.0 g/dL), a small aortic root, or sequential stenoses in parallel (coexistent left ventricular outflow tract and valvular obstruction). The calculation of aortic valve area with echocardiography is highly dependent on accurate measurement of the diameter of the left ventricular outflow

Table 2.—Criteria for Determining Severity of Aortic Stenosis

Severity	Mean gradient, mm Hg	Aortic valve area, cm^2
Mild	< 25	> 1.5
Moderate	25-50	1.0-1.5
Severe	> 50	< 1.0
Critical	> 80	< 0.7

tract. Thus, special attention must be used when diagnosing severe aortic stenosis in patients with small valve areas but relatively low mean gradients. In these instances, correlation with clinical findings is essential.

If the clinical findings are not consistent with the Doppler echocardiographic results, cardiac catheterization is recommended for further hemodynamic assessment. Cardiac catheterization should consist of the simultaneous measurement of two pressures, one in the left ventricle and one in the aorta, from which a mean gradient can be calculated. A "pull-back" tracing from the left ventricle to the aorta may be used in patients with normal sinus rhythm but is not accurate in patients with irregular rhythms or low-output states. The use of simultaneous left ventricular and femoral artery pressures is not accurate for assessing aortic valve gradient, because there may be a significant difference between central aortic pressure and femoral artery pressure. At the time of cardiac catheterization, cardiac output should be assessed for calculation of valve area, preferably by the Fick method. Thermodilution or green dye curves are used, but these tests have inherent limitations in patients with irregular heart rhythms or low-output states. Coexistent mitral or aortic regurgitation may cause errors in calculation of valve area by cardiac catheterization.

- If atrial fibrillation is present on electrocardiography, suspect mitral valve disease.
- A mean aortic valve gradient greater than 50 mm Hg on Doppler echocardiography should be considered indicative of severe aortic stenosis.
- The major pitfall of Doppler echocardiography is underestimation of the aortic valve gradient.

Natural History and Treatment

The natural history of aortic stenosis is well known. After symptoms occur in a patient with severe aortic stenosis, there is a rapidly progressive downhill course, with a 2- to 3-year mortality of 50%. Therefore, it has been recommended that aortic valve replacement be performed in all patients with severe aortic stenosis who have symptoms. Aortic valve replacement has a low perioperative mortality of less than 5% in young, healthy patients and results in significant improvement of longevity.

Before aortic valve surgery, a complete hemodynamic assessment of the aortic valve with either Doppler echocardiography or cardiac catheterization is required (see below). Left ventricular function and concomitant mitral valve disease should be assessed. Coronary angiography should be performed in older patients who have risk factors for coronary artery disease, but it usually is not required in men younger than 40 years or women younger than 50 years without risk factors. Aortic valve replacement should be performed in all patients with severely symptomatic aortic stenosis, regardless of concomitant left ventricular function. If significant mitral regurgitation is present, the degree of regurgitation should be evaluated intraoperatively after replacement of the aortic valve to determine the need for mitral valve repair or replacement, unless there is intrinsic disease of the mitral valve apparatus.

In the 1990s, an increasing number of elderly patients are presenting with severe aortic stenosis. The risk of aortic valve replacement increases with age and concomitant medical problems. In patients older than 80 years, operative mortality can be as high as 30%. When percutaneous aortic balloon valvuloplasty was introduced 10 years ago, it was thought to be a way of avoiding high operative mortality in elderly patients. By inflating one or more large balloons across the aortic valve from a percutaneous route, a modest decrease in gradient and a significant improvement in symptoms could be achieved in elderly critically ill patients. However, follow-up has demonstrated a high rate of restenosis (> 60% at 6 months and nearly 100% at 2 years), with no decrease in mortality rate after the procedure. Therefore, percutaneous aortic balloon valvuloplasty is used only 1) for critically ill elderly patients who are not candidates for surgical intervention or 2) as a "bridge" in critically ill patients before aortic valve replacement.

- Aortic valve replacement is indicated for patients with symptoms of severe aortic stenosis, regardless of the left ventricular ejection fraction.
- Coronary angiography may not be required preoperatively in younger patients without risk factors for coronary artery disease.

- Percutaneous aortic balloon valvuloplasty is reserved only for critically ill patients as a "bridge" to surgery.

Controversial Issues in the Management of Patients With Aortic Stenosis

Asymptomatic Patients With Severe Aortic Stenosis

Treatment of asymptomatic patients with severe aortic stenosis is a matter of controversy. Advocates of "prophylactic" aortic valve replacement in asymptomatic patients recommend that the procedure be done to prevent sudden death. Recently, several longitudinal studies have shown that the incidence of sudden death in patients who are truly asymptomatic is low. It has been stated that "the most common cause of death in patients with asymptomatic severe aortic stenosis is an operation." Although no hard data support any plan of approach, it is reasonable to follow, closely and serially, asymptomatic patients as long as exercise tolerance is good and left ventricular systolic function is preserved. Exercise testing may be performed carefully to document exercise tolerance and the hemodynamic response to exercise. Surgery should be performed at the onset of symptoms or left ventricular systolic dysfunction. Patients with very high gradients and critical aortic stenosis (gradients > 80 to 90 mm Hg and valve areas < 0.5 cm^2) or those who have limited exercise tolerance may be at higher risk. Surgical treatment may be offered sooner in these patients, especially if there is a low operative risk.

Definition of "Severe" Aortic Stenosis

The definition of severe aortic stenosis varies. Valve areas less than 0.5, less than 0.7, and less than 1.0 cm^2 and a valve area indexed to body surface area less than 0.5 cm^2/m^2 have all been used as criteria for "severe" aortic stenosis. Valve area, especially from a single measurement, should not be used as the sole determinant for the severity of stenosis. The reproducibility of valve area may vary as much as 0.4 to 0.6 cm^2. A valve area for a large man may have a different hemodynamic consequence than the same valve area for a small woman, supporting the concept that valve area should be corrected for body surface area. Studies have shown that the natural history of symptomatic patients with "moderate" aortic stenosis (valve area, 0.7 to 1.2 cm^2) is comparable to the classic natural history of symptomatic patients with "severe" aortic stenosis. The message is that patients should not be treated on the basis of a single determination of valve area in isolation from clinical signs and symptoms. Numerous factors, such as clinical presentation, exercise tolerance, mean gradient, and left ventricular function, should be considered when determining need for aortic valve surgery.

Low-Output/Low-Gradient Aortic Stenosis

Patients may present with low-output/low-gradient aortic stenosis, that is, with a mean aortic valve gradient less than 30 mm Hg and the calculated valve area in the range of "severe" aortic stenosis ($< 1.0 \text{ cm}^2$ or $< 0.5 \text{ cm}^2/\text{m}^2$). These patients may have critical end-stage aortic stenosis in which ventricular function has deteriorated because of progressive afterload on the left ventricle. Aortic valve replacement will result in symptomatic improvement, increased longevity, and return of left ventricular systolic function. However, there may be other patients with a combination of mild calcific valvular aortic stenosis and concomitant left ventricular dysfunction due to another cause. In these patients, the "calculated aortic valve area" is low because the stroke volume is not sufficient to open completely the mildly stenotic aortic valve.

It has been difficult to differentiate these two subsets of patients. Several areas under investigation to separate these two include 1) systolic time intervals ("pseudonormal" ejection time in severe aortic stenosis), 2) the use of dobutamine stress to normalize cardiac output, and 3) "diagnostic" percutaneous aortic balloon valvuloplasty.

Mitral Stenosis

Cause

Most cases of mitral stenosis have a rheumatic cause. The rheumatic process causes "immobility" and thickening of the mitral valve leaflets, with fusion of the commissures. Leaflet calcification and subvalvular fusion occur in the late stages of the disease. In rare instances, the cause may be a congenital abnormality of the mitral valve or a parachute mitral valve. Cor triatriatum is an abnormality that simulates mitral stenosis. In this condition, a thin membrane across the left atrium obstructs pulmonary venous inflow. Left atrial myxoma and pulmonary vein obstruction may also present with signs and symptoms similar to those of mitral stenosis.

Pathophysiology

The pathophysiology of mitral stenosis is related to the increase in left atrial pressure from obstruction across the mitral valve. This increased pressure is reflected onto the pulmonary circulation, causing symptoms of dyspnea, orthopnea, and paroxysmal nocturnal dyspnea.

Unless mitral stenosis is severe, patients do not have symptoms at rest; however, with exercise or the onset of atrial fibrillation, left atrial pressure increases. This is due to the very slow filling from the left atrium to the left ventricle during the shortened diastolic filling period.

In long-standing severe mitral stenosis, secondary pulmonary hypertension may occur and lead to right ventricular failure and tricuspid regurgitation. Symptoms of angina pectoris are rare but may be due to right ventricular hypertrophy and ischemia of the right ventricle. The left ventricle is not affected in pure mitral stenosis.

Pathologically, rheumatic mitral stenosis results in commissural fusion. Secondary effects of the long-standing rheumatic process may involve progressive calcification and fibrosis of the mitral valve leaflets. The rheumatic process can also affect the subvalvular apparatus, leading to shortened and fibrotic chordae.

- The differential diagnosis of mitral stenosis should include cor triatriatum, atrial myxoma, and pulmonary vein obstruction.
- The hallmark of mitral stenosis is commissural fusion.
- The left ventricle is not affected in pure mitral stenosis.

Clinical Presentation

The presentation of mitral stenosis is related to the increase in left atrial pressure, which produces symptoms of dyspnea. The early course of the disease—before the development of symptoms—may last for decades, and symptoms then begin insidiously, with mild dyspnea only on exertion. Frequently, patients are not aware of progressive limitations in exercise because their activity level has decreased imperceptibly over the years. With a severe increase in left atrial pressure, paroxysmal nocturnal dyspnea and orthopnea occur. High pulmonary venous pressures may cause distention of the bronchial veins, and rupture of these veins may result in hemoptysis. Stasis occurs in the enlarged left atrium, especially in the presence of atrial fibrillation, and produces a nidus for thrombus formation. Systemic embolic events are seen in approximately one-third of patients with atrial fibrillation and mitral stenosis and may be the presenting event before the diagnosis of mitral stenosis is made.

Classically, the physical examination of a patient with mitral stenosis consists of a loud first heart sound, an opening snap, and a diastolic rumble. The interval between aortic valve closure and the opening snap is related to left atrial pressure and, thus, can be used to determine the severity of mitral stenosis. Patients with severe mitral stenosis have

A_2-OS intervals shorter than 60 to 70 ms, and those with mild mitral stenosis have A_2-OS intervals longer than 100 to 110 ms. The intensity and duration of the diastolic rumble increase as the gradient across the mitral valve increases. However, because of differences in body habitus and chest cavity, severe mitral stenosis may be present with a barely audible diastolic rumble. If the mitral valve is pliable and noncalcified, the first heart sound will be loud and snappy and the opening snap will be very prominent. With progressive calcification and fibrosis of the leaflets, the first heart sound may diminish in intensity and the opening snap may disappear. The intensity of the pulmonic component of the second heart sound is important to note in determining the severity of coexistent pulmonary hypertension. In patients who do not have a diastolic rumble on initial auscultation, increasing heart rate by mild exercise (sit-ups or step-ups) may bring out a diastolic rumble.

Echocardiography

The standard for diagnosis and determination of the severity of mitral stenosis is two-dimensional/Doppler echocardiography. On two-dimensional echocardiography, the typical hockey-stick deformity of the mitral valve leaflets is easily visualized on the parasternal long-axis view. Commissural fusion and narrowing of the mitral valve opening area are seen on the short-axis view. In patients with adequate echocardiographic images, the area of the mitral valve can be determined planimetrically from the short-axis view if the plane of the two-dimensional view is at the tip of the mitral valve leaflets. Two-dimensional echocardiography is also important in identifying the morphology of the mitral valve leaflets and the subvalvular apparatus.

A grading system has been assigned to determine suitability for mitral valve repair based on two-dimensional features of the following: 1) leaflet thickening, 2) leaflet calcification, 3) leaflet mobility, and 4) subvalvular fusion. Each of the four morphological features is assigned a score from 1 to 4, with 1 being the least involvement and 4, the most severe involvement. The mitral score is the sum of these four numbers. A score of 8 or less is indicative of a pliable noncalcified valve that should be suitable for balloon valvuloplasty or commissurotomy. Alternatively, a score of 10 or greater indicates a calcified fibrotic valve with subvalvular fusion that may not be appropriate for valve repair. Calcification of the commissures may also preclude adequate valve repair.

Determining the severity of obstruction across the mitral valve requires measuring the mean mitral valve gradient and calculating mitral valve area. By conventional criteria, mild mitral stenosis is present when the mean gradient is less than 5 mm Hg; moderate stenosis, 5 to 10 mm Hg; and severe stenosis, greater than 10 mm Hg. These values apply to patients with normal cardiac output and heart rates within the physiologic range of 60 to 90 beats/min. Previously, cardiac catheterization was needed to determine the mitral valve gradient. However, Doppler echocardiography can measure the mean mitral valve gradient accurately and reproducibly. Doppler determination of mitral valve mean gradient is more accurate than that of conventional cardiac catheterization, when using pulmonary artery wedge pressure and left ventricular pressures.

The mean mitral valve gradient depends not only on the degree of obstruction but also on flow and the diastolic filling period. A calculated mitral valve area incorporates all these factors. By convention, an area less than 1.0 cm^2 indicates severe mitral stenosis; 1.0 to 1.5 cm^2, moderate stenosis; and greater than 1.5 cm^2, mild stenosis (Table 3). The hydraulic Gorlin equation has been the standard for calculating mitral valve area (MVA) in cardiac catheterization laboratories.

$$MVA = \frac{1{,}000 \text{ x CO}}{38 \text{ x HR x DFP x } \sqrt{\Delta P}}$$

where CO = cardiac output, DFP = diastolic filling period, and HR = heart rate.

The Gorlin equation has limitations and is not applicable at low or high cardiac outputs. It is erroneous with concomitant mitral regurgitation. In addition, the determination of cardiac output by cardiac catheterization can be misleading, especially in the presence of atrial fibrillation and concomitant tricuspid regurgitation.

Doppler echocardiography uses the concept of a diastolic half-time to estimate mitral valve area. The diastolic half-time, initially described at cardiac catheterization, is the time it takes for the maximal mitral gradient to decrease by 50%. It is inversely related to valve area. In most patients, an accurate measurement of mitral valve area (MVA) can be obtained from the rate of velocity decrease during early and mid-diastole, as assessed on the transmitral velocity curve.

$$t_{1/2} = DT \text{ x } 0.29$$

$$MVA = \frac{220}{t_{1/2}}$$

Table 3.—Criteria for Determining Severity of Mitral Stenosis

Severity	Gradient, mm Hg	Mitral valve area, cm^2
Mild	< 5.0	> 1.5
Moderate	5.0-10.0	1.0-1.5
Severe	> 10.0	< 1.0

where $t_{1/2}$ = half-time and DT = deceleration time.

There are limitations to using the diastolic half-time, especially when abnormalities of left atrial and left ventricular compliance exist. In these instances, the mitral valve area (MVA) should be calculated with the continuity equation:

$$MVA = \frac{LVOT_{TVI} \times LVOT_{area}}{MV_{TVI}}$$

where LVOT = left ventricular outflow tract, MV = mitral valve, and TVI = time velocity integral.

- Doppler echocardiography is more accurate than cardiac catheterization for determining the mean mitral valve gradient.
- Suitability for valvuloplasty should be assessed with two-dimensional echocardiography and based on the mitral score and appearance of the commissures.
- The continuity equation for mitral valve area should be used when the area derived from the half-time does not correlate with the mean transmitral gradient.

Natural History and Treatment

Mitral stenosis is a disease of plateaus. There is a period of 1 to 2 decades after the onset of rheumatic fever before signs of mitral stenosis appear. This is followed by another period of 1 to 2 decades before mild symptoms occur. Mild symptoms of dyspnea on exertion may be present for another 1 to 2 decades. During this time, the onset of atrial fibrillation may cause further decompensation, but this can be treated by rate control. Finally, severe New York Heart Association class III or IV symptoms develop. Indications for mitral valve replacement include a combination of severe mitral stenosis and New York Heart Association functional class III-IV symptoms, with significant limitation of lifestyle. With the advent of percutaneous mitral balloon valvuloplasty, it may be reasonable to perform balloon valvuloplasty earlier

if the patient is a good candidate for this procedure from the morphological standpoint.

In determining the need for intervention, it is necessary to correlate the symptoms with the gradient and, subsequently, mitral valve area. Some patients may have significant symptoms but a mitral valve gradient and mitral valve area that are consistent with only a mild-to-moderate degree of mitral stenosis (gradient < 10 mm Hg and/or mitral valve area > 1.5 cm^2). What may be a mild degree of obstruction for one patient may be a significant degree of obstruction for another.

In patients whose symptoms are out of proportion to the calculated mitral valve indices, the hemodynamic response to exercise should be measured. Previously, this was assessed at catheterization of the right and left sides of the heart with exercise. However, exercise Doppler echocardiography can provide all the information required. For this, the patient undergoes a treadmill or supine bicycle exercise test until symptoms occur. Mean mitral valve gradient and pulmonary artery systolic pressure should be measured at peak exercise. If the mean gradient dramatically increases more than 20 to 25 mm Hg concomitant with symptoms, the patient should be considered symptomatic on the basis of the mitral valve disease. Alternatively, if symptoms occur and the mitral valve gradient does not increase to those levels, another cause for the symptoms must be pursued. In patients with a mitral valve mean gradient that does not correlate with mitral valve area, other Doppler estimates of mitral valve area must be considered, including the continuity equation or proximal isovelocity surface area calculations.

The operations for mitral stenosis have consisted of closed commissurotomy, open commissurotomy, and mitral valve replacement. Closed commissurotomy was an effective procedure used before the institution of cardiopulmonary bypass. Through a lateral thoracotomy, the surgeon would attempt to split the commissural fusion with a finger or dilator. This was successful in most patients with noncalcified valves but was inadequate for those with calcified fibrotic valves and subvalvular fusion. With the advent of cardiopulmonary bypass, open commissurotomy became the procedure of choice. This requires a median sternotomy and cardiopulmonary bypass. The surgeon directly inspects the mitral valve apparatus and incises the commissures under direct vision, with chordal reconstruction if necessary. For patients with a mitral valve not believed to be suitable for commissurotomy, mitral valve replacement is performed.

Recently, percutaneous mitral balloon valvuloplasty has become an acceptable alternative to mitral valve surgery in selected patients. Fused commissures can be split with one or more large balloons inflated across the mitral valve. This can produce hemodynamic improvement comparable to that of both closed and open commissurotomy. Percutaneous mitral balloon valvuloplasty requires expertise, including the capability for performing a transseptal puncture. However, in experienced hands, the results are excellent and comparable to those of surgery, with the valve area typically increasing from 1.0 to 2.0 cm^2. In several randomized trials comparing mitral balloon valvuloplasty with closed and open surgical commissurotomy, the acute results and long-term outcome have been comparable in young patients with pliable valves. Potential complications, such as systemic embolus, severe mitral regurgitation, and left ventricular perforation, can be avoided by preoperative assessment of

mitral valve morphology and documentation of lack of atrial thrombus by transesophageal echocardiography. In selected patients, percutaneous mitral balloon valvuloplasty should be considered not only in those with New York Heart Association class III or IV symptoms but also in those with class II symptoms who have high resting gradients or pulmonary hypertension.

- Mitral stenosis is a disease of plateaus.
- Exercise hemodynamics should be performed in patients with symptoms out of proportion to calculated mitral valve gradient and area.
- Percutaneous mitral balloon valvuloplasty may be the procedure of choice for patients with mitral stenosis and a noncalcified pliable mitral valve.

Appendix

ACC/AHA Recommendations for Valvular Disease[*][†]

Recommendations for Echocardiography in Aortic Stenosis

Indication	Class
1. Diagnosis and assessment of severity of AS	I
2. Assessment of LV size, function, and/or hemodynamics	I
3. Reevaluation of patients with known AS with changing symptoms or signs	I
4. Assessment of changes in hemodynamic severity and ventricular function in patients with known AS during pregnancy	I
5. Reevaluation of asymptomatic patients with severe AS	I
6. Reevaluation of asymptomatic patients with mild to moderate AS and evidence of LV dysfunction or hypertrophy	IIa
7. Routine reevaluation of asymptomatic adult patients with mild AS having stable physical signs and normal LV size and function	III

From the ACC/AHA Guidelines for the Clinical Application of Echocardiography.

Recommendations for Cardiac Catheterization in Aortic Stenosis

Indication	Class
1. Coronary angiography before AVR in patients at risk for CAD	I
2. Assessment of severity of AS in symptomatic patients when AVR is planned or when noninvasive tests are inconclusive or there is a discrepancy with clinical findings regarding severity of AS or need for surgery	I
3. Assessment of severity of AS before AVR when noninvasive tests are adequate and concordant with clinical findings and coronary angiography is not needed	IIb
4. Assessment of LV function and severity of AS in asymptomatic patients when noninvasive tests are adequate	III

[*]From J Am Coll Cardiol 32:1486-1588, 1998. By permission of the American College of Cardiology.
[†]The abbreviations used in the recommendations are listed at the end of the Appendix.

Recommendations for Aortic Valve Replacement in Aortic Stenosis

Indication	Class
1. Symptomatic patients with severe AS	I
2. Patients with severe AS undergoing coronary artery bypass surgery	I
3. Patients with severe AS undergoing surgery on the aorta or other heart valves	I
4. Patients with moderate AS undergoing coronary artery bypass surgery or surgery on the aorta or other heart valves	IIa
5. Asymptomatic patients with severe AS and	
LV systolic dysfunction	IIa
Abnormal response to exercise (e.g., hypotension)	IIa
Ventricular tachycardia	IIb
Marked or excessive LV hypertrophy ($\geq$ 15 mm)	IIb
Valve area < 0.6 cm^2	IIb
6. Prevention of sudden death in asymptomatic patients with none of the findings listed under indication 5	III

Recommendations for Aortic Balloon Valvotomy in Adults With Aortic Stenosis

Indication	Class
1. A "bridge" to surgery in hemodynamically unstable patients who are at high risk for AVR	IIa
2. Palliation in patients with serious comorbid conditions	IIb
3. Patients who require urgent noncardiac surgery	IIb
4. An alternative to AVR	III

Recommendations for Anticoagulation in Mitral Stenosis

Indication	Class
1. Patients with atrial fibrillation, paroxysmal or chronic	I
2. Patients with previous embolic event	I
3. Patients with severe MS and left atrial dimension $\geq$ 55 mm by echocardiography*	IIb
4. All other patients with MS	III

*Based on grade C recommendation given this indication by American College of Chest Physicians Fourth Consensus Conference on Antithrombotic Therapy. The Working Group of the European Society of Cardiology recommended a lower threshold of left atrial dimension (> 50 mm) for recommending anticoagulation.

Recommendations for Cardiac Catheterization in Mitral Stenosis

Indication	Class
1. Perform percutaneous mitral balloon valvotomy in properly selected patients	I
2. Assess severity of MR in patients being considered for percutaneous mitral balloon valvotomy when clinical and echocardiographic data are discordant	IIa
3. Assess pulmonary artery, left atrial, and LV diastolic pressures when symptoms and/or estimated pulmonary artery pressure are discordant with the severity of MS by 2-D and Doppler echocardiography	IIa
4. Assess hemodynamic response of pulmonary artery and left atrial pressures to stress when clinical symptoms and resting hemodynamics are discordant	IIa
5. Assess mitral valve hemodynamics when 2-D and Doppler echocardiographic data are concordant with clinical findings	III

Recommendations for Percutaneous Mitral Balloon Valvotomy

Indication	Class
1. Symptomatic patients (NYHA functional class II, III, or IV), moderate or severe MS (MVA ≤ 1.5 cm^2),* and valve morphology favorable for percutaneous balloon valvotomy in the absence of left atrial thrombus or moderate to severe MR	I
2. Asymptomatic patients with moderate or severe MS (MVA ≤ 1.5 cm^2)* and valve morphology favorable for percutaneous balloon valvotomy who have pulmonary hypertension (pulmonary artery systolic pressure > 50 mm Hg at rest or 60 mm Hg with exercise) in the absence of left atrial thrombus or moderate to severe MR	IIa
3. Patients with NYHA functional class III-IV symptoms, moderate or severe MS (MVA ≤ 1.5 cm^2),* and a nonpliable calcified valve who are at high risk for surgery in the absence of left atrial thrombus or moderate to severe MR	IIa
4. Asymptomatic patients, moderate or severe MS (MVA ≤ 1.5 cm^2)* and valve morphology favorable for percutaneous balloon valvotomy who have new onset of atrial fibrillation in the absence of left atrial thrombus or moderate to severe MR	
5. Patients in NYHA functional class III-IV, moderate or severe MS (MVA ≤ 1.5 cm^2), and a nonpliable calcified valve who are low-risk candidates for surgery	IIb
6. Patients with mild MS	III

*The committee recognizes that there may be variability in the measurement of MVA and that the mean transmitral gradient, pulmonary artery wedge pressure, and pulmonary artery pressure at rest or during exercise should also be taken into consideration.

Recommendations for Mitral Valve Repair for Mitral Stenosis

Indication	Class
1. Patients with NYHA functional class III-IV symptoms, moderate or severe MS (MVA ≤ 1.5 cm^2),* and valve morphology favorable for repair if percutaneous mitral balloon valvotomy is not available	I
2. Patients with NYHA functional class III-IV symptoms, moderate or severe MS (MVA) ≤ 1.5 cm^2,* and valve morphology favorable for repair if a left atrial thrombus is present despite anticoagulation	I
3. Patients with NYHA functional class III-IV symptoms, moderate or severe MS (MVA ≤ 1.5 cm^2),* and a nonpliable or calcified valve with the decision to proceed with either repair or replacement made at the time of the operation	I
4. Patients in NYHA functional class I, moderate or severe MS (MVA ≤ 1.5 cm^2),* and valve morphology favorable for repair who have had recurrent episodes of embolic events on adequate anticoagulation	IIb
5. Patients with NYHA functional class I-IV symptoms and mild MS	III

*The committee recognizes that there may be a variability in the measurement of MVA and that the mean transmitral gradient, pulmonary artery wedge pressure, and pulmonary artery pressure at rest or during exercise should also be considered.

Recommendations for Mitral Valve Replacement for Mitral Stenosis

Indication	Class
1. Patients with moderate or severe MS (MVA ≤ 1.5 cm^2)* and NYHA functional class III-IV symptoms who are not considered candidates for percutaneous balloon valvotomy or mitral valve repair	I
2. Patients with severe MS (MVA ≤ 1 cm^2)* and severe pulmonary hypertension (pulmonary artery systolic pressure > 60 to 80 mm Hg) with NYHA functional class I-II symptoms who are not considered candidates for percutaneous balloon valvotomy or mitral valve repair	IIa

*The committee recognizes that there may be a variability in the measurement of MVA and that the mean transmitral gradient, pulmonary artery wedge pressure, and pulmonary artery pressure should also be considered.

Abbreviations

ACC/AHA	American College of Cardiology/American Heart Association
AS	aortic stenosis
AVR	aortic valve replacement
CAD	coronary artery disease
LV	left ventricular
MR	mitral regurgitation
MS	mitral stenosis
MVA	mitral valve area
NYHA	New York Heart Association

Suggested Review Reading

1. ACC/AHA guidelines for the management of patients with valvular heart disease. A report of the American College of Cardiology/American Heart Association. Task Force on Practice Guidelines (Committee on Management of Patients With Valvular Heart Disease). *J Am Coll Cardiol* 32:1486-1588, 1998.
Guidelines for valvular heart disease written by a select group of cardiologists who have expertise in valvular heart disease. It is the first of its kind and considers in detail the pathophysiology, presentation, evaluation, and treatment of valvular heart disease. This is an excellent reference that covers all aspects of valvular heart disease.

2. Ben Farhat M, Ayari M, Maatouk F, et al: Percutaneous balloon versus surgical closed and open mitral commissurotomy: seven-year follow-up results of a randomized trial. *Circulation* 97:245-250, 1998.
A long-term follow-up study of a randomized trial of percutaneous mitral balloon valvuloplasty versus closed commissurotomy and open commissurotomy performed in young patients with pliable mitral valve leaflets. The results of mitral balloon valvuloplasty are comparable with those of open heart surgery. This supports the usefulness of mitral balloon valvuloplasty in patients with pliable mitral valve leaflets.

3. Carabello BA, Green LH, Grossman W, et al: Hemodynamic determinants of prognosis of aortic valve replacement in critical aortic stenosis and advanced congestive heart failure. *Circulation* 62:42-48, 1980.
A classic article that describes the determinants of prognosis in patients with critical aortic stenosis and congestive heart failure. Patients who had gradients < 30 mm Hg had a very poor outcome. These are the patients with the "low output low gradient" state, in which the aortic valve areas are calculated to be "severe." However, in these patients, calculation of aortic valve area may be erroneous because the ventricle may not have enough power to open the valve. These patients may actually have mild aortic stenosis and concomitant left ventricular systolic dysfunction.

4. Connolly HM, Oh JK, Orszulak TA, et al: Aortic valve replacement for aortic stenosis with severe left ventricular dysfunction. Prognostic indicators. *Circulation* 95:2395-2400, 1997.
Description of the prognosis of patients with left ventricular dysfunction who undergo aortic valve replacement. In the modern era, the mortality is < 10%, especially in patients with a high gradient.

5. Frank S, Johnson A, Ross J Jr: Natural history of valvular aortic stenosis. *Br Heart J* 35:41-46, 1973.
The classic article describing the natural history of valvular aortic stenosis. With the onset of symptoms, the decrease in survival is significant, with a 2-year mortality rate of 50%.

6. Gorlin R, Gorlin SG. Hydraulic formula for calculation of the area of the stenotic mitral valve, other cardiac valves, and central circulatory shunts (part 1). *Am Heart J* 41:1-29, 1951.
The classic article describing the Gorlin equation used for calculating aortic valve area by cardiac catheterization.

7. Hatle L, Brubakk A, Tromsdal A, et al: Noninvasive assessment of pressure drop in mitral stenosis by Doppler ultrasound. *Br Heart J* 40:131-140, 1978.
A classic article describing the usefulness of Doppler echocardiography in assessing the mean gradient across the mitral valve in mitral stenosis.

8. Nishimura RA, Holmes DR Jr, Reeder GS: Percutaneous balloon valvuloplasty. *Mayo Clin Proc* 65:198-220, 1990.
A review article describing the usefulness of percutaneous balloon valvuloplasty in patients with aortic and mitral stenosis.

9. Orrange SE, Kawanishi DT, Lopez BM, et al: Actuarial outcome after catheter balloon commissurotomy in patients with mitral stenosis. *Circulation* 95:382-389, 1997.
A study of a large number of patients who were followed for more than 7 years after percutaneous mitral balloon valvotomy. It supports the concept that the procedure can be performed at low risk with an excellent long-term outcome.

10. Otto CM, Burwash IG, Legget ME, et al: Prospective study of asymptomatic valvular aortic stenosis. Clinical, echocardiographic, and exercise predictors of outcome. *Circulation* 95:2262-2270, 1997.
A prospective study using Doppler echocardiography to describe the progression of asymptomatic valvular aortic stenosis. The rate of progression is highly variable. Progression occurs most rapidly with more severe aortic stenosis.

11. Pellikka PA, Nishimura RA, Bailey KR, et al: The natural history of adults with asymptomatic, hemodynamically significant aortic stenosis. *J Am Coll Cardiol* 15:1012-1017, 1990.
Patients with moderate to moderately severe aortic stenosis without symptoms were followed for years. Although some patients eventually required aortic valve replacement, there was no sudden death in the absence of preceding symptoms. Asymptomatic patients with moderately severe aortic stenosis do not necessarily need to undergo operation until the onset of symptoms.

12. Roberts WC, Perloff JK: Mitral valvular disease. A clinicopathologic survey of the conditions causing the mitral valve to function abnormally. *Ann Intern Med* 77:939-975, 1972.
A classic article describing the lesions of mitral stenosis. It describes the thickening, calcification, and fibrosis of the leaflets with subvalvular fusion.

13. Ross J Jr: Afterload mismatch and preload reserve: a conceptual framework for the analysis of ventricular function. *Prog Cardiovasc Dis* 18:255-264, 1976.
An excellent overview of ventricular function in patients with valvular heart disease. It describes changes that occur

in ejection fraction caused by changes in preload and after-load induced by valvular lesions. Also described is the underlying pathophysiologic response of the left ventricle to valvular lesions.

14. Selzer A: Changing aspects of the natural history of valvular aortic stenosis. *N Engl J Med* 317:91-98, 1987.
This classic article is an overview of the changing aspects of natural history of valvular aortic stenosis. It describes the emergence of an older population with senile degenerative aortic stenosis as the most common presentation of aortic stenosis in the 1980s and 1990s.

15. Selzer A, Cohn KE: Natural history of mitral stenosis: a review. *Circulation* 45:878-890, 1972.
A classic article on the natural history of mitral stenosis. Patients with mitral stenosis have a disease of plateaus. After the onset of rheumatic fever and before the onset of symptoms, there is a long asymptomatic period. After the onset of mild symptoms, there is another long period before onset of severe symptoms.

Questions

Multiple Choice (choose the one best answer)

1. A 32-year-old woman presents with gradually increasing dyspnea on exertion for 2 years. Her daily activity is now limited. She has a history of rheumatic fever and was told of a heart murmur during an insurance examination at age 21. She has no other medical problems and does not take any medication. Examination findings:

   Blood pressure 110/70 mm Hg; pulse 70 and regular

   Jugular venous pressure normal; carotid pulse, no delay

   LV tapping in quality

   Loud S_1; normal S_2

   High-pitched early diastolic opening snap 80 ms from aortic component of S_2

   2/6 holodiastolic rumbling murmur

   ECG: Sinus rhythm with left atrial enlargement

   Chest radiography: Clear lungs, with straightening of the left border of the heart

   What would you do at this time?

   a. Observation only
   b. Transthoracic echocardiography
   c. Transesophageal echocardiography
   d. Catheterization of the right and left sides of the heart with exercise
   e. Pulmonary angiography

2. The echocardiogram of the patient in question 1 shows a normal left ventricle, with moderate dilatation of the left atrium. There is a mobile noncalcified mitral valve with diastolic valve doming. The aortic and tricuspid valves are normal.

   Doppler echocardiography: Mean transmitral gradient = 6 mm Hg

   Pressure half-time = 180 ms

   Tricuspid regurgitation velocity = 2.5 m/s

   What is the next step in management?

   a. Transesophageal echocardiography
   b. Catheterization of the right and left sides of the heart
   c. Exercise Doppler echocardiography
   d. Pulmonary angiography
   e. Treatment with β-blockers

3. Exercise Doppler echocardiography is performed in the patient in questions 1 and 2. The patient performs only to 50% of her predicted functional aerobic capacity before having to stop because of dyspnea. At peak exercise, the following is obtained:

   Mean transmitral gradient = 22 mm Hg

Tricuspid regurgitation velocity = 3.8 m/s
Heart rate = 140 beats/min

What would you do at this time?

a. Transesophageal echocardiography, then percutaneous mitral balloon valvuloplasty
b. Mitral valve replacement
c. Pulmonary angiography
d. Catheterization of the right and left sides of the heart
e. Treatment with β-blockers

4. A 67-year-old man has class III dyspnea on exertion. Examination reveals tardus +2 of the carotid arterial waveform and a late peaking systolic ejection murmur. There is a moderate left ventricular lift. The aortic component of the second heart sound is present but reduced in intensity. Echocardiography reveals a normal left ventricle, calcified aortic valve, and a mean aortic valve gradient of 18 mm Hg, with an aortic valve area of 1.2 cm^2. What would you do?

a. Catheterization of the right and left sides of the heart, with coronary angiography
b. Dobutamine Doppler echocardiography
c. Exercise test
d. Repeat echocardiography in 9 months
e. Observation

5. A 64-year-old woman has class III symptoms of dyspnea on exertion. She has a long history of a heart murmur (since adolescence) but no symptoms until the last 5 years. On examination, she has a loud P$_2$, a 2/6 holosystolic murmur at the left sternal border, and a 2/6 long diastolic rumble at the apex. Echocardiography reveals a mildly dilated left ventricle and left atrium, with an ejection fraction of 60%. A heavily calcified mitral valve is present. Doppler transmitral gradient is 20 mm Hg, with a mitral valve area of 1.9 cm^2. Mild mitral regurgitation is detected. What would you do?

a. Coronary angiography, then mitral valve replacement
b. Transesophageal echocardiography to look for mitral regurgitation
c. Consider percutaneous mitral balloon valvuloplasty
d. Continuity equation for mitral valve area
e. Catheterization of the right and left sides of the heart

6. A 22-year-old man is asymptomatic but comes for evaluation of a heart murmur. There is a thrill in the carotid arteries, with a 3/6 long systolic ejection murmur in the aortic area with a mid peak. A soft 1/6 diastolic

decrescendo murmur is present. Echocardiography reveals moderate left ventricular hypertrophy, with an ejection fraction of 65%. There is a normal-appearing 3-cusp aortic valve with mild regurgitation and a 4.5-m/s jet across the aortic valve on Doppler echocardiography. No systolic anterior motion of the mitral valve is present. What would you do next?

a. Catheterization of the right and left sides of the heart
b. Aortic valve replacement
c. Observation, with yearly echocardiography
d. Repeat Doppler echocardiography with amyl nitrite
e. Transesophageal echocardiography

7. A 72-year-old man has severe class IV congestive heart failure. He had coronary artery bypass grafting 10 years ago. He recently was found to have a poor ejection fraction (20%) and aortic stenosis. Doppler echocardiography reveals a mean gradient of 17 mm Hg and aortic valve area of 0.5 cm^2. What is the next step?

a. Aortic valve replacement
b. Percutaneous aortic balloon valvuloplasty
c. Afterload reduction
d. Catheterization of the right and left sides of the heart
e. Doppler echocardiography with dobutamine infusion

8. A 64-year-old woman has class III dyspnea on exertion. She has known mitral stenosis from rheumatic heart disease and long-standing hypertension. Echocardiography reveals mild left ventricular hypertrophy with an ejection fraction of 65%, a moderately enlarged left atrium, and a calcified mitral valve. Doppler echocardiography reveals a mean transmitral gradient of 4 mm Hg, a mitral valve area of 1.9 cm^2, and a tricuspid regurgitation velocity of 4.2 m/s. What is the next step in management?

a. Right and left heart catheterization
b. Mitral valve replacement
c. Percutaneous mitral balloon valvuloplasty after transesophageal echocardiography
d. Dobutamine stress test
e. Observation with yearly echocardiography

9. A 24-year-old woman, 1 month pregnant, has a heart murmur. She is not symptomatic. On examination, she has a regular rhythm at a rate of 80 beats/min and a loud first heart sound with a crisp opening snap about 70 ms from the aortic component of the second heart sound. An early-to-mid diastolic rumble is present.

Two-dimensional Doppler echocardiography reveals mitral stenosis with a pliable valve, a mean gradient of 6 mm Hg, a mitral valve area of 1.8 cm^2, and a tricuspid regurgitation velocity of 2.8 m/s. What would you do now?

a. Transesophageal echocardiography
b. Transesophageal echocardiography, then percutaneous mitral balloon valvuloplasty
c. Low-dose β-blocker
d. Catheterization of the right and left sides of the heart
e. Mitral valve replacement

10. A 58-year-old man has had a heart murmur for 20 years. He was asymptomatic until 1 week ago, when severe dyspnea suddenly developed. He was in atrial fibrillation, which was converted to sinus rhythm, with resolution of his symptoms. Catheterization (performed elsewhere) showed a left ventricular pressure of 190/10 mm Hg, aortic pressure of 150/70 mm Hg, and cardiac output of 4.0 L/min, with normal coronary arteries. What is the next step in management?

a. Aortic valve replacement
b. Echocardiography and blood test
c. Observation with yearly echocardiography
d. Exercise test
e. Repeat catheterization

11. Which of the following is not associated with supravalvular aortic stenosis?

a. Elfin facies
b. Hypercalcemia
c. Peripheral pulmonic stenosis
d. Aortic dissection
e. Thrill in right carotid artery

Answers

1. Answer b

Two-dimensional/Doppler echocardiography is the diagnostic modality of choice for evaluating a patient with mitral stenosis. Two-dimensional echocardiography is able to define the presence and morphology of the mitral valve, and Doppler echocardiography is able to evaluate the severity of stenosis.

2. Answer c

The patient has symptoms of significant dyspnea on exertion. However, the mean transmitral gradient is only 6 mm Hg. The symptoms are out of proportion to the resting hemodynamics. Therefore, it would be appropriate to exercise the patient to the point of production of symptoms and to measure the gradient again to determine whether the mitral stenosis is the cause of her symptoms.

3. Answer a

When this patient exercises, her mean gradient increases significantly to > 20 mm Hg and significant pulmonary hypertension develops. This indicates that mitral stenosis is the cause of her symptoms, despite the relatively low resting mean gradient. The patient would benefit from intervention. Because she has a pliable noncalcified valve, percutaneous mitral balloon valvuloplasty can be performed with low risk and a high success rate. Transesophageal echocardiography should be performed first to rule out the presence of left atrial thrombus, which would prohibit the procedure.

4. Answer a

The patient has findings of severe aortic stenosis on clinical examination. However, the echocardiographic findings are consistent with only mild aortic stenosis. A major limitation of Doppler echocardiography is that it may underestimate the severity of aortic stenosis if the Doppler jet is not parallel with the stenotic jet. Therefore, catheterization to remeasure the gradient and output would be appropriate. Alternatively, if one suspected that Doppler echocardiography did not properly define the severity of stenosis, echocardiography could be repeated.

5. Answer a

The patient has severe symptoms of dyspnea, with findings of pulmonary hypertension on examination as well as mitral stenosis and mitral regurgitation. The Doppler echocardiogram demonstrates a valve area of 1.9 cm², indicating that the severity of stenosis is only mild. However, the mean gradient is very high, indicating that the combination of regurgitation and stenosis of the mitral valve is causing a significant increase in left atrial pressure. Therefore, this patient needs mitral valve replacement. Coronary angiography should be performed first. Further diagnostic testing of hemodynamics is not needed.

6. Answer e

This young man has findings of left ventricular outflow tract obstruction. The physical examination and Doppler examination indicate severe obstruction to outflow, but on two-dimensional echocardiography the aortic valve is normal. This patient most likely has discrete subvalvular aortic stenosis. This should be defined with transesophageal echocardiography.

7. Answer e

This patient has a "low output, low gradient" aortic stenosis. The valve area is calculated to be in the "severe" range. This could be due to one of two things. It could be severe end-stage critical aortic stenosis, in which left ventricular function has deteriorated because of long-standing pressure overload. However, it could also be due to a mild degree of aortic stenosis and severe left ventricular dysfunction from another cause. The aortic valve area would be low because the left ventricle does not have enough power to open the valve. In this case, dobutamine stimulation would be indicated. The dobutamine could be used to normalize cardiac output. If the gradient increases to levels consistent with severe aortic stenosis, aortic valve operation should be performed. However, with normalization of cardiac output,

there may not be an increase in mean gradient and mild aortic stenosis would be diagnosed.

8. Answer a

The woman has severe symptoms of dyspnea, with findings of severe pulmonary hypertension. However, her mitral stenosis is only mild; therefore, there is a discrepancy between the severity of mitral valve disease, symptoms, and pulmonary hypertension. In this situation, catheterization should be performed to determine the absolute pressure of the left atrium (or pulmonary artery wedge pressure) as well as left ventricular diastolic pressure. This patient may have either primary pulmonary hypertension or severe diastolic dysfunction.

9. Answer c

Women with mitral stenosis generally tolerate pregnancy well, despite the increased heart rate and volume overload that occur with pregnancy. Percutaneous mitral balloon valvotomy is indicated only if the patient goes into heart failure during pregnancy. Low-dose β-blockade to keep the heart rate down is indicated to prevent an increase in left atrial pressure.

10. Answer b

The patient has findings of aortic stenosis (outside catheterization). However, he developed atrial fibrillation, which is unusual for isolated aortic stenosis. Other causes of the atrial fibrillation should be considered, such as mitral valve disease or hyperthyroidism. Therefore, this patient should have echocardiography and a sensitive thyroid-stimulating hormone test.

11. Answer d

Aortic dissection is not associated with supravalvular aortic stenosis. These patients may have elfin facies, hypercalcemia, peripheral pulmonic stenosis, and a thrill in the right carotid artery.

Notes

Chapter 24

Valvular Regurgitation

Barry L. Karon, M.D.
Maurice Enriquez-Sarano, M.D.

Mitral Regurgitation

The mitral valve is a complicated structure that requires the correct functioning of the valve leaflets, valve commissures, mitral annulus, papillary muscles, chordae tendineae, and left ventricle for competence. Mitral regurgitation results from failure of one or more of the components of normal mitral valve competence. The presentation and management depend on the underlying cause, duration, regurgitant severity, patient symptoms (including objective exercise tolerance), and left ventricular size and systolic function.

Anatomy

There are three basic mechanisms of mitral regurgitation.

1. Alteration of Mitral Leaflets, Commissures, or Annulus

Rheumatic Fever
Rheumatic mitral valve disease may deform valves, shorten chordae, or fuse commissures and lead to pure mitral regurgitation or predominant regurgitation in combination with stenosis.

Mitral Valve Prolapse
Mitral valve prolapse is the most common cause of isolated severe mitral regurgitation. The posterior leaflet is affected more frequently and severely than the anterior leaflet.

Mitral annular dilatation and calcification and myxomatous changes of chordae tendineae may be associated. The likelihood of mitral valve prolapse resulting in significant mitral regurgitation increases with age and is greater in men than in women. Prolapse may occur alone or in association with other conditions, including Marfan syndrome, Ehlers-Danlos syndrome, and thoracic skeletal abnormalities.

Mitral Annulus Calcification
Isolated mitral annulus calcification is usually age-related but may occur in young patients with hypertension, hypertrophic obstructive cardiomyopathy, chronic renal failure, or aortic stenosis.

Infective Endocarditis
Infective endocarditis may damage valve leaflets by perforation or a vegetation that interferes with coaptation. Anatomical abnormalities may persist even after the active infection has been eradicated.

Congenital
A congenital cleft of the anterior mitral leaflet often is associated with primum atrial septal defect, but it can exist in isolation without other features of a persistent atrioventricular canal.

Rare Causes of Mitral Incompetence
Other, uncommon, causes of mitral leaflet abnormalities

include endomyocardial fibrosis, carcinoid disease with right-to-left shunting or bronchial carcinoid-secreting adenomas, ergotamine toxicity, radiation therapy, trauma, rheumatoid arthritis, systemic lupus erythematosus (Libman-Sacks lesions), and diet-drug toxicity.

.

2. Defective Tensor Apparatus

Abnormal Chordae Tendineae
Ruptured chordae are responsible for a significant percentage of cases of mitral regurgitation. Rupture may be idiopathic, a complication of endocarditis, a result of myxomatous degeneration in the setting of mitral valve prolapse, or a result of blunt or direct penetrating thoracic trauma.

Papillary Muscle Dysfunction
Myocardial ischemia or infarction can cause papillary muscle dysfunction (without rupture). The posteromedial papillary muscle is more vulnerable to ischemia or infarction than the anterolateral papillary muscle because of its single end-artery vascular supply. Nonischemic causes of papillary muscle dysfunction include dilated cardiomyopathy, myocarditis, and hypertension.

Myocardial infarction (either transmural or subendocardial) can cause rupture of a papillary muscle. It usually occurs in the first week after infarction at a time when the inflammatory cell response is maximal and most frequently involves the posteromedial papillary muscle. Rarely, chest trauma can cause papillary muscle rupture, usually with coexistent myocardial or ventricular septal rupture.

3. Alterations of Left Ventricular and Left Atrial Size and Function
Global or regional left ventricular enlargement may alter the position and axis of contraction of the papillary muscles in addition to causing dilatation of the mitral ring. Progressive left atrial and ventricular enlargement associated with any type of chronic mitral regurgitation, in turn, leads to more mitral regurgitation by further altering the geometry of the chamber.

Mitral regurgitation in hypertrophic obstructive cardiomyopathy results both from the Venturi effect (systolic anterior motion of the mitral leaflets or chordae or both) and abnormal papillary muscle position.

- Understanding the mechanism of mitral regurgitation helps define the natural history and optimal treatment.

- Mitral prolapse is the most common cause of isolated severe mitral regurgitation.
- Ischemia can cause either dysfunction or rupture of papillary muscle. The posteromedial papillary muscle is affected most often because of its single end-artery blood supply.
- Left ventricular enlargement and abnormal contractile function are common causes of significant mitral regurgitation.

Pathophysiology of Mitral Regurgitation
Mitral regurgitation has three pathophysiologic stages.

1. Acute Stage
In acute severe mitral regurgitation, there is a sudden volume overload on an unprepared left ventricle and left atrium (Fig. 1). The left ventricle responds with increased sarcomere stretch and augmented left ventricular stroke volume via the Frank-Starling stretch mechanism. However, the larger volume increases left ventricular diastolic pressure, which in turn increases left atrial pressure. Because left atrial compliance is normal in the acute state, the large regurgitant volume markedly increases left atrial pressure, which causes pulmonary congestion, edema, and dyspnea.

The sudden opening of a new low-pressure pathway for systolic ejection decreases left ventricular afterload, permitting more complete volume ejection from the ventricle. Although total left ventricular stroke volume increases, forward stroke volume decreases. The combination of increased preload, decreased afterload, and increased left ventricular contractile function increases the measured ejection fraction to between 60% and 75%.

When new-onset mitral regurgitation is not severe in quantity, the same pathophysiology is operative, although significant pulmonary congestion or dyspnea is uncommon. Affected patients enter the chronic compensated phase silently and may have a more benign natural history.

2. Chronic Compensated Stage
In the chronic compensated stage (Fig. 2), left ventricular volume overload elongates individual myocytes, causing compensatory eccentric left ventricular hypertrophy and increasing left ventricular end-diastolic volume. The Frank-Starling mechanism continues to augment total stroke volume. The left atrium dilates, thus increasing its compliance. Although the dilated left atrium decreases ventricular afterload, the increased left ventricular radius increases afterload. Thus, the net effect is that left ventricular afterload is

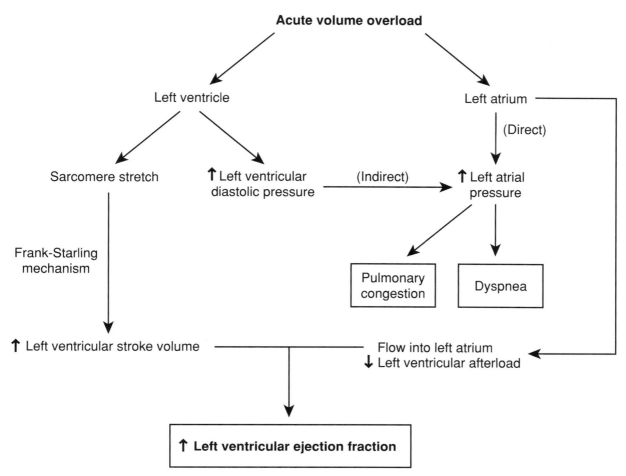

Fig. 1. Acute severe mitral regurgitation.

unchanged. The combination of increased end-diastolic volume, augmented contraction, and unchanged afterload continues to result in a high ejection fraction. The dilated left ventricle and atrium allow the regurgitant volume to be accommodated at lower filling pressures, thereby minimizing symptoms of pulmonary congestion.

3. Chronic Decompensated Stage

Eventually, left ventricular contractile function declines, and the chronic decompensated stage of mitral regurgitation begins (Fig. 3). This downward spiral includes an increase in end-systolic volume as left ventricular function decreases. Left ventricular filling pressures increase and cause pulmonary congestion. Increased ventricular pressure further dilates the left ventricle, increasing systolic wall stress and afterload. The increased afterload further reduces ventricular systolic function, thus completing the downward cycle. As end-diastolic and end-systolic volumes increase, the ejection fraction may be in the 50% to 60%

"normal" range. In patients with severe mitral regurgitation, an ejection fraction less than 60% is probably abnormal and indicative of ventricular dysfunction.

The time during which patients progress from compensated to decompensated mitral regurgitation depends on the severity of the regurgitation (which itself can change over time), variables that affect afterload and ventricular contractility, and individual, poorly understood, patient characteristics.

- Acute severe mitral regurgitation is characterized by normal-sized chambers, high ejection fraction, and pulmonary congestion.
- Chronic compensated severe mitral regurgitation is typified by few symptoms, enlargement of the left ventricle and atrium, and high ejection fraction.
- A "normal range" ejection fraction in the setting of severe mitral regurgitation usually implies left ventricular systolic dysfunction.

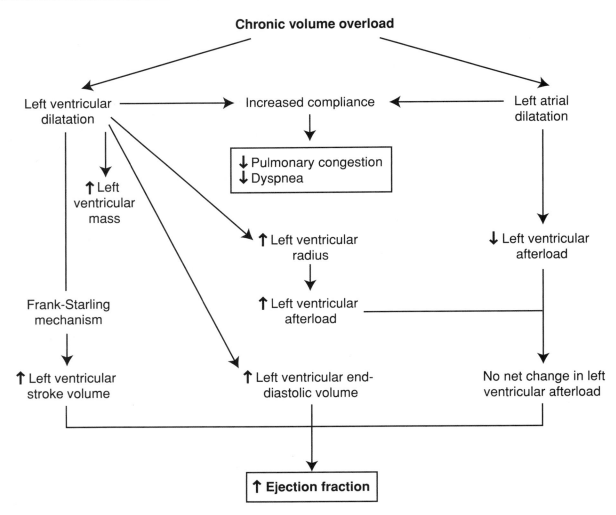

Fig. 2. Chronic compensated mitral regurgitation.

Clinical Syndrome of Mitral Regurgitation

Acute Mitral Regurgitation

Acute mitral regurgitation usually results from infective endocarditis, infarction, ischemic heart disease, trauma, or chordal rupture. If acute mitral regurgitation is severe, severe pulmonary congestion is expected. The high left atrial pressure and left ventricular end-diastolic pressure account for the third and fourth heart sounds. The systolic murmur of mitral regurgitation in this acute condition may be short, soft, or completely absent. Rarely, there may be only a small left ventricular-to-atrial pressure gradient (because left atrial pressure has increased close to that of the left ventricle). This may result in the absence of an audible murmur and Doppler color flow evidence of mitral regurgitation (indicating almost no turbulence in the regurgitant flow).

Chronic Mitral Regurgitation

Patients with chronic mitral regurgitation may have a prolonged asymptomatic interval. However, adverse ventricular changes may develop during this period. Once symptoms arise, the low cardiac output symptoms of fatigue and generalized weakness predominate early. As left ventricular function deteriorates, exertional dyspnea, orthopnea, and paroxysmal nocturnal dyspnea become more prominent.

At this stage, examination of the precordium reveals a brief, laterally displaced, and enlarged apical impulse. A ventricular filling impulse may be palpable. The presence of an apical thrill indicates severe mitral regurgitation. As ventricular systolic function deteriorates, the duration of the apical impulse increases.

Auscultation may reveal single or multiple nonejection

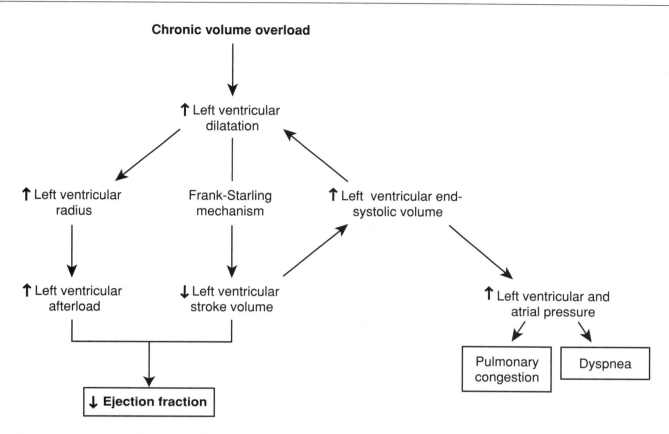

Chronic volume overload

↑ Left ventricular dilatation

↑ Left ventricular radius

Frank-Starling mechanism

↑ Left ventricular end-systolic volume

↑ Left ventricular afterload

↓ Left ventricular stroke volume

↑ Left ventricular and atrial pressure

Pulmonary congestion

Dyspnea

↓ **Ejection fraction**

Fig. 3. Chronic decompensated mitral regurgitation.

clicks whose timing may be varied by maneuvers. An accentuated pulmonic component of the second heart sound indicates pulmonary hypertension. Aortic closure may be early because of decreased duration of forward flow, causing persistent wide splitting of the second heart sound (however, the duration of the murmur often obscures the second heart sound, making the splitting hard to detect). An apical third heart sound is common, but fourth heart sounds are unusual because of the flaccidity of the left atrium.

A holosystolic murmur is the hallmark of mitral regurgitation. The intensity of the murmur does not necessarily correlate with the severity of the regurgitant flow. Although the murmur frequently radiates to the axilla, a primary posterior leaflet abnormality will direct the regurgitant flow anteriorly and the radiation may be toward the aortic area. Characteristically, the mitral regurgitant murmur is constant despite different cycle lengths; this feature helps, at the bedside, to distinguish it from aortic outflow murmurs. The presence of a short diastolic apical rumble in the absence of mitral stenosis implies high diastolic transmitral flow and severe mitral regurgitation. Coexistent mitral stenosis also causes a diastolic apical rumble. Inhalation of amyl nitrite increases the intensity and duration of the diastolic rumble if mitral stenosis is present but decreases them if the rumble is solely due to severe mitral regurgitation. An opening snap, if present, also indicates mitral stenosis.

- Acute severe mitral regurgitation may have a short or soft murmur because of the low left ventricular-to-atrial pressure gradient.
- Nonspecific fatigue and weakness may represent the early symptoms of chronic severe mitral regurgitation.
- The duration of the apical impulse in chronic severe mitral regurgitation is related to left ventricular systolic function.
- A fourth heart sound is infrequent in chronic severe mitral regurgitation.
- Posterior leaflet prolapse often produces a murmur that radiates to the aortic area.
- The failure of a mitral regurgitant murmur to change with variable cycle lengths distinguishes it from an outflow tract murmur.
- Amyl nitrite distinguishes the diastolic rumble of mixed mitral stenosis and regurgitation from that due to isolated severe mitral regurgitation.

Evaluation of Mitral Regurgitation

Electrocardiography

No electrocardiographic (ECG) findings are diagnostic of mitral regurgitation. The ECG may show atrial fibrillation; left atrial enlargement is expected if sinus rhythm persists. Left ventricular hypertrophy and nonspecific ST-segment and T-wave changes are also common.

Chest Radiography

Significant chronic mitral regurgitation causes the left ventricular and left atrial enlargement seen on chest radiographs. Left atrial enlargement might be recognized as straightening of the left border of the heart, an atrial double density, or elevation of the left main-stem bronchus. Pulmonary venous congestion may be present in any stage of mitral regurgitation. Note that none of the above findings are specific for mitral regurgitation.

Echocardiography

Echocardiography assesses the morphology of the mitral valve, annulus, commissures, and papillary muscles. Assessment of the severity of mitral regurgitation is performed with an integrated Doppler and two-dimensional echocardiographic examination (Table 1). A flail mitral valve leaflet usually is associated with severe mitral regurgitation. In some cases, transesophageal echocardiography is required to better assess the anatomy of the mitral valve and its supporting structures, to inspect the atria for thrombus, and to gather supplemental data used in qualitative and quantitative measures of regurgitation severity. Echocardiography also evaluates the impact of mitral regurgitation on left ventricular and atrial size and function, in addition to right ventricular function and hemodynamics.

Radionuclide angiography and magnetic resonance imaging can measure ejection fraction and regurgitant volumes, but their role in routine patient management is unproved.

Cardiac Catheterization

Left ventriculography is used primarily when noninvasive data are discordant or technically limited or differ from the clinical perception of the severity of mitral regurgitation or ventricular function. Angiographic grading of mitral regurgitation is dependent on the volume and injection rate of the contrast agent, catheter position, hemodynamics at the time of injection, and volume of the left atrium in addition to the severity of valve regurgitation. Calculations of the invasively derived regurgitant fraction are also subject to

Table 1.—Doppler Indicators of Severe Mitral Regurgitation*

Color jet area ($> 8.0 \text{ cm}^2$; $> 1/3$ LA area)
Wide vena contracta (color flow)
Regurgitant volume (> 60 mL)[†]
Regurgitant fraction ($> 55\%$)[†]
ERO ($> 0.35 \text{ cm}^2$)[†]
Pulmonary vein PW Doppler flow profile (systolic flow reversal)
CW Doppler signal intensity (dense)
Transmitral PW flow velocity (E > 1.5 m/s)

CW, continuous-wave; E, early transmitral flow; ERO, effective regurgitant orifice area; LA, left atrium; PW, pulsed-wave.
*Measurements indicative of severe regurgitation are in parentheses.
[†]Can be measured by volumetric Doppler, proximal isovelocity surface area method, or a combination of these, including two-dimensional measures.

the above limitations. The presence or absence of prominent "v" waves on a pulmonary wedge hemodynamic tracing depends not only on mitral regurgitant flow at the time of the study but also on the compliance of the left atrium.

- There are no ECG or chest radiographic findings pathognomonic of mitral regurgitation.
- Echocardiography is invaluable for assessing the cause and severity of mitral regurgitation and its effects on the size and function of the left ventricle, left atrium, and right ventricle.
- Left ventriculography is most useful when noninvasive data are discordant or technically limited or differ from the clinical impression of the severity of mitral regurgitation or ventricular function.

Mitral Valve Prolapse

Mitral valve prolapse differs in some ways from the other causes of mitral regurgitation. The systolic billowing of a portion of the mitral leaflet into the left atrium may cause an audible click. If the prolapse is significant, mitral regurgitation results. This condition is dynamic; the timing of the click and murmur varies with preload and afterload. Maneuvers that decrease the ventricular preload (Valsalva maneuver, standing) cause prolapse, and the click and murmur occur earlier in the cardiac cycle. The converse is true with maneuvers that increase preload.

The unique saddle-shaped anatomy of the mitral valves was not well described until the late 1980s, and in some patients an incorrect diagnosis of mitral valve prolapse was made with echocardiography before this was fully appreciated.

The natural history of most cases of mitral valve prolapse is benign, although progression to severe mitral regurgitation is more prevalent in men than women and with advancing age. Rare complications of mitral valve prolapse such as endocarditis, severe rhythm disturbances, and strokes occur predominantly in patients with thickened valve leaflets.

Patients with mitral valve prolapse and severe mitral regurgitation are managed similarly to other patients with severe mitral regurgitation. If the regurgitation is mild, patients should be reassured and followed clinically for any changes in either symptoms or physical findings. Antibiotic prophylaxis is advised for patients with a click-and-murmur incompetence or a click and echocardiographic findings of significant leaflet thickening or regurgitation.

Patients with mitral valve prolapse and palpitations or increased adrenergic tone, atypical chest pain, anxiety, or fatigue should be counseled to minimize their use of exogenous stimulants and may benefit from β-adrenergic blocker therapy. Aspirin is advised for transient ischemic events in the setting of mitral valve prolapse if no other cause is found.

Natural History of Mitral Regurgitation

The natural history of *acute* mitral regurgitation is dependent on its cause and severity. Patients with papillary muscle rupture or severe regurgitation from an unstable mitral prosthesis have a poor short-term outlook without operation. Those with acute regurgitation from endocarditis have a variable course depending on the response to antibiotic treatment. Patients with abrupt chordal rupture have a natural history dependent primarily on the severity of regurgitation.

Patients with *chronic* mitral regurgitation have a clinical course characterized by an initial compensated phase followed by progressive left ventricular dysfunction. A "typical" time course for progression to ventricular dysfunction cannot be stated because of wide individual variability and uncertainty about the duration of disease at the time of the initial examination of the patient. Studies of patients not eligible for cardiac operation are confounded by selection bias. In addition, there have been changes in the causes of mitral regurgitation, and most patients currently manifest degenerative rather than inflammatory disease.

Occasionally, acute worsening of mitral regurgitation in the setting of chronic regurgitation is experienced, and in these cases, chordal rupture, infective endocarditis, a new atrial arrhythmia, or superimposed ischemia should be suspected.

Recent work indicates that in patients with flail leaflets who do not undergo operation, the natural history is one of significant early mortality, morbidity, and near certainty of the need for mitral operation in the long term. Patients who were even transiently in New York Heart Association functional class III or IV have a high mortality rate (Fig. 4 through 6).

- The natural history of acute mitral regurgitation depends on its cause.
- The time course of progressive left ventricular dysfunction in chronic mitral regurgitation is variable and unpredictable.
- Acute worsening of mitral regurgitation suggests chordal rupture, infection, new arrhythmia, or ischemia.

Outcome After Surgical Correction of Mitral Regurgitation (the Unnatural History)

Operation is the treatment of choice for patients with severe mitral regurgitation. The timing of operation depends on the expected operative risk, the degree of ventricular dysfunction (if any), and the long-term morbidity associated with valvular prostheses and obligate anticoagulation should the valve be unrepairable. Current surgical practice is to operate on patients with severe mitral regurgitation before the development of heart failure or ventricular dysfunction, if possible.

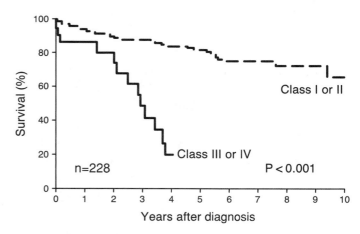

Fig. 4. Long-term survival with medical treatment for mitral regurgitation, according to New York Heart Association class. The New York Heart Association class was not available for one patient. (From *N Engl J Med* 335:1417-1423, 1996. By permission of the Massachusetts Medical Society.)

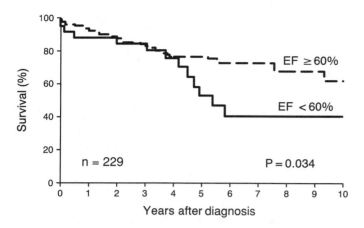

Fig. 5. Long-term survival with medical treatment for mitral regurgitation, according to ejection fraction (EF). (From *N Engl J Med* 335:1417-1423, 1996. By permission of the Massachusetts Medical Society.)

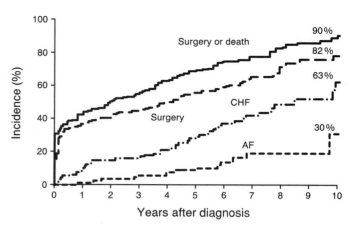

Fig. 6. Incidence of atrial fibrillation (AF), congestive heart failure (CHF), mitral valve surgery, and surgery or death in patients with isolated mitral regurgitation due to flail leaflet. A total of 175 patients were initially at risk for atrial fibrillation, and 229 were initially at risk for the other end points. Values are mean event rates at 10 years. (From *N Engl J Med* 335:1417-1423, 1996. By permission of the Massachusetts Medical Society.)

Left ventricular dysfunction is a major source of poor postoperative congestive heart failure and survival. The preoperative ejection fraction is the best predictor of long-term mortality, congestive heart failure, and postoperative left ventricular function. The end-systolic dimension is also a significant predictor of postoperative left ventricular function. Severe preoperative symptoms are associated with a worse long-term survival and increased incidence of heart failure, even after correcting for other determinants of outcome. Atrial fibrillation of more than 3 months in duration preoperatively is associated with a high risk of postoperative arrhythmia persistence and the resultant necessity of long-term anticoagulation.

Treatment of Acute Severe Mitral Regurgitation

Patients with *acute* severe mitral regurgitation may be hemodynamically stable or unstable at presentation. Any patient with hemodynamic instability requires rapid evaluation and therapy with intravenous vasodilators (usually sodium nitroprusside), intravenous inotropes, and, perhaps, intra-aortic balloon counterpulsation. Patients presenting with acute regurgitation often have a ruptured papillary muscle or an unstable mitral prosthesis, and repair or replacement of the mitral valve generally is indicated because long-term medical therapy is ineffective.

Other therapies for mitral regurgitation include antibiotics if endocarditis is present and antianginal drugs or angioplasty or stenting in some cases of ischemic papillary muscle dysfunction. In endocarditis, operation is often delayed

in the hope of sterilizing the mitral valve bed because ongoing active infection puts the new valve at peril of prosthetic endocarditis. Patients with endocarditis should be considered for urgent surgical intervention if progressive heart failure, infection unresponsive to antibiotics, intracardiac abscess, or recurrent systemic embolization develops despite therapy.

Treatment of Chronic Nonischemic Mitral Regurgitation

All patients with mitral regurgitation should be instructed in dental hygiene and the use of antibiotic prophylaxis against infective endocarditis. If their regurgitation is mild or moderate in severity, any contributing underlying disease (such as coronary artery disease, left ventricular enlargement and dysfunction) should be optimally treated.

The available short-term hemodynamic studies of medical therapy in small groups of patients (without matched control groups) with severe mitral regurgitation do not allow us to reach scientific conclusions about the role of medical therapy in these patients. There are no data to indicate that diuretics or vasodilator therapy (or both) provide morbidity or mortality benefit; in fact, some investigators fear that such treatment may either mask symptoms or promote ventricular decompensation.

Accordingly, every patient with severe mitral regurgitation should be considered for valve operation. In addition to an accurate understanding of the amount of regurgitation, both the mechanism of regurgitation and the status of the left ventricle (end-systolic dimension, ejection fraction) must be known. Other considerations include whether the valve is likely to be repairable and comorbid conditions that would increase the operative risk (Table 2).

There is a subgroup of high-risk patients with severe ventricular dysfunction (ejection fraction < 35% or cardiac index < 1.5 L/min per m^2) who are at increased risk for perioperative death or congestive heart failure. Mitral valve repair (instead of replacement) should be performed, if possible, in this high-risk subgroup because of its better preservation of ventricular function (Fig. 7).

Mitral valve repair should be performed preferentially to replacement whenever possible because studies have now shown repair to be a favorable predictor of operative mortality, late survival, and postoperative ejection fraction on multivariate analysis. Intraoperative transesophageal echocardiography supplements the surgeon's assessment of the success of repair. Mitral regurgitation that is non-rheumatic, noninfective, and nonischemic is most amenable to repair. Significant calcification reduces the likelihood of successful repair (Table 3). Posterior leaflet disease is repaired more successfully than anterior leaflet or bileaflet lesions. Whenever mitral valve replacement is performed, preservation of the annular-chordal structures should be attempted.

Figures 8 and 9 show postoperative survival according to preoperative ejection fraction and New York Heart Association class.

Surgical Treatment of Mitral Regurgitation Due to Ischemia or Cardiomyopathy

Patients with severe secondary mitral regurgitation due to prior infarctions or dilated cardiomyopathy may remain severely symptomatic despite maximal medical therapy. Recent studies have shown significant short- and interme-diate-term symptomatic improvement in these patients with mitral annular rings.

- Patients with acute severe mitral regurgitation and hemo-dynamic instability require rapid evaluation, aggressive stabilization, and early valve operation.
- Patients with acute severe mitral regurgitation who are hemodynamically stable should have semielective cardiac operation.
- Indications for valve operation in endocarditis include progressive heart failure, resistance to antibiotics, intra-cardiac abscess, or recurrent systemic embolization despite therapy.

Table 2.—Indication for Operation in Severe Mitral Regurgitation

Definite indications
  NYHA functional class III or IV
  Ejection fraction < 60%
  Ejection fraction ≥ 60% but with serially progressive decline
  Left ventricular end-systolic diameter > 45 mm or end-systolic volume index > 50 mL/m^2
Emerging indications*
  Flail leaflet
  LA dimension > 45 mm
  Paroxysmal or recent-onset atrial fibrillation
  Abnormal end-systolic volume or ejection fraction response to exercise
  Rest PA pressure > 50 mm Hg (or > 60 mm Hg with exercise)

LA, left atrial; NYHA, New York Heart Association; PA, pulmonary artery.
*In the absence of the indications listed above.

- Patients with severe chronic mitral regurgitation who are in New York Heart Association class III or IV, have an ejection fraction less than 60%, have an end-systolic diam-eter more than 45 mm, or have an end-systolic volume more than 50 mL/m^2 should undergo valve surgery, if not otherwise contraindicated.
- Emerging indications for mitral valve replacement include flail leaflet, paroxysmal or recent-onset atrial fibrillation, and pulmonary hypertension.
- Patients with impaired ventricular function are better served by valve repair than replacement.
- Successful valve repair is less likely in cases that are rheumatic, ischemic, or due to infection, when prolapse is anterior or bileaflet, or when significant calcification is present.

Aortic Regurgitation

Aortic regurgitation may result from intrinsic structural abnor-malities of the aortic valve or the ascending aorta or both.

Anatomy

Intrinsic Valvular Disease
Rheumatic fever causes mild aortic regurgitation during the

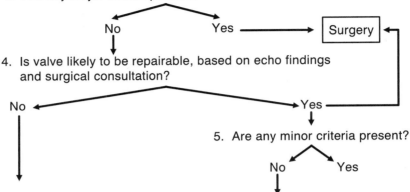

1. Suspect severe MR in a patient eligible for operation
2. Confirm severe MR by quantitative echo assessment
3. Are any major criteria present?

No   Yes ——————→ Surgery

4. Is valve likely to be repairable, based on echo findings and surgical consultation?

No   Yes

5. Are any minor criteria present?

No   Yes

6. Repeat clinical assessment and echo every 6-12 months

7. Have any major criteria appeared or has the EF declined over serial measurements?

No

Return to no. 6

8. Repeat clinical assessment and echo every 6-12 months

9. Have any major or minor criteria appeared or has the EF declined over serial measurements?

No

Return to no. 8

Yes

Surgery

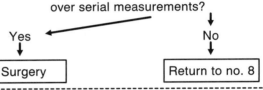

Major criteria
- Class III or IV heart failure (at any time)
- EF < 60%
- End-systolic diameter > 45 mm
- End-systolic volume index > 50 mL/m²

Minor criteria:
- Any symptoms of heart failure or suboptimal exercise tolerance test
- Flail mitral leaflet
- Left atrial dimension > 45 mm
- Paroxysmal atrial fibrillation
- Abnormal exercise end-systolic volume index or EF

Fig. 7. Algorithm for treatment of severe chronic mitral regurgitation (MR). echo, echocardiographic; EF, ejection fraction.

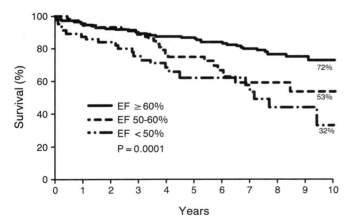

Fig. 8. Late survival of operative survivors according to preoperative echocardiographic ejection fraction (EF). (From Circulation 90:830-837, 1994. By permission of the American Heart Association.)

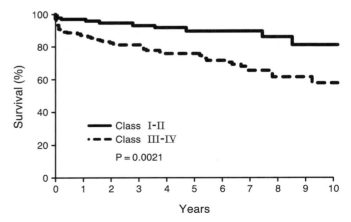

Fig. 9. Survival in patients with preoperative echocardiographic ejection fraction of 60% or more, according to preoperative symptoms. Survival was significantly worse if severe symptoms were present before operation. (From Circulation 90:830-837, 1994. By permission of the American Heart Association.)

Table 3.—Recommendations for Mitral Valve Surgery in Nonischemic Severe Mitral Regurgitation

Indication	Class
1. Acute symptomatic MR in which repair is likely	I
2. Patients with NYHA functional class II, III, or IV symptoms with normal LV function defined as ejection fraction > 60% and end-systolic dimension < 45 mm	I
3. Symptomatic or asymptomatic patients with mild LV dysfunction, ejection fraction 50% to 60%, and end-systolic dimension 45 to 50 mm	I
4. Symptomatic or asymptomatic patients with moderate LV dysfunction, ejection fraction 30% to 50%, or end-systolic dimension 50 to 55 mm	I
5. Asymptomatic patients with preserved LV function and atrial fibrillation	IIa
6. Asymptomatic patients with preserved LV function and pulmonary hypertension (pulmonary artery systolic pressure > 50 mm Hg at rest or > 60 mm Hg with exercise)	IIa
7. Asymptomatic patients with ejection fraction 50% to 60% and end-systolic dimension < 45 mm and asymptomatic patients with ejection fraction > 60% and end-systolic dimension 45 to 55 mm	IIa
8. Patients with severe LV dysfunction (ejection fraction < 30% or end-systolic dimension > 55 mm) in whom chordal preservation is highly likely	IIa
9. Asymptomatic patients with chronic MR with preserved LV function in whom mitral valve repair is highly likely	IIb
10. Patients with MVP and preserved LV function who have recurrent ventricular arrhythmias despite medical therapy	IIb
11. Asymptomatic patients with preserved LV function in whom significant doubt about the feasibility of repair exists	III

LV, left ventricular; MR, mitral regurgitation; MVP, mitral valve prolapse; NYHA, New York Heart Association.
From *J Am Coll Cardiol* 32:1486-1588, 1998. By permission of the American College of Cardiology.

first episodes, but with time the leaflets fibrose, shorten, and contract, resulting in malalignment and loss of coaptation. There usually is associated aortic stenosis due to commissural fusion. It is uncommon to have rheumatic aortic disease without coexistent mitral disease.

The most common congenital cause of aortic regurgitation in adults is a bicuspid valve with malcoaptation or diastolic prolapse of a cusp or both. In addition, chronic progressive aortic regurgitation also may be associated with ventricular septal defects (due to weakening of the neighboring supporting aortic annulus) or subaortic stenosis (causing turbulent high-velocity jets that hit and damage the aortic leaflets).

Infective endocarditis usually involves previously abnormal valves and leads to tissue destruction, vegetation interference with proper alignment of the commissures during closure, or invasion and structural distortion of the aortic valve annulus. Even after medical eradication of infection, regurgitation may progress because of contracture of healing cusps.

Collagen vascular diseases usually affect the aortic root,

but they also can affect the cusps themselves. The associated valvulitis leads to contracture of leaflets, with central regurgitation. Perforation of leaflets is less common.

Senile degenerative aortic valve disease is usually important clinically because of aortic stenosis, but some degree of aortic regurgitation, especially in early stages, is often seen. Significant regurgitation often occurs after either operative decalcification or percutaneous balloon valvuloplasty for aortic stenosis.

Diseases of the Ascending Aorta

Acute destruction of the aortic root disrupts the supporting structures of the valve and results in regurgitation. Aortic dissection longitudinally cleaves the aortic intima or media with a dissecting column of blood and occurs most often in patients with idiopathic dilatation of the ascending aorta, hypertension, or Marfan syndrome. It also can be associated with pregnancy, result from blunt chest trauma, or follow acute aortitis complicating aortic valve infective endocarditis.

Many diseases are associated with chronic dilatation of the aortic root, and they cause regurgitation by stretching the valve cusps. These diseases include 1) Marfan syndrome, usually associated with progressive aortic dilatation as a result of cystic medial necrosis; 2) progressive idiopathic aortic dilatation with cystic medial necrosis; 3) senile dilatation and annuloaortic ectasia of unknown cause; 4) syphilitic aortitis developing 15 to 25 years after the initial infection and sparing the sinuses of Valsalva; and 5) connective tissue disorders (rheumatoid arthritis, ankylosing spondylitis, Reiter syndrome, relapsing polychondritis, giant cell arteritis, and Whipple disease). Marfan syndrome, progressive idiopathic aortic dilatation, and some of the connective tissue disorders also can affect the mitral leaflets as well as the proximal conducting system.

- It is essential to know whether a patient's aortic regurgitation is due to valvular disease or proximal aortic disease or both.
- Many causes of aortic regurgitation often have associated mitral valve abnormalities: endocarditis, rheumatic fever, collagen vascular disease, or Marfan syndrome.

Pathophysiology of Aortic Regurgitation

Acute or subacute significant aortic regurgitation causes the abrupt introduction of a large volume of blood into a noncompliant left ventricle, thus increasing left ventricular end-diastolic and pulmonary venous pressures and leading to dyspnea or pulmonary edema.

In chronic aortic regurgitation, compensatory left ventricular changes occur over time. The excess volume load causes stretching and elongation of myocardial fibers, which in turn increase wall stress. Wall stress is normalized by sarcomere replication and hypertrophic thickening of the ventricular walls. Thus, although the ratio of wall thickness to cavity radius remains essentially normal, left ventricular mass increases (eccentric hypertrophy).

Initially, ventricular enlargement increases the ejection fraction through the Frank-Starling mechanism. However, further enlargement exhausts preload reserve, and the ejection fraction decreases to the "normal" range. Eventually, ejection fraction decreases further, whereas end-systolic volume increases. This end-systolic volume increase is a sensitive index of myocardial dysfunction. When the ventricle can dilate no further, diastolic pressure increases and results in dyspnea, another sign of decompensation.

During exercise, the volume of aortic regurgitation tends to decrease because of decreased systemic vascular resistance and shortened diastolic period. However, there also are increases in venous return that the enlarged left ventricle

may not be able to handle, thus causing a relative decrease in output (exertional fatigue) or increase in end-diastolic pressure (dyspnea) or both.

Patients with chronic aortic regurgitation may experience anginal symptoms despite normal coronary arteries. Mechanisms include increase in total myocardial oxygen consumption (increased left ventricular myocardial mass and wall tension), decreased subendocardial perfusion gradient due to compressed intramyocardial coronary arterioles, decreased central aortic diastolic driving pressure, and diminished coronary arteriolar vasodilatory reserve.

- Acute severe aortic regurgitation is characterized by normal left ventricular size, high ejection fraction, and dyspnea or pulmonary edema.
- Chronic compensated aortic regurgitation is typified by minimal symptoms and left ventricular enlargement.
- Decompensation is characterized by symptoms (initially with exertion) and decreasing ejection fraction.

Clinical Syndrome of Aortic Regurgitation

Acute aortic regurgitation usually is due to aortic dissection or infective endocarditis. In these circumstances, the manifestations of the underlying process usually predominate. Because compensatory cardiac mechanisms cannot develop, significant dyspnea occurs as a consequence of high left ventricular end-diastolic and pulmonary venous pressures. A murmur may be minimal because of the abrupt increase in left ventricular end-diastolic pressure and rapidly diminishing aortic-left ventricular diastolic pressure gradient. Peripheral manifestations (which are caused by rapid volume runoff into the left ventricle) may be absent because of acutely high ventricular diastolic pressures.

In chronic aortic regurgitation, the first symptom the patient often notices is an uncomfortable awareness of overactivity of the heart and neck vessels because of the forceful heartbeat associated with the high pulse pressure. Exertional dyspnea is a symptom of left ventricular failure.

Inspection of the patient may reveal nodding of the head (de Musset sign), visible capillary pulsation in the nail beds during gentle pressure on the edge of the nail (Quincke sign), features of Marfan syndrome, or stigmata of infective endocarditis.

Hemodynamically severe aortic regurgitation generally causes a widened pulse pressure more than 100 mm Hg with a diastolic pressure less than 60 mm Hg. Pulse pressure may not accurately reflect the severity of aortic regurgitation in young patients with compliant vessels or in patients with accompanying left ventricular failure and increased left ventricular end-diastolic pressure. Other signs of high-volume systolic ejection of blood with rapid diastolic runoff include a sharp, rapid carotid upstroke, followed by abnormal collapse (Corrigan pulse), a "pistol-shot" sound heard over the femoral artery (Duroziez murmur), or a biphasic bruit heard during mild compression of the femoral artery with the stethoscope. The jugular venous pulse and pressure are generally normal in isolated aortic regurgitation unless a dilated ascending aorta compresses the superior vena cava.

The apical impulse in chronic aortic regurgitation is diffuse, hyperdynamic, and displaced inferiorly and leftward. A third heart sound may be palpated. A diastolic thrill at the base of the heart signifies severe aortic regurgitation, whereas a systolic thrill at the base signifies a large systolic stroke volume.

Severe aortic regurgitation may cause partial diastolic closure of the mitral valve, decreasing the intensity of the first heart sound. An early systolic ejection click can signify either a bicuspid aortic valve or a large stroke volume entering a dilated aortic root. The second heart sound may be normal or abnormal (if the aortic valve does not close properly). A third heart sound may be present even without significant ventricular dysfunction, because of the rapid early diastolic filling of the ventricle by the sum of the transmitral and aortic regurgitant blood flow.

The characteristic auscultatory finding is a high-pitched diastolic decrescendo murmur best heard along the left sternal border. If it is most audible at the right sternal border, significant aortic root dilatation is suggested. The murmur is heard best with the diaphragm of the stethoscope, with the patient leaning forward with breath held in full expiration. The duration of the murmur, rather than its loudness, correlates best with the severity of regurgitation. When the murmur is musical or cooing, a cusp fenestration or perforation is suspected. A coexistent aortic systolic murmur does not necessarily imply the presence of aortic stenosis and may be a functional flow murmur due to the ejection of an abnormally high volume of blood during systole. The carotid upstroke helps define coexistent aortic stenosis. In significant aortic regurgitation, an additional diastolic apical rumbling (Austin Flint) murmur may be detected. Amyl nitrite inhalation softens an Austin Flint murmur but makes the rumbling murmur of mitral stenosis louder. Late in the course of disease, ventricular dilatation causes mitral annular dilatation and resultant mitral regurgitation.

- There may be few typical physical findings in *acute* aortic regurgitation.
- In patients with aortic regurgitation, "wide pulse pressure" implies low diastolic pressure in addition to the large difference between systolic and diastolic pressures.
- Physical findings in severe aortic regurgitation include a long diastolic murmur, apical diastolic rumble, enlarged and displaced apex, and peripheral findings of high output and rapid runoff.

Evaluation of Aortic Regurgitation

Acute, subacute, and mild chronic aortic regurgitation are not necessarily associated with ECG abnormalities. Chronic moderate or severe aortic regurgitation usually causes features of left ventricular hypertrophy, but a significant minority of such patients may not have ventricular hypertrophy by voltage criteria.

Chronic significant aortic regurgitation, with its associated enlargement of the left ventricle, increases the radiographic cardiothoracic ratio. The ascending aorta may be dilated, but it can appear normal because the most proximal portion of the ascending aorta is hidden within the cardiac silhouette

Echocardiography visualizes the ascending aorta and the aortic valve and measures left ventricular size and function (Table 4). Findings may include aortic leaflet prolapse, diastolic vibration of the anterior mitral leaflet, or premature closure of the mitral valve. Assessment of the severity of aortic regurgitation involves an integrated assessment of left ventricular size in conjunction with a comprehensive Doppler investigation (Table 5). Transesophageal echocardiography images the thoracic aorta more completely and provides superior identification of aortic valvular vegetations or infectious complications involving the aortic leaflets or annulus. Often, however, it adds little information about the severity of regurgitation.

An algorithm for management of severe chronic aortic regurgitation is shown in Figure 10.

Other noninvasive imaging methods, including cine magnetic resonance imaging, cine computed tomography, and radionuclide angiography, allow measurement of regurgitant flow, ventricular dimensions, and myocardial function. Of these, radionuclide angiography is the best studied and the most widely available (Table 6).

Noninvasive assessment of the cause and severity of aortic regurgitation is usually sufficient. Aortic root angiography is still appropriate, however, in patients in whom noninvasive testing was technically inadequate or gave results

Table 4.—Recommendations for Echocardiography in Aortic Regurgitation

Indication	Class
1. Confirm presence and severity of acute AR	I
2. Diagnosis of chronic AR in patients with equivocal physical findings	I
3. Assessment of cause of regurgitation (including valve morphology and aortic root size and morphology)	I
4. Assessment of LV hypertrophy, dimension (or volume), and systolic function	I
5. Semiquantitative estimate of severity of AR	I
6. Reevaluation of patients with mild, moderate, or severe regurgitation with new or changing symptoms	I
7. Reevaluation of LV size and function in asymptomatic patients with severe regurgitation (recommended timing of reevaluation is given in Figure 10)	I
8. Reevaluation of asymptomatic patients with mild, moderate, or severe regurgitation and enlarged aortic root	I
9. Yearly reevaluation of asymptomatic patients with mild to moderate regurgitation with stable physical signs and normal or near-normal LV chamber size	III

AR, aortic regurgitation; LV, left ventricular.
From *J Am Coll Cardiol* 32:1486-1588, 1998. By permission of the American College of Cardiology.

discordant with clinical findings (Table 7). Exercise testing also may be valuable for determining functional capacity (Table 8).

- Echocardiography assesses the cause and severity of aortic regurgitation in addition to left ventricular size and function.

Table 5.—Doppler Indicators of Severe Aortic Regurgitation*

AR color jet diameter/LVOT diameter in parasternal long-axis view (> 60%)

AR color jet area/LVOT area in parasternal short-axis view (> 60%)

AR pressure half-time by CW Doppler (< 250 ms)

Transmitral PW Doppler diastolic profile (restrictive or premature flow cessation)

Flow reversal by PW Doppler in proximal descending thoracic aorta (holodiastolic)

CW Doppler signal intensity (dense)

Regurgitant volume (> 60 mL)[†]

Regurgitant fraction (> 55%)[†]

AR, aortic regurgitation; CW, continuous-wave; LVOT, left ventricular outflow tract; PW, pulsed wave.
*Measurements indicative of severe regurgitation are in parentheses.
[†]Can be measured by volumetric Doppler, proximal isovelocity surface area method, or combination of techniques, including two-dimensional volume measures.

- Transesophageal echocardiography is a useful adjunct for anatomical assessment but adds much less to the quantitative assessment of aortic regurgitation.
- Echocardiographic assessment of the severity of regurgitation should not rely exclusively on color flow data.
- Aortography is indicated when noninvasive data are discordant, technically limited, or differ from the clinical impression of regurgitant severity.

Natural History of Aortic Regurgitation
In patients with significant *acute* aortic regurgitation, dyspnea and heart failure usually develop (Table 9). Their clinical course is dictated by the cause of the acute regurgitation. Patients with aortic dissection have high mortality without operation. Those with aortic valve endocarditis who have severe aortic regurgitation may require early surgical replacement of the valve.

In comparison, patients with *chronic* severe aortic regurgitation and normal left ventricular function may remain asymptomatic for long periods. However, once they become symptomatic, the long-term prognosis is poor, especially after a first episode of congestive heart failure. Patients who are asymptomatic but have resting left ventricular systolic dysfunction usually become symptomatic within 3 years after evaluation.

- The cause of acute aortic regurgitation dictates its natural history.
- Patients with impaired resting systolic function and severe

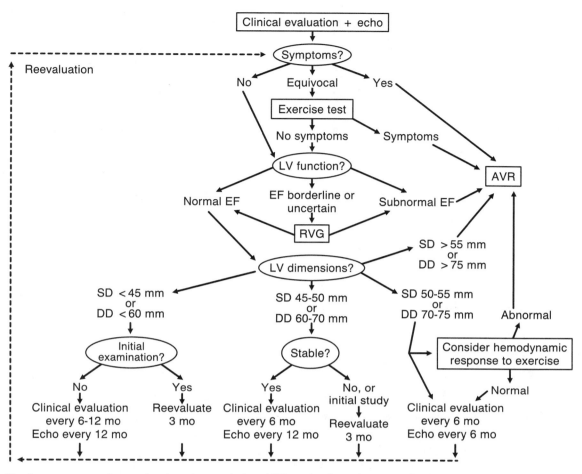

Fig. 10. Algorithm for management of severe chronic aortic regurgitation. AVR, aortic valve replacement; DD, end-diastolic dimension; echo, echocardiography; LV, left ventricular; RVG, radionuclide ventriculography; SD, end-systolic dimension. (From *J Am Coll Cardiol* 32:1486-1588, 1998. By permission of the American College of Cardiology.)

Table 6.—Recommendations for Radionuclide Angiography in Aortic Regurgitation

Indication	Class
1. Initial and serial assessment of LV volume and function at rest in patients with suboptimal echocardiograms or equivocal echocardiographic data*	I
2. Serial assessment of LV volume and function at rest when serial echocardiograms are not used*	I
3. Assessment of LV volume and function in asymptomatic patients with moderate to severe regurgitation when echocardiographic evidence of declining LV function is suggestive but not definitive*	I
4. Confirmation of subnormal LV ejection fraction before recommending surgery in an asymptomatic patient with borderline echocardiographic evidence of LV dysfunction*	I
5. Assessment of LV volume and function in patients with moderate to severe regurgitation when clinical assessment and echocardiographic data are discordant*	I
6. Routine assessment of exercise ejection fraction	IIb
7. Quantification of AR in patients with unsatisfactory echocardiograms	IIb
8. Quantification of AR in patients with satisfactory echocardiograms	III
9. Initial and serial assessment of LV volume and function at rest in addition to echocardiography	III

AR, aortic regurgitation; LV, left ventricular.

*In centers with expertise in cardiac magnetic resonance imaging (MRI), cardiac MRI may be used in place of radionuclide angiography for these indications.

From *J Am Coll Cardiol* 32:1486-1588, 1998. By permission of the American College of Cardiology.

Table 7.—Recommendations for Cardiac Catheterization in Chronic Aortic Regurgitation

Indication	Class
1. Coronary angiography before AVR in patients at risk for CAD	I
2. Assessing severity of regurgitation when noninvasive tests are inconclusive or discordant with clinical findings regarding severity of regurgitation or need for surgery	I
3. Assessing LV function when noninvasive tests are inconclusive or discordant with clinical findings regarding LV dysfunction and need for surgery in patients with severe AR	I
4. Assessment of LV function and severity of regurgitation before AVR when noninvasive tests are adequate and concordant with clinical findings and coronary angiography is not needed	IIb
5. Assessment of LV function and severity of regurgitation in asymptomatic patients when noninvasive tests are adequate	III

AR, aortic regurgitation; AVR, aortic valve replacement; CAD, coronary artery disease; LV, left ventricular.
From *J Am Coll Cardiol* 32:1486-1588, 1998. By permission of the American College of Cardiology.

Table 8.—Recommendations for Exercise Testing in Chronic Aortic Regurgitation*

Indication	Class
1. Assessment of functional capacity and symptomatic responses in patients with a history of equivocal symptoms	I
2. Evaluation of symptoms and functional capacity before participation in athletic activities	IIa
3. Prognostic assessment before AVR in patients with LV dysfunction	IIa
4. Exercise hemodynamic measurements to determine the effect of AR on LV function	IIb
5. Exercise radionuclide angiography for assessing LV function in asymptomatic or symptomatic patients	IIb
6. Exercise echocardiography or dobutamine stress echocardiography for assessing LV function in asymptomatic or symptomatic patients	III

*These recommendations differ from the ACC/AHA Guidelines for Exercise Testing. The committee believes that indications 1, 2, and 3 above warrant a higher recommendation than IIb.
AR, aortic regurgitation; AVR, aortic valve replacement; LV, left ventricular.
From *J Am Coll Cardiol* 32:1486-1588, 1998. By permission of the American College of Cardiology.

aortic regurgitation usually become symptomatic within 3 years after evaluation; symptoms herald poor long-term prognosis without operation.

Treatment of Aortic Regurgitation

The most important predictor of outcome after aortic valve replacement is preoperative resting left ventricular function. Patients with a normal preoperative ejection fraction have a longer postoperative survival than those whose preoperative ejection fraction was reduced. Other variables that are predictive of postoperative survival are indicated in Table 10.

Thus, the current management approach to chronic aortic regurgitation is as follows. All patients with aortic regurgitation should practice antibiotic prophylaxis against endocarditis. The indications for operation are listed in Table 11.

Surgical treatment is expected to improve both survival and the likelihood of postoperative ventricular improvement. Other patients should be followed serially, with clinical monitoring of symptoms and objective measures of ventricular function and exercise capacity. If a decrease in ventricular function, a marked increase in ventricular size, or a decrease in exercise capacity is detected, operation is advised.

Aortic valve replacement is the usual operation for patients with aortic regurgitation. Pulmonary valve autografts (Ross procedure) and aortic valve repair should be used only by surgeons who are experienced in both selecting appropriate patients and performing these procedures.

Short-term studies of pharmacologic treatment have shown short-term improvement in left ventricular volume, ejection fraction, mass, and wall stress using hydralazine,

Table 9.—Natural History of Aortic Regurgitation

Asymptomatic patients with normal LV systolic function	
Progression to symptoms or LV dysfunction	< 6%/year
Progression to asymptomatic LV dysfunction	< 3.5%/year
Sudden death	< 0.2%/year
Asymptomatic patients with LV systolic dysfunction	
Progression to cardiac symptoms	> 25%/year
Symptomatic patients	
Mortality rate	> 10%/year

LV, left ventricular.
From *J Am Coll Cardiol* 32:1486-1588, 1998. By permission of the American College of Cardiology.

nifedipine, and enalapril (Table 12). One study in a small number of patients demonstrated that the group treated with nifedipine had less progression to need for valve replacement than the group treated with digoxin. It is not known which vasodilator should be used in which patients. However, because chronic aortic regurgitation is a condition of high afterload, vasodilator therapy is reasonable and has been recommended for 1) patients with severe aortic regurgitation with symptoms of left ventricular dysfunction but in whom operation is not possible and 2) asymptomatic patients without severe left ventricular dilatation or ventricular dysfunction.

- Patients with aortic regurgitation should practice antibiotic prophylaxis.

Table 10.—Predictors of Poor Postoperative Outcome* in Aortic Regurgitation

End-systolic diameter > 55 mm by echocardiography
End-systolic volume index > 90 mL/m^2 by radionuclide angiography
Poor treadmill exercise time
Higher New York Heart Association functional class preoperatively
Left ventricular systolic dysfunction > 18 months' duration

*Reduced survival, persistent left ventricular dysfunction, or postoperative congestive heart failure.

Table 11.—Indications for Operation in Severe Aortic Regurgitation

NYHA functional class III or IV
Progressive LV dilatation, declining ejection fraction or exercise tolerance
Concomitant angina and severe AR
Mild to moderate LV dysfunction (EF < 50%)
Severe LV dilatation (EDD > 75 mm, ESD > 55 mm; consider lower threshold for small stature)

AR, aortic regurgitation; EDD, end-diastolic diameter; EF, ejection fraction; ESD, end-systolic diameter; LV, left ventricular; NYHA, New York Heart Association.

- Operation is the treatment of choice for patients with symptoms or impaired exercise tolerance due to valvular regurgitation, impaired ventricular systolic function, or significant increase in ventricular end-systolic dimensions.
- Vasodilator therapy is appropriate for any patient with severe aortic regurgitation who is not a surgical candidate.

Tricuspid Regurgitation

Clinically significant tricuspid regurgitation is rarely an isolated lesion.

Anatomy and Etiology
The six parts of the tricuspid apparatus are necessary for proper function: leaflets, chordae, papillary muscles, annulus, right ventricle, and right atrium.

Right Ventricular, Right Atrial, and Tricuspid Annular Dilatation
The most common cause of tricuspid regurgitation is dilatation of the right ventricle and tricuspid annulus because of chronic left-sided valvular disease or heart failure. It less commonly is due to cor pulmonale, isolated or predominant right ventricular myocardial infarction, or pulmonary hypertension caused by pulmonary vascular disease.

Abnormal Tricuspid Valve Leaflets, Chordae, and Papillary Muscles
Isolated lesions of the tricuspid valve are unusual. Congenital abnormalities include Ebstein anomaly and tricuspid valve prolapse. Tricuspid valve prolapse often coexists with mitral

Table 12.—Recommendations for Vasodilator Therapy for Chronic Aortic Regurgitation

Indication	Class
1. Chronic therapy in patients with severe regurgitation who have symptoms or LV dysfunction when surgery is not recommended because of additional cardiac or noncardiac factors	I
2. Long-term therapy in asymptomatic patients with severe regurgitation who have LV dilatation but normal systolic function	I
3. Long-term therapy in asymptomatic patients with hypertension and any degree of regurgitation	I
4. Long-term ACE inhibitor therapy in patients with persistent LV systolic dysfunction after AVR	I
5. Short-term therapy to improve the hemodynamic profile of patients with severe heart failure symptoms and severe LV dysfunction before proceeding with AVR	I
6. Long-term therapy in asymptomatic patients with mild to moderate AR and normal LV systolic function	III
7. Long-term therapy in asymptomatic patients with LV systolic dysfunction who are otherwise candidates for valve replacement	III
8. Long-term therapy in symptomatic patients with either normal LV function or mild to moderate LV systolic dysfunction who are otherwise candidates for valve replacement	III

ACE, angiotensin-converting enzyme; AR, aortic regurgitation; AVR, aortic valve replacement; LV, left ventricular.
From *J Am Coll Cardiol* 32:1486-1588, 1998. By permission of the American College of Cardiology.

valve prolapse or an atrial septal defect (or both).

Acquired lesions that affect the tricuspid valve include rheumatic valvulitis, infective endocarditis, and carcinoid syndrome. Iatrogenic causes include transvenous pacemaker, catheters, and repeated right ventricular biopsy in heart transplant recipients, which may interfere with normal leaflet closure, traumatize subvalvular support structures, or even perforate the leaflets. Other uncommon acquired lesions are listed in Table 13.

● Tricuspid regurgitation most often is due to right ventricular enlargement. This usually is due to left-sided heart disease and less commonly to pulmonary parenchymal or pulmonary vascular disease.

Pathophysiology of Tricuspid Regurgitation
In the absence of tricuspid regurgitation, flow from the venae cavae continues into the right atrium during ventricular systole. Tricuspid regurgitation decreases the amount of returning blood. If valvular regurgitation is severe enough, the amount of blood returning to the right atrium is markedly decreased, thus limiting cardiac output. Additionally, increased venous pressure in the systemic circulation leads to fluid extravasation.

Clinical Syndrome of Tricuspid Regurgitation
Tricuspid regurgitation is generally well tolerated in the absence of pulmonary hypertension. However, with

pulmonary hypertension, regurgitant volume increases and cardiac output decreases significantly. Right-sided heart failure is characterized by exertional dyspnea, fatigue, ascites, uncomfortable congestive hepatomegaly and enteropathy, and edema.

Common physical findings include atrial fibrillation, increased jugular venous pressure with prominent "v" waves, a palpable right ventricular impulse, liver enlargement, ascites, and edema. The severity and chronicity of disease influence how many of these findings are present.

Auscultation reveals a pansystolic murmur heard along the left sternal border or subxiphoid region. The murmur is

Table 13.—Acquired Valvular Lesions Associated With Tricuspid Regurgitation

Rheumatic fever
Infective endocarditis
Carcinoid disease
Iatrogenic cause
Trauma
Radiation
Hypereosinophilic syndrome
Systemic lupus erythematosus
Rheumatoid arthritis
Other connective tissue disorders
Tumors

more intense when pulmonary hypertension is present. The intensity of the murmur increases with inspiration, because of augmented right ventricular filling (Carvallo sign), but this finding is lost in right ventricular failure when the ventricle can no longer increase its filling and stroke volume during inspiration. When there is significant right ventricular enlargement, it occupies the anterior surface of the heart, making the murmur more prominent at the apex and, thus, difficult to distinguish from mitral regurgitation. Tricuspid regurgitation murmur intensity may vary more with varying R-R intervals than the murmur of mitral regurgitation. Inhalation of amyl nitrite increases the murmur of tricuspid regurgitation by increasing venous return and decreases the murmur of mitral regurgitation by decreasing systemic vascular resistance. A coexistent diastolic flow rumble may signify either severe tricuspid regurgitation or coexistent tricuspid stenosis; the behavior of the "y" descent in the jugular veins helps to distinguish between the two.

In advanced stages of right-sided heart failure, weight loss, cachexia, cyanosis (right-to-left shunting across a patent foramen ovale), and jaundice may develop.

- Right-sided heart failure is characterized by exertional dyspnea, fatigue, ascites, edema, and symptoms referable to congested abdominal viscera.
- Physical findings of severe tricuspid regurgitation include large "v" waves, right ventricular impulse, pulsatile liver, and diastolic rumble at the left parasternal border.
- The murmur of tricuspid regurgitation is dynamic with respiration (until right ventricular failure ensues), radiates to the apex with right ventricular enlargement, and increases in intensity with amyl nitrite inhalation.

Evaluation of Tricuspid Regurgitation

ECG does not establish the presence or severity of tricuspid regurgitation, but it provides insight into any electrical and structural abnormalities that might coexist with tricuspid regurgitation. Atrial enlargement is suggested by either a right or a biatrial enlargement pattern or by atrial fibrillation. Complete or incomplete right bundle branch block and right ventricular hypertrophy also may be seen. However, because most cases of severe tricuspid regurgitation are due to left-sided heart disease, ECG is often dominated by changes related to the process on the left side of the heart.

Chest radiographic evidence of right atrial enlargement or pleural effusion suggests high pressure in the right atrium. This might result from significant tricuspid regurgitation,

but it also can be seen in tricuspid stenosis or high right ventricular diastolic pressure from any cause. Right ventricular enlargement causes filling-in of the retrosternal air space on a lateral chest film. In severe right-sided failure with ascites, the hemidiaphragms may be displaced upward.

Echocardiography assesses the presence, severity, and mechanism of tricuspid regurgitation; the size and function of the right ventricle; and right-sided systolic pressure. An integrated approach to the assessment of regurgitant severity is necessary and includes not just color flow extent but also appearance of the tricuspid valve, size of the right ventricle and atrium, strength of the regurgitant jet Doppler spectral profile, antegrade diastolic velocities through the tricuspid valve, size and respiratory behavior of the inferior vena cava and hepatic veins, and pulsed-wave Doppler profiling of the hepatic vein and superior vena cava flow pattern. In general, transesophageal echocardiography allows greater image resolution than transthoracic echocardiography, but it does not always provide a better image of the tricuspid valve, because the tricuspid valve is in the far field relative to the esophagus.

Catheterization and right ventriculography are rarely needed for information about regurgitation severity, right ventricular pressure, and systolic function. However, catheterization allows measurement of pulmonary resistance and responsiveness to pharmacologic intervention. The use of more flexible catheters usually does not influence the amount of tricuspid regurgitation during right ventriculography. Catheterization of the right side of the heart is indicated whenever clinical and echocardiographic assessments of right-sided systolic pressures are discordant or when pulmonary vascular resistance and responsiveness need to be measured.

Ultrafast computed tomography and magnetic resonance imaging techniques can be used to assess right ventricular size and function, but these methods are not universally available; their role in day-to-day assessment of tricuspid regurgitation has not been defined.

- Echocardiography assesses the mechanism and severity of tricuspid regurgitation, right ventricular function, and pressures on the right side of the heart.

Natural History of Tricuspid Regurgitation

Because isolated significant tricuspid regurgitation is rare, its natural history is unknown. When significant tricuspid regurgitation accompanies left-sided heart disease or systemic disease, the natural history is determined by the primary disease.

Treatment of Tricuspid Regurgitation

Severe tricuspid regurgitation without pulmonary hypertension requires treatment when clinical right-sided heart failure or right ventricular systolic dysfunction is identified. Initial treatment includes sodium restriction and diuretics; digitalis is used when there is right ventricular systolic dysfunction. Surgical treatment depends on the mechanism of the regurgitation; annular dilatation is treated with annuloplasty, whereas valve lesions require either valve repair (usually with annuloplasty) or replacement (Table 14).

Significant tricuspid regurgitation with pulmonary hypertension usually is due to left-sided heart disease, and the best treatment is aimed at the primary disease. If it is approached surgically (as in mitral valve disease), treatment of the tricuspid regurgitation depends on whether it is functional or organic. Preoperative and intraoperative echocardiography are important adjuncts to the surgeon's decision making. Although organic tricuspid disease usually requires either valve replacement or annuloplasty plus repair, functional regurgitation is usually treated initially with annuloplasty alone, followed by surgical or intraoperative transesophageal echocardiographic assessment (or both) of residual regurgitation before the patient comes off bypass.

Significant tricuspid regurgitation with pulmonary hypertension due to pulmonary vascular or parenchymal disease is treated with diuretics, sodium restriction, and treatment of the primary disease.

Patients with infective endocarditis confined to the tricuspid valve (usually intravenous drug addicts) may require tricuspid valvectomy, followed by antibiotic therapy sufficient to eradicate the infection. Later, they can undergo tricuspid valve replacement after the surgical bed is sterile.

Pulmonary Regurgitation

Pulmonary valve regurgitation is highly prevalent on the basis of color flow Doppler evaluation in clinically normal subjects. However, it usually is not clinically significant in adults.

Etiology

Common causes of pulmonary regurgitation include dilatation of the annulus due to either pulmonary hypertension or idiopathic dilatation of the pulmonary artery. Less common causes include rheumatic valvulitis, infective endocarditis, carcinoid disease, and trauma (including iatrogenic causes, such as pulmonary artery catheters). Congenital lesions may be isolated or associated with other cardiac anomalies.

Pathophysiology of Pulmonary Regurgitation

If chronic and severe enough, isolated pulmonary regurgitation causes right ventricular volume overload. Pulmonary hypertension hastens this process and can precipitate right-sided heart failure.

Clinical Syndrome of Pulmonary Regurgitation

Isolated severe pulmonary regurgitation is uncommon, and,

Table 14.—Recommendations for Surgery for Tricuspid Regurgitation

Indication	Class
1. Annuloplasty for severe TR and pulmonary hypertension in patients with mitral valve disease requiring mitral valve surgery	I
2. Valve replacement for severe TR due to disease or abnormal tricuspid valve leaflets not amenable to annuloplasty or repair	IIa
3. Valve replacement or annuloplasty for severe TR with mean pulmonary artery pressure < 60 mm Hg when symptomatic	IIa
4. Annuloplasty for mild TR in patients with pulmonary hypertension due to mitral valve disease requiring mitral valve surgery	IIb
5. Valve replacement or annuloplasty for TR with pulmonary artery systolic pressure < 60 mm Hg in the presence of a normal mitral valve, in asymptomatic patients, or in symptomatic patients who have not received a trial of diuretic therapy	III

TR, tricuspid regurgitation.
From *J Am Coll Cardiol* 32:1486-1588, 1998. By permission of the American College of Cardiology.

thus, the clinical presentation usually is related to the manifestations of the underlying disease process. If right-sided heart failure has ensued, symptoms of fatigue, dyspnea, edema, ascites, and passive enteric congestion (early satiety, postcibal fullness) are variably present.

Hyperdynamic left parasternal pulsations indicate right ventricular enlargement, with maintained systolic function. Systolic dysfunction is accompanied by a sustained parasternal impulse. Pulmonary artery dilatation may be palpable in the second left intercostal space.

A loud pulmonic second sound indicates pulmonary hypertension, but this may be absent if pulmonary leaflet coaptation is limited. Widened splitting of the second heart sound indicates prolonged right ventricular stroke time (mechanical) or right bundle branch block (electrical) or both. Gallop sounds may be present on the right side.

The murmur of pulmonary regurgitation in the absence of pulmonary hypertension is often inaudible. When present, it is low-pitched, brief, and diamond-shaped, and it is intensified by either inspiration or inhalation of amyl nitrite. However, when pulmonary pressures are increased, the murmur becomes high-pitched and resembles the murmur of aortic regurgitation (Graham Steell murmur). The presence of other findings of pulmonary hypertension (and the absence of other findings of severe aortic regurgitation) provides bedside clues to the true cause of the murmur.

Evaluation of Pulmonary Regurgitation

As with tricuspid regurgitation, the ECG in pulmonary regurgitation usually is dominated by findings related to the primary left-sided heart disease. In uncommon cases in which pulmonary regurgitation is primary, the ECG might suggest right atrial volume or pressure overload with right atrial enlargement, an rSr´ or rsR configuration in the right precordial leads, or evidence of right ventricular hypertrophy.

Chest radiography shows enlargement of the pulmonary artery and right ventricle (often with enlargement of the right atrium as well), but echocardiography is the most definitive imaging method. It allows assessment of the size and systolic function of the right ventricle, anatomy of the pulmonary valve and artery, degree of pulmonary regurgitation, and systolic and diastolic pressures in the pulmonary arteries. Transesophageal echocardiography (especially multiplane) may provide superior imaging of the pulmonary valve and proximal pulmonary arteries (the left pulmonary artery may be shielded by the carina).

Treatment of Pulmonary Regurgitation

Treatment usually is aimed at the disease responsible for pulmonary hypertension, which in turn is augmenting the pulmonary regurgitant volume. Less commonly, operation is necessary for lesions causing primary pulmonary regurgitation, such as infective endocarditis and carcinoid syndrome. Dilatation and failure of the right ventricle are treated with diuretics and digoxin. Afterload reduction can help treat pulmonary hypertension, but there is risk of decreasing systemic resistance more than pulmonary resistance, thus precipitating cardiogenic shock. Therefore, such therapy should be applied carefully and sometimes only in an inpatient, monitored setting.

An appendix of echocardiographic findings in valvular regurgitation follows.

Echocardiography in Mitral Regurgitation

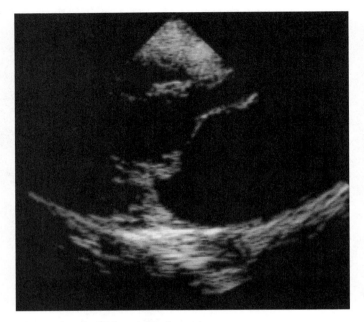

Fig. 11. Anterior leaflet mitral valve prolapse.

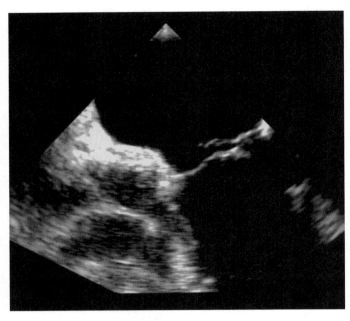

Fig. 12. Flail mitral leaflet. Transesophageal echocardiogram.

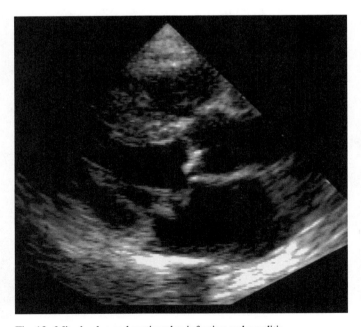

Fig. 13. Mitral valve and aortic valve infective endocarditis.

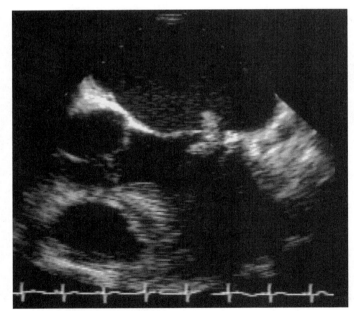

Fig. 14. Mitral valve infective endocarditis. Transesophageal echocardiogram.

Echocardiography in Mitral Regurgitation

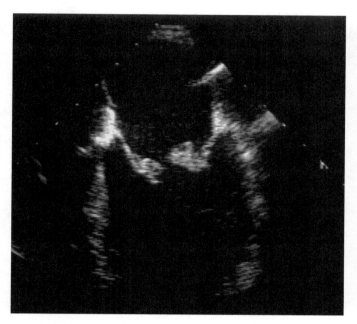

Fig. 15. Libman-Sacks mitral valve endocarditis. Transesophageal echocardiogram.

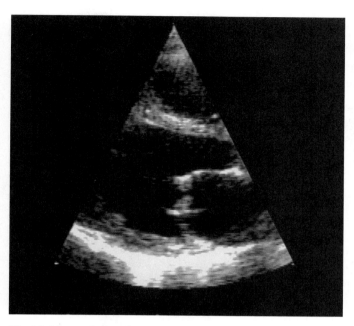

Fig. 16. Libman-Sacks mitral valve endocarditis.

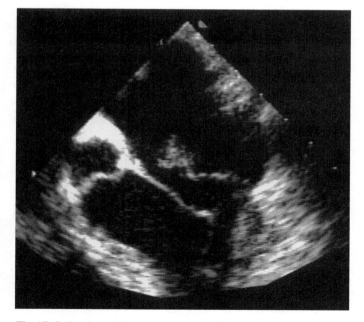

Fig. 17. Ischemic papillary muscle rupture. Transesophageal echocardiogram.

Echocardiography in Aortic Regurgitation

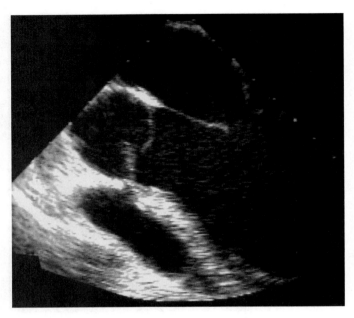

Fig. 18. Aortic valve prolapse. Transesophageal echocardiogram.

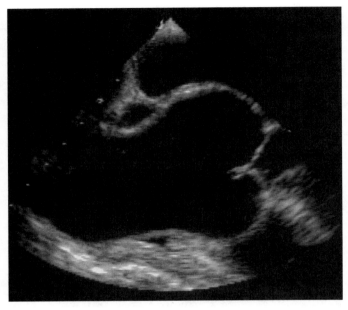

Fig. 19. Aortic root aneurysm. Transesophageal echocardiogram.

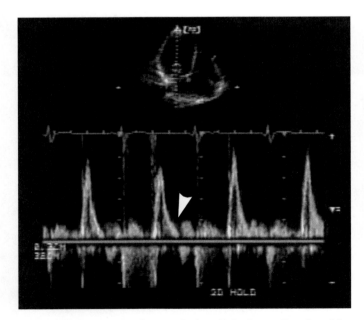

Fig. 20. Acute severe aortic regurgitation. Pulsed-wave Doppler of the mitral valve shows short deceleration with premature flow cessation (*arrowhead*) indicative of increased left ventricular end-diastolic pressure.

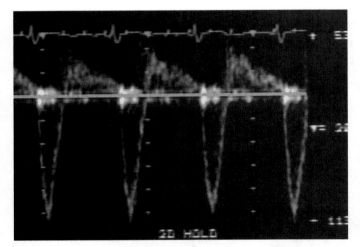

Fig. 21. Acute severe aortic regurgitation. Holodiastolic flow reversal in descending thoracic aorta.

Echocardiography in Tricuspid Regurgitation

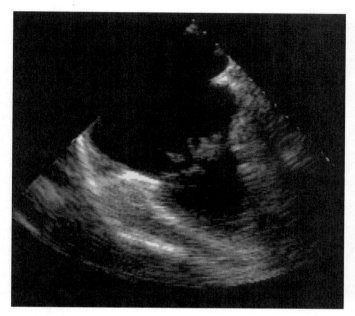

Fig. 22. Tricuspid valve infective endocarditis. Transesophageal echocardiogram.

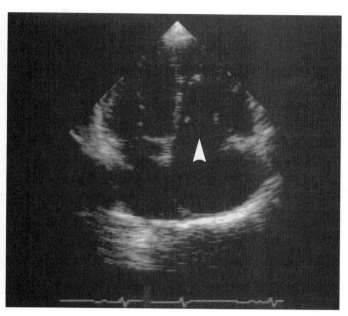

Fig. 23. "Fixed" open tricuspid valve of carcinoid tricuspid disease (note mitral valve closed, systole).

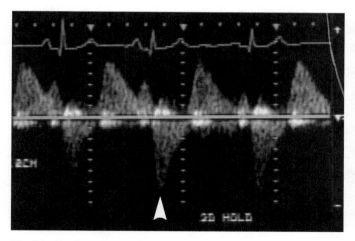

Fig. 24. Continuous-wave Doppler echocardiogram in severe tricuspid regurgitation due to carcinoid syndrome. This results in greatly increased right atrial pressure (note truncated tricuspid regurgitation signal).

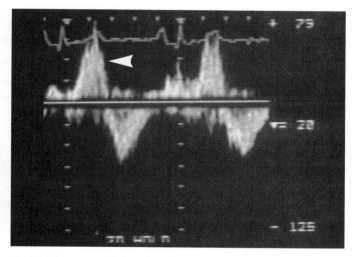

Fig. 25. Flow reversal in hepatic vein due to severe tricuspid regurgitation. Pulsed-wave Doppler echocardiogram.

Suggested Review Reading

1. ACC/AHA guidelines for the management of patients with valvular heart disease. A report of the American College of Cardiology/American Heart Association Task Force on Practice Guidelines (Committee on Management of Patients with Valvular Heart Disease). *J Am Coll Cardiol* 32:1486-1588, 1998.
This is a comprehensive, referenced summary of regurgitant valvular lesions and many issues related to valvular heart disease.

2. Bach DS, Bolling SF: Early improvement in congestive heart failure after correction of secondary mitral regurgitation in end-stage cardiomyopathy. *Am Heart J* 129:1165-1170, 1995.
These authors present the first series of patients (9 consecutive) who underwent mitral valve repair for secondary mitral regurgitation in end-stage cardiomyopathy. They had no operative deaths and at short-term follow-up reported uniform symptom improvement and statistically significant improvements in ejection fraction and cardiac output.

3. Bolling SF, Pagani FD, Deeb GM, et al: Intermediate-term outcome of mitral reconstruction in cardiomyopathy. *J Thorac Cardiovasc Surg* 115:381-386, 1998.
Forty-eight patients with severe ischemic or dilated cardiomyopathy underwent mitral valve repair with low operative mortality and significant symptomatic improvement.

4. Bonow RO: Asymptomatic aortic regurgitation: indications for operation. *J Card Surg* 9 (Suppl 2):170-173, 1994.
This excellent review of the literature guides most of our decisions about operating on patients with asymptomatic aortic regurgitation.

5. Bonow RO, Lakatos E, Maron BJ, et al: Serial long-term assessment of the natural history of asymptomatic patients with chronic aortic regurgitation and normal left ventricular systolic function. *Circulation* 84:1625-1635, 1991.
This classic work defines the impact of left ventricular function and dimensions in determining patient outcome and therefore patient management. Both echocardiography and radionuclide angiography were used, and 104 consecutive patients were followed for a mean of 8 years.

6. Bonow RO, Nikas D, Elefteriades JA: Valve replacement for regurgitant lesions of the aortic or mitral valve in advanced left ventricular dysfunction. *Cardiol Clin* 13:73-83; 85, 1995.
The data regarding valvular operation in patients with significant ventricular dysfunction are reviewed. The study concluded that although risks are higher when ventricular dysfunction is present, operation for aortic regurgitation can almost always be done, whereas there still are limits to when operation for mitral regurgitation should be attempted.

7. Carabello BA: Mitral valve regurgitation. *Curr Probl Cardiol* 23:202-241, 1998.
Mitral regurgitation is thoroughly reviewed. There is a particularly good review of the mechanism of systolic dysfunction in patients entering the chronic decompensated stage of the disease.

8. Carabello BA, Crawford FA Jr: Valvular heart disease. *N Engl J Med* 337:32-41, 1997.
This is a succinct review of stenotic and regurgitant lesions of the left-sided cardiac valves. The diagram of the pathophysiologic stages of mitral regurgitation is worth reviewing.

9. Connolly HM, Nishimura RA, Smith HC, et al: Outcome of cardiac surgery for carcinoid heart disease. *J Am Coll Cardiol* 25:410-416, 1995.
This is a review of the Mayo Clinic experience with valvular operation in 26 patients with carcinoid heart disease. Perioperative mortality was high, but survivors had significant symptomatic improvement. Operation is recommended when cardiac symptoms become severe. Comments are given about the choice of tricuspid prosthesis and management of the pulmonary valve.

10. Cooper HA, Gersh BJ: Treatment of chronic mitral regurgitation. *Am Heart J* 135:925-936, 1998.
This is an excellent review of the current literature and issues in the management of chronic mitral regurgitation, including an algorithm for management.

11. Devlin WH, Starling MR: Outcome of valvular heart disease with vasodilator therapy. *Compr Ther* 20:569-574, 1994.
The pathophysiology and natural history of aortic and mitral regurgitation are reviewed, and the results are given

for trials using vasodilators for both acute and chronic forms of left-sided valvular regurgitation.

12. Enriquez-Sarano M, Orszulak TA, Schaff HV, et al: Mitral regurgitation: a new clinical perspective. *Mayo Clin Proc* 72:1034-1043, 1997.
The authors summarize their body of work regarding operation for mitral regurgitation and advocate an aggressive approach in managing patients with mitral regurgitation.

13. Enriquez-Sarano M, Schaff HV, Orszulak TA, et al: Congestive heart failure after surgical correction of mitral regurgitation. A long-term study. *Circulation* 92:2496-2503, 1995.
Long-term follow-up data are given for 576 survivors of mitral valve operation for mitral regurgitation. Postoperative congestive heart failure was common and portended a poor survival. Most postoperative congestive heart failure was due to myocardial dysfunction and was independently predicted by preoperative ejection fraction, coronary artery disease, and functional class.

14. Enriquez-Sarano M, Schaff HV, Orszulak TA, et al: Valve repair improves the outcome of surgery for mitral regurgitation. A multivariate analysis. *Circulation* 91:1022-1028, 1995.
The outcomes in 195 patients undergoing valve repair are compared with the outcomes in 214 patients receiving valve replacement for organic mitral regurgitation. Valve repair conferred an independent benefit on overall survival, operative mortality, late survival, and postoperative ejection fraction. An accompanying editorial raises a question of whether the high percentage of ball-cage prosthetic valves may have played a role in these results.

15. Enriquez-Sarano M, Tajik AJ, Schaff HV, et al: Echocardiographic prediction of survival after surgical correction of organic mitral regurgitation. *Circulation* 90:830-837, 1994.
This study retrospectively reviewed 266 patients who had mitral valve operation for mitral regurgitation and both preoperative and postoperative evaluation of ejection fraction by echocardiography. Postoperative left ventricular dysfunction (ejection fraction < 50%) was associated with a poor prognosis and could be independently predicted by preoperative ejection fraction and systolic dimension. The authors recommended consideration of surgical correction at an earlier stage instead of waiting for left ventricular

enlargement and a decrease in systolic function. An accompanying editorial also emphasizes the role of echocardiography in delineating the mechanism of mitral regurgitation.

16. From the Centers for Disease Control and Prevention. Cardiac valvulopathy associated with exposure to fenfluramine or dexfenfluramine: US Department of Health and Human Services interim public health recommendations, November 1997. *JAMA* 278:1729-1731, 1997.
This article provides interim recommendations regarding patient management, recognizing that the certainty and magnitude of the association between fenfluramine and dexfenfluramine and valvular disease are still under evaluation.

17. Gaasch WH, Sundaram M, Meyer TE: Managing asymptomatic patients with chronic aortic regurgitation. *Chest* 111:1702-1709, 1997.
This is a comprehensive, recent review of the subject, including pathophysiology, ventricular remodeling, natural history, and treatment options.

18. Klodas E, Enriquez-Sarano M, Tajik AJ, et al: Surgery for aortic regurgitation in women. Contrasting indications and outcomes compared with men. *Circulation* 94:2472-2478, 1996.
The sex differences in the manifestation of severe aortic regurgitation in a retrospective series of patients are described.

19. Levine HJ, Gaasch WH: Vasoactive drugs in chronic regurgitant lesions of the mitral and aortic valves. *J Am Coll Cardiol* 28:1083-1091, 1996.
This article reviews the use of vasodilators in both acute and chronic settings and ventricular remodeling and the interaction between vasodilators and this process.

20. Lin M, Chiang HT, Lin SL, et al: Vasodilator therapy in chronic asymptomatic aortic regurgitation: enalapril versus hydralazine therapy. *J Am Coll Cardiol* 24:1046-1053, 1994.
The authors followed 76 patients with nonrheumatic aortic regurgitation for 1 year. Both the enalapril and the hydralazine regimens decreased left ventricular wall stress, but only enalapril reduced left ventricular mass and volume and suppressed the renin-angiotensin system. The study postulated (but was not set up to examine) that enalapril might favorably influence the natural history of the disease.

21. Ling LH, Enriquez-Sarano M, Seward JB, et al: Clinical outcome of mitral regurgitation due to flail leaflet. *N Engl J Med* 335:1417-1423, 1996.

The authors retrospectively reviewed 229 patients with isolated mitral regurgitation due to a flail mitral leaflet and compared the group undergoing operation with the 86 patients who were treated medically. The medically treated group had higher mortality and more heart failure, and either operation or death was virtually inevitable. The authors concluded that early operation should be considered in all such patients. The accompanying editorial takes a more conservative view.

22. Ling LH, Enriquez-Sarano M, Seward JB, et al: Early surgery in patients with mitral regurgitation due to flail leaflets: a long-term outcome study. *Circulation* 96:1819-1825, 1997.

Two groups (surgical, medical) with flail mitral leaflets were compared to assess the effect of initial treatment strategy in long-term (6-15 years) follow-up. Although the surgical group was younger, more symptomatic, and more likely to be in atrial fibrillation, the surgical strategy was associated with improved overall survival and a lower incidence of cardiovascular deaths and congestive heart failure.

23. Otto CM: Aortic valve insufficiency: changing concepts in diagnosis and management. Cardiologia 41:505-513, 1996.

This article reviews the management approach to aortic regurgitation, emphasizing the role of echocardiography and Doppler in diagnosis and assessment.

24. Pagani FD, Monaghan HL, Deeb GM, et al: Mitral valve reconstruction for active and healed endocarditis. *Circulation* 94(Suppl II):II-133-II-138, 1996.

The role of mitral valve repair for mitral regurgitation due to infective endocarditis is discussed.

25. Roberts WC: A unique heart disease associated with a unique cancer: carcinoid heart disease. *Am J Cardiol* 80:251-256, 1997.

Carcinoid heart disease with primarily right-sided cardiac valvular involvement is reviewed; aspects are devoted to evaluation and treatment.

26. Robiolio PA, Rigolin VH, Harrison JK, et al: Predictors of outcome of tricuspid valve replacement in carcinoid heart disease. *Am J Cardiol* 75:485-488, 1995.

This is a review of the Duke experience with 8 surgical patients and is also a recent literature review. Like the Mayo study, it noted high surgical mortality rates but potential for significant symptom palliation and long-term survival in surgical survivors.

27. Scognamiglio R, Rahimtoola SH, Fasoli G, et al: Nifedipine in asymptomatic patients with severe aortic regurgitation and normal left ventricular function. *N Engl J Med* 331:689-694, 1994.

The authors randomized 143 patients to receive either nifedipine (40 mg a day) or digoxin (0.25 mg a day). After 6-year follow-up, 34% of the digoxin group but only 15% of the nifedipine group had gone on to aortic valve replacement (mostly because of a decrease in systolic function). Postoperatively, most of the patients had normalization of ventricular function (including all nifedipine-treated patients who had operation).

28. Tornos MP, Olona M, Permanyer-Miralda G, et al: Clinical outcome of severe asymptomatic chronic aortic regurgitation: a long-term prospective follow-up study. *Am Heart J* 130:333-339, 1995.

This study followed 101 patients for an average of 55 months. The authors concluded that the prognosis for these patients is good, that development of asymptomatic ventricular dysfunction is uncommon, and that operation can be safely postponed until either symptoms or ventricular dysfunction develops.

29. Freed LA, Levy D, Levine RA, et al: Prevalence and clinical outcome of mitral-valve prolapse. *N Engl J Med* 341:1-7, 1999.

30. Gilon D, Buonanno FS, Joffe MM, et al: Lack of evidence of an association between mitral-valve prolapse and stroke in young patients. *N Engl J Med* 341:8-13, 1999.

31. Nishimura RA, McGoon MD: Perspectives on mitral-valve prolapse (editorial). *N Engl J Med* 341:48-50, 1999.

The two articles and the accompanying editorial show the benign nature of mitral valve prolapse using contemporary echocardiographic diagnostic standards.

Questions

Multiple Choice (choose the one best answer)
A 60-year-old man presents for a general medical examination. He is totally asymptomatic and has a normal physical activity, but a 3/6 systolic murmur is heard over the precordium, at the base of the heart and at the apex. (This information applies to questions 1-4.)

1. Among the following diagnoses, which is the *least* likely to produce this murmur?
   a. Aortic stenosis
   b. Mitral regurgitation due to prolapse of the posterior leaflet
   c. Mitral regurgitation due to prolapse of the anterior leaflet
   d. Ventricular septal defect
   e. Hypertrophic obstructive cardiomyopathy

2. If this patient has mitral regurgitation, the following signs suggest severe mitral regurgitation, *except*:
   a. Third heart sound
   b. Increased first heart sound
   c. Systolic thrill
   d. A systolic murmur intensity of 4/6 or more
   e. A diastolic rumble

Dynamic maneuvers are performed during clinical examination.
3. None of these statements applies to mitral regurgitation *except*: The mitral regurgitation murmur intensity
   a. Decreases with methoxamine
   b. Decreases with amyl nitrite
   c. Increases with post-extrasystolic potentiation
   d. Increases with expiration
   e. Decreases in the left lateral decubitus position

An echocardiogram is obtained and shows the presence of mitral regurgitation.
4. What is the most frequent cause of mitral regurgitation leading to surgery in the United States?
   a. Rheumatic disease
   b. Mitral valve prolapse
   c. Endocarditis
   d. Mitral annular calcification
   e. Ischemic mitral regurgitation

5. All the following signs are suggestive of severe mitral regurgitation, except:
   a. A jet 8 cm^2 or more by color flow imaging
   b. A blunted pulmonary venous systolic flow
   c. A short mitral deceleration time
   d. An enlarged left atrium
   e. An increased mitral E velocity

6. In patients with mitral valve prolapse, dynamic changes during systole may be observed, *except*:
   a. The regurgitation begins later in systole in the standing position
   b. The effective regurgitant orifice increases late in systole
   c. The regurgitant volume peaks in mid-systole
   d. The systolic jet area may increase with exercise
   e. The regurgitation begins during systole at a fixed left ventricular volume independently of dynamic maneuvers

Echocardiography shows severe mitral regurgitation as a result of mitral valve prolapse with a flail leaflet.
7. Ten years after diagnosis, in patients with severe mitral regurgitation due to flail leaflets treated conservatively, the following event rates are observed, *except*:
   a. Endocarditis in less than 20%
   b. Atrial fibrillation in more than 20%
   c. Congestive heart failure in more than 50%
   d. Mortality not different from expected
   e. Thromboembolism in less than 20%

8. The treatment of patients with mitral regurgitation is based on the following evidence obtained from the literature:
   a. In severe mitral regurgitation, angiotensin-converting enzyme inhibitors improve survival
   b. In severe mitral regurgitation, nifedipine allows safe delay of surgery
   c. Valve repair restores normal left ventricular function
   d. Endocarditis prophylaxis is not necessary in patients with mild to moderate mitral regurgitation
   e. Chordal preservation is used in valve replacement to minimize the risk of left ventricular dysfunction

Mitral regurgitation also may be due to ischemic heart disease.
9. All the following statements apply to ischemic mitral regurgitation, *except*:
   a. Moderate or severe mitral regurgitation may be present without murmur

b. Mitral regurgitation is associated with decreased long-term survival

c. The mechanism of ischemic mitral regurgitation is mostly valve prolapse

d. It is more frequent after inferior than anterior myocardial infarction

e. The degree of ischemic mitral regurgitation may be overestimated by color flow imaging

After surgery for mitral regurgitation, left ventricular dysfunction may be observed.

10. All the following statements apply to left ventricular dysfunction after surgery for organic mitral regurgitation, *except*:
    a. It is a frequent cause of postoperative heart failure
    b. It can be predicted by preoperative left ventricular ejection fraction
    c. It occurs less after mitral valve repair than replacement
    d. It can be predicted by preoperative left ventricular end-systolic diameter
    e. It is mostly due to associated coronary artery disease

11. The widely accepted indications for surgery in patients with severe mitral regurgitation are the following, *except*:
    a. Symptoms of New York Heart Association class III or IV
    b. Transient congestive heart failure
    c. Left ventricular ejection fraction less than 60%
    d. Left ventricular end-diastolic diameter 60 mm or more
    e. Left ventricular end-systolic diameter 45 mm or more

A 52-year-old woman is referred for shortness of breath. Her clinical examination shows a 2/6 diastolic murmur along the left sternal border. (This information applies to questions 12-14.)

12. If this patient has aortic regurgitation, the following signs suggest severe aortic regurgitation, *except*:
    a. A loud fourth heart sound
    b. A decreased first heart sound
    c. A blood pressure of 150/60 mm Hg
    d. A diastolic murmur intensity of 3/6 or more
    e. An apical diastolic rumble

13. In patients with a barely audible diastolic murmur and heart failure, what sign is suggestive that severe aortic regurgitation is the cause of the heart failure?

a. A third heart sound
b. A murmur of functional mitral regurgitation
c. An increased second heart sound
d. A blood pressure of 130/45 mm Hg
e. A decreased first heart sound

Echocardiography shows the presence of aortic regurgitation.

14. What, among the following, is the most frequent cause of aortic regurgitation leading to surgery in the United States?
    a. Rheumatic disease
    b. Bicuspid aortic valve
    c. Endocarditis
    d. Syphilis
    e. Degenerative aortic valve disease with or without annuloaortic ectasia

15. All the following signs are consistent with severe aortic regurgitation, *except*:
    a. A jet width/outflow tract diameter of 40% by color flow imaging
    b. A holodiastolic reversal in the descending aorta
    c. A regurgitant fraction of 50%
    d. A left ventricular end-diastolic diameter of 65 mm
    e. A regurgitant orifice of 20 mm^2

16. All the following are determinants of a large regurgitant volume in patients with aortic regurgitation, *except*:
    a. Tachycardia
    b. Large regurgitant orifice
    c. High regurgitant velocity
    d. Bradycardia
    e. Increased left ventricular compliance

17. An echocardiogram shows an ascending aortic aneurysm without dissection. What clinical sign should have led to the suspicion of the aneurysm of the aorta?
    a. Increased first heart sound
    b. Increased second heart sound
    c. Asymmetric blood pressure
    d. Systolic hypertension
    e. Decreased femoral pulses

18. In asymptomatic patients with severe aortic regurgitation, the following outcomes have been demonstrated in the literature, *except*:

a. A left ventricular end-diastolic diameter of 70 mm or more is predictive of future progression to aortic surgery

b. A left ventricular end-systolic diameter of 50 mm or more is predictive of future progression to aortic surgery

c. A left ventricular end-diastolic diameter of 80 mm or more is associated with sudden death

d. After aortic valve replacement, mortality is in excess of expected because of the presence of the prosthetic valve

e. An ejection fraction less than 50% may return to normal with prompt operation

19. The treatment of patients with aortic regurgitation is based on the following evidence obtained from the literature:

a. In severe aortic regurgitation, angiotensin-converting enzyme inhibitors improve survival

b. In severe aortic regurgitation, nifedipine allows safe delay of surgery

c. Valve repair restores normal left ventricular function

d. Endocarditis prophylaxis is not necessary in patients with mild to moderate aortic regurgitation

e. Digoxin is a standard treatment of severe aortic regurgitation

20. The widely accepted indications for surgery in patients with severe aortic regurgitation are the following, *except*:

a. Symptoms of New York Heart Association class III or IV

b. Transient congestive heart failure

c. Left ventricular ejection fraction less than 50%

d. Left ventricular end-diastolic diameter of 80 mm or more

e. Left ventricular end-systolic diameter of 45 mm or more

Answers

1. Answer c

Aortic stenosis, mitral regurgitation due to prolapse of the posterior leaflet, and hypertrophic obstructive cardiomyopathy may all produce murmurs that can be heard with equal intensity from the base to the apex. The ventricular septal defect murmur is heard over the precordium. The murmur of mitral regurgitation due to prolapse of the anterior leaflet is typically maximum at the apex and radiates to the axilla following the jet's tract.

2. Answer b

All of the signs cited are signs of severe mitral regurgitation, but the increased first heart sound has no relationship to the degree of mitral regurgitation and may be heard in rheumatic mitral disease.

3. Answer b

The murmur of mitral regurgitation decreases with amyl nitrite, which decreases both preload and afterload, but it increases with methoxamine and in the left lateral decubitus position and does not change after extrasystole or expiration.

4. Answer b

The lesion most frequently leading to surgery for mitral regurgitation in the United States is mitral valve prolapse with or without flail leaflet in more than half of the cases. Rheumatic disease represents around 10% of the cases of pure mitral regurgitation and endocarditis, a little less. Ischemic mitral regurgitation is the second most frequent lesion leading to surgery for pure mitral regurgitation, representing 20% to 30% of cases. Mitral annular calcification may be associated with mitral valve prolapse, but isolated, it most often causes mild regurgitation.

5. Answer c

All of these signs are consistent with severe mitral regurgitation, although each has been criticized, but the mitral inflow deceleration time is unrelated to the degree of regurgitation.

6. Answer a

In mitral valve prolapse, the standing position, by decreasing left ventricular filling, increases the time of systole during which the prolapse is present, bringing the click and beginning of regurgitation earlier in systole. This change is related to the fact that the prolapse and the regurgitation occur at a fixed ventricular volume irrespective of the maneuvers performed. Use of the proximal isovelocity surface area (PISA) method has shown that the regurgitant orifice increases throughout systole but that the regurgitant volume peaks in mid-systole, before the regurgitant orifice is maximal, as a result of the maximal ventriculoatrial gradient in mid-systole. The jet area of mitral regurgitation may increase during exercise because of increased regurgitant volume or velocity.

7. Answer d

All event rates are accurate but the 10-year survival in patients with flail leaflets treated conservatively is lower than the expected survival in the general population of the same age and sex.

8. Answer e

Neither angiotensin-converting enzyme inhibitors nor nifedipine has been shown to have the ascribed effects. Endocarditis prophylaxis is necessary in mild, moderate, and severe mitral regurgitation. Valve repair does not normalize the left ventricular dysfunction but provides better function than valve replacement, which is best when combined with chordal preservation, if needed.

9. Answer c

Ischemic mitral regurgitation may be silent, in particular in acute myocardial infarction, bears a negative prognostic implication, is more frequent in inferior myocardial infarction, and may be overestimated by color flow imaging because it is usually a central regurgitation in an enlarged atrium leading to spuriously large jets. It is most usually not due to mitral valve prolapse but to regional remodeling due to apical displacement of papillary muscles and annular enlargement.

10. Answer e

Left ventricular dysfunction is the most common cause of postoperative heart failure and can be predicted by preoperative left ventricular ejection fraction and end-systolic diameter. It can be prevented in part by valve repair. Overall, postoperative heart failure after mitral valve surgery occurs most often in patients without associated coronary disease.

But flow-limiting coronary artery disease increases the risk of heart failure.

11. Answer d

The widely accepted indications for surgery in mitral regurgitation are all those listed except that regarding the end-diastolic diameter, which has no bearing on outcome with either medical or surgical treatment.

12. Answer a

A soft first heart sound consistent with premature closure of the mitral valve, a high-intensity murmur, a high blood pressure differential with low diastolic blood pressure, and an apical diastolic rumble consistent with functional mitral stenosis due to the aortic regurgitation are all signs of severe aortic regurgitation. A loud or soft fourth heart sound has no relationship to the degree of aortic regurgitation.

13. Answer d

In patients with heart failure of any cause, a third heart sound, a murmur of functional mitral regurgitation, and a soft first heart sound are commonly observed. An increased second heart sound is unrelated to the degree of mitral regurgitation. Persistent peripheral signs of aortic regurgitation despite the heart failure, such as bounding arteries, increased blood pressure differential, and decreased diastolic pressure, are particularly suggestive of severe aortic regurgitation as the cause of the heart failure.

14. Answer e

Degenerative disease with dystrophic valves, enlarged annulus, and possibly aortic ectasia is the most frequent cause of aortic regurgitation leading to surgery, followed by congenitally abnormal valves.

15. Answer e

A large regurgitant jet, a prolonged diastolic reversal in the descending aorta, a high regurgitant fraction, and an enlarged left ventricle are all consistent with severe aortic regurgitation. A regurgitant orifice less than $25 \ mm^2$ is more consistent with moderate than severe aortic regurgitation.

16. Answer a

The main determinant of a large regurgitant volume is a large regurgitant orifice. Increased driving force as observed with high regurgitant velocity and compliant left ventricle contributes to a high regurgitant volume. Bradycardia, by prolonging diastole, increases the regurgitant volume for any given regurgitant orifice. Tachycardia tends to decrease the regurgitant volume for any given regurgitant orifice.

17. Answer b

An increased second heart sound may be due to the amplifying effect of an enlarged aorta and is suggestive of an ascending aortic aneurysm in patients with aortic regurgitation.

18. Answer d

In asymptomatic patients with severe aortic regurgitation, the predictors of the need for future surgery have been underscored in the literature. Patients with New York Heart Association class I or II symptoms who have operation for aortic regurgitation have, despite the prosthetic valve, a normal expected survival. This result has led some authors to suggest that this early symptomatic phase represents the preferred timing for surgery.

19. Answer b

Nifedipine has been shown to delay the occurrence of predefined indications of surgery (symptoms of left ventricular dysfunction) without an excess rate of postoperative complications. Angiotensin-converting enzyme inhibitors have not been shown to improve survival. The effect of valve repair on left ventricular function is undocumented. Endocarditis prophylaxis is necessary in moderate as well as in severe aortic regurgitation. Digoxin has no known beneficial effect but may be detrimental because of bradycardia in severe aortic regurgitation.

20. Answer e

Class III or IV symptoms, transient heart failure, or left ventricular dysfunction should lead to prompt consideration of surgery. Severe left ventricular enlargement appears to be associated with the occurrence of sudden death and does not preclude an excellent postoperative result and, therefore, is a widely accepted indication for surgery. A moderate increase of end-systolic diameter is not a common indication for surgery. If it is 55 mm or more, it remains a disputed predictor of postoperative outcome.

Notes

Chapter 25

Prosthetic Heart Valves

Fletcher A. Miller, Jr., M.D.
Nalini Rajamannan, M.D.
Martha Grogan, M.D.
Joseph G. Murphy, M.D.

Prosthetic valves only approximate normal human valve hemodynamics and carry the risk of unique complications, such as structural failure, thrombosis, hemolysis, and infections. Understanding the various types of prostheses and the risk of complications associated with each is important for the Cardiology Board Examination as well as for the clinical practice of cardiology.

Valve Types

Valvular prostheses are classified as mechanical and bioprosthetic valves. Mechanical valves are subdivided into caged-ball, tilting-disk, and bileaflet. Bioprosthetic valves are subdivided into stented heterografts, homografts, and stentless heterografts (Plate 1). The homograft and stentless heterograft valves are designed for implantation in the aortic or pulmonic positions. All the other valve types can be implanted in any valve position.

Specific types of prosthetic valves that have been implanted in patients in the last 25 years are listed in Table 1.

Each of the different types of prostheses is manufactured in several different sizes, ranging from 19 to 33 mm in diameter. Aortic prostheses are generally available in odd-numbered sizes from 19 through 31 and mitral and tricuspid prostheses, in odd-numbered sizes from 23 through 33. The size refers to the external sewing-ring diameter in millimeters. The size of the prosthetic valve greatly influences its hemodynamics, particularly in the aortic position.

Starr-Edwards Valve

The currently available Starr-Edwards valves have a cage that is constructed from the alloy Stellite 21 and a Silastic poppet (ball) that is specially cured to prevent lipid accumulation (which can result in ball variance). The struts of the modern Starr-Edwards prosthesis are not covered with cloth.

Medtronic-Hall Valve

The Medtronic-Hall valve has a tilting disk made of pyrolytic carbon. The valve housing is machined from a single block of titanium and is composed of the valve ring with a sigmoid strut, which projects into the center of the ring and passes through a hole in the center of the disk. The tilting disk is supported by a smaller strut and two lugs, which also project from the ring. The disk tilts to an opening angle of 75° for aortic prostheses and 70° for mitral prostheses.

Björk-Shiley Valve

The Björk-Shiley valve also has a disk made of pyrolytic carbon. The standard disk is planar on one side and convex on the other. This disk is restrained by an inlet and an outlet strut. In 1978, the struts were modified and the disk was changed to a convexoconcave profile (the C-C model). This new model was available in versions that tilted to 60° and to 70° of opening angle. Only 60° valves have been implanted in the U.S. Subsequently, the Björk-Shiley C-C model was found to be subject to fractures of the outlet strut, with disk escape (see below). Later, a model with a modified

Table 1.--Types of Prosthetic Heart Valves*

Bioprostheses
    Porcine (stented)
        Hancock I
        Hancock II
        Hancock MO (modified orifice)
        Carpentier-Edwards
        C/E Duraflex
        Medtronic Intact
        Bioimplant
    Pericardial
        Ionescu-Shiley
        Carpentier-Edwards pericardial
        Mitroflow
    Homograft
    Porcine (stentless)
Mechanical prostheses
    Caged-ball
        Starr-Edwards
        Braunwald-Cutter
        Smeloff-Cutter
        Magovern-Cromie
    Tilting-disk
        Björk-Shiley
        Björk-Shiley convexoconcave
        Medtronic-Hall
        Lillihei-Kaster
        Omniscience
        Sorin
    Bileaflet
        St. Jude Medical
        Carbomedics
        Duromedics

*Boldface indicates valves most likely to be encountered in modern practice.

outlet strut was developed. With this model, the entire ring and struts are machined from one piece (i.e., there are no welds). This is referred to as the "monostrut valve."

St. Jude Medical Valve

The most widely used mechanical prosthesis is the St. Jude Medical, a bileaflet valve. The housing and the leaflets are manufactured entirely from pyrolytic carbon. The leaflets move in a slot with complex opening and closing motions that are a combination of sliding and tilt. The leaflets open to a nearly parallel position (85°). The closing angle varies from 120° to 130°, depending on valve size, with valves ≤ 25 mm having the smaller closing angle. Other examples of bileaflet prostheses include Carbomedics and Duromedics valves.

Heterograft Valves

For all porcine heterograft prostheses, a pig aortic valve is used whether the valve is implanted in the aortic, pulmonic, mitral, or tricuspid position. The pig aortic valve is mounted on flexible stents, which are covered with Dacron. The leaflets are fixed with glutaraldehyde. For earlier generation valves, a high-pressure technique was used for applying the glutaraldehyde fixative. This resulted in compression of the leaflets, which theoretically would provide better hemodynamics. Electron microscopy has shown that this high-pressure fixation results in destruction of the natural collagen architecture of the leaflets and likely contributes to valve degeneration. Therefore, with modern porcine valves, the glutaraldehyde is applied at low or no pressure. Currently, efforts are under way to treat tissue prostheses with chemicals that will delay calcification. An example is the Medtronic Intact porcine valve, which is treated with toluidine blue. The blue dye occupies sites that normally would be occupied by calcium. It is hoped that this will delay calcification. Experience has shown that toluidine blue leeches out with time. Newer anticalcification agents, which bond irreversibly, are being intensely investigated.

Heterograft valves have also been constructed from pericardium sutured to flexible, cloth-covered stents. The Ionescu-Shiley valve was one of the original pericardial valves. A design flaw predisposed this valve to sudden rupture of the cusps. Currently, the Baxter pericardial valve is being used, but it is too early to ascertain its long-term durability.

Homograft Valves

Homografts are valves harvested from cadavers and cryopreserved. They frequently are used in the setting of infective endocarditis. Homografts have a low thromboembolic potential and superb hemodynamics; however, their durability is less than that of native valves. The original homograft valves were fixed with glutaraldehyde. A disastrous rate of degenerative calcification was observed with these valves. The current variety of homograft valve is fresh frozen and has proved to be very durable, with outstanding hemodynamic performance (Plate 2). Homografts are prepared with the valve and entire ascending aorta or with the valve and pulmonary artery (Plate 3). The surgeon can trim the homograft specimen, using as much of it as necessary (i.e., the entire ascending aorta can be used along with the valve in cases that involve significant root abnormality). As with all human donor tissue, availability of homograft valves is a limiting factor.

Two stentless porcine aortic prostheses have been approved by the U.S. Food and Drug Administration. As with homografts, the Medtronic Freestyle porcine prosthesis includes not only the valve but also the pig ascending aorta (Plate 3). The surgeon trims the specimen as indicated for each case. This stentless aortic porcine prosthesis may be fashioned so that the porcine aortic sinuses are sutured inside the recipient aortic sinuses (the "cylinder within a cylinder" technique). In this case, the prosthesis is sutured both proximally and distally. This implantation technique, which can also be used with homografts, creates a unique echocardiographic appearance. The Toronto SPV, manufactured by St. Jude Medical, is already trimmed for subcoronary implantation (Plate 3).

Principles of Prosthetic Valve Selection

Similar early and late mortality rates have been reported for mechanical and tissue valves. Because valve durability is less with bioprostheses, the need for reoperation is higher than with mechanical valves. Mechanical valves have a higher thrombogenicity and a higher anticoagulation-related bleeding rate than tissue valves.

Mechanical valves are the prosthesis of choice (Table 2), with the following exceptions:

1. Bioprostheses function well in the tricuspid position and deteriorate more slowly than comparable valves in the mitral or aortic position. When right ventricular size is normal, mechanical valves in the tricuspid position have a high rate of thrombosis in spite of adequate anticoagulation. Mechanical tricuspid prostheses can be used successfully for patients with large right ventricles, as in the Ebstein anomaly.

2. Very elderly patients who are unlikely to outlive their valve should receive a tissue valve. Tissue valves deteriorate more slowly in elderly patients, and the risk of anticoagulation-associated bleeding is higher for this group of patients.

3. Patients with a history of bleeding disorders should receive tissue valves.

4. Poorly compliant patients, patients unwilling to take warfarin long-term, patients living in developing or remote locations without access to anticoagulation monitoring, alcoholics, and intravenous drug abusers are poor candidates for mechanical valves.

Bioprosthetic valves have a high failure rate in patients receiving hemodialysis and in young and adolescent patients. Hypercalcemia and chronic renal failure are contraindications to tissue valves.

Mechanical valves should be used in patients receiving anticoagulation treatment for other reasons, such as atrial fibrillation.

Women with critical valve disease who desire pregnancy pose a therapeutic problem. Warfarin increases the risk of fatal fetal bleeding and is teratogenic. Bioprostheses have a lower durability in young women and a second valve

Table 2.—Factors Affecting Choice of Valve for Individual Patient*

Factor	Ball valve	Bileaflet or tilting-disk valve	Porcine valve	Pericardial valve	Homograft or stentless porcine prosthesis[†]
Young age	+	+	...	...	±
Small annulus	...	+	...	+	+
Pregnancy desired	...	...	+	+	+
Bleeding history	...	...	+	+	+
Atrial fibrillation	+	+	...	...	...
Poor anticoagulation compliance	...	...	+	+	+

*+, Valve possesses this quality.

[†]For aortic valve replacement in young athletes, the valve of choice may be a homograft or stentless porcine; this is also the valve of choice for aortic valve replacement with active endocarditis.

Modified from Giuliani ER, Gersh BJ, McGoon MD, Hayes DL, Schaff HV (editors): *Mayo Clinic Practice of Cardiology*. Third edition. Mosby, 1996, p 1494. By permission of Mayo Foundation.

operation will almost always be required if a tissue valve is implanted. Also, pregnancy is associated with an increased risk of thromboembolism.

Ross Procedure

A pulmonary autograft is the transplantation of a patient's own pulmonary valve and main pulmonary artery to the aortic position, with reimplantation of the coronary arteries. A homograft is placed in the pulmonary position (Ross procedure). This procedure usually is performed in children and adolescents. The advantages of the procedure are 1) durability is better than with tissue valves, 2) anticoagulation is not required, and 3) the valve and root continue to grow if the patient is a child or adolescent. The procedure is technically demanding.

Complications of Prosthetic Valves

> Accurate diagnosis and management of prosthetic valve dysfunction are expected of Examination candidates.

Prosthetic valves have specific complications (Table 3).

Perivalvular Leak

Perivalvular regurgitation is always abnormal (Plate 4). The clinical significance is determined by the volume of regurgitation or the presence of mechanical hemolysis (or both). Pathologic transvalvular regurgitation must be distinguished from the normal regurgitation that is "built into" various prosthetic valves. All prosthetic valves have associated closing volume regurgitation. This is the volume of blood displaced by the occluder when it closes (Plate 5). Tilting-disk and bileaflet prostheses also have a built-in leakage volume. This is true transvalvular regurgitation that travels between the disk or leaflets and the housing and also between closed bileaflets (Plate 6). This leakage volume serves to wash the surface of the disk or leaflets. Earlier models that were designed without any leakage volume have an unacceptably high incidence of valve thrombosis. Closing volume depends on occluder size, length of travel, and speed of closure. Leakage volume depends on the size of the gap between the occluder and the rim of the housing. It increases with valve size and with decreasing heart rate. In the extreme, the sum of closing and leakage volumes may be as great as 10 mL per beat.

Table 3.--Complications of Prosthetic Valves

1. Structural deterioration of the valve leading to stenosis and/or regurgitation
2. Nonstructural dysfunction—an abnormality, not intrinsic to the valve, resulting in stenosis and/or regurgitation (exclusive of infection and thrombosis)
   Pannus
   Suture entrapment
   Paravalvular leak
   Inappropriate sizing (patient-prosthesis mismatch)
   Clinically important hemolytic anemia
3. Thromboembolism
   Neurologic deficit
   Peripheral emboli
   Acute myocardial infarction after operation, if coronary arteries are known to be normal
4. Valve thrombosis
5. Anticoagulation-related hemorrhage
6. Prosthetic valve endocarditis

- Perivalvular leak is always abnormal.
- "Built in" transvalvular leakage should be less than 10 mL per beat.

Structural Failure of Prosthetic Valves

Structural deterioration is most common for bioprostheses. Degenerative calcification most often results in leaflet tears with transvalvular regurgitation, but it may also result in stenosis. Nonstructural lesions such as pannus and suture entrapment are most common with mechanical prostheses, whereas perivalvular leaks are common with either mechanical valves or bioprostheses. Clinically important hemolytic anemia is usually the result of perivalvular regurgitation, particularly if the regurgitant jet is directed against prosthetic material. Inappropriate sizing (termed "patient-prosthesis mismatch" by Rahimtoola) can occur with any of the types of prostheses. Regardless of valve type, size-19 valves are often significantly stenotic, even when functioning normally according to their specifications.

Currently, the most common structural dysfunction of mechanical prostheses is fracture of the outlet strut of the Björk-Shiley C-C prosthesis. The risk of outlet strut fracture is significantly higher for 70° C-C valves than for 60° C-C valves. Only 60° C-C valves have been implanted in the U.S. The risk of strut fracture is highest for large valve sizes (29,

31, and 33 mm). The largest valves are estimated to have a potential strut fracture rate as high as 280/10,000 valves implanted.

- Outlet strut fracture of Björk-Shiley C-C valve is the commonest structural dysfunction of mechanical valves.

Thromboembolism

Thromboembolism is a common problem of all prostheses, although it is significantly more common with mechanical valves than with bioprostheses. It is also more common with mitral than with aortic prostheses. Thromboembolism should be clearly distinguished from valve thrombosis. The latter can result in thromboembolism, but it also has the potential for acute and severe hemodynamic disturbance due to entrapment of the moving parts with either severe stenosis or severe regurgitation.

Prosthetic Valve Endocarditis

Prosthetic valve endocarditis can occur with any of the various prostheses. With mechanical prostheses, vegetations form on the sewing ring. With bioprostheses, vegetations can occur on the ring or on the cusps. In either case, the infection is difficult to eradicate without replacing the prosthesis. Perivalvular extension of infection, such as valve-ring abscess formation, is a dreaded and all-too-common complication of prosthetic valve endocarditis. Staphylococci are the most common isolate from patients with early-onset prosthetic valve infection, with *Staphylococcus epidermidis* accounting for a substantial percentage of the cases. Streptococci are the predominant microorganism causing late-onset prosthetic valve infection.

- Valve-ring abscess is a common complication of prosthetic valve endocarditis.

Diagnosis of Prosthetic Valve Dysfunction

Patient History

When evaluating a patient who has a prosthetic valve, the exact valve type, size, and model should be noted. If the patient is unaware of this information, it is contained on the identification card. The valve size, in millimeters, usually precedes an A or M (which indicates aortic or mitral models, respectively) in the serial number.

Ask whether they are taking antiplatelet agents and/or receiving anticoagulation. If they are taking warfarin, the adequacy of anticoagulation should be assessed by checking their International Normalized Ratio (INR) over a period of months. Ask about bleeding, symptoms consistent with embolic events, and symptoms suggesting endocarditis. If a patient has been aware of valve clicks, ask about any sudden changes, because the loss of valve clicks may indicate valve thrombosis.

Establish whether the patient is in sinus rhythm or atrial fibrillation, because the latter increases the incidence of thromboembolic events. Ask about the patient's functional status, and look for symptoms of left-sided and right-sided heart failure. Patients with aortic prostheses should also be questioned about angina and exertional syncope or near-syncope, just as patients with native aortic stenosis would be questioned.

- In patients with mechanical heart valves, always determine whether they have a history of atrial fibrillation.

Physical Examination

Typically, there is a brief systolic ejection murmur across normal aortic prostheses. Normal mitral prostheses may create a brief and low-grade apical rumble (Table 4). This is particularly true for mitral bioprostheses. The bioprostheses create normal closing sounds (i.e., normal-sounding heart sounds). They do not create opening clicks. Caged-ball mechanical prostheses have prominent opening and closing clicks, whereas tilting-disk and bileaflet prostheses have prominent closing clicks, but muffled hard-to-hear opening sounds.

- Loss of expected valve sounds is an important sign of mechanical valve thrombosis.

The examination of patients with prosthetic valve stenosis or regurgitation is similar to that of patients with corresponding native-valve lesions. This includes a decreased aortic-closure-to-mitral-opening interval in patients with prosthetic mitral valve stenosis. This finding is singled out because it is particularly easy to elicit in patients with certain types of prostheses, particularly those with the caged-ball variety of mitral prosthesis.

Radiography

The sewing ring of most prostheses can be visualized on standard P-A and lateral chest radiographs. Heterograft stents are radiopaque, as are many of the mechanical valve occluders. For patients with valvular prostheses, however,

Table 4.—Auscultatory Findings in Patients With Normally Functioning Prosthetic Heart Valves

Prosthesis	Aortic	Mitral
Starr-Edwards ball valve	Sharp opening sound at S_1*	Sharp opening sound 70-150 ms after S_2
	Sharp closing sound at S_2	Sharp closing sound at S_1
	Ball "rattles" during systole	Ball "rattles" during diastole
	SEM	SEM
Björk-Shiley	Soft opening sound at S_1	Soft opening sound 70-150 ms after S_2
	Sharp closing sound at S_2	Sharp closing sound at S_1
	SEM	
Heterograft	SEM	Diastolic rumble[†]

SEM, systolic ejection murmur.

*Absence of opening or closing sounds with mechanical prosthesis usually signifies severe prosthesis dysfunction.

[†]Should be brief; if prolonged, indicates bioprosthetic obstruction or prosthesis-patient mismatch.

Modified from Rahimtoola SH, Chandraratna PAN: Valvular heart disease. In *Clinical Medicine*. Vol 6. *Cardiovascular Diseases*. Edited by JA Spittell Jr. Harper & Row, Publishers, 1982, chap 15, pp 1-51. By permission of Lippincott Williams & Wilkins.

the standard chest radiograph is most useful in demonstrating signs of heart failure, such as pulmonary venous hypertension.

For valves with radiopaque occluders, fluoroscopy can be used to measure the opening and closing angles. Valve thrombosis will result in a significantly reduced opening or closing motion (or both). The fluoroscopic appearance is useful not only for diagnosing prosthetic valve thrombosis but also for assessing the efficacy of thrombolytic therapy.

Currently, fluoroscopy is the only method available for diagnosing strut fracture of the Björk-Shiley C-C prosthesis. However, once the fracture has occurred—and thus is identifiable on fluoroscopy—the patient's condition is extremely serious.

Echocardiography

Echocardiography provides a complete hemodynamic assessment of valvular prostheses in most clinical situations. This has revolutionized the diagnostic approach to patients with suspected prosthetic valve dysfunction.

Aortic Prostheses

Complete echocardiographic assessment of prosthetic aortic valves includes measurement of peak systolic velocity, mean gradient, and effective orifice area (EOA). In addition, the presence or absence of regurgitation is noted, and the regurgitation is characterized as normal (i.e., closing volume and/or leakage volume) or pathologic. An attempt is made to separate pathologic regurgitation into perivalvular or transvalvular, according to the origin of the jet. Semiquantitative and quantitative measures are used to characterize the amount of regurgitation.

Gradients across prosthetic valves are determined by the simplified Bernoulli equation:

$$\Delta P = 4v^2$$

The mean systolic gradient is calculated electronically by measuring instantaneous gradients at multiple points along the Doppler time-velocity curve, summing them, and dividing by the number of points sampled. The gradient across a prosthetic valve will be underestimated if the Doppler beam is oriented at an angle greater than 20° from the major axis of blood flow through the valve; thus, multiple acoustic windows, including apical and periapical, right parasternal, subcostal, suprasternal, and right supraclavicular, are used.

Effective Orifice Area of Prosthetic Valves

The EOA for prosthetic valves is determined with the continuity equation (Table 5). This means that the volume of flow through the left ventricular outflow tract (LVOT) is equivalent to the volume of flow through the effective orifice of the aortic prosthesis. Volume flow through the LVOT (i.e., stroke volume) is calculated by multiplying the cross-sectional area of the LVOT by the time velocity integral (TVI) of flow through the outflow tract. The cross-sectional area is obtained by measuring the diameter of the LVOT in systole, from the two-dimensional image, and assuming circular geometry. The TVI of the LVOT is obtained by integrating the time-velocity spectrum from pulsed-wave Doppler with the sample volume positioned in the LVOT. Similarly, flow through the prosthesis EOA is given by the product of the orifice area times the TVI of flow at the orifice. The latter is measured from the continuous-wave Doppler signal across the prosthesis, the same signal that is used to measure the mean gradient.

In contrast to the Gorlin method, the continuity method is valid regardless of the degree of prosthetic aortic regurgitation (because the regurgitant volume crosses both the LVOT and the prosthesis).

Table 5.—Calculation of Effective Orifice Area (EOA)

Flow Through LVOT = Flow Through Prosthesis EOA
(LVOT Area) x (LVOT TVI) = (EOA) x (Prosthesis TVI)

This can be rearranged as follows:

$$EOA = \frac{(LVOT\ area)\ x\ (LVOT\ TVI)}{(Prosthesis\ TVI)}$$

(where LVOT is left ventricular outflow tract and TVI is time velocity integral)

In our experience, the average mean gradient was 13 to 15 mm Hg for heterograft, Björk-Shiley, St. Jude Medical, and Medtronic-Hall prostheses. The average mean gradient was significantly greater for Starr-Edwards aortic prostheses (23 mm Hg) and was significantly lower for homograft prostheses (8 mm Hg). However, it is important to be aware of patient-to-patient variability. With all valve types, except homografts, there are individuals with normally functioning prostheses with mean gradients as high as 35 to 45 mm Hg. In general, these patients have small prostheses, and these high gradients are due to patient-prosthesis mismatch. These patients may have EOAs less than 1.0 cm². Particularly because of this variability in mean gradient and EOA among patients with normal prosthetic valve function, it is mandatory that a baseline echocardiographic and Doppler examination be performed on each patient soon after implantation. This effectively "fingerprints" the individual prosthesis and serves as a baseline for comparison, should symptoms develop consistent with prosthetic valve dysfunction.

Pitfalls of Echocardiographic Assessment of Prosthetic Heart Valves

1. Falsely large or small measurements of the LVOT diameter will cause over- or underestimation of the prosthesis EOA. The prosthesis sewing ring must be visualized clearly to measure LVOT diameter. In rare cases in which this measurement cannot be made confidently, it is acceptable to approximate the measurement with the external diameter of the sewing ring (i.e., the valve size). It has been shown that this approximation will slightly overestimate the actual EOA.

2. Placement of the pulsed-wave sample volume too close to the prosthesis sewing ring will result in an inaccurately large LVOT TVI and, hence, an inaccurately large

stroke volume. This will result in overestimation of the prosthesis EOA. When the LVOT diameter and TVI are measured, the heart rate should be noted. The measurements should be used to calculate cardiac output. If the calculated cardiac output appears to be inconsistent with the patient's left ventricular systolic function, the LVOT diameter and TVI should be remeasured.

3. The prosthesis TVI can be underestimated through an angulation error, identical to that described above for measurement of the mean gradient.

4. If an inappropriately low-velocity spectrum is used to measure the prosthesis TVI, the EOA will be overestimated.

Assessment of Prosthetic Aortic Valve Incompetence

Semiquantitation of aortic regurgitation is performed by using information from two-dimensional imaging, spectral Doppler, and color flow imaging. The degree to which color flow signals of regurgitation fill the LVOT in diastole is determined. In addition, the intensity of high-velocity signals in the continuous-wave spectrum of aortic regurgitation, the pressure half-time of the continuous-wave signal, the amount of diastolic flow reversal in the descending thoracic aorta (obtained by pulsed-wave Doppler), and the size of the left ventricle (from two-dimensional imaging) are assessed. If a patient has a native mitral valve that is competent, the aortic regurgitant volume and regurgitant fraction can be calculated by comparing forward flow through the LVOT with forward flow across the mitral annulus.

Assessment of Prosthetic Mitral and Tricuspid Valves

Mitral and tricuspid prostheses are assessed more easily by Doppler hemodynamics because the optimal window for interrogation is always apical or periapical. Complete assessment requires measurement of the peak early velocity (E velocity), the velocity with atrial contraction (A velocity) for patients in sinus rhythm, the pressure half-time, EOA, and the presence and degree of regurgitation. The velocities and mean gradient are measured from the continuous-wave Doppler signal. Although the EOA can be calculated from the pressure half-time for obstructed prostheses, this method tends to overestimate the EOA for normally functioning prostheses. Therefore, it is preferable to report the pressure half-time independently and to calculate the EOA by the continuity method. As with aortic prostheses, the LVOT stroke volume is divided by the prosthesis TVI to obtain the EOA. However, this method cannot be used with mitral or tricuspid prostheses if there is significant aortic regurgitation or significant prosthesis regurgitation; under these circumstances, continuity of flow will no longer exist. In such cases, the pressure half-time should be reported and the EOA should not be calculated.

Because mitral and tricuspid prostheses create reverberations and acoustic shadowing within the atria, visualization of regurgitant jets by surface echocardiography is always suboptimal. However, important clues to significant regurgitation may be found on the surface examination. These include an increased E velocity with normal pressure half-time, a dense continuous-wave regurgitant signal, and color Doppler signals of flow convergence on the ventricular side of the regurgitant orifice. Transesophageal echocardiography provides complete visualization of color jets due to prosthetic mitral or tricuspid regurgitation. It also allows sampling of the left and right upper pulmonary veins for systolic flow reversal.

In our series of normal mitral prostheses, the average mean gradient was in the 4- to 5-mm Hg range for heterograft, tilting-disk, bileaflet, and caged-ball prostheses. There were occasional normal valves with mean gradients as high as 10 mm Hg. For normal tricuspid prostheses, the mean gradient averages 2 to 3 mm Hg, with mean gradients of outliers as high as 5.5 mm Hg. For all Doppler hemodynamic calculations, at least three cardiac cycles should be averaged for patients in sinus rhythm and at least five cycles for those in atrial fibrillation. For tricuspid prostheses, 10 cycles must be averaged, even for patients in sinus rhythm, because of significant variation in mean gradient with the respiratory cycle.

Transesophageal Echocardiography

Most prosthetic valve hemodynamic information is available from surface echocardiography. Similarly, the amount of prosthetic aortic regurgitation usually can be assessed by the surface examination. Complete visualization of mitral and tricuspid prosthesis regurgitant jets requires transesophageal echocardiography, which is also indicated if it is necessary to determine the mechanism of regurgitation or stenosis. Because transesophageal echocardiography is sensitive enough to detect normal closing volume and leakage volume, the echocardiographer must be aware of the normal patterns for each type of prosthesis.

For patients with clinically significant prosthetic valve dysfunction, an echocardiographic examination usually can obviate the need for invasive hemodynamics before surgical replacement.

Laboratory Tests and Hemolysis

For patients with prosthetic valves who are receiving long-term anticoagulation therapy, the INR should be checked at least monthly. Also, the hemoglobin value should be checked periodically, because a decrease could be due to bleeding. Also, keep in mind that a decreased hemoglobin value may result from significant hemolysis. This is a mechanical, intravascular hemolytic process. Sheared red blood cells will appear as schistocytes on a peripheral blood smear. The level of serum haptoglobin will approach zero, and the level of lactate dehydrogenase will increase. There usually is a compensatory increase in reticulocytes. The loss of iron in the urine, in the form of hemosiderin, produces iron deficiency.

Invasive Hemodynamics

The diagnosis of prosthetic valve dysfunction seldom requires an invasive procedure. Catheters should not be passed across mechanical aortic prostheses; thus, measurement of aortic prosthesis gradients requires a transseptal approach. If both mitral and aortic prostheses are present, measurement of the gradients requires not only transseptal puncture but also left ventricular puncture. For mitral prostheses, it is always necessary to measure the gradient using a transseptal approach, with direct measurement of left atrial pressure, rather than depending on pulmonary artery wedge pressure. The latter nearly always results in significant overestimation of the gradient, even when the phase delay is taken into account. When measuring prosthetic aortic valve gradients invasively, it is important to remember that the distal catheter must be placed as close to the vena contracta as possible. Otherwise, the gradient will be underestimated because of the phenomenon of pressure recovery.

Primary Prevention of Valve Dysfunction

Anticoagulation

The intensity of anticoagulation must be tailored for each patient, taking into account age, bleeding risk, and gait stability. Generally, a higher target INR range is used for mitral prostheses or multiple prostheses than for isolated aortic valve replacement. Significant left ventricular dysfunction, atrial fibrillation, and previous history of embolism are other factors that warrant a higher target INR.

For caged-ball prostheses and for older generation tilting disks, such as Björk-Shiley, a target INR range of 2.5 to 3.5 is used for aortic prostheses and 3.0 to 4.0 for mitral prostheses. For bileaflet prostheses and newer generation tilting disks, such as Medtronic-Hall, the typical target range for aortic prostheses is 2.0 to 3.0, whereas a range of 2.5 to 3.5 is used for mitral replacements.

Patients with bioprostheses generally receive anticoagulation treatment with warfarin for the first 3 months until endothelialization occurs and then with aspirin alone. The target range for both aortic and mitral bioprostheses is typically 2.0 to 3.0 during the initial 3 months. In patients with chronic atrial fibrillation, warfarin treatment should be continued indefinitely, which removes the major advantage for bioprostheses. Therefore, mechanical prostheses should be selected for most patients with chronic atrial fibrillation.

Antiplatelet therapy, such as aspirin (81 mg/day), should be used in conjunction with warfarin for Starr-Edwards valves, older generation tilting disk valves, and when the patient has had coronary artery bypass grafting in addition to valve replacement. Also, aspirin should be added to warfarin whenever the patient experiences embolism despite a satisfactory INR.

Endocarditis Prophylaxis

The 1997 recommendations of the American Heart Association/American College of Cardiology for antibiotic prophylaxis of prosthetic valves are included in the chapter on Infections of the Heart.

Management of Prosthetic Valve Complications

Replacement of a dysfunctional prosthetic valve carries a significantly higher surgical risk in comparison with initial valve replacement. Therefore, with most chronic or subacute problems, one should be conservative when deciding whether to replace a dysfunctional prosthesis. Definite indications for surgery include 1) severe prosthetic stenosis or regurgitation with resultant symptoms and/or ventricular dysfunction, 2) transfusion-dependent hemolysis, 3) recurrent emboli despite adequate anticoagulation/antiplatelet therapy, and 4) prosthetic valve endocarditis with hemodynamic compromise, persistent fever despite adequate antibiotic therapy, perivalvular extension of infection, or large mobile vegetations seen on transesophageal echocardiography.

Valve thrombosis may be treated with thrombolytic therapy or with surgery. Thrombolytic therapy should be the first-line treatment for thrombosis of right-sided prostheses. For left-sided prostheses, thrombolytic therapy carries a significant risk of embolism and stroke. Nevertheless, many patients with thrombosed left-sided valves will also have a very high operative mortality. In these cases, it is best for the cardiologist and cardiac surgeon to arrive jointly at a decision, which will depend heavily on the estimated risk of replacing the thrombosed valve.

Questions

Multiple Choice (choose the one best answer)

1. Which of the following mechanical prostheses has the highest rate of structural deterioration?
   a. Björk-Shiley C-C (convexoconcave) valve
   b. Carbomedics valve
   c. St. Jude Medical valve
   d. Medtronic-Hall valve
   e. Björk-Shiley standard valve

2. On echocardiographic evaluation of an aortic Medtronic-Hall prosthesis, the following measurements were obtained: left ventricular outflow tract (LVOT) diameter, 1.9 cm; LVOT time velocity integral (TVI), 22 cm; and prosthesis TVI, 120 cm. The effective orifice area (EOA) is approximately:
   a. 0.63 cm^2
   b. 0.4 cm^2
   c. 0.52 cm^2
   d. 0.8 cm^2
   e. 1.2 cm^2

3. A 43-year-old woman had acute onset of shortness of breath and lightheadedness. She had a history of rheumatic fever at age 11 and mitral valve surgery at age 31. On physical examination, she was pale and tachypneic. Heart rate was 98 beats/min and regular, with a low-volume pulse. Blood pressure was 88/40 mm Hg. There were bilateral pulmonary rales with associated hepatosplenomegaly, lower extremity edema, and elevated jugular venous pressure. A new murmer was present. The next step in your evaluation should be:
   a. Cardiac catheterization
   b. Fluoroscopy
   c. Transthoracic echocardiography
   d. Transesophageal echocardiography

4. The patient had an abnormality shown on the accompanying transesophageal echocardiogram. Your next management step should include:
   a. Thrombolytic agent
   b. Antibiotics given intravenously
   c. Referral for emergency cardiac surgery
   d. High-dose intravenous heparin therapy

5. You would recommend the following anticoagulation treatment for a patient with a mitral tilting-disk prosthetic heart valve who has had a large embolic stroke:
   a. Continue full anticoagulation after the stroke to avoid

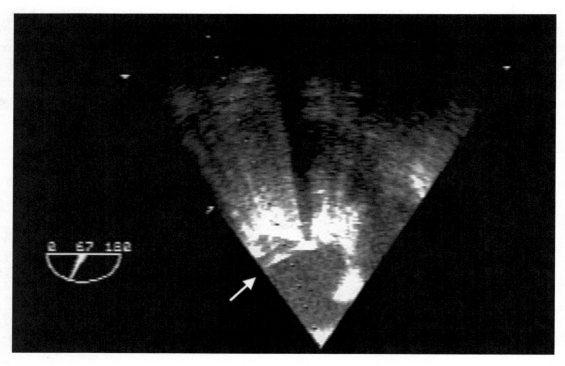

Question 4

additional embolic events

b. Wait 4-6 weeks to start anticoagulation to avoid hemorrhagic conversion of the cerebral infarct or intracranial bleeding

c. Restart full anticoagulation in 5-7 days if computed tomographic brain scan shows a nonhemorrhagic cerebral infarct

d. Observation until all neurologic symptoms have resolved before restarting full anticoagulation

6. In patients with mechanical prosthetic heart valves who become pregnant while receiving anticoagulation treatment with warfarin, warfarin should always be discontinued because of the risks of embryopathy.
   a. True
   b. False

7. Exposure to warfarin in the first trimester includes all the following complications *except*:
   a. Nasal hypoplasia
   b. Microcephaly
   c. Mental retardation
   d. Limb deformities
   e. Optic neuropathy

8. Which of the following valves has a built-in leakage volume?
   a. Stented heterograft
   b. Caged-ball
   c. Homograft
   d. Bileaflet
   e. Stentless heterograft

9. The Ross procedure is:
   a. Replacement of a mechanical valve for a bioprosthethic valve in the tricuspid position
   b. Transposition of the pulmonic valve into the aortic position
   c. Indicated for elderly patients with aortic stenosis who are poorly compliant with medication regimens
   d. Indicated for patients with the Ebstein anomaly

10. All the following are associated with hemolysis caused by a prosthetic valve *except*:
    a. Increased number of reticulocytes
    b. Increased serum level of lactate dehydrogenase
    c. Increased serum level of haptoglobin
    d. Increased urine level of hemosiderin
    e. Schistocytes on a peripheral blood smear

11. Which of the following *least* influences mean gradient for a mechanical prosthesis?
    a. Prosthesis type
    b. Prosthesis position
    c. Prosthesis size
    d. Prosthesis regurgitation
    e. Length of time the prosthetic valve has been implanted

12. Patients with a recent history of rheumatic carditis who have undergone valve replacement still have an increased incidence of recurrent rheumatic carditis and thus should have antibiotic prophylaxis.
    a. True
    b. False

Answers

1. Answer a

The convexoconcave Björk-Shiley valve, especially in the larger annulus sizes, has been associated with an increased risk of in vivo strut fracture.

2. Answer c

$$EOA = \frac{(LVOT\ area) \times (LVOT\ TVI)}{Prosthesis\ TVI}$$

$$= \frac{\pi r^2 \times (LVOT\ TVI)}{Prosthesis\ TVI}$$

$$= \frac{\pi(0.95)^2 \times 22}{120}$$

$$= 0.52\ cm^2$$

3. Answer c

Transthoracic echocardiography should be performed initially and if adequate views of her prosthetic valve are not obtained, transesophageal echocardiography.

4. Answer c

5. Answer c

6. Answer b

7. Answer d

Limb deformities are not associated with warfarin therapy.

8. Answer d

Bileaflet valves, of which St. Jude Medical is the best known, have a built-in leakage volume that serves to "clean" the leaflet surface and reduce thrombus formation on the valve surface.

9. Answer b

10. Answer c

The serum level of haptoglobin decreases with intravascular hemolysis.

11. Answer e

In the absence of prosthetic or ventricular dysfunction, the mean gradient across a prosthesis does not change significantly with time since implantation.

12. Answer a

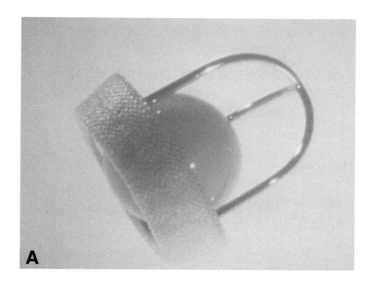

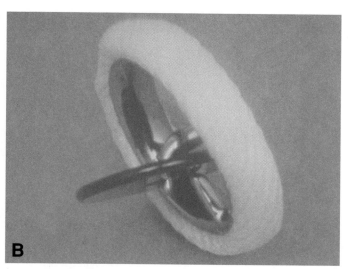

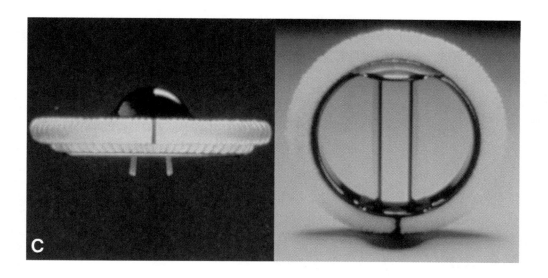

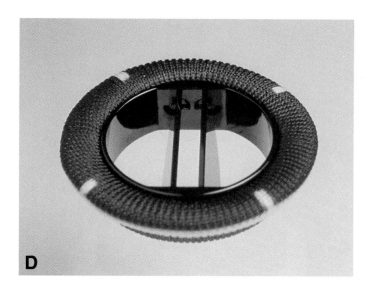

Plate 1. Mechanical prostheses. *A*, Starr-Edwards prosthesis in closed position. *B*, Medtronic-Hall prosthesis in fully open position (central strut fits through hole in disk; open disk creates major and minor orifices). *C* and *D*, St. Jude Medical and Carbomedics bileaflet prostheses in fully open position (there are two large orifices and a smaller central orifice).

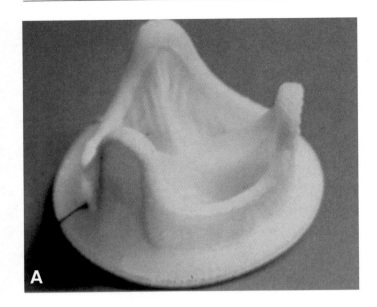

Elgiloy orifice ring and stents; porcine leaflets; Teflon cuff

Flexible stents

High profile

Durability limited by calcification

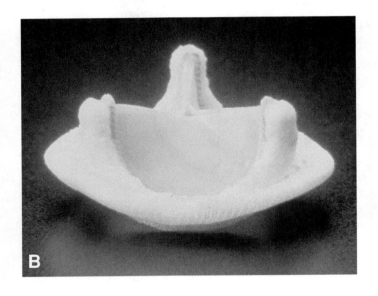

Plate 2. Stented heterograft prostheses. *A*, Carpentier-Edwards standard valve. Porcine aortic valve is frame-mounted and glutaraldehyde-preserved. *B*, Carpentier-Edwards pericardial valve.

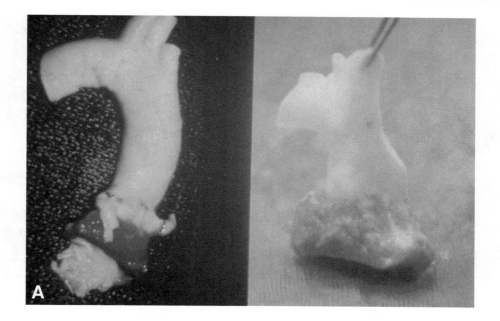

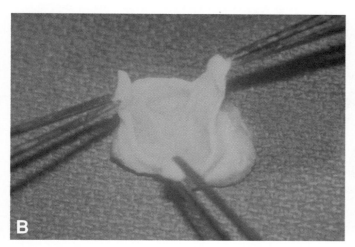

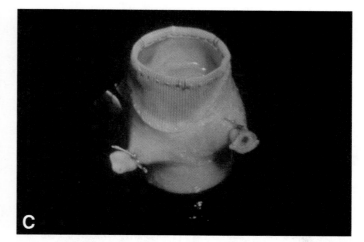

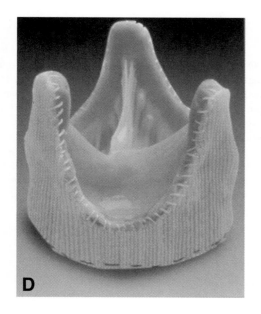

Plate 3. Stentless bioprostheses. *A*, Aortic and pulmonary homografts. *B*, Aortic homograft scalloped for subcoronary implantation. *C*, Medtronic Freestyle porcine aortic prosthesis. It may be used as root replacement or root inclusion or trimmed for subcoronary implantation. *D*, Toronto SPV valve (St. Jude Medical) is manufactured for subcoronary implantation.

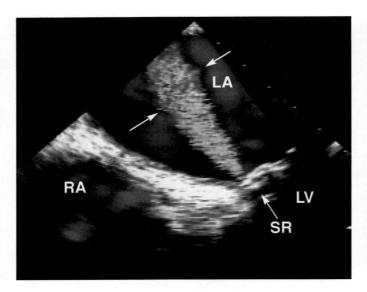

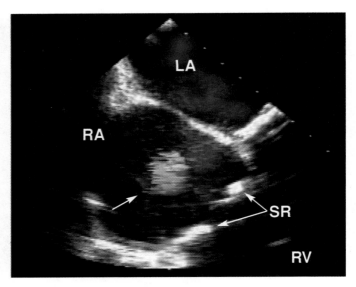

Plate 4. Transesophageal echocardiography, horizontal plane view from a patient with a Starr-Edwards mitral prosthesis who had symptoms of congestive failure and a murmur of mitral regurgitation. Soon after the transducer was introduced into the esophagus, a relatively narrow periprosthetic jet (*arrows*) originating around the medial portion of the sewing ring (*SR*) was identified. Note the mosaic appearance. This jet would certainly explain the systolic murmur, but its size seems insufficient to explain the patient's congestive symptoms. LA, left atrium; LV, left ventricle; RA, right atrium. (From Freeman WK, Seward JB, Khandheria BK, et al: *Transesophageal Echocardiography*. Little, Brown and Company, 1994, p 280. By permission of Mayo Foundation.)

Plate 5. Transesophageal echocardiography, horizontal plane, four-chamber view. Normal Starr-Edwards tricuspid prosthesis. In this systolic frame, the poppet and cage are not visible in the right ventricle. The ball-shaped, low-velocity color map (*arrow*) in the right atrium (*RA*) represents the volume of blood that is displaced as the poppet moves to its closed position against the sewing ring. This color array is therefore referred to as the prosthetic "closing volume." *LA*, left atrium; *RV*, right ventricle; *SR*, sewing ring. (From Freeman WK, Seward JB, Khandheria BK, et al: *Transesophageal Echocardiography*. Little, Brown and Company, 1994, p 279. By permission of Mayo Foundation.)

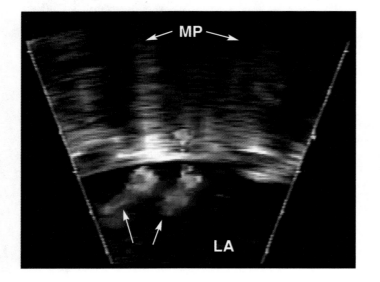

Plate 6. Omniplane transesophageal echocardiographic evaluation, with color flow imaging, of a normal Lillihei-Kaster mitral prosthesis (*MP*). This tilting-disk valve has a normal, small amount of transvalvular regurgitation. Note the two separate jets (*arrows*) in the left atrium (*LA*). Besides their small size, these jets clearly represent very mild regurgitation, because they are uniformly red (nonturbulent). Very few blood cells are traveling at higher velocities (i.e., above the Nyquist limit); therefore, minimal color aliasing is seen within these jets. (From Freeman WK, Seward JB, Khandheria BK, et al: *Transesophageal Echocardiography*. Little, Brown and Company, 1994, p 281. By permission of Mayo Foundation.)

Chapter 26

Pulmonary Hypertension

Michael D. McGoon, M.D.

Diagnosis of Pulmonary Hypertension

The pulmonary vascular bed is normally a low-pressure, low-resistance circulation with compliant, thin-walled vessels (Table 1).

Pulmonary hypertension refers to any condition in which pulmonary artery pressure at rest consistently exceeds 35 mm Hg systolic, 15 mm Hg diastolic, or 25 mm Hg mean. Pulmonary hypertension is also present if exertional mean pulmonary artery pressure is more than 35 mm Hg while rest values are normal. Clinically significant pulmonary hypertension is usually associated with substantially higher pulmonary artery pressures, ranging from 50 to 150 mm Hg systolic. Pulmonary artery pressure (PA) is related to pulmonary vein pressure (PV), pulmonary artery blood flow (Qp), and pulmonary vascular resistance (Rp):

$$Qp \text{ (L/min per m}^2) = \frac{PA - PV \text{ (mm Hg)}}{Rp \text{ (U·m}^2)}$$

$$\left(\text{flow} = \frac{\text{driving pressure}}{\text{resistance}} \right)$$

- Pulmonary hypertension is by definition a pulmonary artery systolic pressure more than 35 mm Hg.

Table 1.—Comparison of Pulmonary and Systemic Circulations

	Circulation	
	Pulmonary	Systemic
Arterial pressure, mm Hg	22/10 (mean, 13)	120/80 (mean, 90)
Capillary pressure, mm Hg	6-9 (7)	10-30 (17)
Venous pressure, mm Hg	1-4 (2)	0-10 (6)
Arterial M:D ratio, %	3-8 (5)	15-25 (20)
Venous M:D ratio, %	2-5 (3)	3-6 (4)
Vascular resistance, U·m2	1-4 (3)	10-25 (15)
Blood flow, L/min	5	5

M:D ratio, ratio of thickness of media to external diameter of the vessel.
From Giuliani ER, Gersh BJ, McGoon MD, Hayes DL, Schaff HV (editors): *Mayo Clinic Practice of Cardiology.* Third edition. Mosby, 1996, p 1816. By permission of Mayo Foundation.

Etiology of Pulmonary Hypertension

Five types of pulmonary hypertension are identified on the basis of cause:

1. Pulmonary venous hypertension

An atlas illustrating treatment for (plate 2) and pathologic conditions associated with pulmonary hypertension is at the end of the chapter (Plates 1-10).

2. Chronic hypoxia with secondary vasoconstriction of the pulmonary vascular bed
3. Pulmonary artery obstruction
4. Left-to-right shunts with increased flow across the pulmonary vascular bed
5. Idiopathic, or primary, from multiple presumed causes

Pulmonary Venous Hypertension

Pulmonary venous hypertension is the most common form of pulmonary hypertension and is usually due to left-sided heart disease (valvular, coronary, or myocardial) (Table 2). It results from obstruction to blood flow downstream from the small pulmonary veins. The hypertension and pulmonary vascular lesions are reversible if the obstructing lesion is removed, although months to years may be required for a relatively normal functional and morphologic state to return.

The histopathologic findings of pulmonary venous hypertension reflect the back pressure caused by the obstructive lesion on the pulmonary vessels and right ventricle (Table 3). There is often superimposed constriction of arteriolar vessels.

The clinical characteristics of pulmonary venous hypertension depend on the stage of evolution of the hypertension:

Table 2.—Causes of Pulmonary Venous Hypertension

Location	Condition
Aorta	Coarctation
	Supravalvular aortic stenosis
Left ventricle	Left ventricular failure of any cause
	Aortic stenosis
	Aortic regurgitation
	Congenital subaortic stenosis
	Hypertrophic cardiomyopathy
	Constrictive pericarditis
	Restrictive cardiomyopathy
	Dilated cardiomyopathy
	Mitral stenosis
	Mitral regurgitation
Left atrium	Ball-valve thrombus
	Myxoma
	Cor triatriatum
Pulmonary veins	Congenital pulmonary vein stenosis
	Mediastinitis
	Mediastinal fibrosis
	Mediastinal neoplasm

Table 3.—Histopathology of Pulmonary Venous Hypertension

Location	Histopathologic feature
Right ventricle	Hypertrophy with or without dilatation
Pulmonary arteries	Medial hypertrophy
	Eccentric intimal proliferation or fibrosis
	Dilatation and shallow intimal atheromas of elastic arteries
Pulmonary capillaries	Engorged with blood
Pulmonary veins	Engorged with blood
	Medial hypertrophy of veins and venules ("arterialization")
	Eccentric intimal fibrosis
Other	Edema of pleura and interlobular septa
	Dilatation of pleural and septal lymphatics
	Alveolar edema
	Microhemorrhages and hemosiderosis

the stage of passive back pressure or the stage of reactive pulmonary arteriolar vasoconstriction (Table 4). In the absence of mitral valve disease, left atrial and left ventricular pressure equalize during diastole. This pressure is transmitted to the pulmonary venous circulation. If left ventricular end-diastolic pressure is significantly increased from any cause, pulmonary artery pressure must increase to enable forward blood flow to occur.

- Pulmonary venous hypertension is the most common form of pulmonary hypertension.

Hypoxic Pulmonary Hypertension

In chronic pulmonary parenchymal diseases and other conditions of chronic low oxygen saturation, hypoxia-induced pulmonary vasoconstriction and anatomical destruction of the vascular bed cause high pulmonary resistance and hypertension (Table 5), and ultimately right ventricular failure (cor pulmonale). The nonfibrotic lesions may regress if the chronic alveolar hypoxia is reversed.

The mechanisms by which these conditions produce pulmonary hypertension include vasoconstriction induced by

Table 4.—Clinical Profile of Pulmonary Venous Hypertension

Stage of pulmonary hypertension	Clinical feature
Passive	Dyspnea
	Pulmonary edema (orthopnea, paroxysmal nocturnal dyspnea)
	Hemoptysis
Arteriolar vasocon- striction	Dyspnea
	Fatigue
	Cough
	Right ventricular failure
	Tricuspid regurgitation
	Hepatomegaly
	Peripheral edema

alveolar hypoxia, ventilation-perfusion mismatch leading to decreased saturation, secondary erythrocytosis, and structural loss of vascular bed.

The histopathologic findings in hypoxic pulmonary hypertension are primarily related to the underlying disease (Table 6), as well as to the secondary pulmonary hypertension.

The clinical profile of chronic hypoxic pulmonary hypertension is dominated by the underlying cause. In some cases of otherwise indeterminate pulmonary hypertension, however, a concerted effort must be made to diagnose the presence of restrictive lung disease or obstructive sleep apnea. Bronchitic disorders ("blue bloaters") are more frequently associated with pulmonary hypertension than is emphysema ("pink puffers"). Chronic exposure to high altitude may cause a hypoxic type of pulmonary hypertension.

- The clinical profile of chronic hypoxic pulmonary hypertension is dominated by the underlying cause.

Arterial Obstructive Pulmonary Hypertension

This category of pulmonary hypertension is important to recognize because it includes several diagnoses that are potentially reversible but require conscientious evaluation in order to detect (Table 7).

Chronic major vessel thromboembolism is a treatable entity that may produce severe pulmonary hypertension

Table 5.—Causes of Hypoxic Pulmonary Hypertension

Long-term dwelling at a high altitude
Restrictive respiratory dysfunction
    Obesity
    Kyphoscoliosis
    Neuromuscular disorders
    Severe pleural fibrosis
    Lung resection
Chronic upper airway obstruction
    Congenital webs
    Enlarged tonsils
    Obstructive sleep apnea
Chronic lower airway obstruction
    Chronic bronchitis
    Asthmatic bronchitis
    Bronchiectasis
    Cystic fibrosis
    Emphysema
Chronic diffuse parenchymal disease
    Interstitial fibrosis
    Pneumoconioses
    Granulomatous disease
    Alveolar filling disorders
    Connective tissue disorders (scleroderma, rheumatoid lung)

Table 6.—Histopathology of Hypoxic Pulmonary Hypertension

Location	Histopathologic feature
Right ventricle	Hypertrophy with or without dilatation
Pulmonary arteries	Medial hypertrophy
	Eccentric intimal proliferation or fibrosis
	Longitudinal smooth muscle bundles within intima, media, or adventitia of muscular arteries
	Organized thrombus or retracted fibroelastic plugs may be present
	Dilatation and shallow intimal atheromas of elastic arteries
Other	Parenchymal abnormalities of chronic obstructive pulmonary disease

Table 7.—Causes of Arterial Obstructive Pulmonary Hypertension

Thrombotic disease
    Sickle cell disease
    Coagulation disorders
Embolic disease
    Chronic thromboemboli
    Tumor emboli
    Schistosomiasis
    Connective tissue disorders
    Lupus
    Systemic sclerosis

even in the absence of a clear history of acute pulmonary hypertension.

The persistence of large-vessel thromboemboli after acute or recurrent pulmonary embolism produces pulmonary hypertension by anatomical obstruction of arteries and by promoting ongoing platelet activation with release of vasoconstrictor substances, such as thromboxane and serotonin. In situ thrombosis may occur in pulmonary hypertension from other causes or as a component of primary pulmonary hypertension (Table 8).

The clinical profile of chronic thromboembolic pulmonary hypertension may mimic that of primary pulmonary hypertension, with symptoms of dyspnea, chest pain, and syncope.

● The persistence of large-vessel thromboemboli after acute or recurrent pulmonary embolism produces pulmonary hypertension by anatomical obstruction of arteries and by promoting ongoing platelet activation with release of vasoconstrictor substances.

Table 8.—Histopathology of Arterial Obstructive Pulmonary Hypertension

Location	Histopathologic feature
Right ventricle	Hypertrophy with or without dilatation
Pulmonary arteries	Organized, recanalized, endothelialized thrombi in main, lobar, or segmental arteries
	Dilatation and shallow intimal atheromas of elastic arteries
Other	May be associated with evidence of prior deep vein thrombosis

Pulmonary Hypertension Due to Left-to-Right Shunts

The development of established pulmonary hypertension not responsive to vasodilators indicates that the underlying lesion has become irreparable and that pulmonary hypertension would now persist even after anatomical repair of the lesion (Table 9). This continuing pulmonary hypertension in the absence of a shunt after repair would lead to intolerably high right ventricular pressures and the death of the patient.

Medial hypertrophy and intimal proliferation are potentially reversible after operation, but more complex higher-grade lesions are generally considered to be histopathologic hallmarks that are contraindications to operation (Table 10).

Patients with pulmonary hypertension due to left-to-right shunting initially have high pulmonary blood flow followed by increased pulmonary vascular resistance and eventual reversal of the shunt (Eisenmenger complex). Clinically, this results in the cyanosis and polycythemia characteristic of this type of pulmonary hypertension, as well as dyspnea, clubbing, and hemoptysis.

● Patients with pulmonary hypertension due to left-to-right shunting initially have high pulmonary blood flow followed by increased pulmonary vascular resistance and eventual reversal of the shunt (Eisenmenger complex).

Primary Pulmonary Hypertension

Idiopathic, or primary, pulmonary hypertension is pulmonary hypertension of undetermined cause. It is a rare disease; the annual incidence is approximately 2 per million (500 new patients per year in the United States). It is

Table 9.—Causes of Pulmonary Hypertension Associated With Left-to-Right Shunts

Extracardiac shunts
    Patent ductus arteriosus
    Aortopulmonary window
    Rupture of aortic sinus
Intracardiac shunts
    Ventricular septal defect
    Atrial septal defect

Table 10.—Histopathology of Pulmonary Hypertension Due to Left-to-Right Shunts

Location	Histopathologic feature
Right ventricle	Hypertrophy with or without dilatation
Pulmonary arteries	Medial hypertrophy
	Extension of smooth muscle into arterioles
	Intimal cell proliferation
	Concentric intimal fibrosis
	Fibrinoid degeneration ("necrotizing arteritis")[*]
	Dilatation lesions[*]
	Plexiform lesions[*]
	Dilatation and shallow intimal atheromas of elastic arteries

[*]Higher-grade lesions, contraindications to operation.

Table 11.—Types of Primary Pulmonary Hypertension

Pulmonary arteriopathy
    Plexogenic
    Thrombotic
Pulmonary veno-occlusive
Pulmonary capillary hemangiomatosis

more common in women than men by a factor of about 2:1, and the female preponderance is greater among blacks (4:1). The mean age of patients at diagnosis is 35 years, ranging from infancy to 80s. Familial clusters have been reported in about 6% of cases.

Primary pulmonary hypertension exists in three histologic subtypes (Table 11). Plexogenic pulmonary hypertension is identified in about 28% of patients presenting with pulmonary hypertension of unknown cause. Although thrombotic or thromboembolic histologic findings occur more often (56%), it is unclear whether this subtype is 1) primary pulmonary hypertension with thrombosis in situ or secondary thromboemboli from engorged systemic veins or a failing right ventricle or 2) clinically occult pulmonary embolism resulting in pulmonary hypertension. Veno-occlusive disease constitutes the remaining 16%, and capillary hemangiomatosis is very rare (Table 12).

By definition, the cause of primary pulmonary hypertension is unknown (Table 13). Probably, the clinical entity represents a "final common pathway" for multiple undetected underlying substrates (Fig. 1).

Some clinical conditions have been identified with an increased prevalence of clinical primary pulmonary hypertension. The use of appetite suppressants has been linked to an increased risk for development of primary pulmonary hypertension. Persons who have taken dexfenfluramine for 6 months or more have 23 times the risk for development of clinically apparent primary pulmonary hypertension.

Nevertheless, the absolute risk from this exposure remains low (about 1 in 20,000). Pulmonary hypertension can be associated with portal hypertension (portopulmonary hypertension), but it is generally characterized as more hyperdynamic with a higher cardiac output and lower systemic resistance than pure primary pulmonary hypertension. Connective tissue diseases occasionally exhibit pulmonary hypertension, especially CREST syndrome (calcinosis cutis, Raynaud phenomenon, esophageal dysfunction, sclerodactyly, telangiectasia), scleroderma, and overlap syndromes. More rarely, pulmonary hypertension may develop in patients with systemic lupus erythematosus. In 40% of patients who have primary pulmonary hypertension without other evidence of connective tissue disease, the antinuclear antibody (ANA) titer is 1:80 dilutions or more. Patients with human immunodeficiency virus may exhibit clinical and histopathologic findings essentially identical to those of primary pulmonary hypertension; the incidence is as high as 0.5%, significantly higher than that in the general population. Finally, primary pulmonary hypertension has been identified in other family members of at least 6% of patients with the disease, and specific chromosome loci have been mapped by linkage analysis in some families with primary pulmonary hypertension.

- Primary pulmonary hypertension is more common in women (2:1), and familial clusters occur in 6% of cases.

Diagnostic Procedures in Pulmonary Hypertension

Physical Examination

The physical examination provides valuable clues about the presence, severity, and underlying cause of pulmonary hypertension. Its critical role is as both a screening and a diagnostic tool. The important components of the physical examination in relation to pulmonary hypertension are provided in Tables 14 through 16.

Table 12.—Histopathology of Primary Pulmonary Hypertension

Type of primary pulmonary hypertension	Histopathologic feature
Plexogenic arteriopathy	
Right ventricle	Hypertrophy with or without dilatation
Pulmonary arteries	Medial hypertrophy (Plate 1*A*)
	Extension of smooth muscle into arterioles
	Intimal proliferation (Plate 1*B*)
	Concentric intimal fibrosis (Plate 1*C*)
	Fibrinoid degeneration
	Dilatation lesions (Plate 1*D*)
	Plexiform lesions (Plate 1*E*)
	Dilatation and shallow intimal atheromas of elastic arteries
Thrombotic primary arteriopathy	
Right ventricle	Hypertrophy with or without dilatation
Pulmonary arteries	Medial hypertrophy less severe than in other forms
	Dilatation and shallow intimal atheromas of elastic arteries
	Recent thrombi in elastic arteries
	Organized thrombi in elastic arteries appearing as luminal webs or fibrocalcific pads
Pulmonary veno-occlusive disease	
Right ventricle	Hypertrophy with or without dilatation
Pulmonary arteries	Medial hypertrophy
	Dilatation and shallow intimal atheromas of elastic arteries
	Arteries may be dilated
	Eccentric and concentric nonlaminar intimal fibrosis
Pulmonary capillaries	Congestion
Pulmonary veins	Organized and recanalized thrombi in veins and venules
	Medial hypertrophy
Other	Edema of pleura and interlobular septa
	Dilatation of pleural and septal lymphatics
	Alveolar edema
	Microhemorrhages and hemosiderosis
Pulmonary capillary hemangiomatosis	
Right ventricle	Hypertrophy with or without dilatation
Pulmonary arteries	Medial hypertrophy
	Dilatation and shallow intimal atheromas of elastic arteries
Pulmonary capillaries	Proliferation of thin-walled microvessels infiltrating the interstitium, lung parenchyma, pleura, and walls of pulmonary veins
Pulmonary veins	Medial expansion due to microvessel infiltration and fibrous luminal obstruction
Other	Alveolar hemosiderin-laden macrophages

Chest Radiography

The chest radiograph shows central pulmonary and right ventricular enlargement. Findings specific to advanced pulmonary hypertension include a prominent pulmonary trunk and hilar pulmonary arteries, "pruning" of the peripheral pulmonary arteries, and obliteration of the retrosternal clear space by the enlarged, anteriorly situated right ventricle (Fig. 2). Other findings may reflect possible underlying disease, such as pulmonary venous congestion (pulmonary venous hypertension, pulmonary veno-occlusive disease), hyperinflation (chronic obstructive pulmonary disease), or kyphosis (restrictive pulmonary disease).

- Radiographic findings specific to advanced pulmonary hypertension include a prominent pulmonary trunk and hilar pulmonary arteries, "pruning" of the peripheral

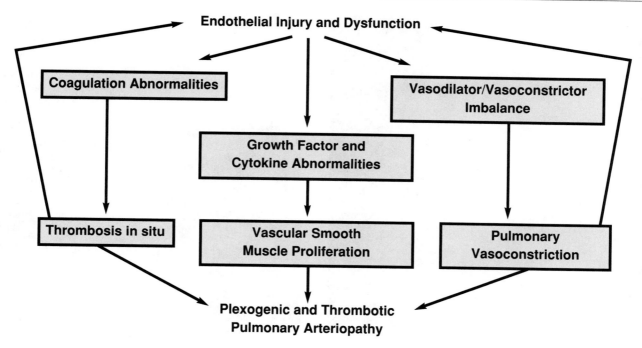

Fig. 1. Pathophysiologic pathways involved in primary pulmonary hypertension.

Table 13.—Possible Causes of Primary Pulmonary Hypertension

Proposed mechanism	Evidence
Occult thromboembolism or in situ thrombosis	Pathologic studies
	Response to anticoagulation
Genetic factors	Family clusters
Connective tissue disorder	High incidence of positive ANA
	Occasional Raynaud phenomenon
	Similarities with PSS-related pulmonary hypertension
Exogenous toxins	Examples: aminorex fumarate, toxic rapeseed oil, *Crotalaria*, L-tryptophan, dexfenfluramine
Inadequate hepatic detoxi-fication mechanisms	Occasional association with cirrhosis and portal hypertension
Hormonal factors	Female preponderance
	Possible oral contraceptive role
Vasospasm, chronic or recurrent	Occasional Raynaud phenomenon
	Occasional vasodilator benefit

ANA, antinuclear antibody; PSS, progressive systemic sclerosis.
From Giuliani ER, Gersh BJ, McGoon MD, Hayes DL, Schaff HV (editors): *Mayo Clinic Practice of Cardiology*. Third edition. Mosby, 1996, p 1831. By permission of Mayo Foundation.

pulmonary arteries, and obliteration of the retrosternal clear space.

Electrocardiography

The electrocardiogram in pulmonary hypertension shows evidence of right ventricular hypertrophy and right atrial enlargement. Criteria for right ventricular hypertrophy are right-axis deviation; a tall R wave and small S wave with R/S ratio > 1 in lead V_1; qR complex in lead V_1; rSR′ pattern in lead V_1; a large S wave and small R wave with R/S ratio < 1 in lead V_5 or V_6; or S_1, S_2, S_3 pattern. ST-T wave depression and inversion are often present in the right precordial leads. Right atrial enlargement is seen as a tall R wave (≥ 2.5 mm) in leads II, III, and aVF and frontal P axis of 75° or more (Fig. 3).

- The electrocardiogram in pulmonary hypertension shows evidence of right ventricular hypertrophy and right atrial enlargement.

Echocardiography

Doppler echocardiographic criteria can estimate pulmonary arterial systolic, diastolic, and mean pressures. Systolic pressure is extrapolated from right ventricular pressure in the absence of pulmonary stenosis. Right ventricular pressure is determined with continuous-wave Doppler

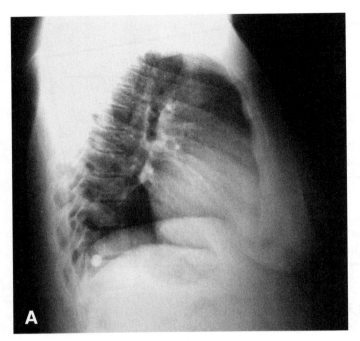
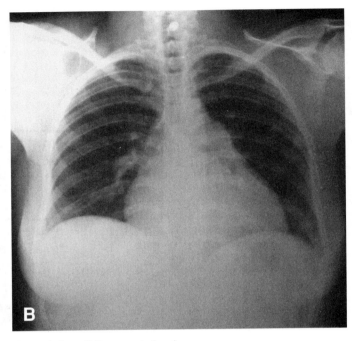

Fig. 2. Chest radiographs from patient with primary pulmonary hypertension. *A*, Lateral view. *B*, Posteroanterior view.

echocardiography to measure the retrograde velocity across the tricuspid valve (Fig. 4). The tricuspid pressure gradient is derived from the modified Bernoulli equation:

$$\Delta P_{TV} = 4V_{TR}^2$$

in which ΔP_{TV} = maximal systolic pressure gradient across the tricuspid valve and V_{TR} = peak Doppler signal velocity of the regurgitant jet across the tricuspid valve.

The addition of estimated right atrial pressure (RAP) yields right ventricular systolic pressure (RVSP):

$$\Delta P_{TV} + RAP = RVSP$$

Pulsed-wave Doppler analysis of central laminar flow in the distal right ventricular outflow tract or proximal main pulmonary artery can determine the mean pulmonary artery pressure by measuring pulmonary acceleration time and applying a regression equation.

End-diastolic pulmonary regurgitant velocity can be measured with continuous-wave Doppler echocardiography (Fig. 5). Pulmonary artery diastolic pressure (PADP) corresponds to the regurgitant pressure gradient across the pulmonary valve plus the right atrial (i.e., right ventricular end-diastolic) pressure (RAP):

$$\Delta P_{PV} = 4V_{PR}^2$$
$$\Delta P_{PV} + RAP = PADP$$

in which ΔP_{PV} = end-diastolic pressure gradient across the pulmonary valve and V_{PR} = regurgitant Doppler signal velocity across the pulmonary valve at end-diastole.

Echocardiographic imaging also can provide information about right ventricular size and function and disclose underlying causes such as left-sided lesions or shunt. Echocardiographic hallmarks of pulmonary hypertension

Table 14.—Physical Signs That *Indicate* Pulmonary Hypertension

Sign	Implication
Accentuated pulmonary component of S_2 (audible at apex)	High pulmonary pressure increases force of pulmonary valve closure
Early systolic click	Sudden interruption of opening of pulmonary valve into high-pressure artery
Midsystolic ejection murmur	Turbulent transvalvular pulmonary outflow
Left parasternal lift	High right ventricular pressure and hypertrophy present
Increased jugular "a" waves	High right ventricular filling pressure

From Giuliani ER, Gersh BJ, McGoon MD, Hayes DL, Schaff HV (editors): *Mayo Clinic Practice of Cardiology.* Third edition. Mosby, 1996, p 1826. By permission of Mayo Foundation.

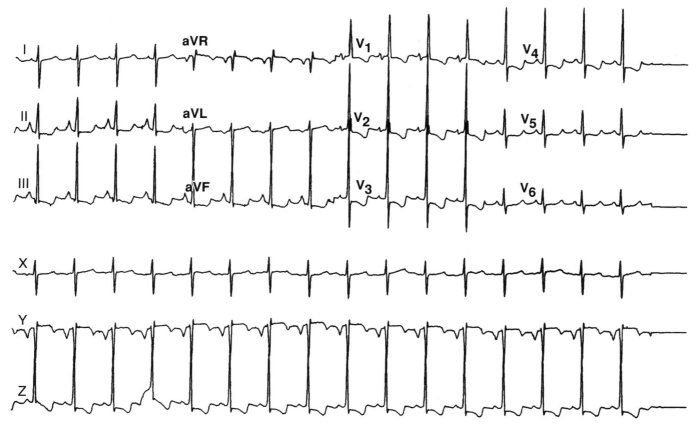

Fig. 3. Electrocardiogram from 28-year-old woman with primary pulmonary hypertension.

Table 15.—Physical Signs That *Indicate Severity* of Pulmonary Hypertension

Sign	Implication
Moderate to severe pulmonary hypertension	
Diastolic murmur	Pulmonary regurgitation
Holosystolic murmur that increases with inspiration	Tricuspid regurgitation
Increased jugular v waves	Tricuspid regurgitation
Hepatojugular reflux	Tricuspid regurgitation
Pulsatile liver	Tricuspid regurgitation
Advanced pulmonary hypertension with right ventricular failure	
Right ventricular S_3	Right ventricular dysfunction
Marked distention of jugular veins	Right ventricular dysfunction or tricuspid regurgitation or both
Hepatomegaly	Right ventricular dysfunction or tricuspid regurgitation or both
Peripheral edema	Right ventricular dysfunction or tricuspid regurgitation or both
Ascites	Right ventricular dysfunction or tricuspid regurgitation or both
Low blood pressure, diminished pulse pressure, cool extremities	Reduced cardiac output, peripheral vasoconstriction

From Giuliani ER, Gersh BJ, McGoon MD, Hayes DL, Schaff HV (editors): *Mayo Clinic Practice of Cardiology.* Third edition. Mosby, 1996, p 1827. By permission of Mayo Foundation.

Table 16.—Physical Signs That Detect Possible *Underlying Cause or Associations* of Pulmonary Hypertension

Sign	Implication
Central cyanosis	Hypoxemia, right-to-left shunt
Clubbing	Congenital heart disease
Cardiac auscultatory findings, including systolic murmurs, diastolic murmurs, opening snap, and gallop	Congenital or acquired heart or valvular disease
Rales, dullness, or decreased breath sounds	Pulmonary congestion or effusion or both
Fine rales, accessory muscle use, wheezing, protracted expiration, productive cough	Pulmonary parenchymal disease
Obesity, kyphoscoliosis, enlarged tonsils	Possible substrate for disordered ventilation
Sclerodactyly, arthritis, rash	Connective tissue disorder
Peripheral venous insufficiency or obstruction	Possible venous thrombosis

From Giuliani ER, Gersh BJ, McGoon MD, Hayes DL, Schaff HV (editors): *Mayo Clinic Practice of Cardiology.* Third edition. Mosby, 1996, p 1827. By permission of Mayo Foundation.

include a systolic "notch" in the M-mode opening contour of the pulmonary valve leaflet (Fig. 6), right ventricular enlargement, flattened interventricular septum, and a small D-shaped, normally contractile left ventricle on two-dimensional echocardiography (Fig. 7).

- Echocardiography can noninvasively estimate pulmonary artery systolic pressure from $RAP + 4V^2_{TR}$ and pulmonary artery diastolic pressure from $RAP + 4V^2_{PR}$.

Radionuclide Studies

Ventilation-perfusion lung scanning is useful for determining whether pulmonary hypertension has a thromboembolic cause. The presence of an unmatched segmental perfusion defect requires searching for potentially treatable chronic thromboembolism (Fig. 8).

Pulmonary Artery Imaging

A segmental (or greater) perfusion defect on ventilation-perfusion lung scanning warrants further investigation to assess the possibility of thromboembolic pulmonary

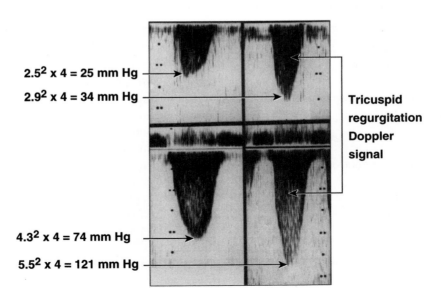

$2.5^2 \times 4 = 25$ mm Hg

$2.9^2 \times 4 = 34$ mm Hg

Tricuspid regurgitation Doppler signal

$4.3^2 \times 4 = 74$ mm Hg

$5.5^2 \times 4 = 121$ mm Hg

Fig. 4. Continuous-wave Doppler echocardiography signals of varying degrees of tricuspid regurgitant velocity which are used to estimate right ventricular systolic pressure.

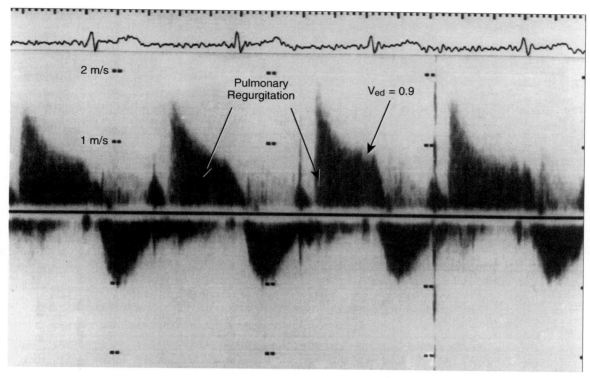

Fig. 5. Continuous-wave Doppler signal of pulmonary regurgitation. The regurgitant velocity at end-diastole (V_{ed}) is used to estimate pulmonary artery diastolic pressure. An end-diastolic velocity of 0.9 m/s corresponds to an estimated pressure gradient of $4\,(.9^2) = 3.24$. If the right atrial pressure is 14 mm Hg, then the pulmonary artery diastolic pressure is $3 + 14 = 17$ mm Hg.

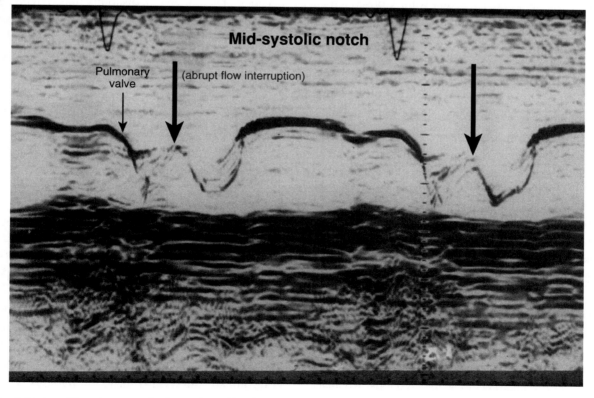

Fig. 6. M-mode tracing of the pulmonary valve in a patient with pulmonary hypertension.

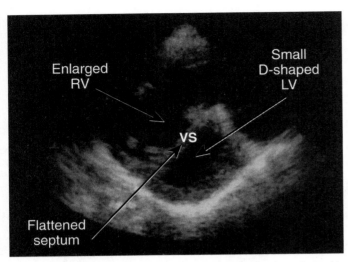

Fig. 7. Still frame of two-dimensional echocardiogram of a patient with severe primary pulmonary hypertension. LV, left ventricle; RV, right ventricle; VS, ventricular septum.

hypertension, because significant remediable chronic thromboembolism may be present despite a minimally abnormal scan. Pulmonary angiography has been regarded as the definitive examination of pulmonary intraluminal anatomy. However, in thromboembolic pulmonary hypertension, chronic thrombi may have organized and become an integral component of the vascular wall. Consequently, angiography may underestimate the degree of vascular obstruction by proximal clots.

Alternative imaging methods that have shown promise in enhancing the diagnosis of pulmonary thromboembolic disease are magnetic resonance imaging, angioscopy, intravascular ultrasonography, and electron beam computed tomography (Fig. 9). Electron beam and spiral computed tomography are becoming the imaging methods of choice in many centers for the diagnosis of proximal vessel pulmonary emboli.

- A segmental (or greater) perfusion defect on ventilation-perfusion lung scanning warrants further investigation to assess the possibility of thromboembolic pulmonary hypertension.

Hemodynamic Studies

Direct hemodynamic assessment with invasive studies may be required for confirmation and quantitation of pulmonary artery pressure (PAP) and for evaluation of the acute hemodynamic response to pharmacologic interventions. Capillary wedge pressure (CWP) measurements and cardiac output

(CO) determination allow calculation of pulmonary artery resistance (Rp):

$$Rp = (PAP - CWP)/CO$$

Pulmonary Biopsy

Open or thoracoscopic lung biopsy carries substantial risk and seldom provides information that affects therapy.

Clinical Course

The clinical course of primary pulmonary hypertension is generally one of inexorable progression toward death. Among patients who do not undergo heart-lung transplantation or treatment with an effective vasodilator, actuarial survival is about 72% at 1 year, 55% at 2 years, 48% at 3 years, 36% at 4 years, and 30% at 5 years. The usual causes of death are right ventricular failure (63%), pneumonia (7%), and sudden death (7%).

Various indicators appear to have predictive value for survival (Table 17) (Fig. 10).

Among patients with Eisenmenger complex with an equal degree of pulmonary hypertension, survival is likely to be much longer than that of patients with primary pulmonary hypertension, perhaps as long as 2 or more decades. Their degree of disability due to hypoxemia may be considerable, however. Survival in patients with cor pulmonale due to ventilatory disease is variable and is determined by complications related to the specific pulmonary defect.

- Among patients with Eisenmenger complex with an equal degree of pulmonary hypertension, survival is likely to be much longer than that of patients with primary pulmonary hypertension.

Treatment

If possible, the underlying cause of pulmonary hypertension should be addressed and removed or treated as specifically as possible (Table 18).

Some patients with primary pulmonary hypertension benefit from vasodilators. High doses of calcium blockers (nifedipine, amlodipine, or diltiazem, *not* verapamil) appear to improve long-term pulmonary hemodynamics (Fig. 11) and survival (Fig. 12) in patients who have an initial hemodynamic response. Potent very short-acting

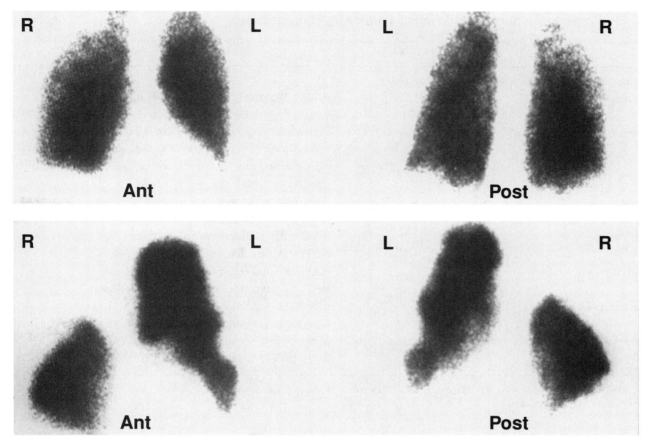

Fig. 8. Perfusion lung scans, showing diffuse inhomogeneity of perfusion, especially apically, suggestive of primary pulmonary hypertension (*Top*) and segmental and subsegmental defects consistent with chronic major vessel thromboembolic pulmonary hypertension (*Bottom*). Ant, anterior; L, left; Post, posterior; R, right.

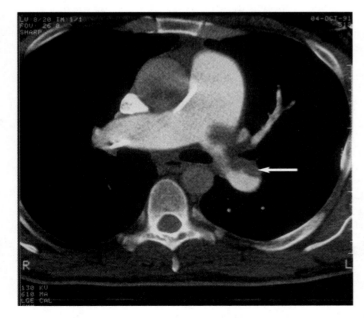

Fig. 9. Cardiac computed tomography scan, showing thrombus in the left main pulmonary artery (*arrow*).

vasodilators (Table 19) predict whether a patient has sufficient vasodilatory capability to warrant an attempt at long-term therapy with calcium blockers. Use of calcium blockers must be initiated during hemodynamic monitoring in an intensive care unit or catheterization laboratory in order to assess acute efficacy and allow early detection of adverse effects, particularly systemic hypotension. Epoprostenol (prostacyclin, prostaglandin I_2), one of 90 prostaglandins synthesized from arachidonic acid, is a powerful vasodilator and one of the strongest endogenous inhibitors of platelet aggregation; it is synthesized mainly in endothelial cells. Evidence suggests that at least one component of pulmonary hypertension is an abnormally low ratio of epoprostenol in relation to the endogenous vasoconstrictor thromboxane A_2 (Fig. 13).

Two randomized, controlled studies have confirmed that infusion of epoprostenol in patients with symptomatic primary pulmonary hypertension improves survival, exercise duration, subjective well-being, and hemodynamics (Fig. 14).

Table 17.—Predictors of Survival in Primary Pulmonary Hypertension

Category	Observation
Pulmonary vascular resistance and pulmonary arterial mean pressure (PA_m)	PA_m < 55 mm Hg: median survival, 48 mo
	PA_m ≥ 85 mm Hg: median survival, 12 mo
Response to vasodilator therapy	Patients in whom pulmonary arteriolar resistance decreases with short-term administration of vasodilators tend to survive longer, and this benefit may be independent of subsequent treatment status
	Treatment with vasodilators may also enhance survival
New York Heart Association (NYHA) functional classification	NYHA I-II: median survival, 58.6 mo
	NYHA III: median survival, 31.5 mo
	NYHA IV: median survival, 6 mo
Right atrial pressure (RAP)	RAP > 20 mm Hg: median survival, 1 mo
	RAP < 10 mm Hg: median survival, 46 mo
Cardiac index (CI)	CI < 2.0 L · m^2/min: median survival, 17 mo
	CI ≥ 4.0 L · m^2/min: median survival, 43 mo
Pulmonary arterial (mixed venous) oxygen saturation (SvO_2)	SvO_2 < 63%: mean 3-year survival, 17%
	SvO_2 ≥ 63%: mean 3-year survival, 55%

From Giuliani ER, Gersh BJ, McGoon MD, Hayes DL, Schaff HV (editors): *Mayo Clinic Practice of Cardiology*. Third edition. Mosby, 1996, p 1832. By permission of Mayo Foundation.

Because of a half-life of only several minutes in the circulation, epoprostenol must be infused continuously and chronically. The usual starting dosage is 2 to 8 ng/kg per minute; in most patients the dosage must be increased gradually over time to maintain benefit. The administration of epoprostenol requires an indwelling central venous catheter (such as a Hickman catheter) and portable external infusion pump (Plate 2).

Anticoagulation with warfarin is recommended for patients with primary pulmonary hypertension because coagulation disorders have been detected in some patients, histopathologic examinations show a high prevalence of thrombosis in situ of the pulmonary arterioles, and high right ventricular pressures may promote deep vein thrombosis. In addition, retrospective studies have suggested a survival benefit for patients treated with warfarin (Fig. 15).

• All patients with primary pulmonary hypertension should receive anticoagulation unless there are strong patient-specific contraindications.

Other components of therapy for primary pulmonary

hypertension include oxygen supplementation, diuretics for fluid retention, and digoxin for inotropic support of the failing right ventricle. Percutaneous atrial blade septostomy has been reported to improve symptoms due to right ventricular failure, but it exacerbates systemic hypoxemia. With single- and double-lung transplantation for primary pulmonary hypertension, the 1-year survival rate is 70% to 75%.

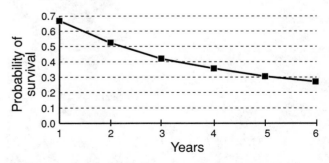

Fig. 10. Probability of survival for a patient with primary pulmonary hypertension and a cardiac index of 1.88 L/min per m^2, right atrial pressure of 10 mm Hg, and mean pulmonary artery pressure of 61 mm Hg.

Table 18.—Treatment of Pulmonary Hypertension, by Cause

Category	Treatment
Pulmonary venous hypertension	Remove underlying cause if possible
	Mitral valve surgery
	Left ventricular afterload reduction
Chronic obstructive lung disease, parenchymal lung disease	Oxygen
	Lung transplantation
	Vasodilator
	Consider lung reduction procedure
	Consider phlebotomy
	Consider anticoagulation
	Consider diuretic
Obesity, obstructive sleep apnea, hypoventilation	Positive airway pressure (CPAP, BiPAP)
	Respiratory stimulants (medroxyprogesterone)
	Weight reduction
Restrictive lung disease	Oxygen
Skeletal	BiPAP
Fibrotic	Vasodilators
Neuromuscular	Anticoagulation
	Lung transplantation (fibrotic)
	Consider phrenic nerve stimulation (neuromuscular)
High altitude	Oxygen
	Lower altitude
Vascular	Thromboendarterectomy
	Inferior vena cava filter
	Anticoagulation
	Vasodilators
	Oxygen
Intracardiac shunt	Lung transplantation with repair of intracardiac defect
	Heart-lung transplantation

BiPAP, bilevel positive airway pressure; CPAP, continuous positive airway pressure.

Table 19.—Dosing Strategies for Assessment of Pulmonary Arterial Vasodilator Capacity*

Drug	Route	Initial dosage	Increments	Step duration	Maximal dosage
Epoprostenol	Intravenous	2 ng/kg per min	2 ng/kg per min	10 min	16 ng/kg per min
Adenosine	Intravenous	50-100 µg/kg per min	50 µg/kg per min	2 min	350 µg/kg per min
Acetylcholine	Intravenous	1 mg/min	1-2 mg per min	10 min	10 mg/min
Nitric oxide	Inhaled	20 ppm in air	20 ppm in air	5 min	80 ppm in air
Nifedipine	Oral	10-20 mg	20 mg	1 hour	200 mg cumulative
Diltiazem	Oral	60 mg	60 mg	1 hour	600 mg cumulative

*A decrease in pulmonary arterial pressure or resistance by 20% to 30% in response to administration of a maximally tolerated dose of a short-acting vasodilator warrants a trial of treatment with a calcium channel blocker.

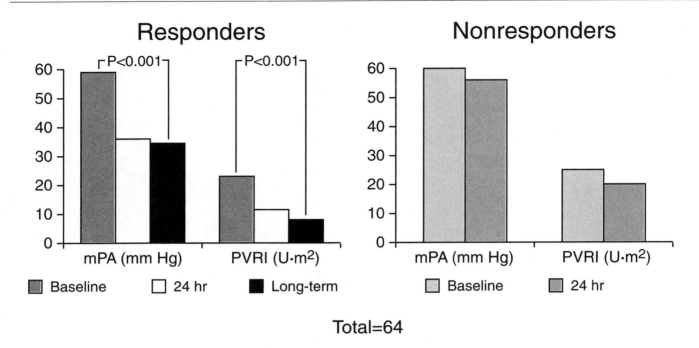

Fig. 11. Approximately 25% of patients with primary pulmonary hypertension have an acute hemodynamic benefit from administration of calcium blockers, and this effect is maintained with long-term treatment. However, the remaining three-fourths of patients fail to respond. mPA, main pulmonary artery; PVRI, pulmonary vascular resistance index. (Data from *N Engl J Med* 327:76-81, 1992.)

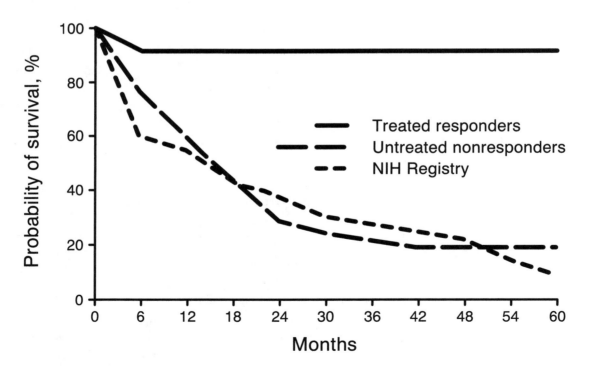

Fig. 12. Patients who respond to calcium blockers and have long-term treatment have better survival than those who fail to respond or are untreated (*P* < 0.003, responders vs. other groups). NIH, National Institutes of Health. (From *N Engl J Med* 327:76-81, 1992. By permission of Massachusetts Medical Society.)

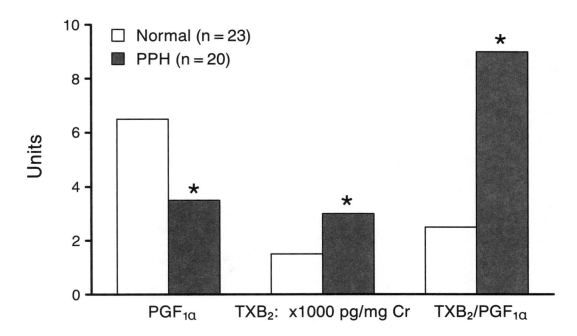

Fig. 13. Compared with patients who have normal pulmonary artery pressure, patients with primary pulmonary hypertension (PPH) have lower urinary levels of epoprostenol metabolites (prostaglandin $F_{1\alpha}$, $PGF_{1\alpha}$) and higher levels of thromboxane metabolites (TXB_2), suggesting a vasoconstrictor predisposition. *Differences between groups were significant ($P < 0.05$). (Data from *N Engl J Med* 327:70-75, 1992.)

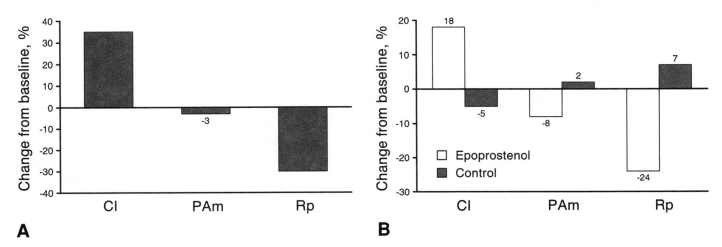

Fig. 14. *A*, Average acute pulmonary hemodynamic response in all patients in two studies of epoprostenol in primary pulmonary hypertension, *B*, Average change in hemodynamic variables among patients with primary pulmonary hypertension who were treated with epoprostenol for 12 weeks and patients who did not receive epoprostenol. CI, cardiac index; PAm, mean pulmonary artery pressure; Rp, pulmonary resistance. (Data from *Ann Intern Med* 112:485-491, 1990 and *Ann Intern Med* 121:409-415, 1994.)

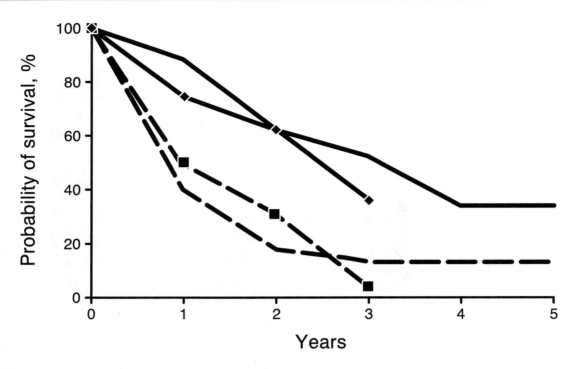

Fig. 15. Patients who receive warfarin (solid lines) have longer survival than those who do not (broken lines). (Data from *Circulation* 70:580-587, 1984 [lines with squares] and *N Engl J Med* 327:76-81, 1992.)

Suggested Review Reading

1. Abenhaim L, Moride Y, Brenot F, et al: Appetite-suppressant drugs and the risk of primary pulmonary hypertension. *N Engl J Med* 335:609-616, 1996.
This carefully performed case-control study demonstrated an increased risk of development of primary pulmonary hypertension in patients who took appetite suppressants.

2. Barst RJ, Rubin LJ, McGoon MD, et al: Survival in primary pulmonary hypertension with long-term continuous intravenous prostacyclin. *Ann Intern Med* 121:409-415, 1994.
Patients who were treated with chronic epoprostenol infusion had longer survival than matched patients in the National Institutes of Health registry of primary pulmonary hypertension.

3. Bjornsson J, Edwards WD: Primary pulmonary hypertension: a histopathologic study of 80 cases. *Mayo Clin Proc* 60:16-25, 1985.
This large autopsy series demonstrated that most patients with primary pulmonary hypertension have a thrombotic variant, whereas fewer have classic plexiform lesions and only a small minority have pulmonary veno-occlusive disease.

4. Christman BW, McPherson CD, Newman JH, et al: An imbalance between the excretion of thromboxane and prostacyclin metabolites in pulmonary hypertension. *N Engl J Med* 327:70-75, 1992.
Patients with primary pulmonary hypertension or secondary pulmonary hypertension have an excess of thromboxane derivative in relation to epoprostenol compared with normal patients or those with obstructive pulmonary disease without pulmonary hypertension.

5. D'Alonzo GE, Barst RJ, Ayres SM, et al: Survival in patients with primary pulmonary hypertension. Results from a national prospective registry. *Ann Intern Med* 115:343-349, 1991.
This study describes the survival outcome of patients with primary pulmonary hypertension who were enrolled in a large National Institutes of Health registry in the mid-1980s.

6. Fuster V, Steele PM, Edwards WD, et al: Primary pulmonary hypertension: natural history and the importance of thrombosis. *Circulation* 70:580-587, 1984.
This retrospective study of more than 100 patients suggests that the use of warfarin improves survival outcome.

7. Galie N, Ussia G, Passarelli P, et al: Role of pharmacologic tests in the treatment of primary pulmonary hypertension. *Am J Cardiol* 75:55A-62A, 1995.
This is a good summary of strategies for assessing the vasodilator response of the pulmonary vasculature in order to determine optimal treatment.

8. Kuo PC, Plotkin JS, Johnson LB, et al: Distinctive clinical features of portopulmonary hypertension. *Chest* 112:980-986, 1997.
This article distinguishes the characteristic hemodynamic features of patients with primary pulmonary hypertension, portopulmonary hypertension, and chronic liver disease. Patients with portopulmonary hypertension characteristically have a higher cardiac output and lower systemic vascular resistance than those with primary pulmonary hypertension.

9. McGoon MD: Medical treatment of pulmonary hypertension. *Cardiologia* 40:561-577, 1995.
This is a general review of treatment strategies and their rationales.

10. McLaughlin VV, Genthner DE, Panella MM, et al: Reduction in pulmonary vascular resistance with long-term epoprostenol (prostacyclin) therapy in primary pulmonary hypertension. *N Engl J Med* 338:273-277, 1998.
Long-term treatment of primary pulmonary hypertension with epoprostenol leads to further reduction of pulmonary resistance compared with what was found at the time of acute vasodilator testing with adenosine. This suggests that vascular remodeling occurs in some patients.

11. Morse JH, Jones AC, Barst RJ, et al: Mapping of familial primary pulmonary hypertension locus (PPH1) to chromosome 2q31-q32. *Circulation* 95:2603-2606, 1997.
This is a report of a chromosome locus potentially associated with primary pulmonary hypertension.

12. Petitpretz P, Brenot F, Azarian R, et al: Pulmonary hypertension in patients with human immunodeficiency virus infection. Comparison with primary pulmonary hypertension. *Circulation* 89:2722-2727, 1994.
This article describes 20 patients with pulmonary hypertension in the setting of human immunodeficiency virus infection, suggesting that clinically and pathologically it is similar to primary pulmonary hypertension.

13. Rich S, Kaufmann E, Levy PS: The effect of high doses of calcium-channel blockers on survival in primary pulmonary hypertension. *N Engl J Med* 327:76-81, 1992.
Patients who exhibited a vasodilator response to calcium channel blockade demonstrated excellent survival when treated with calcium channel blockers for up to 5 years. Among the untreated group, survival was better in those who were treated with warfarin, but overall the group who did not receive calcium blockers had an inferior probability of survival compared with those who did receive calcium blockers.

14. Rubin LJ: Primary pulmonary hypertension. *N Engl J Med* 336:111-117, 1997.
This is a good general review.

15. Rubin LJ, Mendoza J, Hood M, et al: Treatment of primary pulmonary hypertension with continuous intravenous prostacyclin (epoprostenol). Results of a randomized trial. *Ann Intern Med* 112:485-491, 1990.
This large randomized study (81 patients) found that treatment of primary pulmonary hypertension with epoprostenol resulted in somewhat better hemodynamics, improved symptoms and exercise capacity, and markedly better survival over 12 weeks.

16. Shapiro SM, Oudiz RJ, Cao T, et al: Primary pulmonary hypertension: improved long-term effects and survival with continuous intravenous epoprostenol infusion. *J Am Coll Cardiol* 30:343-349, 1997.
This single-center follow-up study confirmed better survival among patients treated with epoprostenol.

Questions

Multiple Choice (choose the one best answer)

1. A 43-year-old woman has a tricuspid regurgitant velocity of 4.4 m/s, an enlarged, moderately hypocontractile right ventricle, normal valves, and normal left ventricular size and function. She complains of fatigue and breathlessness while doing household work. Which of the following is an appropriate next step?
   a. Urgent outpatient initiation of high-dose nifedipine or diltiazem
   b. Stress radionuclide myocardial perfusion study and coronary angiography if the perfusion study is markedly abnormal
   c. Pulmonary function testing, ventilation-perfusion scintigraphy, transesophageal echocardiography with bubble contrast, and determination of antinuclear antibody titer
   d. Surgical consultation for tricuspid annuloplasty
   e. Initiation of chronic intravenous epoprostenol

A 34-year-old woman from Minnesota has a pulmonary artery pressure (PAP) of 99/48 (mean 63) mm Hg at right heart catheterization, and the thermodilution cardiac index (CI) is 2.1 L/min per m². Right atrial pressure (RAP) is 16 mm Hg, right ventricular pressure (RVP) is 102/16 mm Hg, and pulmonary capillary wedge pressure (PCWP) is 14 mm Hg. Previous evaluation has disclosed no evidence of thromboembolism, connective tissue or liver disease, sleep apnea, intracardiac shunt, or ventilatory lung disease.

2. The transpulmonary gradient is:
   a. 2 mm Hg
   b. 51 mm Hg
   c. 63 mm Hg
   d. 49 mm Hg
   e. 86 mm Hg

3. The patient's pulmonary artery resistance index is:
   a. 30 U/m²

b. Not possible to calculate without knowing the body surface area
   c. 23 U
   d. 30 U
   e. 23 U $\cdot$ m²

4. The likely diagnosis is:
   a. Primary pulmonary hypertension
   b. Pulmonary veno-occlusive disease
   c. Right ventricular cardiomyopathy
   d. Schistosomiasis
   e. Pulmonary arteriovenous malformations

5. The appropriate next step is:
   a. Acute vasodilator testing with intravenous epoprostenol
   b. Acute vasodilator testing with intravenous adenosine
   c. Acute vasodilator testing with inhaled nitric oxide
   d. Any of the above
   e. None of the above

6. The percentage of patients with primary pulmonary hypertension who have another family member with primary pulmonary hypertension is approximately:
   a. 0.6%
   b. 6%
   c. 0.06%
   d. 16%
   e. 61%

7. The best indicator of a loud P_2 is:
   a. It is palpable
   b. It is associated with a right ventricular S_4 gallop
   c. It is associated with an early systolic ejection click
   d. It is associated with paradoxical splitting of S_2
   e. It is audible at the apex

8. A 48-year-old man in New York Heart Association class III who has primary pulmonary hypertension undergoes an acute vasodilator study with epoprostenol. The results are as follows:

	Pressure, mm Hg			Cardiac output, L/min	Blood pressure, mm Hg
	Mean right atrial	Pulmonary artery	Mean pulmonary capillary wedge		
Baseline	12	82/40 (mean 54)	12	3.5	122/72
Peak drug dose	11	79/38 (mean 50)	15	5.0	108/61

The pulmonary arterial resistance changed by:
a. 8%
b. -8%
c. -42%
d. -33%
e. 33%

9. The recommended treatment strategy in view of these results is:
a. Initiate chronic infusion of epoprostenol
b. Trial of high-dose nifedipine, diltiazem, or amlodipine
c. Comfort care only
d. No specific treatment necessary in view of the excellent prognostic category
e. Angiotensin-converting enzyme inhibitors

10. Epoprostenol infusion has been shown to do all *except*:
a. Lengthen survival in patients with primary pulmonary hypertension
b. Improve exercise tolerance in patients with primary pulmonary hypertension
c. Reduce pulmonary edema in patients with pulmonary veno-occlusive disease
d. Lower pulmonary resistance in patients with primary pulmonary hypertension
e. Attenuate symptoms in patients with primary pulmonary hypertension

11. A pulmonary valve peak regurgitant velocity of 3.0 m/s, end-diastolic regurgitant velocity of 1.0 m/s, and a right ventricular outflow tract velocity of 2.0 m/s in a patient with a mean right atrial pressure (RAP) of 20 mm Hg indicate a pulmonary artery diastolic pressure (PADP) of:
a. 24 mm Hg
b. 56 mm Hg
c. 36 mm Hg
d. 4 mm Hg
e. Insufficient data to calculate

12. Which of the following statements is correct?
a. A negative history for acute thromboembolism obviates further evaluation of chronic thromboembolic pulmonary hypertension
b. A ventilation-perfusion scan with 3 or fewer subsegmental defects or 1 or zero segmental defects essentially excludes chronic thromboembolism as a cause of pulmonary hypertension
c. Optimal treatment of chronic major vessel pulmonary thromboembolism is local infusion of urokinase followed by lifelong anticoagulation and inferior vena cava filter
d. Fast computed tomography fails to detect more than 50% of surgically remediable chronic pulmonary thromboemboli identified by pulmonary angiography
e. Pulmonary thromboendarterectomy is the treatment of choice for chronic major vessel pulmonary thromboembolism

Answers

1. Answer c

The Doppler study, right ventricular function, and symptoms indicate the presence of significant pulmonary hypertension. A diagnosis of an underlying secondary disease or a diagnosis by exclusion of primary pulmonary hypertension should be made. The proper diagnosis will determine whether a right heart hemodynamic study is required and which treatment strategy to pursue.

2. Answer d

Transpulmonary gradient (TPG) = mean PAP - PCWP = 63 - 14 = 49.

3. Answer e

Pulmonary artery resistance index = TPG/CI = 49/2.1 = 23.3. The units are based on U = PA/cardiac output (CO) = mm Hg/(L/min), and CI = (L/min)/m^2. Thus, indexed units are PA/CO per m^2 = PAP $\cdot$ m^2/CO = U $\cdot$ m^2.

4. Answer a

The patient has pulmonary arterial hypertension without an identifiable cause. The PCWP is not particularly high, which argues against pulmonary veno-occlusive disease. Right ventricular dysfunction alone would not increase PAP. Schistosomiasis is a rare cause of pulmonary hypertension in the United States. Right-to-left shunting through pulmonary arteriovenous malformations would not be expected to cause pulmonary hypertension.

5. Answer d

For a patient with primary pulmonary hypertension undergoing a right heart hemodynamic study, assessment of the response to potent short-acting vasodilators is important in determining treatment strategy.

6. Answer b

7. Answer e

If the P$_2$ is audible at the apex, it is loud.

8. Answer c

(54 - 12)/3.5 = 12; (50 - 15)/5 = 7; 12 - 7 = 5; 5/12 = 42% decrease in pulmonary arterial resistance.

9. Answer b

A significant decrease (> 20% to 30%) in pulmonary resistance warrants a trial of calcium channel blocker treatment initially before starting epoprostenol therapy.

10. Answer c

Epoprostenol can provoke pulmonary edema in pulmonary veno-occlusive disease if the pulmonary arterioles dilate in the absence of any decrease in pulmonary venous resistance.

11. Answer a

The relevant value is the end-diastolic pulmonary valve regurgitant velocity (v): PADP = 4v^2 + RAP = (4 x 1^2) + 20 = 24 mm Hg.

12. Answer e

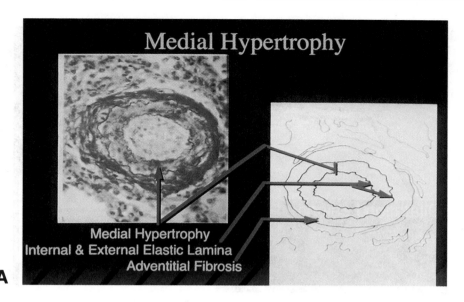

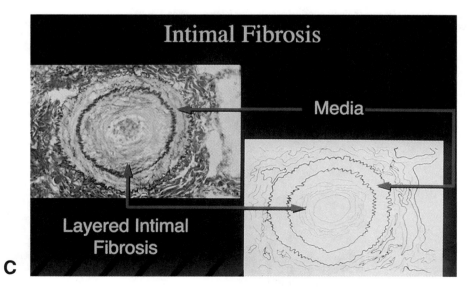

Plate 1

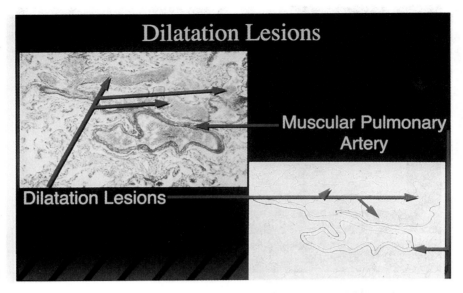

Plate 1 (continued). Histopathology of primary pulmonary hypertension.

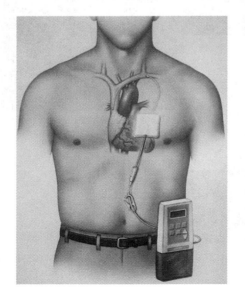

Plate 2. Patient with central venous catheter and portable infusion pump for administration of epoprostenol.

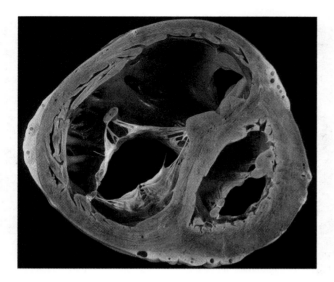

Plate 3. Right ventricular hypertrophy and dilatation in pulmonary hypertension.

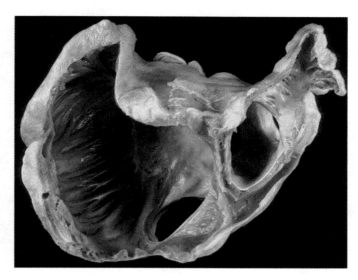

Plate 4. Right atrial dilatation and normal left atrium.

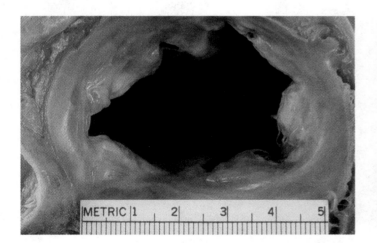

Plate 5. Tricuspid regurgitation due to annular dilatation in chronic pulmonary hypertension.

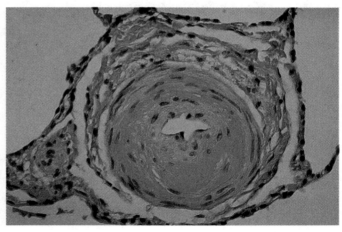

Plate 6. Fibrinoid degeneration in a pulmonary arteriole in pulmonary hypertension. (x100.)

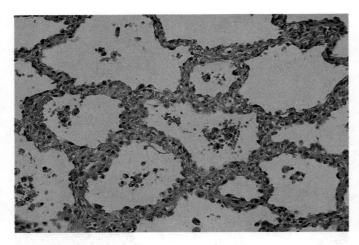

Plate 7. Thick alveolar walls in chronic pulmonary venous hypertension. (x50.)

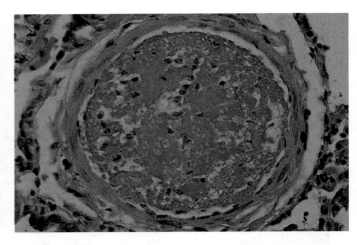

Plate 8. Pulmonary arteriole occluded by fresh thrombus in thromboembolic pulmonary hypertension.

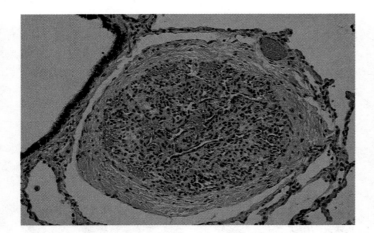

Plate 9. Plexiform lesion in pulmonary arteriole in pulmonary hypertension.

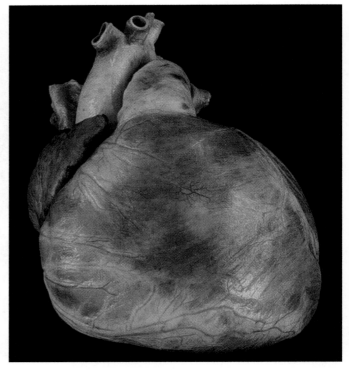

Plate 10. Right ventricular hypertrophy and enlargement in primary pulmonary hypertension (anterior view).

Chapter 27

Pulmonary Embolism

Udaya B. S. Prakash, M.D.

Epidemiology of Pulmonary Embolism

Pulmonary embolism (PE) is common in hospitalized patients, with a prevalence of about 1%. Although is it the immediate cause of death in about 10% of patients who die in U.S. hospitals, it is detected in 30% of routine autopsies. The correct antemortem diagnosis is made in less than 1/3 of cases. Note that the mortality from PE has not diminished in the last 20 years.

PE and deep vein thrombosis (DVT) are closely linked, with the incidence in the U.S. of DVT of the legs and PE estimated to be about 270,000 cases/year, of which about 2/3 are new cases and 1/3 are recurrent disease. Patients who die of PE die rapidly, usually within 2 hours after the embolism.

DVT is the cause of PE in more than 80% of patients, and the risk of fatal PE depends on the extent of the DVT. The risk of PE from untreated proximal DVT is 50%, and the mortality from untreated PE is 8%. Chronic pulmonary hypertension as a complication of recurrent PE occurs in approximately 2,500 patients/year in the U.S.

- PE is a common problem in hospitalized patients that frequently is *not* adequately diagnosed.
- Consider PE in *all* patients with lung problems.
- Adequate prophylaxis against DVT/PE is frequently omitted in high-risk patients.
- Risk of PE from untreated DVT is 50%.
- Risk of death from untreated PE is 8%.

Etiology of PE

The most important factor responsible for PE is DVT of the lower extremities. DVT results from the triad of Virchow: venous stasis, injury to venous intima, and coagulation disorders. The primary or secondary coagulation disorders are listed in Table 1.

Factor V Leiden Mutation
Factor V Leiden mutation has been shown not to be a significant risk factor for acute DVT in patients undergoing hip or knee replacement surgery. However, it is associated with increased risk of thromboembolic disease, particularly in men older than 60 years, men with hyperhomocystinemia, and women taking oral contraceptives. Routine screening for factor V Leiden mutation is not indicated in patients with suspected DVT or PE, nor is it indicated for family members of patients with known factor V Leiden mutation.

Lower Limb DVT
Although most (> 95%) PEs arise from thrombi in the lower

An atlas illustrating lesions associated with pulmonary embolism is found at the end of the chapter (Plates 1-8).

Table 1.—Coagulation Disorders That Predispose to the Development of Deep Vein Thrombosis (DVT) and Pulmonary Embolism (PE)

Primary hypercoagulable states	Secondary hypercoagulable states
Activated protein C resistance* (factor V Leiden carriers)	Cancer
	Postoperative states (stasis)
Antithrombin III deficiency[†]	Lupus anticoagulant syndrome
Protein-C deficiency[†]	Increased factor VII and fibrinogen
Protein-S deficiency[†]	
Fibrinolytic abnormalities	Pregnancy
Hypoplasminogenemia	Nephrotic syndrome
Dysplasminogenemia	Myeloproliferative disorders
tPA release deficiency	Disseminated intravascular coagulation
Increased tPA inhibitor	
Dysfibrinogenemia	Acute stroke
Homocystinuria	Hyperlipidemias
Heparin cofactor deficiency	Diabetes mellitus
Increased histidine-rich glycoprotein	Paroxysmal nocturnal hemoglobinuria
	Behcet disease and vasculitides
	Anticancer drugs (chemotherapy)
	Heparin-induced thrombocytopenia
	Oral contraceptives
	Obesity

tPA, tissue plasminogen activator.

*Prevalence of factor V Leiden in patients with DVT is 16%; presence of V Leiden is associated with a 40% risk of recurrent DVT (*N Engl J Med* 336:399-403, 1997).

[†]Prevalence of these protein deficiencies in patients with DVT is 5% to 10%.

Modified from *Ann Intern Med* 119:819-827, 1993. By permission of the American College of Physicians.

extremities, DVT is detected in only 40% of cases of PE, and even among patients with fatal PE, DVT has been identified clinically in only about 50%. Most patients with PE have lower extremity DVT that is asymptomatic. Approximately 45% of femoral and iliac DVTs embolize to the lungs. Other sources of pulmonary emboli include thrombi from the upper extremities, right ventricle, and indwelling catheters.

- 20% of calf-only DVTs propagate to the thigh and iliac veins.
- 10% of cases of superficial thrombophlebitis are complicated by DVT.

- Varicose veins do not increase the risk of developing DVT.
- Leiden factor V mutation is associated with increased risk of thromboembolic disease in men older than 60 years.
- Approximately 45% of femoral and iliac DVTs embolize to the lungs.

Upper Limb DVT

Upper extremity DVT should also be considered when the source of PE is not identified. Central venous catheters, thrombophilic states, and a previous leg vein thrombosis are statistically associated with upper extremity DVT. PE occurs in 36% of patients with upper limb DVT. DVT of the upper extremity is associated with higher morbidity and mortality than DVT of the lower extremity.

Incidence of DVT With Specific Conditions

The incidence of DVT without prophylaxis in various clinical circumstances is as follows: major abdominal surgery, 14% to 33%; thoracic surgery, 25% to 60%; post-myocardial infarction, 20% to 40%; congestive heart failure, 70%; stroke with paralysis, 50% to 70%; postpartum, 3%; and trauma, 20% to 40%. The risks of DVT in other surgical patients who do not receive prophylaxis are listed in Table 2.

Carcinoma and DVT

Idiopathic DVT, particularly when recurrent, may indicate the presence of neoplasm in 10% to 20% of patients. The risk of diagnosis of cancer is significantly increased only during the first 6 months after the diagnosis of DVT or PE. The occurrence of thromboembolism in patients with cancer portends a poor prognosis. Among those with a diagnosis of cancer within 1 year after thromboembolism, 40% will have distant metastases at the time of the diagnosis of cancer.

- DVT is detected in only 40% of all cases of PE.
- Most patients with PE have DVT of the lower extremities.
- Idiopathic DVT, when recurrent, may indicate neoplasm in up to 20% of patients.
- Risk of DVT: thoracic surgery, 25%-60%; hip surgery, 50%-75%; post-myocardial infarction, 20%-40%; congestive heart failure, 70%; and stroke with paralysis, 50%-70%.

Table 2.—Deep Vein Thrombosis (DVT) Risk Without Prophylaxis in Surgical Patients

Type of surgery	Specific factors	Risk of DVT, %
General	Age > 40 yr	16-42
	Age > 60 yr	46-61
	Cancer resection	40-59
Gynecologic	Procedure duration < 30 min, age < 40 yr, benign disease	< 3
	Minor procedure, age 40-70 yr	10
	Major procedure, age 40-70 yr	0-40
	Cancer resection	35
Urologic	Open prostatectomy	28-42
	TURP	10
	Other procedures	31-58
Neurologic	Craniotomy	18-40
	Laminectomy	4-25
Orthopedic	Total hip arthroplasty	40-78
	Hip fracture	48-75
	Tibial fracture	45
	Knee procedure	57

TURP, transurethral resection of the prostate.

From *J Crit Illness* 13:486-499, 1998. By permission of Cliggott Publishing Company.

Diagnosis of DVT

DVT is diagnosed in only 50% of clinical cases. A diagnosis based on physical examination alone is unreliable.

Homans Sign

Homans sign (pain and tenderness on dorsiflexion of the ankle) is a poor physical sign for the diagnosis of DVT and is elicited in fewer than 40% of patients with proven DVT. A false-positive Homans sign occurs in 30% of high-risk patients.

Noninvasive Investigations

Impedance plethysmography (IPG) and duplex ultrasonography together are the most commonly used noninvasive tests and have a diagnostic accuracy of 90% to 95% in detecting iliac and femoral DVTs. Their accuracy in the diagnosis of calf vein thrombosis is unreliable. Serial (daily) IPG and/or duplex ultrasonography is recommended for high-risk patients because of a 15% detection rate of DVT after an initial negative study. It is safe to withhold anticoagulation if the results of simplified compression ultrasonography are normal at presentation and on a repeated test 5 to 7 days later.

Invasive Venography

Invasive venography is the best diagnostic test for DVT. In patients in whom recurrent DVT is suspected, venography may help differentiate a new thrombosis from an old one. Algorithmic approaches to the diagnosis of initial and recurrent DVTs are shown in Figures 1 and 2.

- DVT is diagnosed clinically in only 50% of cases.
- Impedance plethysmography plus ultrasonography are up to 95% accurate for detection of iliac and femoral DVT.
- Serial venous studies are important in high-risk chronically hospitalized patients.

Clinical Features

Tachypnea and tachycardia are observed in nearly all patients with PE. Other common (> 75% of patients) symptoms include dyspnea and/or pleuritic pain. Less common symptoms (< 25% of patients) are hemoptysis, pleural friction rub, and wheezing. The differential diagnosis of PE includes myocardial infarction, pneumonia, congestive cardiac failure, pericarditis, esophageal spasm, asthma, exacerbation of chronic obstructive lung disease, intrathoracic malignancy, rib fracture, pneumothorax, pleurisy from any cause, pleurodynia, anxiety, and nonspecific skeletal pains. Acute cor pulmonale occurs if more than 65% of the pulmonary circulation is obstructed by emboli.

- Acute cor pulmonale occurs when > 65% of the pulmonary vasculature is obstructed by pulmonary emboli.

Diagnostic Tests

Clinical examination, ECG, chest radiography, blood gas abnormalities, and increased plasma D-dimer values, although helpful, have low specificity and sensitivity for

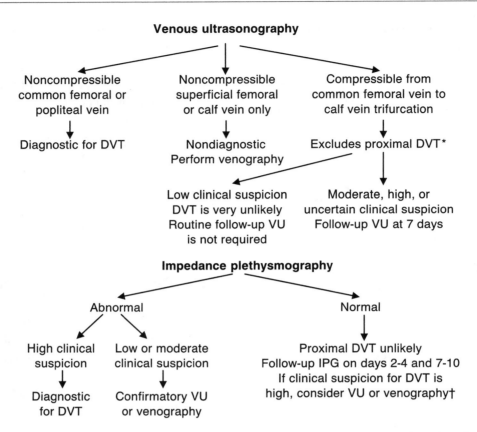

Fig. 1. Approaches to diagnosing a first symptomatic deep vein thrombosis (DVT) with venous ultrasonography (VU) or impedance plethysmography (IPG). *Follow-up venous ultrasonography after 7 days is recommended in all pregnant patients. If clinical suspicion of iliac DVT is high (e.g., if the entire leg is swollen or if the patient has back pain), venography or impedance plethysmography should be done. †In pregnant patients, if symptoms and signs of DVT are confined to below the knee or if intraluminal filling defects are found on limited venography (with abdominal shielding), radiologic examination of the iliac veins is not necessary. (From *Ann Intern Med* 128:663-677, 1998. By permission of the American College of Physicians.)

the diagnosis of PE. Clinical suspicion is the most important factor in steering clinicians toward appropriate tests to diagnose PE.

Chest Radiography in PE
The commonest chest radiographic abnormality in PE is diaphragmatic elevation (about 60% of patients), followed by pulmonary infiltrates in 30%, focal oligemia in 10% to 50%, pleural effusion in 20%, and an enlarged pulmonary artery in 20%. Chest radiographs are normal in 30% of patients with PE.

- Chest radiographs are normal in 30% of patients with PE.

Electrocardiography
The commonest electrocardiographic (ECG) abnormalities in PE are nonspecific changes (noted in 80% of patients), ST and T changes in 65%, S wave in lead I and Q wave in lead III (S_1Q_3) in 15%, right bundle branch

block in 12%, and left axis deviation in 12%. Nonspecific T-wave inversion in the precordial leads is commonly seen and is the ECG sign best correlated with the severity of PE.

- The classic pattern of S wave in lead I and Q wave in lead III (S_1Q_3) is seen in only 15% of patients with PE.
- T-wave inversion in precordial leads is the ECG sign best correlated with the severity of PE.

Arterial Blood Gases
Both the PaO_2 and $P(A-a)O_2$ gradient may be normal in up to 20% of patients with PE. The $(A-a)O_2$ gradient shows a linear correlation with the severity of the PE, but a normal $(A-a)O_2$ does not exclude PE. In the Prospective Investigation of Pulmonary Embolism Diagnosis (PIOPED) study, about 20% of patients with angiographically documented PE had a normal $P(A-a)O_2$ gradient (≤ 20 mm Hg). Most patients with acute PE demonstrate hypocapnia.

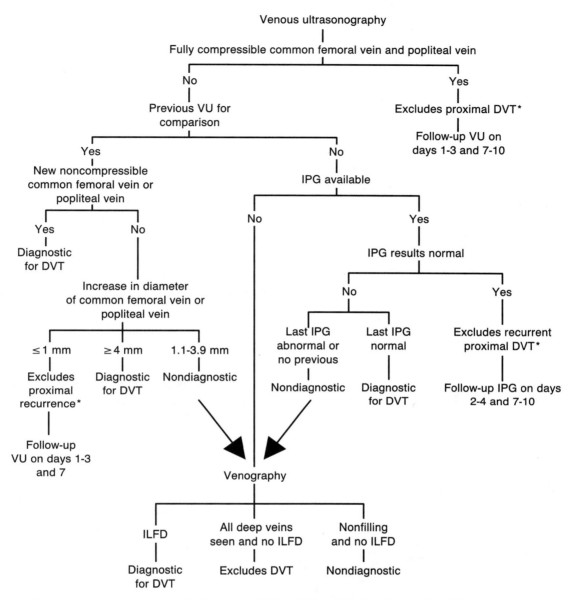

Fig. 2. Approach to the diagnosis of recurrent deep vein thrombosis (DVT). ILFD, intraluminal filling defect; IPG, impedance plethysmography; VU, venous ultrasonography. *If clinical suspicion for DVT is high, venography should be considered. (From *Ann Intern Med* 128:663-677, 1998. By permission of the American College of Physicians.)

- P(A-a)O$_2$ gradient linearly correlates with the severity of PE.
- Of patients with PE, 20% have a normal P(A-a)O$_2$ gradient (≤ 20 mm Hg).

D-Dimer Test

D-Dimer, a specific fibrin degradation product, may be increased in patients with DVT and PE. A high level of D-dimer is a very nonspecific finding and has no positive predictive value for PE. Normal levels of D-dimer alone do not reliably exclude DVT or PE in the absence of imaging studies.

- Normal levels of D-dimer do not reliably exclude DVT or PE in the absence of imaging studies.
- Elevated D-dimer level has no positive predictive value for pulmonary embolism.

Echocardiography

Echocardiography identifies thrombi in the right side of the heart in up to 15% of patients with PE. A mobile right-heart thrombus-in-transit has a 98% risk of acute PE and a 1-week mortality of 50%. In patients with major PE, echocardiographic detection of a patent foramen ovale identifies a high risk of death and arterial thromboembolic complications. Transesophageal echocardiography has a sensitivity of 97% and a specificity of 86% for the diagnosis of centrally located pulmonary arterial thrombi. Echocardiography is also helpful in assessing the presence of secondary pulmonary hypertension caused by recurrent PE.

Ventilation-Perfusion Lung Scan

The ventilation-perfusion (V/Q) lung scan is commonly used in the diagnosis of PE. In patients with proven DVT, many physicians recommend the V/Q lung scan to exclude asymptomatic PE. A high-probability lung scan has a sensitivity of 41% and a specificity of 97%. The likelihood of PE in a scan that shows "high probability" is 90% (Fig. 3).

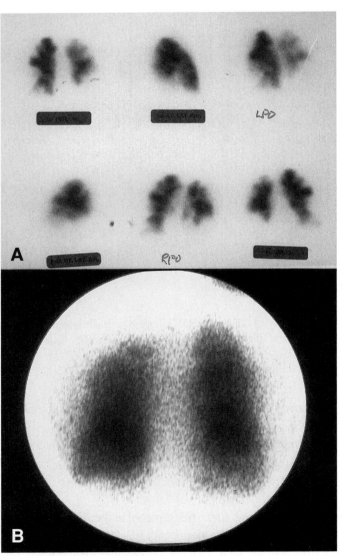

Fig. 3. Ventilation-perfusion scan showing multiple bilateral perfusion defects (*A*) even though the ventilation scan is normal (*B*). This was interpreted as showing a high probability of pulmonary embolism.

A "low-probability" lung scan excludes the diagnosis of PE in more than 85% of patients. A normal lung scan excludes PE in 100%. An "intermediate-" or "indeterminate-probability" scan is associated with pulmonary embolism in 21% to 30% of patients. Therefore, patients with an "intermediate-probability" lung scan usually require pulmonary angiography or other imaging modalities. A negative or normal perfusion-only scan (excluding ventilation scan) rules out PE with a very high probability. Intermediate scans are encountered in 60% of patients with chronic obstructive lung disease. In the PIOPED study, only 41% of patients with angiographically proven PE had a high-probability V/Q scan; therefore, 59% of patients with acute PE had either a low-probability or intermediate-probability scan. Both ventilation and perfusion scans are not necessary in all patients with suspected PE. If the initial perfusion scan is normal, no ventilation scan is needed. The algorithmic approach shown in Figure 4 is recommended to simplify the steps to take after obtaining the results of the V/Q scan.

- High-probability scan = 90% probability of PE.
- Intermediate-probability scan = 30% probability of PE.
- Low-probability scan = 15% probability of PE.
- Normal scan excludes PE in 100% of patients.

Ultrafast Computed Tomography

Computed tomography (CT) permits ultrafast scanning of pulmonary arteries during the injection of contrast material into peripheral veins. The overall sensitivity and specificity of CT in the diagnosis of PE in the central pulmonary arteries (main through segmental) are 94% and 94%, respectively (Fig. 5 and 6). The sensitivity is low (13%) for the detection of PE in the subsegmental pulmonary arteries. Overall, CT is better than the V/Q scan in the diagnosis of PE.

- A normal contrast-enhanced CT does not exclude distal PE, particularly in subsegmental arteries.

Magnetic Resonance Imaging

The role of magnetic resonance imaging (MRI) in the diagnosis of DVT and PE is undergoing validation. MRI has shown a sensitivity of 100% and a specificity of 95% for detecting DVT of pelvic and thigh veins and 85% and 98%, respectively, in the calf veins.

Pulmonary Angiography

Invasive pulmonary angiography is the best diagnostic test (Fig. 7). It should be performed within 24 to 48 hours if

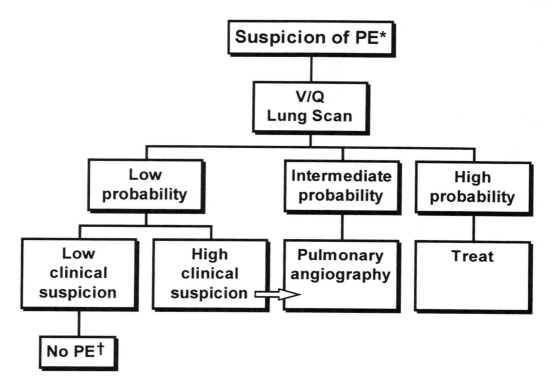

Fig. 4. Diagnostic and therapeutic approach after obtaining the ventilation-perfusion (V/Q) lung scan in patient suspected to have pulmonary embolism (PE). *As soon as the suspicion of PE is aroused, heparin bolus is administered, unless contraindicated, before diagnostic studies are performed, including blood gas analysis, chest radiography, electrocardiography, and V/Q scan. †Continued follow-up is necessary and serial impedance plethysmography with duplex ultrasonography of the lower extremities may be required if the patient is at high risk for development of deep vein thrombosis of the lower extremities. Active anticoagulation with heparin or warfarin is not a contraindication to pulmonary angiography.

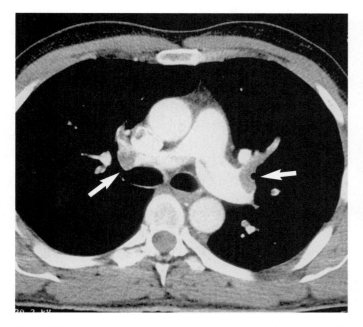

Fig. 5. Ultrafast computed tomography showing large pulmonary emboli occluding major pulmonary arteries bilaterally (*arrows*).

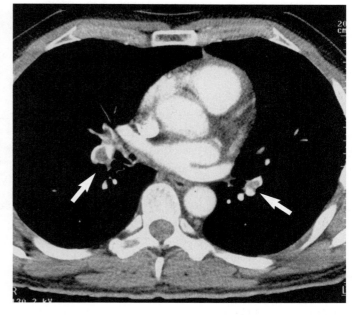

Fig. 6. Ultrafast computed tomography showing occlusion of the lobar and segmental pulmonary arteries bilaterally (*arrows*).

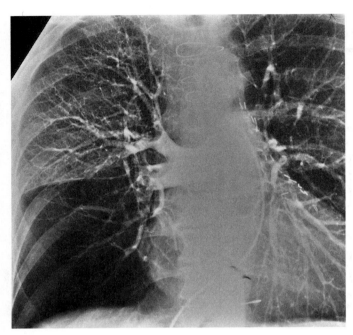

Fig. 7. Pulmonary angiogram showing almost total occlusion of the pulmonary arteries to the right middle and lower lobes.

the diagnosis is considered. False-negative results are observed in 1% to 2% of pulmonary angiographic studies.

- Major and minor complications from pulmonary angiography = 1% and 2%; mortality = 0.5%.
- Pulmonary angiography followed by therapy with tPA is associated with a 14% risk of major hemorrhage.

Treatment of Pulmonary Embolus

The treatment for uncomplicated PE is the same as that for DVT and is described below. For acute disease, treatment with heparin and warfarin can be initiated simultaneously unless warfarin is otherwise contraindicated. An overlap period of 4 or 5 days is recommended. Heparin (80 U/kg) is administered as a bolus, followed by a maintenance dose of 18 U/kg per hour intravenously. The dose should be adjusted to maintain an activated partial thromboplastin time (aPTT) greater than 1.5 times the control value. Low-molecular-weight heparin at home has been shown to be as effective as unfractionated heparin in the hospital for the treatment of DVT. It should be noted, however, that in the U.S., low-molecular-weight heparin has not been approved (as of 1999) for outpatient or inpatient treatment of DVT or PE.

- In acute DVT and PE, treatment with heparin and warfarin

can be initiated simultaneously.

- Heparin dose: bolus = 80 U/kg; maintenance = 18 U/kg per hour.

Long-term anticoagulant therapy can be maintained with either heparin or warfarin. Heparin is indicated when warfarin is contraindicated. The usual dose of heparin is 5,000 to 10,000 U subcutaneously twice daily. However, the dose should be adjusted on the basis of aPTT. Weight-based heparin dosage is not reliable for maintenance therapy by the subcutaneous route. Low-molecular-weight heparin, 30 mg twice daily subcutaneously, has been used in patients with difficulty in monitoring aPTT. A study comparing 510 patients with symptomatic DVT assigned to low-molecular-weight heparin therapy (fixed-dose subcutaneously) to 511 patients with symptomatic DVT assigned to unfractionated heparin therapy (adjusted-dose subcutaneously) observed recurrent DVT in 5.3% of the former group and 4.9% (not significant) in the latter. The risk of major hemorrhage was 3.1% versus 2.3% (not significant). Furthermore, low-molecular-weight heparin has been shown to be as effective and safe as unfractionated heparin in the treatment of acute PE without increasing the risk of major bleeding.

Warfarin is recommended at a dosage to achieve an International Normalized Ratio (INR) of 2 to 3.

- aPTT in uncomplicated cases, 1.5 to 2.0 times control value.
- INR in uncomplicated cases of PE, 2-3.

Most studies indicate that uncomplicated DVT and PE should be treated with anticoagulants for 6 months. Recurrent and complicated cases (coagulopathies, etc.) may require lifelong anticoagulation, maintenance of higher aPTT or PT levels, and other measures such as plication of the inferior vena cava. A study reported that among 111 patients randomly selected to receive only 6 months of warfarin after a second episode of either DVT or PE, 21% developed recurrent DVT or PE. In contrast, a recurrence rate of 2.6% was noted among 116 patients who received therapy indefinitely for a second episode of either DVT or PE.

- Recurrence of DVT or PE after 6 months of therapy, 9.5%.
- Recurrence of DVT or PE after 6 weeks of therapy, 18%.
- 6 months of warfarin after a second episode of DVT or PE, 21% recurrence.
- Warfarin indefinitely after a second episode of DVT or PE, 2.6% recurrence.

Thrombolysis

Thrombolytic agents (streptokinase, urokinase, and tPA) are used to treat massive PE and massive iliofemoral thrombosis. Several studies have shown the superiority of thrombolytic agents over heparin in the treatment of PE (Table 3). The 1-year mortality among those treated with anticoagulation alone and those treated with thrombolytic agents was 19% and 9%, respectively, in the PIOPED study. Some physicians recommend venography (for DVT) or pulmonary angiography (for PE) before therapy with thrombolytic agents. However, in patients with high-probability V/Q scans, the likelihood of PE is 96%; therefore, pulmonary angiography is not absolutely necessary.

In patients who have pulmonary angiography before receiving tPA, the risk for major bleeding is 14%, in comparison with 4% for those receiving tPA after a noninvasive diagnostic procedure. Ideally, thrombolytic agents are administered within 24 hours after PE. Dosages for different agents are as follows: streptokinase, loading dose of 250,000 IU infused over 30 minutes, followed by maintenance dose of 100,000 U/hr for up to 24 hours; urokinase, loading dose of 4,400 IU/kg, infused over 10 minutes, followed by continuous infusion of 4,400 IU/kg per hour for 12 to 24 hours; and tPA, a total dose of 100 mg intravenously over a 2-hour period. Heparin infusion is begun or resumed if aPTT is less than 80 seconds after thrombolytic therapy. The contraindications to thrombolytic therapy are listed in Table 4.

- Thrombolytic agents should be given within 24 hours after PE.

Table 3.—Complications of Heparin Versus Thrombolytic Agents in Acute Pulmonary Embolism (PE): Analysis of Eight Trials

	Heparin (216 patients)	Thrombolytic agents (237 patients)
Overall mortality	13 (6%)	11 (4.6%)*
Fatal hemorrhage	0	4 (1.7%)†
Recurrent PE	24 (11%)	13 (5.5%)†
Death due to recurrent PE	5 (2.3%)	1 (0.4%)†

*$P = 0.11$ (not significant).
†$P < 0.01$.

From *J Respir Dis* 18:474-486, 1997. By permission of Cliggott Publishing Company.

- One-year mortality: anticoagulant alone, 19%; thrombolytic drug, 9%.
- Heparin therapy is necessary following thrombolytic therapy.

Bleeding Complications

Among patients receiving chronic warfarin therapy, the cumulative incidence of fatal bleeding is 1% at 1 year and 2% at 3 years. Presence of malignant disease at initiation of warfarin therapy is significantly associated with major hemorrhage. Among patients with PE treated with thrombolytic agents, the risk of intracranial bleeding is about 1%.

Drugs that prolong the effect of warfarin include salicylate, heparin, estrogen, antibiotics, clofibrate, quinidine, and cimetidine. Drugs that decrease the effect of warfarin include rifampin and barbiturates. This is only a partial list of drugs that interfere with warfarin metabolism.

Inferior Vena Caval Interruption

Inferior vena caval interruption is aimed at preventing PE while maintaining blood flow through the inferior vena cava. Inferior vena caval plication or insertion of a filter into the inferior vena cava is indicated in recurrent DVT in a patient who recently had a massive PE, presence of

Table 4.—Contraindications to Thrombolytic Therapy in Venous Thromboembolism

Absolute
    Intracranial disorders (neoplasms, vascular accidents, hemorrhagic stroke, aneurysm)
    Intracranial or intraspinal surgery or trauma within the preceding 2 months
    Operation, obstetric delivery, or organ biopsy within the preceding 10 days
    Active internal bleeding within the preceding 6 months
    Bleeding diathesis
    Severe hypertension (systolic blood pressure > 200 mm Hg or diastolic blood pressure > 110 mm Hg)
    Recent trauma (including cardiopulmonary resuscitation)
Relative
    Pregnancy
    Infective endocarditis
    Pericarditis
    Diabetic hemorrhagic retinopathy or other hemorrhagic ophthalmic conditions

From *J Respir Dis* 18:474-486, 1997. By permission of Cliggott Publishing Company.

bleeding disorder or other contraindication to anticoagulant therapy, or failure of anticoagulant therapy. The routine use of an inferior vena caval filter in patients with cancer and DVT or PE is not recommended.

Inferior vena caval plication or filter placement does not replace anticoagulant therapy; many patients require both. Anticoagulant therapy after filter insertion is aimed at preventing DVT at the insertion site, inferior vena caval thrombosis, cephalad propagation of clot from an occluded filter, and propagation or recurrent DVTs of the lower extremities. Most inferior vena caval filters are inserted through the internal jugular vein. Five types of filters are available in the U.S.: the Greenfield filter (Fig. 8), titanium Greenfield filter, Simon-Nitinol filter, bird's-nest filter, and LGM or Vena Tech filter, although none is ideal. A review of the literature noted the following indications for the Greenfield filter: complication from or contraindication to anticoagulants in about 60% of patients, failure of anticoagulants in 8%, and prophylaxis or miscellaneous reasons in about 30%.

PE occurs in 2.5% of patients even after insertion of an inferior vena caval filter. The complications of filter insertion include DVT at the insertion site (2%), change in position after insertion (migration, tilting in up to 50%), perforation of the inferior vena cava (15% to 24%, but most are radiologically diagnosed and have no clinical problems), obstruction of the inferior vena cava below the filter (6%), and edema of the lower extremities (5%). Infections from filter insertion are extremely rare. Most complications are clinically insignificant, and the mortality rate from inferior vena caval filters is 0.12%.

- Inferior vena caval plication does not replace chronic anticoagulant therapy.
- Recurrent PE occurs in fewer than 2.5% of patients after filter insertion.
- Inferior vena caval plication does not affect mortality from PE.
- Complications: DVT (2%), migration (50%), perforation of inferior vena cava (24%), and edema of legs (5%).

Prophylaxis of DVT and PE

In 1994, only 52% of high-risk hospitalized patients in the U.S. received adequate prophylaxis against DVT or PE. Prophylaxis includes early ambulation after surgery or immobilization, intermittent pneumatic compression of the lower extremities, active and passive leg exercises, and low-dose heparin subcutaneously (10,000-15,000 U/day). Approaches

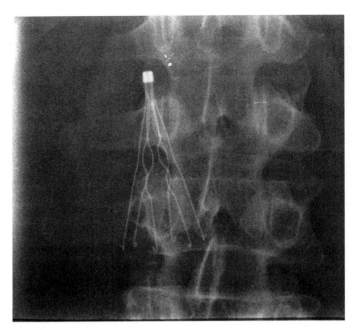

Fig. 8. A properly placed inferior vena caval filter in a patient with recurrent pulmonary emboli and secondary pulmonary hypertension.

to the prevention of DVT are listed in Table 5. Low-dose heparin reduces the incidence of DVT from 25% to 8%. Low-dose heparin is given 5,000 U preoperatively and then every 8 to 12 hours postoperatively. Low-molecular-weight heparin has been approved in the U.S. for prophylaxis against DVT and PE following total hip arthroplasty and total knee arthroplasty. A postoperative, fixed-dose low-molecular-weight heparin (enoxaparin, 30 mg subcutaneously every 12 hours) is more effective than adjusted-dose warfarin (INR 2-3) in preventing DVT after total hip or knee arthroplasty. Low-molecular-weight heparin has a rapid onset of action and may supersede standard heparin in the future. It is safe and approximately 50% more effective than unfractionated (standard) heparin. Because of a more predictable dose response to low-molecular-weight heparin, routine laboratory monitoring of anticoagulation is not needed. The advantages of low-molecular-weight heparin and recommended doses for the prevention and treatment of thromboembolism are shown in Table 6.

- Low-molecular-weight heparin is approved for DVT and PE prophylaxis after total hip arthroplasty.
- Low-molecular-weight heparin therapy does not require aPTT measurement.
- Heparin-induced thrombocytopenia is reduced with low-molecular-weight heparin.

Table 5.—Approaches to the Prevention of Venous Thromboembolism

Condition or procedure	Prophylaxis
General surgery	Unfractionated heparin, 5,000 U 2-3 times daily
	Enoxaparin, 40 mg/day SC
	Dalteparin, 2,500 or 5,000 U/day SC
	Nadroparin, 3,100 U/day SC*
	Tinzaparin, 3,500 U/day SC, with or without graduated-compression stockings*
Total hip replacement	Warfarin (target INR, 2.5)[†]
	Intermittent pneumatic compression
	Enoxaparin, 30 mg SC twice daily[‡]
	Danaparoid, 750 U SC twice daily
Total knee replacement	Enoxaparin, 30 mg SC twice daily[‡]
	Ardeparin, 50 U/kg SC twice daily
Neurosurgery	Graduated-compression stockings and intermittent pneumatic compression, with or without unfractionated heparin, 5,000 U twice daily
Trauma (non-brain)	Enoxaparin, 30 mg SC twice daily
Thoracic surgery	Graduated-compression stockings, intermittent pneumatic compression, and unfractionated heparin, 5,000 U 3 times daily
Uncomplicated coronary artery bypass grafting	Graduated-compression stockings, with or without unfractionated heparin, 5,000 U 2-3 times daily
General medical condition requiring hospitalization	Graduated-compression stockings, intermittent pneumatic compression, or unfractionated heparin, 5,000 U 2-3 times daily
Condition requiring hospitalization in the intensive care unit	Graduated-compression stockings and intermittent pneumatic compression, with or without unfractionated heparin, 5,000 U 2-3 times daily
Pregnancy[§]	Dalteparin, 5,000 U/day SC
	Enoxaparin, 40 mg/day SC

INR, International Normalized Ratio; SC, subcutaneously.

*This drug has not been approved for use by the Food and Drug Administration.

[†]Warfarin is started the night before surgery, usually in a dose of 5 mg.

[‡]In Europe, the customary approach to prophylaxis in patients undergoing joint replacement is to give 40 mg of enoxaparin the night before surgery and then 40 mg once daily thereafter.

[§]Prophylaxis is used in women with a history of idiopathic pulmonary embolism or deep venous thrombosis.

From *N Engl J Med* 339:93-104, 1998. By permission of the Massachusetts Medical Society.

Table 6.—Advantages of Low-Molecular-Weight Heparins and Recommended Doses for the Prevention and Treatment of Thrombosis

Indication	Advantages of low-molecular-weight heparins	Recommended doses*
Prevention		
General surgery	At least as effective as low-dose unfractionated heparin but can be given once daily and cause fewer hematomas at injection sites	Low risk[†]
		Dalteparin, 2,500 U 1-2 hr before surgery and once daily after surgery
		Enoxaparin, 2,000 U 1-2 hr before surgery and once daily after surgery
		Nadroparin, 3,100 U 2 hr before surgery and once daily after surgery
		Tinzaparin, 3,500 U 2 hr before surgery and once daily after surgery
		High risk[‡]
		Dalteparin, 5,000 U 10-12 hr before surgery and once daily after surgery
		Enoxaparin, 4,000 U 10-12 hr before surgery and once daily after surgery

Table 6 (continued)

Indication	Advantages of low-molecular-weight heparins	Recommended doses*
Orthopedic surgery	More effective than low-dose unfractionated heparin; more effective than warfarin in patients undergoing total knee replacement; no monitoring required	Ardeparin, 50 U/kg twice daily starting 12-14 hr after surgery Dalteparin, 5,000 U 8-12 hr before surgery and once daily starting 12 hr after surgery Enoxaparin, 3,000 U twice daily starting 12-24 hr after surgery or 4,000 U once daily starting 10-12 hr before surgery Nadroparin, 40 U/kg starting 2 hr before surgery and once daily after surgery for 3 days; the dose is then increased to 60 U/kg once daily Tinzaparin, 50 U/kg 2 hr before surgery and once daily after surgery or 75 U/kg once daily starting 12-24 hr after surgery
Acute spinal injury	Apparently effective, whereas low-dose unfractionated heparin is not, and higher doses of unfractionated heparin cause excessive bleeding	Enoxaparin, 3,000 U twice daily
Multiple trauma	More effective than unfractionated heparin	Enoxaparin, 3,000 U twice daily
Medical conditions	As effective as low-dose unfractionated heparin but can be given once daily	Dalteparin, 2,500 U once daily Enoxaparin, 2,000 U once daily
Treatment		
Venous thrombo-embolism	At least as safe and effective as unfractionated heparin but can be given subcutaneously without laboratory monitoring, thereby allowing out-of-hospital treatment	Dalteparin, 100 U/kg twice daily Enoxaparin, 100 U/kg twice daily Nadroparin, 90 U/kg twice daily Tinzaparin, 175 U/kg once daily
Unstable angina	At least as effective as unfractionated heparin but can be given subcutaneously without monitoring	Dalteparin, 100 U/kg twice daily Enoxaparin, 100 U/kg twice daily

*Doses are shown in anti-factor Xa units. Low-molecular-weight heparins are given subcutaneously for both prophylaxis and treatment. The prophylactic doses recommended for each low-molecular-weight heparin preparation are slightly different, but a common rationale underlies these regimens. Lower doses are used for low-risk general surgical or medical patients, whereas higher doses are used for high-risk general surgical or orthopedic surgical patients. When relatively large doses of low-molecular-weight heparins are started preoperatively, the dose is given 10 to 12 hours before surgery, to avoid excessive intra-operative bleeding. Lower doses of low-molecular-weight heparins can be given 1 to 2 hours before surgery. The doses used for the treatment of venous thromboembolism or for unstable angina are higher than those used for prophylaxis, and similar regimens are used for each of the low-molecular-weight heparins.

†Low-risk general surgical patients are those undergoing uncomplicated abdominal or pelvic surgery lasting 30 minutes or more.

‡High-risk general surgical patients are those undergoing abdominal or pelvic surgery for cancer or those with previous venous thromboembolism.

From *N Engl J Med* 337:688-698, 1997. By permission of the Massachusetts Medical Society.

Complications of Pulmonary Embolism

Pulmonary infarction occurs in fewer than 10% of patients with PE. Pulmonary infarction and hemorrhage occur more frequently in patients with disseminated intravascular coagulation. Complications of pulmonary infarction include secondary infection, cavitation, pneumothorax, and hemothorax. Recurrent PE is a common cause of secondary pulmonary hypertension. Mechanical obstruction of one-half to two-thirds of the pulmonary vascular bed by emboli is necessary for this complication to develop (see below).

- Pulmonary infarction occurs in < 10% of patients with PE.
- PIOPED study: recurrent pulmonary embolism in 8% of patients.
- Secondary pulmonary hypertension occurs in 0.5%.

Special Forms of Embolism

Recurrent Pulmonary Embolism
Chronic thromboembolic pulmonary hypertension (CTEPH) develops in 0.1% to 0.5% of patients (or 500 to 2,500 patients in the U.S.) with PE. Many patients with the initial diagnosis of primary pulmonary hypertension are subsequently found to have CTEPH. The underlying causes for the development of recurrent PE are the same as those for acute PE. CTEPH develops in some patients even though the occurrence of recurrent PE cannot be documented. Multiple PEs may not be the cause of CTEPH in some patients. Chronic recurrent in situ thrombosis initiated by the first PE may be responsible for these cases.

Fewer than 50% of patients have a history compatible with a previous episode of DVT or PE. Lupus anticoagulant is present in about 10% of patients with CTEPH, and 1% have deficiencies of either antithrombin III, protein C, or protein S. CTEPH develops in many patients without underlying coagulopathy because of either a delayed or missed diagnosis of PE or inadequate anticoagulation for previously documented DVT or PE. Lung biopsy specimens from patients with CTEPH show plexiform lesions, suggesting that factors other than obstructive PE may have a role in the onset of CTEPH. Indeed, the degree of angiographic obstruction correlates poorly with the degree of pulmonary hypertension.

- Recurrent PE leads to development of CTEPH in up to 0.5% of patients.
- Plexiform lesions occur in CTEPH.

- Lupus anticoagulant is present in 10% of patients with CTEPH.
- Antithrombin-III, protein-C, or protein-S deficiencies occur in about 1% of patients with CTEPH.

Clinically, many patients remain asymptomatic ("honeymoon period") despite extensive PE. When symptoms develop, they are similar to those of primary pulmonary hypertension. Clinical findings may include the presence of low-pitched flow murmurs or bruit, systolic or diastolic, in areas of partial stenosis caused by intra-arterial clots and fibrotic bands; these flow murmurs/bruits are present in 20% of patients. Usually, chest radiographic findings are unremarkable. The diffusing capacity of the lung for carbon monoxide is either normal (in many patients) or reduced (in a small proportion); a normal value does not exclude CTEPH. A mild-to-moderate restrictive defect is noted in 20% of patients. $P(\text{A-a})\text{O}_2$ is usually widened and PaO_2 decreases with exercise in most patients. In almost all patients with CTEPH, at least one segmental or larger perfusion defect (with corresponding ventilation mismatch) is observed. However, the V/Q scan underestimates the extent of central pulmonary vascular obstruction.

- Honeymoon (asymptomatic) period despite extensive PE in many patients.
- Low-pitched flow murmurs or bruit, systolic or diastolic, over lung fields in 20% of patients.
- Diffusing capacity of the lung for carbon monoxide: either normal or reduced (in a few); a normal value does not exclude CTEPH.
- Mild-to-moderate restrictive pulmonary dysfunction in 20% of patients.

Pulmonary thromboendarterectomy (PTEA) may be used to treat CTEPH, with an overall mortality of about 10% and perioperative mortality of 5%. An atrial septal defect or patent foramen ovale is encountered in about 25% of patients undergoing PTEA. Selection criteria for PTEA include thrombi accessible to a surgical approach, pulmonary vascular resistance (PVR) greater than 300 dynes/s/cm^{-5}, and absence of significant coexisting disease. Complications of PTEA include reperfusion pulmonary edema, aortic dissection, cerebrovascular accident, and mediastinal hemorrhage. Symptomatic improvement may occur over a period of up to 12 months. Long-term anticoagulation and inferior vena caval filter placement are indicated in all patients who undergo PTEA.

- PTEA: overall mortality, 10%; perioperative mortality, 5%.
- PTEA selection criteria: thrombi accessible to PTEA, PVR > 300 dynes/s/cm^{-5}, and absence of coexisting disease.
- Atrial septal defect or patent foramen ovale is detected in 25% of patients undergoing PTEA.
- Life-long anticoagulation is indicated after PTEA.

Massive PE

In most patients, the degree of hypoxia and its acuteness and effect on hemodynamics as well as the underlying cardiopulmonary disease determine the "massive" nature, rather than the volume of emboli that occlude the pulmonary vasculature (Fig. 9). Massive PE is associated with mortality rates estimated at 10% within 1 hour after the occurrence of PE and 85% in the first 6 hours. The sudden onset of severe dyspnea, syncope, and hemodynamic collapse and clinical detection of acute right ventricular failure (increased jugular venous pressure, right-sided S$_3$, parasternal lift or heave) and hypoxia in a high-risk patient should suggest the possibility. Massive PE may acutely increase right atrial pressure and open a patent foramen ovale, with a resultant right-to-left shunt and worsening hypoxia. A more serious complication is paradoxic embolization into the systemic circulation. Chest radiography may demonstrate acute oligemia. Electrocardiograms are more likely to exhibit S$_1$Q$_3$ and new incomplete right bundle branch block in massive PE than in nonmassive PE. The diagnostic and therapeutic approaches are similar to those in nonmassive PE, but thrombolytic therapy is more important in this group of patients. Acute pulmonary embolectomy is seldom required. Hemodynamic stabilization, oxygenation, and close follow-up in the intensive care unit are indicated.

- Mortality in massive pulmonary embolism: 10% within 1 hour, 85% within 6 hours.
- Important signs of massive pulmonary embolism: sudden dyspnea, syncope, shock, and acute right ventricular failure.

Sickle-Cell Disease

Pulmonary vascular occlusion is a serious complication in sickle-cell disease, sickle-cell-hemoglobin C disease, and S-β-thalassemia. Pulmonary vascular occlusion or embolism is the result of in situ thrombosis occurring in small pulmonary arterioles and is the consequence of sludging of misshapen and

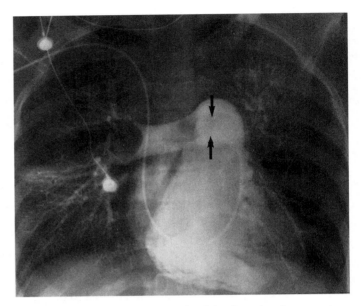

Fig. 9. Massive pulmonary embolism involving the main pulmonary artery (*arrows*). Reduced perfusion of contrast agent into the right upper lobe arteries is evident.

distorted erythrocytes following deoxygenation-induced polymerization. Pulmonary vascular occlusion is uncommon in children, but it seems to occur more frequently in the later stages of pregnancy in women with sickle-cell disease and hemoglobin C disease. Therapy includes supplemental oxygen, antibiotics (for infection), and hydroxyurea. Chronic anticoagulant therapy does not seem to have any benefit.

- The regular type of PE *does not* occur with increasing frequency in sickle-cell disease.
- Pulmonary vascular occlusion occurs because of in situ thrombosis in pulmonary arterioles.
- Pulmonary vascular occlusion results from sludging of misshapen and distorted erythrocytes.
- Differentiating pulmonary vascular occlusion from acute chest syndrome can be difficult.

Air Embolism

Small amounts of air that enter the venous system are usually absorbed and produce no clinical problems. Significant air embolism has been observed after injury or procedures in the head and neck area, thoracic cage, cardiothoracic bypass, introduction of catheters and needles in the neck veins, acute decompression sickness, and procedures requiring air insufflation. Massive air embolism may lead to life-threatening acute pulmonary hypertension and death. The frothy air-blood mixture, churned in the chambers on the right side of the heart, cannot navigate the pulmonary capillary network, and when it reaches the capillary network, it induces hypoxia. Therapeutic measures include immediately placing the patient in the left lateral decubitus position (to prevent air entrance into the pulmonary arteries) and hyperbaric oxygen therapy.

- Massive air embolism may lead to acute pulmonary hypertension and death.

Paradoxic Embolism

Parodoxic embolism is venous thrombosis that causes systemic embolization through a right-to-left shunt. The presence of a right-to-left shunt, either intracardiac or extracardiac, is necessary for paradoxic embolism to occur. A patent foramen ovale occurs in about 30% of the normal population but is not suspected clinically in most of the patients. In a review of patients with a patent foramen ovale and arterial occlusion, two-thirds had DVT, and of these, two-thirds of the DVTs were silent.

- Venous-to-arterial embolization through a right-to-left shunt.
- Paradoxic embolism does not cause PE but may result from it.

Hereditary Hemorrhagic Telangiectasia (Osler-Weber-Rendu Disease)

This is an important cause of paradoxic embolism that occurs via the intrapulmonary right-to-left shunt caused by pulmonary arteriovenous malformation or fistula. It is an autosomal dominantly inherited disorder characterized by telangiectasia of the skin and mucous membranes and intermittent bleeding from vascular abnormalities. Hereditary hemorrhagic telangiectasia is the most common cause of pulmonary arteriovenous malformation, and 20% of the patients with the disorder have pulmonary lesions. Most of the pulmonary arteriovenous malformations are located in the lower lobes and are multiple in 30% of patients. Brain and systemic abscesses as a result of paradoxic embolism are serious complications. Neurologic complications are seen in 30% of patients, and brain abscess develops in 1%. Pulmonary angiographic examination is necessary to confirm the diagnosis in virtually all patients.

- Hereditary hemorrhagic telangiectasia: paradoxic embolism occurs commonly.
- Neurologic complications in 30% of patients and brain abscess in 1%.
- Brain abscess can be the initial manifestation in hereditary hemorrhagic telangiectasia.
- Almost all pulmonary arteriovenous malformations should be treated.
- Pulmonary embolotherapy is the initial treatment of choice.

Suggested Review Reading

1. ACCP Consensus Committee on Pulmonary Embolism: Opinions regarding the diagnosis and management of venous thromboembolic disease. *Chest* 113:499-504, 1998.
This consensus report addresses clinically relevant questions on the diagnosis and treatment of deep vein thrombosis and pulmonary embolism. The statement is based on information from the literature.

2. Alley MT, Shifrin RY, Pelc NJ, et al: Ultrafast contrast-enhanced three-dimensional MR angiography: state of the art. *Radiographics* 18:273-285, 1998.
A state-of-the-art review on the role of ultrafast breath-hold contrast material-enhanced three-dimensional magnetic resonance (MR) angiography in the diagnosis of pulmonary embolism and other structures and diseases.

3. Bassiri AG, Haghighi B, Doyle RL, et al: Pulmonary tumor embolism. *Am J Respir Crit Care Med* 155:2089-2095, 1997.
A review of the topic provides detailed information on pathologic and clinical manifestations and the diagnostic approach to patients with tumor emboli involving pulmonary arteries.

4. Birdwell BG, Raskob GE, Whitsett TL, et al: The clinical validity of normal compression ultrasonography in outpatients suspected of having deep venous thrombosis. *Ann Intern Med* 128:1-7, 1998.

A study of 405 consecutive outpatients suspected of having a first episode of deep venous thrombosis observed that it is safe to withhold anticoagulation if the results of simplified compression ultrasonography are normal at presentation and on a single repeated test done 5 to 7 days later.

5. The Columbus Investigators: Low-molecular-weight heparin in the treatment of patients with venous thromboembolism. *N Engl J Med* 337:657-662, 1997.

A comparison study of 510 patients with symptomatic deep vein thrombosis assigned to low-molecular-weight heparin therapy (fixed-dose subcutaneously) and 511 patients with symptomatic deep vein thrombosis assigned to unfractionated heparin therapy (adjusted-dose subcutaneously) observed recurrent deep vein thrombosis in 5.3% and 4.9% (not significant), respectively.

6. Decousus H, Leizorovicz A, Parent F, et al: A clinical trial of vena caval filters in the prevention of pulmonary embolism in patients with proximal deep-vein thrombosis. *N Engl J Med* 338:409-415, 1998.

A study of 400 patients with proximal deep vein thrombosis who were at risk for pulmonary embolism observed that the initial beneficial effect of vena caval filters for the prevention of pulmonary embolism was counterbalanced by an excess of recurrent deep vein thrombosis, without any difference in mortality.

7. Douketis JD, Ginsberg JS, Holbrook A, et al: A reevaluation of the risk for venous thromboembolism with the use of oral contraceptives and hormone replacement therapy. *Arch Intern Med* 157:1522-1530, 1997.

A literature search led the authors to estimate that users of non-third-generation oral contraceptives have a less than 3-fold increase in the risk for venous thromboembolism compared with nonusers and that the risk for venous thromboembolism is possibly higher with the use of third-generation oral contraceptives.

8. Douketis JD, Kearon C, Bates S, et al: Risk of fatal pulmonary embolism in patients with treated venous thromboembolism. *JAMA* 279:458-462, 1998.

A literature review of 25 studies in which patients with symptomatic deep vein thrombosis (DVT) or pulmonary embolism (PE) were treated 5 to 10 days with heparin and 3 months with oral anticoagulants (1966-1997) showed that among patients with DVT, the rate of fatal PE during anticoagulant therapy was 0.4%; following anticoagulant therapy, it was 0.3 per 100 patient-years. The case-fatality rate of recurrent DVT or PE during anticoagulant therapy was 8.8%; following anticoagulant therapy, it was 5.1%. Among patients with PE, the rate of fatal PE during anticoagulant therapy was 1.5%; following anticoagulant therapy, it was 0 per 265 patient-years. The case-fatality rate of recurrent DVT or PE among patients presenting with PE was 26.4%.

9. Fennerty T: The diagnosis of pulmonary embolism. *BMJ* 314:425-429, 1997.

A review of clinical, diagnostic, and therapeutic aspects of pulmonary embolism.

10. Ferrari E, Imberg A, Chevalier T, et al: The ECG in pulmonary embolism. Predictive value of negative T waves in precordial leads—80 case reports. *Chest* 111:537-543, 1997.

A study of 80 consecutive patients hospitalized for pulmonary embolism observed that T-wave inversion in the precordial leads was the most common abnormality (68%) and represented the ECG sign best correlated to the severity of the pulmonary embolism. The subepicardial ischemic pattern was an even stronger marker of severity when it appeared as early as the first day, and its reversibility before the sixth day indicated a good outcome or high level of therapeutic efficacy.

11. Geerts WH, Jay RM, Code KI, et al: A comparison of low-dose heparin with low-molecular-weight heparin as prophylaxis against venous thromboembolism after major trauma. *N Engl J Med* 335:701-707, 1996.

This study compared low-dose heparin (136 patients) and a low-molecular-weight heparin (129 patients) in a randomized clinical trial in 344 patients with trauma. Among those who received low-dose heparin, 60 (44%) developed deep vein thrombosis. Among those who received enoxaparin, 40 (31%) had deep vein thrombosis. The authors concluded that low-molecular-weight heparin was more effective than low-dose heparin in preventing venous thromboembolism after major trauma.

12. Ginsberg JS: Management of venous thromboembolism. *N Engl J Med* 335:1816-1828, 1996.

A review of the various aspects of management of venous thromboembolism.

13. Goldhaber SZ: Contemporary pulmonary embolism thrombolysis. *Chest* 107 (Suppl 1):45S-51S, 1995. *Discussion of thrombolytic therapy in pulmonary embolism. The author indicates that the current (1995) estimate is that no more than 10% of patients with pulmonary embolism receive thrombolysis in the United States. The author concludes that thrombolysis can be applied with a 2-week "time window," without mandatory angiography in many cases, via a brief infusion through a peripheral vein, and without special laboratory tests.*

14. Goldhaber SZ: Pulmonary embolism. *N Engl J Med* 339:93-104, 1998.
A state-of-the-art review of pulmonary embolism, with 139 references.

15. Goldhaber SZ, Grodstein F, Stampfer MJ, et al: A prospective study of risk factors for pulmonary embolism in women. *JAMA* 277:642-645, 1997.
A prospective study of a group of 112,822 women aged 30 to 55 years with 1,619,770 person-years of follow-up documented 280 cases of pulmonary embolism, of which 125 were primary. Obesity, cigarette smoking, and hypertension were independent predictors of pulmonary embolism. The relative risk of primary pulmonary embolism was 1.9 for women currently smoking 25 to 34 cigarettes per day and 3.3 for those smoking 35 cigarettes or more daily as compared with "never smokers." High serum levels of cholesterol and diabetes did not appear to be related to primary pulmonary embolism.

16. Hingorani A, Ascher E, Hanson J, et al: Upper extremity versus lower extremity deep venous thrombosis. *Am J Surg* 174:214-217, 1997.
A review of records of patients with deep venous thrombosis of the upper extremity and lower extremity observed pulmonary embolism in 17% of the former and 8% of the latter group. The 6-month mortality in the former group was 48% compared with 13% mortality in the latter. The authors concluded that deep venous thrombosis of the upper extremity is associated with a higher morbidity and mortality than deep venous thrombosis of the lower extremities.

17. Kanter DS, Mikkola KM, Patel SR, et al: Thrombolytic therapy for pulmonary embolism. Frequency of intracranial hemorrhage and associated risk factors. *Chest* 111:1241-1245, 1997.
Analysis of data from 312 patients from five previously reported studies of pulmonary embolism thrombolysis noted that intracranial hemorrhage (up to 14 days after pulmonary embolism thrombolysis) occurred in six (1.9%) patients; two of six intracranial hemorrhages were fatal.

18. Kasper W, Konstantinides S, Geibel A, et al: Management strategies and determinants of outcome in acute major pulmonary embolism: results of a multicenter registry. *J Am Coll Cardiol* 30:1165-1171, 1997.
Multicenter (204) study of 1,001 consecutive patients observed that echocardiography was the most frequently performed diagnostic procedure (74%), and lung scan or pulmonary angiography was performed in 79% of clinically stable patients but in only 32% of those with circulatory collapse at presentation. Thrombolytics were given to 48% of patients despite the presence of contraindications in 40%. In-hospital mortality was 8.1% among the stable patients, 25% among those with cardiogenic shock, and 65% among patients requiring cardiopulmonary resuscitation. Major bleeding was reported in 9.2% of patients; cerebral bleeding was uncommon (0.5%). Recurrent pulmonary embolism occurred in 17%.

19. Kearon C, Hirsh J: Management of anticoagulation before and after elective surgery. *N Engl J Med* 336:1506-1511, 1997.
A review of the management of patients who require anticoagulation before and after elective surgical procedures.

20. Kearon C, Julian JA, Newman TE, et al: Noninvasive diagnosis of deep venous thrombosis. McMaster Diagnostic Imaging Practice Guidelines Initiative. *Ann Intern Med* 128:663-677, 1998.
A detailed review of various noninvasive diagnostic methods used in deep vein thrombosis. The information gathered was based on a literature review of pertinent studies.

21. Konstantinides S, Geibel A, Kasper W, et al: Patent foramen ovale is an important predictor of adverse outcome in patients with major pulmonary embolism. *Circulation* 97:1946-1951, 1998.
This prospective study of 139 consecutive patients with major pulmonary embolism used contrast echocardiography and diagnosed patent foramen ovale in 48 patients (35%). These patients had a death rate of 33% as opposed to 14% in patients with a negative echo-contrast examination (P = 0.015).

22. Koopman MMW, Prandoni P, Piovella F, et al: Treatment of venous thrombosis with intravenous unfractionated heparin administered in the hospital as compared with subcutaneous low-molecular-weight heparin administered at home. *N Engl J Med* 334:682-687, 1996.

Based on a study of 198 patients assigned to adjusted-dose intravenous standard heparin administered in the hospital and 202 patients assigned to fixed-dose subcutaneous low-molecular-weight heparin administered at home, the authors concluded that in patients with proximal-vein thrombosis, treatment with low-molecular-weight heparin at home is feasible, effective, and safe.

23. Krivec B, Voga G, Zuran I, et al: Diagnosis and treatment of shock due to massive pulmonary embolism: approach with transesophageal echocardiography and intrapulmonary thrombolysis. *Chest* 112:1310-1316, 1997.

Report of 24 patients who were admitted with the diagnosis of massive pulmonary embolism. The authors observed that transesophageal echocardiography had a sensitivity of 92% and a specificity of 100% in the diagnosis of massive pulmonary embolism. They concluded that this test enables physicians to make the diagnosis and to deliver immediate intrapulmonary thrombolytic therapy. An accompanying editorial (Chest 112:1158-1159) provides an overview.

24. Levine M, Gent M, Hirsh J, et al: A comparison of low-molecular-weight heparin administered primarily at home with unfractionated heparin administered in the hospital for proximal deep-vein thrombosis. *N Engl J Med* 334:677-681, 1996.

Based on a study of 253 patients assigned to adjusted-dose intravenous standard heparin administered in the hospital and 247 patients assigned to subcutaneous low-molecular-weight heparin (1 mg/kg twice daily) administered at home, the authors concluded that in patients with proximal-vein thrombosis, low-molecular-weight heparin can be used safely and effectively at home.

25. Litin SC, Heit JA, Mees KA: Use of low-molecular-weight heparin in the treatment of venous thromboembolic disease: answers to frequently asked questions. *Mayo Clin Proc* 73:545-551, 1998.

A concise review provides answers to many frequently asked questions about the role of low-molecular-weight heparin in the treatment of venous thromboembolic diseases.

26. Lualdi JC, Goldhaber SZ: Right ventricular dysfunction after acute pulmonary embolism: pathophysiologic factors, detection, and therapeutic implications. *Am Heart J* 130:1276-1282, 1995.

A review of pathophysiologic changes that occur in the right ventricle after acute pulmonary embolism. The authors conclude that the concept of "hemodynamic instability" after pulmonary embolism should be expanded to include right ventricular dilatation and wall motion abnormalities, even among normotensive patients.

27. Manganelli D, Palla A, Donnamaria V, et al: Clinical features of pulmonary embolism. Doubts and certainties. *Chest* 107 (Suppl 1):25S-32S, 1995.

The authors describe clinical features of pulmonary embolism based on their review of the literature and their own experience.

28. Matsumoto AH, Tegtmeyer CJ: Contemporary diagnostic approaches to acute pulmonary emboli. *Radiol Clin North Am* 33:167-183, 1995.

A review of imaging procedures deployed in the diagnosis of pulmonary embolism. Topics include ventilation-perfusion scan, fast computed tomography, magnetic resonance imaging techniques, and pulmonary angiography.

29. Mayo JR, Remy-Jardin M, Muller NL, et al: Pulmonary embolism: prospective comparison of spiral CT with ventilation-perfusion scintigraphy. *Radiology* 205:447-452, 1997.

Prospective study to compare spiral computed tomography (CT) to ventilation-perfusion scan showed that the sensitivity of spiral CT is greater than that of ventilation-perfusion scan; the interobserver agreement was better with spiral CT.

30. Meaney JF, Weg JG, Chenevert TL, et al: Diagnosis of pulmonary embolism with magnetic resonance angiography. *N Engl J Med* 336:1422-1427, 1997.

This study compared gadolinium-enhanced pulmonary magnetic resonance angiography (MRA) with pulmonary angiography (PA) for diagnosing pulmonary embolism in 30 consecutive patients with suspected pulmonary embolism. PA detected pulmonary embolism in 8 patients and MRA diagnosed pulmonary embolism in all 5 lobar emboli and 16 of 17 segmental emboli identified on PA. Compared with PA, MRA had high sensitivity and specificity (3 sets of readings had sensitivities of 100%, 87%, and 75% and specificities of 95%, 100%, and 95%) for the diagnosis of pulmonary embolism.

31. Montgomery KD, Geerts WH, Potter HG, et al: Thromboembolic complications in patients with pelvic trauma. *Clin Orthop* 329:68-87, 1996.
Based on a review of the literature, the authors estimate that the incidence of deep vein thrombosis in patients with pelvic fractures is 35% to 60% and the incidence of symptomatic pulmonary embolism is 2% to 10%. The authors state that the cornerstone of effective management is prophylaxis and propose an algorithm for the management of thromboprophylaxis in patients with pelvic trauma.

32. Morehead RS, Tzouanakis AE, Berger R: Preventing VTE: a guide to nonpharmacologic therapies. *J Crit Illness* 13:486-499, 1998.
A review of various nonpharmacologic therapies to prevent venous thromboembolism. Provides an overview of key clinical trials.

33. Morpurgo M, Schmid C: The spectrum of pulmonary embolism. Clinicopathologic correlations. *Chest* 107 (Suppl 1):18S-20S, 1995.
Description of pathophysiologic and clinical findings in 92 postmortem cases of massive or submassive pulmonary embolism; only 28% were diagnosed pre-mortem.

34. Perez Gutthann S, Garcia Rodriguez LA, Castellsague J, et al: Hormone replacement therapy and risk of venous thromboembolism: population based case-control study. *BMJ* 314:796-800, 1997.
This population-based case-control study from England of a cohort of 347,253 women (50 to 79 years old) without major risk factors for venous thromboembolism observed that the adjusted odds ratio of venous thromboembolism for current use of hormone replacement therapy compared with non-users was 2.1. This increased risk was restricted to first-year users, with odds ratios of 4.6 during the first 6 months and 3.0 from 6 to 12 months after starting treatment.

35. Perrier A, Buswell L, Bounameaux H, et al: Cost-effectiveness of noninvasive diagnostic aids in suspected pulmonary embolism. *Arch Intern Med* 157:2309-2316, 1997.
According to this literature data-based cost-effectiveness analysis of noninvasive diagnostic aids in suspected pulmonary embolism observed, strategies combining D-dimer (> 500 μg/L) and ultrasonography with lung scan were most cost-effective.

36. Prandoni P, Polistena P, Bernardi E, et al: Upper-extremity deep vein thrombosis. Risk factors, diagnosis, and complications. *Arch Intern Med* 157:57-62, 1997.
Of 58 consecutive patients with signs and symptoms suggestive of upper-extremity deep vein thrombosis (UEDVT), venography confirmed UEDVT in 27 patients (47%). Central venous catheters, thrombophilic states, and a previous leg vein thrombosis were statistically significantly associated with UEDVT. Pulmonary embolism occurred in 36% of the patients.

37. Price DT, Ridker PM: Factor V Leiden mutation and the risks of thromboembolic disease: a clinical perspective. *Ann Intern Med* 127:895-903, 1997.
A MEDLINE search-based review of case-control and prospective cohort studies provides a detailed perspective on the prevalence and risks for thromboembolic disease in persons with factor V Leiden mutation.

38. Robinson KS, Anderson DR, Gross M, et al: Ultrasonographic screening before hospital discharge for deep venous thrombosis after arthroplasty: the Post-Arthroplasty Screening Study. A randomized, controlled trial. *Ann Intern Med* 127:439-445, 1997.
This double-blind, randomized, controlled trial of 1,024 patients undergoing elective total hip or knee arthroplasty who received warfarin prophylaxis observed that the use of warfarin prophylaxis during hospitalization results in a very low rate of symptomatic deep vein thrombosis or pulmonary embolism after hospital discharge.

39. Rosenow EC III: Venous and pulmonary thromboembolism: an algorithmic approach to diagnosis and management. *Mayo Clin Proc* 70:45-49, 1995.
An algorithm for assessing patients with possible venous and pulmonary thromboembolism is presented; decisions about proceeding with various studies are based primarily on the clinician's degree of suspicion for the presence of pulmonary thromboembolism and the findings on a ventilation-perfusion scan.

40. Ryan DH, Crowther MA, Ginsberg JS, et al: Relation of factor V Leiden genotype to risk for acute deep venous thrombosis after joint replacement surgery. *Ann Intern Med* 128:270-276, 1998.

A study of 825 patients hospitalized for hip or knee replacement surgery observed that the factor V Leiden mutation is not a significant risk factor for the development of acute deep vein thrombosis. The incidence of acute deep vein thrombosis was 31% in patients with the mutation and 26% in those without.

41. Schulman S, Granqvist S, Holmstrom M, et al: The duration of oral anticoagulant therapy after a second episode of venous thromboembolism. *N Engl J Med* 336:393-398, 1997.

A comparison of 6 months versus indefinite anticoagulation for the treatment of a second episode of either venous thromboembolism or pulmonary embolism showed that the recurrence rate is higher (21%) after 6 months of therapy, compared with a recurrence rate of 2.6% for those who received therapy indefinitely.

42. Siddique RM, Siddique MI, Rimm AA: Trends in pulmonary embolism mortality in the US elderly population: 1984 through 1991. *Am J Public Health* 88:478-480, 1998.

This study determined race-, age- and sex-specific trends in 30-day pulmonary embolism mortality rates among Medicare beneficiaries with a primary or secondary discharge diagnosis of pulmonary embolism from 1984 to 1991 (n = 391,991). For a primary diagnosis of pulmonary embolism, mortality rates declined by 15.2% and 16.0%, respectively, for white male patients 65 to 74 years old and 75 years or older. There was a corresponding decline in mortality rates for white women. For a secondary diagnosis of pulmonary embolism, mortality rates declined by 14.7% and 9.8%, respectively, for white males 65 to 74 years old and 75 years or older. The decline in white mortality rate revealed in this study did not translate, in all cases, to groups of black patients.

43. Silverstein MD, Heit JA, Mohr DN, et al: Trends in the incidence of deep vein thrombosis and pulmonary embolism: a 25-year population-based study. *Arch Intern Med* 158:585-593, 1998.

Population-based study of patients in Olmsted County, Minnesota, observed that the overall average age- and sex-adjusted annual incidence of venous thromboembolism was 117 per 100,000 (deep vein thrombosis, 48 per 100,000; pulmonary embolism, 69 per 100,000), with higher age-adjusted rates among males and females (130 vs 110 per 100,000, respectively).

44. Simonneau G, Sors H, Charbonnier B, et al: A comparison of low-molecular-weight heparin with unfractionated heparin for acute pulmonary embolism. *N Engl J Med* 337:663-669, 1997.

In this comparative study of symptomatic pulmonary embolism, 308 patients were treated with low-molecular-weight heparin (once-daily fixed-dose subcutaneously) and 308 patients received unfractionated heparin (adjusted-dose intravenously). Low-molecular-weight heparin was as effective and safe as unfractionated heparin. The risk of major bleeding was similar in the two treatment groups throughout the study.

45. Sorensen HT, Mellemkjaer L, Steffensen FH, et al: The risk of a diagnosis of cancer after primary deep venous thrombosis or pulmonary embolism. *N Engl J Med* 338:1169-1173, 1998.

This study observed that the risk of diagnosis of cancer is significantly increased only during the first 6 months after the diagnosis of deep vein thrombosis or pulmonary embolism and that the risk of cancer diagnosis declined rapidly to a constant level 1 year after the thrombotic event. Among those with a diagnosis of cancer within 1 year after thromboembolism, 40% had distant metastases at the time of the diagnosis of cancer. The authors concluded that an aggressive search for a hidden cancer in a patient with a primary deep vein thrombosis or pulmonary embolism is not warranted.

46. Stein PD, Henry JW: Clinical characteristics of patients with acute pulmonary embolism stratified according to their presenting syndromes. *Chest* 112:974-979, 1997.

Prospective Investigation of Pulmonary Embolism Diagnosis (PIOPED) study to evaluate clinical characteristics in pulmonary embolism noted that 12% of patients had neither dyspnea nor tachypnea. A normal ECG was seen in 46%, a $PaO_2 > 80$ mm Hg in 27%, and a high-probability V/Q lung scan in 32%.

47. Traill ZC, Gleeson FV: Venous thromboembolic disease. *Br J Radiol* 71:129-134, 1998.

A review of the role of spiral computed tomography in the diagnosis of venous thromboembolic disease. Discussion includes the limitations of previous methods of investigation.

48. Turkstra F, Kuijer PM, van Beek EJ, et al: Diagnostic utility of ultrasonography of leg veins in patients suspected of having pulmonary embolism. *Ann Intern Med* 126:775-781, 1997.

A prospective cohort study of 397 consecutive inpatients and outpatients in whom pulmonary embolism was suspected noted that the overall sensitivity of compression ultrasonography for deep vein thrombosis in patients with pulmonary embolism was 29% and the specificity was 97%. The authors concluded that diagnostic value of compression ultrasonography for the detection of deep vein thrombosis in patients suspected of having pulmonary embolism is limited.

49. Tuttle-Newhall JE, Rutledge R, Hultman CS, et al: Statewide, population-based, time-series analysis of the frequency and outcome of pulmonary embolus in 318,554 trauma patients. *J Trauma* 42:90-99, 1997.
Of 318,554 patients, 952 (0.30%) had a recorded diagnosis of pulmonary embolism (PE), and the mortality rate for patients with PE (26%) was 10 times higher than that for those without PE (2.6%). Age was a significant predictor of the risk of PE: 0.05% for patients < 55 years and 0.7% in those ≥ 55 years. The rate of PE was highest in patients with injuries of the extremities, 0.53%.

50. van Beek EJ, Kuijer PM, Buller HR, et al: The clinical course of patients with suspected pulmonary embolism. *Arch Intern Med* 157:2593-2598, 1997.
Among 243 patients with proven pulmonary embolism, recurrent pulmonary embolism occurred in approximately 5 patients (2.5%) who were treated for a previous episode. Fatal bleeding complications attributable to the use of anticoagulants were encountered in 1%. Mortality at 6 months was 17%; death was related to (recurrent) pulmonary embolism in 5%.

51. van den Belt AG, Sanson BJ, Simioni P, et al: Recurrence of venous thromboembolism in patients with familial thrombophilia. *Arch Intern Med* 157:2227-2232, 1997.
A literature review showed that the annual incidence of a first recurrent venous thromboembolism in patients with antithrombin or protein-S deficiency ranged from 13% to 17% and 14% to 16%, respectively, and that the annual incidence of recurrent venous thromboembolism is high during the first years after a first episode but seems to decline thereafter.

52. Wagenvoort CA: Pathology of pulmonary thromboembolism. *Chest* 107 (Suppl 1):10S-17S, 1995.
A review of pathologic findings in both acute and chronic pulmonary thromboembolism. The author states that the thrombotic arteriopathy is often associated with pulmonary hypertension and is characterized by irregular, nonlaminar, often obliterative, intimal fibrosis.

53. Ward R, Jones D, Haponik EF: Paradoxical embolism. An underrecognized problem. *Chest* 108:549-558, 1995.
A review of paradoxic embolism as it relates to patent foramen ovale, which is encountered in 27% to 35% of the normal population. The authors conclude that the primary therapy for patients with paradoxic embolism is anticoagulation, with thrombolytics considered for carefully selected persons. The authors caution that there is little published information about long-term treatment and outcome.

54. Weitz JI: Low-molecular-weight heparins. *N Engl J Med* 337:688-698, 1997.
A detailed review of low-molecular-weight heparin. Discussion includes mechanisms of action, pharmacokinetics, comparisons of different low-molecular-weight heparins, and complications.

Questions

Multiple Choice (choose the one best answer)

1. Factor V Leiden mutation is a significant risk factor for the development of deep vein thrombosis and pulmonary embolism. Factor V Leiden mutation is not a significant risk factor for the development of venous thrombosis and pulmonary embolism in which *one* of the following patients?
   a. Patients undergoing hip or knee replacement surgery
   b. Men older than 60 years
   c. Men with hyperhomocystinemia
   d. Women taking contraceptives
   e. A patient with recurrent deep vein thrombosis and/or pulmonary embolism

2. Which one of the following is not an independent risk factor for the development of pulmonary embolism in women?
   a. Chronic oral contraceptive use
   b. High serum level of cholesterol and diabetes mellitus
   c. Obesity
   d. Cigarette smoking
   e. Hypertension

3. Which one of the following statements about deep vein thrombosis/pulmonary embolism and malignancy is not true?
   a. In patients with deep vein thrombosis/pulmonary embolism, the risk of the diagnosis of cancer is increased only during the first 6 months after the diagnosis of deep vein thrombosis/pulmonary embolism
   b. Deep vein thrombosis/pulmonary embolism in elderly subjects may indicate occult neoplasm in 20%
   c. Occurrence of deep vein thrombosis/pulmonary embolism in patients with cancer does not affect the prognosis
   d. An aggressive search for underlying cancer is not indicated in most patients with deep vein thrombosis/pulmonary embolism
   e. If cancer is diagnosed within 1 year after the diagnosis of deep vein thrombosis/pulmonary embolism, 40% of such patients will have distant metastases at the time of the diagnosis of cancer

4. A 68-year-old previously healthy man is evaluated for acute chest pain of 4 days' duration. Clinical examination elicits calf tenderness on the left. Pulmonary embolism is suspected. Electrocardiography is performed. Which one of the following is *not* true regarding electrocardiographic changes in pulmonary embolism?
   a. Nonspecific changes are noted in 80% of patients
   b. T-wave inversion in the precordial leads is the most common abnormality
   c. The pattern of S wave in lead I and Q wave in lead III is present in 15%
   d. T-wave inversion in the precordial leads has no prognostic significance
   e. Right bundle branch block occurs in 12%

5. A 56-year-old woman has a history of left calf pain and pleuritic right chest pain of 6 days' duration. Physical examination findings suggest deep vein thrombosis complicated by pulmonary embolism. Among the following test results obtained in this patient, which one is *not* compatible with the diagnosis of pulmonary embolism?
   a. $P(A\text{-}a)O_2$ gradient of 18 mm Hg
   b. Normal electrocardiogram
   c. Normal plasma D-dimer level
   d. Normal chest radiograph
   e. Normal perfusion lung scan

6. A 78-year-old man with a previous history of inadequately treated deep vein thrombosis presents with pleuritic right chest pain of 2 days' duration. Physical examination reveals normal calves without edema, redness, or tenderness. Lung examination reveals a pleural friction rub on the right side of the chest. Which one of the following is most likely to help diagnose pulmonary embolism in this patient?
   a. Transesophageal echocardiography
   b. Magnetic resonance imaging of the thorax
   c. Bronchoscopic ultrasonography of the pulmonary arteries
   d. Ventilation/perfusion lung scan
   e. Ultrafast computed tomography of the chest

7. Which one of the following statements about anticoagulant therapy for treatment of pulmonary embolism is *incorrect*?
   a. Treatment with heparin and warfarin can be initiated simultaneously
   b. Low-molecular-weight heparin therapy is as effective as unfractionated heparin therapy

c. A prothrombin time INR of 2 to 3 is recommended for patients with uncomplicated pulmonary embolism

d. There is no difference in long-term outcome between the 6-week and 6-month therapy

e. Frequent monitoring of aPTT is not necessary if low-molecular-weight heparin is used

8. Which one of the following statements about thrombolytic agents in the treatment of pulmonary embolism is *incorrect*?

a. Less than 15% of patients with pulmonary embolism receive thrombolytic therapy

b. One-year mortality among those treated with thrombolytic agents is less than among those treated with anticoagulants

c. Pulmonary embolism must be documented by pulmonary angiography before thrombolytic therapy

d. Risk of intracranial bleeding is higher in those treated with thrombolytic agents than in those treated with anticoagulants

e. Adequacy of thrombolytic therapy is monitored with thrombin time

9. Which one of the following statements about inferior vena caval filter placement or plication to prevent pulmonary embolism is *incorrect*?

a. Long-term anticoagulant therapy is required after inferior vena caval plication

b. Recurrent pulmonary embolism does not occur after inferior vena caval plication

c. There is no "ideal" inferior vena caval filter

d. Routine plication of the inferior vena cava is not recommended in patients with cancer and deep vein thrombosis

e. Inferior vena caval filter therapy prevents pulmonary embolism but leads to an excess of recurrent deep vein thrombosis

10. A 59-year-old woman has a 3-year history of progressive dyspnea. Evaluations reveal significant hypoxemia after exercise and moderately increased pulmonary artery pressure (60 mm Hg by echocardiography). She has a history of several episodes of deep vein thrombosis that were inadequately treated. Which one of the following diagnostic tests is *least* likely to provide useful information for the management of this patient?

a. Lung biopsy to identify plexiform lesions

b. Measurement of lupus anticoagulant

c. Assessment for deficiencies of antithrombin III, protein C, or protein S

d. Pulmonary function tests

e. Pulmonary angiography

Answers

1. Answer a

A study of 825 patients hospitalized for hip or knee replacement surgery reported that the factor V Leiden mutation is not a risk factor for the development of acute deep vein thrombosis (*Ann Intern Med* 128:270-276, 1998).

2. Answer b

A prospective study of a group of 112,822 women 30 to 55 years old with 1,619,770 person-years of follow-up documented showed that obesity, cigarette smoking, and hypertension were independent predictors of pulmonary embolism. High serum cholesterol levels and diabetes were not related to pulmonary embolism (*JAMA* 277:642-645, 1997).

3. Answer c

The occurrence of deep vein thrombosis/pulmonary embolism in patients with cancer portends poor prognosis. One study reported that the risk of diagnosis of cancer is significantly increased only during the first 6 months after the diagnosis of deep vein thrombosis or pulmonary embolism and that the risk of cancer diagnosis declined rapidly to a constant level 1 year after the thrombotic event. Among those with a diagnosis of cancer within 1 year after thromboembolism, 40% had distant metastases at the time of the diagnosis of cancer (*N Engl J Med* 338:1169-1173, 1998).

4. Answer d

A study of 80 consecutive patients hospitalized for pulmonary embolism observed that T-wave inversion in the precordial leads was the most common abnormality (68%) and represented the electrocardiographic sign best correlated with the severity of pulmonary embolism. The subepicardial ischemic pattern was an even stronger marker of severity when it appeared as early as the first day, and its reversibility before the sixth day indicated a good outcome or high level of therapeutic efficacy (*Chest* 111:537-543, 1997).

5. Answer e

A normal perfusion lung scan excludes pulmonary embolism in more than 96% of patients. In the Prospective Investigation of Pulmonary Embolism Diagnosis (PIOPED) study, 20% of patients with angiographically documented pulmonary embolism had a normal $P(A-a)O_2$ gradient (≤ 20 mm Hg). The study also noted that 12% of patients had neither dyspnea nor tachypnea; a normal electrocardiogram was seen in 46% and a $PaO_2 > 80$ mm Hg, in 27% (*Chest* 112:974-990, 1997).

6. Answer e

Overall sensitivity and specificity of computed tomography in the diagnosis of pulmonary embolism in the central pulmonary arteries (main through segmental) are 94% and 94%, respectively. Prospectively, studies have shown that the sensitivity and interobserver agreement of spiral computed tomography are greater than those of ventilation-perfusion scan (*Radiology* 205:447-452, 1997). Transesophageal echocardiography has been reported to have high sensitivity and specificity for the diagnosis of massive pulmonary embolism (*Chest* 112:1310-1316, 1997).

7. Answer d

A randomized controlled trial with a 2-year follow-up of 897 patients showed that in patients with a first episode of either condition, those who received 6 months of therapy had fewer recurrences than those who had only 6 weeks of treatment (9.5% vs. 18.1%). Another study has shown that low-molecular-weight heparin is as effective as unfractionated heparin for treatment of pulmonary embolism (*N Engl J Med* 337:663-669, 1997).

8. Answer c

Pulmonary angiography is not needed in all patients selected for thrombolytic therapy. Fewer than 10% of patients in the PIOPED trial received thrombolytic therapy. Analysis of data from 312 patients from five previously reported studies of pulmonary embolism thrombolysis noted that intracranial hemorrhage (up to 14 days after pulmonary embolism thrombolysis) occurred in 6 (1.9%) of patients; two of six intracranial hemorrhages were fatal (*Chest* 107 [Suppl]:45S-51S, 1995).

9. Answer b

Pulmonary embolism occurs in 2.5% of patients even after insertion of an inferior vena caval filter. The routine use of inferior vena caval filters in patients with cancer and deep vein thrombosis is not recommended. Inferior vena caval plication does not replace anticoagulant therapy; many patients require both. A study of 400 patients with proximal deep vein thrombosis who were at risk for pulmonary embolism observed that the initial beneficial effect of vena caval filters for the prevention of pulmonary embolism was counterbalanced by an excess of recurrent deep vein thrombosis, without any difference in mortality (*N Engl J Med* 338:409-415, 1998).

10. Answer a

Plexiform lesions, although more common in primary pulmonary hypertension, also occur in chronic thromboembolic pulmonary hypertension, which this patient has. Lupus anticoagulant is present in 10% of patients with chronic thromboembolic pulmonary hypertension, and antithrombin-III, protein-C, or protein-S deficiencies occur in < 1% of patients with this disease.

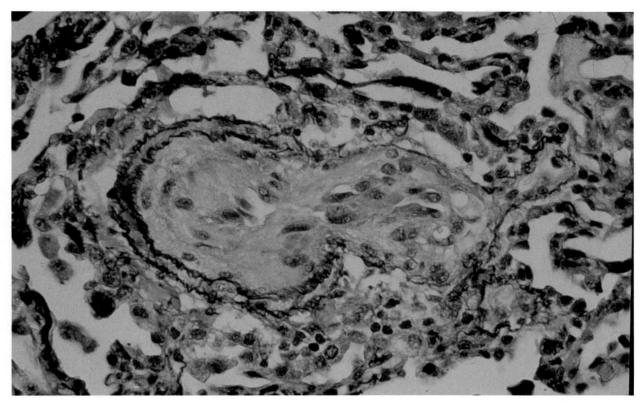

Plate 1. Pulmonary arteriolar obstruction in thromboembolic pulmonary hypertension (lung tissue; x100).

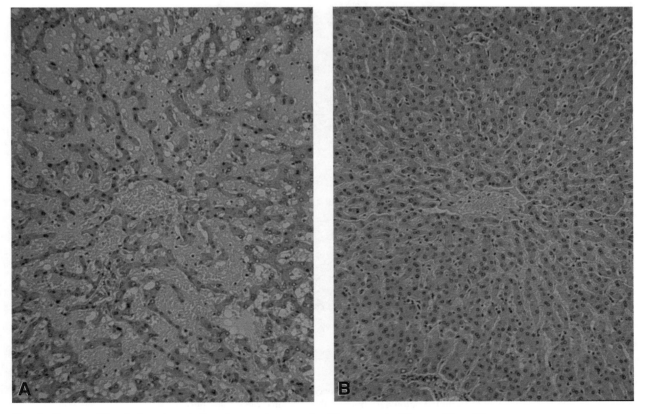

Plate 2. Congested liver in thromboembolic pulmonary hypertension (A) compared with normal liver (B).

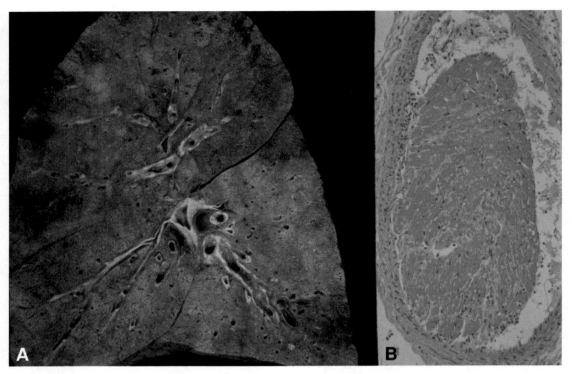

Plate 3. *A*, Gross lung specimen showing multiple pulmonary emboli with pulmonary infarctions. *B*, Histologic section showing thrombus in a pulmonary vessel.

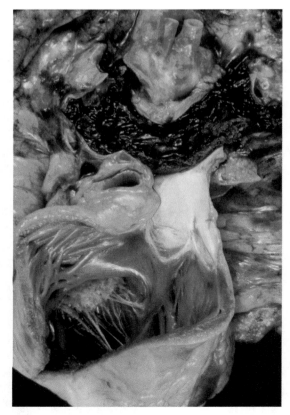

Plate 4. Massive fatal pulmonary embolus occupying the right and left pulmonary trunks. The pulmonary valve and pulmonary outflow tract are seen inferiorly.

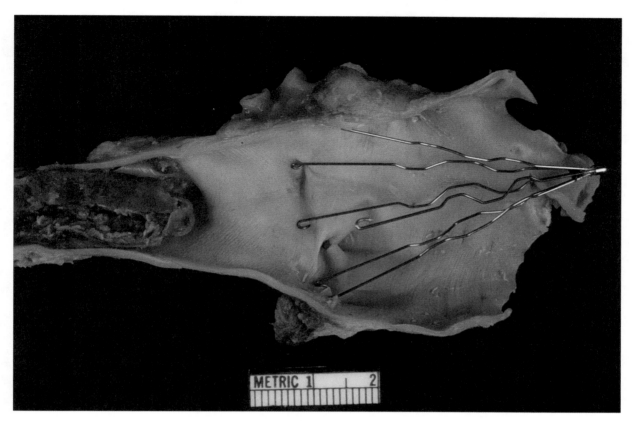

Plate 5. Greenfield inferior vena cava filter with occluding thrombus after pelvic irradiation for uterine cancer.

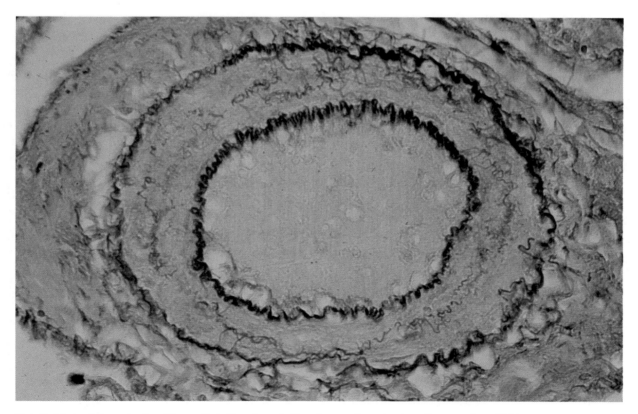

Plate 6. Moderate hypertrophy of the media in thromboembolic pulmonary hypertension. (Lung section; x100.)

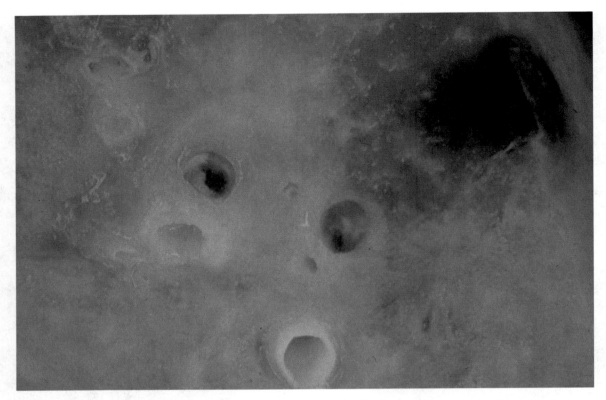

Plate 7. Acute pulmonary embolus with lung infarction in a person who had head trauma from a motor vehicle accident.

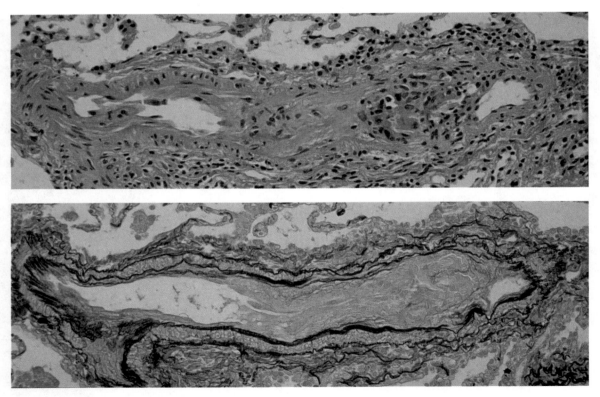

Plate 8. Lung biopsy specimens of thromboembolic pulmonary hypertension with organized arterial thrombus formation. Plexiform lesions are not present. (x50.)

Chapter 28

Infections of the Heart

Robin Patel, M.D.
James M. Steckelberg, M.D.

Native Valve Infective Endocarditis

Epidemiology

From 10,000 to 15,000 new cases of infective endocarditis are diagnosed annually in the U.S. Although the total number of cases of endocarditis is relatively constant, the spectrum of underlying cardiac conditions and etiologic organisms has changed during the last decade. The median age of patients with infective endocarditis has gradually increased, and currently, more than one-half of all patients are older than 54 years, with the mean age of those with enterococcal endocarditis even higher.

Infective endocarditis is uncommon in children and is usually associated with underlying structural congenital heart disease, surgical repair of congenital heart disease, or nosocomial catheter-related bacteremia, especially in infants. According to a recent study, complex congenital heart disease and unrepaired ventricular septal defect are the most common underlying lesions in children. Blood cultures should be performed before antibiotics are prescribed for a febrile patient with congenital heart disease unless a well-defined focus of infection is present. Indiscriminate use of antibiotics may delay the diagnosis of infective endocarditis or retard recovery of a causative organism.

- Although the total number of cases of endocarditis is relatively stable, the spectrum of underlying conditions and

causal organisms has changed during the last decade.
- Complex congenital heart disease and unrepaired ventricular septal defect are the most common underlying cardiac lesions predisposing to infective endocarditis in children.

Overall, men are affected more commonly than women by infective endocarditis, with an incidence rate of 2.5:1. Chronic rheumatic valvular disease has been supplanted by mitral valve prolapse with regurgitation and degenerative aortic valve disease as the leading cardiac conditions underlying bacterial endocarditis in adults. A new form of endocarditis (nosocomial endocarditis) due to therapeutic modalities (intravenous catheters, hyperalimentation lines, pacemakers, dialysis shunts, etc.) has emerged. A high proportion of cases, particularly right-sided endocarditis, continue to occur in intravenous drug users. The need for surgical intervention is increasing compared with that in previous years.

The heart valve most commonly involved in infective endocarditis is the mitral valve (Plate 1), followed by the aortic valve. Isolated aortic valve endocarditis is increasing in frequency and is more common in men than in women. Congenitally bicuspid aortic valve is an important underlying condition, especially in older men. The mitral valve is involved in more than 85% of cases of infective endocarditis on valves previously damaged by rheumatic fever. When

We would like to acknowledge Walter R. Wilson, M.D., for the generous provision of patient photographs in Figure 2 and Plates 1-13.

only the mitral valve is involved, women outnumber men by 2:1. The tricuspid valve rarely is involved (0% to 6%), except in intravenous drug users, and the pulmonary valve even less so (< 1%). Both right- and left-sided endocarditis is present in 0% to 4% of patients.

● The heart valve most commonly affected by endocarditis is the mitral valve, followed by the aortic, tricuspid, and pulmonary valves.

Congenital heart disease (patent ductus arteriosus, ventricular septal defect, coarctation of the aorta, bicuspid aortic valve, tetralogy of Fallot, and, rarely, pulmonic stenosis) underlies 6% to 24% of cases of endocarditis. Surgical closure of ventricular septal defect decreases the risk of infective endocarditis. Endocarditis is extremely rare in secundum atrial septal defects. Many other conditions (syphilitic heart disease, arterial fistulas, hemodialysis shunts or fistulas, intracardiac pacemaker wires, and intracardiac prostheses) also predispose to endocarditis. Patients with hypertrophic obstructive cardiomyopathy (HOCM) are also at risk for infective endocarditis, especially those with hemodynamically severe forms of the disease (high peak systolic pressure gradient and high prevalence of symptoms). Either the mitral or aortic valve, or both valves, may be involved. New murmurs develop in 36% of patients with HOCM complicated by infective endocarditis, and this physical finding correlates with a high mortality rate.

● Endocarditis is extremely rare in secundum atrial septal defects.
● Patients with HOCM and high gradients are at high risk for endocarditis.

Infective endocarditis is associated with mitral prolapse syndrome, especially in patients with mitral valve prolapse and valvular redundancy. After infective endocarditis develops in patients with mitral valve prolapse, the symptoms and signs are more subtle and the mortality rates less than in left-sided infective endocarditis of other types.

Recently, several cases of endocarditis have been reported in solid organ transplantation recipients: *Corynebacterium jeikeium*, *Pseudallescheria boydii*, *Candida* species, and *Aspergillus flavus* endocarditis in liver transplant recipients, cytomegalovirus and *Staphylococcus epidermidis* endocarditis in heart transplant recipients, and *Staphylococcus aureus* and *Candida albicans* endocarditis in heart-lung transplant recipients.

In patients with bacteremia due to *S. aureus*, certain factors identify a high probability of infective endocarditis. These include the absence of a primary site of infection, community acquisition of the infection, metastatic sequelae, and valvular vegetations detected with echocardiography.

● Mitral valve prolapse with regurgitation and degenerative aortic valve disease are the most common predisposing lesions for infective endocarditis.

Pathogenesis

The development of infective endocarditis requires the occurrence of several events (Fig. 1). The valve surface must first be damaged to produce a suitable site for bacterial attachment and colonization. Typically, this damage is caused by blood flow turbulence, which leads to the deposition of platelets and fibrin and the formation of "nonbacterial thrombotic endocarditis." Hemodynamic factors contribute to the usual localization of the lesions of infective endocarditis downstream from a regurgitant flow. Infective endocarditis characteristically occurs on the atrial surface of the mitral valve and on the ventricular surface of the aortic valve when associated with valvular insufficiency. Lesions with high degrees of turbulence (small ventricular septal defects with jet lesions, valvular stenoses) readily create conditions that lead to bacterial colonization, whereas defects with large surface areas (large ventricular septal defects), low flow (ostium secundum atrial septal defects), or attenuation of turbulence (chronic congestive heart failure with atrial fibrillation) are rarely implicated in infective endocarditis.

● Infective endocarditis characteristically occurs on the atrial surface of the mitral valve and on the ventricular surface of the aortic valve.

After the formation of the lesion in nonbacterial thrombotic endocarditis, bacteria must reach the site and adhere to the lesion. Transient bacteremia may occur sporadically or when a mucosal surface heavily colonized with bacteria is traumatized, as with dental extractions and other dental procedures and with gastrointestinal, urologic, and gynecologic procedures. The degree of bacteremia is proportional to the trauma produced by the procedure and the number of organisms inhabiting the area. The microorganisms that are isolated reflect the resident microbial flora. Less than one-half of the cases of bacterial endocarditis can be attributed to an identifiable invasive procedure (estimates range from 4% to 49%).

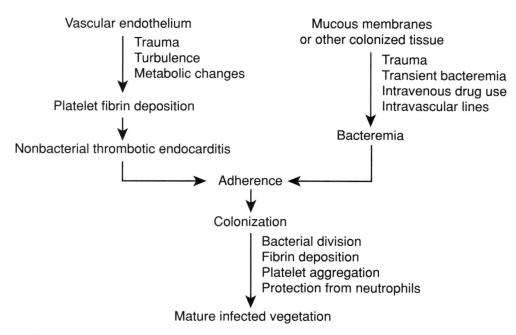

Fig. 1. Pathogenesis of infective endocarditis. (Modified from Mandell GL, Bennett JE, Dolin R [editors]: *Principles and Practice of Infectious Diseases.* Fourth edition. Churchill Livingstone, 1995, p 742. By permission of the publisher.)

Certain strains of bacteria appear to have a selective advantage in adhering to platelets, fibrin, or valvular endothelium. Thus, they produce disease with a lower inoculum than other strains.

After colonization of the valve occurs and a critical mass of adherent bacteria develops, the vegetation enlarges by additional deposition of platelet/fibrin and continued proliferation of bacteria. Platelets may also have a role in host defense within the cardiac vegetation during infective endocarditis.

● Less than one-half of the cases of bacterial endocarditis can be attributed to an identifiable invasive procedure.

Infective endocarditis causes the stimulation of both humoral and cellular immunity, as manifested by hypergammaglobulinemia, splenomegaly, and the presence of macrophages in peripheral blood. Rheumatoid factor (anti-IgG, IgM antibody) develops in about one-half of the patients with infective endocarditis of more than 6 weeks' duration. Antinuclear antibodies may also occur in infective endocarditis and contribute to musculoskeletal manifestations, low-grade fever, and pleuritic pain. Circulating immune complexes have been found in high titer in virtually all patients with infective endocarditis and are found with increased frequency in connection with a long duration of illness, extravalvular manifestations, hypocomplementemia,

and right-sided infective endocarditis. Concentrations decrease and become undetectable with successful therapy. Patients with infective endocarditis and circulating immune complexes may develop a diffuse glomerulonephritis. Immune complexes and complement are deposited subepithelially along the glomerular basement membrane to form a "lumpy-bumpy" pattern. Some of the peripheral manifestations of infective endocarditis, such as Osler nodes, may also result from the deposition of circulating immune complexes (positive cultures from aspirates from Osler nodes may also be noted). In some diffuse purpuric lesions in infective endocarditis, immune complex deposits (IgG, IgM, and complement) may be detected in dermal blood vessels.

● The vascular endothelium is damaged most often by turbulent blood flow; platelets and fibrin are deposited; the nonbacterial thrombotic endocarditis lesion is seeded during a bacteremic episode, and a mature vegetation develops.
● Circulating immune complexes have been found in high titer in virtually all patients with infective endocarditis.

Pathologic Changes

Pathologic changes of infective endocarditis are shown in Table 1. The classic vegetation is located along the line of closure of the valve leaflet. Vegetations may be single or multiple, vary from a few millimeters to several centimeters in size, and vary in color, consistency, and gross appearance. Destruction of the underlying valve may be present. With treatment, healing occurs by fibrosis and, occasionally, calcification. In acute cases, the vegetation is larger, softer, and more friable and may be associated with more suppuration, more necrosis, and less healing than that in subacute cases. Infection may lead to perforation of the valve leaflet or rupture of the chordae tendineae, interventricular septum, or papillary muscle. Endocarditis, especially *S. aureus* endocarditis, may produce valve-ring abscesses, with fistula formation into the myocardium or pericardial sac. Aneurysms of the valve leaflet or sinus of Valsalva are also seen. Valvular stenosis may result from large vegetations. Myocarditis, myocardial infarction, and pericarditis may be present. Myocardial abscesses are associated with *S. aureus* endocarditis, high fever, rapid onset of congestive heart failure, and conduction disturbances. Embolic phenomena are common in infective endocarditis; major embolic episodes occur in at least one-third of cases. Embolic phenomena most frequently involve the cerebral, renal, splenic, or coronary circulation. Emboli and immune complex deposition contribute

Table 1.—Pathologic Findings in Infective Endocarditis

Location	Manifestation	Comment
Central nervous system	Cerebral emboli	
	Cerebral infarction	
	Arteritis	
	Abscess	
	Mycotic aneurysm	
	Intracerebral or subarachnoid hemorrhage	
	Encephalomalacia	
	Cerebritis	
	Meningitis	
Spleen	Splenic infarct	
	Splenic abscess	
	Splenic enlargement	Pathologic findings include hyperplasia of lymphoid follicles, increase in secondary follicles, proliferation of reticuloendothelial cells, scattered focal necrosis
Lung	Pulmonary emboli	Associated with right-sided infective endocarditis
	Pleural effusion	
	Empyema	
Skin	Petechiae	
	Osler nodes	Consist of arteriolar intimal proliferation with extension to venules and capillaries, which may be accompanied by thrombosis and necrosis; diffuse perivascular infiltrate consisting of neutrophils and monocytes surrounds dermal vessels; immune complexes may be seen in dermal vessels
	Janeway lesions	Consist of bacteria, neutrophilic infiltration, necrosis, and subcutaneous hemorrhage; secondary to septic emboli; subcutaneous abscesses on histologic examination
Eye	Roth spots	Consist of lymphocytes surrounded by edema and hemorrhage in nerve fiber layer of retina

to the extracardiac manifestations of infective endocarditis and may involve virtually any organ system. When large emboli occlude major vessels, consider fungal endocarditis, marantic endocarditis, or an intracardiac myxoma.

- *S. aureus* is frequently associated with valve-ring abscesses and myocardial abscess.

Renal Complications of Infective Endocarditis

Abscess, infarction, or glomerulonephritis may be found in the kidney in infective endocarditis (Plates 2 and 3). Glomerulonephritis may be a focal, local, or segmental process characterized by endothelial and mesangial proliferation, hemorrhage, neutrophilic infiltration, fibrinoid necrosis, crescent formation, and healing by fibrosis. However, diffuse glomerulonephritis, consisting of generalized cellular hyperplasia in all glomerular tufts, may also be seen. Less commonly, membranoproliferative glomerulonephritis, characterized by marked mesangial proliferation and by splitting of the glomerular basement membrane, may be found.

- Glomerulonephritis may be a focal, local, or segmental process.

Mycotic Aneurysms

Mycotic aneurysms may develop during active infective endocarditis, occasionally months to years after successful therapy. They may arise by 1) direct bacterial invasion of the arterial wall, with subsequent abscess formation or rupture (or both); 2) septic or bland embolic occlusion of the vasa vasorum; or 3) immune complex deposition, with resultant injury to the arterial wall. Mycotic aneurysms tend to occur at bifurcation points and are found in the cerebral vessels (especially the peripheral branches of the middle cerebral artery), but they also occur in the abdominal aorta, sinus of Valsalva, ligated patent ductus arteriosus, and in splenic, coronary, pulmonary, and superior mesenteric arteries. Importantly, mycotic aneurysms often are silent clinically until rupture occurs.

- Central nervous system mycotic aneurysms usually are silent clinically until rupture occurs.

Clinical Manifestations

Clinical manifestations of infective endocarditis are listed in Table 2. Fever is the most common manifestation but is not present in all patients. Approximately 50% of all patients with infective endocarditis become afebrile within 3 days after initiation of appropriate antimicrobial therapy, and ~75% and ~90% become afebrile after 1 and 2 weeks of treatment, respectively. Prolonged fever is associated with *S. aureus* (particularly if treated with vancomycin rather than a β-lactam), gram-negative bacilli, fungi, culture-negative endocarditis, microvascular phenomena, embolization of major vessels, myocardial abscess, peripheral complications, tissue infarction, the need for cardiac surgery, a higher mortality rate, pulmonary emboli, drugs, and nosocomial infection. In patients with prolonged fever, abdominal computed tomography (CT) may be helpful to rule out splenic abscess, and transesophageal echocardiography may be helpful in excluding valve-ring abscess.

Heart murmurs occur in most patients but may be absent with right-sided or mural infection. The classic changing murmur or new murmur is uncommon but may be seen with acute staphylococcal disease. More than 90% of patients who demonstrate a new regurgitant murmur will develop congestive heart failure (the leading cause of death in infective endocarditis). Pericarditis is rare, and when present, it usually is accompanied by myocardial abscess formation as a complication of *S. aureus* infection.

- Prolonged fever is associated with *S. aureus*.
- More than 90% of patients who demonstrate a new regurgitant murmur will develop congestive heart failure.

Peripheral Lesions in Endocarditis

Osler nodes are small, painful nodular lesions usually found on the pads of the fingers or toes and occasionally on the thenar eminence (Plate 4). They range in size from 2 to 15 mm and are frequently multiple. They disappear in a matter of hours to days. These nodes are not specific for infective endocarditis. Janeway lesions are hemorrhagic, macular, painless plaques with a predilection for the palms or soles (Plate 5). They persist for several days and are thought to be embolic in origin. Roth spots are oval pale retinal lesions surrounded by hemorrhage (Plate 6). They usually are near the optic disk. They are not specific for infective endocarditis. Musculoskeletal manifestations of infective endocarditis include proximal oligo- or monoarticular arthralgias, lower extremity mono- or oligoarticular arthritis, low back pain, and diffuse myalgias. Splinter hemorrhages and palatal or conjunctival petechiae may occur but are not specific for infective endocarditis (Plates 7-9).

- Osler nodes are small, painful nodular lesions usually found on the pads of the fingers or toes.

**Table 2.—Clinical Manifestations of Infective
Endocarditis**

Symptom	Physical finding
Fever	Fever
Chills	Heart murmur
Weakness	Changing murmur
Dyspnea	New murmur
Sweats	Embolic phenomena
Anorexia	Skin manifestations--Osler nodes,
Weight loss	petechiae, Janeway lesions
Malaise	Splenomegaly
Cough	Septic complications--pneumonia,
Skin lesions	meningitis, etc.
Stroke	Mycotic aneurysms
Nausea	Clubbing
Vomiting	Retinal lesions
Headache	Signs of renal failure
Myalgia	Arthritis--reactive or infectious
Arthralgia	Mucosal petechiae (e.g., palate,
Edema	conjunctiva)
Chest pain	Splinter hemorrhages
Abdominal pain	
Delirium	
Coma	
Hemoptysis	
Back pain	

Modified from Mandell GL, Bennett JE, Dolin R (editors): *Principles and Practice of Infectious Diseases.* Fourth edition. Churchill Livingstone, 1995, p 748. By permission of the publisher.

- Janeway lesions are hemorrhagic, macular, painless plaques with a predilection for the palms or soles.

Embolic Events

Major embolic episodes are an important complication of infective endocarditis. Splenic artery emboli with infarction may result in left upper quadrant abdominal pain (with radiation to the left shoulder), splenic or pleural rubs, or left pleural effusion. Renal infarctions may be associated with microscopic or gross hematuria. Retinal artery emboli are rare and may be manifested by a complete, sudden loss of vision. Pulmonary emboli arising from right-sided endocarditis are a common feature in intravenous drug users. Coronary artery emboli usually arise from the aortic valve and may result in septic myocarditis with arrhythmias or myocardial infarction. Major vessel emboli (femoral, brachial, popliteal, or radial arteries) are more frequent in fungal endocarditis.

Major cerebral emboli affect 10% to 30% of patients with infective endocarditis and may result in hemiplegia, sensory loss, ataxia, aphasia, or alteration in mental status.

- Splenic artery emboli with infarction may result in left upper quadrant abdominal pain (with radiation to the left shoulder).
- Renal infarctions may be associated with microscopic or gross hematuria.

Neurologic Complications

Neurologic manifestations occur in one-third of patients with infective endocarditis. Up to 50% of these patients present with neurologic signs and symptoms as heralding features of their illness. Mycotic aneurysms of the cerebral circulation occur in 2% to 10% of patients (Fig. 2). Typically, these aneurysms are single, small, and peripheral and may lead to devastating subarachnoid hemorrhage. Other neurologic features include seizures, severe headache, visual changes, choreoathetoid movements, mononeuropathy, cranial nerve palsies, and toxic encephalopathy.

- Neurologic manifestations occur in one-third of patients with infective endocarditis.

Infective Endocarditis in Intravenous Drug Addicts

The risk for the development of endocarditis among intravenous drug addicts is as high as 5% per patient per year and may be considerably higher in patients who previously had prosthetic valve replacement or in those with rheumatic valvular heart disease. Acute infection accounts for the majority of hospital admissions among intravenous drug addicts, and infective endocarditis is found in ~10% of these episodes. In a febrile intravenous drug addict, infective endocarditis is frequently difficult to differentiate from other infections. Cocaine use, visualization of vegetations with echocardiography, and presence of embolic phenomena are among the most reliable indicators of infective endocarditis in febrile parenteral drug users. In this group of patients, two-thirds have no clinical evidence of preexisting underlying heart disease, and there is a predilection for infection of the tricuspid valve. The predominance of right-sided endocarditis in intravenous drug addicts is presumed to be due to the injection of both drug and adjunctive compounds used to dilute the active agent, resulting in endocardial damage of the tricuspid (and pulmonic) valves. In these patients, tricuspid valve infection may result in pleuritic chest pain,

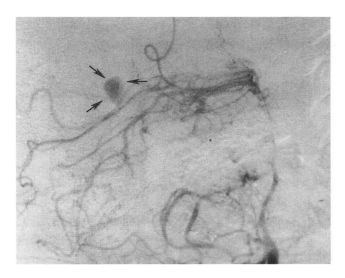

Fig. 2. Mycotic aneurysm (*arrows*).

cough, and hemoptysis, with chest radiographic findings of infiltrates and effusions. Signs of tricuspid insufficiency are present in a small proportion of these cases. The microbiology of endocarditis associated with intravenous drug addicts differs from that of nonaddicts, with a higher prevalence of gram-negative, fungal, and staphylococcal organisms being identified, plus regional variabilities in the spectrum of the causative agent. The course of acute *S. aureus* endocarditis in parenteral drug addicts tends to be less severe than in nonaddicts, although this may not be true in patients infected with the human immunodeficiency virus (HIV).

- Changing murmurs or new murmurs are important findings in endocarditis but are uncommon.
- Cutaneous manifestations of endocarditis include petechiae, Osler nodes, and Janeway lesions.

Laboratory Findings in Infective Endocarditis
Several hematologic abnormalities may be noted in infective endocarditis. Anemia is seen in ~75% of patients and typically is a mild normochromic normocytic anemia with a low serum concentration of iron and a low iron-binding capacity. Thrombocytopenia occurs less frequently. Leukocytosis is seen in about one-third of patients and typically is mild; leukopenia is occasionally noted, especially in conjunction with splenomegaly. Large mononuclear cells (histiocytes) may be noted in peripheral blood, especially in blood from an earlobe puncture. The erythrocyte sedimentation rate is increased in 75% of

patients. Hypergammaglobulinemia with accompanying bone marrow plasmacytosis, a positive rheumatoid factor, hypocomplementemia, a false-positive VDRL test, and a false-positive Lyme serologic test may occur in endocarditis. Circulating immune complexes as well as mixed-type cryoglobulins may also be detected. The results of urinalysis usually are normal but may reveal proteinuria, microscopic hematuria, red blood cell casts, gross hematuria, pyuria, white blood cell casts, or bacteriuria.

- A false-positive VDRL test and a false-positive Lyme serologic test may occur in endocarditis.

Blood Culture
Blood culture is the most important laboratory test for diagnosing infective endocarditis. The bacteremia of infective endocarditis typically is continuous and low grade. When bacteremia is present, the first two blood cultures will yield the etiologic agent in more than 90% of cases. At least three blood culture sets should be obtained during the first 24 hours. More cultures may be necessary if the patient has received antibiotics in the preceding 2 weeks. Nutritionally variant streptococci (*Abiotrophia adiacens*, *Abiotrophia defectiva*) require supplementation of the culture media with either L-cysteine or pyridoxal phosphate (vitamin B_6). In patients who have received antibiotics, blood cultures in hypertonic media may allow detection of organisms with defective cell walls; alternatively, removal of antibiotics from the blood with a resin device may facilitate recovery of microorganisms. Some unusual organisms, such as *Brucella* species and members of the HACEK group (see below), are slow-growing, requiring that cultures be held for extended incubation (4 weeks). Special culture techniques or media may be required for some organisms (e.g., *Legionella* species). Serologic studies are necessary for the diagnosis of Q fever, murine typhus, brucellosis, legionellosis, and psittacosis. Blood culture results are negative in more than 50% of cases of fungal endocarditis. The lysis-centrifugation blood culture method may be useful in detecting some cases of fungal endocarditis.

When embolization to major vessels occurs, embolectomy should be performed and the material examined with stains and culture for fungi.

- Blood culture is the most important test for diagnosing infective endocarditis.
- Blood cultures are negative in more than 50% of cases of

fungal endocarditis.

- Endocarditis is often associated with anemia and an increased erythrocyte sedimentation rate.
- At least three blood culture sets should be obtained during the first 24 hours.

Echocardiography

Echocardiography is widely used to assist in the diagnosis and management of infective endocarditis. The characteristic finding is shaggy dense irregular echoes distributed nonuniformly on one or more leaflets. The average size of vegetations is similar on the aortic and mitral valves. Tricuspid valve vegetations are significantly larger, but pulmonic valve vegetations are usually smaller. Negative findings on transesophageal echocardiography decrease the likelihood that endocarditis is present but do not exclude the diagnosis.

Echocardiography is extremely valuable in assessing local complications of infective endocarditis. Overall, the presence or absence of the vegetations or their size does not accurately predict future embolic events. Also, vegetation size has no definite relationship to the incidence of heart failure, the risk of death during the acute phase of infective endocarditis, or the final outcome.

Transesophageal echocardiography is more sensitive than conventional transthoracic echocardiography in the detection of intracardiac vegetations and perivalvular abscess, but it does not improve the diagnostic accuracy of transthoracic echocardiography in the detection of vegetations associated with right-sided endocarditis in intravenous drug abusers.

The development of a new atrioventricular block or bundle branch block seen on electrocardiography is 88% specific as a predictor of perivalvular abscess. The degree of mitral valve preclosure in patients with aortic insufficiency, as determined by echocardiography, correlates with increased left ventricular end-diastolic pressure and the severity of hemodynamic compromise.

CT of the head is indicated in all patients with endocarditis and neurologic symptoms. Infarction, hemorrhage, or abscess usually can be differentiated by this technique. Cerebral angiography should be considered for all patients with neurologic symptoms not readily explained with CT to exclude intracranial mycotic aneurysm.

- Transesophageal echocardiography is more sensitive than conventional transthoracic echocardiography in the detection of intracardiac vegetations and perivalvular abscess.

Diagnostic Criteria

The Duke diagnostic criteria for infective endocarditis are listed in Table 3A, and the definitions of the diagnostic terms are given in Table 3B.

Microbiology

Streptococcal Endocarditis

Streptococci are the most common causative agents of infective endocarditis (Table 4). Of these, the viridans streptococci are the most common subgroup. The cure rate of nonenterococcal streptococcal endocarditis exceeds 90%, although complications may be seen in more than 30% of cases. An association of *Streptococcus bovis* bacteremia with carcinoma of the colon and other lesions of the gastrointestinal tract has been shown; colonoscopy and/or barium enema should be performed when this organism is isolated from blood cultures. Enterococcal infective endocarditis typically affects either older men after genitourinary tract manipulation or younger women after an obstetric procedure. More than 40% of patients with enterococcal endocarditis have no underlying heart disease, although more than 95% develop a heart murmur during the course of the illness. Classic peripheral manifestations are uncommon. Enterococcal bacteremias are increasing in frequency. Factors that suggest that a patient with enterococcal bacteremia may have infective endocarditis include the absence of other organisms on blood culture, no identifiable extracardiac focus of infection, preexistent valvular heart disease or heart murmur, and community acquisition.

Streptococcus pneumoniae is a rare cause of infective endocarditis; however, when present, it typically has a fulminant course and often is associated with perivalvular abscess formation or pericarditis (or both). In *S. pneumoniae* infective endocarditis, the aortic valve is typically involved and many such patients have a history of alcohol abuse. Concurrent meningitis is present in ~70% of patients. Infective endocarditis due to nutritionally variant streptococci typically is indolent in onset and associated with previous heart disease. Therapy is difficult because of systemic embolization and frequent relapse.

Group B streptococci have been included as a cause of infective endocarditis, especially in recent times. Risk factors for group B streptococcal infective endocarditis in adults include diabetes mellitus, carcinoma, alcoholism, liver failure, elective abortion, and intravenous drug use. Group B streptococci have been associated with villous adenomas of the colon. The mortality of this type of infection approach-

Table 3A.—Duke Criteria for Diagnosis of Infective Endocarditis

Definite infective endocarditis
> Pathologic criteria
>> Microorganisms: demonstrated by culture or histology in a vegetation, or in a vegetation that has embolized, or in an intracardiac abscess, *or*
>> Pathologic lesions: vegetation or intracardiac abscess present, confirmed by histology showing active endocarditis
> Clinical criteria, using specific definitions for these terms as listed in Table 3*B*
>> 2 major criteria *or*
>> 1 major and 3 minor criteria *or*
>> 5 minor criteria

Possible infective endocarditis
> Findings consistent with infective endocarditis that fall short of "Definite" but not "Rejected"

Rejected
> Firm alternate diagnosis explaining evidence of infective endocarditis, *or*
> Resolution of infective endocarditis syndrome with antibiotic therapy for 4 days or less *or*
> No pathologic evidence of infective endocarditis at surgery or autopsy, with antibiotic therapy for 4 days or less

Table 3B.—Definition of Terms Used in the Diagnostic Criteria

Major criteria
> Positive blood culture for infective endocarditis
>> Typical microorganisms for infectious endocarditis from two separate blood cultures
>>> Viridans streptococci, *S. bovis*, HACEK group, *or*
>>> Community-acquired *S. aureus* or enterococci, in the absence of a primary focus, *or*
>> Persistently positive blood culture, defined as microorganism consistent with infective endocarditis from:
>>> Blood cultures drawn more than 12 hours apart *or*
>>> All of three, or majority of four or more, separate blood cultures, with first and last drawn at least 1 hr apart
> Evidence of endocardial involvement
>> Positive echocardiogram for infective endocarditis
>>> Oscillating intracardiac mass on valve or supporting structures or in the path of regurgitant jets or on iatrogenic devices, in the absence of an alternative anatomical explanation, *or*
>>> Abscess *or*
>>> New partial dehiscence of prosthetic valve *or*
>> New valvular regurgitation (worsening or changing of preexisting murmur not sufficient)

Minor criteria
> Predisposition: predisposing heart condition *or* intravenous drug use
> Fever: ≥ 38.0°C (100.4°F)
> Vascular phenomena: arterial embolism, septic pulmonary infarcts, mycotic aneurysm, intracranial hemorrhage, Janeway lesions
> Immunologic phenomena: glomerulonephritis, Osler nodes, Roth spots
> Microbiologic evidence: positive blood culture but not meeting major criterion as noted above *or* serologic evidence of active infection with organism consistent with infective endocarditis
> Echocardiogram: consistent with infective endocarditis but not meeting major criterion as noted above

HACEK, *Haemophilus* spp, *Actinobacillus actinomycetemcomitans*, *Cardiobacterium hominis*, *Eikenella corrodens*, and *Kingella* spp.
From *Am J Med* 96:200-209, 1994. By permission of Excerpta Medica.

Table 4.—Etiologic Agents of Native Valve Infective Endocarditis

Agent	Cases, %			
	Nonintravenous drug users		Intravenous drug addicts	
Streptococci	60-80		27	
Viridans streptococci		30-40		15
Enterococci		5-18		2
Other streptococci		15-25		10
Staphylococci	20-35		66	
S. aureus		10-27		66
Coagulase-negative staphylococci		1-3		0
Gram-negative aerobic bacilli	1.5-13		2	
Fungi	2-4		1-20	
Miscellaneous bacteria	< 5		1	
Mixed infections	1-2		1	
"Culture negative"	<5-24		2	

Nonintravenous drug users from Mandell GL, Bennett JE, Dolin R (editors): *Principles and Practice of Infectious Diseases*. Fourth edition. Churchill Livingstone, 1995, p 753. By permission of the publisher. Intravenous drug addicts modified from *Arch Intern Med* 155:1641-1648, 1995. By permission of the American Medical Association.

es 50%. A similar clinical picture with a destructive process, left-sided predominance, frequent complications, and high mortality has been observed with group G streptococci. *S. anginosus* is a rare cause of infective endocarditis, but it is notable because it has a predilection for suppurative complications involving the brain and liver; perinephric, myocardial, and other abscesses; cholangitis; peritonitis; pericarditis; and empyema more characteristic of *S. aureus* infections.

- Streptococci are the most common causative agents of infective endocarditis.
- The cure rate of nonenterococcal streptococcal endocarditis is more than 90%.
- More than 40% of patients with enterococcal endocarditis have no underlying heart disease

Staphylococcal Endocarditis

Staphylococci are the second most common cause of infective endocarditis. Of the staphylococci, *S. aureus* is the most common cause of native valve infective endocarditis (Plate 10). *S. aureus* may attack normal heart valves in addition to diseased ones. The course of *S. aureus* infective endocarditis typically is fulminant when it involves the mitral or aortic valve, with widespread metastatic infection and a 40% chance of death. Myocardial abscesses, purulent pericarditis, valve-ring abscesses, and peripheral foci of suppuration (lung, brain, spleen, kidney, etc.) are common

with *S. aureus* infective endocarditis. Approximately one-third of patients with *S. aureus* endocarditis experience neurologic manifestations, with approximately two-thirds of this group presenting with neurologic symptoms and one-third developing neurologic symptoms after initiation of antimicrobial therapy. The most frequent neurologic presentation is unilateral hemiparesis. In intravenous drug addicts, *S. aureus* is the most frequent cause of infective endocarditis, but the disease tends to be less severe than that in nonaddicted patients. Children with endocarditis due to *S. aureus* are more likely than those with infections due to viridans streptococci to have prolonged fever, secondary fever, and complications and to require surgery. Recently, infective endocarditis caused by methicillin-resistant *S. aureus* has been noted, especially in intravenous drug addicts. Although coagulase-negative staphylococci are an important cause of prosthetic valve endocarditis, they are seen less frequently in native valve endocarditis.

- Staphylococci are the second most common cause of infective endocarditis.
- In intravenous drug addicts, S. aureus is the most frequent cause of infective endocarditis.

Gram-Negative Endocarditis

Gram-negative bacilli may also cause infective endocarditis. Typically, the gram-negative bacilli involved are fastidious organisms such as those belonging to the HACEK group (see below), although occasionally the Enterobacteriaciae may be involved. Persons addicted to narcotics, prosthetic valve recipients, and patients with cirrhosis appear to be at increased risk for gram-negative bacillary endocarditis. Congestive heart failure is common in this group of patients, and the prognosis is poor, with the mortality rate approaching 80%. Of the Enterobacteriaciae, *Salmonella* species are associated with valvular perforation or destruction (or both), atrial thrombi, myocarditis, and pericarditis. Other Enterobacteriaciae, such as *Escherichia coli*, *Citrobacter* species, *Klebsiella* species, *Enterobacter* species, *Proteus* species, and *Providencia* species, have also been reported to cause infective endocarditis. Notably, several cases of infective endocarditis due to *Serratia marcescens* have been noted in intravenous drug users. Typically, this infection has involved the aortic and mitral valves, with large vegetations and near-total occlusion of the valve orifice in the absence of significant underlying valvular destruction.

Pseudomonas species infective endocarditis has also been noted in intravenous drug addicts. These organisms usually affect normal valves. Major embolic phenomena, inability to sterilize valves, neurologic complications, ring and annular abscesses, splenic abscesses, bacteremic relapses, and rapidly progressive congestive heart failure are common. Ecthyma gangrenosum is seen occasionally. *Pseudomonas aeruginosa* endocarditis has been associated with the use of pentazocine and tripelennamine. *Neisseria gonorrhoeae* occasionally causes infective endocarditis and typically follows an indolent course, with aortic valve involvement, large vegetations, associated valve-ring abscesses, congestive heart failure, and nephritis. A high frequency of late complement component deficiencies has been noted in patients with gonococcal endocarditis. Occasionally, other *Neisseria* species and *Moraxella catarrhalis* may cause infective endocarditis, but they typically produce infection on abnormal or prosthetic heart valves.

- Persons addicted to narcotics, prosthetic valve recipients, and patients with cirrhosis appear to be at increased risk for gram-negative bacillary endocarditis.
- *Pseudomonas aeruginosa* endocarditis has been associated with the use of pentazocine and tripelennamine.

HACEK Endocarditis

Members of the HACEK group of organisms include *Haemophilus* species, *Actinobacillus actinomycetem-*comitans, *Cardiobacterium hominis*, *Eikenella corrodens*, and *Kingella* species. Infective endocarditis due to the HACEK group of organisms (normal inhabitants of the human oropharynx) has been reported in patients who have dental infections and a history of dental procedures and in intravenous drug users who have "cleaned" the injection site with saliva. The clinical syndrome produced by this group of infectious agents is characterized by a lengthy course (2 weeks to 6 months before diagnosis), large friable vegetations, frequent emboli, and the development of congestive heart failure, with eventual valve replacement. All the HACEK group of organisms are fastidious and may require 2 to 3 weeks for primary isolation, although a recent study showed that blood cultures became positive in a mean of 3 days.

Other Agents

Other, miscellaneous bacteria may also be associated with infective endocarditis, including *Corynebacterium* species, *Listeria* species, and *Erysipelothrix* species (associated with mammal or fish exposure and alcoholism), *Bacillus* species, *Tropheryma whippelii* (the causative agent of Whipple's disease), and anaerobic bacteria. *Bartonella henselae*, the causative agent of cat-scratch disease, along with *Bartonella quintana*, both of which cause bacillary angiomatosis and peliosis hepatis especially in HIV-infected persons, have recently been associated with endocarditis in homeless persons with alcoholism and patients in inner-city settings. The microbiology of infective endocarditis in intravenous drug users is distinct from that in nonintravenous drug users (Table 4).

Fungal Endocarditis

During the last few decades, a marked increase in the number of cases of fungal endocarditis has occurred because of the increase in the number of open heart operations and in the number of immunocompromised patients and drug users, the extensive use of broad-spectrum antibiotics, prolonged hospitalizations, and the use of indwelling central venous catheters or hyperalimentation. *Candida parapsilosis* and *Candida tropicalis* predominate in intravenous drug users, and *C. albicans* and *Aspergillus* species cause most cases of fungal infective endocarditis in nonintravenous drug users. Fungal endocarditis carries a poor prognosis because of large bulky vegetations, the tendency for fungal invasion of the myocardium, widespread systemic septic emboli, poor penetration of antifungal agents into the vegetation, the low toxic-therapeutic ratio of the available antifungal agents, and the lack of consistent fungicidal activity with these compounds (Plates 11-13). Surgical intervention is almost always required. In patients with *Aspergillus* infective endocarditis, most blood cultures will be negative, in contrast to the continuous bacteremia seen in bacterial endocarditis. Other accessible features (e.g., emboli, cutaneous lesions, and oropharyngeal lesions) should be examined and cultured for fungi in suspected settings. Valvular vegetations are not always seen on echocardiography, and clinical manifestations of endocarditis are not always present in *Aspergillus* endocarditis. Rarely, fungi other than *Candida* and *Aspergillus* may be associated with infective endocarditis.

Culture-Negative Endocarditis

Culture-negative endocarditis accounts for a small proportion of cases (< 5%). It may occur because of several factors: 1) slow growth of fastidious organisms such as members of the HACEK group of organisms, nutritionally variant streptococci, or *Brucella* species; 2) recent administration of antimicrobial agents; 3) fungal endocarditis; 4) endocarditis caused by intracellular parasites such as *Bartonella* species, *Chlamydia* species, and perhaps viruses; or 5) noninfectious (marantic) or alternative diagnoses (Table 5). *Bartonella* species are slow-growing gram-negative bacteria that may require a month or longer for culture isolation. Organisms may be detected by plating sediment from lysis-centrifugation blood culture system onto chocolate media and incubating the latter under conditions of increased carbon dioxide and humidity for 30 days or longer. If valvular tissue is available, Warthin-Starry staining may show pleomorphic organisms. Molecular techniques and serology may also be useful.

Coxiella burnetii, the agent of Q fever, may also cause endocarditis. It occurs most commonly in males, and most patients have underlying heart disease. Typically, the presentation of Q-fever endocarditis is chronic, with a history of an influenza-like illness 6 to 12 months previously. Risk factors include exposure to sheep, cattle, rabbits, or parturient cats. Most commonly, the aortic valve is involved, and there may be associated hepatosplenomegaly, hepatitis, thrombocytopenia, hypergammaglobulinemia, and immune complex glomerulonephritis. Because the isolation of *C. burnetii* poses hazards to laboratories, the diagnosis is often made with serologic studies. Valve replacement is often necessary for cure.

- In patients with *Aspergillus* infective endocarditis, most blood cultures will be negative.
- *Coxiella burnetii*, the agent of Q fever, may also cause endocarditis.

- Viridans streptococci are the most common agent of native valve endocarditis in nonintravenous drug users.
- *S. aureus* is the most common agent of endocarditis in intravenous drug users.

Antimicrobial Therapy of Infective Endocarditis

Several principles govern the therapy of infective endocarditis. 1) The selection of antimicrobial agents to be used must be based on microbial susceptibility testing after isolation of the causative microbe. 2) Generally, parenteral antimicrobial agents are preferred because of the erratic absorption of oral agents, although some recently available oral agents (e.g., fluoroquinolines) may be suitable for treatment in highly selected cases. 3) Generally, treatment requires prolonged administration of antimicrobial agents. 4) Bactericidal agents or antibiotic combinations that produce synergistic, rapidly bactericidal effects are used. 5) When aminoglycosides are used for treatment, the concentration of antibiotic in the serum should be measured periodically because these agents have a low toxic-therapeutic ratio, especially in elderly patients and in those with renal disease. Peak and trough concentrations should be measured and the dose adjusted accordingly. Regimens for treatment of infective endocarditis are shown in Table 6.

- Penicillin-susceptible viridans streptococcal endocarditis may be treated with a 2-week course of penicillin G and gentamicin.
- Enterococcal endocarditis must be treated with a cell-wall active agent to which the organism is susceptible and an aminoglycoside when high-level resistance is not present.

Anticoagulation does not prevent embolization related to infective endocarditis. In patients with infective endocarditis in whom anticoagulation is needed for an underlying condition (e.g., prosthetic heart valves, mitral stenosis with atrial fibrillation), anticoagulation treatment should be given. Persistent or recurrent fever despite appropriate antimicrobial therapy may be due to pulmonary or systemic emboli or drug hypersensitivity; however, the most common cause is extensive infection of the valve ring or adjacent structures.

- Anticoagulation does not prevent embolization related to infective endocarditis.

Table 5.—Clues to the Diagnosis of Culture-Negative Endocarditis

Epidemiologic clues
  Travel to endemic areas—*Coxiella burnetii, Brucella* spp.
  Exposure to animals or their products—*C. burnetii, Chlamydia psittaci, Brucella* spp., *Bartonella henselae*
  Risk factors for fungal endocarditis
  Travel to areas endemic for demographic fungi
  Intravenous drug use—fungi, *Corynebacterium* spp.
  Homeless persons, chronic alcoholism, human immunodeficiency virus—*Bartonella* spp.
  Underlying immunocompromised host—*Listeria* spp., *Corynebacterium* spp., *Legionella* spp.
  Poor dental hygiene—HACEK group, nutritionally variant streptococci
Echocardiographic clues
  Large vegetations—HACEK group, fungi
  Vegetations with "fingerlike projections"—*Chlamydia* spp.
Clinical clues
  Periodontal disease, emboli—nutritionally variant streptococci, HACEK group
  Underlying neoplasm (atrial myxoma, adenocarcinoma, lymphoma, rhabdomyosarcoma, carcinoid tumor)—noninfective
    endocarditis
  Underlying autoimmune disease (rheumatic heart disease, systemic lupus erythematosus)—Libman-Sacks endocarditis,
    antiphospholipid syndrome, polyarteritis nodosa, Behçet disease, noninfective endocarditis
  Postvalvular operation—noninfectious process (e.g., thrombus, suture(s), other postvalvular surgical change)
  Miscellaneous conditions associated with noninfective endocarditis (e.g., eosinophilic heart disease, ruptured mitral chordae,
    myxomatous degeneration)

HACEK, *Haemophilus* spp, *Actinobacillus actinomycetemcomitans, Cardiobacterium hominis, Eikenella corrodens*, and *Kingella* spp.

Enterococcal Endocarditis

Enterococci deserve special mention because of their relative or absolute resistance to certain antimicrobial agents. Most enterococci are inhibited—but not killed—by clinically relevant concentrations of all effective antibiotics used singly. However, penicillin, ampicillin, or vancomycin in combination with certain aminoglycoside antibiotics exerts a synergistic bactericidal effect on these organisms. The degree of resistance of enterococci to aminoglycosides is highly variable. A minimal inhibitory concentration greater than or equal to 2,000 µg streptomycin/mL or 500 µg gentamicin/mL is considered the dividing point between low-level and high-level resistance of enterococci to these agents. Enterococci that are highly resistant to an aminoglycoside are not synergistically killed when that aminoglycoside is combined with either penicillin or vancomycin. For enterococci that do not exhibit high-level resistance to streptomycin or gentamicin, either aminoglycoside provides synergistic killing when combined with penicillin or vancomycin.

Because high-level resistance to gentamicin and streptomycin is encoded by separate genes, strains of enterococci that cause endocarditis should be screened with both compounds, and an aminoglycoside to which the strain is not highly resistant should be used for treatment. If endocarditis is caused by a strain of enterococci that exhibits high-level resistance to both gentamicin and streptomycin, the addition of an aminoglycoside to a cell-wall active agent will not be beneficial. Instead, prolonged treatment (8 to 12 weeks) with high doses of penicillin or ampicillin may cure ~50% of these patients. Surgical intervention should be considered for those in whom therapy fails. Along with the increasing incidence of aminoglycoside resistance, both penicillin and vancomycin resistance have been seen in enterococci.

All enterococcal strains that cause endocarditis must be screened to define antimicrobial resistance patterns. For enterococci with intrinsic high-level resistance to penicillin (minimal inhibitory concentrations > 16 µg/mL), vancomycin is the agent of choice for synergistic therapy, but for organisms resistant to penicillin because of β-lactamase production, either ampicillin-sulbactam sodium or vancomycin may be combined with an aminoglycoside for bactericidal synergistic therapy. For organisms resistant to both penicillin and vancomycin, the optimal treatment is unknown. No regimen of choice has emerged. Surgical intervention may be required.

• Most enterococci are inhibited—but not killed—by clinically relevant concentrations of all effective antibiotics used singly.

Methicillin-susceptible staphylococcal endocarditis is treated with nafcillin or, alternatively, cefazolin or vancomycin for 4 to 6 weeks, with aminoglycosides optional for the first 3 to 5 days of treatment. The combination of nafcillin plus gentamicin, in comparison with nafcillin alone, results in a more rapid rate of eradication of *S. aureus* bacteremia in the setting of infective endocarditis, but it does not improve mortality and is associated with increased nephrotoxicity. Importantly, in intravenous drug addicts with right-sided *S. aureus* endocarditis without evidence of renal failure, extrapulmonary metastatic infectious complications, aortic or mitral valve involvement, meningitis, or infection by methicillin-resistant *S. aureus*, 2 weeks of treatment with nafcillin plus tobramycin may be effective. In methicillin-susceptible staphylococcal endocarditis, a β-lactam agent is more effective than vancomycin. For selected intravenous drug users with right-sided *S. aureus* endocarditis, oral therapy with a 28-day course of ciprofloxacin and rifampin may be effective. In patients with infective endocarditis caused by methicillin-resistant *S. aureus* or methicillin-resistant coagulase-negative staphylococcus, vancomycin is the therapy of choice.

Regimens for treating endocarditis caused by HACEK microorganisms are listed in Table 6. Fungal endocarditis is treated with a combination of medical and surgical approaches. The mainstay of antifungal drug therapy is amphotericin B; however, this agent is associated with significant toxicity. After 1 to 2 weeks of treatment with amphotericin B, surgery should be considered. If isolated tricuspid endocarditis is present (as in an intravenous drug user), total tricuspid valvulectomy may be sufficient. Rarely, removal of the vegetation alone is curative. Valve replacement is necessary for left-sided fungal endocarditis. The duration of antifungal therapy after surgery varies. Oral antifungal agents (e.g., fluconazole, itraconazole) are not recommended as first-line agents for fungal endocarditis. Fluconazole as a single agent may, however, be considered as a therapeutic agent for candidal endocarditis under certain circumstances (e.g., when both surgery and amphotericin B are contraindicated and the organism is sensitive to fluconazole).

Q-fever endocarditis is usually treated with prolonged courses (at least 3 years) of doxycycline and trimethoprim-sulfamethoxazole, rifampin, or a quinolone. Valve replacement is often required. The long-term prognosis is guarded.

Therapy for culture-negative endocarditis is controversial. Recommended empiric antimicrobial therapy for patients with apparent culture-negative endocarditis is outlined in Table 7.

Cardiac Surgery in Infective Endocarditis
Indications for cardiac surgical intervention in patients with active native valve infective endocarditis are outlined in Table 8.

If organisms are found at surgery (e.g., with Gram's stain, positive cultures, or in annular abscesses), late complications are more frequent. In contrast to left-sided infective endocarditis, in which congestive heart failure is the usual indication for surgical intervention, persistent infection is the usual indication for surgery in right-sided infective endocarditis. Most of these patients are intravenous drug users with endocarditis caused by organisms that are difficult to eradicate with antimicrobial therapy alone. Currently, tricuspid valvulectomy or resection of the vegetation with valvuloplasty is the procedure of choice for refractory right-sided endocarditis. A recently described alternative is transplantation of a cryopreserved mitral homograft into the tricuspid position. Valve replacement and a second operation are indicated only when medical management fails to adequately control the hemodynamic manifestations and the patient has ceased to use illicit drugs.

Prosthetic Valve Endocarditis

Prosthetic valve endocarditis has been reported to occur in up to 10% of patients during the lifetime of the prosthesis. For mechanical prostheses, the incidence peaks in the first few weeks after valve replacement and then decreases to a stable low incidence rate during subsequent months to years. The risk of infection for mechanical and bioprosthetic valves is not significantly different. There is no difference in the risk of prosthetic valve endocarditis between patients with mitral or aortic prostheses. Prosthetic valve endocarditis has been classified arbitrarily as "early" when it occurs within the first 60 days after implantation and "late" when it occurs after 60 days. Classically, it was thought that "early" cases were acquired at the time of implantation and "late" cases thereafter. Subsequently, it was shown that many cases of prosthetic valve endocarditis that occur during the first year after surgery are acquired at the time of implantation. Some investigators have recommended that the time limit for early disease be extended to 6 months or even 1 year.

Table 6.—Antimicrobial Treatment in Adults With Infective Endocarditis

Causative agent	Antibiotic	Dosage and route	Duration of treatment, wk	Comments
I. Native valve endocarditis				
Viridans streptococci and *Streptococcus bovis* penicillin-susceptible (MIC, < 0.2 mg/mL)	1) Aqueous crystalline penicillin G *or*	12-18 million U/24 hr IV continuously or 6 equally divided doses	4	Preferred in most patients older than 65 yr and in those with impaired CN VIII or renal function
	Ceftriaxone	2 g once daily IV or IM*	4	
	2) Aqueous crystalline penicillin G *with*	12-18 million U/24 hr IV continuously or 6 equally divided doses	2	When obtained 1 hr after 20-30 min IV infusion or IM injection, serum concentration of genta-
	Gentamicin†	1 mg/kg IM or IV every 8 hr	2	micin of ~3 µg/mL is desirable; trough concentration should be < 1 µg/mL
	3) Vancomycin‡	30 mg/kg per 24 hr IV in two equally divided doses, not to exceed 2 g/24 hr unless serum levels are monitored	4	Vancomycin is recommended for patients allergic to β-lactams
Viridans streptococci and *S. bovis* relatively resistant to penicillin (MIC, 0.1-0.5 µg/mL)	1) Aqueous crystalline penicillin G *with*	18 million U/24 hr IV continuously or 6 equally divided doses	4	Cefazolin or other first-generation cephalosporins may be substituted for penicillin in patients
	Gentamicin†	1 mg/kg IM or IV every 8 hr	2	with penicillin hypersensitivity not of the immediate type
	2) Vancomycin‡	30 mg/kg per 24 hr IV in 2 equally divided doses, not to exceed 2 g/24 hr unless serum levels are monitored	4	Vancomycin is recommended for patients allergic to β-lactams
Enterococci (and viridans streptococci with penicillin MIC > 0.5 µg/mL, nutritionally variant viridans streptococci)	1) Aqueous crystalline penicillin G *with*	18-30 million U/24 hr IV either continuously or 6 equally divided doses	4-6	4-wk therapy recommended for patients with symptoms < 3 mo duration; 6-wk therapy
	Gentamicin	1 mg/kg IM or IV every 8 hr	4-6	for patients with symptoms > 3 mo duration
	2) Ampicillin *with*	12 g/24 hr IV either continuously or 6 equally divided doses	4-6	
	Gentamicin	1 mg/kg IM or IV every 8 hr	4-6	
	3) Vancomycin‡ *with*	30 mg/kg per 24 hr IV in 2 equally divided doses, not exceeding 2 g/24 hr unless serum levels are monitored	4-6	Vancomycin is recommended for patients allergic to β-lactams; cephalosporins are not
	Gentamicin	1 mg/kg IM or IV every 8 hr	4-6	acceptable alternatives for patients allergic to penicillin

Table 6 (continued)

Causative agent	Antibiotic	Dosage and route	Duration of treatment, wk	Comments
Staphylococci-penicillin-susceptible	Aqueous crystalline penicillin G	20 million U/24 hr IV either continuously or 6 equally divided doses	4-6	
Staphylococci-methicillin-susceptible	1) Nafcillin or oxacillin *with*	2 g IV every 4 hr	4-6	Benefit of additional aminoglycosides has not been established
	Optional addition of gentamicin*	1 mg/kg IM or IV every 8 hr	3-5 days	
	2) Cefazolin (or other first-generation cephalosporin in equivalent dosages) *with*	2 g IV every 8 hr	4-6	For β-lactam-allergic patients, cephalosporins should be avoided in those with immediate-type hypersensitivity to penicillin
	Optional addition of gentamicin[†]	1 mg/kg IM or IV every 8 hr	3-5 days	
Staphylococci-methicillin-resistant	Vancomycin[‡]	30 mg/kg per 24 hr IV in 2 equally divided doses, not exceeding 2 g/24 hr unless serum levels are monitored	4-6	
HACEK microorganisms	1) Ceftriaxone	2 g once daily IV or IM*	4	Cefotaxime sodium or other third-generation cephalosporins may be substituted
	2) Ampicillin[§] *with*	2 g IV every 4 hr or 12 g/24 hr IV continuously		
	Gentamicin	1 mg/kg body weight (not exceeding 80 mg) IM or IV every 8 hr		
II. Prosthetic valve endocarditis				
Staphylococci-methicillin-resistant	Vancomycin[‡]	30 mg/kg per 24 hr IV in 2 or 4 equally divided doses, not exceeding 2 g/24 hr unless serum levels are monitored	≥6	
	with Rifampin and	300 mg orally every 8 hr	≥6	Rifampin increases amount of warfarin sodium required for antithrombotic therapy
	Gentamicin	1.0 mg/kg IM or IV every 8 hr	2	
Staphylococci-methicillin-sensitive	Nafcillin or oxacillin *with*	2 g IV every 4 hr	≥6	First-generation cephalosporins or vancomycin should be used in patients allergic to β-lactams. Cephalosporins should be avoided in patients with immediate-type hypersensitivity to penicillin or with methicillin-resistant staphylococci
	Rifampin and	300 mg orally every 8 hr	≥6	
	Gentamicin	1.0 mg/kg IM or IV every 8 hr	2	

Table 6 (continued)

Causative agent	Antibiotic	Dosage and route	Duration of treatment, wk	Comments
Streptococci-nonentero-coccal-penicillin-susceptible (MIC, ≤ 0.1 µg/mL)	1) Aqueous crystalline penicillin G *with*	20 million U/day IV in divided doses every 4 hr	6	
	Gentamicin	1 mg/kg body weight (not exceeding 80 mg) IV or IM q8h	2	
	2) Cephalothin	2.0 g IV every 4 hr	6	
	3) Cefazolin	2.0 g IV every 8 hr	6	
Diphtheroids-gentamicin-susceptible (MIC, ≤ 4 µg/mL)	1) Aqueous crystalline penicillin G *with*	20 million U/day in divided doses every 4 hr	6	
	Gentamicin	1 mg/kg body weight (not exceeding 80 mg) IV or IM every 8 hr	6	
	2) Vancomycin	30 mg/kg body weight IV in divided doses every 12 hr or 6 hr	6	
Diphtheroids-gentamicin-resistant (MIC, > 4 µg/mL)	1) Vancomycin	30 mg/kg body weight IV in divided doses every 12 hr or 6 hr	6	
	2) Ampicillin[§]	2 g IV every 4 hr	6	
HACEK microorganisms	1) Ceftriaxone	2 g once daily IV or IM[*]	6	Cefotaxime or other third-generation cephalo-sporins may be substituted
	2) Ampicillin[§] *with*	2 g IV every 4 hr or 12 g/24 hr IV continuously	6	
	Gentamicin	1 mg/kg body weight (not exceeding 80 mg) IM or IV every 8 hr	6	

CN, cranial nerve; HACEK, *Haemophilus* spp, *Actinobacillus actinomycetemcomitans*, *Cardiobacterium hominis*, *Eikenella corrodens*, and *Kingella* spp; IV, intravenous; IM, intramuscular; MIC, minimal inhibitory concentration.

[*]Patients should be informed that IM injection of ceftriaxone is painful.

[†]Dosing of gentamicin on an mg/kg basis will produce higher serum concentrations in obese than in lean patients. Thus, in obese patients, dosing should be based on ideal body weight. (Ideal body weight for men is 50 kg + 2.3 kg/in. over 5 ft and for women, 45.5 kg + 2.3 kg/in. over 5 ft.) Relative contraindications to use of gentamicin are age > 65 yr and renal or CN VIII impairment. Other potentially nephrotoxic agents (e.g., nonsteroidal anti-inflammatory drugs) should be used cautiously in patients receiving gentamicin.

[‡]Vancomycin dosage should be decreased in patients with impaired renal function. Vancomycin given on an mg/kg basis will produce higher serum concentrations in obese than in lean patients. Thus, in obese patients, dosing should be based on ideal body weight. Each dose of vancomycin should be infused over at least 1 hr to reduce risk of histamine-release "red man" syndrome.

[§]Ampicillin should not be used if laboratory tests show β-lactamase production.

Modified from *JAMA* 274:1706-1713, 1995. By permission of the American Medical Association.

The mortality associated with prosthetic valve endocarditis is 30% to 80% in the early form and 20% to 40% in late postsurgical endocarditis, with an adverse prognosis associated with a new or changing murmur, new or worsening heart failure, persistent fever despite appropriate antibiotics, new conduction abnormalities that are often associated with myocardial abscess, renal insufficiency, *S. aureus* as the causative agent, and neurologic complications.

- Prosthetic valve endocarditis has been reported to occur in up to 10% of patients during the lifetime of the prosthesis.
- Prosthetic valve endocarditis has been classified arbitrarily as "early" when it occurs within the first 60 days after implantation and "late" when it occurs after 60 days.

Pathogenesis of Prosthetic Valve Endocarditis

Early *S. epidermidis* prosthetic valve endocarditis is thought to result from valve contamination during the perioperative period. This may occur at the time of surgery or in the immediate postoperative period when the prosthetic valve and sewing ring are not yet endothelialized and are susceptible to microbial colonization. Bacteria or fungi originating from intraoperative sources, infected intravascular catheters, cardiac pacemakers, or pressure-monitoring devices may seed the prosthesis. Bacteremia may result from postoperative infections at extracardiac sites. Nosocomial bacteremia is an important risk factor for prosthetic valve endocarditis. Another potential (but uncommon) source of infection is contamination of the prosthesis before implantation (e.g., contamination of glutaraldehyde-fixed porcine prosthetic valves with *Mycobacterium chelonei*). Early prosthetic valve endocarditis is associated with surgeons in training, a history of previous endocarditis, coma, prolonged mechanical ventilation, deep postoperative wound infections, postoperative jaundice, and ventricular arrhythmias.

The pathogenesis of late prosthetic valve endocarditis appears similar to that of native valve endocarditis, with microorganisms from a transient bacteremia localizing on a prosthesis or area of damaged endothelium. This is reflected in the much higher proportion of infection due to viridans streptococci in late disease. Even late prosthetic valve endocarditis caused by *S. epidermidis* or other organisms that typically cause early prosthetic valve endocarditis may result from a delayed onset of the infection acquired in the perioperative period.

Valve-Ring Abscess

Valve-ring abscess is a serious complication of prosthetic valve endocarditis and is seen with mechanical and bioprosthetic valves. Valve-ring abscesses occur where infection involves the sutures used to secure the sewing ring to the periannular tissue; this may result in dehiscence of the valve. The clinical finding of a new perivalvular leak in a patient with prosthetic valve endocarditis is presumptive evidence of a valve-ring abscess. Extension of the abscess beyond the valve ring may result in myocardial abscess formation, septal perforation, or purulent pericarditis. In addition to sewing-ring abscesses, prosthetic valve endocarditis of the bioprosthesis may cause leaflet destruction, with

Table 7.—Empiric Antimicrobial Therapy for Patients With Apparent Culture-Negative Endocarditis

Clinical setting	Antimicrobial therapy	Alternative regimen
Acute onset		
Native valve	Nafcillin plus an aminoglycoside	Vancomycin hydrochloride plus an aminoglycoside
Subacute onset		
Native valve	Ampicillin-sulbactam plus an aminoglycoside	Vancomycin-ceftriaxone sodium and an aminoglycoside
Prosthetic valve	Vancomycin plus an aminoglycoside plus rifampin (consider broader coverage for gram-negative bacilli)	
Intravenous drug use	Nafcillin plus an aminoglycoside (consider broader coverage for gram-negative bacilli)	Vancomycin plus an aminoglycoside

From *Mayo Clin Proc* 72:532-542, 1997. By permission of Mayo Foundation for Medical Education and Research.

Table 8.—Indications for Cardiac Surgery in Patients With Native Valve Infective Endocarditis

Accepted indications
    Congestive heart failure and hemodynamic instability
        Valvular incompetence or stenosis
    Unresponsive infection
        Fungal endocarditis
        Gram-negative bacillus endocarditis
        Persistent bacteremia
        Paravalvular invasion and abscess
Relative indications
    Systemic emboli
    Staphylococcus aureus infection
    Echocardiographically demonstrable vegetations
    Relapse

From *Mediguide® to Infect Dis* 9 issue 3:1, 1989. By permission of Lawrence DellaCorte Publications.

resulting valvular incompetence. Large vegetations occasionally obstruct blood flow and lead to functional valvular stenosis or a combination of stenosis and insufficiency. This complication appears to be more common in mitral prosthetic valve endocarditis than in aortic disease. Extracardiac pathologic features classically associated with native valve endocarditis may also be seen in prosthetic valve endocarditis. Immune complex-mediated glomerulonephritis manifested by an abnormal urinalysis with or without increased serum levels of creatinine has been described in patients with prosthetic valve endocarditis. Bioprosthetic valve endocarditis may involve only the valve cusps, the sewing ring, or both.

The strongest predictor of mortality in prosthetic valve endocarditis is renal dysfunction; other risk factors include patient's age, time to diagnosis, and mode of management.

- Early prosthetic valve endocarditis results from valve contamination during the perioperative period.
- Late prosthetic valve endocarditis results more often from transient bacteremia.

Clinical Manifestations of Prosthetic Valve Endocarditis

Symptoms and signs of prosthetic valve endocarditis include fever, new or changing murmurs, systemic emboli, petechiae, splenomegaly, peripheral signs (Osler nodes, Janeway lesions, Roth spots), anemia, hematuria, and leukocytosis. Clinical evidence of systemic embolization is reported in about 40%

of patients. New or changing cardiac murmurs are reported in up to 56% of patients with prosthetic valve endocarditis. Regurgitant murmurs reflect the hemodynamic consequences of valvular insufficiency due to a perivalvular leak, whereas muffling of heart sounds or stenosis murmurs result from occlusion or malfunction of the prosthetic valve.

- New or changing murmurs are not present in all patients with prosthetic valve endocarditis.
- Persistently positive blood cultures are the hallmark of prosthetic valve endocarditis.

Laboratory Findings in Prosthetic Valve Endocarditis

Anemia, hematuria, and leukocytosis may be seen in prosthetic valve endocarditis. As in native valve endocarditis, blood culture is the most important laboratory test used to make the diagnosis of prosthetic valve endocarditis. Importantly, not all instances of bacteremia occurring after valve replacement indicate prosthetic valve endocarditis. Prosthetic valves seem relatively resistant to colonization by gram-negative bacilli, and prosthetic valve endocarditis is rare after transient gram-negative bacteremia. If gram-negative bacteremia clears after an extracardiac source is removed, patients who have no other manifestations of prosthetic valve endocarditis can usually be given a short course (2 weeks) of antibiotics intravenously. If, however, bacteremia fails to resolve or the source of infection is not apparent, patients should be assumed to have prosthetic valve endocarditis. Because gram-positive bacteria are more adherent, their presence in blood cultures often reflects colonization of the prosthetic device. However, if there is doubt about the significance of a positive blood culture (e.g., a single blood culture growing coagulase-negative staphylococci in the absence of clinical manifestations), antimicrobial therapy may reasonably be withheld while additional culture results are being obtained.

Transthoracic echocardiography is less useful in the diagnosis of prosthetic valve endocarditis than in native valve endocarditis, because the echoes generated by the prosthesis may mask subtle abnormalities such as small vegetations. Transesophageal echocardiography is more sensitive than transthoracic echocardiography for the detection of vegetations and valvular complications. Nonetheless, transesophageal echocardiography is only 36% sensitive for detecting perivalvular abscess in patients with prosthetic valve endocarditis. Myocardial damage from ischemia, due to coronary artery flow impairment, myocardial abscess, or pericarditis, may cause various arrhythmias or conduction defects in patients with prosthetic valve endocarditis.

CT (or magnetic resonance imaging) of the head is indicated in all patients with prosthetic valve endocarditis and neurologic symptoms. Infarction, hemorrhage, or abscess usually can be differentiated by this technique. In addition, cerebral angiography should be considered in all patients with neurologic symptoms not readily explained by CT findings to exclude the possibility of an intracranial mycotic aneurysm.

- Transesophageal echocardiography is recommended for diagnosis of prosthetic valve endocarditis.
- CT of the head is indicated in patients with prosthetic valve endocarditis and neurologic symptoms.

Diagnostic Criteria

The currently accepted diagnostic criteria for infective endocarditis are outlined in Table 3.

Microbiology

Table 9 lists the microbial causes of prosthetic valve endocarditis. Among cases of prosthetic valve endocarditis, coagulase-negative staphylococci are the dominant cause of endocarditis occurring in the first postoperative year. The organisms causing prosthetic valve endocarditis more than 12 months after valve implantation differ from those causing this condition during the first year and are similar to those associated with native valve endocarditis (except for nosocomial and drug abuse-associated infective endocarditis). During this late postoperative period, the predominant causes of infection are streptococci, coagulase-negative staphylococci, enterococci, S. aureus, and members of the HACEK group of organisms. A broad range of bacteria have also caused sporadic cases of prosthetic valve endocarditis. Corynebacterium species cause prosthetic valve endocarditis that occurs within the first 6 postoperative months and are notable because of their relative resistance to many antimicrobial agents (other than vancomycin) and their fastidious growth requirements. In addition, various unusual organisms have been reported as the etiologic agents for specific cases of prosthetic valve endocarditis, including Nocardia asteroides, Bacillus cereus, Listeria monocytogenes, and Legionella species.

Fungi not only account for a significant number of cases of prosthetic valve endocarditis but are associated with high case fatality rates. Candida species followed by Aspergillus species are the two most common fungi that cause prosthetic valve endocarditis. Fungal vegetations formed on prosthetic valves are bulky and may partially occlude the orifice or embolize and occlude medium-sized arteries. Notably, patients with prosthetic heart valves who develop nosocomial candidemia are at risk for either having or developing candidal prosthetic valve endocarditis months or years later. Late-onset candidemia and lack of an identifiable portal of entry should heighten concern about candidal prosthetic valve endocarditis in such patients. Patients with prosthetic valve endocarditis caused by Legionella species, mycobacteria, and fungi other than Candida species commonly have negative blood cultures at presentation when routine techniques are used. Similarly, in patients with prosthetic valve endocarditis due to C. burnetii, blood cultures are negative. This diagnosis is suggested by serologic testing and confirmed by isolation of the organism from the prosthesis itself.

- Coagulase-negative staphylococci are the most common cause of prosthetic valve endocarditis in the first postoperative year.

Treatment

Antimicrobial therapy is based on laboratory identification of the etiologic microorganism and in vitro susceptibility testing. Bactericidal antibiotics are necessary. Recommended antibiotic regimens are listed in Table 6. Many isolates of coagulase-negative staphylococci isolated from patients with prosthetic valve endocarditis are resistant to oxacillin. For methicillin-resistant staphylococcal infection on prosthetic valves, treatment with a combination of vancomycin, rifampin, and gentamicin is recommended. Fungal prosthetic valve endocarditis requires combined medical and surgical therapy. For Candida endocarditis, high doses of amphotericin B given intravenously in combination with oral flucytosine are often used. For culture-negative prosthetic valve endocarditis, vancomycin plus gentamicin should be used. When prosthetic valve endocarditis is considered but the level of clinical suspicion is low, 3 or 4 blood specimens should be obtained by separate venipunctures for culture and the patient observed. If valve replacement is imminent, it is reasonable to initiate empirical antimicrobial therapy with vancomycin and gentamicin. The diagnosis of prosthetic valve endocarditis can usually be confirmed or excluded at the time of valve replacement.

- For methicillin-resistant staphylococcal infection on prosthetic valves, treatment with a combination of vancomycin,

Table 9.—Microbial Causes of Prosthetic Valve Endocarditis

Organism	No. of cases for 1975-1982		
	< 2 mo[*]	> 2-12 mo[*]	> 12 mo[*]
Coagulase-negative staphylococci	22	19	10
Staphylococcus aureus	2	3	5
Gram-negative bacilli	2	1	1
Streptococci (nonenterococcal)	0	1	12
Enterococci	0	2	4
Pneumococci	0	0	0
Diphtheroids	4	0	1
Fungi	2	2	1
Fastidious gram-negative coccobacilli (including HACEK organisms)	0	1	7
Others	3	2	1
Culture negative	3	3	2
Total	38	34	44

HACEK, *Haemophilus* spp, *Actinobacillus actinomycetemcomitans*, *Cardiobacterium hominis*, *Eikenella corrodens*, and *Kingella* spp.
[*]Time of onset after surgery.
Modified from Bisno AL, Waldvogel FA (editors): *Infections Associated With Indwelling Medical Devices.* Second edition. ASM Press, 1994, p 218. By permission of the publisher.

rifampin, and gentamicin is recommended.

- For culture-negative prosthetic valve endocarditis, vancomycin plus gentamicin should be used.

After initiation of antimicrobial therapy, blood should be cultured daily for the first few days and weekly thereafter until the completion of therapy. Usually, blood cultures will be sterile within 3 to 5 days after appropriate antimicrobial therapy is initiated. After the completion of therapy, blood should be cultured weekly for 1 month. A relapse necessitates reinstitution of antimicrobial therapy, retesting of the microorganism for antimicrobial susceptibility, and consideration of valve replacement. Occasionally, relapse may be due to persistent infection at an extracardiac site, including infection of the intravenous catheter used to administer the antimicrobial agent; careful consideration should be given to the possibility of an occult abscess or mycotic aneurysm.

Indications for cardiac surgery in patients with prosthetic valve endocarditis are listed in Table 10. Some of these indications are not absolute but rather serve to prompt careful consideration of surgical therapy. Moderate to severe congestive heart failure (New York Heart Association functional class III or IV) associated with prosthesis dysfunction is a commonly accepted indication for surgery. Few patients with this degree of prosthetic valve endocarditis-induced heart failure are alive 6 months after medical treatment, whereas combined surgical and medical treatment has resulted in survival rates of up to 64%.

Patients with relapse of prosthetic valve endocarditis after appropriate antibiotic therapy have been found to have invasive perivalvular infection; they are more likely to survive prosthetic valve endocarditis if treated surgically. Although several investigators favor surgical therapy for prosthetic valve endocarditis caused by *S. aureus* or coagulase-negative staphylococci, this is not a uniformly accepted indication for surgical treatment. Rather than being an indication for surgery, the potential for additional systemic emboli is often viewed as a factor that in combination with other considerations might help to justify surgery. In fact, a recent review noted that recurrent emboli are rare in patients with prosthetic valve endocarditis who are receiving appropriate antimicrobial therapy. Patients with culture-negative endocarditis who continue to experience fever during empiric antibiotic therapy are candidates for surgical intervention. Surgery will allow a definitive microbiologic diagnosis and development of specific, effective antimicrobial therapy. Also, some of these patients will be found to have fungal endocarditis or unrecognized invasive infection that warrants surgery. The association of vegetation size with risk of systemic embolization is controversial, but some have suggested that echocardiographically detected left-sided vegetations larger than 10 mm pose 1) a significantly increased risk of systemic embolization and 2) a greater need for valve-replacement surgery than cases in which either no or smaller vegetations are detected.

- Patients with culture-negative endocarditis who continue to experience fever during empiric antibiotic therapy are candidates for surgical intervention.
- Medical therapy alone is appropriate for some patients with prosthetic valve endocarditis.

The timing of cardiac surgery in patients with prosthetic valve endocarditis must be individualized. The hemodynamic status of the patient is the most important consideration in determining the timing of operation. As in patients with native valve endocarditis, the likelihood of those with

Table 10.—Indications for Cardiac Surgery in Patients With Prosthetic Valve Endocarditis

Moderate to severe heart failure due to prosthesis dysfunction (incompetence or obstruction)
Invasive and destructive perivalvular infection
    Partial valve dehiscence
    New or progressive conduction system disturbances
    Fever persisting 10 or more days during appropriate antibiotic therapy
    Purulent pericarditis
    Sinus of Valsalva aneurysm or intracardiac fistula
Uncontrolled bacteremic infection during therapy
Infection caused by selected organisms
    Fungi
    Staphylococcus aureus*
    Coagulase-negative staphylococci*
Relapse after appropriate antimicrobial therapy
Persistent fever during therapy for culture-negative prosthetic valve endocarditis in absence of other causes of fever
Recurrent arterial emboli*

*Relative indication.
From Bisno AL, Waldvogel FA (editors): *Infections Associated With Indwelling Medical Devices.* Second edition. ASM Press, 1994, p 233. By permission of the publisher.

prosthetic valve endocarditis surviving valve replacement is inversely related to the severity of the patient's heart failure at the time of operation. Thus, although in theory it may be desirable to control infection with antibiotic therapy preoperatively, this must not be attempted at the expense of progressive destruction of perivalvular tissue and further deterioration in the patient's hemodynamic status. Longer periods of antibiotic therapy preoperatively do not correlate with inability to recover bacteria from intraoperative cultures or with a more favorable outcome. Renal dysfunction preoperatively is one of the most important predictors of both increased operative mortality and overall long-term poor prognosis. Renal failure is often associated with advanced decompensated heart failure and low cardiac output.

- The hemodynamic status of the patient is the most important consideration in determining the timing of operation.

In selected patients with prosthetic valve endocarditis, the results of treatment with antibiotics alone are comparable to the results of combined surgical and medical therapy; for these patients, medical therapy is recommended. Included in this subgroup are patients with late-onset prosthetic valve endocarditis (12 months or more postoperatively) who are infected with less virulent organisms (viridans streptococci, enterococci, and fastidious gram-negative coccobacilli) and who do not develop complicated endocarditis.

Careful anticoagulation therapy has been advocated for patients with mechanical prosthetic valve endocarditis involving prostheses that usually would warrant maintenance of anticoagulation. Retrospective data suggest that the risk of central nervous system complications is higher among patients not receiving adequate anticoagulation therapy than among those receiving adequate anticoagulation therapy. Although a recent examination of this issue failed to confirm this benefit of anticoagulation therapy, increased risk of hemorrhagic stroke was not associated with anticoagulation therapy. Anticoagulation should be reversed temporarily if a patient experiences a hemorrhagic central nervous system event. Anticoagulation is not recommended for prosthetic valve endocarditis involving devices that under usual circumstances do not require anticoagulation therapy.

Prophylaxis of Infective Endocarditis

Prophylaxis for infective endocarditis is advised for patients who have an underlying cardiac condition that places them at increased risk for endocarditis and who are undergoing a procedure that carries a risk of transient bacteremia due to an organism that causes endocarditis. Endocarditis prophylaxis is recommended in high-risk and, in most cases, moderate-risk patients; it is not required in low-risk patients (Table 11).

Mitral valve prolapse is common and represents a spectrum of disease. The need for endocarditis prophylaxis for this condition is controversial. A clinical approach to determine the need for prophylaxis in persons with suspected mitral valve prolapse is shown in Figure 3. Mitral valve prolapse is often an abnormality of volume status, adrenergic state, or growth phase and not of valve structure or function. When normal valves prolapse without leaking, as in patients with one or more systolic clicks but no murmurs and no Doppler-demonstrated mitral regurgitation, the risk of endocarditis is not increased above that of the normal population. Therefore, antibiotic prophylaxis against bacterial endocarditis is not necessary. This is because it is

Table 11.—Cardiac Conditions Associated With
Endocarditis*

Endocarditis Prophylaxis Recommended

High-risk category
  Prosthetic cardiac valves, including bioprosthetic and
    homograft valves
  Previous bacterial endocarditis
  Complex cyanotic congenital heart disease (e.g., single
    ventricle states, transposition of the great arteries,
    tetralogy of Fallot)
  Surgically constructed systemic pulmonary shunts or
    conduits
Moderate-risk category
  Most other congenital cardiac malformations (other than
    above and below)
  Acquired valvar dysfunction (e.g., rheumatic heart
    disease)
  Hypertrophic cardiomyopathy
  Mitral valve prolapse with valvar regurgitation and/or
    thickened leaflets

Endocarditis Prophylaxis Not Recommended

Negligible-risk category (no greater risk than the general
  population)
  Isolated secundum atrial septal defect
  Surgical repair of atrial septal defect, ventricular septal
    defect, or patent ductus arteriosus (without residua
    beyond 6 mo)
  Previous coronary artery bypass graft surgery
  Mitral valve prolapse without valvar regurgitation
  Physiologic, functional, or innocent heart murmurs
  Previous Kawasaki disease without valvar dysfunction
  Previous rheumatic fever without valvar dysfunction
  Cardiac pacemakers (intravascular and epicardial) and
    implanted defibrillators

*Please consult the original table for references to the sources of the data.
From *JAMA* 277:1794-1801, 1997. By permission of the American Medical
Association.

not the abnormal valve motion but the jet of mitral insufficiency that creates the shear force and flow abnormalities that increase the likelihood of bacterial adherence on the valve during bacteremia. However, patients with prolapsing and leaking mitral valves, evidenced by audible clicks and murmurs of mitral regurgitation or by Doppler-demonstrated mitral insufficiency, should receive prophylactic treatment with antibiotics. Similarly, patients with myxomatous mitral valve degeneration with regurgitation should receive

endocarditis prophylaxis. Because older age and male sex have been shown to be risk factors for the development of endocarditis, men older than 45 years with mitral valve prolapse, even without a consistent systolic murmur, may warrant prophylaxis even in the absence of resting regurgitation.

Some experts believe that an audible nonejection click even without a murmur may identify patients with a potential for intermittent regurgitation and, thus, a risk of developing endocarditis. Although there are insufficient data on this issue, an isolated click may be an indication for more thorough evaluation of valve morphology and function, including Doppler echocardiographic imaging or auscultation during maneuvers that elicit or augment mitral regurgitation.

The American Heart Association has identified common procedures for which prophylaxis is recommended or not recommended according to the perceived degree of risk (Table 12). The recommended antimicrobial regimens for infective endocarditis prophylaxis are outlined in Tables 13 and 14. Some specific recommendations also apply to patients with prosthetic heart valves. Some experts have suggested that the criteria for using endocarditis prophylaxis should be downgraded, but this is controversial.

Before elective valve replacement, the dental health of every patient should be evaluated and any necessary dental work completed under close observation and with appropriate antibiotic coverage.

The number of organisms in the mouth and gingival crevices can be decreased temporarily by local irrigation with an antiseptic solution such as iodinated glycerol. Some dental experts recommend routine use of this measure before dental extractions.

Occasionally, a patient may be taking an antibiotic when going to see a physician or dentist. If the patient is taking an antibiotic normally used for endocarditis prophylaxis, it is prudent to select a drug from a different class rather than to increase the dose of the current antibiotic. In particular, antibiotic regimens used to prevent the recurrence of acute rheumatic fever are inadequate for the prevention of bacterial endocarditis. Persons who take an oral penicillin for secondary prevention of rheumatic fever or for other purposes may have viridans streptococci in their oral cavities that are relatively resistant to penicillin, amoxicillin, or ampicillin. In such cases, clindamycin, azithromycin, or clarithromycin should be selected for endocarditis prophylaxis. Because of possible cross-resistance with cephalosporins, this class of antibiotic should be avoided. If possible, one could delay the procedure until at least 9 to 14 days after

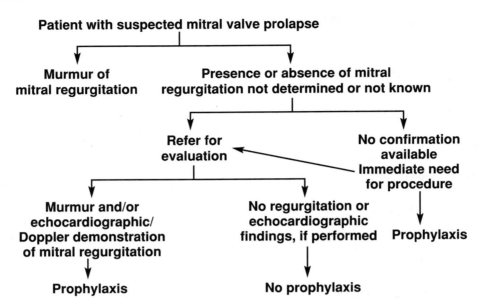

Fig. 3. Clinical approach to determination of need for prophylaxis in patients with suspected mitral valve prolapse. (From *JAMA* 277:1794-1801, 1997. By permission of the American Medical Association.)

completion of the antibiotic to allow the usual oral flora to be reestablished.

- Patients receiving a low dose of penicillin for rheumatic fever prophylaxis should not receive penicillin for endocarditis prophylaxis.

Pacemaker Infections

Pacemaker infections complicate 3.6% and 2% of epicardial and transvenous pacemaker placements, respectively. Infections can involve either the pocket in which the generator sits or the electrode leads or both, with or without concomitant bacteremia and, less commonly, with endocarditis. Generally, medical centers at which an experienced, dedicated team places all the devices have a much lower infection rate than those at which implantation is performed by several and less experienced teams. Risk factors for infection include the presence of diabetes mellitus, steroid use, underlying malignancy, overlying dermatologic disorders (especially pustular disorders), hematoma formation within the pocket, urgent placement or frequent replacement of the generator, and inexperience of the implantation team.

The most common location for pacemaker infections is the subcutaneous generator box pocket. Most such infections present soon after pacemaker implantation but may not become evident for 2 years or longer. The pathogenesis of generator box infections is thought to be contamination of the device by skin flora at the time of implantation. Wound infection or erosion of the box through the overlying skin may also lead to microbial contamination and subsequent infection. Infection can manifest with either local signs overlying the pocket itself (or the wires' tract) with or without any systemic findings or, less commonly, as an indolent systemic infection without any local findings. Early infections, those usually defined as occurring less than 60 days from implantation, typically present with acute symptoms (fever, leukocytosis, and local signs over the pocket such as pain, purulence, and overlying skin erythema). The primary source of the infection is the surgical wound and, consequently, involves skin flora. *S. aureus* is the most commonly recovered bacterium, with coagulase-negative staphylococci being the next most common. Late infections typically are more indolent and occult, with a paucity of local signs and symptoms. Coagulase-negative staphylococci tend to be more common in this group. The other major category of pacemaker infection is involvement of the epicardial or transvenous electrodes. This usually results from the direct spread of a microorganism along the wires of an infected generator box, but hematogenous seeding is seen occasionally. Isolated lead infections may present similarly to generator box infections and may or may not be accompanied by fever, bacteremia, and pulmonary lesions. Again, staphylococci are involved in most cases of infection of pacemaker leads.

Table 12.—Recommendations for Prophylaxis During Various Procedures That May Cause Bacteremia*

Endocarditis Prophylaxis Recommended

Dental Procedures[†]
  Dental extractions
  Periodontal procedures including surgery, scaling and
    root planing, probing, and recall maintenance
  Dental implant placement and reimplantation of avulsed
    teeth
  Endodontic (root canal) instrumentation or surgery only
    beyond the apex
  Subgingival placement of antibiotic fibers or strips
  Initial placement of orthodontic bands but not brackets
  Intraligamentary local anesthetic injections
  Prophylactic cleaning of teeth or implants where bleeding
    is anticipated

Other Procedures
  Respiratory tract
    Tonsilectomy and/or adenoidectomy
    Surgical operations that involve respiratory mucosa
    Bronchoscopy with a rigid bronchoscope
  Gastrointestinal tract[‡]
    Sclerotherapy for esophageal varices
    Esophageal stricture dilation
    Endoscopic retrograde cholangiography with biliary
      obstruction
    Biliary tract surgery
    Surgical operations that involve intestinal mucosa
  Genitourinary tract
    Prostatic surgery
    Cystoscopy
    Urethral dilation

Endocarditis Prophylaxis *Not* Recommended

Dental Procedures
  Restorative dentistry[§] (operative and prosthodontic) with
    or without retraction cord[//]
  Local anesthetic injections (nonintraligamentary)
  Intracanal endodontic treatment; post placement and
    buildup
  Placement of rubber dams
  Postoperative suture removal
  Placement of removable prosthodontic or orthodontic
    appliances
  Taking of oral impressions
  Fluoride treatments
  Taking of oral radiographs
  Orthodontic appliance adjustment
  Shedding of primary teeth
Other Procedures
  Respiratory tract
    Endotracheal intubation
    Bronchoscopy with a flexible bronchosope, with or

  without biopsy[¶]
  Tympanostomy tube insertion
Gastrointestinal tract
  Transesophageal echocardiography[¶]
  Endoscopy with or without gastrointestinal biopsy[//]
Genitourinary tract
  Vaginal hysterectomy[¶]
  Vaginal delivery[¶]
  Cesarean section[¶]
  In uninfected tissue:
    Urethral catheterization
    Uterine dilatation and curettage
    Therapeutic abortion
    Sterilization procedures
    Insertion or removal of intrauterine devices
Other
  Cardiac catheterization, including balloon angioplasty
  Implanted cardiac pacemakers, implanted
    defibrillators, and coronary stents

*Please consult the original table for references to the sources of the data.
[†]Prophylaxis is recommended for patients with high- and moderate-risk cardiac conditions.
[‡]Prophylaxis is recommended for high-risk patients; optional for medium-risk patients.
[§]This includes restoration of decayed teeth (filling cavities) and replacement of missing teeth.
[//]Clinical judgment may indicate antibiotic use in selected circumstances that may create significant bleeding.
[¶]Prophylaxis is optional for high-risk patients.
From *JAMA* 277:1794-1801, 1997. By permission of the American Medical Association.

Table 13.—Prophylactic Regimens for Dental, Oral, Respiratory Tract, or Esophageal Procedures*

Situation	Agent	Regimen[†]
Standard general prophylaxis	Amoxicillin	Adults: 2.0 g; children: 50 mg/kg orally 1 hr before procedure
Unable to take oral medications	Ampicillin	Adults: 2.0 g intramuscularly (IM) or intravenously (IV); children: 50 mg/kg IM or IV within 30 min before procedure
Allergic to penicillin	Clindamycin *or*	Adults: 600 mg; children: 20 mg/kg orally 1 hr before procedure
	Cefalexin[‡] or cefadroxil[‡] *or*	Adults: 2.0 g; children: 50 mg/kg orally 1 hr before procedure
	Azithromycin or clarithromycin	Adults: 500 mg; children: 15 mg/kg orally 1 hr before procedure
Allergic to penicillin and unable to take oral medications	Clindamycin *or*	Adults: 600 mg; children: 20 mg/kg IV within 30 min before procedure
	Cefazolin[‡]	Adults: 1.0 g; children: 25 mg/kg IM or IV within 30 min before procedure

*Please consult the original table for references to the sources of the data.
[†]Total children's dose should not exceed adult dose.
[‡]Cephalosporins should not be used in persons with immediate-type hypersensitivity reaction (urticaria, angioedema, or anaphylaxis) to penicillins.
From *JAMA* 277:1794-1801, 1997. By permission of the American Medical Association.

Table 14.—Prophylactic Regimens for Genitourinary and Gastrointestinal (Excluding Esophageal) Procedures*

Situation	Agents[†]	Regimen[‡]
High-risk patients	Ampicillin plus gentamicin	Adults: ampicillin 2.0 g intramuscularly (IM) or intravenously (IV) plus gentamicin 1.5 mg/kg (not to exceed 120 mg) within 30 min of starting the procedure; 6 hr later, ampicillin 1 g IM/IV or amoxicillin 1 g orally Children: ampicillin 50 mg/kg IM or IV (not to exceed 2.0 g) plus gentamicin 1.5 mg/kg within 30 min of starting the procedure; 6 hr later, ampicillin 25 mg/kg IM/IV or amoxicillin 25 mg/kg orally
High-risk patients allergic to ampicillin/amoxicillin	Vancomycin plus gentamicin	Adults: vancomycin 1.0 g IV over 1-2 hr plus gentamicin 1.5 mg/kg IV/IM (not to exceed 120 mg); complete injection/infusion within 30 min of starting the procedure Children: vancomycin 20 mg/kg IV over 1-2 hr plus gentamicin 1.5 mg/kg IV/IM; complete injection/infusion within 30 min of starting the procedure
Moderate-risk patients	Amoxicillin or ampicillin	Adults: amoxicillin 2.0 g orally 1 hr before procedure, or ampicillin 2.0 g IM/IV within 30 min of starting the procedure Children: amoxicillin 50 mg/kg orally 1 hr before procedure, or ampicillin 50 mg/kg IM/IV within 30 min of starting the procedure
Moderate-risk patients allergic to ampicillin/amoxicillin	Vancomycin	Adults: vancomycin 1.0 g IV over 1-2 hr; complete infusion within 30 min of starting the procedure Children: vancomycin 20 mg/kg IV over 1-2 hr; complete infusion within 30 min of starting the procedure

*Please consult the original table for references to the sources of the data.
[†]Total children's dose should not exceed adult dose.
[‡]No second dose of vancomycin or gentamicin is recommended.
From *JAMA* 277:1794-1801, 1997. By permission of the American Medical Association.

Whereas staphylococci are the predominant organisms recovered from pacemaker infections, gram-negative bacilli, yeast, anaerobes, and atypical mycobacteria have been recovered. Polymicrobial cultures are obtained 25% of the time. Patients are often bacteremic (up to 28%) in either presentation, even in the absence of systemic findings. Thus, despite the usual recovery of staphylococci from the wound, it is wise to culture blood, the pacemaker pocket, and any other wounds before initiating treatment with antibiotics. A definitive diagnosis of pacemaker infection depends on isolation of an etiologic microorganism from the pacemaker pocket or from the bloodstream. Transesophageal echocardiography may demonstrate vegetations in cases of infection of pacemaker leads.

Treatment of pacemaker infections remains controversial. All the hardware should be removed in both generator box and electrode infections, especially when these disorders are accompanied by bacteremia. A complication rate of 51% has been noted when functionless pacer electrodes are left in place after partial system removal for infection. However, occasional cures of generator box infections with parenteral antibiotics and local irrigation alone have been reported. Reported mortality rates for retained infected wires have ranged from 28% to 60%. Percutaneous removal of the wires generally is successful with the techniques of extraction available. Again, operator experience is essential for success and surgical backup is mandatory in the event of a complication (e.g., laceration or rupture of the right atrium or ventricle, tricuspid valve, pericardium, or venous system).

Parenteral antimicrobial agents must be chosen on the basis of identification and susceptibility of the isolated pathogen. The optimal duration of therapy is unknown, but it has been suggested that a 6-week course of antimicrobial therapy be administered in cases of pacemaker lead infections. Most centers use a single-step reimplantation strategy instead of a dual step (placing a temporary pacing system for a period of time during antibiotic therapy before placing a permanent device). If any foreign material is left in place, the use of long-term suppressive therapy should be considered, although this practice is of unproven efficacy.

Endocarditis prophylaxis is not recommended in patients with cardiac pacemakers.

- Staphylococci are the most common cause of pacemaker infections.
- When possible, all the hardware should be removed in pacemaker infections.

Implantable Cardioverter Defibrillator Infection

Implantable cardioverter defibrillator infections complicate 1% to 2% of implantable cardioverter defibrillator placements. In patients receiving epicardial implantable cardioverter defibrillator systems, the highest risk of infection has been observed in those undergoing concomitant cardiovascular surgery. The placement of a subcutaneous defibrillation patch is a risk factor for subsequent implantable cardioverter defibrillator infection. Infections may develop any time following implantable cardioverter defibrillator implantation, with a mean time to development of infection (after implantation) of approximately 6 months. Staphylococci are the predominant pathogens involved in implantable cardioverter defibrillator infections, with *S. aureus* accounting for approximately 25% of such infections and coagulase-negative staphylococci accounting for another 25%. The rest are caused by miscellaneous pathogens similar to those seen in pacemaker infections. Bacteremia may or may not be present in cases of implantable cardioverter defibrillator infections. The optimal management of infection of implantable cardioverter defibrillators is not well defined, but many authors have suggested that explantation of the whole implantable cardioverter defibrillator system is required along with a course of antimicrobial therapy.

Chagas Disease

Trypanosoma cruzi, the etiologic agent of American trypanosomiasis (or Chagas disease), is transmitted by various species of blood-sucking reduviid insects, or kissing bugs (Plate 14). Transmission to a human host occurs when mucous membranes, the conjunctiva, or breaks in the skin are contaminated with bug feces containing the infectious forms. Transmission of *T. cruzi* also occurs through blood transfusion and by congenital transmission. The insect vector necessary for natural transmission of *T. cruzi* is found from the southern half of the U.S. to southern Argentina. Despite the presence of *T. cruzi*-infected insects in many parts of the southern and western U.S., transmission of the agent to humans in the U.S. is rare, probably because of the relatively high housing standards and low overall vector density. The mean age at the time of infection in areas of intense transmission is 4 years. Currently, it is estimated that 16 to 18 million people are infected with *T. cruzi* and that up to 50,000 people die each year of Chagas disease. Most of the infected people are asymptomatic. The mean age at onset of the cardiac and gastrointestinal tract symptoms of chronic Chagas disease is 35 to 45 years. Several million people have immigrated to the U.S. from areas in which Chagas disease is endemic. Thus, physicians in the U.S. need to be familiar with Chagas disease not only in this immigrant population but also because transfusion-associated transmission of *T. cruzi* has been reported in the U.S. and Canada.

After the bite of the reduviid bug, acute Chagas disease may develop in a small proportion of patients. A chagoma, which consists of an injured area with erythema and swelling accompanied by local lymph node involvement, may be seen. Romaña's sign—the classic sign of acute Chagas disease—consists of painless edema of the palpebrae and periocular tissues and may appear when the conjunctiva is the portal of entry. These initial local signs are followed by fever, malaise, anorexia, and edema of the face and lower extremities. Generalized lymphadenopathy and mild hepatosplenomegaly may also occur. Meningeal encephalitis and severe myocarditis may rarely be seen (Plate 15).

Chronic Chagas disease becomes apparent years or even decades after the initial infection. The heart is the organ most commonly involved, and symptoms include rhythm disturbances, congestive heart failure, and thromboembolism (Plate 16). The cardiomyopathy that develops often affects primarily the right ventricle, and the classic signs of right-sided heart failure are frequently present. After congestive heart failure develops, death often occurs in a matter of months. Although some patients have both cardiomyopathy and arrhythmias, most do not. The clinical course is frequently complicated by emboli to the brain or other areas. Other findings of chronic Chagas disease include megaesophagus and megacolon. Heart transplantation in patients with end-stage Chagas cardiac disease is controversial because of postoperative reactivation of the infection. Gross examination of the hearts of chronic chagasic patients who died of heart failure reveals marked bilateral ventricular enlargement, often involving the right side of the heart more than the left side. Thinning of the ventricular walls is common, as are apical aneurysms and mural thrombi. Widespread lymphocytic infiltration is present, accompanied by diffuse interstitial fibrosis and atrophy of myocardial cells. Parasites are rarely seen. Dense fibrosis and chronic inflammatory lesions are common in the conduction system of chronic chagasic hearts.

The diagnosis of Chagas cardiac disease may be made by obtaining a history of residence in an area in which transmission occurs (or receipt of a blood transfusion in an endemic area), accompanied by the detection of IgG antibodies that bind specifically to parasite antigens in the serum. Indirect immunofluorescence, complement fixation, enzyme-linked immunoadsorbent, and radioimmunoprecipitation assays may be used. Direct detection of the parasite is rarely used.

Currently, two drugs are used to treat patients infected with *T. cruzi*: nifurtimox and benznidazole. However, both of them appear to be useful only in acute Chagas disease. The treatment of patients with chronic chagasic heart disease is supportive.

- Transfusion-associated transmission of *T. cruzi* has been reported in the U.S. and Canada.
- Chagas disease is caused by *T. cruzi*.
- The most commonly affected organ in chronic Chagas disease is the heart.
- Antimicrobial therapy is not effective in chronic chagasic heart disease.

Heart Involvement in Patients With Human Immunodeficiency Virus Infection

Myocardial Involvement at Autopsy

Premortem signs and symptoms underestimate the incidence of cardiac involvement in patients dying of acquired immunodeficiency syndrome (AIDS). Autopsy studies have demonstrated myocarditis in up to 77% of patients with AIDS. This myocarditis usually is mild and focal, but myocardial fibrosis and atrophy may also be observed. Cardiac chamber abnormalities observed at autopsy include ventricular hypertrophy and ventricular dilatation. Right ventricular dilatation is observed most frequently in patients with pulmonary complications of AIDS, such as *Pneumocystis carinii* pneumonia. This right ventricular dilatation may occur alone, may be seen in association with right ventricular hypertrophy, or may be seen in combination with left ventricular dilatation.

- Autopsy studies have demonstrated myocarditis in up to 77% of patients with AIDS.

Pericardial Involvement at Autopsy

Pericardial involvement is described at autopsy in up to one-third of patients with AIDS and includes serous pericarditis, nonspecific fibrinous pericarditis, tuberculous pericarditis, and pericardial inflammation accompanying infiltration of the pericardium with Kaposi sarcoma.

Kaposi sarcoma involvement of the heart is observed in up to 8% of postmortem examinations of patients who die of this complication of AIDS. Kaposi sarcoma may involve the pericardium, myocardium, valvular endothelium, and coronary arteries. Lymphomatous involvement of the heart may also be seen.

- Pericardial involvement is described at autopsy in up to one-third of patients with AIDS.

Endocardial Involvement at Autopsy

Nonbacterial thrombotic endocarditis is described in up to 6% of autopsies. Opportunistic organisms are identified in the myocardium in up to 13% of cases. These include *Toxoplasma gondii*, *Cryptococcus neoformans*, *Mycobacterium* species, and *Candida* species. These organisms may or may not be associated with microscopic evidence of surrounding myocardial inflammation, although myocardial abscesses have been reported.

S. aureus is the most common pathogen causing infective endocarditis in HIV-infected patients. The clinical presentation of endocarditis in these patients is similar when compared with patients who do not carry the virus. However, the sequelae may be more clinically severe in patients who have lower CD4 counts, and a higher mortality has been identified in those with CD4 counts less than 200/mm^3. Retrospective clinical studies have implicated an apparent higher rate of recurrence and inpatient mortality in patients with HIV who have endocarditis than in those without HIV. Prospective studies involving injection drug addicts correlated the presence of HIV infection and a lower CD4 count with the subsequent risk of developing endocarditis.

The rare, newly described entity of *Bartonella quintana* endocarditis appears to represent a true opportunistic infection, arising because of failure of cellular immunity. The treatment is erythromycin.

Clinical Manifestations

Clinical manifestations of cardiac involvement in patients with HIV infection are shown in Table 15. From 6% to 7% of patients with HIV infection have clinically significant cardiac disease manifested by cardiac tamponade, dilated cardiomyopathy, ventricular arrhythmias, or sudden cardiac death. Cardiac disease as a primary cause of death occurred in 1% to 6% of patients reported from 1981 to 1988. An incidence of heart failure of 2.1% has been described in patients infected with HIV. There appears to be an association between the severity of cardiac dysfunction and the magnitude of depression of CD4 counts. Global left ventricular dysfunction may be seen in patients who are asymptomatic from the cardiac standpoint and who do not have a third heart sound gallop. Evidence of left ventricular dysfunction on a single echocardiographic study does not portend an especially poor prognosis; in contrast, a persistently low left ventricular ejection fraction on serial studies is associated with a poor prognosis.

Up to 38% of patients with AIDS demonstrate pericardial effusion. Although usually silent, clinical symptoms of chest pain may be due to pericarditis. Cardiac tamponade has been described in several cases and may be secondary to involvement of the pericardium by Kaposi sarcoma. Pulmonary hypertension may also be noted, usually in patients with multiple pulmonary infections but occasionally in those without any preceding pulmonary infection.

Specific signs of cardiovascular involvement—such as the presence of an enlarged cardiac silhouette on a radiograph, the development of a pericardial friction rub, the clinical features of congestive heart failure with a third heart sound gallop, pulmonary edema, or the development of a pathologic murmur—are all findings that should initiate a cardiovascular diagnostic work-up.

Table 15.—Clinical Manifestations of Cardiac Involvement in Patients With Human Immunodeficiency Virus Infection

Myocardial involvement
    Asymptomatic ventricular dysfunction
    Dilated cardiomyopathy/heart failure
    Inflammatory myocarditis
    Right ventricular hypertrophy/dilatation
Pericardial involvement
    Pericardial effusion
    Pericarditis
    Cardiac tamponade
Endocardial involvement
    Infective endocarditis
    Nonbacterial thrombotic endocarditis
Conduction system involvement
    Nonspecific repolarization abnormalities
    Bundle branch block
    Atrioventricular block
    Supraventricular and ventricular arrhythmias
    Abnormal results on signal-averaged electrocardiogram
    Sudden cardiac death

From *Heart Dis Stroke* 3:388-394, 1994. By permission of the American Heart Association.

Symptomatic cardiac arrhythmias have been described premortem in patients dying of AIDS. They usually occur in patients with histologic evidence of myocarditis. Sudden cardiac death has also been reported in patients dying of AIDS, including polymorphous ventricular tachycardia culminating in ventricular fibrillation in a patient with active lymphocytic myocarditis proven on endomyocardial biopsy.

Pathogenesis

The pathogenesis of cardiac involvement in patients infected with HIV is incompletely understood but has been postulated to be due to direct myocardial injury from HIV, inflammatory myocarditis, immune-mediated processes and malnutrition, opportunistic cardiac infections (e.g., cytomegalovirus, herpes simplex virus, *Toxoplasma gondii*, *Cryptococcus neoformans*, *Aspergillus* species, *Candida* species, *Mycobacterium* species, *Coccidioides immitis*), neoplastic involvement (e.g., Kaposi sarcoma and lymphoma), and chemotherapeutic toxicity (e.g., zidovudine, didanosine, zalcitabine, foscarnet, and interferon alfa).

- Premortem signs and symptoms underestimate the incidence of cardiac involvement in patients dying of AIDS.
- Cardiac findings in patients dying of AIDS include myocarditis, pericarditis, ventricular wall and/or chamber abnormalities, myocardial involvement with Kaposi sarcoma, cardiac invasion from lymphoma, nonbacterial thrombotic endocarditis, infective endocarditis, and cardiac infection with opportunistic organisms.
- There appears to be an association between the severity of cardiac dysfunction and the magnitude of depression of CD4 counts.

Suggested Review Reading

1. Mugge A: Echocardiographic detection of cardiac valve vegetations and prognostic implications. *Infect Dis Clin North Am* 7:877-898, 1993.
The use of echocardiography is discussed vis-à-vis 1) diagnosis of endocarditis (visualization of vegetations), 2) demonstration of endocarditis-related complications (e.g., valvular destruction, myocardial abscess), and 3) identification of patients at risk (e.g., arterial embolism).

2. Wilson WR, Karchmer AW, Dajani AS, et al: Antibiotic treatment of adults with infective endocarditis due to streptococci, enterococci, staphylococci, and HACEK microorganisms. *JAMA* 274:1706-1713, 1995.
This article provides guidelines for the treatment of endocarditis in adults caused by viridans streptococci and other streptococci, enterococci, staphylococci, and fastidious gram-negative bacilli of the HACEK group.

3. DeWitt DE, Paauw DS: Endocarditis in injection drug users. *Am Fam Physician* 53:2045-2049, 1996.
This article discusses clinical manifestations of diagnosis and therapy of endocarditis in injection drug users.

4. Acar J, Michel PL, Varenne O, et al: Surgical treatment of infective endocarditis. *Eur Heart J* 16 (Suppl B):94-98, 1995.
This review presents a synopsis of indications for and optimal timing of surgical treatment of infective endocarditis.

5. Dajani AS, Taubert KA, Wilson W, et al: Prevention of bacterial endocarditis. Recommendations by the American Heart Association. *JAMA* 277:1794-1801, 1997.

Updates recommendations by the American Heart Association published in 1990 for the prevention of bacterial endocarditis in individuals at risk for this disease. Major changes in the updated recommendations include 1) emphasis that most cases of endocarditis are not attributable to an invasive procedure; 2) cardiac conditions are stratified into high-, moderate-, and negligible-risk categories based on potential outcome if endocarditis develops; 3) procedures that may cause bacteremia and for which prophylaxis is recommended are more clearly specified; 4) an algorithm was developed to define more clearly when prophylaxis is recommended for patients with mitral valve prolapse; 5) for oral or dental procedures, the initial amoxicillin dose is reduced to 2 g, a follow-up antibiotic dose is no longer recommended, erythromycin is no longer recommended for penicillin-allergic patients, but clindamycin and other alternatives are offered; and 6) for gastrointestinal or genitourinary procedures, the prophylactic regimens have been simplified.

6. Martin JM, Neches WH, Wald ER: Infective endocarditis: 35 years of experience at a children's hospital. *Clin Infect Dis* 24:669-675, 1997.
The authors review the predisposing conditions, the presenting signs and symptoms, as well as the risk factors and bacterial etiologies in children with infective endocarditis, focusing on hospital course and outcome.

7. Berbari EF, Cockerill FR III, Steckelberg JM: Infective endocarditis due to unusual or fastidious microorganisms. *Mayo Clin Proc* 72:532-542, 1997.
In this article, the authors review the microbiologic and clinical features of infective endocarditis due to fastidious organisms and provide recommendations for diagnosis and treatment.

8. Klug D, Lacroix D, Savoye C, et al: Systemic infection related to endocarditis on pacemaker leads: clinical presentation and management. *Circulation* 95:2098-2107, 1997.
This article reviews the clinical manifestations, diagnosis, and management of endocarditis related to pacemaker lead infection.

9. Tischler MD, Vaitkus PT: The ability of vegetation size on echocardiography to predict clinical complications: a meta-analysis. *J Am Soc Echocardiogr* 10:562-568, 1997.
The results of this meta-analysis support the hypothesis that echocardiographically detected left-sided vegetations > 10 mm pose 1) a significantly increased risk of systemic embolization and 2) a greater need for valve-replacement surgery than cases where either no or small vegetations are detected.

10. Lindner JR, Case RA, Dent JM, et al: Diagnostic value of echocardiography in suspected endocarditis. An evaluation based on the pretest probability of disease. *Circulation* 93:730-736, 1996.
The use and clinical application of echocardiography as a diagnostic tool in endocarditis is extensively reviewed in this paper, with emphasis placed on clinical stratification as to the pretest likelihood of disease prior to the selection of diagnostic interventions. The use of transthoracic and transesophageal echocardiographic techniques is discussed.

11. Smith PN, Vidaillet HJ, Hayes JJ, et al: Infections with nonthoracotomy implantable cardioverter defibrillators: can these be prevented? *Pacing Clin Electrophysiol* 21:42-55, 1998.

12. Strom BL, Abrutyn E, Berlin JA, et al: Dental and cardiac risk factors for infective endocarditis. A population-based, case-control study. *Ann Intern Med* 129:761-769, 1998.
This study showed that dental treatment did not seem to be a risk factor for infective endocarditis and that few cases of infective endocarditis would be preventable with antibiotic prophylaxis. This is a controversial issue.

13. Durack DT: Antibiotics for prevention of endocarditis during dentistry: time to scale back? *Ann Intern Med* 129:829-831, 1998.
This editorial suggests that endocarditis prophylaxis should be downgraded to "not recommended" for most dental procedures except extractions and gingival surgery (including implant placement) and for most underlying cardiac conditions except prosthetic valves and previous endocarditis. When any one or more of these four high-risk factors is present, prophylaxis should follow the American Heart Association guidelines (Table 12). This is a controversial issue.

Questions

Multiple Choice (choose the one best answer)

1. Which of the following is an indication for infective endocarditis prophylaxis in a patient undergoing sclerotherapy for esophageal varices?
   a. Previous bacterial endocarditis
   b. Isolated secundum atrial septal defect
   c. Previous coronary artery bypass graft surgery
   d. Prosthetic knee joint
   e. Cardiac pacemaker

2. The treatment of choice for a patient with native mitral valve endocarditis caused by methicillin-susceptible *Staphylococcus aureus* is:
   a. Nafcillin or oxacillin with or without gentamicin
   b. Vancomycin
   c. Ceftriaxone
   d. Cefotaxime
   e. Gentamicin

3. Cutaneous manifestations of infective endocarditis include all the following *except*:
   a. Janeway lesions
   b. Osler nodes
   c. Erythema marginatum
   d. Petechiae

4. The most common cause of infective endocarditis in intravenous drug users is:
   a. Viridans streptococci
   b. *Enterococcus faecium*
   c. *Staphylococcus aureus*
   d. *Candida parapsilosis*
   e. *Kingella kingae*

5. Indications for surgical intervention during active infective endocarditis include all the following *except*:
   a. Systemic emboli
   b. Fungal endocarditis
   c. Congestive heart failure and hemodynamic instability
   d. Paravalvular invasion and abscess
   e. Right-sided *Staphylococcus aureus* endocarditis

6. Which of the following is true about the treatment of infective endocarditis?
   a. When enterococci resistant to both penicillin G and vancomycin cause endocarditis, no medical therapy is reliably effective
   b. Cefazolin may be used to treat enterococcal endocarditis
   c. Oral agents such as fluconazole and itraconazole are the treatment of choice for fungal endocarditis
   d. A high dose of intravenous penicillin alone is effective in curing enterococcal endocarditis caused by penicillin-susceptible enterococci

7. Which of the following is true of Chagas disease?
   a. Most commonly, transmission occurs by the bite of a blood-sucking reduviid bug
   b. Nifurtimox and benznidazole are useful for treatment of chronic chagesic cardiac disease
   c. The heart is the organ most commonly involved by chronic Chagas disease
   d. The diagnosis of Chagas disease may be made easily by the isolation of the organisms from blood cultures

8. Culture-negative endocarditis commonly occurs for all the following reasons *except*:
   a. Q-fever endocarditis
   b. *Escherichia coli* endocarditis
   c. Fungal endocarditis
   d. Nutritionally variant streptococcal endocarditis
   e. *Bartonella quintana* endocarditis

9. A 28-year-old homeless man in Seattle, Washington, presents with a 2-month history of fever and night sweats. Examination is significant for heart murmur compatible with aortic insufficiency. Three sets of blood cultures are negative after 48 hours. The patient has not recently received antimicrobial therapy. The most likely diagnosis is endocarditis caused by:
   a. *Bartonella quintana*
   b. *Staphylococcus aureus*
   c. *Enterococcus faecium*
   d. *Pseudomonas aeruginosa*
   e. *Aspergillus fumigatus*

10. The HACEK group of organisms includes all the following *except*:
    a. *Eikenella corrodens*
    b. *Cardiobacterium hominis*
    c. *Haemophilus aphrophilus*
    d. *Helicobacter pylori*
    e. *Actinobacillus actinomycetemcomitans*

Answers

1. Answer a

Certain underlying conditions such as previous bacterial endocarditis are associated with a relatively high risk of infective endocarditis. In contrast, other disorders such as isolated atrial septal defect, previous coronary artery bypass graft surgery, prosthetic joints, and cardiac pacemakers are associated with very low or negligible risk (Table 11).

2. Answer a

In methicillin-susceptible staphylococcal endocarditis, a beta-lactam agent is more effective than vancomycin.

3. Answer c

Janeway lesions, Osler nodes, and petechiae are all cutaneous manifestations of infective endocarditis. Erythema marginatum is seen in association with rheumatic fever.

4. Answer c

Staphylococcus aureus is the most common cause of infective endocarditis in injection drug users.

5. Answer e

Indications for cardiac surgery in patients with endocarditis are shown in Table 8. *S. aureus* right-sided endocarditis typically responds to antimicrobial therapy alone.

6. Answer a

When enterococci resistant to both penicillin G and vancomycin cause endocarditis, no medical therapy is reliably effective.

7. Answer c

Trypanosoma cruzi, the etiologic agent of American trypanosomiasis, or Chagas disease, is transmitted by various species of blood-sucking reduviid bugs. Nifurtimox and benznidazole may be useful in the treatment of acute Chagas disease but show minimal usefulness in the treatment of chronic Chagas disease. The diagnosis of chronic Chagas disease is usually made by detecting IgG antibodies that bind to parasite antigens in the serum of patients.

8. Answer b

Culture-negative endocarditis may occur with fungal endocarditis, and with slow-growing fastidious organisms such as nutritionally variant streptococci, *Coxiella burnetii* (the causative agent of Q-fever), and *Bartonella quintana*; *E. coli* generally is not a cause of culture-negative endocarditis.

9. Answer a

Bartonella quintana has recently been associated with endocarditis in homeless persons with alcoholism and in patients in inner-city settings. *Bartonella* spp. are slow-growing gram-negative bacteria that may require a month or longer for culture isolation.

10. Answer d

Members of the HACEK group of organisms include *Haemophilus paraphrophilus*, *H. parainfluenzae*, *H. aphrophilus*, *Actinobacillus actinomycetemcomitans*, *Cardiobacterium hominis*, *Eikenella corrodens*, *Kingella kingae*, *K. dentrificans*, and *K. indologenes*. *Helicobacter pylori* is not part of the HACEK group of organisms and is not associated with endocarditis.

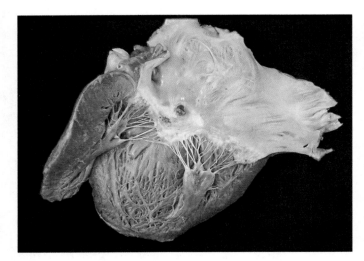

Plate 1. Infective endocarditis involving the mitral valve.

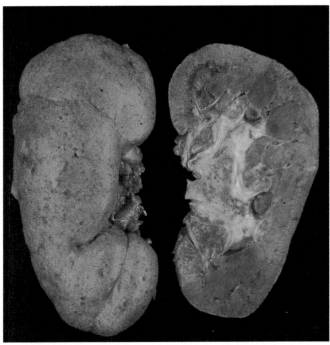

Plate 2. Gross appearance of kidney in *S. aureus* endocarditis.

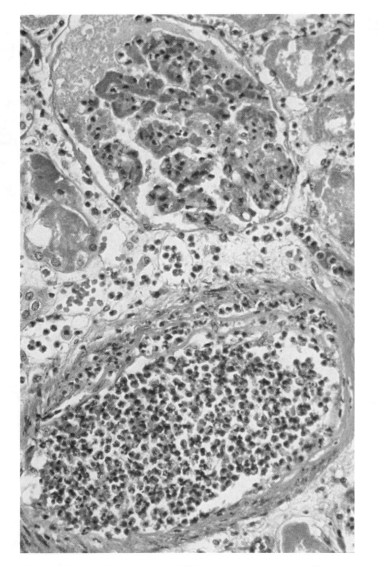

Plate 3. Microscopic appearance of kidney in *S. aureus* endocarditis.

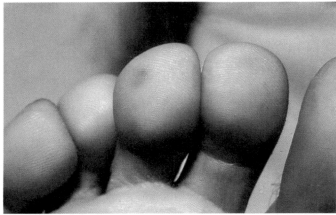

Plate 4. Osler node.

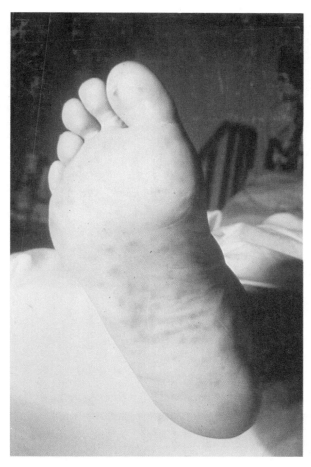

Plate 5. Janeway lesions.

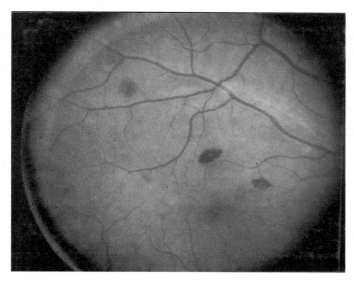

Plate 6. Roth spots.

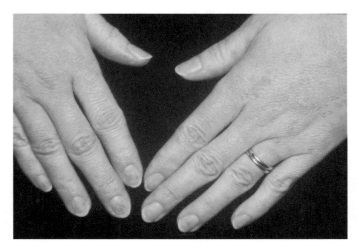

Plate 7. Splinter hemorrhages.

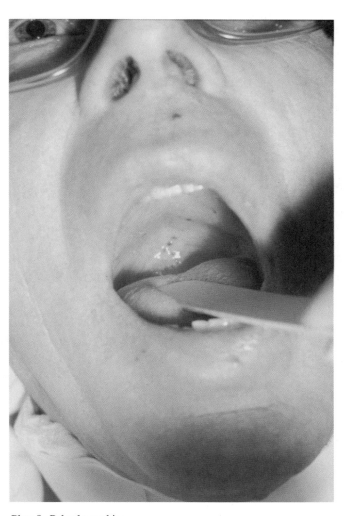

Plate 8. Palatal petechiae.

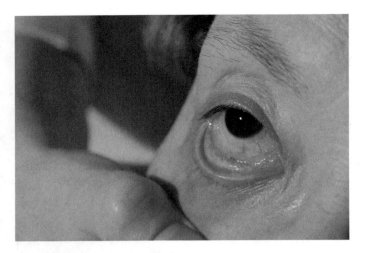

Plate 9. Conjunctival petechiae.

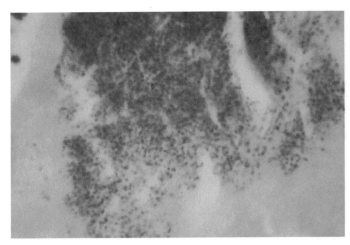

Plate 10. Gram stain of *S. aureus* vegetation from a patient with infective endocarditis.

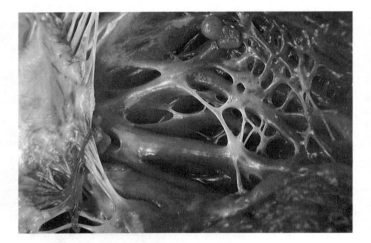

Plate 11. Gross appearance of the heart from a patient with *Aspergillus* infective endocarditis.

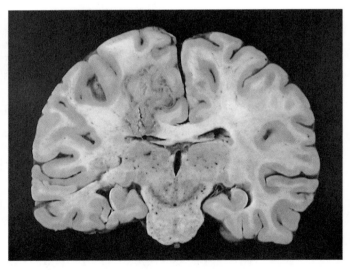

Plate 12. Brain abscess caused by *Aspergillus* species in a patient with *Aspergillus* infective endocarditis. (From same patient as in Plate 11.)

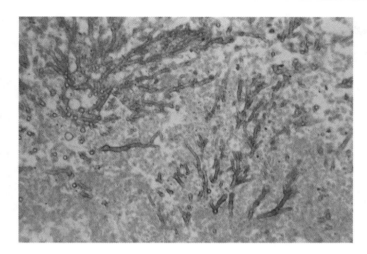

Plate 13. Microscopic appearance of the brain abscess shown in Plate 12.

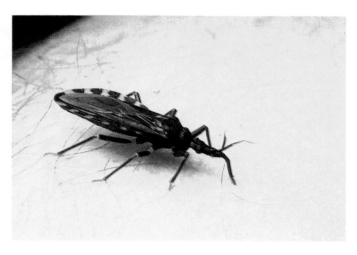

Plate 14. Reduviid bug. (From Peters W, Gilles H: *A Colour Atlas of Tropical Medicine and Parasitology*. Second edition. Wolfe Medical Publications, 1981, p 77. By permission of the authors.)

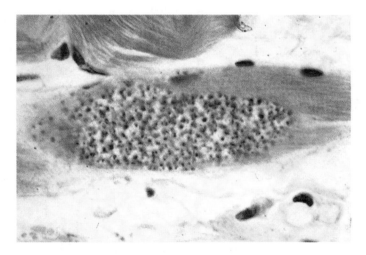

Plate 15. Amastigotes in heart muscle in Chagas disease. After a stage of initial parasitemia associated with fever, trypomastigotes pass to the cardiac muscle and smooth muscle lining the intestinal tract. Here, they transform to the amastigote stage in which they multiply to form pseudocysts. In the heart, this is associated with severe myocarditis, especially in the early stages of the infection. (From Peters W, Gilles H: *A Colour Atlas of Tropical Medicine and Parasitology*. Second edition. Wolfe Medical Publications, 1981, p 79. By permission of the authors.)

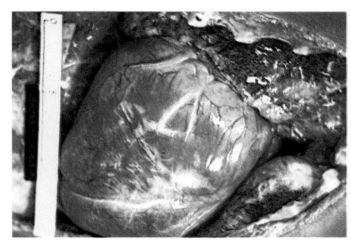

Plate 16. Cardiomegaly associated with Chagas' disease. The heart shows gross enlargement and dilatation. The dilatation of the right atrium and both ventricles is marked in this specimen. (From Peters W, Gilles H: *A Colour Atlas of Tropical Medicine and Parasitology*. Second edition. Wolfe Medical Publications, 1981, p 81. By permission of the authors.)

Notes

Chapter 29

Dilated Cardiomyopathy

A. Jamil Tajik, M.D.
Joseph G. Murphy, M.D.

> Cardiomyopathy is an important topic to review for the Cardiology Examinations. Special attention should be paid to the physical signs and possible causes of dilated cardiomyopathy.

The diagnosis and management of heart failure are discussed further in Chapters 5 and 6. Myocarditis is reviewed in Chapter 31. Systolic and diastolic ventricular function are reviewed in Chapters 3 and 4.

Cardiomyopathies are diseases of heart muscle associated with cardiac dysfunction (1995 World Health Organization [WHO]/International Society and Federation of Cardiology Definition of Cardiomyopathy). They are classified as either dilated cardiomyopathy (DCM) or hypertrophic cardiomyopathy (HCM) on the basis of ventricular morphology or as restrictive cardiomyopathy (RCM) primarily on the basis of a characteristic hemodynamic pathophysiology. Arrhythmic right ventricular cardiomyopathy is a rare type of cardiomyopathy associated with sudden death in young patients.

Prevalence of Cardiomyopathy

DCM is the most common type of cardiomyopathy, with an estimated prevalence in the general population of 40 to 50 cases per 100,000. HCM is about one-fifth as common, and RCM and arrhythmogenic right ventricular cardiomyopathy are extremely rare.

Characteristic Features of Cardiomyopathies

The characteristic features of each of the main types of cardiomyopathy can readily be identified with two-dimensional and Doppler echocardiography on the basis of chamber size, wall thickness, and systolic and diastolic function of the left ventricle (Table 1).

DCM consists of an enlarged left ventricular cavity with depressed systolic function. HCM is characterized by a small-to-normal size left ventricular cavity, massive hypertrophy of the myocardium, and hyperdynamic systolic function. The major abnormality in RCM is diastolic dysfunction of the myocardium.

It is important to remember that there is some overlap among the types of cardiomyopathies (Fig. 1). End-stage HCM may exhibit ventricular dilatation and have features of both HCM and DCM. Some cases of HCM in which the ventricular walls are only mildly thickened may mimic the restrictive hemodynamic profile of RCM. RCM may also exhibit some degree of ventricular dilatation; this is referred to as "minimally dilated restrictive cardiomyopathy."

An atlas illustrating the pathologic features of dilated cardiomyopathy is found at the end of the chapter.

Table 1.—Comparison of Dilated, Hypertrophic, and Restrictive Cardiomyopathies

| Feature | Cardiomyopathy | | |
	Dilated	Hypertrophic	Restrictive
Cavity size	Enlarged	Small	Normal
Wall thickness	Normal	Marked	Normal
Systolic function	Severely depressed	Hyperdynamic	Normal/reduced
Diastolic function	Abnormal	Abnormal	Abnormal
Other		Outflow tract obstruction	

Although each type of cardiomyopathy has a pure form, some degree of clinical overlap can exist among these entities.

Dilated Cardiomyopathy

Definition

The WHO defined dilated cardiomyopathy as myocardial disease "characterized by dilatation and impaired contraction of the left ventricle or both left and right ventricles. It may be idiopathic, familial/genetic, viral and/or immune, alcoholic/toxic, or associated with recognized cardiovascular disease in which the degree of myocardial dysfunction is not explained by the abnormal loading conditions or the extent of ischemic damage. The histologic findings are frequently nonspecific. Presentation is usually with heart failure, which is often progressive. Arrhythmias, thromboembolism, and sudden death are common and may occur at any stage."

Features

The macroscopic pathologic features of DCM are distinct and almost identical in all patients: four-chamber dilatation is usual and thrombi are frequent in the apices of both ventricular chambers. Left ventricular wall thickness is entirely normal, but left ventricular mass is markedly increased in tandem with the increased ventricular diastolic dimension. There also is a concomitant increase in right ventricular size. In clinical practice, patients may present in the early stage of the disease with only left ventricular dilatation, followed later

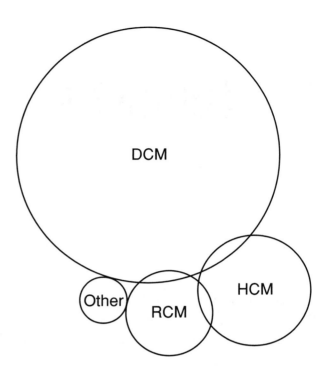

Fig. 1. Overlap of features of the types of cardiomyopathy. DCM, dilated cardiomyopathy; HCM, hypertrophic cardiomyopathy; RCM, restrictive cardiomyopathy. Other forms of cardiomyopathy include right ventricular dysplasia of idiopathic origin.

by left atrial dilatation, and finally with dilatation of all four cardiac chambers. Right ventricular dilatation in DCM carries a poor prognosis. DCM occurs more frequently in males than females (about 3:1) and is more common in African-Americans than in whites (the ratio is about 2.5:1). Patients with DCM frequently have a history of an increase in alcohol intake and systemic hypertension. Echocardiographically, DCM has similar features in all patients: marked dilatation of the left ventricular cavity, normal wall thickness, and globally reduced systolic function. Regional wall motion abnormalities can be superimposed on DCM even if no flow-limiting coronary disease is present. Regional wall motion abnormalities do not exclude a diagnosis of idiopathic DCM. Anginal pain does not occur in DCM, and its presence should lead to a search for coronary artery disease.

- Regional wall motion abnormalities do not exclude a diagnosis of idiopathic DCM.

Etiology of Dilated Cardiomyopathy

The most important causes of DCM are listed in Table 2. It is important to remember the reversible forms of heart disease

Table 2.—Important Causes of Dilated Cardiomyopathy

Post-chemotherapy (doxorubicin)
Acquired immunodeficiency syndrome
Infiltrative disease (hemochromatosis)
Peripartum cardiomyopathy
Associated with muscular dystrophy
Tachycardia-induced
Alcohol-induced

Table 3.—Prognostic Factors in Dilated Cardiomyopathy That Predict Poor Survival

Abnormal ventricular function
    Decreased ejection fraction is the most powerful prognostic indicator in dilated cardiomyopathy
    Increased left ventricular size (assessed by the cardiothoracic ratio on chest radiography or, more accurately, by left ventricular end-diastolic dimension on echocardiography)
    Right ventricular dilatation is an independent predictor of poor survival in cardiomyopathy
Functional class
    Poor New York Heart Association functional class
    Maximal oxygen uptake < 12 mL/kg per minute on cardiopulmonary exercise testing
Electrocardiography
    Left bundle branch block
    Asymptomatic nonsustained ventricular tachycardia
Clinical features
    Clinical left or right heart failure
    Syncope
Endocrine activation and electrolyte levels
    Hyponatremia (serum sodium concentration < 135 mmol/L)
    Increased plasma concentrations of norepinephrine, atrial natriuretic factor, and renin
Hemodynamic
    High (> 18 to 20 mm Hg) left ventricular end-diastolic pressure or pulmonary capillary wedge pressure used as a surrogate for left ventricular end-diastolic pressure
    Low cardiac output (cardiac index < 2.5 L/min per m^2)
    Pulmonary hypertension (pulmonary artery systolic pressure > 35 mm Hg)
Cardiac biopsy
    Loss of intracellular cardiac myofilaments
    Persistence of enteroviral RNA

may mimic idiopathic DCM. One of these is tachycardia-induced cardiomyopathy, which may be seen in patients with recurrent supraventricular tachycardia or atrial fibrillation of long duration. By treating the arrhythmia, left ventricular dysfunction can be reversed. Patients with very frequent premature ventricular contractions may also develop left ventricular dysfunction. Successful suppression of the premature ventricular contractions may allow ventricular function to normalize. Another reversible form of cardiomyopathy is hibernating myocardium, which is discussed in Chapter 48.

Infiltrative diseases, in particular hemochromatosis, may cause a DCM that improves with reduction in iron overload. In spite of being an infiltrative cardiomyopathy, hemochromatosis does not produce thickened ventricular walls as amyloidosis does. Phlebotomy performed weekly in patients with hemochromatosis-induced cardiomyopathy results in marked improvement of ventricular function and decrease in left ventricular size. In contrast, amyloid heart disease, another infiltrative disease, is not reversible.

- In patients with a dilated, poorly functioning left ventricle, always check the serum levels of iron and ferritin, a fat aspirate for amyloid, and protein electrophoresis.

The incidence of a familial form of DCM is up to 20% of all cases of DCM. Family members of patients with DCM should have echocardiographic screening even if asymptomatic.

The prognostic factors in DCM predictive of poor survival are listed in Table 3.

Specific Cardiomyopathies*

The term "specific cardiomyopathies" is now used to describe heart muscle diseases that are associated with specific cardiac or systemic disorders. These were previously defined as specific heart muscle diseases.

Ischemic cardiomyopathy presents as dilated cardiomyopathy with impaired contractile performance not explained by the extent of coronary artery disease or ischemic damage.

Valvular cardiomyopathy presents with ventricular dysfunction that is out of proportion to the abnormal loading conditions.

Hypertensive cardiomyopathy often presents with left

ventricular hypertrophy in association with features of dilated or restrictive cardiomyopathy with cardiac failure.

Inflammatory cardiomyopathy is defined by myocarditis in association with cardiac dysfunction. Myocarditis is an inflammatory disease of the myocardium and is diagnosed by established histologic, immunologic, and immunohistochemical criteria. Idiopathic, autoimmune, and infectious forms of inflammatory cardiomyopathy are recognized. Inflammatory myocardial disease is involved in the pathogenesis of dilated cardiomyopathy and other cardiomyopathies (e.g., Chagas disease, human immunodeficiency virus, enterovirus, adenovirus, and cytomegalovirus).

Metabolic cardiomyopathy includes the following categories: endocrine (e.g., thyrotoxicosis, hypothyroidism, adrenal cortical insufficiency, pheochromocytoma, acromegaly, and diabetes mellitus), familial storage disease and infiltrations (e.g., hemochromatosis, glycogen storage disease, Hurler syndrome, Refsum syndrome, Niemann-Pick disease, Hand-Schüller-Christian disease, Fabry-Anderson disease, and Morquio-Ullrich disease), deficiency (e.g., disturbances of potassium metabolism, magnesium deficiency, and nutritional disorders such as kwashiorkor, anemia, beri-beri, and selenium deficiency), amyloid (e.g., primary, secondary, familial, and hereditary cardiac amyloidoses), familial Mediterranean fever, and senile amyloidosis.

General system disease includes connective tissue disorders (e.g., systemic lupus erythematosus, polyarteritis nodosa, rheumatoid arthritis, scleroderma, and dermatomyositis). Infiltrations and granulomas include sarcoidosis and leukemia.

Muscular dystrophies include Duchenne, Becker-type, and myotonic dystrophies.

Neuromuscular disorders include Friedreich ataxia, Noonan syndrome, and lentiginosis.

Sensitivity and toxic reactions include reactions to alcohol, catecholamines, anthracyclines, irradiation, and miscellaneous. Alcoholic cardiomyopathy may be associated with a heavy alcohol intake. Currently, we cannot define a causal versus a conditioning role of alcohol or apply precise diagnostic criteria.

Peripartal cardiomyopathy may first manifest in the peripartum period. This is probably a heterogeneous group.

*This section is from *Circulation* 93:841-842, 1996. By permission of the American Heart Association.

Arrhythmogenic Right Ventricular Dysplasia/Arrhythmogenic Right Ventricular Cardiomyopathy

Arrhythmogenic right ventricular dysplasia (ARVD), also known as "arrhythmogenic" or "isolated" right ventricular cardiomyopathy, is a rare form of cardiomyopathy frequently associated with sustained or nonsustained ventricular tachycardia and sudden death, frequently precipitated by exercise. The WHO defined arrhythmogenic right ventricular cardiomyopathy as myocardial disease characterized by "progressive fibrofatty replacement of right ventricular myocardium, initially with localized and later global right and some left ventricular involvement, with relative sparing of the septum. Familial disease is common, with autosomal dominant inheritance and incomplete penetrance; a recessive form is described. Presentation with arrhythmias and sudden death is common, particularly in the young."

The disorder has both a familial form mapped to chromosome 14 and a sporadic form. Males predominate in all reported series. The clinical presentation can be hemodynamic, with right heart failure, or arrhythmogenic, with sudden death, or ventricular tachycardia, with left bundle branch block morphology reflecting a right ventricular origin.

The baseline ECG shows T-wave inversion in leads V_1-V_3. Imaging studies of the right ventricle show a dilated hypokinetic chamber.

Treatment is usually placement of an automatic implantable cardioverter-defibrillator and/or amiodarone.

Questions

Multiple Choice (choose the one best answer)

1. All the following are true about the β-adrenergic system in idiopathic dilated cardiomyopathy *except*:
   a. β_1-receptor density in the myocardium is decreased
   b. β_2-receptor density in the myocardium is decreased
   c. Inhibitory myocardial G_1 protein is increased
   d. β_2-receptor uncoupling is increased
   e. The inotropic response to β-agonists is decreased

2. The following characteristic histologic findings are seen on light microscopy in idiopathic dilated cardiomyopathy *except*:
   a. Myocyte hypertrophy
   b. Myocyte atrophy
   c. Myofilament loss
   d. Lymphocytic infiltration associated with adjacent myocyte necrosis
   e. Normal intramural arteries and capillaries

3. Prognostic factors in patients with idiopathic dilated cardiomyopathy include all the following *except*:
   a. Plasma level of norepinephrine
   b. Atrial natriuretic factor level
   c. Presence of hyponatremia
   d. Preceding viral illness
   e. Left ventricular ejection fraction

Answers

1. Answer b

The significant changes in the myocardial adrenergic receptors in idiopathic dilated cardiomyopathy include a decrease in myocardial β_1-receptor density and an uncoupling of β_2-receptors, probably related to an increase in inhibitory G protein (G_1) levels. In heart failure and dilated cardiomyopathy, there is a decreased response to administered β-agonists because of a decrease in the number of β_2-receptors. The number of β_1-receptors is normal.

2. Answer d

Lymphocytic infiltration associated with adjacent myocyte necrosis is characteristic of myocarditis, not dilated cardiomyopathy. The intramural vessels are normal on light microscopy. Both myocyte atrophy and hypertrophy may be seen.

3. Answer d

Poor prognostic factors in idiopathic dilated cardiomyopathy include increased levels of plasma norepinephrine, atrial natriuretic factor, hyponatremia, and left ventricular ejection fraction. A history of a viral illness does not have a prognostic effect.

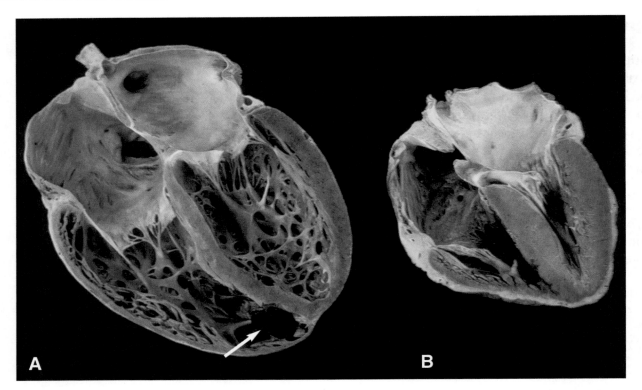

Plate 1. Comparison of heart with dilated cardiomyopathy (*A*) and normal heart (*B*). In *A*, note dilatation of all four chambers and thrombus (*arrow*) in the right ventricle.

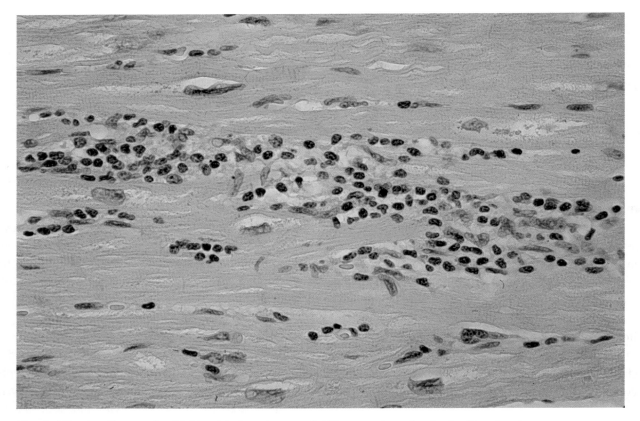

Plate 2. Dilated cardiomyopathy. Right ventricular endomyocardial biopsy specimen showing focal lymphocytes.

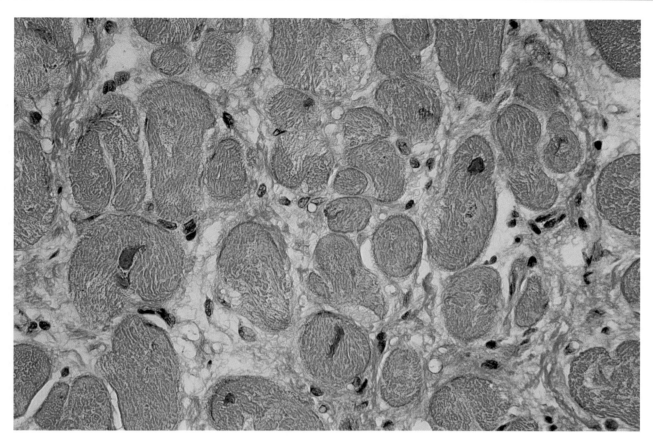

Plate 3. Right ventricular endomyocardial biopsy showing moderate pericellular fibrosis in dilated cardiomyopathy.

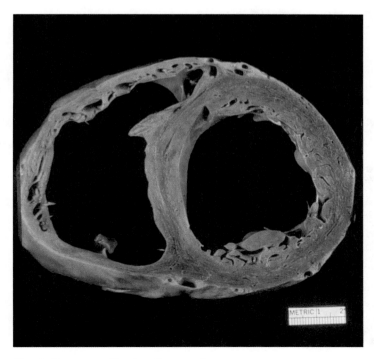

Plate 4. Postpartum dilated cardiomyopathy.

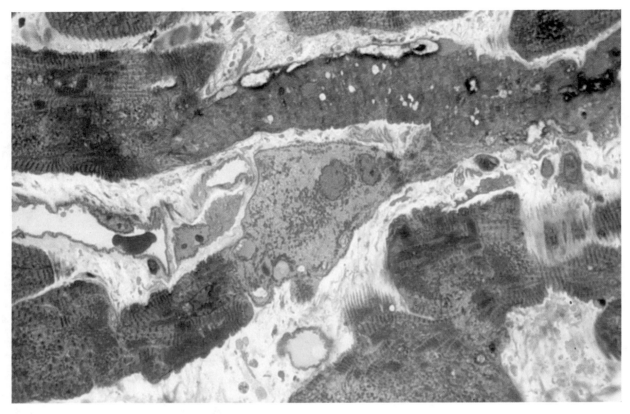

Plate 5. Doxorubicin cardiotoxicity.

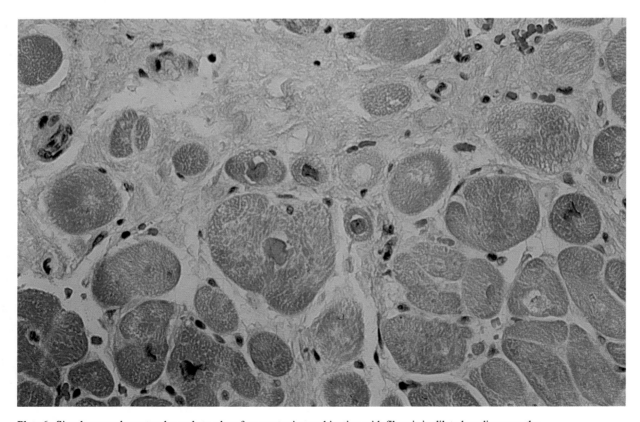

Plate 6. Simultaneous hypertrophy and atrophy of myocytes in combination with fibrosis in dilated cardiomyopathy.

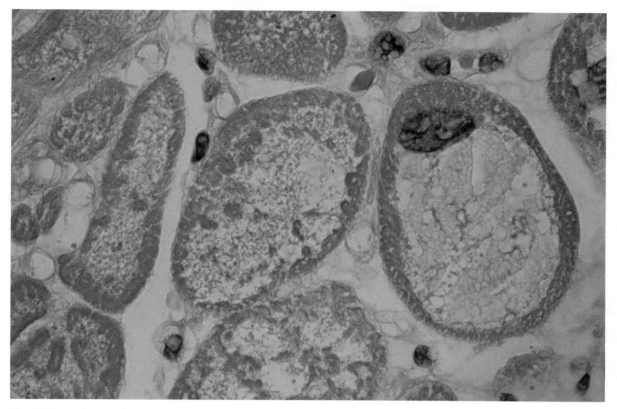

Plate 7. Loss of contractile elements in dilated cardiomyopathy.

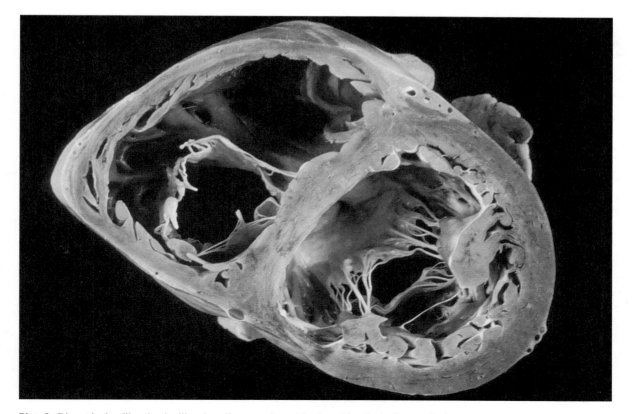

Plate 8. Biventricular dilatation in dilated cardiomyopathy, with tricuspid and mitral regurgitation.

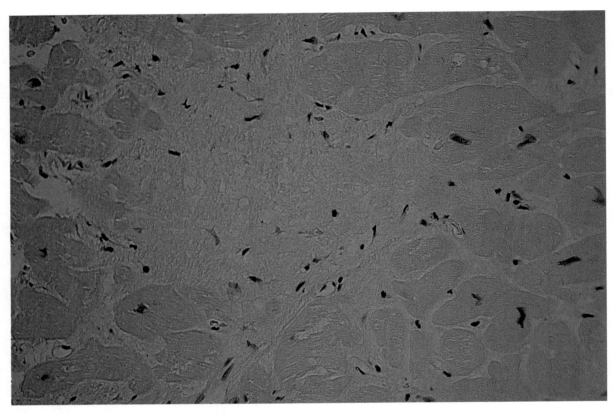

Plate 9. Patchy replacement fibrosis in dilated cardiomyopathy.

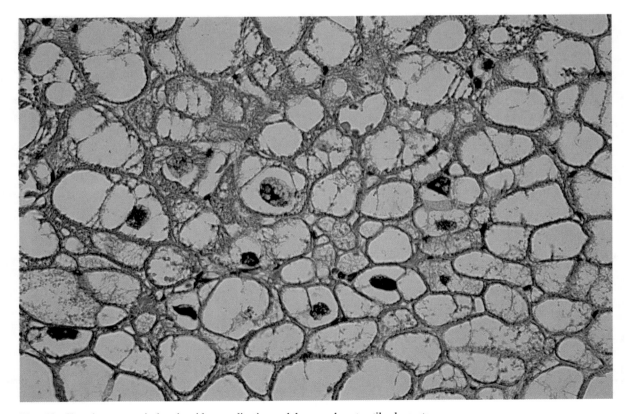

Plate 10. Chronic myocyte ischemia with vacuolization and decreased contractile elements.

Chapter 30

Hypertrophic and Restrictive Cardiomyopathies

A. Jamil Tajik, M.D.
Joseph G. Murphy, M.D.

Hypertrophic Cardiomyopathy

Definition

The World Health Organization (WHO) defined hypertrophic cardiomyopathy (HCM) as "left and/or right ventricular hypertrophy, which is usually asymmetric and involves the interventricular septum. Typically, the left ventricular volume is normal or reduced. Systolic gradients are common. Familial disease with autosomal dominant inheritance predominates. Mutations in sarcomeric contractile protein genes cause disease. Typical morphological changes include myocyte hypertrophy and disarray surrounding areas of increased loose connective tissue. Arrhythmias and premature sudden death are common. HCM is also defined as inappropriate ventricular hypertrophy without a cardiac or systemic cause."

Diagnosis of HCM

HCM typically produces marked asymmetric hypertrophy of the left ventricle, frequently localized to the ventricular septum (Fig. 1-3). HCM may be distinguished from the "athletic heart" by careful echocardiographic measurements. In HCM, left ventricular septal wall thickness is typically greater than 15 mm, the left atrium is dilated (> 4 cm), and the left ventricular end-diastolic diameter is less than 45 mm. In the athletic heart, the dimensions are less than 15 mm for the septum, less than 4 cm for the left atrium, and

greater than 45 mm for left ventricular end-diastolic diameter. In the athletic heart, left ventricular hypertrophy is always concentric and regresses after training stops, usually within 3 months. Diastolic function is always normal in the athletic heart. In HCM, the electrocardiogram (ECG) is generally very abnormal and beyond the voltage increase due to the increased ventricular mass seen in the athletic heart. Diastolic function is always abnormal in HCM and is a hallmark of the condition.

HCM may be associated with massive hypertrophy of the myocardium (wall thickness of 45 to 50 mm). The size of the left ventricular cavity is normal to small, and diastolic relaxation is impaired, whereas systolic function is usually hyperdynamic. Dynamic left ventricular outflow tract obstruction may be present because of a combination of narrowing of the outflow tract, systolic anterior motion of the mitral valve leaflet, and the muscular sphincter action of the outflow tract.

In HCM, the papillary muscles may be hypertrophied, malpositioned, and misoriented. Secondary left atrial dilatation is usually a consequence of left ventricular diastolic dysfunction and mitral regurgitation. Right ventricular hypertrophy may also be present (Fig. 3).

The stimulus for the development of HCM is not known: one speculation is that it is a disorder of intracellular calcium metabolism and another is that it is due to a neural crest disorder.

An atlas illustrating the macroscopic and microscopic features of hypertrophic and restrictive cardiomyopathies is found at the end of the chapter (Plates 1-14).

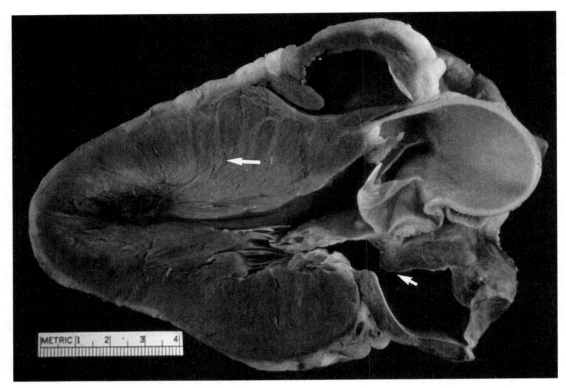

Fig. 1. Autopsy specimen of hypertrophic cardiomyopathy showing marked septal hypertrophy (*long arrow*), a small left ventricular cavity, and a moderately dilated left atrium (*short arrow*).

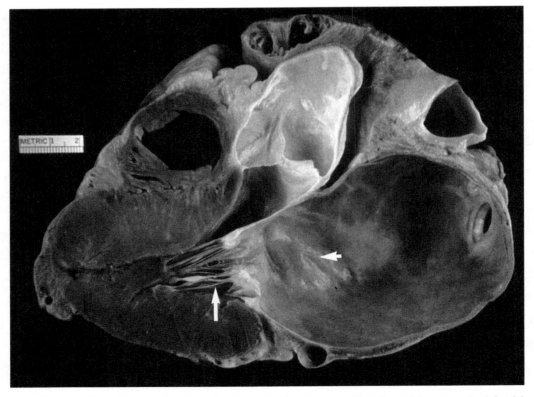

Fig. 2. Autopsy specimen of hypertrophic cardiomyopathy with predominant apical involvement of the left ventricle and massive left atrial enlargement (*short arrow*). Also, the papillary muscles are malpositioned and misoriented (*long arrow*).

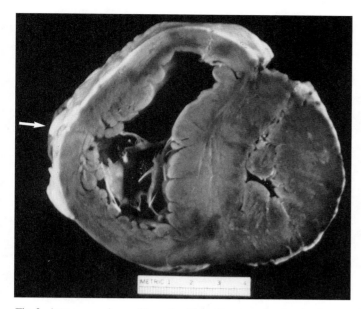

Fig. 3. Autopsy specimen of hypertrophic cardiomyopathy showing hypertrophy of the inferior wall and right ventricle (*arrow*) in addition to that of the septum and anterolateral wall.

Table 1.—Mutations in Genes for Cardiac
Sarcomeric Proteins Causally Linked to
Hypertrophic Cardiomyopathy (HCM)

Sarcomeric protein	Chromosome
β-Myosin heavy chain	14
Cardiac troponin T	1
Cardiac troponin I	19
Regulatory myosin light chains	3
	12
HCM with Wolff-Parkinson-White syndrome	7
α-Tropomyosin	15
Cardiac myosin-binding protein C	11

Genetic Abnormalities in HCM

HCM is frequently a hereditary disorder, with transmission to first-degree relatives in 50% of cases. Genetically as well as phenotypically, HCM is an extremely heterogeneous disease. The trait is usually inherited as an autosomal dominant disorder. Mutations in the genes for cardiac sarcomeric proteins have been causally linked to HCM (Table 1). Other suggested genetic abnormalities include polymorphism of the angiotensin-converting enzyme gene and mitochondrial DNA abnormalities. Troponin T mutations have a high risk of sudden death even in the absence of the usual ventricular hypertrophy seen in HCM. To date, the largest number of mutations have been identified in the β-myosin heavy chain gene on chromosome 14.

Variants of Hypertrophic Cardiomyopathy

The most common location of ventricular hypertrophy in HCM is subaortic, septal, and anterior wall hypertrophy, frequently accompanied by endocardial friction lesions from systolic anterior motion of the mitral valve against the ventricular septum (Fig. 4).

Asymmetric hypertrophy of the left ventricle, predominantly of the septum and anterior wall of the left ventricle, is present in 70% of patients with HCM. The basal septal hypertrophy variant is seen in about 15% to 20% of patients; the patients in this subgroup are frequently hypertensive and elderly. Concentric left ventricular hypertrophy is seen

in about 8% to 10% of patients. Apical or lateral wall hypertrophy variants are extremely uncommon in the Western world (< 2%). In Japan, apical HCM is more common and occurs in up to 25% of persons with HCM. The apical variant of HCM is usually accompanied by characteristic giant T-wave inversion across the lateral precordial leads (Fig. 5) and a spade-like left ventricular cavity on ventriculography during diastole. Apical HCM is not associated with an intraventricular gradient and usually has mild symptoms and a more benign clinical course.

Endocardial plaque formation or thickening of the subaortic portion of the ventricular septum is frequently seen in the obstructive variant of the disease (HOCM). In addition to subaortic obstruction, there may be diffuse hypertrophy of the septum and papillary muscles at the midventricular level, resulting in combined midventricular obstruction. Two-dimensional echocardiography is the optimal imaging modality for delineation of this HOCM variant and in selecting patients for referral for myotomy/myectomy. The midcavity variant of HOCM must be identified preoperatively in patients selected for myotomy/myectomy to allow the surgeon to extend the incision further apically than normal to relieve the midventricular component of obstruction. The HCM variant in which hypertrophy is localized to the apex of the heart can also be visualized with echocardiography, as can the concentric and diffuse variants. The precise HCM variant present will determine the pathophysiologic findings as well as influence patient management.

Hypertensive Hypertrophic Cardiomyopathy

Elderly women may present with a condition called "hypertensive HCM" that simulates HCM. It is an

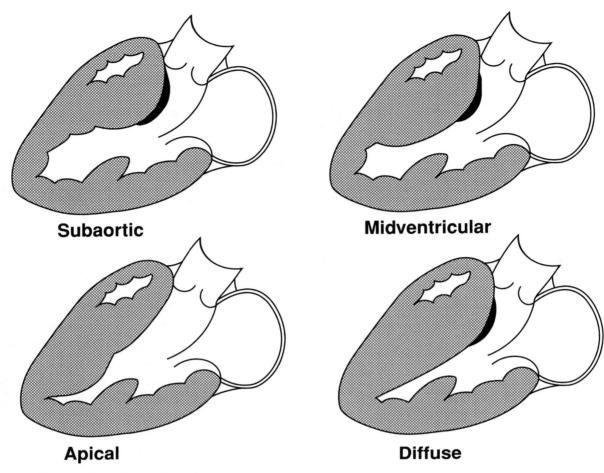

Subaortic

Midventricular

Apical

Diffuse

Fig. 4. Diagram of hypertrophic cardiomyopathy variants.

extreme ventricular response to untreated or poorly treated hypertension. Hypertensive HCM is associated with concentric left ventricular hypertrophy, a relatively small left ventricular cavity, and, in some patients, angulation of the septum. Mitral annular calcification and mitral regurgitation may also be prominent. Patients usually present with increasing dyspnea. The prognosis for hypertensive HCM is generally better than that for non-hypertensive HCM.

HCM may also be associated with Friedreich ataxia, lentiginosis, pheochromocytoma, neurofibromatosis, and generalized lipodystrophy. Cardiac amyloidosis and glycogen storage disease may simulate the massive ventricular hypertrophy of HCM, but they usually have low or normal ECG voltages.

- Genetically and phenotypically, HCM is an extremely heterogeneous disease.
- The papillary muscle may be malpositioned and misoriented in HCM.

Pathophysiology of Hypertrophic Cardiomyopathy

The pathophysiologic mechanisms in HCM are complex and vary from patient to patient. Traditionally, dynamic left ventricular outflow tract obstruction has been considered as the cause of symptoms in patients, but it should be remembered that diastolic dysfunction, myocardial ischemia (even in the presence of normal coronary arteries), mitral regurgitation, and arrhythmias are also important in producing the symptoms of dyspnea, angina, syncope, embolism, and congestive heart failure (Fig. 6).

Left Ventricular Outflow Tract Gradient in HCM

Left ventricular outflow tract obstruction is dynamic in nature and dependent on both the loading conditions and the contractile state of the left ventricle. Outflow obstruction is increased in the presence of a decreased ventricular preload, decreased ventricular afterload, or increased ventricular contractility. The series of pathophysiologic events that contribute to the obstruction has been described as "eject-obstruct-leak."

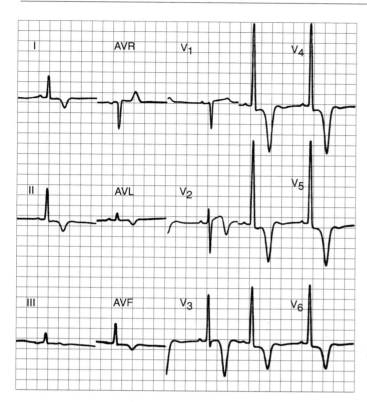

Fig. 5. ECG of patient with apical hypertrophic cardiomyopathy variant with deeply inverted T waves in chest leads V$_2$-V$_6$ and limb leads II, III, and aVL.

The hypertrophied septum bulges into the left ventricular outflow tract during early systole and together with a hyperdynamic ventricular ejection leads to an initial increase in the velocity of blood flow in the left ventricular outflow tract and mild obstruction. This, in turn, produces a Venturi effect, by which the anterior mitral valve leaflets and chordae are sucked into the outflow tract, further increasing the degree of obstruction. Finally, the mitral valve apparatus becomes so distorted that it causes an eccentric jet of mitral regurgitation in mid-late systole. This degree of mitral regurgitation in some patients may be severe and contribute substantially to symptoms of heart failure.

The ventricular outflow obstruction may be present at rest or may be provoked by exercise, maneuvers (Valsalva), or drugs (amyl nitrite), or may even be absent. About 30% to 50% of patients with HCM do not have any outflow obstruction, either at rest or with provocation. Many patients have only a mild gradient in the resting state but may develop severe obstruction, with gradients greater than 100 mm Hg with provocative maneuvers or exercise.

Diastolic Dysfunction in HCM
Diastolic dysfunction is thought to be one of the major pathophysiologic mechanisms present in all patients with HCM, frequently leading to diastolic heart failure. Marked abnormalities of both ventricular relaxation and chamber stiffness may be present. Multiple abnormal loads are imposed on the left ventricle, including contraction loads (from outflow obstruction) and relaxation loads as well as nonuniformity of relaxation. The thick, hypertrophied ventricular muscle causes abnormalities of passive filling because of the increased stiffness of the left ventricle.

Arrhythmias in HCM
Arrhythmias also contribute to the pathophysiology of HCM. Atrial arrhythmias are common and may cause severe hemodynamic deterioration from loss of atrial contraction as well as from rapid heart rates. Ventricular ectopy is a common finding on Holter monitoring. Sustained ventricular tachycardia and fibrillation are the most likely mechanisms of syncope and sudden death in these patients. Patients with HCM are very dependent on normal atrial function for filling of the stiff hypertrophied left ventricle. Cardiac output may decrease as much as 40% if atrial fibrillation occurs, leading to rapid deterioration of the patient's symptoms.

Histology of Hypertrophic Cardiomyopathy
The characteristic histologic abnormalities in HCM are myocardial fiber disarray, endocardial plaques, and abnormal relaxation of the bizarre and diversely oriented myocardial fibers (Fig. 6). Ventricular myocyte disarray also occurs with the left ventricular hypertrophy of aortic stenosis, congenital heart disease, and severe systemic hypertension. Because of ventricular hypertrophy and intimal hyperplasia of intramural coronary arteries and endothelial dysfunction, myocardial perfusion defects are frequently seen in HCM even in patients with normal epicardial coronary arteries. Spontaneous myocardial infarction may occur in patients with HCM without plaque rupture or critical coronary artery stenosis.

Clinical Presentations of Hypertrophic Cardiomyopathy
HCM may be newly diagnosed at any age from early childhood to advanced old age. The clinical presentation of HCM varies widely (Fig. 7). Patients may be completely asymptomatic, with the diagnosis made on the basis of a heart murmur, abnormal ECG, or a screening echocardiogram in competitive athletes or relatives of a patient with known HCM.

Even patients with massive hypertrophy of the heart can be completely asymptomatic until they present with sudden cardiac death. (HCM is the leading cause of sudden

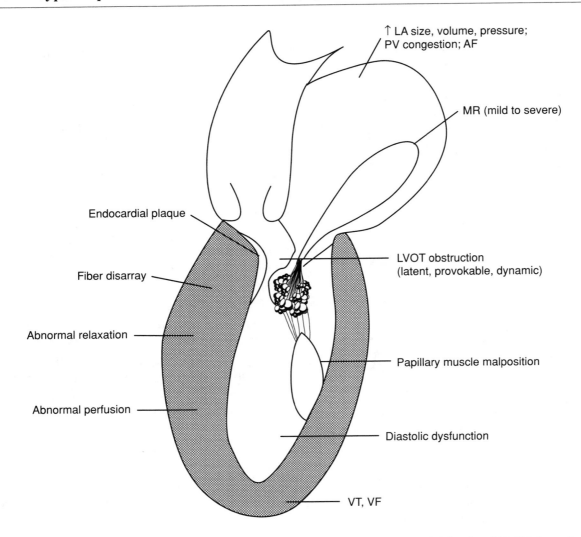

Fig. 6. Spectrum of abnormal findings in hypertrophic cardiomyopathy. AF, atrial fibrillation; LA, left atrium; LVOT, left ventricular outflow tract; MR, mitral regurgitation; PV, pulmonary vein; VF, ventricular fibrillation; VT, ventricular tachycardia.

Fig. 7. Spectrum of clinical presentations of hypertrophic cardiomyopathy.

death in competitive athletes.)

The typical triad of symptoms in HCM includes dyspnea on exertion, angina, and presyncope or syncope. Patients with atrial fibrillation may also present with systemic embolism.

The dyspnea in HCM is due to increased left atrial pressure, which can result from abnormal left ventricular diastolic function, outflow tract obstruction, or significant mitral regurgitation. Angina pectoris is common even in the absence of epicardial coronary artery disease and is related to an abnormal myocardial oxygen supply/demand mismatch due to the hypertrophied left ventricular walls, increased arteriolar compressive wall tension caused by diastolic relaxation abnormalities, and endothelial dysfunction. Syncope may be due to arrhythmias or a sudden increase in outflow tract obstruction. Patients with HCM frequently have abnormal autonomic function, and vasodepressor syncope may be part of the mechanism of syncope.

- Diastolic dysfunction is frequent in HCM.
- Patients with HCM may have abnormal autonomic function.

Physical Examination in Hypertrophic Cardiomyopathy

Physical examination findings are always abnormal when there is obstruction of the outflow tract, but in non-obstructive HCM the abnormal results may be less obvious. The hallmark of the physical examination in HCM is the finding of severe myocardial hypertrophy. This is detected by palpation of the left ventricular apex, which is localized but markedly sustained. There frequently is a palpable presystolic impulse of the augmented atrial contraction present (palpable S_4). In the presence of outflow obstruction, there is a "triple ripple." The jugular venous pressure may be slightly increased, with a prominent "a" wave indicating abnormal diastolic function of the right side of the heart. The carotid pulse has a rapid upstroke due to the hyperdynamic systolic function and rapid ventricular emptying.

In the presence of ventricular outflow tract obstruction, the carotid upstroke has a distinctive "jerky" bifid quality (spike-and-dome pulse), and the left ventricle may have a triple impulse. The spike is the initial rapid ventricular emptying phase, whereas the dome corresponds to the onset of ventricular obstruction, followed by the more gradual increase in ventricular pressure to overcome the gradient.

The triple-ripple apical impulse is classic for HCM but is rarely observed. A bifid apex or double apical impulse is more common. The first impulse is the large atrial kick (atrial boost, presystolic boost), and the next impulse is a sustained left ventricular apical impulse. The atrial kick is due to a forceful atrial systole secondary to atrial hypertrophy in response to the chronically elevated left ventricular diastolic pressure and mitral regurgitation. In addition to an S_4 gallop, there may be an S_3 gallop. Previously, it was thought that a dilated chamber was necessary for an S_3 gallop, but both S_3 and S_4 gallops are frequent in HCM, even in the absence of left ventricular dilatation.

A harsh systolic ejection murmur is heard across the entire precordium and radiates to the apex and base of the heart but not the neck. In many instances, a separate mitral regurgitation murmur may be auscultated. Both murmurs respond in a similar manner to examination maneuvers that change the loading conditions of the left ventricle. During the strain phase of the Valsalva maneuver or squat-to-stand maneuver, there is an increase in the intensity of the murmur(s) because of decreased venous return.

The murmur of HCM is increased by maneuvers that decrease left ventricular end-diastolic volume (decreased venous return and afterload, increased contractility, and vasodilators, inotropes, dehydration, and the Valsalva maneuver). The murmur decreases with squatting, passive leg raising, negative inotropes such as β-blockers, disopyramide, and any maneuver that increases left ventricular end-diastolic volume.

- An S_3 gallop may occur in HCM in the absence of heart failure or left ventricular dilatation.

Cardiac arrhythmias are frequent and partly explain the occurrence of sudden death in patients with HCM.

When ventricular outflow obstruction occurs, it frequently is accompanied by mitral regurgitation. The severity of mitral regurgitation is related to the degree of outflow tract obstruction and varies from mild to severe. The combination of mitral regurgitation and severe ventricular diastolic dysfunction causes the left atrium to enlarge uniformly, resulting in an increase in left atrial size, volume, and pressure, which leads to the typical symptoms of pulmonary venous congestion and may also result in atrial fibrillation.

- The severity of mitral regurgitation is related to the degree of outflow tract obstruction.

Echocardiography in Hypertrophic Cardiomyopathy

Two-Dimensional Echocardiography

Two-dimensional and Doppler echocardiography are the standard tests for the diagnosis and evaluation of HCM. Two-dimensional echocardiography is able to visualize and characterize the site and extent of the hypertrophy of the myocardium. Although in the majority of cases the hypertrophy is classically asymmetric septal hypertrophy with anterolateral extensions, it can also be diffuse concentric hypertrophy or localized to specific areas such as the apex or free wall of the left ventricle. Systolic anterior motion of the mitral valve is frequently present when there is outflow tract obstruction.

Doppler Echocardiography

Doppler echocardiography is used to study the pathophysiology of HCM. A dynamic outflow obstruction can be diagnosed and accurately quantitated by a continuous-wave Doppler examination across the outflow tract. The Bernoulli equation is used to obtain the peak systolic gradient from the peak velocity. If there is no significant outflow gradient at rest, amyl nitrite or a Valsalva maneuver is used to elicit a dynamic outflow gradient. Coexistent mitral regurgitation can be diagnosed and semiquantitated with color-flow imaging. Diastolic filling of the left ventricle can also be characterized using the mitral as well as the pulmonary venous flow velocity curves.

It is important to establish whether HCM is the obstructive or nonobstructive variant. To diagnose the nonobstructive variant, provocative maneuvers must be used. The Valsalva maneuver and inhalation of amyl nitrite are used to exclude the presence of latent obstruction; occasionally, isoproterenol is infused. When obstruction is present, the site and severity should be quantitated and defined, the associated mitral regurgitant severity should be defined, and the diastolic ventricular dysfunction should be assessed.

Doppler is used to quantitate and localize the level and severity of obstruction. It is important to distinguish between the mitral regurgitant signal and the signal due to the intra-cavitary obstruction. The typical appearance of the HCM Doppler signal is late-peaking and frequently referred to as "dagger-shaped" (Fig. 8). To distinguish the HCM signal from mitral regurgitation, look for the aortic closure signal. The mitral regurgitant signal in HCM may be late-peaking, but it continues until mitral valve forward flow begins in diastole, while the left ventricular outflow obstruction signal ends with aortic valve closure. Doppler-derived gradients in patients with HCM correlate well with catheter-derived gradients during simultaneous examinations.

Cardiac catheterization is not necessary to diagnose HCM or to evaluate the severity of left ventricular outflow tract obstruction or mitral regurgitation. Catheterization may be used to optimize hemodynamics during dual-chamber pacing for HCM.

- The typical appearance of the HCM Doppler signal is a late-peaking signal frequently referred to as "dagger-shaped."

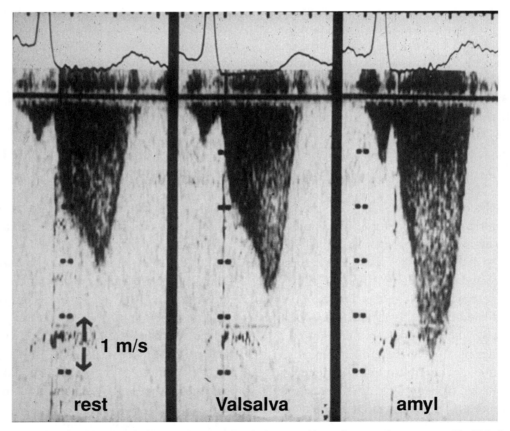

Fig. 8. Doppler "dagger-shaped" late-peaking signal of intracavitary gradient in hypertrophic cardiomyopathy accentuated by Valsalva response and by inhaled amyl nitrite. At rest, the velocity is 3.0 m/s (gradient, 36 mm Hg) and increases to 3.5 m/s (gradient, 50 mm Hg) during Valsalva and to 4.7 m/s (gradient, 88 mm Hg) after inhalation of amyl nitrite.

• The Brockenbrough response is a classic hemodynamic function in HCM (Fig. 9).

Diastolic Dysfunction in Hypertrophic Cardiomyopathy

Diastolic function is very abnormal in HCM, with the most prominent pattern being abnormal relaxation, prolonged deceleration time, systolic pulmonary venous dominance flow, and reduced diastolic forward flow (Fig. 10 and Table 2). There also can be a pseudonormal or restrictive pattern mitral inflow signal. In patients with marked septal hypertrophy, mild free-wall hypertrophy, and a normal-appearing mitral inflow signal, be alert for a pseudonormal mitral inflow signal.

There is another abnormal Doppler signal that may be seen in some patients with HCM; during the isovolumic relaxation period, a prominent flow velocity signal may be seen. In typical HCM, in which the base and mid-ventricle are markedly hypertrophied and the apex is relatively spared, the apex, as usual, relaxes before the base. Thus, at end-systole, when both the mitral and aortic valves are closed and the left ventricle is relaxing, the apex relaxes before the base. Hence, the end-systolic blood volume contained at the base is shifted toward the apex during the isovolumic phase and produces a transient signal. The opposite sequence of events and "flow" signal occurs in patients with apical and midventricular obstruction variants.

Diseases That Imitate Hypertrophic Cardiomyopathy

In the early stages of amyloid heart disease, ventricular dysfunction may be absent and systolic function is normal, even somewhat hyperdynamic, and can mimic HCM on two-dimensional echocardiography. Always look for electrocardiographic and echocardiographic concordance of left ventricular hypertrophy (Fig. 11 and 12). If there are thickened walls on echocardiography and low voltages on ECG, it is very unlikely to be HCM but probably cardiac amyloidosis mimicking HCM.

Natural History of Hypertrophic Cardiomyopathy

The natural history of HCM is highly variable. Early studies reported a mortality of 3% per year, increasing to 6% to 8% per year in the presence of nonsustained ventricular tachycardia. Sudden death is more common in adolescents with HCM, about 6% per year. The prognosis of patients with HCM in a community-based population study as well as for older patients is more benign. Several clinical features portend a poorer prognosis, including younger age, male sex, positive family history of sudden death, and history of syncope (Fig. 13). Severe hypertrophy on echocardiography also portends a poorer prognosis, although there are many patients who died suddenly and autopsy showed only mild hypertrophy. In the future, genetic markers may become the test of choice for identifying high-risk subgroups.

The differences in prognosis of HCM associated with different genetic mutations of the β cardiac myosin heavy chain are important. Mutations of the arginine gene are associated with a worse prognosis than those of the leucine gene (Fig. 14 and Table 3).

Management of Hypertrophic Cardiomyopathy

General Principles

There are several general guidelines for management of HCM. All first-degree relatives should undergo screening with echocardiography, and younger affected members of the family should have genetic counseling if they plan to

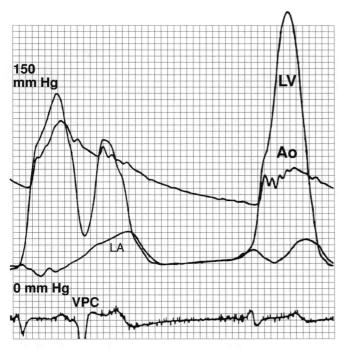

Hypertrophic cardiomyopathy following a ventricular premature (VPC) beat

Fig. 9. Brockenbrough response shows an increase in left ventricular (LV) systolic pressure, a decrease in ascending aortic (Ao) systolic pressure, and an increase in the gradient between the LV and ascending aorta. Note that there is also a decrease in the height of pulse pressure in the ascending aorta (systolic-diastolic blood pressure).

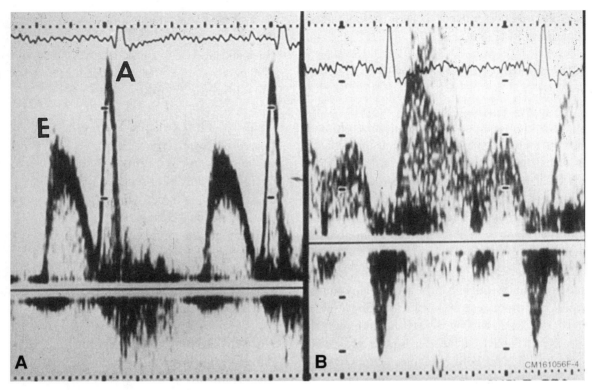

Fig. 10. Abnormal diastolic function in hypertrophic cardiomyopathy. *A*, Abnormal left ventricular relaxation with tall A- and small E-wave velocity and prolonged deceleration time (290 ms). *B*, Pulmonary venous flow is dominant in systole. Reduced diastolic forward flow; note large atrial reversal wave.

Table 2.—Diastolic Dysfunction in Hypertrophic Cardiomyopathy

Abnormal relaxation pattern
"Pseudonormal" pattern
Restrictive pattern
Prolonged isovolumic relaxation time and isovolumic
  relaxation "flow"

have a family. Patients should avoid competitive athletics or other types of strenuous activity. Antibiotics should be given prophylactically according to the AHA guidelines before medical and dental procedures to prevent infective endocarditis. Dehydration should be avoided. Holter monitoring should be performed for 48 hours to detect ventricular arrhythmias and for risk stratification.

β-*Blockers, Calcium Blockers, Disopyramide*

For patients with obstructive cardiomyopathy and symptoms, first-line drug therapy should be β-blockade with large dosages in the range of 200 to 400 mg propranolol or equivalent per day. Selective β-blockers lose their selectivity at high doses

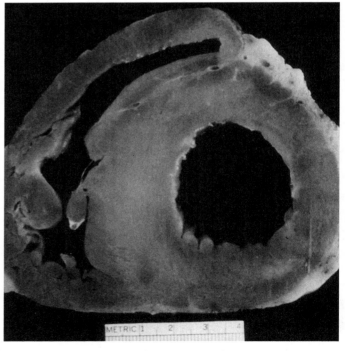

Fig. 11. Autopsy specimen of amyloid heart disease mimicking hypertrophic cardiomyopathy.

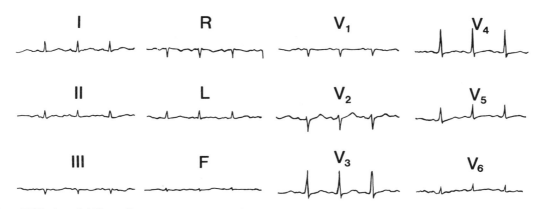

Fig. 12. Low-voltage ECG of amyloid heart disease.

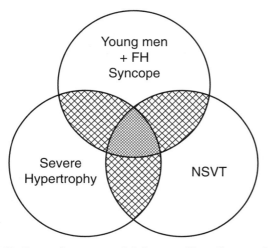

Fig. 13. Predictors of poor prognosis in hypertrophic cardiomyopathy. FH, family history; NSVT, nonsustained ventricular tachycardia.

so there is little to be gained by using a β_1 selective β-blocker. β-blockers relieve symptoms in about 50% of patients by slowing the heart rate, which allows a longer diastolic filling time and decreases myocardial oxygen consumption, thus reducing myocardial ischemia and left ventricular outflow tract obstruction through a direct negative inotropic effect. If this does not adequately decrease the intraventricular gradient and control symptoms, calcium channel blockers may be added, usually verapamil in dosages of 240 to 320 mg per day. Care must be taken when prescribing calcium channel blockers for patients with large outflow tract obstruction, because acute hemodynamic deterioration may occur because of peripheral vasodilatation. In general, most patients are treated with combined β-blocker and calcium channel blocker therapies. Disopyramide, a class I antiarrhythmic agent with strong negative inotropic properties, may also be used to treat HCM, especially in patients with outflow tract obstruction, but

it frequently causes urinary retention in men and dry mouth. Disopyramide does not improve the diastolic dysfunction characteristic of HCM.

For patients with severe symptoms unresponsive to medical therapy, the treatment options are dual-chamber pacing, surgical myectomy, or alcohol septal ablation.

Surgery for HCM

Septal myotomy/myectomy is a well-proven therapy that can abolish the outflow tract gradient and provide excellent long-term relief if done at a medical center skilled at performing this procedure. The mortality associated with the operation is low, particularly in young patients. For patients younger than 40, the mortality is less than 1% in our series (Table 4). Surgical mortality increases to 10% to 15% for patients older than 65. With surgery, the outflow tract gradient is decreased markedly and mitral regurgitation is abolished or decreased. Although it is likely that survival of the surgically treated HCM patients is better than that of the medically treated patients, this conclusion is not based on randomized studies. The natural history of attrition in HCM is 3% to 4% per year, and patients who have had myotomy/myectomy have an attrition rate of about 1.7% to 2.0% per year. Surgery should be considered in patients with a high resting outflow tract gradient (> 50 mm Hg) or in those with HCM refractory to medical therapy. Sudden death is not eliminated by surgery, but the incidence is certainly reduced. Aortic incompetence is rarely seen after myotomy/myectomy.

Strategies to prevent sudden death in high-risk patients with HCM are evolving. Patients who have experienced an out-of-hospital arrest or have documented sustained ventricular tachycardia should undergo implantation of an automatic defibrillator. It is less clear what to do for asymptomatic

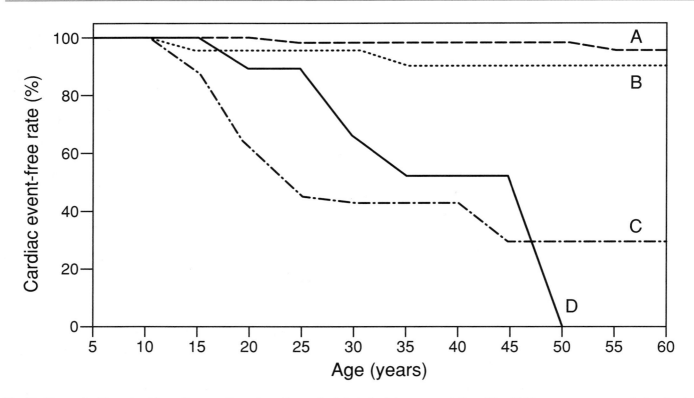

Fig. 14. Prognosis of hypertrophic cardiomyopathy varies with genetic defect. Arginine gene mutations (C and D) have a worse prognosis than leucine gene mutations (A and B). (From *Circulation* 89:22-32, 1994. By permission of the American Heart Association.)

Table 3.—Mutations and Survival in Hypertrophic Cardiomyopathy

Premature death (at mean age of 35 yr)
    Arginine 403 → glutamine
    Arginine 719 → glutamine
    Arginine 719 → tryptophan
"Normal" life expectancy
    Leucine 908 → valine
    Glycine 256 → glutamine

Table 4.—Results of Myotomy/Myectomy at the Mayo Clinic for Hypertrophic Cardiomyopathy

Mortality < 5% overall
    Patients younger than 40 years, < 1%
    Higher in older patients with other disease
Substantial decrease in gradient
Substantial decrease in mitral regurgitation

patients who, on the basis of clinical factors and Holter monitoring, are at high risk for sudden death. Electrophysiologic testing may have a role in better defining the prognosis of these high-risk patients. Low-dose amiodarone reduces the risk of sudden death in patients with HCM and nonsustained ventricular tachycardia.

- Care must be taken when prescribing calcium channel blockers for patients with large outflow tract obstruction, because acute hemodynamic deterioration may occur.
- The indicators of poor prognosis in HCM are a severe degree of ventricular hypertrophy, young age at presen-

tation, male sex, a positive family history, history of syncope, and sustained or nonsustained ventricular tachycardia that is clinically apparent or documented on Holter monitoring.

Dual Chamber Pacing in HCM

A more recent method of managing symptomatic patients with HCM is dual-chamber pacing (Fig. 15). With dual-chamber pacing, there frequently is a substantial reduction in the gradient (usually by about 50%) in the early follow-up period, and this is maintained throughout long-term follow-up. In addition to this acute effect of pacing in reducing the

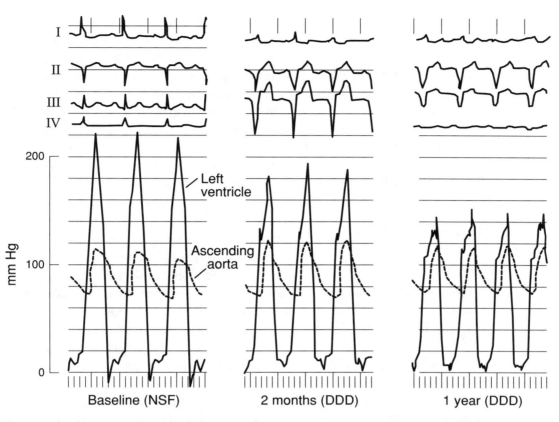

Fig. 15. Effect of dual-chamber pacing (DDD) on intraventricular gradient in hypertrophic cardiomyopathy at 2 months and 1 year. (From *Circulation* 90:2731-2742, 1994. By permission of the American Heart Association.)

gradient, it probably has a chronic remodeling effect that further decreases the gradient (Fig. 15 and 16).

Ideal candidates for dual-chamber pacing should be symptomatic, have resting obstruction (chronotropic incompetence is an additional indication), and be elderly (i.e., patients with higher operative risks) (Table 5).

Potential Mechanisms of Benefit of Pacing in HCM*
Comprehension of how pacing produces benefit in HCM is evolving and is partially speculative. A variety of mechanisms may be involved:

1. Right ventricular apical pacing and maintenance of atrioventricular (AV) synchrony appear to produce an abnormal pattern of septal contraction. This reduces early systolic bulging of the hypertrophic subaortic septum in the left ventricular outflow tract and diminishes Venturi forces that produce systolic anterior motion of the anterior mitral valve leaflet. AV pacing increases the left ventricular outflow tract width during systole by decreasing the regional septal ejection fraction.

2. Modification of the ventricular activation sequence

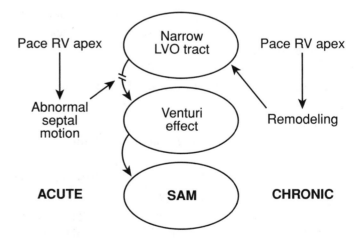

Fig. 16. Possible mechanisms of the benefit of dual-chamber pacing in hypertrophic cardiomyopathy. LVO, left ventricular outflow; RV, right ventricle; SAM, systolic anterior motion of the mitral valve.

may reduce systolic (hyper)contractility analogous to the effect of β-blockers or other negative inotropes. Careful hemodynamic study has demonstrated a rightward shift of the left ventricular end-systolic pressure-volume relationship in hypertrophied hearts

Table 5.—Candidates for Dual Chamber Pacing

Good candidates
  Subaortic obstruction ($\geq$ 30 mm Hg at rest; $\geq$ 55 mm Hg
    provokable)
  Coexisting chronotropic incompetence
Poor candidates
  Rapid native atrioventricular conduction (? candidates for
    radio-frequency ablation)
  Abnormal mitral valve anatomy with significant
    mitral regurgitation
  Primary diastolic dysfunction
Age considerations, operative risk, coronary artery disease

during VDD pacing. This increases end-systolic volume at any given end-systolic pressure, thus reducing intraventricular pressure gradients and myocardial work.

3. Pacing may decrease mitral regurgitation if it is due to systolic anterior motion of the anterior mitral valve leaflet.

4. Diastolic function may favorably alter during pacing in HOCM, although substantial evidence also suggests that it is affected adversely, especially at shorter AV delays.

5. Left ventricular hypertrophy has been reported to regress during pacing, but there are evidence and interpretations to the contrary.

Practical Aspects of Pacing in HOCM

Patient selection
  Inclusion criteria:
  1. Symptomatic despite adequate conventional medications
  2. Left ventricular outflow tract gradient > 30 mm Hg at rest or > 50 mm Hg with provocation
  3. Prominent basal interventricular septal hypertrophy
  4. Modestly severe functional mitral regurgitation
  5. Bradycardic indications for pacing
  6. High risk or refusal to consider surgery
  Exclusion criteria:
  1. Isolated apical hypertrophy or midcavitary obstruction only
  2. Significant mitral regurgitation due to structural valvular abnormalities
  3. Fixed subvalvular aortic obstruction
  4. Chronic or frequent paroxysmal atrial fibrillation

Optimizing AV Interval

There are substantial interindividual differences in optimal AV interval for maximal benefit. The pacemaker should be programmed appropriately with the assistance of invasive and/or Doppler hemodynamic measurements at different AV interval settings. It is essential that ventricular stimulation occur at all heart rates, rather than ventricular activation via the AV node. This may require the use of concomitant medications to slow AV nodal conduction. Negative AV hysteresis, rate adaptive AV delay, pace/sense AV offset, and high upper rate limits should be considered to ensure complete ventricular capture in all circumstances. The need for short AV intervals is somewhat counterbalanced by the fact that as AV delay becomes too short, atrial contraction occurs against closed AV valves and compromises LV filling in a very preload-dependent population. To achieve full ventricular capture while avoiding excessively short AV intervals, radiofrequency ablation or modification of the AV node has been reported as a viable option.

Use of Acute Temporary Pacing Studies

A trend to omit acute hemodynamic studies is emerging because of considerations of cost, inconvenience, and a degree of insensitivity to long-term hemodynamic and symptomatic results. Advantages of acute studies, however, are that they more precisely define the optimal AV interval prospectively, assess the effect of pacing on mitral regurgitation, identify occasional patients who have adverse hemodynamic effects from pacing, and permit the systematic accumulation of data which will be important to further understanding the effect and role of pacing in these patients.

Ventricular Pacing Site

Apical lead position gives best hemodynamic and clinical results.

Device Selection

DDD or DDDR pacemakers are required. Programming features that include a wide range of AV intervals, rate-adaptive AV delay, and automatic AV delay adjustment after paced versus sensed atrial events are desirable.

Role of Pacing Versus Surgical Myectomy

Myectomy has an established high level of efficacy with low morbidity and mortality in experienced hands. Although pacing is a reasonable first choice in some patients because it is minimally invasive, proceeding to surgery should not be delayed too long in patients who are both symptomatic and good candidates for surgery. No randomized comparison between pacing versus surgery (or versus placebo) has been reported. If longer term follow-up with pacing therapy should suggest the hemodynamic benefits are less sustained than currently suspected, then consideration may favor the surgical approach earlier. Myectomy should be considered early in patients who are young, active, have more severe symptoms, and do not have significant surgical risk factors. If a trial of pacing is used, failure to demonstrate substantial hemodynamic and especially subjective symptomatic or objective functional improvement within 3 months warrants early consideration of surgery. Pacing helps in HCM by optimizing AV delay and reducing systolic anterior motion of the mitral valve and the left ventricular outflow tract gradient.

*Modified from McGoon M: Syllabus for Mayo Cancun Cardiology meeting.

- Pacing helps in HCM by optimizing AV delay and reducing systolic anterior motion of the mitral valve and the left ventricular outflow tract gradient.
- The indication for myotomy/myectomy is symptomatic HCM refractory to medical treatment.
- Ideal candidates for dual-chamber pacing should be symptomatic and have resting obstruction.

Alcohol Septal Ablation

This technique uses a controlled myocardial infarction of the basal ventricular septum to reduce the intraventricular gradient. The first septal artery is occluded with a balloon catheter and alcohol is injected distally. The role of this procedure in HCM is being evaluated.

Restrictive Cardiomyopathy

Definition and Etiology

Restrictive cardiomyopathy (RCM), a rare form of cardiomyopathy, is the least well understood cardiomyopathy. The WHO defined RCM as myocardial disease "characterized by restrictive filling and reduced diastolic volume of either or both ventricles with normal or near-normal systolic function and wall thickness. Increased interstitial fibrosis may be present. It may be idiopathic or associated with other disease (e.g., amyloidosis; endomyocardial disease with or without hypereosinophilia)" It may be difficult to distinguish RCM from constrictive pericarditis, hence its

clinical importance. The primary abnormality in RCM is ventricular diastolic dysfunction (Table 6). With diastolic dysfunction, the increase in pressure per unit ventricular blood volume during filling of the ventricles is greater, and this is reflected onto the pulmonary circulation and causes symptoms of shortness of breath and congestive heart failure. Also, because the ventricle cannot fill to meet the preload requirements, stroke volume is decreased despite normal systolic function. At the end stage of disease, there eventually may be decompensation of systolic function.

The cause of primary RCM is not known (Table 7 and Table 8). The two major categories are idiopathic RCM (nonobliterative RCM) and endomyocardial fibrosis (obliterative RCM). Idiopathic RCM is seen mainly in the U.S. and is caused by progressive fibrosis of the myocardium. Nontropical endomyocardial fibrosis is very rare and may be the end stage of eosinophilic syndromes in which an intracavitary thrombus fills the left ventricular apex and restricts filling of the ventricles. Fibrosis may also extend to involve the atrioventricular valves and cause valvular regurgitation. Two different forms of endomyocardial fibrosis are described: an active inflammatory eosinophilic myocarditis in the temperate zones and chronic endomyocardial fibrosis in the tropic zones.

Other diseases that cause infiltration of the myocardium and have a presentation and pathophysiology similar to that of primary RCM include amyloidosis, sarcoidosis, hemochromatosis, and chronic renal failure. Signs and symptoms similar to those of RCM may develop in patients after mediastinal radiation therapy or after heart transplantation.

- The primary abnormality in RCM is diastolic dysfunction.
- Endomyocardial fibrosis is probably an end stage of eosinophilic syndromes.

Clinical Presentation of Restrictive Cardiomyopathy

Patients with RCM usually present with severe symptoms of failure of the right side of the heart and low output state.

Table 6.—Definition of Restrictive Cardiomyopathy

Restrictive cardiomyopathy—a cardiomyopathy characterized by

    Normal-sized ventricular chambers

    Variable reduction in systolic function

    Restrictive diastolic function (atrial enlargement)

Table 7.—Primary Forms of Restrictive Cardiomyopathy

Obliterative (thrombus-filled ventricles)
    Endomyocardial fibrosis
    Hypereosinophilic syndrome (Löffler's)
Nonobliterative
    Primary restrictive cardiomyopathy
    Senile restrictive disease

Fatigue, shortness of breath, edema, and ascites are the most common complaints. Atrial arrhythmias are common, and atrial fibrillation may be present. Bilateral pleural effusions may contribute to the symptoms of shortness of breath. The major differential diagnosis of RCM is constrictive pericarditis.

Physical Examination in Restrictive Cardiomyopathy

The physical examination findings in RCM are remarkable for increased venous pressure with rapid X and Y descents in the jugular venous pressure waveform. The carotid upstroke has a low volume, consistent with the low output state. The precordium is usually normal. Murmurs of mitral and/or tricuspid valve regurgitation may be present. Nearly always, a loud diastolic filling sound (S_3) is present. Edema and ascites are frequently present in advanced cases.

Echocardiography in Restrictive Cardiomyopathy

The imaging modality of choice for diagnosing RCM is echocardiography. In most instances, a two-dimensional echocardiogram shows normal left ventricular size and function and marked dilatation of both atria (Fig. 17 and Table 9). Doppler echocardiography shows features of "restriction to filling," indicating a marked decrease in chamber compliance. This is seen as a high E-to-A ratio, with a short deceleration time on the mitral inflow velocities, and as a low systolic-to-diastolic flow ratio of the pulmonary venous flow velocities.

After RCM has been diagnosed, the underlying cause should be determined if possible. Blood tests such as iron studies, special protein studies, levels of angiotensin converting enzymes, and peripheral blood smears may provide a clue to the diagnosis. If the diagnosis remains equivocal after echocardiography and blood tests, endomyocardial biopsy may be helpful.

Table 8.—Causes of Restrictive Cardiomyopathy

Primary (idiopathic) restrictive cardiomyopathy
Eosinophilic endomyoardial disease and endomyocardial fibrosis
Infiltrative cardiomyopathies
    Amyloid heart disease
    Hemochromatosis
    Glycogen storage disease
    Fabry disease
    Mucopolysaccharidoses
    Sarcoidosis
Scleroderma
Post-heart transplantation
Post-mediastinal irradiation
Pseudoxanthoma elasticum
Doxorubicin and daunorubicin chemotherapy
Carcinoid heart disease
Malignant disease with encasement of the heart from pericardial metastases
Associated with the eosinophilia-myalgia syndrome due to toxic contamination of L-tryptophan dietary supplements

• RCM is a disease characterized by normal-sized ventricular chambers with marked biatrial dilatation.

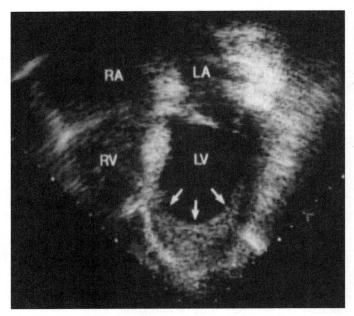

Fig. 17. Echocardiogram of obliterative variant of restrictive cardiomyopathy. The left ventricular (LV) apex is obliterated by a combination of fresh thrombus and fibrosis (*arrows*). This patient had hypereosinophilic syndrome. LA, left atrium; RA, right atrium; RV, right ventricle.

Table 9.—Features of Restrictive Cardiomyopathy

Dilated atria
Normal-sized ventricles
Variable decrease in systolic function
Severe diastolic dysfunction

In contrast to dilated cardiomyopathy and HCM, left ventricular cavity size and wall thickness are normal in RCM, and systolic function may be normal or slightly reduced. The characteristic hemodynamics of RCM are the "square root" sign in the ventricular pressure tracing and a shortened deceleration time in the mitral inflow signal.

Clinically, RCM is also mimicked by amyloid heart disease, but the two are distinguished clearly by two-dimensional echocardiography. In amyloid heart disease, the thickness of the wall of the left ventricle is increased and may have a "scintillating" appearance; thickening and regurgitation of all four valves and pericardial effusions are common (Fig. 18). In RCM, the dimensions and wall thickness of the ventricular cavities are normal, but the atria are markedly enlarged (Fig. 19). Histologically, there are fibrosis and fibrous tissue replacement of the myocardial cells. In amyloid heart disease, the myocardium is thickened and has an abnormal texture (Fig. 20). Two-dimensional echocardiography can clearly distinguish amyloid heart disease from primary restrictive disease and pericardial constriction.

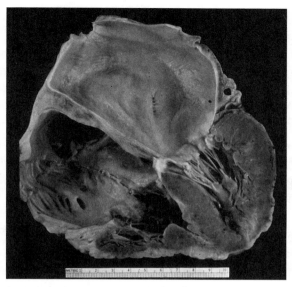

Fig. 19. Autopsy specimen of restrictive cardiomyopathy. The size of the left ventricular cavity and the thickness of its wall are normal; however, the atria are markedly dilated.

Frequently, the major diagnostic dilemma is to distinguish idiopathic RCM from constrictive pericarditis, because both may present with right heart failure out of proportion to myocardial systolic dysfunction or valvular abnormalities. Computed tomography or magnetic resonance imaging of the pericardium may be helpful by showing a thickened, calcified pericardium in constrictive pericarditis and a normal pericardium in RCM. Respiratory changes in Doppler flow velocities are useful in distinguishing between restriction

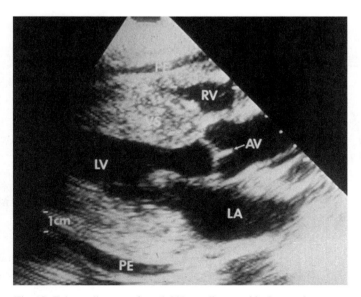

Fig. 18. Echocardiogram of amyloid heart disease with abnormal myocardial texture ("scintillating granular myocardium") and wall thickening. AV, aortic valve; PE, pericardial effusion. Other abbreviations as in Figure 17.

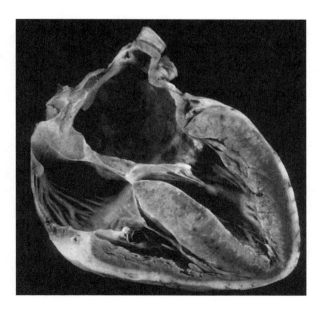

Fig. 20. Autopsy specimen of amyloid heart disease. Note the diffusely thickened walls of the left ventricle and the dilatation of the left atrium.

and constriction type pathophysiology, being present in constriction and absent in restriction.

The square root sign on hemodynamic tracings is common to both RCM and constrictive pericarditis (Fig. 21 and 22). To distinguish between constrictive pericarditis and RCM, respiratory-related dissociation must be demonstrated between intracavitary and intrathoracic pressures as well as exaggerated ventricular interaction (Table 10). These two points can be demonstrated clearly echocardiographically (two-dimensional/Doppler) and by cardiac catheterization.

Eosinophilic Endomyocardial Disease

Severe prolonged eosinophilia of any cause (allergic, autoimmune, parasitic, leukemic, or idiopathic) can lead to eosinophilic infiltration of the myocardium. Eosinophilic degranulation results in myocardial damage through the action of major basic and cationic proteins. This disease, also called Löffler syndrome, in its late stages is associated with dense endomyocardial fibrosis, intraventricular thrombus formation, and obliteration of the ventricular cavity. End-stage cardiac structure is similar to that of a condition called "endomyocardial fibrosis" found almost exclusively in equatorial Africa and, less frequently, in Asia and South America.

The treatment of Löffler syndrome consists of correctly identifying the condition before end-stage fibrosis occurs; the administration of corticosteroids, cytotoxic agents, and interferon to suppress the intense eosinophilic infiltration of the myocardium; and conventional heart failure medications. Anticoagulation with warfarin is important to reduce systemic embolization from ventricular thrombi.

Endomyocardial Fibrosis

Tropical endomyocardial fibrosis is a common form of RCM that occurs in equatorial Africa, Asia, and South America. Because most patients with this condition also have heavy parasite loads, it was thought for many years that endomyocardial fibrosis represented an end stage of eosinophilic endomyocardial disease in response to an allergic/immune reaction to parasitosis. This is now considered incorrect because patients with the tropical form of endomyocardial fibrosis do not exhibit eosinophilia. The prognosis for endomyocardial fibrosis is poor, but surgical removal of fibrotic disease and valve repair or replacement may be helpful.

Treatment of Restrictive Cardiomyopathy

Treatment of the underlying condition is rarely possible, except for hemochromatosis-associated disease that may respond to chelation therapy and, possibly, sarcoidosis-associated disease that may respond to corticosteroid therapy. Diuretics are helpful to treat congestive symptoms, but a high ventricular filling pressure is needed to maintain cardiac output in the setting of restrictive physiology. Dehydration and overdiuresis should be avoided. Calcium channel blockers and β-blockers probably have harmful effects in RCM.

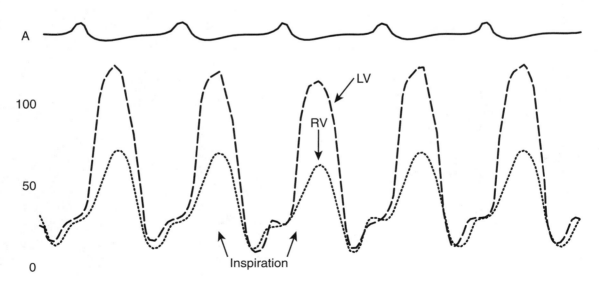

Fig. 21. Hemodynamic tracing of restrictive cardiomyopathy. LV, left ventricle; RV, right ventricle. (From *Circulation* 79:357-370, 1989. By permission of the American Heart Association.)

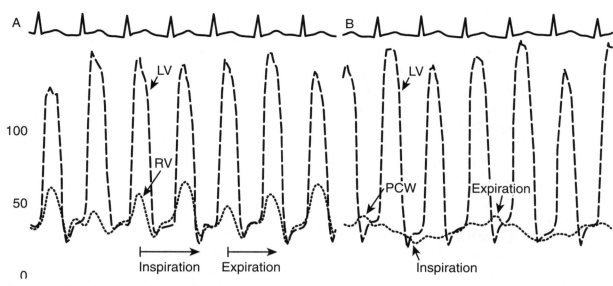

Fig. 22. Hemodynamic tracing of constrictive pericarditis. *A*, LV and RV tracing; *B*, LV and PCW tracing. LV, left ventricle; PCW, pulmonary capillary wedge; RV, right ventricle. (From *Circulation* 79:357-370, 1989. By permission of the American Heart Association.)

Heart rate control of atrial fibrillation, which is frequently associated with restrictive cardiomyopathy, is important. The drug of choice is digoxin. Inotropic agents or vasodilators are of unproven use in this condition. Heart transplantation should be considered for patients with refractory symptoms who are otherwise suitable candidates.

Table 10.—Hemodynamics of Constrictive Pericarditis

The hemodynamics in constrictive pericarditis reflect
  Dissociation between intracavitary and intrathoracic pressures
  Ventricular interaction

Suggested Reading List

1. Corrado D, Basso C, Schiavon M, et al: Screening for hypertrophic cardiomyopathy in young athletes. *N Engl J Med* 339:364-369, 1998.
The results show that hypertrophic cardiomyopathy was an uncommon cause of death in these young competitive athletes and suggest that the identification and disqualification of affected athletes at screening before participation in competitive sports may have prevented sudden death.

2. Kushwaha SS, Fallon JT, Fuster V: Restrictive cardiomyopathy. *N Engl J Med* 336:267-276, 1997.
Excellent review of restrictive cardiomyopathy.

3. Niimura H, Bachinski LL, Sangwatanaroj S: Mutations in the gene for cardiac myosin-binding protein C and late-onset familial hypertrophic cardiomyopathy. *N Engl J Med* 338:1248-1257, 1998.
The clinical expression of mutations in the gene for cardiac myosin-binding protein C is often delayed until middle age or old age. Delayed expression of cardiac hypertrophy and a favorable clinical course may hinder recognition of the heritable nature of mutations in the cardiac myosin-binding protein C gene. Clinical screening in adult life may be warranted for members of families characterized by hypertrophic cardiomyopathy.

4. Spirito P, Seidman CE, McKenna WJ, et al: The management of hypertrophic cardiomyopathy. *N Engl J Med* 336:775, 1997.
Excellent review of the management of hypertrophic cardiomyopathy.

5. Yetman AT, McCrindle BW, MacDonald C, et al: Myocardial bridging in children with hypertrophic cardiomyopathy—a risk factor for sudden death. *N Engl J Med* 339:1201-1209, 1998.
Myocardial bridging is associated with a poor outcome in children with hypertrophic cardiomyopathy. The observations reported in this paper suggest that bridging is associated with myocardial ischemia.

Questions

Multiple Choice (choose the one best answer)

1. All the following features favor a diagnosis of hypertrophic cardiomyopathy (HCM) instead of athletic heart *except*:
   a. Left ventricular cavity size, as determined by echocardiography, greater than 55 mm
   b. Left atrial enlargement
   c. Abnormal left ventricular diastolic function on Doppler echocardiography
   d. Family history of sudden cardiac death at an age younger than 40 years
   e. No regression of left ventricular hypertrophy with deconditioning

2. Syncope and/or presyncope is common in patients with hypertrophic cardiomyopathy (HCM). All the following statements are correct regarding this symptom in HCM *except*:
   a. Syncopal symptoms correlate poorly with outflow tract gradients
   b. HCM is associated with a higher than expected occurrence of bypass tracts (Wolff-Parkinson-White syndrome)
   c. Hypotension frequently occurs during head-up tilt table testing in patients with HCM
   d. Rapid atrial arrhythmias may cause rapid hemodynamic deterioration in patients with HCM
   e. The commonest mechanism of post-exercise-induced syncope in HCM is decreased venous return in association with sympathetic stimulation of the heart leading to a critical increase in outflow tract gradient and a precipitous decrease in cardiac output leading to syncope

3. All the following statements are correct about hypertension-associated hypertrophic cardiomyopathy (HCM) *except*:
   a. Occurs at an older age and in a greater proportion of women than non-hypertension-induced HCM
   b. Is commonly associated with heart failure
   c. Is commonly associated with angina pectoris
   d. Is associated with a lower rate of sudden death than non-hypertension-associated HCM
   e. Responds well symptomatically to blood pressure reduction by afterload-reducing agents

4. Mitral regurgitation is frequently present in hypertrophic cardiomyopathy (HCM). The following statements are true *except*:
   a. The severity of mitral regurgitation correlates with outflow tract gradient
   b. Most mitral regurgitation in HCM occurs in late systole
   c. Mitral valve replacement with a low-profile prosthetic valve may in itself improve left ventricular outflow tract obstruction
   d. The commonest site for endocarditis in patients with HCM is on the mitral valve or the point of apposition of the mitral valve and the septum
   e. Is frequently associated with the presence of a cleft mitral valve

Answers

1. Answer a

Differentiation between an athletic heart and hypertrophic cardiomyopathy may be a problem. Features that favor HCM include left ventricular wall thickness greater than 16 mm in men and 14 mm in women, no regression of left ventricular hypertrophy with the cessation of athletic training, and abnormal left ventricular filling indices on Doppler echocardiography. A family history of sudden cardiac death at an early age or a definitive diagnosis of HCM in family members also favors HCM. Other features suggestive of HCM include atrial enlargement, a diastolic left ventricular size less than 45 mm, nonsymmetric patterns of ventricular hypertrophy, and bizarre ECG patterns.

Features that favor an athletic heart include left ventricular wall thickness less than 12 mm and a left ventricular cavity size greater than 55 mm on echocardiography.

2. Answer e

Syncope or presyncope is most likely due to cardiac arrhythmias in patients with HCM and correlates poorly with outflow tract gradients. Other causes of syncope/presyncope in patients with HCM include activation of ventricular baroreceptors by exercise, leading to bradycardia and hypotension, reciprocating tachycardias across bypass tracts and hemodynamic deterioration secondary to atrial arrhythmias because of the abnormal dependence of the hypertrophied ventricle on atrial filling to achieve adequate cardiac output.

3. Answer e

The HCM variant associated with hypertension usually occurs in elderly women and is characterized by a small ventricular cavity and often a sigmoid-shaped septum. It generally has a more benign prognosis than non-hypertension-associated HCM, but it may cause both heart failure and angina pectoris. Afterload-reducing agents and diuretics are contraindicated, and β-blockers are the drugs of choice if there is no contraindication to their use.

4. Answer e

Mitral regurgitation in HCM is multifactorial in cause but correlates well in severity with the degree of left ventricular outflow tract obstruction. Ostium primum atrial septal defect but not HCM is associated with a cleft mitral value. Mitral valve replacement—"Cooley operation"—may abolish systolic anterior motion of the mitral valve and improve left ventricular outflow tract obstruction.

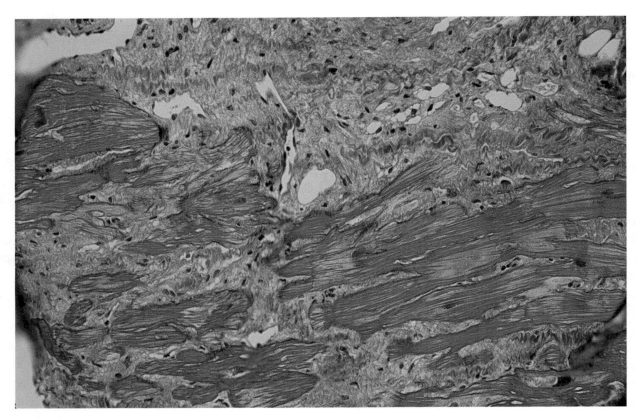

Plate 1. Right ventricular endomyocardial biopsy specimen showing eosinophilic restrictive cardiomyopathy (16% eosinophils).

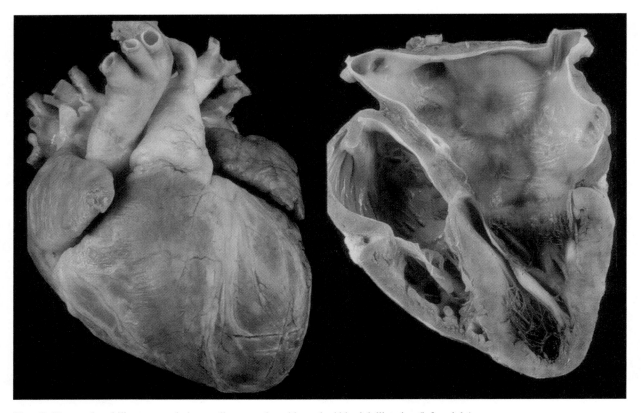

Plate 2. Non-eosinophilic type restrictive cardiomyopathy with marked biatrial dilatation (left > right).

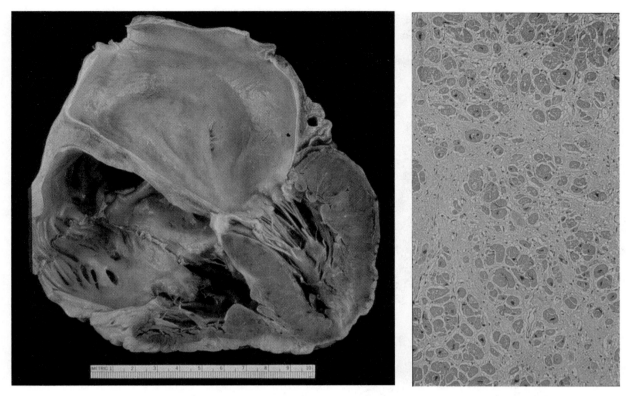

Plate 3. *Left*, Four-chamber view of primary non-eosinophilic restrictive cardiomyopathy. *Right*, Myocardial biopsy specimen.

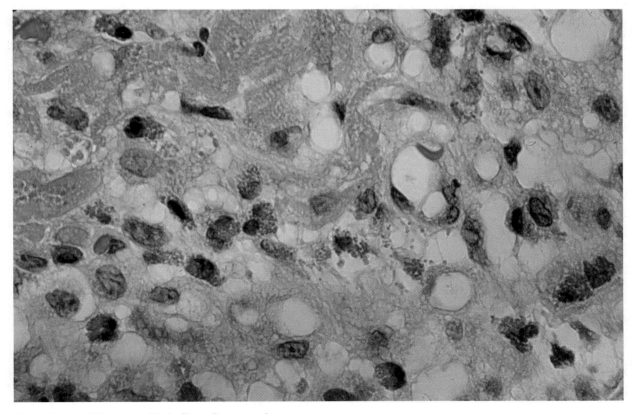

Plate 4. Eosinophilic myocarditis in Churg-Strauss syndrome.

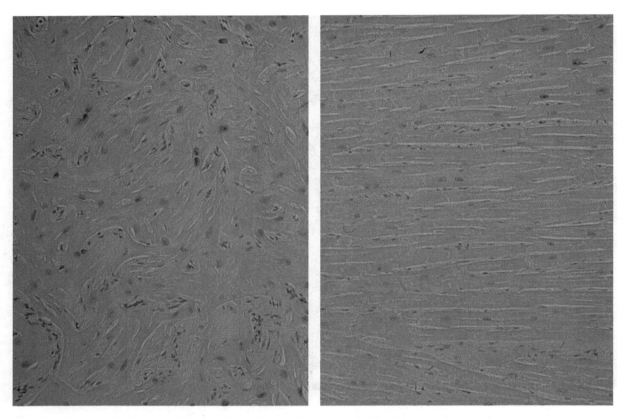

Plate 5. *Left*, myocardial disarray in hypertrophic cardiomyopathy compared with, *right*, normal myocardium.

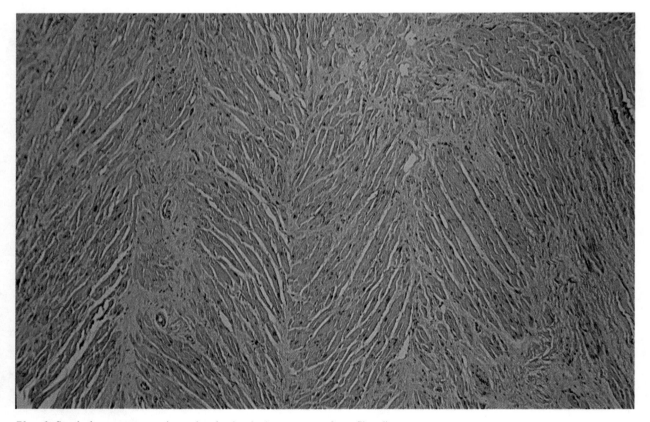

Plate 6. Surgical myectomy specimen showing herringbone pattern of myofiber disarray.

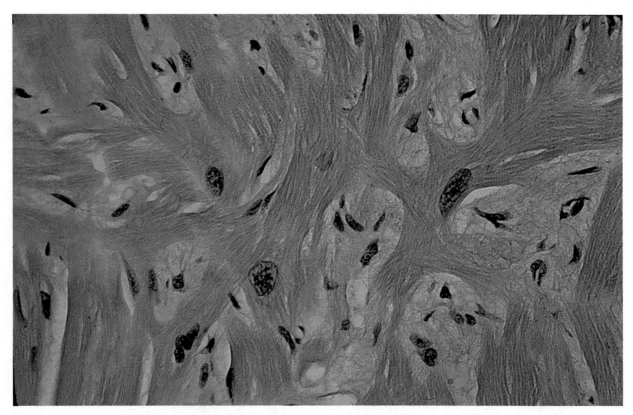

Plate 7. Myofiber disarray in hypertrophic cardiomyopathy.

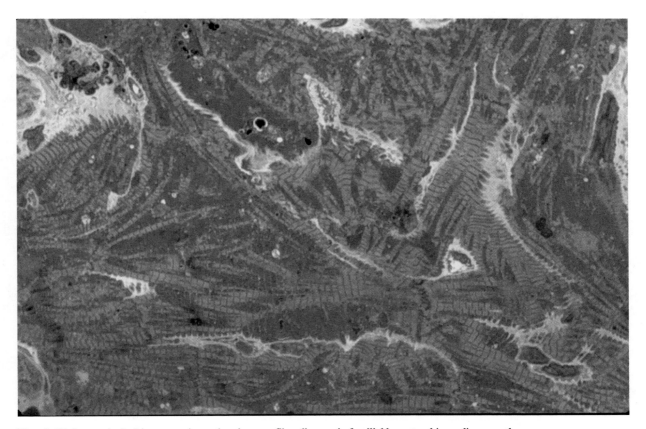

Plate 8. Right ventricular biopsy specimen showing myofiber disarray in familial hypertrophic cardiomyopathy.

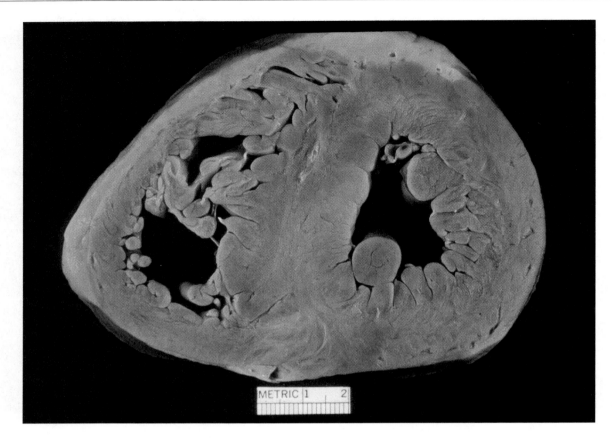

Plate 9. Hypertrophic cardiomyopathy (short-axis view).

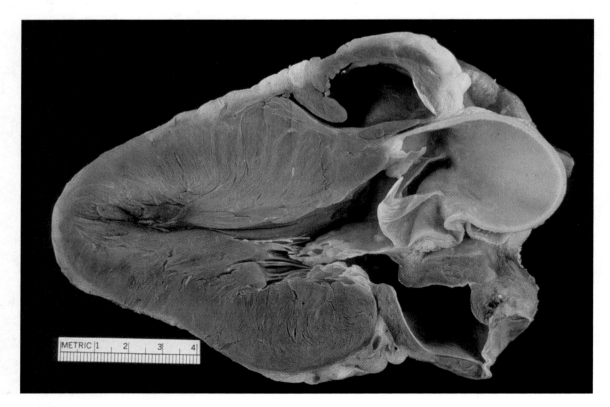

Plate 10. Hypertrophic cardiomyopathy complicated by sudden death (long-axis view).

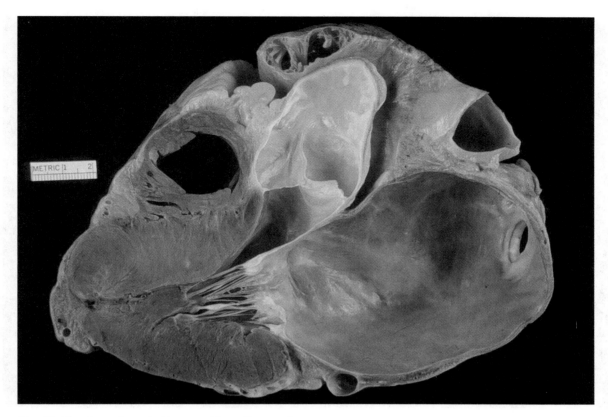

Plate 11. Nonobstructive apical hypertrophic cardiomyopathy.

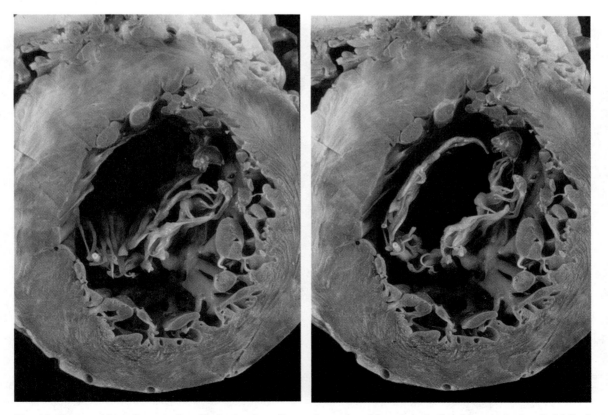

Plate 12. Hypertrophic cardiomyopathy with simulated systolic anterior motion of the anterior leaflet of the mitral valve. *Left*, Mitral valve closed in systole. *Right*, Mitral valve open in diastole, with systolic anterior motion of the anterior leaflet.

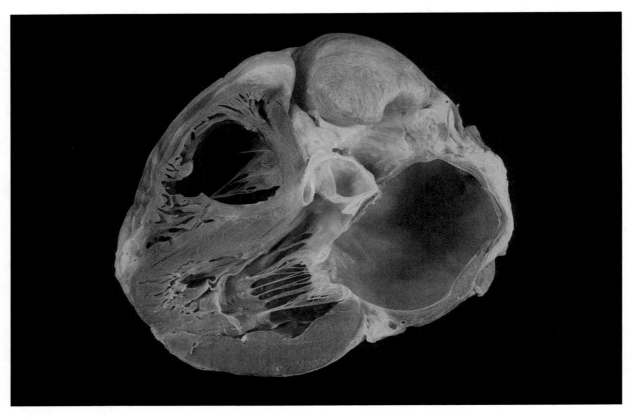

Plate 13. End-stage hypertrophic cardiomyopathy showing biventricular dilation (long-axis view).

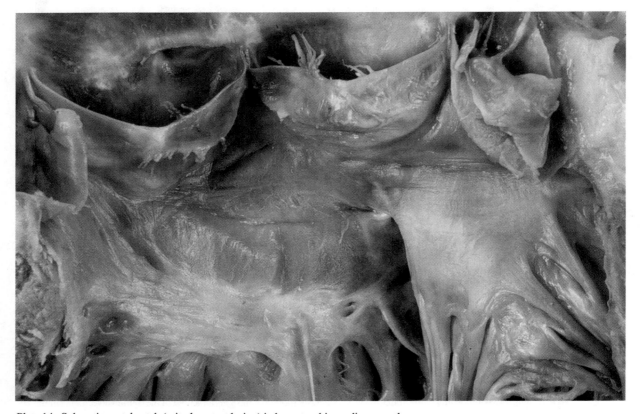

Plate 14. Subaortic septal patch (mitral contact lesion) in hypertrophic cardiomyopathy.

Chapter 31

Myocarditis

Leslie T. Cooper, Jr., M.D.

Myocarditis is present histologically when myocyte damage is associated with inflammatory cells, generally lymphocytes and macrophages (Plate 1). Clinically, the most common presentation of myocarditis is the onset of congestive heart failure in an otherwise healthy young person. Occasionally, the presentation may be that of sudden death, acute myocardial infarction, new atrial or ventricular arrhythmias, or complete heart block. The important causes of myocarditis are listed in Table 1. Regardless of the severity of the acute illness, most patients with viral myocarditis have improvement over several months, although in a proportion the disease progresses to dilated cardiomyopathy and chronic congestive heart failure. Many infectious agents, toxins, and systemic inflammatory disorders have been associated with myocarditis, but most of them are rarely encountered in a general cardiology practice.

Viral, or Idiopathic, Myocarditis

Viral myocarditis, also called "idiopathic" or "lymphocytic myocarditis," is the most common form of acute myocarditis among North American adults. Viral myocarditis is a rare cause of acute heart failure, but it is an important cause of dilated cardiomyopathy. The incidence of histologic myocarditis at autopsy is as high as 5%, suggesting that most cases of myocarditis are subclinical or unrecognized

by physicians. Active myocarditis is defined in the widely accepted Dallas Criteria as "an inflammatory infiltrate of the myocardium with necrosis and/or degeneration of adjacent myocytes..." (Table 2). The nature of the specific immune response that results in myocardial damage is controversial, but several aspects are clinically important because they form the rationale for clinical trials of immunosuppressive therapy. Macrophages and T lymphocytes form the majority of the cellular infiltrate and produce cytokines, including tumor necrosis factor-α (TNF-α). The hypothesis that certain T-helper cells and proinflammatory cytokines are the mechanism for the development of myocardial dysfunction forms the rationale for treatment directed against T-lymphocytes and proinflammatory cytokines. Immunosuppressive agents investigated for the treatment of myocarditis include prednisone, cyclosporine, azathioprine, immune globulin, anti-lymphocyte monoclonal antibodies, and vesnarinone (Tables 3-14).

> Coxsackie B virus, an enterovirus, and adenoviruses are associated with lymphocytic myocarditis.

Clinical Presentation

Although the spectrum of infectious agents that may cause myocardial dysfunction, tachyarrhythmias, or heart block is very broad, many of these viral, bacterial, rickettsial, fungal,

Table 1.—Common Causes of Myocarditis

Associated disorder or agent	Clinical clues	Diagnostic method
Viral/Coxsackie B	Flu-like prodrome	Endomyocardial biopsy
Acute rheumatic fever	Jones criteria	Throat culture, antistreptolysin O titer
Lyme disease	History of tick bite	Serology
Doxorubicin/anthracycline	Previous cancer treatment	Clinical, endomyocardial biopsy
Chagas disease	Travel to Central or South America	Serology
Peripartum cardiomyopathy*	Last trimester or first 6 mo postpartum	Clinical

*Reviewed in Heart Disease in Pregnancy chapter.

and spirochetal infections have clinical clues that lead to a specific diagnostic evaluation. A typical patient with acute myocarditis is relatively young and otherwise healthy. The Myocarditis Treatment Trial enrolled 111 patients with a mean age of 42 years; 62% were males. Myocarditis is diagnosed less commonly in the elderly. This may be due to a lower biopsy rate or to a more or less virulent course in this population. The majority of affected persons reported a flu-like prodrome.

- Myocarditis usually presents as subacute congestive heart failure in an otherwise healthy person.
- Median age of persons affected is about 42 years.
- Most patients report a flu-like prodrome.
- Left ventricular function usually improves over several months.
- Myocarditis is an important cause of dilated cardiomyopathy.

Most cases of myocarditis probably are subclinical; however, symptomatic persons generally have had a recent onset of dyspnea, orthopnea, or paroxysmal nocturnal dyspnea. It is important to remember that a small proportion of patients with myocarditis may present with ventricular or atrial arrhythmia, heart block, or sudden death. Acute focal myocarditis may mimic acute myocardial infarction. Rarely, myocarditis may present with arterial or venous thromboembolism.

> In a 20- to 50-year-old person with few cardiac risk factors who presents with acute myocardial infarction and normal findings on coronary angiography, consider the diagnosis of acute focal myocarditis.

Physical Examination in Myocarditis

The physical examination findings in patients with myocarditis are those of acute decompensated congestive heart failure. Patients are usually tachycardic, and the apex may be diffuse and displaced laterally. S_1 may be soft and there may be an S_3, S_4, or both.

Certain findings may suggest a specific cause. Enlarged lymph nodes may suggest systemic sarcoidosis. A pruritic, maculopapular rash may suggest a hypersensitivity reaction, often to a drug. Sustained ventricular tachycardia in the setting of rapidly progressive congestive heart failure suggests giant cell myocarditis. Erythema marginatum, polyarthralgia, chorea, and subcutaneous nodules constitute the other Jones Criteria major manifestations of acute rheumatic fever. Diagnosis of a specific myocarditis by physical examination alone is rare, because the physical findings are those of acute heart failure.

Table 2.—Dallas Criteria for the Diagnosis of Lymphocytic Myocarditis*

First biopsy
  Active myocarditis (with or without fibrosis)
  Borderline myocarditis (not diagnostic and requiring further biopsy)
  No evidence of myocarditis
Subsequent biopsies
  Ongoing (persistent) myocarditis
  Resolving (healing) myocarditis
  Resolved (healed) myocarditis

*The histologic diagnosis of active myocarditis requires an inflammatory infiltrate with necrosis and/or degeneration of adjacent myocytes without evidence of Chagas disease or features of ischemic heart disease.

Table 3.—Viral Myocarditis

Cause	Clinical features	Pathologic findings	Comments
Coxsackievirus	See text	Lymphocytic infiltrate with myocyte necrosis	Sensitivity of endomyocardial biopsy is about 35%
Influenza	Tachycardia, ECG abnormalities, dyspnea, anginal chest pain, congestive failure, complete heart block, and death	Myocarditis present in one-third of fatal cases; biventricular dilatation, subendocardial and subepicardial hemorrhage, and mononuclear perivascular inflammation	Treat type A with amantadine
Cytomegalovirus	Symptomatic disease rare; pericardial effusion occasionally present	Focal lymphocytic infiltration and fibrosis	
Poliomyelitis	Often found in fatal cases; cardiovascular collapse, heart failure, and pulmonary edema		Immunization effective, maintain proper oxygenation and pulmonary function
Infectious mononucleosis	ECG changes common, cardiac symptoms unusual, congestive heart failure or death rare	Myocardial infiltrates of atypical lymphocytes and necrosis	Consider treatment with corticosteroids
Human immunodeficiency virus	Pericarditis, arrhythmias, ECG abnormalities, and dilated cardiomyopathy	Lymphocytic myocarditis, opportunistic myocardial infections, and ventricular dilatation	Consider opportunistic infections and malignancy
Viral hepatitis	Usually transient; ECG abnormalities of bradycardia, ventricular premature complexes, ST-T change; congestive failure and sudden death in severe cases	Focal necrosis and inflammation; petechial hemorrhage, including hemorrhage into conduction system	
Mumps	Clinical and cardiac involvement uncommon, ST- and T-wave abnormalities more frequent	Cardiac dilatation and hypertrophy, mural thrombi, interstitial fibrosis and infiltration of mononuclear cells and focal necrosis, possible relationship of maternal mumps and fetal endocardial fibroelastosis	
Rubeola	Transient ECG abnormalities, rare congestive heart failure	Perivascular lymphocyte infiltrate	
Varicella	Rare bundle-branch block, conduction defects, heart failure, and sudden death; nonsustained ventricular tachycardia and fibrillation	Intranuclear inclusion bodies within myocardial cells, interstitial edema, cellular infiltrates, and myonecrosis	

Table 3 (continued)

Cause	Clinical features	Pathologic findings	Comments
Variola and vaccinia	Myocarditis rare but may be fatal, myocarditis may follow vaccination by 2 weeks	Mononuclear infiltrate, interstitial edema, and necrosis	Variola now eradicated and immunization no longer recommended; myocarditis after vaccination has responded to steroids
Arbovirus (chikungunya, dengue)	Myocarditis frequent; chest pain, dyspnea, palpitations, murmurs, gallops, and cardiomegaly; ST-T abnormalities, supraventricular and ventricular arrhythmias, and sudden death; chronicity	Embolization	
Respiratory syncytial viruses	Rare congestive failure, complete heart block, and arrhythmias		
Herpes simplex virus		Chronic interstitial inflammation and fibrosis	Treat with adenine arabinoside or acyclovir, but effectiveness not proved
Adenovirus	Myocarditis rare	Dilated right and left ventricles, mononuclear infiltrate	
Yellow fever virus	Hepatitis, gastrointestinal bleeding, cardiovascular collapse, and bradycardia inappropriate to the fever	Pericardial petechial hemorrhages and myocyte degeneration	
Rabies	Rare tachycardia, gallop rhythm, and hypotension	Diffuse interstitial infiltrate, myocardial necrosis	

ECG, electrocardiographic.
Modified from Giuliani ER, Gersh BJ, McGoon MD, Hayes DL, Schaff HV (editors): *Mayo Clinic Practice of Cardiology*. Third edition. Mosby, 1996, p 643-644. By permission of Mayo Foundation.

Diagnostic Evaluation of Suspected Myocarditis

The electrocardiogram (ECG) in myocarditis frequently shows sinus tachycardia with nonspecific ST-segment and T-wave abnormalities. Occasionally, myocarditis may present with ECG changes suggestive of acute myocardial infarction. Intraventricular conduction delay is common. In a small proportion of patients, various degrees of heart block may occur, although high-grade heart block requiring pacemaker implantation occurred in approximately 1% of the Myocarditis Treatment Trial subjects. Both supraventricular and nonsustained ventricular arrhythmias are common.

Echocardiography may show either diffuse ventricular hypokinesia or, less commonly, regional wall motion abnormalities. Occasionally, an arrhythmia presentation with normal left ventricular function is seen. Wall motion abnormalities may be global or segmental. Cavity size may be increased or normal. In addition, there may be diastolic relaxation abnormalities. In the Myocarditis Treatment Trial, the ejection fraction increased from about 25% to 35% by 28 weeks of treatment, with or without immunosuppressive treatment. In short, echocardiography is useful to exclude other causes of heart failure such as valvular heart disease, congenital heart disease, or amyloidosis and to define left ventricular function for serial comparisons. No specific echocardiographic findings establish the diagnosis of myocarditis in patients with acute congestive heart failure.

Table 4—Rickettsial Myocarditis

Cause	Clinical features	Pathologic findings	Comments
Scrub typhus (*R. tsutsugamushi*)	Myocarditis common, usually mild, and resolves without sequelae; occasional fatalities	Focal panvasculitis of small blood vessels with proliferative endothelial changes and perivascular round cell infiltrate	Antibiotic therapy
Rocky Mountain spotted fever (*R. rickettsii*)	Peripheral vascular collapse	Interstitial mononuclear myocarditis; immunofluorescent demonstration of rickettsia in myocardial capillaries, venules, and arterioles	Antibiotic therapy
Q fever (*R. burnetii*)	Endocarditis and pericarditis dominate picture; ECG ST and T changes and ventricular arrhythmias	Pericardial petechial hemorrhage, scattered necrosis and fibrosis of myocardium	Antibiotic therapy

ECG, electrocardiographic.

From Giuliani ER, Gersh BJ, McGoon MD, Hayes DL, Schaff HV (editors): *Mayo Clinic Practice of Cardiology.* Third edition. Mosby, 1996, p 647. By permission of Mayo Foundation.

Endomyocardial Biopsy

Right ventricular endomyocardial biopsy is the reference standard for the diagnosis of acute myocarditis (Table 15). Although the specificity of endomyocardial biopsy for lymphocytic myocarditis is high at 79%, the sensitivity is only about 35% when compared with the clinical standard of improved left ventricular function over time. The incidence of positive right ventricular biopsy findings on specimens from patients with suspected myocarditis ranges from 0% to 67%. In the Myocarditis Treatment Trial only 214 of 2,233 patients (10%) with heart failure and suspected myocarditis had diagnostic biopsy findings. The low incidence of diagnostic biopsy findings may be due to several factors, including the true incidence of myocarditis, sampling error from small biopsy specimens, and the limitations of routine histologic techniques for detecting inflammation.

The technique of endomyocardial biopsy may affect the interpretation of the histologic findings (Fig. 1). A minimum of 4, and preferably 8, biopsy specimens should be obtained. Care should be taken to avoid crush injury to the specimen. If clinically indicated, specimens should be specifically stained to test for fungi or acid-fast bacilli. A normal myocardial biopsy specimen and a specimen with diffuse myocarditis by the Dallas Criteria are shown in Plate 1.

Recently, many clinicians have questioned the role of routine endomyocardial biopsy in the diagnosis of lymphocytic myocarditis. This is based in part on evidence from the Myocarditis Treatment Trial, which demonstrated a lack of efficacy of immunosuppression, thus obviating a specific histologic diagnosis in the absence of effective treatment for myocarditis.

Various serologic tests have been proposed to aid in the diagnosis of acute myocarditis. A promising test with high specificity is cardiac troponin I. In patients with clinically suspected myocarditis, cardiac troponin I levels were increased in 34% of patients with biopsy-proven myocarditis compared with 11% of those without biopsy-proven myocarditis (estimated sensitivity, 34%; specificity, 89%). Cardiac troponin I was increased more frequently than creatine kinase MB subunits (CK-MB) in patients with myocarditis, presumably because of the long window for detecting elevation of cardiac troponin I. Therefore, a positive cardiac troponin I test is useful to diagnose myocarditis in the proper clinical setting.

Antimyosin scintigraphy, a noninvasive technique, has been used to identify patients with cardiomyocyte necrosis. A comparison of antimyosin scintigraphic results with endomyocardial biopsy findings of myocarditis revealed a high sensitivity (91% to 100%) and negative predictive value (93% to 100%). The specificity (31% to 44%) and positive predictive value (28% to 33%) were low. Compared with clinical improvement suggestive of reversible left ventricular dysfunction, antimyosin scintigraphy had a high sensitivity (82% to 94%) but low specificity (25% to 42%).

Table 5.—Bacterial Myocarditis, *Mycoplasma pneumoniae*, and Psittacosis

Cause	Clinical features	Pathologic findings	Comments
Diphtheria	Heart block, bradycardia, ventricular arrhythmias		
Tuberculosis	Heart block, heart failure	Caseating granulomas	
Streptococci	Acute myocarditis, distinct from rheumatic carditis; may accompany scarlet fever; conduction abnormalities and arrhythmia uncommon, and sudden death rare	Interstitial infiltrate of mononuclear cells and polymorphonuclear cells, bacteria sometimes detectable in the heart	Antibiotic therapy
Meningococci	Myocardium commonly involved, especially in fatal cases; pericardial effusions, heart block, congestive heart failure, and death	Interstitial myocarditis and hemorrhagic myocardial lesions	Antibiotic therapy
Brucellosis	Endocarditis, conduction system disturbance	Tuberculoid granulomas	Antibiotic therapy
Clostridia		Gas bubbles in myocardium, organisms may be in tissues or intramural coronary arteries, myocardial abscess formation and purulent pericarditis	Antibiotic therapy
Staphylococci	May be associated with endocarditis or overwhelming sepsis	Multiple abscesses, may complicate myocardial infarction, cardiac perforation	
Melioidosis	May mimic myocardial infarction	Abscess formation	Antibiotic therapy
Mycoplasma pneumoniae	Myalgias and ST-T-wave abnormalities in up to one-third of patients, usually associated with pneumonia, may require intensive care, may result in permanent sequelae		Antibiotic therapy
Psittacosis	Congestive heart failure; pericarditis; fever, chest pain, tachycardia, hypotension, and emboli	Inclusion bodies and plasma cells, subendocardial hemorrhage	Antibiotic therapy

Modified from Giuliani ER, Gersh BJ, McGoon MD, Hayes DL, Schaff HV (editors): *Mayo Clinic Practice of Cardiology*. Third edition. Mosby, 1996, pp 647-648. By permission of Mayo Foundation.

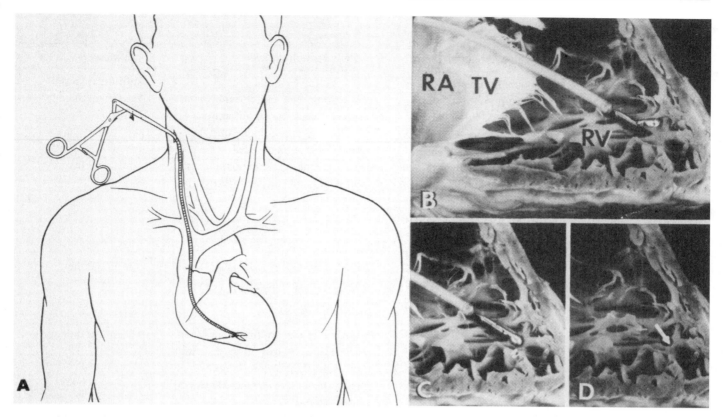

Fig. 1. Right ventricular endomyocardial biopsy. *A*, Diagram showing ease of access to right ventricular apex via right internal jugular vein. *B* to *D*, Autopsy specimen used to simulate biopsy procurement, with bioptome jaws opened around a trabecula carnea (*B*), jaws closed (*C*), and appearance of biopsy site (*arrow*) (*D*). RA, right atrium; RV, right ventricle; TV, tricuspid valve. (From *Mayo Clin Proc* 57:407-418, 1982. By permission of Mayo Foundation.)

Table 6.—Spirochetal Myocarditis

Cause	Clinical features	Pathologic findings	Comments
Syphilis	Arrhythmias and heart block	Myocarditis found in congenital syphilis; gummas may be found in myocardium, valves, and conduction system	Antibiotic therapy
Leptospirosis (Weil's disease)	ST and T abnormalities and arrhythmias with conduction defects, congestive heart failure rare	Interstitial inflammation and subepicardial hemorrhage	Antibiotic therapy
Relapsing fever (*Borrelia*)	Tachyarrhythmias, AV conduction defects, hypotension, and heart failure	Petechiae and interstitial infiltrate	Antibiotic therapy
Lyme disease	Tick-borne, AV conduction defects, myocarditis, pericarditis	Thought to be immune-mediated	Antibiotic therapy

AV, atrioventricular.

From Giuliani ER, Gersh BJ, McGoon MD, Hayes DL, Schaff HV (editors): *Mayo Clinic Practice of Cardiology*. Third edition. Mosby, 1996, p 649. By permission of Mayo Foundation.

Table 7.—Fungal Myocarditis

Cause	Clinical features	Pathologic findings	Comments
Candidiasis	Immunocompromised host		Antifungal therapy
Aspergillosis	Immunocompromised host	Endocarditis frequent, thrombosis of coronary vessels with infarction, invasion by fungus aided by elaboration of oxalic acid	Antifungal therapy
Cryptococcosis	Patients with malignancy; congestive heart failure and cardiomegaly; ventricular arrhythmias, first-degree AV block, and T-wave abnormalities	Cardiac dilatation, granuloma formation with giant cells and fibrosis	Antifungal therapy
Histoplasmosis	Cardiac involvement rare; endocarditis and pericarditis; arrhythmias and T-wave abnormalities	Granulomas with *Histoplasma capsulatum* in phagocytes	Antifungal therapy
Actinomycosis	Myocarditis rare; right and left heart failure	Extension of disease from thorax via pericardium or, less often, hematogenous spread; abscesses contain organism and are surrounded by granulation tissue	Antifungal therapy
Blastomycosis	Third and fourth decades of life; tachycardia, systolic murmur, dyspnea, cyanosis, and peripheral edema	Spreads from mediastinal lymph nodes, to pericardium, to myocardium, to endocardium, or by hematogenous miliary seeding; mural thrombi may form; caseation with tubercles and giant cells	Antifungal therapy
Coccidioidomycosis	Pericarditis may be present	Myocarditis, focal interstitial and perivascular infiltrate, granulomas sometimes containing fungi	Antifungal therapy
Mucormycosis	Cardiac involvement rare	Septic thrombosis, myocarditis, mycotic valvular thrombi	Antifungal therapy

Modified from Giuliani ER, Gersh BJ, McGoon MD, Hayes DL, Schaff HV (editors): *Mayo Clinic Practice of Cardiology.* Third edition. Mosby, 1996, p 650. By permission of Mayo Foundation.

Thus, negative findings on antimyosin scintigraphy can reasonably exclude active myocarditis in a population of patients with suspected myocarditis. However, the applicability of this technology is limited by the availability of antimyosin antibody and low specificity. Promising techniques for diagnosing and localizing myocarditis include gadolinium-enhanced magnetic resonance imaging and novel echocardiographic techniques.

A reasonable diagnostic strategy for a young patient with new onset of heart failure of unknown cause is the following:

1. Exclude treatable causes of heart failure, including congenital, valvular, and coronary artery disease, by echocardiography and coronary angiography.
2. Consider a cardiac troponin I test: positive results would confirm acute myocarditis.
3. Consider antimyosin scintigraphy: negative findings would exclude active myocarditis.
4. Consider endomyocardial biopsy if the patient has a history or clinical course suggestive of a specific myocardial procress such as sarcoidosis or giant cell myocarditis.

Table 8.—Protozoal Myocarditis

Cause	Clinical features	Pathologic findings	Comments
Chagas disease	History of travel to endemic region, megaesophagus	Apical aneurysm	*
Toxoplasmosis	Immunocompromised host	May have toxoplasmic cysts, diffuse or focal myocarditis	*
African trypanosomiasis (*T. gambiense* and *T. rhodesiense*)	CNS (somnolence) dominates, Q-T prolongation and T-wave abnormalities common, cardiomegaly and congestive heart failure	Myocardial granulomas or diffuse interstitial infiltrates; primary arteritis and valvulitis	*
Malaria	May have chest pain and rarely heart failure	Capillary thrombosis and occlusion by parasites; interstitial infiltrates and hemorrhage	*
Leishmaniasis (kala-azar)		Myocarditis and suppurative pericarditis, intracellular plasmatocytes with Leishman-Donovan bodies	*
Balantidiasis (*Balantidium coli*)		Subacute myocarditis, cardiac dilatation, and pericardial effusion; parasites within coronary vessels and myocardium	*
Sarcosporidiosis	Rare in humans	Sarcocysts in muscle fibers	*

CNS, central nervous system.

*For current information regarding antiparasitic treatment, the reader is advised to consult the Centers for Disease Control, Atlanta, Georgia, or a comparable source.

Modified from Giuliani ER, Gersh BJ, McGoon MD, Hayes DL, Schaff HV (editors): *Mayo Clinic Practice of Cardiology*. Third edition. Mosby, 1996, p 653. By permission of Mayo Foundation.

Treatment Options: the Myocarditis Treatment Trial

The Myocarditis Treatment Trial was a prospective, randomized, double-blinded, placebo-controlled trial of prednisone plus cyclosporine or azathioprine for the treatment of biopsy-proven lymphocytic myocarditis in persons with congestive heart failure. There was no benefit to immunosuppression over placebo in survival or left ventricular ejection fraction. The mean left ventricular ejection fraction increased from 24% to 35% in both groups, and the actuarial mortality (death or transplantation) was 56% by 4 years regardless of immunosuppression. This survival is similar to that for patients with dilated cardiomyopathy. Because of these data, enthusiasm for immunosuppression in lymphocytic myocarditis has waned. However, there are theoretical grounds for immunosuppressive treatment, and trial design limitations in the Myocarditis Treatment Trial limit the applicability of its conclusions to all patients with myocarditis. An uncontrolled study of intravenous immunoglobulin showed improvement in ejection fraction and New York Heart Association class, and a randomized trial of intravenous immunoglobulin for lymphocytic myocarditis is under way.

● The Myocarditis Treatment Trial showed no benefit to immunosuppression with prednisone plus cyclosporine or azathioprine in patients with lymphocytic myocarditis.

Treatment for myocarditis in patients with heart failure may include an angiotensin-converting enzyme inhibitor at a dose equivalent to captopril (50 mg 3 times daily if tolerated), a relatively low dose of a diuretic such as furosemide, and digoxin. Heart block and tachyarrhythmias may be treated with standard agents, including a pacemaker, although this is not often needed. The condition of most patients with lymphocytic myocarditis improves clinically over a few months, although in some the disease eventually progresses to dilated cardiomyopathy.

Table 9.—Helminthic Myocarditis

Cause	Clinical features	Pathologic findings	Comments
Trichinosis	Associated encephalitis	Diagnosis by muscle biopsy	*
Echinococcosis	Seen in sheep-raising regions	Large ventricular cysts that may calcify or rupture	*
Schistosomiasis	Cor pulmonale frequent, direct myocardial involvement infrequent	Ova in myocardium or coronary arteries with coronary thrombosis and myocardial infarction, inflammatory myocarditis and perivasculitis	Cardiac toxicity may also result from antimony derivatives used in treatment of schistosomiasis*
Heterophyiasis	Chronic congestive heart failure; uncommonly, sudden death	Interstitial edema, capillary thrombosis, ova in myocardium, ova attached to mitral valve result in thickening and calcification	*
Cysticercosis	Cardiac involvement uncommon, ECG abnormalities, congestive heart failure occasionally	Intense tissue reaction resulting in cysts around degenerative larvae, cysts may calcify	*
Visceral larva migrans (*Toxocara canis*)	Consider in young children with pica, congestive heart failure and death reported	Granulomas in myocardium	*
Filariasis	Congestive heart failure, eosinophilia	Pericardial effusion, endocarditis	*

ECG, electrocardiographic.
*For current information regarding antiparasitic treatment, the reader is advised to consult the Centers for Disease Control, Atlanta, Georgia, or a comparable source.
Modified from Giuliani ER, Gersh BJ, McGoon MD, Hayes DL, Schaff HV (editors): *Mayo Clinic Practice of Cardiology*. Third edition. Mosby, 1996, p 654. By permission of Mayo Foundation.

> The condition of most patients with lymphocytic myocarditis improves clinically over several months with treatment for congestive heart failure, although in some the disease eventually progresses to dilated cardiomyopathy.

Sarcoidosis and Giant Cell Myocarditis

Two unusual myocardial disorders important to consider when evaluating a younger patient with heart failure are cardiac sarcoidosis and giant cell myocarditis. Cardiac sarcoidosis occurs clinically in about 5% of patients with systemic sarcoidosis. Higher rates have been reported from autopsy series. Isolated cardiac sarcoidosis may present with ventricular tachycardia, heart block, or congestive heart failure. The diagnosis may be made on the basis of endomyocardial biopsy findings that show characteristic

noncaseating granuloma (Plate 2) or it may be presumed if there is a tissue diagnosis from an extracardiac source with cardiomyopathy of unknown origin. According to published case reports, sarcoidosis may respond to corticosteroid treatment. If cardiac sarcoidosis is suspected, consider endomyocardial biopsy. If the diagnosis is established, consider steroid treatment.

> Lymphocytic myocarditis and giant cell myocarditis cannot be distinguished on the basis of the patient's age, gender, or presenting symptoms. Unlike lymphocytic myocarditis, giant cell myocarditis generally causes progressive left ventricular failure complicated by arrhythmias. Giant cell myocarditis is associated with worse survival than lymphocytic myocarditis.

Giant cell myocarditis is an unusual but devastating disease that generally affects otherwise healthy persons

Table 10.—Hypersensitivity Myocarditis

Drug	Symptoms	Mode of death	Pathology
Methyldopa	Shortness of breath, malaise, headache, fever, cerebrovascular accident	Sudden	Myocarditis, vasculitis, hepatitis
Sulfonamides (sulfadiazine, sulfisoxazole, sulfamethoxypyridazine, carbutamide)	Fever, shortness of breath	Sudden	Myocarditis, petechial hemorrhages, vasculitis, granulomas
Penicillin, ampicillin	Rash, congestive heart failure	Sudden	Myocarditis, granulomas, pericarditis, myocardial infarction
Phenylbutazone	Shortness of breath, fever, rash, chest pain, hypotension	Sudden	Myocarditis, hepatitis, myocardial giant cells, perivascular granulomas, fibrinoid degeneration, pericarditis
Oxyphenbutazone	Congestive heart failure	Sudden	Myocarditis
Chlortetracycline	Fever, tachycardia		Interstitial and perivascular infiltrates
Chloramphenicol		Sudden	Myocarditis, hepatitis
Streptomycin	Chest pain, fever, rash	Sudden	Myocarditis, petechial hemorrhage, pericardial effusion
p-Aminosalicylic acid	Heart failure, hypotension, ventricular irritability		
Phenytoin	Epistaxis	Sudden	Myocarditis
Carbamazepine	Jaundice, fever, rash	Sudden	Myocarditis
Indomethacin	Cardiac arrest, fever	Brain damage	Myocarditis
Spironolactone with hydrochlorothiazide	Low back pain, fever	Sudden	Myocarditis
Acetazolamide	Fever, rash	Uremia	Myocarditis, hepatitis
Amitriptyline		Sudden	Myocarditis
Phenindione			Myocarditis
Interleukin-2	Congestive heart failure; may occur within days after therapy initiated		Myocarditis

From Giuliani ER, Gersh BJ, McGoon MD, Hayes DL, Schaff HV (editors): *Mayo Clinic Practice of Cardiology.* Third edition. Mosby, 1996, p 661. By permission of Mayo Foundation.

of either sex. Similar to patients with lymphocytic myocarditis, the mean age is 42 years; however, the median survival from the onset of symptoms is only 5.5 months (Plate 3 and Fig. 2). Because of the poor survival rate, a biopsy-proven diagnosis prompts consideration of immunosuppression and early evaluation for cardiac transplantation. Preliminary data suggest that combination immunosuppressive therapy that includes cyclosporine and prednisone may prolong time to death or transplantation. Despite a 25% incidence of post-transplantation recurrence detected with biopsy, 5-year survival after transplantation is about 71%, which is comparable to survival after transplantation for cardiomyopathy.

Hypersensitivity and Eosinophilic Myocarditis

Occasionally, a drug-related hypersensitivity reaction may involve the myocardium. The clinical presentation

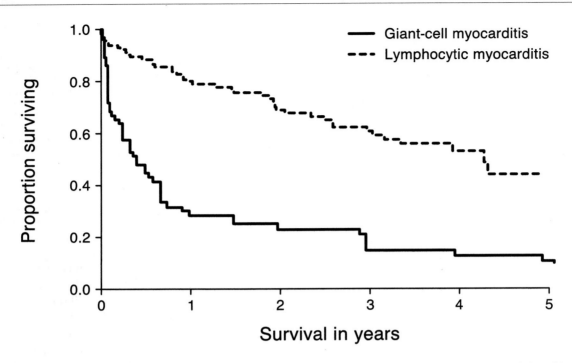

Fig. 2. Kaplan-Meier survival curve for patients with giant-cell myocarditis. (From *N Engl J Med* 336:1860-1866, 1997. By permission of the Massachusetts Medical Society.)

Table 11.—Cardiac Toxicity Due to Chemicals

Chemical	Signs and symptoms	Mode of cardiac death	Cardiac pathology
Hydrocarbons	Congestive heart failure, arrhythmias, CNS depression, hepatic injury, dermatitis	Congestive heart failure, sudden death	Myocytolysis
Carbon monoxide	Arrhythmias, angina	Congestive heart failure, sudden death	Subendocardial infarction
Arsenic	Dyspnea, congestive heart failure, ECG changes of ischemia; chronic GI, CNS, hematologic, renal toxicity; arsine gas inhalation may be rapidly fatal	Congestive heart failure	Focal myocardial hemorrhages, pericardial effusion; arsine gas may cause myocardial necrosis
Lead	Chest pain, dyspnea, conduction system abnormalities, CNS and GI symptoms	Congestive heart failure	Myocardial inflammation and fibrosis
Phosphorus	Pulmonary edema, arrhythmias	Congestive heart failure	Myocyte necrosis
Mercury	ST- and T-wave changes, QT prolongation	Congestive heart failure	Myocyte necrosis
Cobalt	Congestive heart failure, arrhythmias	Congestive heart failure, sudden death	Dilated cardiomyopathy
Thallium	Cardiac and pulmonary toxicity, tachycardia, abdominal pain, ataxia, coma, alopecia, neuropathy	Death usually not attributable primarily to cardiac disturbance	Myocardial edema and inflammation

CNS, central nervous system; ECG, electrocardiographic; GI, gastrointestinal.
From Giuliani ER, Gersh BJ, McGoon MD, Hayes DL, Schaff HV (editors): *Mayo Clinic Practice of Cardiology*. Third edition. Mosby, 1996, pp 661-662. By permission of Mayo Foundation.

Table 12.—Cardiac Toxicity Due to Physical Agents

Agent	Signs and symptoms	Mode of cardiac death	Cardiac pathology
Radiation	Acute pericarditis, percardial effusion, ventricular failure; late constrictive pericarditis, coronary disease, restrictive myocardial disease	Acute pericardial disease or congestive heart failure; late constriction, restriction, myocardial infarction	Pericarditis, myocytolysis, fibrosis, coronary disease
Heatstroke	ECG shows sinus tachycardia, ST- and T-wave changes, QT prolongation; CNS manifestations	Shock	Myocardial hemorrhage, right ventricular dilatation
Hypothermia	ECG, ST-segment changes	Shock	Myocardial hemorrhage, chamber dilatation

CNS, central nervous system; ECG, electrocardiography.

From Giuliani ER, Gersh BJ, McGoon MD, Hayes DL, Schaff HV (editors): *Mayo Clinic Practice of Cardiology*. Third edition. Mosby, 1996, p 662. By permission of Mayo Foundation.

Table 13.—Cardiac Toxicity Due to Bites and Stings

Agent	Signs and symptoms	Mode of cardiac death	Cardiac pathology	Therapy
Scorpion venom	Tachycardia, mydriasis, sweating, pulmonary edema, priapism, ECG ST changes and conduction disturbances, neurotoxic symptoms	Sudden	Myocarditis, myocyte necrosis	? Adrenergic blocking agents
Snake venom	ECG ST changes and QRS prolongation, dyspnea	Myocardial infarction, shock	Myocyte necrosis	Antivenom
Black widow spider venom	Arrhythmias, labile blood pressure	Shock		? β-blockers
Wasp venom	Cyanosis, pulmonary edema, chest pain	Shock	Myocardial hemorrhage	
Tick paralysis	Congestive heart failure	Congestive heart failure	Cardiac dilatation	

ECG, electrocardiographic.

From Giuliani ER, Gersh BJ, McGoon MD, Hayes DL, Schaff HV (editors): *Mayo Clinic Practice of Cardiology*. Third edition. Mosby, 1996, p 662. By permission of Mayo Foundation.

is different from that of lymphocytic myocarditis in that the patients generally are older (mean age, 58 years) and are often taking several medications. Drugs commonly associated with hypersensitivity myocarditis include several classes of antibiotics, antihypertensive agents, and antiseizure agents (Table 10). The clinical presentation is often acute, with rash, fever, and liver function test abnormalities commonly, but not always, present. The ECG is similar to that in lymphocytic myocarditis, with sinus tachycardia and nonspecific T-wave abnormalities, although ST-segment elevation may be seen. Chest radiography may show cardiomegaly or normal results. The cardiac presentation is often sudden death, but it may be congestive heart failure or even chest pain.

Although most of the cases have been described at autopsy, hypersensitivity myocarditis may be diagnosed by endomyocardial biopsy or presumed from a classic presentation. The histologic features are often a perivascular infiltrate

Table 14.—Possible Effects of Various Drugs on the Heart

Hypersensitivity myocarditis	Toxic myocarditis	Dilated cardiomyopathy
Acetazolamide	Amphetamines	Amphetamines
p-Aminosalicylic acid	Antihypertensives	Anthracyclines
Amitriptyline	Antimony	Chloroquine
Amphotericin B	Arsenicals	Cobalt
Carbamazepine	Barbiturates	Cocaine
Chloramphenicol	Caffeine	Ephedrine
Diphenylhydantoin	Catecholamines	Ethanol
Diphtheria toxin	Cocaine	Lithium
Horse serum	Cyclophosphamide	
Hydrochlorothiazide	Emetine	**Endocardial fibrosis**
Indomethacin	5-Fluorouracil	Anthracyclines
Isoniazid	Immunosuppressives	Busulfan
Methyldopa	Lithium	Ergotamine
Penicillins	Paraquat	Mercury
Phenindione	Phenothiazines	Methysergide
Phenylbutazone	Plasmocid	Serotonin
Smallpox vaccine	Quinidine	
Spironolactone	Rapeseed oil	**Myocardial fibrosis**
Streptomycin	Theophylline	Cyclosporine[*]
Sulfonamides		
Sulfonylureas		
Tetanus toxoid		
Tetracycline		

*In transplanted hearts only.
From Giuliani ER, Gersh BJ, McGoon MD, Hayes DL, Schaff HV (editors): *Mayo Clinic Practice of Cardiology.* Third edition. Mosby, 1996, p 678. By permission of Mayo Foundation.

rich in eosinophils, with little fibrosis or myocyte necrosis (Plate 4). Occasionally, the histologic features are more typical of lymphocytic, giant cell, or granulomatous myocarditis.

The treatment is to withdraw the offending agent and give a high dose of corticosteroids. Despite these interventions, patients often die. This suggests that more aggressive immunosuppression has a role in treatment. A case has been reported in which the disease responded to treatment with intravenously administered immunoglobulin and a high dose of corticosteroid. No data have been published on the role of cyclosporine or other immunosuppressive therapy.

Chagas Cardiomyopathy

Infection by *Trypanosoma cruzi* may present as an acute myocarditis or as a chronic cardiomyopathy. Chagas cardiac disease is a major cause of cardiomyopathy worldwide and may be seen in immigrants from rural Central and South America. Human infection by *Trypanosoma cruzi* may occur through infection at the site of a reduviid bug bite (family Reduviidae), by congenital transmission, or by blood transfusion. Endemic transmission of Chagas disease is limited to rural Central and South America. In endemic areas, Chagas cardiomyopathy is a leading cause of dilated cardiomyopathy and cardiovascular death. Acute myocarditis occurs in 1% of infections, and chronic Chagas cardiac disease may present with symptoms of congestive heart failure, cardiac arrhythmia, or heart block in 10% to 20% of infected persons. An additional 20% to 30% of infected persons have asymptomatic cardiac involvement.

Usually, the disease is suspected if the person has a strong history of environmental exposure (Table 16). The diagnosis is confirmed by serologic testing or the polymerase chain reaction test. Electrocardiography may show evidence of conduction system disease, including right bundle branch block or left anterior fascicular block. Echocardiography or contrast ventriculography may reveal a left ventricular apical aneurysm, regional wall motion abnormalities, or diffuse cardiomyopathy. Symptoms may be related to congestive heart failure due to left ventricular dysfunction or ventricular arrhythmia.

The best treatment of Chagas cardiomyopathy is prevention. Improvements in housing and use of pesticides may decrease the incidence of infection and, thereby, the incidence of disease. Antiparasitic treatments directed at *Trypanosoma cruzi* may eradicate the disease in cases of acute or subacute infection. Congestive heart failure may be treated symptomatically with afterload-reducing agents, diuretics, and digoxin. Ventricular arrhythmias may respond to electrophysiology-guided treatment. Heart transplantation for Chagas cardiomyopathy has been performed successfully; however, reactivation of *Trypanosoma cruzi* infection is common.

Lyme Myocarditis

Myocarditis occasionally occurs in association with infection by the spirochete *Borrelia burgdorferi* (Lyme disease). Suspect Lyme disease if the patient has travelled to endemic regions or has given a history of tick bite. The presentation may include transient or permanent heart block or cardiac arrhythmia. The diagnosis of Lyme disease is confirmed by serologic testing, but this does not establish the diagnosis of myocarditis. Endomyocardial biopsy may show a lymphocytic myocarditis with prominent plasmacytic component. The organism may be seen with special stains. In a patient with suspected Lyme disease after a tick bite, consider the possibility of coinfection with *Ehrlichia* (ehrlichiosis) or *Babesia* (babesiosis), which can also cause myocarditis. Serologic tests are available for both disorders.

Predictors of Survival in Lymphocytic Myocarditis

In a multivariate analysis, predictors of death or heart transplantation after acute myocarditis included syncope, low ejection fraction, and left bundle branch block.

Table 15.—Causes of Various Histopathologic Forms of Myocarditis in Biopsy Tissues

Lymphocytic	Eosinophilic
Idiopathic	Idiopathic
Viral syndrome	Hypereosinophilia
Polymyositis	Restrictive cardiomy-
Sarcoidosis	opathy
Lyme disease	Asthmatic bronchitis
Mucocutaneous lymph	Churg-Strauss syndrome
node syndrome	Parasitic infestations
(Kawasaki disease)	Drug hypersensitivity
Acquired immunodefic-	
iency syndrome	**Giant cell or granulomatous**
Mycoplasma pneumoniae	Idiopathic
Drug toxicity	Sarcoidosis
	Infective
Neutrophilic or mixed	Rheumatoid
Idiopathic	Rheumatic
Infection	Drug hypersensitivity
Infarction	
Drug toxicity	

From Giuliani ER, Gersh BJ, McGoon MD, Hayes DL, Schaff HV (editors): *Mayo Clinic Practice of Cardiology.* Third edition. Mosby, 1996, p 678. By permission of Mayo Foundation.

Table 16.—Clinical Presentation of North American Patients With Chagas Heart Disease

Feature	Patients	
	No.	%
Atrioventricular block	9	21
Congestive heart failure	8	19
Chest pain	6	14
Conduction abnormality on ECG	8	19
Aborted sudden death	3	7
Sustained ventricular tachycardia	3	7
Embolic event	3	7
Other	2	5
Total	42	

ECG, electrocardiography.
Modified from *N Engl J Med* 325:763-768, 1991. By permission of the Massachusetts Medical Society.

Acute Rheumatic Fever

Acute rheumatic fever is a pancarditis that to varying extents affects the endocardium, myocardium, and pericardium. The incidence of acute rheumatic fever in the U.S. is about 2 cases per 100,000 population, with several recent localized outbreaks. The incidence in Asia, Africa, and South America is estimated at about 100 cases per 100,000 population, an incidence similar to that in the U.S. at the beginning of the 20th century.

Acute rheumatic fever is an unusual immunologic response to a pharyngeal infection with group A streptococci. The risk of rheumatic fever overall is about 3% in those with untreated streptococcal pharyngitis and is related to the presence of certain virulent types of streptococci that induce a strong immune response to M-type mucoid proteins that encapsulate the organism. Patients with HLA-DR 1, 2, 3, and 4 haplotypes are probably at increased risk for rheumatic fever.

Major Manifestations (Mnemonic—RANCH)

Rash—Erythema marginatum is a rare (< 5% of patients), fleeting, nonpruritic rash with irregular borders and a pale center.

Arthritis—Common (75% of patients) large joint inflammation of the knees, ankles, elbows, and wrists that resolves spontaneously without deformity.

Nodules—They are rare (< 5% of patients) and are firm, painless subcutaneous nodules on the extensor surfaces of the wrists and ankles and over tendons and the occipital scalp.

Chorea—Sydenham chorea is rare (< 5% of patients) and consists of involuntary, jerky movements of the face and extremities.

Heart—It is affected in 50% of patients clinically and in more than 90% echocardiographically.

Valvulitis of the mitral leaflets and chordae and the aortic leaflets results in mitral regurgitation, mitral valve prolapse, and, less commonly, aortic incompetence. Tricuspid and pulmonary valve involvement are rare.

Myocarditis associated with early sinus tachycardia, heart failure, and ventricular arrhythmias is a manifestation of acute rheumatic fever and is indistinguishable from myocarditis of other cause.

Another manifestation is pericarditis and, rarely, associated abdominal pain.

Treatment of Acute Rheumatic Fever

Primary and secondary prevention of rheumatic fever and duration of prophylaxis for secondary rheumatic fever are listed in Tables 17-19.

1. For patients with heart failure, bed rest in combination with diuretics, digoxin, and ACE inhibitors.

2. Penicillin—orally, phenoxymethyl penicillin (500 mg three times daily for 10 days), or intramuscularly, benzathine penicillin G (600,000 U once if patient weighs ≤ 27 kg or 1.2 million U if > 27 kg).

3. Aspirin (75 mg/kg daily orally) for mild-moderate carditis and corticosteroids (prednisone, 1 mg/kg daily) for severe carditis.

Table 17.—Primary Prevention of Rheumatic Fever

Agent	Dose	Mode	Duration
Benzathine Penicillin G	600,000 U for patients ≤ 27 kg (60 lb)	Intramuscular	Once
	1,200,000 U for patients > 27 kg (60 lb)		
	or		
Penicillin V (phenoxymethyl penicillin)	Children: 250 mg 2-3 times daily	Oral	10 days
	Adolescents and adults: 500 mg 2-3 times daily		
For individuals allergic to penicillin:			
Erythromycin	20-40 mg/kg daily	Oral	10 days
Estolate	2-4 times daily (maximum 1 g/d)		
Ethylsuccinate	40 mg/kg daily	Oral	10 days
	2-4 times daily (maximum 1 g/d)		
Azithromycin	500 mg on first day	Oral	5 days
	250 mg/d for the next 4 days		

From *J Am Coll Cardiol* 32:1486-1588, 1998. By permission of the American College of Cardiology.

Table 18.—Secondary Prevention of Rheumatic Fever

Agent	Dose	Mode
Benzathine Intramuscular Penicillin G	1,200,000 U every 4 wk (every 3 wk for high-risk* pt such as those with residual carditis)	
Penicillin V	250 mg twice daily *or*	Oral
Sulfadiazine	0.5 g once daily for pt ≤ 27 kg (60 lb) 1.0 g once daily for pt > 27 kg (60 lb)	Oral
For persons allergic to penicillin and sulfadiazine: Erythromycin	250 mg twice daily	Oral

Pt, patients.

*High-risk patients include those with residual rheumatic carditis as well as patients from economically disadvantaged populations.

From Pediatrics 96:758-764, 1995. By permission of the American Academy of Pediatrics.

Table 19.—Duration of Secondary Rheumatic Fever Prophylaxis

Category	Duration
Rheumatic fever with carditis and residual heart disease (persistent valvular disease)	≥ 10 yr since last episode and at least until age 40 yr, sometimes lifelong prophylaxis*
Rheumatic fever with carditis but no residual heart disease (no valvular disease)	10 yr or well into adulthood, whichever is longer
Rheumatic fever without carditis	5 yr or until age 21 yr, whichever is longer

*"Lifelong" prophylaxis refers to patients who are at high risk and likely to come in contact with populations with a high prevalence of streptococcal infection, i.e., teachers, day-care workers.

From Pediatrics 96:758-764, 1995. By permission of the American Academy of Pediatrics.

Suggested Review Reading

1. Anonymous: Jones criteria (revised) for guidance in the diagnosis of rheumatic fever (editorial). *Circulation* 32:664-668, 1965.

2. Aretz HT, Billingham ME, Edwards WD, et al: Myocarditis. A histopathologic definition and classification. *Am J Cardiovasc Pathol* 1:3-14, 1987.
The Dallas Criteria for the diagnosis of lymphocytic myocarditis.

3. Cooper LT Jr, Berry GJ, Shabetai R: Idiopathic giant-cell myocarditis—natural history and treatment. *N Engl J Med* 336:1860-1866, 1997.
Giant cell myocarditis is a rapidly fatal disease that may be diagnosed by endomyocardial biopsy and may respond to immunosuppression with combination immunosuppressive agents. Many of these patients require heart transplantation.

4. Hagar JM, Rahimtoola SH: Chagas' heart disease. *Curr Probl Cardiol* 20:825-924, 1995.
A detailed review of the history, diagnosis, and treatment of Chagas heart disease.

5. Kasper EK, Agema WR, Hutchins GM, et al: The causes of dilated cardiomyopathy: a clinicopathologic review of 673 consecutive patients. *J Am Coll Cardiol* 23:586-590, 1994.
Lymphocytic myocarditis is an important cause of dilated cardiomyopathy.

6. Levy NT, Olson LJ, Weyand C, et al: Histologic and cytokine response to immunosuppression in giant-cell myocarditis. *Ann Intern Med* 128:648-650, 1998.
Giant cell myocarditis is associated with increased tissue cytokine levels that decrease with immunosuppressive treatment. Treatment with monoclonal anti-T-cell antibodies (muromonab-CD3) may be effective in giant cell myocarditis.

7. Mason JW, O'Connell JB, Herskowitz A, et al: A clinical trial of immunosuppressive therapy for myocarditis. *N Engl J Med* 333:269-275, 1995.
A clinical trial of immunosuppression for lymphocytic myocarditis showed no benefit of cyclosporine or azathioprine plus prednisone. The mean ejection fraction increased from 25% to 35% in treatment and control groups. Cardiac mortality was 56% at 4.3 years.

8. Narula J, Khaw BA, Dec GW Jr, et al: Brief report: recognition of acute myocarditis masquerading as acute myocardial infarction. *N Engl J Med* 328:100-104, 1993.
Lymphocytic myocarditis may present as acute myocardial infarction.

9. Narula J, Khaw BA, Dec GW, et al: Diagnostic accuracy of antimyosin scintigraphy in suspected myocarditis. *J Nucl Cardiol* 3:371-381, 1996.
Antimyocin scintigraphy had a high sensitivity (91% to 100%) and negative predictive power (93% to 100%) but low specificity (31% to 44%) and positive predictive power (28% to 33%) for lymphocytic myocarditis.

10. Passarino G, Burlo P, Ciccone G, et al: Prevalence of myocarditis at autopsy in Turin, Italy. *Arch Pathol Lab Med* 121:619-622, 1997.
Lymphocytic myocarditis is present in up to 5% of autopsy cases.

11. Phillips M, Robinowitz M, Higgins JR, et al: Sudden cardiac death in Air Force recruits. A 20-year review. *JAMA* 256:2696-2699, 1986.
Lymphocytic myocarditis may present as sudden death.

12. Smith SC, Ladenson JH, Mason JW, et al: Elevations of cardiac troponin I associated with myocarditis. Experimental and clinical correlates. *Circulation* 95:163-168, 1997.
Cardiac troponin I had an 89% specificity and a 34% sensitivity for the diagnosis of lymphocytic myocarditis.

13. Taliercio CP, Olney BA, Lie JT: Myocarditis related to drug hypersensitivity. *Mayo Clin Proc* 60:463-468, 1985.
Hypersensitivity myocarditis is frequently associated with skin lesions and liver function abnormalities. Endomyocardial biopsy may reveal the diagnosis. Treatment with drug withdrawal, a high dose of corticosteroids, and, perhaps, intravenous immunoglobulin is indicated.

14. Vignola PA, Aonuma K, Swaye PS, et al: Lymphocytic myocarditis presenting as unexplained ventricular arrhythmias: diagnosis with endomyocardial biopsy and response to immunosuppression. *J Am Coll Cardiol* 4:812-819, 1984.
Lymphocytic myocarditis may present as unexplained arrhythmia.

Questions

Multiple Choice (choose the one best answer)

1. A 28-year-old woman lawyer comes to the emergency room complaining of substernal chest pain and severe dyspnea for 3 hours. She has no known risk factors for coronary artery disease and denies illicit drug use. One week earlier, she was evaluated in your office for upper respiratory tract infection and treated with amoxicillin, 250 mg orally 4 times daily. For the last few nights, she has used four pillows because of nocturnal wheezing and dyspnea. She is not pregnant. On examination, she is acutely ill, with tachycardia at 120 beats/min, blood pressure of 154/74 mm Hg, and a respiratory rate of 32. Jugular venous pressure is 12 cm H_2O. Rales are present bilaterally. S_1 is diminished, there are no murmurs, but there is a summation gallop at the left sternal border. The electrocardiogram is shown below. Echocardiography showed severe anterolateral hypokinesis. Coronary angiography showed minimal luminal irregularities. What is your working diagnosis and management?
   a. Severe coronary vasospasm; treat with verapamil
   b. Acute coronary artery thrombosis spontaneously lysed; treat with aspirin and β-blocker and evaluate for thrombophilia
   c. Hypersensitivity reaction; stop amoxicillin treatment, and check peripheral blood smear for eosinophilis
   d. Focal myocarditis; treat with furosemide and an angiotensin-converting enzyme inhibitor and repeat echocardiography in 6 months if her condition improves clinically.
   e. Cocaine use; screen for illicit drugs

2. A 42-year-old fireman comes to your office because he has had progressive dyspnea on exertion for 4 weeks. For the last few days, dyspnea developed when he brushed his teeth or combed his hair. He had been physically active, with no significant past medical history. His only medication is ibuprofen for occasional headaches. On examination, heart rate is 110 beats/min, blood pressure is 110/70 mm Hg, respiratory rate is 28, and jugular venous pressure is 10 cm with hepatojugular reflux, bibasilar rales, and 1+ peripheral edema. S_1 is diminished, with a 2/6 right upper sternal border systolic murmur that varies with respiration. There is an S_3 at the apex. The results of coronary angiography are normal. Echocardiography shows an ejection fraction of 25%, with global hypokinesis. The endomyocardial biopsy specimen revealed lymphocytic myocarditis. What is the best management at this point?
   a. Discuss the seriousness of the condition with the patient and recommend evaluation for cardiac transplantation

28-Year-Old Female

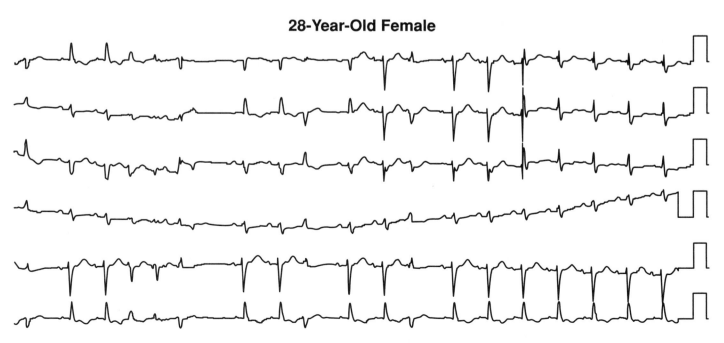

b. Start treatment with prednisone, 1 mg/kg daily, in addition to an angiotensin-converting enzyme inhibitor and a diuretic

c. Start treatment with cyclosporine, 25 mg orally twice daily, and prednisone, 1 mg/kg daily

d. Place prophylactic implantable defibrillator because of the high likelihood of ventricular tachycardia in the next year.

e. Start treatment with angiotensin-converting enzyme inhibitor and diuretic and follow up with serial echocardiography to follow left ventricular function.

3. You are consulted by the intensive care unit service to evaluate a 17-year-old boy for intermittent palpitations and lightheadedness. He was well until 4 weeks ago when he noted decreased exercise tolerance. Echocardiography at that time showed moderate global hypokinesis, with an ejection fraction of 40%. His primary care physician suspected viral myocarditis and treated it with captopril, digoxin, and furosemide. Despite treatment for congestive heart failure, the symptoms progressed. For the last 2 days, the boy has noted brief episodes of lightheadedness associated with a fluttering sensation in his chest. He was admitted this morning with hemodynamically stable monomorphic ventricular tachycardia. Following the restoration of sinus rhythm with lidocaine, his blood pressure is 80/40 mm Hg and the heart rate is 135 beats/min. Currently, he is receiving lidocaine, 2 μg/kg; dobutamine, 10 μg/kg intravenous drip; captopril, 25 mg orally 3 times daily; furosemide, 40 mg intravenously twice daily; and digoxin, 0.25 mg orally daily. He denies any significant past medical history or use of prescription or illegal drugs. You repeat echocardiography at the bedside and find he now has severely decreased left ventricular function and an estimated ejection fraction of 15%. What management strategy is best?

a. Place an implantable defibrillator (AICD) with pacemaker function, because the risk of recurrent ventricular tachycardia and heart block is great

b. Add metolazone to furosemide to improve diuresis, and reassure the family that myocarditis usually improves with the standard treatment for heart failure

c. Empirically treat with cyclosporine and prednisone, because the sensitivity of endomyocardial biopsy is low

d. Initiate heart transplantation evaluation, and perform endomyocardial biopsy

4. A 40-year-old African-American female marathon runner complains of progressive exercise intolerance. She has been in good health except for recent pyelonephritis, for which she is taking trimethoprim-sulfamethoxazole twice daily. For the last 5 days she has had a pruritic maculopapular rash over her legs and arms. On examination, jugular venous pressure is 8 cm H_2O, bibasilar rales are present over both lung fields, S_1 is decreased, and S_4 is detected at the left sternal border. Electrocardiography shows sinus tachycardia at 104 beats/min, with nonspecific T-wave abnormalities in V_1 to V_5. Which of the following would you do next?

a. Perform endomyocardial biopsy to rule out cardiac sarcoidosis, which is a treatable form of heart failure that occurs in higher frequency among African-American women than among Caucasian women.

b. Stop trimethoprim-sulfamethoxazole treatment, and check liver function tests and peripheral blood smear for eosinophils

c. Start treatment with a diuretic, an angiotensin-converting enzyme inhibitor, and digoxin for presumed lymphocytic myocarditis

d. Perform coronary angiography to rule out ischemic cardiomyopathy

5. A 25-year-old immigrant to the U.S. from rural Venezuela presents with dyspnea and palpitations of 3 months' duration. He previously was well except for recurrent fecal impactions thought to be due to colonic dysmotility. Echocardiography showed an apical left ventricular aneurysm and global left ventricular hypokinesis. The most common electrocardiographic abnormalities in this setting are

a. Right bundle branch block with or without left anterior fascicular block

b. Third-degree heart block

c. Atrial fibrillation

d. Ventricular tachycardia

Answers

1. Answer d

The history of antecedent viral syndrome and subacute progression of congestive heart failure is typical for myocarditis. The presentation of myocarditis may occasionally mimic acute myocardial infarction.

2. Answer e

There is no established benefit to immunosuppression in addition to standard treatment for congestive heart failure in patients with lymphocytic myocarditis. A 42-year-old man with symptoms of heart failure for 4 weeks is a typical case of lymphocytic myocarditis. The short-term prognosis is good, particularly if the duration of symptoms is short and the patient is taking few cardiac medications at presentation. Despite New York Heart Association class III symptoms, his risk of death or cardiac transplantation in the next few months is low, and he does not need to be listed for transplantation or have an automatic implantable cardioverter-defibrillator placed.

3. Answer d

Lymphocytic myocarditis usually responds to treatment for congestive heart failure. The patient's rapid deterioration despite appropriate therapy suggests he had a more aggressive myocarditis, possibly giant cell myocarditis. In this setting, endomyocardial biopsy findings positive for giant cell myocarditis would confirm the poor prognosis, facilitate transplantation listing, and allow for counseling about post-transplantation recurrence. Empiric treatment with immunosuppression with the assumption that this is giant cell myocarditis would be a possibility, but the sensitivity of endomyocardial biopsy in giant cell myocarditis is not known.

4. Answer b

Hypersensitivity myocarditis is a serious but unusual drug reaction, although the diagnosis is often not suspected.

5. Answer a

Right bundle branch block with or without left anterior vesicular block is seen in about 50% of patients with Chagas cardiomyopathy. Third-degree heart block occurs in 7% to 8% of patients and atrial fibrillation, in 7% to 10%. Ventricular tachycardia or sudden death occurs in up to 39% of patients.

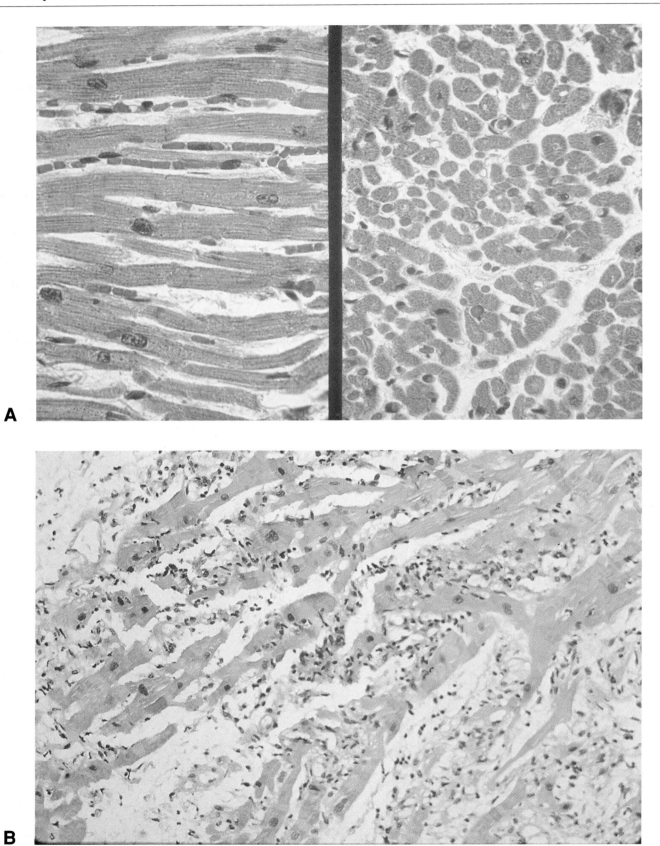

Plate 1. *A*, Normal myocardium in longitudinal (*left*) and cross (*right*) sections. (Courtesy of William D. Edwards, M.D.) *B*, Lymphocytic myocarditis with a mixed inflammatory infiltrate and associated myocyte necrosis. (Courtesy of Henry D. Tazelaar, M.D.)

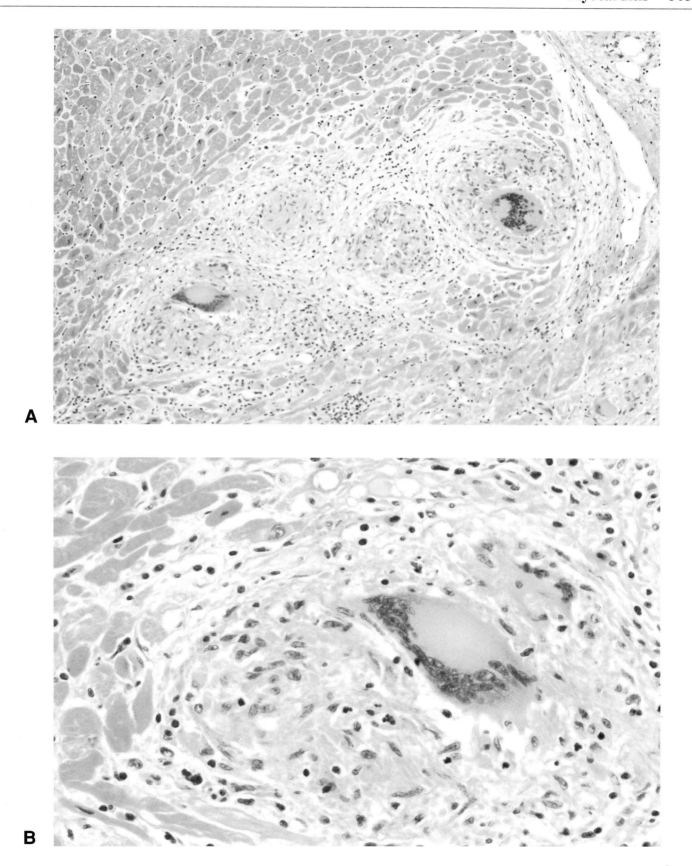

Plate 2. *A*, Cardiac sarcoidosis. Well-formed granuloma with giant cells may be seen without myocyte necrosis. (Original magnification, x125.) *B*, Follicular granuloma in cardiac sarcoidosis. (Original magnification, x400.)

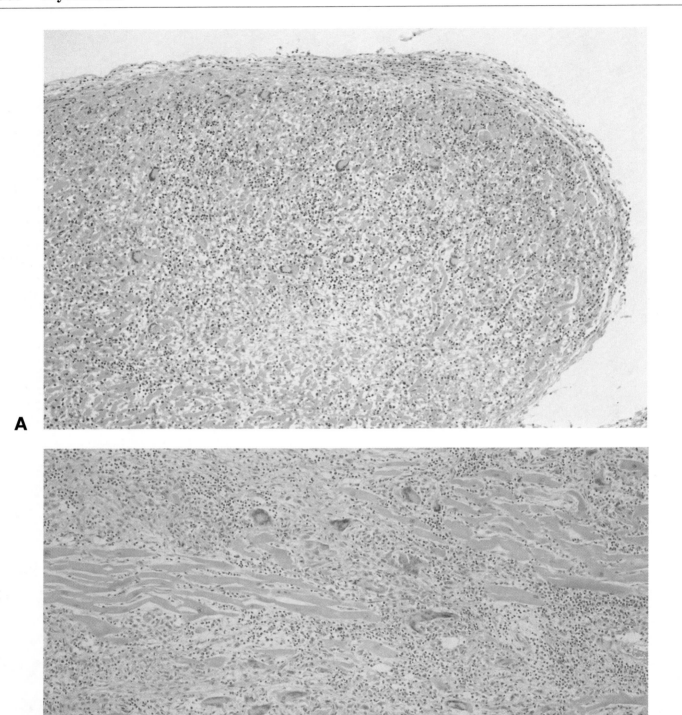

Plate 3. *A*, Idiopathic giant cell myocarditis. Diffuse endomyocardial inflammatory infiltrate with multinucleated giant cells in the absence of granuloma. (Original magnification, x25.) *B*, Widespread mixed inflammatory infiltrate with multinucleated giant cells and myocyte necrosis. (Original magnification, x100.)

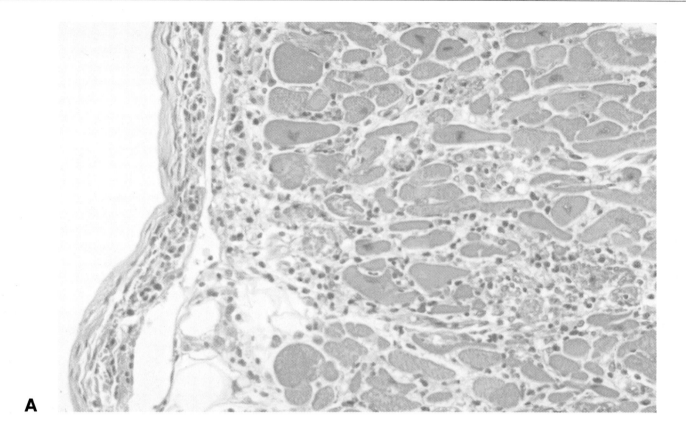

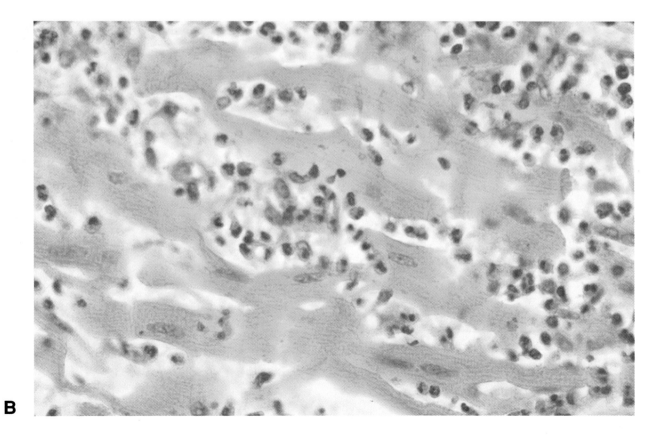

Plate 4. *A* and *B*, Eosinophilic myocarditis demonstrating an interstitial inflammatory infiltrate with prominent eosinophils. (Courtesy of Henry D. Tazelaar, M.D.)

Notes

Chapter 32

Pericardial Diseases

Jae K. Oh, M.D.

Function of the Pericardium

The pericardium provides mechanical protection of the heart and lubricates the heart to reduce the friction between the heart and surrounding structures. The pericardium also has a significant hemodynamic impact on the atria and ventricles. Normally, intrapericardial pressure is equal to intrapleural pressure and is transmitted uniformly throughout the fluid-filled (usually 25 to 50 mL of clear fluid secreted by the visceral pericardium) intrapericardial space. The nondistensible pericardium limits acute distention of the heart. Ventricular volume is greater at any given ventricular filling pressure with the pericardium removed than with the pericardium intact. The pericardium also contributes to diastolic coupling between the two ventricles: the distention of one ventricle alters the filling of the other, an effect that is important in the pathophysiology of cardiac tamponade and constrictive pericarditis. Ventricular interdependence becomes more marked at high ventricular filling pressures.

- The pericardium protects and lubricates the heart.
- The pericardium contributes to diastolic coupling of the right and left ventricles, an effect that is important in tamponade and constrictive pericarditis.

Congenital Absence of the Pericardium

Complete absence of the pericardium is very rare and usually asymptomatic. More commonly, a small portion of the pericardium, usually on the left, is absent. Rarely with extreme cardiac shift to the left, the patient may experience left-sided nonexertional chest pain or prominent cardiac pulsation. This condition usually is diagnosed incidentally on chest radiography and displays marked left-sided shift of the heart without tracheal deviation. Lung tissue is present between the aorta and the main pulmonary artery and between the inferior border of the heart and the left hemidiaphragm. The left ventricular contour is flattened (left upper border) and elongated, giving an appearance of a "snoopy dog" (Fig. 1). The traditional echocardiographic windows demonstrate predominance of the right-sided cardiac chambers and may lead to an erroneous diagnosis of right ventricular volume overload and atrial septal defect. Cardiac motion is exaggerated on echocardiography, especially the posterior wall of the left ventricle. All cardiac structures are shifted to the left, resulting in prominent visualization of the right ventricular cavity and abnormal ventricular septal motion. Congenital absence of the pericardium is associated with atrial septal defect, bicuspid aortic valve, and bronchogenic cysts. Rarely, herniation of cardiac chambers

An Atlas illustrating pericardial disease is found at the end of the chapter (Plates 1-8).

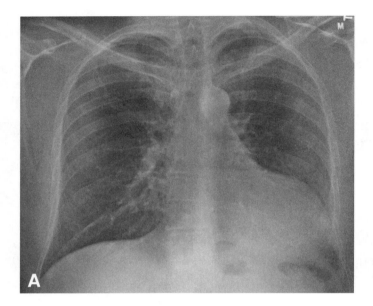 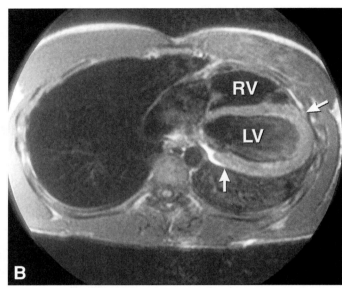

Fig. 1. *A*, Chest radiograph typical of congenital absence of pericardium. *B*, Magnetic resonance scan of chest showing marked cardiac shift to the left due to congenital absence of pericardium. *Arrows*, area of absent pericardium. LV, left ventricle; RV, right ventricle. *B*, from Oh JK, Seward JB, Tajik AJ: *The Echo Manual*. Second edition. Lippincott-Raven Publishers, 1999, p 182. By permission of Mayo Foundation.

through a partial defect of the pericardium may cause sudden death, presumably because of marked ischemia from compression of the coronary artery. Closure of the pericardial defect is necessary in symptomatic patients.

- Congenital absence of the pericardium gives a "snoopy dog" cardiac silhouette on a chest radiograph.
- Congenital absence of the pericardium is associated with atrial septal defect, bicuspid aortic valve, and bronchogenic cysts.
- Partial absence of the pericardium has been linked to sudden death.

Pericardial Cyst

A pericardial cyst is a benign structural abnormality of the pericardium that usually is detected as an incidental mass lesion on chest radiographs in an asymptomatic person (Fig. 2). Most frequently, it is located at the right costophrenic angle, but it may also be found at the left costophrenic angle, hilum, or superior mediastinum. The differential diagnoses are malignant tumors, cardiac chamber enlargement, and diaphragmatic hernia. Two-dimensional echocardiography, computed tomography (CT), or magnetic resonance imaging (MRI) may be used to differentiate pericardial cysts from other solid tumors. In asymptomatic patients, no treatment is necessary.

- Pericardial cyst is usually benign and located at the right costophrenic border.

Acute Pericarditis

The causes of acute pericarditis are numerous. Acute pericarditis usually is self-limited unless caused by malignancy or other systemic disease. Occasionally, acute pericarditis may undergo a transient constrictive phase. The most prominent symptom of acute pericarditis is pleuropericardial chest pain. Because the visceral pericardium is devoid of pain fibers, the parietal pericardium must be inflamed to cause chest pain. Characteristically, the pain is sharp, stabbing, and pleuritic and radiates to the scapula and back. Pericarditic pain may mimic anginal pain, and clinical differentiation may be difficult on the basis of the medical history alone. Patients with acute pericarditis may develop a significant amount of pericardial effusion to the point of hemodynamic compromise, resulting in dyspnea, hypotension, tachycardia, and heart failure. On physical examination, a typical finding is a pericardial friction rub, which is characterized by scratchy high-pitched sounds with three distinct components (coincidental with rapid ventricular filling, ventricular contraction, and atrial contraction). In a subset of patients, however, the pericardial friction rub may have only one component. A pericardial rub usually is heard

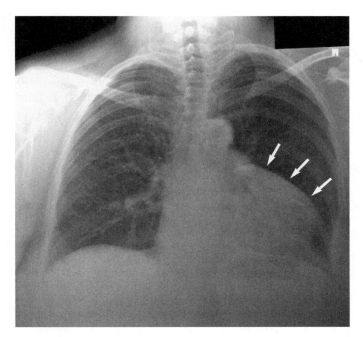

Fig. 2. Chest radiograph of a pericardial cyst (*arrows*).

"concave upward" and is associated with upright T waves. After several days of pericarditis, the ST segment returns to baseline and the T wave flattens and, later, becomes inverted. Another electrocardiographic (ECG) characteristic of pericarditis is depression of the PR segment because of atrial involvement (see lead I on Figure 3). This happens within several days after the onset of pericarditis.

Chest radiographs usually are normal unless the patient has a large amount of pericardial effusion. The most sensitive diagnostic technique for detecting pericardial effusion is echocardiography, which shows an echo-free space around the heart. The absence of pericardial effusion on echocardiography does not exclude the diagnosis of acute pericarditis.

best at the left sternal border, with the patient leaning forward during held expiration. It is common for the rub to disappear when a pericardial effusion develops. A pericardial knock does not occur in acute pericarditis.

Electrocardiography in Acute Pericarditis

The ST-segment elevation in acute pericarditis is different from that in acute myocardial infarction (Fig. 3). ST-segment elevation in pericarditis is more diffuse, involving both limb and precordial leads. ST-segment elevation is

Treatment of Acute Pericarditis

In most patients, acute pericarditis resolves gradually, and treatment is with nonsteroidal anti-inflammatory agent(s), usually aspirin, 650 mg every 4 hours, or indomethacin, 25 to 75 mg three times daily for 7 to 10 days, with gradual tapering. Rarely, recurrent chest pain may develop, for which steroid therapy should be considered. The treatment of pericarditic pain with a steroid may make the patient's pain steroid-dependent. Steroid treatment should be considered only when pericarditic pain does not respond to combinations of nonsteroidal anti-inflammatory agents. Colchicine has been used to treat recurrent pericarditic pain, but a larger study is needed to confirm its efficacy. If the pain continues to limit the patient's activity and lifestyle, pericardiectomy may be required, even in the setting of no hemodynamic embarrassment.

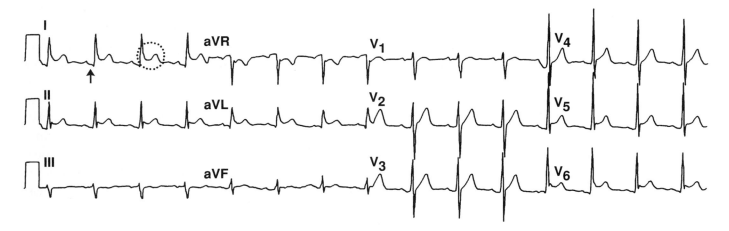

Fig. 3. Electrocardiogram typical of acute pericarditis. *Arrow*, PR depression in lead I. *Circle*, Typical "concave upward" ST-segment elevation.

Transient Constrictive Phase of Acute Pericarditis

About 7% to 10% of patients with acute pericarditis may have a transient constrictive phase. These patients usually have a moderate amount of pericardial effusion, and as the pericardial effusion disappears, the pericardium remains inflamed, thickened, and noncompliant, resulting in constrictive hemodynamics. The patient presents with dyspnea, peripheral edema, increased jugular venous pressure, and, sometimes, ascites, as in patients with chronic constrictive pericarditis. This transient constrictive phase may last 2 to 3 months before it gradually resolves either spontaneously or with treatment with anti-inflammatory agents. When hemodynamics and findings typical of constriction develop in patients with acute pericarditis, initial treatment is indomethacin (Indocin) for 2 to 3 weeks and, if there is no response, to use steroids for 1 to 2 months after being sure the pericarditis is not caused by bacterial infection, including tuberculosis. Constrictive hemodynamics can be diagnosed readily with Doppler echocardiography (see below); resolution of constrictive physiology can be documented clinically and by follow-up echocardiography.

- The classic pericardial rub has three components.
- Acute pericarditis may cause PR-segment depression on the ECG because of inflammation of the atrial wall.
- From 7% to 10% of patients with acute pericarditis may have a transient constrictive phase.

Pericardial Effusion/Tamponade

Pericardial inflammation of any cause may result in a large amount of fluid collecting in the pericardial sac. The pericardium may be filled with blood product (hemopericardium) because of cardiac rupture (injury, iatrogenic, or acute myocardial infarction), aortic dissection, or after cardiac bypass surgery. Pericardial effusion may be related to underlying heart failure or abnormality in lymphatic drainage. When a pericardial effusion develops gradually, so that it does not impair pericardial compliance, the patient may remain asymptomatic, even with a massive amount of pericardial effusion. If the rate of pericardial effusion is rapid, even a small amount (50 to 100 mL) of fluid or blood in the pericardium can cause cardiac tamponade. Cardiac tamponade is the result of a critical elevation of intrapericardial pressure produced by accumulation of pericardial fluid.

Hemodynamics of Pericardial Tamponade

When intrapericardial pressure is increased, atrial pressure is also increased, resulting in impaired venous return. This, in turn, results in systemic venous congestion and reduction in cardiac output (Fig. 4). On physical examination, jugular venous pressure is increased, with prominent systolic x descent and blunted diastolic y descent (Table 1). With pericardial effusion, the precordium is quiet and cardiac sounds are diminished. The Beck triad consists of 1) a decrease in systolic pressure, 2) an increase in systemic venous pressure, and 3) a quiet heart. With reduction in cardiac output, pulse pressure is narrow and systemic venous congestion causes hepatomegaly, peripheral edema, and ascites. In patients with cardiac tamponade, the intrapericardial pressure is increased critically and does not vary with intrapleural pressure. Normally, intrapericardial pressure changes with fluctuations in intrapleural pressure. With inspiration, intrapleural pressure decreases by 5 to 7 mm Hg and similar changes occur in intrapericardial pressure. However, in tamponade, intrapericardial pressure is increased to the level of ventricular diastolic pressures. Both ventricular diastolic pressures equalize with the pericardial pressure. Therefore, left atrial, right atrial, and right ventricular end-diastolic pressure, pulmonary end-diastolic pressure, and pulmonary capillary wedge pressure are equalized within 5 mm Hg of one another.

Intrapericardial and right atrial pressures may not be increased in "low-pressure tamponade," which occurs in the setting of severe hypovolemia. Ventricular filling and stroke volume are affected by relatively normal pressures. Jugular venous distention is absent in this setting.

Pulsus Paradoxus

Pulsus paradoxus is a decrease (> 10 mm Hg) in systolic blood pressure during inspiration. This is due to the underlying mechanism of cardiac tamponade. With increased intrapericardial pressure, normal pressure transmission from the intrapleural to the intrapericardial cavity does not occur. Thus, on inspiration, the driving blood pressure across the pulmonary vascular bed decreases as the lungs expand in inspiration. Pulmonary arteriolar pressure decreases, while left atrial and left ventricular pressure remains relatively fixed. Thus, the decrease in pulmonary venous return to the left heart during inspiration translates into a decrease in left ventricular stroke volume which is detected clinically as pulsus paradoxus. Pulsus paradoxus is characteristic of cardiac tamponade, but it also occurs in other conditions in which there is a significant decrease in forward stroke volume with inspiration, as in patients with acute cor pulmonale

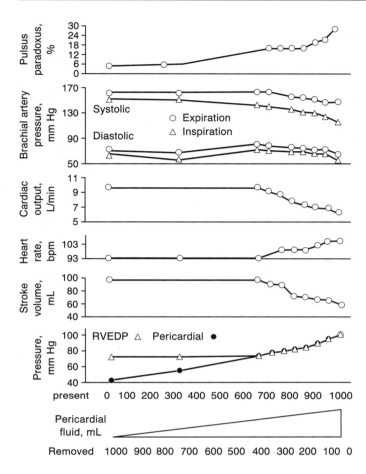

Fig. 4. Hemodynamic changes during pericardial fluid withdrawal in patient with cardiac tamponade. In second frame from top, note the disappearance of pulsus paradoxus.

Table 1.—Comparison of Cardiac Tamponade and Constrictive Pericarditis

	Cardiac tamponade	Constrictive pericarditis
Pulsus paradoxus	Very common	Less common
Kussmaul sign	Absent	May be present
Pericardial knock	Absent	May be present
Jugular venous pressure	Large x descent Small or absent y descent	Normal x descent Large y descent

2. Early diastolic collapse of the right ventricle
3. Late diastolic collapse of the right atrial free wall
4. Plethora of the inferior vena cava with a blunted respiratory change
5. Abnormal ventricular septal motion.

In acute myocardial rupture, clotted blood may be seen in the pericardial sac, highly suggestive of hemopericardium. If there is air in the pericardial sac (pneumopericardium), echocardiographic imaging may be difficult. The Doppler findings in cardiac tamponade are based on the hemodynamic pathophysiology described for pulsus paradoxus. With inspiration, the driving pressure gradient to the left cardiac chamber is decreased so that mitral inflow velocity decreases with inspiration and increases with expiration. Because cardiac volume is relatively fixed with cardiac tamponade, reciprocal changes occur in the right chambers so that increased tricuspid inflow velocity occurs with inspiration and decreased inflow velocity with expiration. With a decrease in filling to the right chambers with expiration, there is significant flow reversal in the hepatic vein with expiration during diastole (Fig. 6 and 7).

Treatment of Cardiac Tamponade

The only effective treatment for cardiac tamponade is the removal of pericardial fluid. The best way to perform pericardiocentesis is with echocardiographic guidance, because it allows the optimal site of the puncture to be located, the depth of the pericardial effusion to be determined, the distance from the puncture site to the effusion to be measured, and the results of the pericardiocentesis to be monitored.

- Pulsus paradoxus is classically seen in pericardial tamponade.

(pulmonary embolism), chronic obstructive lung disease, right ventricular infarction, or asthma.

Echocardiographic Diagnosis of Pericardial Effusion/Tamponade

Chest radiography may show cardiomegaly of globular appearance. The best way to detect pericardial effusion and tamponade is with echocardiography. A small amount of pericardial fluid appears as an echo-free space. As pericardial effusion increases, movement of the parietal pericardium decreases. When there is a large volume of pericardial effusion, the heart may have a swinging motion (Fig. 5) in the pericardial cavity, which is responsible for the ECG manifestation of cardiac tamponade, "electrical alternans." However, the swinging motion may be absent in cardiac tamponade. Other M-mode/2-D echocardiographic findings of tamponade include:

1. Decreased excursion in the E-A slope of the mitral valve

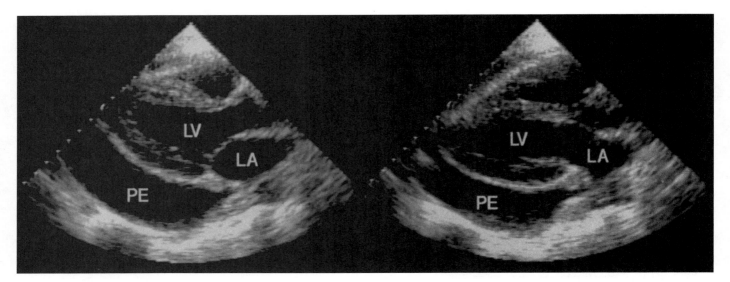

Fig. 5. Parasternal long-axis view over the heart during systole (*left*) and diastole (*right*), showing swinging motion of heart in patient with cardiac tamponade. *LA*, left atrium; *LV*, left ventricle; *PE*, pericardial effusion.

- Elective removal of pericardial fluid should always be guided echocardiographically to reduce complications.

Pericardial Effusion Due to Malignancy

Pericardial effusion due to malignancy is a poor prognostic sign. If cytologic examination demonstrates malignant cells in the pericardial effusion, the prognosis is grim regardless of the patient's underlying type of malignancy. Infrequently, pericardial effusion may be the initial presentation of an underlying malignancy. The tumors that spread most frequently to the pericardium are those of the lung and breast, followed by lymphoma and leukemia. Angiosarcoma is a primary cardiac tumor that presents with pericardial effusion and pericarditis. The pericardial fluid in malignancies is usually bloody, but a bloody effusion is not specific for malignancy. Recurrent pericardial effusion can be treated with repeated pericardiocentesis and sometimes treated with a pigtail catheter left in place for several days for continuous or intermittent drainage of reaccumulated fluid. Instillation of a sclerosing agent into the pericardium is painful and no longer used in our practice.

Pericarditis in Acute Myocardial Infarction

Pericardial effusion occurs in about 20% of patients with acute transmural myocardial infarction, usually associated with a large anterior wall myocardial infarction. The chest pain is different from that of ischemic chest pain and has a pleuritic component and an associated pericardial rub. The presence of a pericardial effusion with or without pericarditic pain after myocardial infarction is not a contraindication for intravenous treatment with heparin. A hemopericardium can occur after myocardial rupture as a complication of acute myocardial infarction and most frequently is associated with a lateral myocardial infarction. Most patients with myocardial rupture develop electromechanical dissociation and do not survive. A subgroup of patients may develop subacute cardiac rupture and present with nausea, vomiting, restlessness, and persistent ECG changes. Rarely, the patient may develop a pseudoaneurysm, in which hemopericardium is contained by the adjacent structures. Although pseudoaneurysm of the left ventricle was considered a surgical emergency, our review suggested that rupture of chronic pseudoaneurysm is rare or of low rate.

Dressler Syndrome

Some patients may develop pericarditis several weeks after myocardial infarction (Dressler syndrome). It is probably mediated immunologically. It is treated initially with nonsteroidal anti-inflammatory agents. Steroid therapy may be needed for a small number of patients with refractory chest pain.

Postcardiotomy Syndrome

Postcardiotomy syndrome is similar to Dressler syndrome,

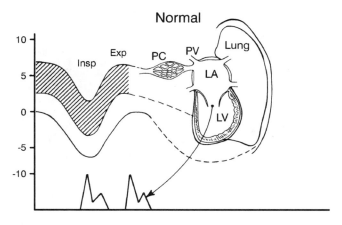

Normal

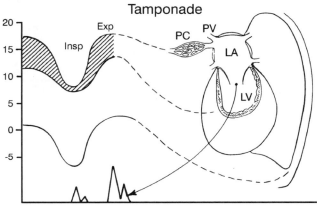

Tamponade

Fig. 6. Diagram of intrathoracic and intracardiac pressure changes with respiration in normal and tamponade physiology. The shaded area indicates left ventricular (LV) filling pressure gradients (difference between pulmonary capillary wedge pressure and LV diastolic pressure). At the bottom of each drawing is a schematic mitral inflow Doppler velocity profile reflecting LV diastolic filling. In tamponade, there is a decrease in LV filling after inspiration (Insp) because the pressure decrease in the pericardium and LV cavity is smaller than that in the pulmonary capillaries (PC). LV filling is restored after expiration (Exp). PV, pulmonary vein. (From Oh JK, Seward JB, Tajik AJ: *The Echo Manual*. Second edition. Lippincott-Raven Publishers, 1999, p 184. By permission of Mayo Foundation.)

and an autoimmune response to cardiac antigens has been implicated in this entity. Postcardiotomy syndrome occurs in about 5% of patients who have a cardiac surgical procedure, with symptoms occurring 3 weeks to 6 months postoperatively. It most likely is related to surgical trauma and irritation by blood products in the mediastinum and pericardium. The initial treatment for this syndrome is with nonsteroidal anti-inflammatory agents, and only in the case of refractory symptoms should systemic steroids be used. Pericardiectomy is rarely required.

Tamponade Related to Aortic Dissection

Cardiac tamponade may occur with proximal aortic dissection. After pericardial tamponade is recognized as a result of aortic dissection, urgent surgical repair of the aortic dissection and tamponade is needed. In this clinical setting, pericardiocentesis may increase blood pressure and cause rupture of the dissected aorta. A recent study showed 60% early mortality for patients with an aortic dissection complicated by cardiac tamponade. All patients who underwent pericardiocentesis died shortly thereafter.

Constrictive Pericarditis

Constrictive pericarditis is characterized by restrictive ventricular filling due to a thickened and calcified pericardium. The pericardium usually contains calcified fibrous scar tissue from an inflammatory process, and in the advanced stage, the scarring may involve the epicardium. The causes of constriction are several, including acute pericarditis, collagen vascular disease, coronary artery bypass surgery, and tuberculosis (Table 2). However, in many patients, the cause may not be identified.

The main clinical features at presentation are dyspnea, peripheral edema, marked systemic venous congestion with hepatomegaly, and ascites. Frequently, patients are evaluated for primary liver disease and may undergo a liver biopsy before constrictive pericarditis is diagnosed. The most prominent findings on physical examination are related to systemic venous congestion, such as distention of the jugular vein (Table 3). Venous pressure often increases with inspiration (Kussmaul sign) because of the inability of the right side of the heart to accept the increased cardiac input with inspiration. Unlike the patients with cardiac tamponade with "x" descent, patients with constrictive pericarditis have rapid "y" descent, which reflects the early diastolic decrease in right ventricular pressure.

With high atrial pressure, rapid filling of the ventricle is accelerated, and this generates the third heart sound known as "pericardial knock," which usually occurs 80 to 120 ms after aortic valve closure (Fig. 8). Other differential diagnoses of a diastolic gallop occurring 80 to 120 ms after aortic valve closure include opening snap of the mitral valve in mitral stenosis (which is followed by a diastolic rumble), tumor plop from atrial myxoma, and a third heart sound related to left ventricular failure.

The correct diagnosis of constrictive pericarditis is crucial

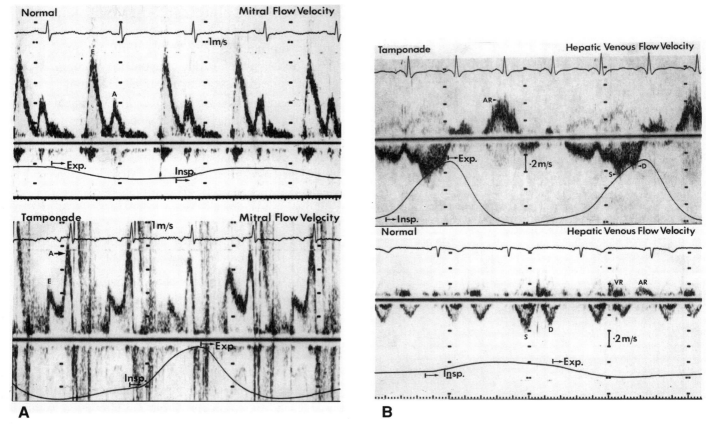

Fig. 7. *A*, Mitral inflow velocity profile typical of a normal subject (*upper*) and a patient with cardiac tamponade (*lower*). *B*, Hepatic venous flow velocity profile in a patient with cardiac tamponade (*upper*, same patient as in A *lower*) and a normal subject (*lower*). Exp, expiration; Insp, inspiration. (From *Mayo Clin Proc* 61:312-324, 1989. By permission of Mayo Foundation for Medical Education and Research.)

because most of the symptoms can be reversed by pericardiectomy. However, the symptoms and clinical findings mimic those of restrictive cardiomyopathy, which is a progressive disease with no effective treatment.

Pericardial Calcification

When constrictive pericarditis is suspected clinically, a chest radiograph, including a left lateral projection, should be reviewed to look for pericardial calcification. Pericardial calcification was commonly seen in patients with tuberculous pericarditis, but currently, it is seen most commonly in patients with idiopathic constrictive pericarditis. If a patient presents with ascites and other clinical evidence of significant systemic venous congestion and a pericardial knock, chest radiographic findings of pericardial calcification make constrictive pericarditis the leading diagnosis, and in this clinical situation, a patient requires surgical exploration and pericardiectomy. No single ECG abnormality is diagnostic of constrictive pericarditis.

Echocardiography in Constrictive Pericarditis

Echocardiography is helpful in diagnosing constrictive pericarditis. The characteristic M-mode/two-dimensional echocardiographic findings include abnormal ventricular septal motion (Fig. 9), increased pericardial thickness or calcification, dilated inferior vena cava with no significant changes with inspiration, and flattening of the left ventricular posterior wall during diastole. However, these findings are neither sensitive nor specific.

Although the underlying pathologic mechanism of constriction is different from that of cardiac tamponade, the hemodynamic events of respiratory variation during left and right ventricular filling are similar in the two conditions. The thickened pericardial layer prevents full transmission of intrapleural pressure changes with respiration to the pericardial and intracardiac cavity, creating respiratory variation in the left-side filling pressure gradient (pressure difference between the pulmonary vein and the left atrium). Therefore, the mitral inflow and pulmonary venous diastolic flow

Table 2.—Causes of Constrictive Pericarditis

Unknown (idiopathic)
Post-acute pericarditis of any cause
Post-cardiac surgery
Uremia
Connective tissue disease (systemic lupus erythematosus, scleroderma, rheumatoid arthritis)
Post-trauma
Drugs (procainamide, hydralazine, methysergide)
Radiation-induced
Neoplastic pericardial disease (melanoma, mesothelioma)
Tuberculosis, fungal infections (histoplasmosis, coccidioidomycosis), parasitic infections
Post-myocardial infarct
Post-Dressler syndrome
Post-purulent pericarditis
Pulmonary asbestosis

Table 3.—Signs and Symptoms of Constrictive Pericarditis

In more than 95% of patients
    Increased jugular venous pressure
    Hepatomegaly
In more than 75% of patients
    Dyspnea
    Edema
    Abdominal swelling (ascites)
    Pleural effusion
    Severe fatigue
In more than 25% of patients
    Pulsus paradoxus
    Palpitations
    Cough
    Abdominal pain
    Orthopnea
In fewer than 25% of patients
    Pericardial knock
    Muscle wasting
    Nausea and vomiting
    Dizziness
In fewer than 5% of patients
    Finger clubbing

velocities decrease immediately after the onset of inspiration and increase with expiration (Fig. 10). Reciprocal changes occur in tricuspid inflow and hepatic venous flow velocity because of the relatively fixed cardiac volume. With decreased filling of the right cardiac chambers on expiration, there are exaggerated diastolic flow reversals and decreased diastolic forward flow in the hepatic vein with the onset of expiration. In contrast, hepatic vein flow reversals are more prominent with inspiration in restrictive cardiomyopathy. However, it is not unusual to see significant diastolic flow reversals in the hepatic vein during both inspiration and expiration in patients with advanced constriction or combined constriction and restriction. A representative Doppler spectrum of constrictive pericarditis is shown in Figure 11. A subgroup of patients with constrictive pericarditis may not have the characteristic respiratory variation of Doppler velocities. Therefore, the absence of respiratory variation in patients with clinical evidence of significant systemic venous congestion does not exclude the diagnosis of constrictive pericarditis, and additional studies should be performed. The typical respiratory variation and Doppler velocities also can occur in other conditions such as chronic obstructive lung disease, right ventricular infarct, sleep apnea, asthma, and pulmonary embolism.

Pericardial Thickness in Constrictive Pericarditis
CT or MRI is best for determining pericardial thickness.

Most patients with constrictive pericarditis present with a thickened pericardium. However, by itself, this finding is not sensitive or specific for constrictive pericarditis. Demonstration of increased pericardial thickness on CT or MRI in patients with significant systemic venous congestion generally indicates constrictive pericarditis. Recently, pericardial thickness has been assessed with transesophageal echocardiography, and the findings correlate well with those of Imatron CT.

Hemodynamic Findings in Constrictive Pericarditis
The hemodynamic findings in constrictive pericarditis include an increase in right atrial pressure and dip-and-plateau configuration of the right and left ventricular diastolic pressure tracings (Fig. 12). Because there is no restriction of early ventricular filling, the "y" descent is quite prominent, corresponding to a prominent early diastolic dip of the ventricular pressure tracing. Right ventricular systolic pressure is usually less than 50 mm Hg, but this finding is not sensitive or specific and cannot be used to differentiate constrictive

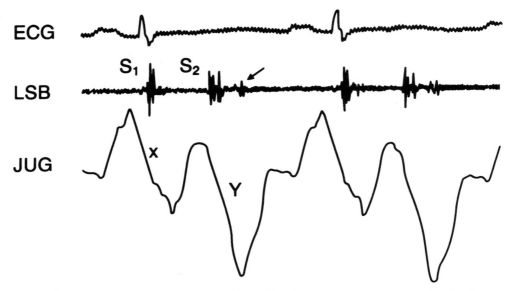

Fig. 8. Simultaneous electrocardiogram (ECG), phonocardiogram (LSB), and jugular venous pressure (JUG) tracing showing the timing of the pericardial knock (*arrow*). (From Tavel ME: *Clinical Phonocardiography and External Pulse Recording*. Fourth edition. Year Book Medical Publishers, 1985, p 378. By permission of Mosby.)

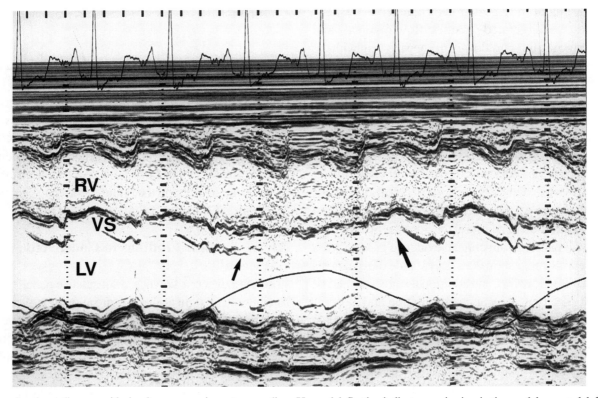

Fig. 9. M-mode echocardiogram with simultaneous respirometer recording. Upward deflection indicates passive inspiration, and downward deflection the onset of expiration. Ventricular septum (*VS*) moves toward the left ventricle (*LV*) with inspiration (*small arrow*) and toward the right ventricle (*RV*) with expiration (*large arrow*). The underlying hemodynamics are explained in the text.

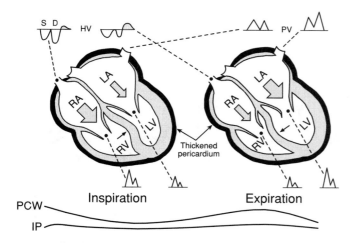

Fig. 10. Diagram of a heart with a thickened pericardium to illustrate the respiratory variation in ventricular filling and the corresponding Doppler features of the mitral valve, tricuspid valve, pulmonary vein (PV), and hepatic vein (HV). These changes are related to discordant pressure changes in the vessels in the thorax, such as pulmonary capillary wedge pressure (PCW) and intrapericardial (IP) and intracardiac pressures. Hatched area under curve indicates the reversal of flow. *Thicker arrows* indicate greater filling. D, diastolic flow; S, systolic flow. LA, left atrium; LV, left ventricle; PCW, pulmonary capillary wedge; RA, right atrium; RV, right ventricle. (From Oh JK, Seward JB, Tajik AJ: *The Echo Manual*. Second edition. Lippincott-Raven Publishers, 1999, p 188. By permission of Mayo Foundation.)

pericarditis from restrictive cardiomyopathy (Fig. 13). The concept of ventricular interdependence and the reciprocal pressure changes in the right and left ventricles with respiration can be used in hemodynamic assessment. Simultaneous left and right ventricular pressure tracings show discordant direction of pressure changes with respiration (Fig. 12). Left ventricular pressure decreases with inspiration and right ventricular pressure increases. An opposite change occurs with expiration. Also, simultaneous left ventricular diastolic pressure and pulmonary capillary wedge pressure show significant reduction in the pressure difference between the pulmonary capillary wedge pressure and the left ventricular diastolic pressure with inspiration in comparison with the difference during expiration (Fig. 12).

- There is no characteristic ECG abnormality that is diagnostic of constrictive pericarditis.
- Remember pericardial constriction in a patient who has nonspecific findings on liver biopsy.
- A subset of patients with constrictive pericarditis may not show the typical respiratory changes in Doppler velocities.

Restriction Versus Constriction

The clinical and hemodynamic profiles of restriction and constriction are similar, despite these conditions having distinctly different pathophysiologic mechanisms (Fig. 13). Both are caused primarily by diastolic filling abnormalities, with preserved global systolic function. The diastolic dysfunction in restrictive cardiomyopathy results from a stiff and noncompliant ventricular myocardium, whereas it is due to a thickened noncompliant pericardium in constrictive pericarditis. Both disease processes limit diastolic filling and result in diastolic heart failure. Pathologically, restriction and constriction may appear similar, with normal-sized ventricles and enlarged atria, but the pericardium is thickened in constriction.

Infiltrative Cardiomyopathy

Infiltrative cardiomyopathy has typical two-dimensional echocardiographic findings and biochemical abnormalities. A prototypical example is cardiac amyloidosis, which is characterized by increased ventricular wall thickness, a granular or sparkling myocardial appearance on echocardiography, and typical amyloid deposits in fat in myocardial biopsy specimens. Also, patients usually (but not always) have monoclonal gammopathy on serum protein electrophoresis. ECG shows a low voltage despite increased left ventricular wall thickness.

Noninfiltrative Restrictive Cardiomyopathy

Noninfiltrative restrictive cardiomyopathy is difficult to diagnose. The myocardium becomes noncompliant with fibrosis and scarring, but systolic function is usually maintained. With limited diastolic filling and increased diastolic pressure, the atria become enlarged. In contrast, myocardial compliance usually is not decreased in patients with constrictive pericarditis. The thickened and sometimes calcified pericardium limits diastolic filling, resulting in hemodynamics that are different from those of restrictive cardiomyopathy. Atrial enlargement in constriction is less prominent than in restrictive cardiomyopathy. When restrictive cardiomyopathy affects both ventricles, clinical signs due to abnormalities of right-sided heart failure are apparent, with increased jugular venous pressure and peripheral edema. An early diastolic gallop sound

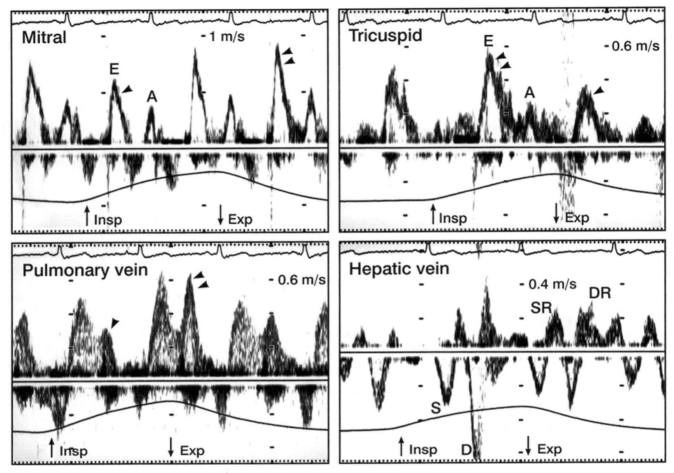

Fig. 11. *A*, Composite of mitral valve, tricuspid valve, pulmonary vein, and hepatic venous flow velocities typically seen in constrictive pericarditis. D, diastolic flow; DR, diastolic flow reversal; Exp, expiration; Insp, inspiration; S, systolic flow; SR, systolic flow reversal. (From Oh JK, Seward JB, Tajik AJ: The Echo Manual. Second edition. Lippincott-Raven Publishers, 1999, p 188. By permission of Mayo Foundation.)

is the rule and, in restriction, often difficult to distinguish from a pericardial knock. ECG and chest radiographic findings are nonspecific, except that a calcified pericardium should point to constrictive pericarditis.

Echocardiographically, it is difficult to distinguish between restriction and constriction only on the basis of M-mode and two-dimensional findings. Both conditions have normal left ventricular systolic function and enlarged atria and inferior vena cava. An increase in ventricular wall thickness, a thickening of the valves, and a small amount of pericardial effusion are typical of cardiac amyloidosis. In constrictive pericarditis, the most striking finding is ventricular septal motion abnormalities, which can be explained on the basis of respiratory variation in ventricular filling. The pericardium usually is thickened, but this may not be obvious on transthoracic echocardiography.

Transesophageal echocardiographic measurement of pericardial thickness correlates well with that measured by electron-beam CT.

Diagnostic Strategy to Differentiate Restrictive Cardiomyopathy From Constrictive Pericarditis

The following diagnostic strategy to differentiate restrictive cardiomyopathy from constrictive pericarditis is recommended:

1. The findings of pulsus paradoxus, calcification of the pericardium (seen on chest radiography), and pericardial knock favor the diagnosis of constrictive pericarditis. Decreased voltage on the ECG may indicate cardiac amyloidosis.

2. Two-dimensional echocardiographic findings of increased left ventricular wall thickness and normal septal

motion in conjunction with enlarged atria suggest restrictive cardiomyopathy. A thickened or calcified pericardium and ventricular septal motion favor constrictive pericarditis.

3. In constriction, there is a typical respiratory variation in ventricular filling (decreased filling of the left ventricle with inspiration and increased filling with expiration and significant hepatic venous flow reversal with expiration because of decreased filling on the right side). Restrictive cardiomyopathy is characterized by the restrictive Doppler physiology, with increased E velocity, decreased A velocity, E/A ratio greater than 2, and shortened deceleration time of E velocity. Hepatic vein diastolic flow reversals occur with inspiration instead of expiration (Fig. 14). A subgroup of patients with constrictive pericarditis may have similar

Doppler findings without respiratory variation. In such cases, the Doppler examination should be repeated after an attempt has been made to reduce preload (head-up tilt position or diuretic therapy). Respiratory Doppler studies may be difficult to perform in patients with atrial fibrillation, but these patients still should have abnormal septal motion and hepatic venous flow velocity changes on Doppler echocardiography. If the diagnosis is still uncertain after a careful clinical examination, review of laboratory data, and two-dimensional Doppler echocardiographic evaluation, additional studies are needed, including CT or MRI, to examine pericardial thickness and cardiac catheterization to look for characteristic discordant respiratory changes in the left and right ventricular pressure tracings.

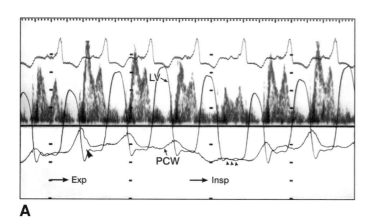
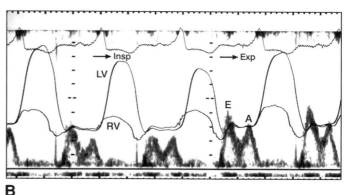

A **B**

Fig. 12. *A*, Simultaneous pressure recordings from the left ventricle (LV) and pulmonary capillary wedge together with mitral inflow velocity on a Doppler echocardiogram. The onset of the respiratory phase is indicated at the bottom. Exp, expiration; Insp, inspiration. With the onset of expiration, pulmonary capillary wedge pressure (PCW) increases much more than LV diastolic pressure, creating a large driving pressure gradient (*large arrowhead*). With inspiration, however, PCW decreases much more than LV diastolic pressure, with a very small driving pressure gradient (*three small arrowheads*). These respiratory changes in the LV filling gradient are well reflected by the changes in the mitral inflow velocities recorded on Dopper echocardiography. *B*, Simultaneous pressure measurements from the LV and right ventricle (RV) together with mitral inflow velocities on Doppler echocardiography. The LV pressure decreases from the second to the third cardiac cycle toward the end of inspiration, but RV systolic pressure increases from the second to the third cardiac cycle. This represents discordant pressure changes with respiration. The increase in RV systolic pressure (third cardiac cycle) follows the decrease in the mitral inflow velocity (second complete mitral inflow velocity recording), indicating that the initial hemodynamic event responsible for respiratory variation in ventricular filling comes from the left side. The typical square root sign and the equalization of diastolic pressure between the LV and RV are well shown in the simultaneous LV and RV pressure tracings. (From Oh JK, Seward JB, Tajik AJ: *The Echo Manual*. Second edition. Lippincott-Raven Publishers, 1999, p 187. By permission of Mayo Foundation.)

	Constriction	Restriction
LVEDP-RVEDP, mm Hg	≤ 5	> 5
RV systolic, mm Hg	≤ 50	> 50
RVEDP/RVSP, mm Hg	≥ 0.33	< 0.3

A

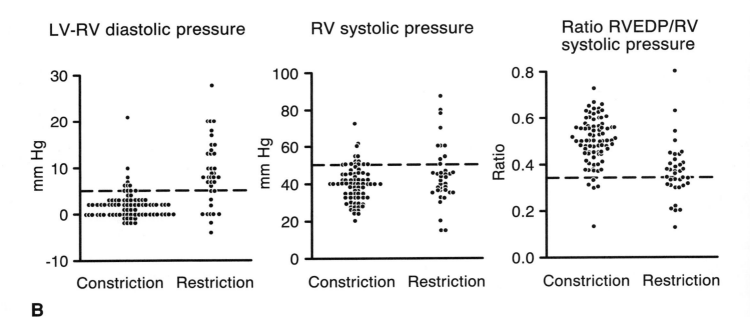

B

Fig. 13. Comparison of constriction and restriction. *A*, Hemodynamics and, *B*, hemodynamic criteria. LV, left ventricle; LVEDP, LV end-diastolic pressure; RV, right ventricle; RVEDP, RV end-diastolic pressure; RVSP, RV systolic pressure. (*B* from *Am Heart J* 122:1431-1441, 1991. By permission of Mosby.)

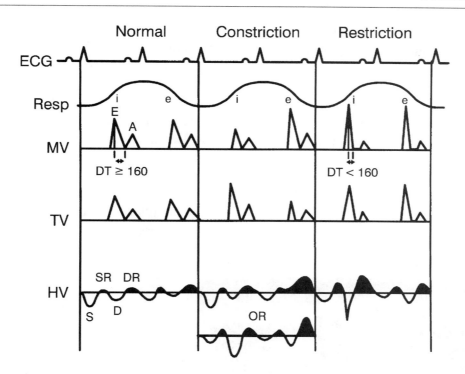

Fig. 14. Comparison of mitral (MV), tricuspid (TV), and hepatic vein (HV) Doppler flow velocities in constrictive pericarditis and restrictive cardiomyopathy. DR, diastolic reversal; DT, deceleration time; e, expiration; ECG, electrocardiogram; i, inspiration; Resp, respiration; SR, systolic reversal. (From Oh JK, Seward JB, Tajik AJ: *The Echo Manual.* Second edition. Lippincott-Raven Publishers, 1999, p 192. By permission of Mayo Foundation.)

Questions

Multiple Choice (choose the one best answer)

1. A 17-year-old male has fatigue. Clinical examination reveals signs of failure of the right side of the heart (i.e., increased jugular venous pressure, mild peripheral edema, hepatomegaly, and a third heart sound). Catheterization of the right side of the heart provided the following data:

Right atrial pressure = 23 mm Hg

Right ventricular pressure = 60/23 mm Hg
Pulmonary capillary wedge pressure = 20 mm Hg
Cardiac index = 1.7 L/min per m^2

The hemodynamic data are consistent with:
a. Restrictive cardiomyopathy
b. Constrictive pericarditis
c. Cardiac tamponade
d. All the above
e. None of the above

2. The patient in question 1 had a two-dimensional Doppler echocardiographic study that showed the following (Figure). The diagnosis is:
   a. Restrictive cardiomyopathy
   b. Constrictive pericarditis
   c. Eisenmenger syndrome
   d. Anomalous pulmonary vein connection
   e. Atrial failure

3. For the patient in questions 1 and 2, the optimal management is:
   a. Verapamil
   b. β-Blocker

c. Pericardiectomy
d. Cardiac transplantation
e. Digoxin

4. A 61-year-old man came to the emergency department because of persistent chest pain after thrombolytic therapy. He was hypotensive, and electrocardiography was performed (Figure). The appropriate next step for his management would be:
   a. Cardiac catheterization
   b. Echocardiography to look for pericardial effusion
   c. Blind pericardiocentesis
   d. Temporary pacemaker

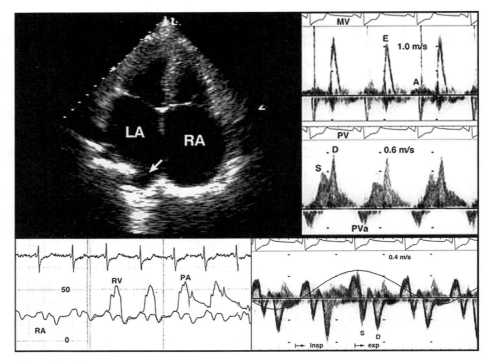

Question 2.
exp, expiration; insp, inspiration; HV, hepatic vein; LA, left atrium; MV, mitral valve; PV, pulmonary valve; RA, right atrium; RV, right ventricle.

Question 4

5. A 44-year-old man had chest pain with pericardial rub. He was treated with a nonsteroidal anti-inflammatory drug. About 2 weeks later, he had increasing dyspnea and fluid retention. Echocardiography did not show pericardial effusion. Which of the following statements is correct?

   a. The problem most likely is a side effect of the non-steroidal anti-inflammatory drug

   b. Constrictive pericarditis is developing

   c. Pericardiectomy is required

   d. The treatment of choice is colchicine

   e. A systemic disease is indicated

6. A simultaneous jugular venous pressure tracing (JVP) and hepatic vein (HV) Doppler recording are shown in the Figure. What other physical finding is expected in this patient?

   a. Pulsus paradoxus

   b. Systolic murmur

   c. Kussmaul sign

   d. Ewart sign

   e. Austin Flint murmur

7. Which of the following statements is always correct in tamponade?

   a. Atrial pressure is increased

   b. Pericardiocentesis is required

   c. Electrocardiography shows electrical alternans

   d. Intrapericardial pressure is higher than atrial pressure

   e. It leads to constriction

8. Which of the following hemodynamic features is typical of restrictive cardiomyopathy?

   a. Discordant left ventricular and right ventricular systolic pressure change

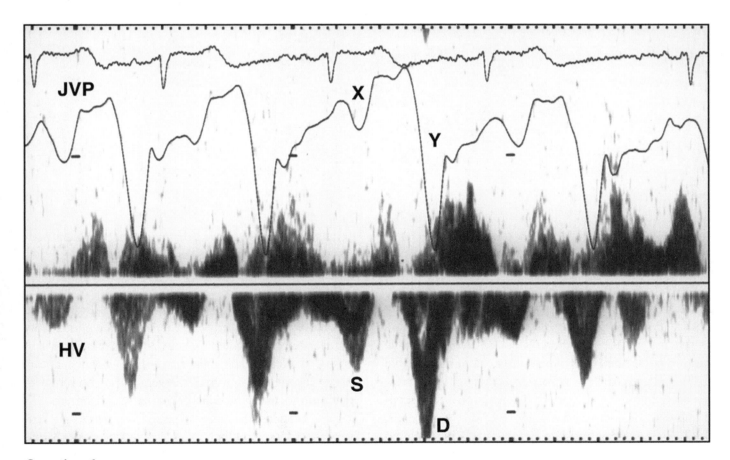

Question 6

Simultaneous jugular venous pressure (JVP) tracing and pulsed-wave Doppler recording of hepatic vein (HV) velocities. There is the characteristic Y descent. *D*, diastolic flow; *S*, systolic flow; *X* and *Y*, jugular venous pressure waveforms. (From Oh JK, Seward JB, Tajik AJ: The Echo Manual. Second edition. Lippincott-Raven Publishers, 1999, p 188. By permission of Mayo Foundation.)

b. Dip-and-plateau ventricular diastolic pressure

c. No significant left ventricular diastolic pressure change with respiration

d. Diastolic hepatic vein flow reversal with expiration

9. Patients with pulsus paradoxus always have which of the following?
   a. Pericardial effusion
   b. Increased interventricular dependence
   c. Electrical alternans
   d. Jugular venous distention
   e. Cardiomegaly

10. A 53-year-old man has ascites, hepatomegaly, and abnormalities in liver function tests. What is your next diagnostic step?
    a. Ultrasonography of the liver
    b. Liver biopsy
    c. Measurement of jugular venous pressure
    d. Echocardiography
    e. Examination of ascitic fluid

11. Which group of patients has the worst prognosis for constrictive pericarditis (CP)?
    a. Radiation-induced CP
    b. Post-bypass CP
    c. CP due to rheumatoid arthritis
    d. CP due to acute pericarditis
    e. Idiopathic CP

12. A 77-year-old woman presents with cough, peripheral edema, pleural effusion, and night sweats. A skin test for tuberculosis was positive, and echocardiography showed effusive constrictive pericarditis. Which of the following statements is not correct for this entity?
    a. Isolation of the tuberculosis organism is required for diagnosis
    b. Treat the patient with antituberculosis medications with the presumptive diagnosis of tuberculosis
    c. Pericardiectomy probably will be required
    d. Corticosteroid therapy may be helpful

Answers

1. Answer d

The hemodynamic data demonstrate increased right atrial pressure, pulmonary capillary wedge pressure, and right ventricular systolic pressure. These hemodynamic data are not specific for one condition. Right ventricular systolic pressure of 60 mm Hg is more consistent with restrictive cardiomyopathy, but the near equalization of right atrial pressure and pulmonary capillary wedge pressure is more consistent with constrictive pericarditis or cardiac tamponade. This question exemplifies the difficulty in differentiating restrictive cardiomyopathy from constrictive pericarditis on the basis of hemodynamic data alone. Therefore, these hemodynamic data are consistent with restrictive cardiomyopathy, constrictive pericarditis, or cardiac tamponade. Thus,

the answer is "all the above." In this setting, more information is needed to establish the correct diagnosis.

2. Answer a

The figure shows the composite of two-dimensional echocardiography, mitral and pulmonary venous flow Doppler velocity, and hepatic vein Doppler velocity as well as hemodynamic tracing. The two-dimensional echocardiographic finding of biatrial enlargement is consistent with either constrictive pericarditis or restrictive cardiomyopathy. Right ventricular dilatation is expected in Eisenmenger syndrome and anomalous pulmonary vein connections. Mitral inflow shows restrictive filling pattern; also, pulmonary venous flow velocity is consistent with restrictive filling pattern. Pulmonary vein atrial flow reversal (PVa) is relatively small, consistent with atrial failure. Hepatic vein

Doppler velocity shows restrictive filling. Diastolic flow reversal is more prominent with inspiration, which is more typical for restrictive cardiomyopathy.

3. Answer d

The treatment of restrictive cardiomyopathy is very difficult. The prognosis for patients with restrictive cardiomyopathy is poor, especially for the pediatric patient population. This 17-year-old male is already symptomatic with restrictive cardiomyopathy, with marked biatrial enlargement and low cardiac output. Most likely, atrial fibrillation and heart failure not responsive to medical treatment will develop in this patient. Optimal management in this case is cardiac transplantation.

4. Answer b

The figure shows sinus tachycardia and diffuse ST-segment elevation. There also is a PR depression in lead I, typical for pericarditis. This patient received thrombolytic therapy because of concern about myocardial infarction, but the electrocardiographic findings are more consistent with pericarditis. Patients with pericarditis also have hypertension, suggesting the possibility of cardiac tamponade. Therefore, the next step for management in this case should be echocardiography to look for pericardial effusion.

5. Answer b

This clinical scenario is typical of transient constrictive pericarditis after acute pericarditis. About 10% of patients with pericarditis develop transient constrictive pericarditis. In this situation, the pericardium becomes inflamed, resulting in constrictive physiology. Computed tomography or magnetic resonance imaging may show thickened pericardium. Treatment should be a high dose of a nonsteroidal anti-inflammatory drug or a short course of corticosteroid therapy, with close clinical follow-up.

6. Answer c

The figure shows a simultaneous jugular venous pressure tracing and hepatic venous Doppler tracing. There is a rapid "y" descent in the jugular venous pressure tracing, which is typical for constrictive pericarditis. Another typical finding in patients with constrictive pericarditis is the Kussmaul sign.

7. Answer d

Atrial pressures are usually increased in patients with cardiac tamponade but may not be increased in patients with low pressure tamponade. Therefore, statement "a" is not always correct. Some patients with cardiac tamponade can be managed without pericardiocentesis. Only a small subset of patients with cardiac tamponade demonstrates electrical alternans, and not all patients with electrical alternans have cardiac tamponade. A small subset of patients with cardiac tamponade have progression to the constrictive stage. However, by definition, cardiac tamponade intrapericardial pressure should always be higher than atrial pressure.

Answer 4

8. Answer b

Although not specific, the dip-and-plateau ventricular diastolic pressure tracing is consistent or compatible with restrictive cardiomyopathy. Choices "a," "c," and "d" are not compatible with restrictive cardiomyopathy but are compatible with constrictive pericarditis.

9. Answer b

Pulsus paradoxus is characterized as more than a 10 mm Hg decrease in systolic blood pressure with inspiration. It is related to decreased left ventricular filling with inspiration, while right ventricular filling increases. In cardiac tamponade, the respiratory change in ventricular filling is related to markedly increased interventricular dependence (increase in right ventricular filling results in a decrease in left ventricular filling).

10. Answer c

It is not uncommon for patients with pericardial disease to have symptoms similar to those of liver disease. What distinguishes pericardial disease from liver disease is the increase in atrial pressure.

11. Answer a

Radiation-induced constrictive pericarditis usually accompanies myocardial disease due to radiation, and the prognosis is worse than that of other causes of constrictive pericarditis.

12. Answer a

Mycobacteria may not be isolated in patients with tuberculous pericarditis. If chest radiography shows findings consistent with tuberculosis or a constellation of findings suggest tuberculosis, the patient needs to be treated with the presumptive diagnosis of tuberculosis.

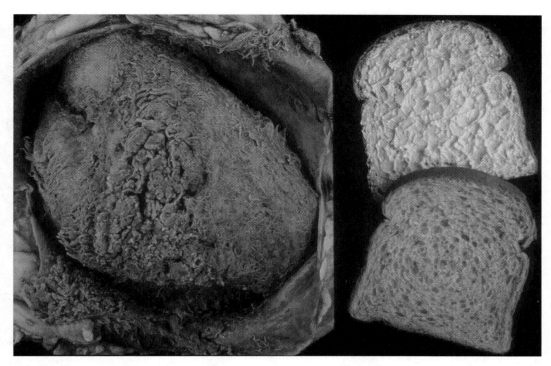

Plate 1. Fibrinous "bread-and-butter" pericarditis.

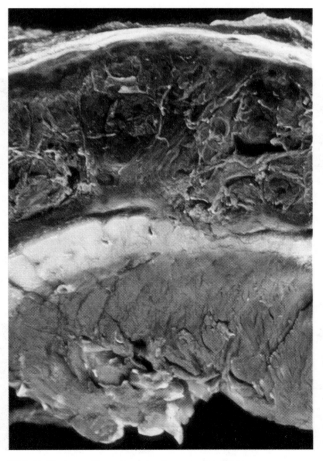

Plate 2. Postoperative organizing hemopericardium.

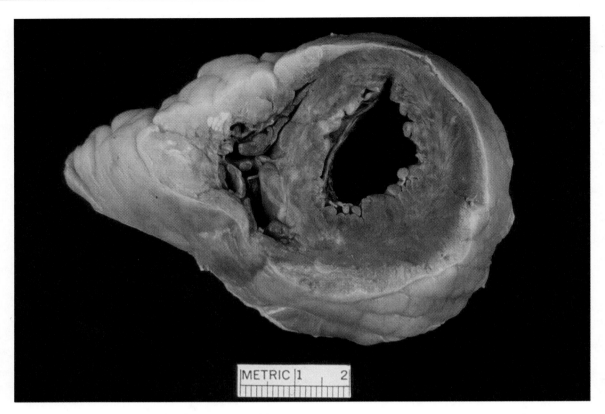

Plate 3. Epicardial fat necrosis of the heart in pancreatitis.

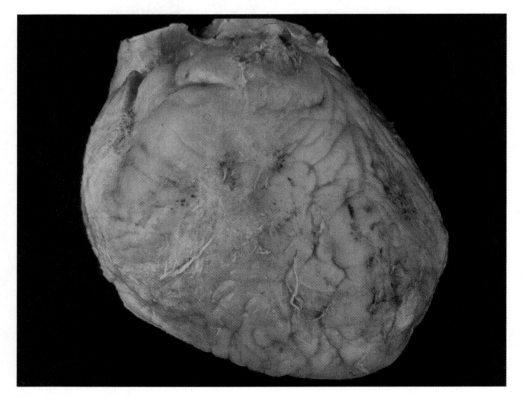

Plate 4. Healed pericarditis due to systemic lupus erythematosus.

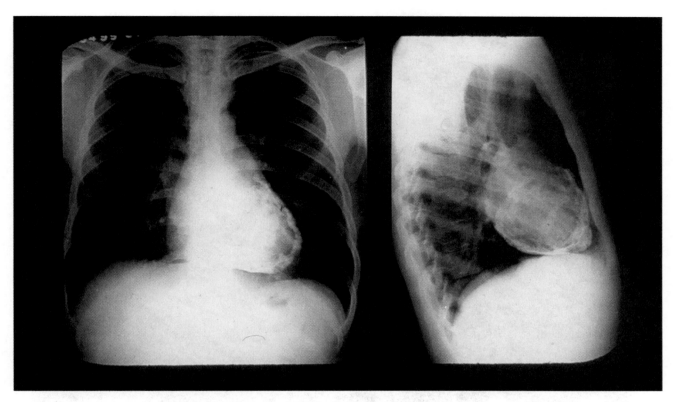

Plate 5. *A*, PA and, *B*, lateral chest radiographs showing a calcified pericardium in constrictive pericarditis.

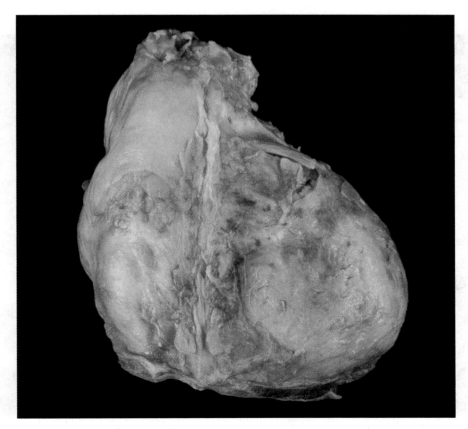

Plate 6. Constrictive pericarditis after coronary artery bypass grafting.

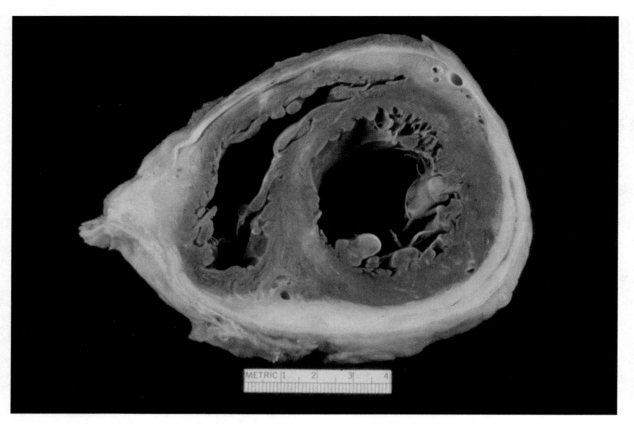

Plate 7. Noncalcific constrictive pericarditis 4 years after coronary artery bypass grafting.

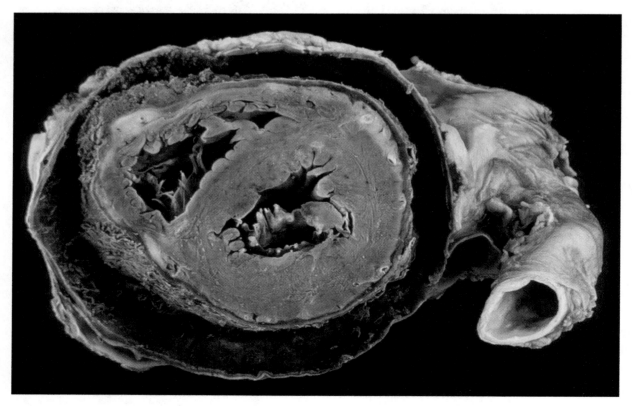

Plate 8. Pericarditis with pericardial effusion.

Chapter 33

Pregnancy and the Heart

Heidi M. Connolly, M.D.

Approximately 2% of pregnancies occur in women who have significant heart disease. Among pregnant women, congenital heart disease is the predominant form of heart disease in developed countries, whereas rheumatic heart disease predominates in developing countries. Heart disease does not preclude successful pregnancy but increases the risk to both mother and baby and requires special management.

> Knowledge of the normal hemodynamic changes that occur during pregnancy and the resultant effect on common cardiovascular diseases is required for the Cardiology Boards.

Physiology

Hemodynamic Changes During Normal Pregnancy

Substantial hemodynamic changes occur during normal pregnancy, including a 20% to 30% increase in red blood cell mass and a 30% to 50% increase in plasma volume. As a result, there is an increase in total blood volume, with a relative anemia (Fig. 1). Heart rate increases about 10 beats/min, with reduction in systemic and pulmonary vascular resistance. Blood pressure decreases slightly during pregnancy. These hemodynamic changes result in a steady increase in cardiac output during pregnancy until the 32nd week, at which time cardiac output plateaus at 30% to 50% above the prepregnancy level (Fig. 2). The pregnant uterus can require up to 18% of cardiac output. Oxygen consumption increases steadily throughout pregnancy and reaches a level of approximately 30% above the prepregnant level by the time of delivery. This increase is due to the metabolic needs of both mother and fetus. During the last half of pregnancy, cardiac output is significantly affected by body position, because the enlarging uterus decreases venous return from the lower extremities. The left lateral position minimizes this reduction in venous return. Normally, the hemodynamic changes that occur during pregnancy are well tolerated by the mother. Heart disease may be manifested initially during pregnancy because of increased cardiac output or because minor preexisting symptoms may be exacerbated.

Cardiac Examination in Normal Pregnancy

During normal pregnancy, there is a brisk and full carotid upstroke, and jugular venous pressure is normal or mildly increased, with prominent "a" and "v" waves. The left ventricular impulse is displaced laterally and enlarged. The first heart sound is louder than normal. The pulmonic second sound may be prominent, and there often is persistent splitting of the second heart sound. A third heart sound is audible in more than 80% of normal pregnant women (Fig. 3). An early peaking ejection systolic murmur is audible in more than 90% of normal pregnant women and is caused by a pulmonary outflow murmur.

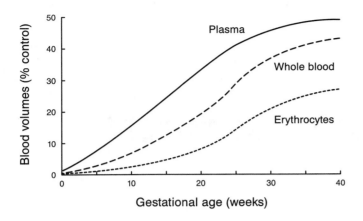

Fig. 1. Hemodynamic changes during normal pregnancy. (From *Am J Physiol* 245:R720-R729, 1983. By permission of the American Physiological Society.)

Venous hums and mammary continuous murmurs are common but without significance. Peripheral edema and venous varicosities are common. Abnormal physical findings include a fourth heart sound, a loud (≥ 3/6) systolic murmur, and a diastolic murmur or fixed splitting of the second heart sound. These do not occur during normal pregnancy in the absence of heart disease.

- Normal physical findings during pregnancy may be misinterpreted as abnormal.

Imaging Studies in Pregnancy

On chest radiographs, the cardiac silhouette is enlarged, with increased vascular markings. On echocardiography, there is a small increase in right and left ventricular volumes. The electrocardiogram shows an increase in heart rate, with a leftward shift of the QRS and T-wave axes because of the upward and horizontal displacement of the heart by the pregnant uterus.

Hemodynamic Changes During Labor and Delivery

With uterine contractions, an additional 300 to 500 mL of blood enters the circulation. This increase in blood volume in conjunction with increased blood pressure and heart rate during labor increases cardiac output. At the time of delivery, cardiac output increases as much as 80% above the prepregnancy level (and may be as great as 9 L/min). Administration of epidural anesthesia decreases cardiac output to about 8 L/min, and the use of general anesthesia decreases it further. Approximately 500 mL of blood is

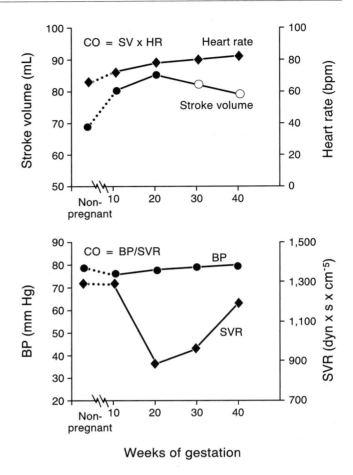

Fig. 2. Cardiac output (CO) can be determined from other variables in at least 3 ways: CO = heart rate (HR) x stroke volume (SV), CO = mean arterial pressure (BP) minus right atrial pressure/systemic vascular resistance (SVR); CO = oxygen (O_2) consumption/arteriovenous (A - V) O_2 difference. The expected values for these variables measured in the supine position during pregnancy are based on information acquired from many studies. (From Alexander RW, Schlant RC, Fuster V [editors]: *Hurst's the Heart, Arteries and Veins*. Ninth edition. Vol. 2. McGraw-Hill, 1998, p 2392. By permission of the publisher.)

lost at the time of vaginal delivery, and approximately 1,000 mL is lost during a normal cesarean section.

Hemodynamic Changes Post Partum

After delivery, venous return increases because of relief from fetal compression on the inferior vena cava. Spontaneous diuresis occurs during the first 24 to 48 hours after delivery; however, it takes about 2 to 4 weeks for hemodynamic values to return to baseline after vaginal delivery and longer after cesarean section.

- Cardiac output increases by 30% to 50% during normal pregnancy.

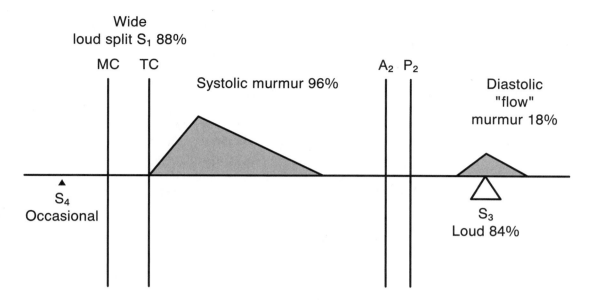

Fig. 3. Normal auscultatory findings during pregnancy. A_2, aortic second sound; MC, mitral valve closure; P_2, pulmonic second sound; TC, tricuspid valve closure.

- Cardiac output increases to about 80% above baseline during labor and delivery.
- Hemodynamics return to baseline 2 to 4 weeks after vaginal delivery and may take up to 6 weeks to return to normal after cesarean section.

Cardiac Disease in Pregnancy

Principles of Management

Antepartum management of women with heart disease should include an anatomical and hemodynamic assessment of any cardiac abnormality to determine the maternal and fetal risks of pregnancy. Doppler echocardiography is ideal for the evaluation of pregnant women with heart disease. When evaluating women with cardiovascular disease, the safety of the mother is always the highest priority. Specific cardiovascular conditions pose an unacceptable risk of death to both mother and baby, and in these situations, pregnancy should be avoided.

Fetal growth and development are monitored with ultrasonography. Fetal heart ultrasonography is also recommended in women with congenital heart disease. Special attention to the woman's hemodynamic response to pregnancy is required. The time and route of delivery should be planned before spontaneous labor to facilitate the delivery and to intervene as appropriate. With few exceptions, vaginal delivery with a facilitated second stage (forceps delivery or vacuum extraction) is preferred for women with heart disease. Cesarean section is indicated for obstetrical reasons and when delivery is required in a patient who is fully anticoagulated with warfarin (Table 1). In addition, cesarean section should be considered for patients with fixed cardiac obstructive lesions and pulmonary hypertension. The optimal anesthesia and analgesia as well as administration of prophylactic treatment for endocarditis should be considered before pregnancy. Invasive hemodynamic monitoring is recommended for severe maternal heart disease. Maternal postpartum care should include early ambulation, attention to neonatal concerns, and consideration of contraception if appropriate.

- Anatomical and hemodynamic assessment of cardiac status antepartum is imperative to determine the maternal and fetal risk of pregnancy.
- Vaginal delivery is the preferred mode of delivery in most women with heart disease.

Prognosis of Heart Disease in Pregnancy

Maternal prognosis during pregnancy is strongly related to New York Heart Association (NYHA) functional class; maternal mortality for women in NYHA class I or II is less than 1%. However, with NYHA class III or IV symptoms, maternal mortality increases to about 7%. Fetal mortality is also strongly related to maternal functional class; the expected fetal mortality rate is 30% for women in NYHA class IV.

Table 1.—Indications for Cesarean Section in Women With Cardiovascular Disease

Obstetrical reasons
Anticoagulation with warfarin
Fixed obstructive cardiac lesions
Pulmonary hypertension

Table 2.—High-Risk Pregnancy

Prosthetic valves
Obstructive lesions, including uncorrected coarctation of the aorta
Marfan syndrome
Hypertrophic obstructive cardiomyopathy
Cyanotic congenital heart disease
Pulmonary hypertension
Systemic ventricular dysfunction (ejection fraction $\leq 35\%$)
Significant uncorrected congenital heart disease

The management of pregnant women in NYHA class I or II should include limiting strenuous exercise, having adequate sleep and rest, maintaining a low-salt diet, avoiding anemia (keep hemoglobin > 11 g), having frequent prenatal examinations (both obstetrical and cardiovascular), and monitoring for arrhythmias. In severely symptomatic women (NYHA class III or IV), pregnancy should be avoided in the first instance; the option of continuing or interrupting the pregnancy should be discussed with the patient. If the patient opts to continue her pregnancy, bed rest is often required during part of the pregnancy, and close cardiac and obstetrical monitoring is mandatory.

Because of the hemodynamic changes that occur during pregnancy, fixed obstructive cardiac lesions or those associated with pulmonary hypertension generally are poorly tolerated (because of inability to increase cardiac output). In contrast, regurgitant lesions are relatively well tolerated (because of the decrease in systemic vascular resistance).

High-risk pregnancy includes women with 1) prosthetic valves; 2) obstructive lesions, including uncorrected coarctation of the aorta; 3) Marfan syndrome; 4) hypertrophic obstructive cardiomyopathy; 5) cyanotic congenital heart disease; 6) pulmonary hypertension; 7) systemic ventricular dysfunction (ejection fraction $\leq 35\%$), or 8) significant uncorrected congenital heart disease (Table 2).

Congenital Heart Disease in Pregnancy

More than ever before, women with congenital heart disease are reaching childbearing age and are considering pregnancy. This is a result primarily of early diagnosis and management of congenital heart disease. In patients with repaired complex congenital heart disease, uncertainty still remains about the ability to conceive, the effects of pregnancy on maternal heart disease, and the effects of heart disease on the fetus. Patients should be counseled about pregnancy and the genetic risk of congenital heart disease in the fetus. Endocarditis prophylaxis is recommended for high-risk patients (for specific recommendations, see chapter "Infections of the Heart").

Cyanosis inhibits fetal growth and development (Fig. 4). Pregnancy in women with severe cyanosis generally is contraindicated. Surgical repair of the underlying cardiac anomaly should be considered before pregnancy if possible (e.g., Ebstein anomaly with right-to-left shunt related to an atrial septal defect).

- Pregnant cyanotic women have a high risk of fetal loss. Also, cyanosis is a recognized handicap to fetal growth, resulting in low birth weight infants.

The incidence of congenital heart disease in the general population is about 1%. Generally, the offspring of women with congenital heart disease have a 5% to 6% incidence of congenital heart disease. Usually, the lesion in the offspring is not the same kind as in the mother, except for syndromes in which the incidence of recurrence with each pregnancy may be up to 50% (e.g., Marfan syndrome, hypertrophic cardiomyopathy).

Fetal echocardiography is used routinely in women with congenital heart disease to detect the presence of congenital heart disease in the fetus.

- Congenital heart disease is the most common form of structural heart disease that affects women of childbearing age in the U.S.
- Congenital heart disease has important implications for both the mother and the fetus.
- The incidence of congenital heart disease in the offspring of women with congenital heart disease is about 5%.

Peripartum Cardiomyopathy

Peripartum cardiomyopathy is defined as congestive heart failure that occurs late in pregnancy or during the early postpartum period (the last trimester or up to 6 months

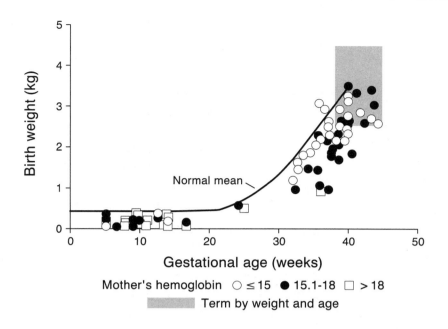

Fig. 4. Severity of maternal cyanosis, as indicated by the hemoglobin level, is related directly to fetal loss (gestational age < 20), prematurity, and infant birth weight. (From Alexander RW, Schlant RC, Fuster V [editors]: *Hurst's the Heart, Arteries and Veins*. Ninth edition. Vol. 2. McGraw-Hill, 1998, p 2401. By permission of the publisher.)

post partum) in the absence of congenital, coronary, or valvular heart disease or another recognized cause of heart failure. Most commonly, it is diagnosed during the first month post partum. The incidence in the U.S. ranges from 1:1,300 to 1:15,000 pregnancies. The incidence is higher in certain parts of Africa because of excess salt intake. Peripartum cardiomyopathy occurs more frequently in twin pregnancies, multiparous women, women older than 30 years, and black women. The cause is unknown, and the prognosis is variable, with 50% of women expected to show improvement in left ventricular function within 6 months after delivery. The management is supportive and includes standard treatment for congestive heart failure. Recurrence with subsequent pregnancies is common, and the risk of recurrence is greater in women with persistent left ventricular dysfunction. Thus, women who have a history of a serious episode of peripartum cardiomyopathy and those with persistent left ventricular dysfunction should be counseled to avoid pregnancy.

- Of women with peripartum cardiomyopathy, 50% have improvement in left ventricular function within 6 months after delivery.
- Because recurrence of peripartum cardiomyopathy is common, repeat pregnancy is contraindicated if a significant episode has occurred or left ventricular dysfunction persists.

Cardiac Contraindications to Pregnancy

There are certain cardiac conditions in which pregnancy should be avoided, and if pregnancy occurs, termination should be considered (Table 3). These include severe pulmonary hypertension (pulmonary artery pressure ≥ 3/4 systemic pressure) and Eisenmenger syndrome. Cardiomyopathy with class III or IV congestive heart failure or left ventricular dysfunction with significant symptoms is another situation in which pregnancy is contraindicated. Any form of severe obstructive cardiac lesion such as aortic stenosis, mitral stenosis, pulmonary stenosis, coarctation, or hypertrophic obstructive cardiomyopathy may result in significant limitations during pregnancy. Intervention before pregnancy is the preferred management option. Marfan syndrome with an aortic root of 40 mm or more is a contraindication to pregnancy, because of the unpredictable risk of aortic dissection and rupture. Severe cyanosis is a relative contraindication to pregnancy, primarily because of adverse fetal outcome. A history of peripartum cardiomyopathy with persistent left ventricular dysfunction or a significant episode of congestive heart failure (or both) is a contraindication for subsequent pregnancy. The risk of recurrence is approximately 50%, and the subsequent episode may be more severe.

Table 3.—Cardiac Contraindications to Pregnancy

Severe pulmonary hypertension

Eisenmenger syndrome

Cardiomyopathy, with class III or IV congestive heart failure

Severe obstructive cardiac lesions

Marfan syndrome, with aortic root ≥ 40 mm

Severe cyanosis

A history of peripartum cardiomyopathy with persistent left ventricular dysfunction and/or a significant episode of congestive heart failure

Cardiovascular Drugs in Pregnancy

The U.S. Food and Drug Administration categorizes drugs according to their potential to cause birth defects. The categories depend on the reliability of documentation of fetal risk and the potential risk-to-benefit ratio. The classifications are as follows:

Class A—No documented fetal risks.

Class B—Animal studies suggest risk, but unconfirmed in controlled human studies (e.g., methyldopa, thiazides, and dipyridamole).

Class C—Animal studies have demonstrated adverse fetal effects, but no controlled human studies (e.g., propranolol, digoxin, hydralazine, heparin, furosemide [Lasix], quinidine, procainamide, and verapamil). These drugs should be given only if the potential benefits justify the risk.

Class D—Evidence of human fetal risk. These drugs should be given only in a life-threatening situation or for a serious disease for which safer drugs either cannot be used or are ineffective. Informed consent is advised when administering these agents during pregnancy (e.g., phenytoin and captopril).

Class X—Documented fetal abnormalities; the drug is contraindicated during part or all of pregnancy (e.g., warfarin).

Pharmacologic Management of Arrhythmias During Pregnancy

Most cardiovascular drugs cross the placenta and are secreted in breast milk. The risk-to-benefit ratio must be considered when administering any medications during pregnancy. Cardiac arrhythmias during pregnancy should be evaluated the same as in a nonpregnant patient and the underlying disease or precipitating factors treated if possible.

Direct Current Cardioversion

Direct current cardioversion may be used safely during pregnancy. This is the treatment of choice for arrhythmias causing hemodynamic compromise during pregnancy. For less urgent situations, pharmacologic management of supraventricular arrhythmias may be required.

Digoxin and Quinidine

Digoxin is thought to be safe for treating arrhythmias except for an increased risk of prematurity and intrauterine growth retardation. Quinidine is a good alternate antiarrhythmic medication. Adverse fetal effects have not been reported when quinidine is given at a therapeutic dose, but toxic doses may induce premature labor. Limited information is available on the use of procainamide and disopyramide during pregnancy, but to date, no adverse fetal effects have been reported.

Amiodarone and Verapamil

The use of amiodarone during pregnancy has been reported in several cases and may result in fetal hypothyroidism. Verapamil has been used in pregnancy for the management of supraventricular arrhythmias, and no adverse effects have been reported. However, it has been recommended that verapamil therapy be discontinued at the onset of labor to prevent dysfunctional labor or postpartum hemorrhage.

β-Blockers

The use of β-blockers during pregnancy has been reported to cause intrauterine growth retardation, apnea at birth, fetal bradycardia, hypoglycemia, and hyperbilirubinemia. Large studies have not confirmed these concerns, and β-blocking agents have been used in a large number of pregnant women without adverse effects. β-Blockers now are thought to be relatively safe and may be used in the treatment of arrhythmias, hypertrophic cardiomyopathy, and hyperthyroidism during pregnancy if clinically indicated. All available β-blockers cross the placenta and are present in human breast milk. These agents can reach significant levels in the fetus or newborn. Therefore, if used during pregnancy, it is appropriate to monitor fetal and newborn heart rate as well as blood glucose and respiratory status after delivery.

Adenosine

Adenosine has been used successfully to treat supraventricular tachycardia during pregnancy. To date, no adverse fetal or maternal effects related to adenosine have been reported.

- Adenosine has been used safely to treat acute supraventricular tachycardia in pregnancy.
- β-Blockers and calcium channel blockers can be used for supraventricular tachycardia prophylaxis in pregnancy, but discontinuation of these agents is advised near the time of delivery.

Pharmacologic Management of Congestive Heart Failure During Pregnancy

The treatment of congestive heart failure is more difficult in pregnant than in nonpregnant women. Conservative measures such as salt restriction and limitation of activity are extremely important. Pharmacologic therapy may be required.

Digoxin and Diuretics

Digoxin can be given safely; however, diuretics impair uterine blood flow and placental perfusion. Initiating diuretic medications during pregnancy is not recommended (unless absolutely necessary). However, the continuation of diuretic therapy initiated before conception does not seem unfavorable. No teratogenetic effects of diuretics have been described; however, cases of neonatal thrombocytopenia, jaundice, hyponatremia, and bradycardia have been reported with the use of thiazides. Therefore, the use of diuretics should be limited to the treatment of severe symptomatic congestive heart failure and selected cases of hypertension.

ACE Inhibitors

The use of angiotensin converting enzyme (ACE) inhibitors is contraindicated during pregnancy. Maternal-fetal transfer of captopril has been documented, and, in animals, exposure to ACE inhibitors during pregnancy has produced prolonged fetal hypotension and death. Also, there is increased risk of early delivery, low birth weight, oligohydramnios, or neonatal anuria and renal failure (or some combination of these). In general, ACE inhibitors should not be used during pregnancy. Currently, insufficient data are available on the use of new angiotensin II blockers during pregnancy.

Nitrates

The use of organic nitrates during pregnancy has been reported in the treatment of hypertension; however, in one case, the decrease in blood pressure with nitroglycerin was associated with fetal heart rate decelerations. Therefore, treatment with nitrates requires further evaluation for the management of pregnancy-related hypertension and congestive heart failure.

- The administration of ACE inhibitors is contraindicated during pregnancy.

Anticoagulants

Hematologic changes that occur during normal pregnancy include an increase in clotting factor concentrations, an increase in platelet adhesiveness, and a decrease in fibrinolysis. These changes result in an overall increased risk of thrombosis or embolism.

Prosthetic Heart Valves

The best type of heart valve prosthesis to use in women of childbearing age who have critical valvular heart disease is debated. Recent data have suggested that premature valve deterioration occurs in bioprosthetic valves during pregnancy, but this has not been documented conclusively or demonstrated experimentally. One report has suggested that reoperation (required for most patients with bioprosthetic valves) carries a higher risk of morbidity and mortality than the risk of anticoagulation during pregnancy.

Pregnant women with a mechanical heart valve have approximately a 10% risk for the development of prosthetic valve thrombosis or other life-threatening complication. There is considerable debate about the best management for a pregnant woman who requires anticoagulation.

Anticoagulation During Pregnancy

Anticoagulation during pregnancy has been referred to as a "double jeopardy," that is, posing significant risk to mother and fetus. Anticoagulation management options during pregnancy include the following:

1. Heparin and warfarin (Coumadin) combination—During the first trimester, stop warfarin treatment as early as possible, preferably before conception, and treat with subcutaneously administered heparin adjusted to the partial thromboplastin time (PTT). The PTT should be 2 to 3 times control (higher than usual). Warfarin treatment should be resumed around 14 to 15 weeks of gestation. Continuation of subcutaneous heparin during pregnancy does not impart adequate anticoagulation in high-risk patients (i.e., women with mechanical valve prostheses) and, thus, is no longer recommended therapy during the second and early third trimester.

2. Warfarin only—Therapeutic warfarin with an international normalized ratio (INR) of 2.5 to 3.5 may be continued throughout pregnancy until the peripartum period. Informed consent must be obtained, and adverse effects, including the risk of warfarin embryopathy and the increased

risk of miscarriage, must be discussed with the patient.

With these anticoagulation options, the pregnant patient should be admitted to the hospital 2 to 4 weeks before term and given PTT-adjusted heparin intravenously. This treatment should be discontinued with the induction of labor and resumed 4 hours after delivery. The peripartum period is a particularly high-risk time for thromboembolic complications.

3. Heparin only—Continuous treatment with PTT-adjusted intravenous heparin throughout pregnancy is rarely advised.

Prolonged heparin therapy (intravenous or subcutaneous) can result in thrombocytopenia, osteoporosis, and alopecia. Erratic absorption of subcutaneously delivered heparin may occur, and frequent monitoring of the PTT to ensure therapeutic anticoagulation is mandatory.

Recent reports have suggested that subcutaneous heparin may not provide sufficient anticoagulation coverage for very high-risk patients (e.g., those with caged-ball or tilting-disk mechanical mitral prosthesis) and that treatment with warfarin be continued during the first trimester of pregnancy (Fig. 5).

Warfarin Embryopathy

Historic reports describe a 30% risk of embryopathy (bone and cartilage abnormalities with chondrodysplasia, nasal hypoplasia, and optic atrophy) with the administration of warfarin during the first trimester. In addition, warfarin therapy during the first trimester carries an increased risk of miscarriage or stillbirth (> 37%); thus, this method of anticoagulation should be used only after the patient has given informed consent. It may be reasonable to administer warfarin to a high-risk patient throughout pregnancy, particularly when the dose is less than 5 mg daily.

The risk associated with warfarin treatment during the second trimester is primarily fetal hemorrhage. During the third trimester, warfarin is hazardous to mother and fetus should preterm labor occur. Warfarin results in fetal anticoagulation because of placental transfer. Cesarean section is recommended in this setting because of the risk of neonatal cerebral hemorrhage and the risk of uncontrolled maternal hemorrhage at the time of placental delivery. Warfarin does not enter breast milk and, thus, can be administered safely to women who breast-feed their infants.

Other Anticlotting Agents in Pregnancy

A low dose of aspirin (81 mg) is safe to use during pregnancy. It is recommended for patients with shunts (e.g.,

atrial septal defect), cyanosis, or a biologic valve prosthesis. However, the antiplatelet effect has not been proved. A low dose of aspirin may also decrease the incidence of preeclampsia. Currently, there is great interest but insufficient data about the appropriate use of low-molecular-weight heparin during pregnancy. Dipyridamole should not be used during pregnancy. Thrombolytic therapy has been safely used during pregnancy but should be avoided when possible.

- Considerable controversy exists about the best method of anticoagulation during pregnancy.
- Use of warfarin during the first trimester is associated with an increased risk of miscarriage and warfarin embryopathy, but it may be the preferred method of anticoagulation for patients with older mechanical mitral prostheses, particularly if the dose is low.

Endocarditis Prophylaxis

The American Heart Association does not recommend endocarditis prophylaxis for patients expected to have an uncomplicated cesarean section or vaginal delivery. However, standard prophylactic treatment with antibiotics given intravenously or intramuscularly is recommended for the placement of a urinary catheter in the presence of urinary tract infection and for vaginal delivery in the presence of vaginal infection.

Our recommendations are more conservative. We recommend the intravenous administration of antibiotics for endocarditis prophylaxis using the gastrointestinal or genitourinary regimen in high-risk cardiac patients because of the risk of undiagnosed infections and the significant patient morbidity and mortality should infective endocarditis occur. Antibiotic therapy should be administered 30 to 60 minutes before delivery is expected and repeated 8 hours later.

Contraception in Patients With Heart Disease

More than 50% of teenagers are sexually active and 10% of the women in the U.S. who are 15 to 19 years old have unplanned pregnancies.

The higher dose estrogen-containing oral contraceptive pill, or "combination pill," has an increased risk of thromboembolic events, pulmonary embolism, and fluid retention; therefore, it should be prescribed with caution

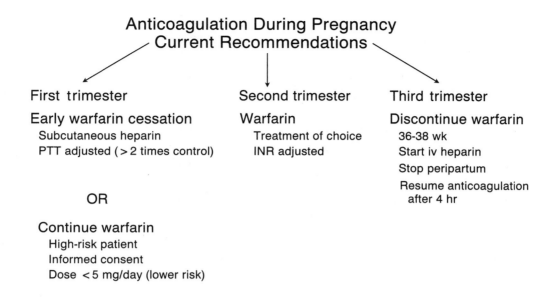

Fig. 5. Anticoagulation options during the 3 trimesters of pregnancy. Treatment must be individualized for each patient. INR, International Normalized Ratio; PTT, partial thromboplastin time.

for women with significant heart disease. Alternative methods include the progesterone-only pill, or "mini pill," which is an option for patients with pulmonary hypertension, right-to-left shunts, or a prosthetic valve. The failure rate of the progesterone-only pill is higher than that of the combination pill and is similar to the failure rate of barrier methods. Also, the progesterone-only pill must be taken at the same time each day. Breakthrough bleeding is common and, when this occurs, contraceptive coverage is not reliable. Barrier methods also have a high failure rate (18% per year) and should be used with caution in patients in whom pregnancy is absolutely contraindicated. An intrauterine device is not suggested for women with heart disease, because of the potential risk of infection. Tubal ligation should be reserved for women in whom pregnancy is absolutely contraindicated and transplantation is not possible. Successful pregnancy has been reported in women after heart-lung transplantation.

Suggested Review Reading

1. Dajani AS, Taubert KA, Wilson W, et al: Prevention of bacterial endocarditis. Recommendations by the American Heart Association. *JAMA* 277:1794-1801, 1997.
The American Heart Association updated guidelines for endocarditis prophylaxis, including recommendations for pregnancy and delivery, are reviewed.

2. Elkayam U, Goodwin TM: Adenosine therapy for supraventricular tachycardia during pregnancy. *Am J Cardiol* 75:521-523, 1995.
Adenosine treatment for supraventricular arrhythmias is reviewed.

3. Pitkin RM, Perloff JK, Koos BJ, et al: Pregnancy and congenital heart disease. *Ann Intern Med* 112:445-454, 1990.
The impact of congenital heart disease on pregnancy is reviewed, as are some of the common congenital lesions encountered during pregnancy.

4. van Hoeven KH, Kitsis RN, Katz SD, et al: Peripartum versus idiopathic dilated cardiomyopathy in young women—a comparison of clinical, pathologic and prognostic features. *Int J Cardiol* 40:57-65, 1993.
Features of peripartum cardiomyopathy are reviewed, including pathogenesis and natural history.

5. Elkayam U, Gleicher N: Cardiac problems in pregnancy. I. Maternal aspects: the approach to the pregnant patient with heart disease. *JAMA* 251:2838-2839, 1984.

6. McAnulty JH, Morton MJ, Ueland K: The heart and pregnancy. *Curr Probl Cardiol* 13:589-665, 1988.
A summary of the normal physiologic changes that occur during pregnancy. Complications, contraindications, and management of cardiovascular problems during pregnancy are also reviewed.

7. Avila WS, Grinberg M, Snitcowsky R, et al: Maternal and fetal outcome in pregnant women with Eisenmenger's syndrome. *Eur Heart J* 16:460-464, 1995.

8. Canobbio MM, Mair DD, van der Velde M, et al: Pregnancy outcomes after the Fontan repair. *J Am Coll Cardiol* 28:763-767, 1996.

9. Clarkson PM, Wilson NJ, Neutze JM, et al: Outcome of pregnancy after the Mustard operation for transposition of the great arteries with intact ventricular septum. *J Am Coll Cardiol* 24:190-193, 1994.

10. Connolly HM, Warnes CA: Ebstein's anomaly: outcome of pregnancy. *J Am Coll Cardiol* 23:1194-1198, 1994.

11. Connolly HM, Warnes CA: Outcome of pregnancy in patients with complex pulmonic valve atresia. *Am J Cardiol* 79:519-521, 1997.

12. Elkayam U, Ostrzega E, Shotan A, et al: Cardiovascular problems in pregnant women with the Marfan syndrome. *Ann Intern Med* 123:117-122, 1995.

13. Presbitero P, Somerville J, Stone S, et al: Pregnancy in cyanotic congenital heart disease. Outcome of mother and fetus. *Circulation* 89:2673-2676, 1994.
The outcome of pregnancy in specific congenital cardiac lesions is reviewed in references 7-13.

14. Arias F, Pineda J: Aortic stenosis and pregnancy. *J Reprod Med* 20:229-232, 1978.

15. Easterling TR, Chadwick HS, Otto CM, et al: Aortic stenosis in pregnancy. *Obstet Gynecol* 72:113-118, 1988.
The outcome of pregnancy with aortic stenosis is reviewed.

16. Elkayam UR: Anticoagulation in pregnant women with prosthetic heart valves: a double jeopardy. *J Am Coll Cardiol* 27:1704-1706, 1996.

17. Melissari E, Parker CJ, Wilson NV, et al: Use of low molecular weight heparin in pregnancy. *Thromb Haemost* 68:652-656, 1992.

18. Salazar E, Izaguirre R, Verdejo J, et al: Failure of adjusted doses of subcutaneous heparin to prevent thromboembolic phenomena in pregnant patients with mechanical cardiac valve prostheses. *J Am Coll Cardiol* 27:1698-1703, 1996.

19. Sbarouni E, Oakley CM: Outcome of pregnancy in women with valve prostheses. *Br Heart J* 71:196-201, 1994.
Controversies about anticoagulation therapy during pregnancy are reviewed.

Questions

Multiple Choice (choose the one best answer)

1. Hemodynamic changes that occur during a normal pregnancy include all the following *except*:
   a. A decrease in systemic vascular resistance
   b. An increase in pulmonary vascular resistance
   c. A minor change in blood pressure
   d. An increase in stroke volume
   e. An increase in heart rate

2. A physical examination in a normal pregnant woman would demonstrate all the following *except*:
   a. An ejection systolic murmur in approximately 90% of the women
   b. A third heart sound in more than 70% of the women
   c. A fourth heart sound in fewer than 10% of the women
   d. A widely split second heart sound
   e. A diastolic murmur in 20% of the women

3. A 36-year-old woman with a mechanical (Björk-Shiley) mitral valve prosthesis is in her 34th week of pregnancy. She takes warfarin and has an INR of 2.5. She presents in labor. Appropriate management of this patient would include all the following *except*:
   a. Discontinue warfarin and start heparin treatment when the INR is less than 2
   b. Try to halt preterm labor with tocolysis
   c. Proceed with vaginal delivery if labor cannot be terminated
   d. Restart heparin and warfarin anticoagulation shortly after delivery, because during the peripartum period the patient is at particularly high risk for a thromboembolic event
   e. Baby aspirin may be administered at this time

4. A 25-year-old woman with a mechanical mitral prosthesis (St. Jude) complains of progressive dyspnea during pregnancy. She is in her 28th week of pregnancy, takes warfarin, and has an INR of 1.9. Physical examination findings include a heart rate of 100 beats/min and elevated jugular venous pressure at 20 cm H_2O. The apical impulse is displaced, and a soft systolic murmur is noted at the apex. Also, there is a diastolic murmur. Mitral prosthetic mechanical sounds are audible but somewhat reduced. There are crackles in both lung bases and on the third heart sound. On transthoracic echocardiography, the mitral prosthesis

is difficult to visualize. However, the mean gradient across the prosthesis is increased at 18 mm Hg. The ejection fraction is normal at 55%. Echocardiography performed before pregnancy demonstrated a mean gradient across the mitral prosthesis of 5 mm Hg, at a heart rate of 70 beats/min. Appropriate treatment options at this time would include all the following *except*:
   a. Emergent cardiovascular surgery
   b. Emergent high-risk obstetric evaluation
   c. Thrombolytic therapy
   d. Administration of both furosemide and heparin
   e. Proceed with cardiac catheterization to measure the mitral valve gradient and coronary angiography

5. A 28-year-old woman 14 weeks pregnant has a murmur and recent dyspnea. Her medical history is positive for a heart murmur, but she has never been evaluated for this. Physical examination findings include a bounding and bifid carotid impulse, a 3-component apical impulse, and a grade 3/6 ejection systolic murmur at the left sternal border that increases after a premature ventricular contraction. Also, a late systolic murmur is noted at the apex. The lungs are clear. Trace peripheral edema is noted. Electrocardiography demonstrates significant left ventricular hypertrophy with a strain pattern. Which of the following statements is correct about the patient's hemodynamic status?
   a. An increase in blood volume will be beneficial to the patient
   b. The decrease in systemic vascular resistance that occurs during pregnancy is beneficial to this patient
   c. The increase in contractility that occurs during pregnancy is beneficial to the patient
   d. The period of highest risk for the patient and fetus is during the first trimester
   e. Cesarean section will result in fewer hemodynamic changes at the time of delivery

6. Appropriate treatment options for the patient described in question 5 would include all the following at this point *except*:
   a. Digoxin
   b. β-Blocker
   c. Regular cardiovascular follow-up during pregnancy
   d. Calcium channel blocker
   e. Surgery if symptoms are not controlled with medical therapy after delivery

7. An 18-year-old woman without known previous cardiovascular disease presents in her third trimester of pregnancy with mild dyspnea. She recently moved to the U.S. from India. She is not taking any medication. Physical examination findings include a heart rate of 100 beats/min and a jugular venous pressure of 15 cm H_2O, with both "a" and "v" waves visible. The apical impulse is in the 5th intercostal space midclavicular line and has a tapping quality. There is a right ventricular lift. An opening snap is noted 90 m/s from the second heart sound and a grade 2/6 diastolic murmur is noted along the left sternal border with presystolic accentuation. There are crackles in both lung bases. All the following statements about this patient's condition are true *except*:
   a. An increase in blood volume during pregnancy may have precipitated the patient's symptoms
   b. The patient's baby is not at increased risk for heart disease
   c. Symptoms may improve with β-blocker therapy
   d. Digoxin can be safely administered
   e. Anticoagulation with warfarin should be started

8. Patients with cyanotic congenital heart disease who are pregnant have increased risk for all the following *except*:
   a. Low-birth-weight infants
   b. Fetal loss
   c. Paradoxical embolus
   d. A 15% chance of congenital heart disease in the baby
   e. Prematurity

9. A 37-year-old woman has dyspnea. She is 3 weeks post partum and had an uncomplicated delivery of her first child. Physical examination findings include a heart rate of 100 beats/min and a jugular venous pressure of 15 cm H_2O, with both "a" and "v" waves. Bilateral crackles are noted at the lung bases. The apical impulse is diffuse and displaced. Also noted are a grade 2/6 systolic murmur at the apex and a third heart sound. On echocardiography, the left ventricle is moderately enlarged and systolic function is reduced, with an estimated ejection fraction of 23%. Mild mitral regurgitation is noted. All the following statements about this patient's condition are true *except*:
   a. Management should be conservative and medical therapy should be instituted immediately
   b. Recurrent problems occur in approximately 50% of subsequent pregnancies

   c. Predisposing factors include the patient's age and that this was her first pregnancy
   d. Future pregnancies are contraindicated if there is persistent cardiovascular abnormality after several months, even in the absence of symptoms
   e. There is a 50% chance of complete resolution of symptoms and left ventricular dysfunction with therapy

10. Contraindications to pregnancy include all the following *except*:
   a. A 27-year-old woman has a previous history of congenital cardiac surgery. She had an atrial septal defect closed at age 19 and feels well. Echocardiography demonstrates enlargement of the cardiac chambers on the right side and a tricuspid regurgitant velocity of 3.9 m/s
   b. A woman with a bicuspid aortic valve with a mean gradient across the valve of 45 mm Hg and no significant aortic regurgitation
   c. A woman with a history of systemic hypertension. Examination demonstrates an ejection click at the left sternal border and a brief systolic murmur. Also, a radiofemoral delay is noted on physical examination
   d. Congenitally corrected transposition of the great vessels in a woman with moderate systemic atrioventricular valve regurgitation and a right ventricular ejection fraction of 45%-50%
   e. A patient with mitral valve prolapse and severe mitral regurgitation. Left ventricular cavity size is moderately enlarged, with borderline systolic function (ejection fraction is 40%). Also, the left atrium is enlarged, and the patient has a history of paroxysmal arrhythmias and dyspnea on exertion

11. A 27-year-old woman has dyspnea, palpitations, fatigue, and a history of heart murmur. There is no evidence of cyanosis on physical examination. There is a marked right ventricular lift and a systolic thrill. Also, the jugular venous pressure is elevated, with a prominent "a" wave. Auscultation demonstrates a grade 5/6 systolic ejection murmur at the second left intercostal space and absence of the pulmonary component of the second heart sound. Results of a pregnancy test are positive. The patient was not aware she was pregnant. Electrocardiography demonstrates right ventricular hypertrophy with strain. The best management option

for this patient at this point includes:

a. Pregnancy is contraindicated and termination is the only reasonable option
b. Conservative observation of the patient during pregnancy
c. Surgical pulmonary valvotomy
d. Institute β-blocker therapy
e. Pulmonary balloon valvuloplasty

12. A 26-year-old woman who is 23 weeks pregnant comes to the emergency room because of palpitations. Appropriate therapy includes all the following *except*:
    a. If hemodynamic compromise exists, direct current cardioversion is the treatment of choice
    b. The monitor demonstrates narrow complex tachycardia, the patient is symptomatic, but the blood pressure is reasonably controlled. The treatment of choice is adenosine
    c. β-Blocker therapy may be safely used during pregnancy for prophylaxis of supraventricular arrhythmias
    d. If the tachycardia demonstrated is wide complex, quinidine may be used for prophylaxis
    e. Treat with calcium channel blockers, because they will not interfere with the patient's pregnancy or delivery

Answers

1. Answer b

Hemodynamic changes that occur during pregnancy include an increase in blood volume and a decrease in systemic and pulmonary vascular resistance. There is a slight decrease in blood pressure during early pregnancy. As a result of these hemodynamic changes, cardiac output typically increases by approximately 40% by the end of pregnancy.

2. Answer e

The common findings of a physical examination in a normal pregnant woman include an elevated jugular venous pressure, with both "a" and "v" waves and bounding carotid pulsation (related to the increase in cardiac output and blood volume); wide splitting of the second heart sound is also common. Other common findings include an ejection systolic murmur audible in about 90% of pregnant women; a third heart sound is also commonly noted. A fourth heart sound or diastolic murmur in a pregnant woman usually indicates an abnormality.

3. Answer c

In a woman who is fully anticoagulated with warfarin, cesarean section is indicated because of the risk of fetal intracranial hemorrhage related to trauma at the time of vaginal delivery. Also, bleeding is difficult to control in women who have vaginal deliveries while receiving warfarin, and the risk of significant hemorrhage is high.

4. Answer e

This is an emergency situation and emergent evaluation by a cardiac surgeon and high-risk obstetrician is required. If the patient is not at a facility where cardiac surgery is an option, thrombolytic therapy should be considered. If transesophageal echocardiography can be performed safely, it may be a reasonable option if the diagnosis of prosthetic valve thrombosis is still in doubt. However, the physical findings and echocardiographic results are consistent with thrombosis of the mechanical prosthesis, and urgent intervention is required to save both the mother and the fetus. It would be appropriate to heparinize and to give furosemide to improve symptoms. Also, thrombolytic therapy, although relatively high risk, has been used safely during pregnancy without adverse effect on the mother or fetus. It must be emphasized that this is a very critical situation and that urgent evaluation and intervention are required. Should surgery be required, it should be performed with obstetrical backup in case fetal compromise occurs during induction of anesthesia or during the operation. Cardiac catheterization likely would not change the management of this patient, based on the above scenario.

5. Answer a

The patient has hypertrophic cardiomyopathy. Reports of pregnancy in hypertrophic cardiomyopathy suggest an optimistic outcome. The hemodynamic alterations that occur during pregnancy usually are well tolerated; the beneficial effect of the increase in blood volume is usually outweighed by the detrimental effect of the decrease in systemic vascular resistance. An increase in contractility is potentially detrimental in this group of patients. The highest risk period for these patients is the peripartum period, and vaginal delivery is preferred when possible. Greater hemodynamic changes occur during a cesarean section delivery than during a normal vaginal delivery.

6. Answer a

The findings in this patient are consistent with hypertrophic obstructive cardiomyopathy. Overall, the hemodynamic changes that occur during pregnancy usually balance in favor of the patient with this disorder; that is, an increase in blood volume is outweighed by the decrease in systemic vascular resistance. Regular cardiovascular follow-up during pregnancy is suggested for women with hypertrophic cardiomyopathy. Data suggest that β-blocker therapy is safe during pregnancy, although therapy may result in lower birth-weight infants and fetal bradycardia. Calcium channel blockers can also be used during pregnancy but may result in dysfunctional uterine contraction at the time of delivery and should be discontinued before the onset of labor. Occasionally, patients with hypertrophic cardiomyopathy present during pregnancy with severe symptoms that cannot be controlled with medical therapy. These patients often have relatively fixed obstruction, and alternative treatment options such as permanent pacemaker implantation or surgical myectomy may be required. Digoxin therapy would not be helpful in this patient and may worsen symptoms.

7. Answer e

The patient has rheumatic mitral stenosis. As a result of the pregnancy-related increase in heart rate and blood volume, she has become symptomatic. Important features in this patient's evaluation include the heart rate of 100 beats/min. Medical therapy is the treatment of choice at this point and likely will improve her symptoms markedly. Although mitral balloon valvuloplasty can be performed, it is not indicated at this time unless the patient has persistent symptoms despite aggressive medical therapy. The treatment of choice would include institution of digoxin and β-blockers to decrease heart rate in order to prolong the diastolic filling period. Anticoagulation is not recommended because the patient is not in atrial fibrillation ("a" waves in the jugular venous pressure) and does not have other significant risk factors for thromboemboli. Also, warfarin increases the risk of intracranial bleeding in the baby and postpartum bleeding in the mother.

8. Answer d

Persons with congenital heart disease have an increased risk of having offspring with congenital heart disease. However, the risk is only about 5%-6%, compared with 1%-2% in the general population. However, certain syndromes, such as Marfan syndrome, hypertrophic cardiomyopathy, and other familial syndromes, are associated with increased risk of heart disease in the offspring. Cyanosis is a recognized retardant to fetal growth and development. Maternal cyanosis results in increased risk of fetal loss, prematurity, and low-birth-weight infants. Most cyanotic patients have a persistent intracardiac right-to-left shunt and, thus, are at high risk for paradoxical emboli.

9. Answer c

The patient has peripartum cardiomyopathy. Predisposing factors include advanced maternal age, twin pregnancy, race (more common in black population), previous history of peripartum cardiomyopathy, and the multiparous state. The management of peripartum cardiomyopathy is usually conservative, with medical therapy. Approximately 50% of the patients have complete resolution of left ventricular dysfunction with appropriate therapy. The chance of recurrence with a subsequent pregnancy is about 50%. If a serious episode of peripartum cardiomyopathy has occurred or if left ventricular dysfunction is persistent after delivery, subsequent pregnancy is contraindicated.

10. Answer d

During pregnancy, a woman with congenitally corrected transposition of the great vessels is at increased risk for development of congestive heart failure. In this case, the woman's right ventricular (systemic ventricular) function, however, is reasonable and she has only moderate atrio-ventricular valve regurgitation. The other patients ("a," "b," "c," and "e") all have significant contraindications to pregnancy. The patient in "a" has significant pulmonary hypertension, which is a contraindication to pregnancy. Further evaluation is required to determine the cause of the pulmonary hypertension. The patient in "b" has significant aortic stenosis, and pregnancy is contraindicated in this setting. The patient in "c" has a medical history and examination findings suggestive of coarctation of the aorta associated with a bicuspid aortic valve. This patient requires further evaluation before pregnancy, and intervention will likely be required. The patient in "e" has severe mitral regurgitation, with evidence of left ventricular dysfunction and symptoms. Although regurgitant lesions are often well tolerated during pregnancy, associated ventricular dysfunction and/or symptoms suggest that the hemodynamic changes that occur during pregnancy are not likely to be well tolerated. Consideration of mitral valve repair before anticipated pregnancy would be suggested.

11. Answer e

This patient is early in her pregnancy and already has symptoms related to her critical pulmonary valve stenosis. To continue the pregnancy, intervention will be required, and pulmonary balloon valvuloplasty is a reasonable option, with appropriate shielding of the abdomen. In the setting of significant dynamic outflow tract obstruction, β-blocker therapy may be required before proceeding with balloon valvuloplasty; however, this needs to be evaluated in each patient.

12. Answer e

Calcium channel blockers can be used during pregnancy; however, there are reports of inadequate labor, and it usually is suggested that calcium channel blocker treatment be stopped before the onset of labor. Adenosine has been used safely during pregnancy for the treatment of supraventricular tachycardia. If there is hemodynamic instability, the treatment of choice is direct current cardioversion. Quinidine and β-blockers may be used in the prophylactic treatment of ventricular and supraventricular arrhythmias during pregnancy.

Notes

Chapter 34

Electrocardiographic Diagnoses

Criteria and Definitions of Abnormalities

Stephen C. Hammill, M.D.
James H. O'Keefe, Jr., M.D.

This chapter is a diagnostic guide for all physicians who evaluate electrocardiograms (ECGs). We hope the criteria are of specific value to persons taking professional examinations in cardiology and internal medicine. The criteria are those used in clinical practice at our institution, and thus they may differ in minor ways from those of the examination bodies. Be sure to check the specific diagnoses available to you on the answer sheet. These criteria are not endorsed by any professional examination body or organization.

Examination Strategy

When reviewing ECGs, be sure to evaluate the tracing systematically for abnormalities of rate, rhythm, and axis and to examine the configuration, duration, and relationship of the P, QRS, and T waves. Most examination ECGs have one to three major findings. The Cardiology Boards emphasize the correct identification of the major diagnoses on the tracing; points are subtracted for important oversights and misdiagnoses. The ancillary minor diagnoses are given minimal or neutral credit.

Systematic Evaluation of an ECG Tracing

1. Standardization and leads shown

   Review for reversed leads, right chest leads, and 1/2 voltage standardization in left ventricular hypertrophy

2. Heart rate: determine separately for QRS and P waves if the rhythm is other than sinus

3. Heart rhythm

4. Cardiac axis

5. Configuration and duration of P, QRS, and T waves

6. Relationship of P wave to QRS complex

7. Intervals:

   PR

   QRS

   QT

8. ECG diagnosis

9. Suggested clinical diagnosis

This chapter lists a score sheet similar to that used in the Cardiology Boards. Minor changes are made to the numbering of the examination answer codes from year to year. We have purposely used letters for our codes to avoid confusion between the numbering scheme of the examination bodies and our criteria. Initially we list all the ECG diagnoses, and in subsequent pages we define our criteria for each diagnosis on the score sheet.

Do not guess the ECG diagnoses on the examination, because wrong diagnoses receive negative credits.

If the ECG looks normal, be aware that it may not be normal. Always double-check for subtle ECG changes, including the delta wave of Wolff-Parkinson-White syndrome, QT interval prolongation, the prominent U waves of hypokalemia, the tall R wave in lead V_1 associated with a posterior wall infarct, and PR segment depression in acute pericarditis.

ECG Diagnoses

1. General Features

   a. Normal ECG
   b. Borderline normal ECG or normal variant
   c. Incorrect electrode placement
   d. Artifact due to tremor

2. Atrial Rhythms

   a. Sinus rhythm
   b. Sinus arrhythmia
   c. Sinus bradycardia (< 60 beats/min)
   d. Sinus tachycardia (> 100 beats/min)
   e. Sinus pause or arrest
   f. Sinoatrial exit block
   g. Ectopic atrial rhythm

   h. Wandering atrial pacemaker
   i. Atrial premature complexes, normally conducted
   j. Atrial premature complexes, nonconducted
   k. Atrial premature complexes with aberrant intraventricular conduction
   l. Atrial tachycardia (regular, sustained, 1:1 conduction)
   m. Atrial tachycardia, repetitive (short paroxysms)
   n. Atrial tachycardia, multifocal (chaotic atrial tachycardia)
   o. Atrial tachycardia with atrioventricular (AV) block
   p. Supraventricular tachycardia, unspecified
   q. Supraventricular tachycardia, paroxysmal
   r. Atrial flutter
   s. Atrial fibrillation
   t. Retrograde atrial activation

3. AV Junctional Rhythms

   a. AV junctional premature complexes
   b. AV junctional escape complexes
   c. AV junctional rhythm, accelerated
   d. AV junctional rhythm

4. Ventricular Rhythms

   a. Ventricular premature complex(es), uniform, fixed coupling
   b. Ventricular premature complex(es), uniform, nonfixed coupling
   c. Ventricular premature complex(es), multiform
   d. Ventricular premature complexes, in pairs (2 consecutive)
   e. Ventricular parasystole
   f. Ventricular tachycardia (≥ 3 consecutive beats)
   g. Accelerated idioventricular rhythm
   h. Ventricular escape complexes or rhythm
   i. Ventricular fibrillation

5. Atrioventricular Interactions in Arrhythmias

   a. Fusion complexes
   b. Reciprocal (echo) complexes
   c. Ventricular capture complexes
   d. AV dissociation
   e. Ventriculophasic sinus arrhythmia

6. AV Conduction Abnormalities

a. AV block, first degree

b. AV block, second degree-Mobitz type I (Wenckebach)

c. AV block, second degree-Mobitz type II

d. AV block, 2:1

e. AV block, third degree

f. AV block, variable

g. Short PR interval (with sinus rhythm and normal QRS duration)

h. Wolff-Parkinson-White pattern

7. Intraventricular Conduction Disturbances

a. Right bundle branch block (RBBB), incomplete

b. RBBB, complete

c. Left anterior fascicular block

d. Left posterior fascicular block

e. Left bundle branch block (LBBB), complete with ST-T waves suggestive of acute myocardial injury or infarction

f. LBBB, complete

g. LBBB, intermittent

h. Intraventricular conduction disturbance, nonspecific type

i. Aberrant intraventricular conduction with supraventricular arrhythmia (specify rhythm)

8. P-Wave Abnormalities

a. Right atrial abnormality

b. Left atrial abnormality

c. Nonspecific atrial abnormality

9. Abnormalities of QRS Voltage or Axis

a. Low voltage, limb leads only

b. Low voltage, limb and precordial leads

c. Left-axis deviation (> -30°)

d. Right-axis deviation (> +100°)

e. Electrical alternans

10. Ventricular Hypertrophy

a. Left ventricular hypertrophy by voltage only

b. Left ventricular hypertrophy by both voltage and ST-T segment abnormalities

c. Right ventricular hypertrophy

d. Combined ventricular hypertrophy

11. Transmural Myocardial Infarction

	Probably acute or recent	Probably old or age indeterminate
Anterolateral	**a.**	**g.**
Anterior	**b.**	**h.**
Anteroseptal	**c.**	**i.**
Lateral or high lateral	**d.**	**j.**
Inferior (diaphragmatic)	**e.**	**k.**
Posterior	**f.**	**l.**

m. Probable ventricular aneurysm

12. ST-, T-, and U-Wave Abnormalities

a. Normal variant, early repolarization

b. Normal variant, juvenile T waves

c. Nonspecific ST- or T-wave abnormalities

d. ST-segment or T-wave abnormalities suggesting myocardial ischemia

e. ST-segment or T-wave abnormalities suggesting myocardial injury

f. ST-segment or T-wave abnormalities suggesting acute pericarditis

g. ST-segment or T-wave abnormalities due to intraventricular conduction disturbance or hypertrophy

h. Post-extrasystolic T-wave abnormality

i. Isolated J-point depression

j. Peaked T waves

k. Prolonged QT interval

l. Prominent U waves

13. Pacemaker Function and Rhythm

a. Atrial or coronary sinus pacing

b. Ventricular demand pacing

c. AV sequential pacing

d. Ventricular pacing, fixed rate (asynchronous)

e. Dual-chamber, atrial-sensing pacemaker

f. Pacemaker malfunction, not constantly capturing

(atrium or ventricle)
g. Pacemaker malfunction, not constantly sensing (atrium or ventricle)
h. Pacemaker malfunction, not firing
i. Pacemaker malfunction, slowing

14. Suggested or Probable Clinical Disorders

a. Digitalis effect
b. Digitalis toxicity
c. Antiarrhythmic drug effect
d. Antiarrhythmic drug toxicity
e. Hyperkalemia
f. Hypokalemia
g. Hypercalcemia
h. Hypocalcemia
i. Atrial septal defect, secundum
j. Atrial septal defect, primum
k. Dextrocardia, mirror image
l. Mitral valve disease
m. Chronic lung disease
n. Acute cor pulmonale, including pulmonary embolus
o. Pericardial effusion
p. Acute pericarditis
q. Hypertrophic cardiomyopathy
r. Coronary artery disease
s. Central nervous system disorder
t. Myxedema
u. Hypothermia
v. Sick sinus syndrome
w. Ebstein's anomaly

Criteria for Score Sheet Diagnosis

1. General Features

a. Normal ECG

- No abnormalities of rhythm, rate, or axis
- The configurations of the P wave, QRS complex, and T wave are within normal limits (Fig. 1)

b. Borderline normal ECG or normal variant

- Early repolarization (see item **12a**)

- Juvenile T waves (see item **12b**)
- S_1, S_2, S_3
  A terminal negative deflection is present in the QRS complexes in the standard limb leads in up to 20% of healthy adults—should be distinguished from abnormal left-axis deviation
- rSR´ or rSr´ in lead V_1 (2.4% of normals)
  1. QRS duration < 0.10 second and < 7 mm in height
  2. r´ amplitude smaller than r or S

c. Incorrect electrode placement
Most commonly:

- Reversal of right and left arm leads (Fig. 2). Resultant ECG mimics dextrocardia in limb leads with P, QRS, and T inversion in limb leads I and aVL. However, the precordial leads remain normal and thus rule out dextrocardia
- Reversal of chest V leads (Fig. 3). There is a sudden decrease in the R-wave amplitude with return in the next V lead.

d. Artifact due to tremor

- Parkinson's tremor simulates atrial flutter with

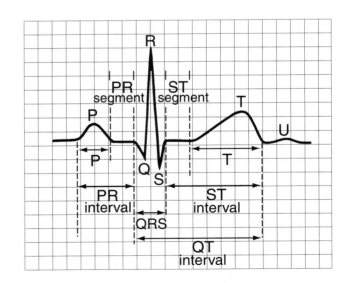

Fig. 1. Components of the scalar electrocardiogram with standard wave labeling (P, Q, R, S, T, U) and clinically useful interval and segment measurements. (From Giuliani ER, Gersh BJ, McGoon MD, Hayes DL, Schaff HV [editors]: *Mayo Clinic Practice of Cardiology.* Third edition. Mosby, 1996, p 76. By permission of Mayo Foundation.)

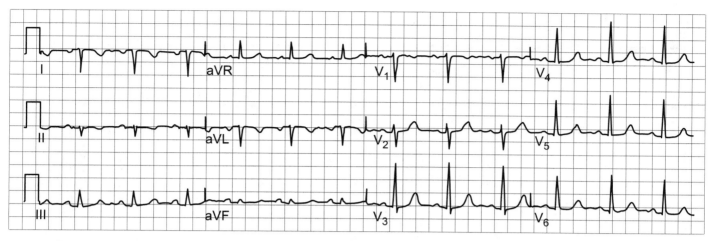

Fig. 2. Reversal of right and left arm leads.

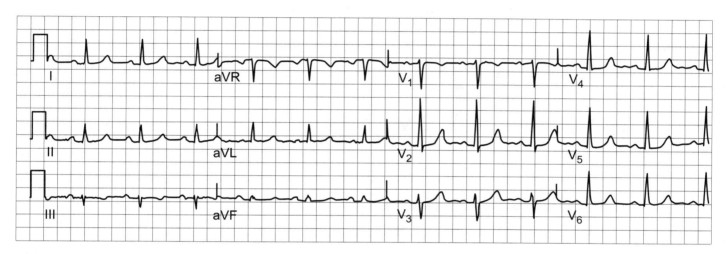

Fig. 3. Reversal of V_2 and V_3 leads in a 61-year-old woman.

rate of approximately 300/min (4 to 6/s) (Fig. 4).
- Physiologic tremor rate is 500/min (7 to 9/s)
- Most prominent in limb leads

2. **Atrial Rhythms**

   a. Sinus rhythm

   - Rate 60 to 100/min
   - P-wave axis normal (15° to 75°)

   b. Sinus arrhythmia
   Requires the following:

   - P-wave morphology and axis normal

- PP interval varies by > 0.16 second or 10%

c. Sinus bradycardia (< 60 beats/min)
Requires the following:

- Rate < 60 beats/min
- Normal P-wave axis
Note: If rate < 40/min, consider 2:1 sinoatrial exit block

d. Sinus tachycardia (> 100 beats/min)
Requires the following:

- Rate > 100 beats/min
- Normal P-wave axis

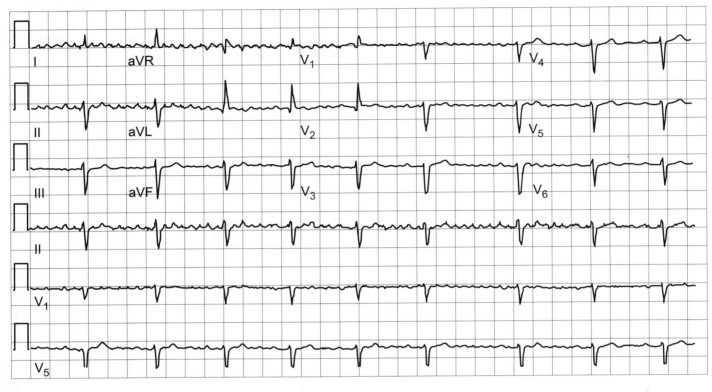

Fig. 4. Parkinson's tremor causing artifact.

Note: P amplitude often increases and PR interval shortens with increasing rate

e. Sinus pause or arrest

Pause > 2.0 seconds without a P wave

Note: The differential diagnosis includes the following:

- Sinus arrhythmia—phasic, gradual PP interval change
- Sinoatrial exit block—pause is multiple (2 times, 3 times, etc.) of usual PP interval
- Nonconducted atrial premature complexes—look for P wave deforming the preceding T wave
- Sinus arrest

f. Sinoatrial exit block

- First- and third-degree not detectable on surface ECG
- Second-degree

- Type I (Mobitz I)—Group beating with shortening of the PP interval, constant PR interval, and a PP pause that is less than twice the normal PP interval
- Type II (Mobitz II)—Constant PP interval followed by a dropped P wave, the pause being a near multiple of the normal PP interval. Interval of pause may be slightly less than twice the normal PP interval but usually within 0.10 second

g. Ectopic atrial rhythm

Requires all the following:

- P-wave axis or morphology different from sinus rhythm
- Rate < 100 beats/min
- PR interval > 0.11 second

Note: Low atrial focus may activate atrium retrogradely (P inverted II, III, aVF) but PR interval > 0.11 second, distinguishing it from AV junctional rhythm

h. Wandering atrial pacemaker
Requires the following:
- Rate < 100 beats/min
- Varying P waves with ≥ 3 morphologic patterns

i. Atrial premature complexes, normally conducted
Suggested by:

- Premature P wave in relation to normal sinus rhythm
- P wave usually abnormal in configuration
- PR interval may be normal, increased, or decreased
- Post-extrasystolic pause is noncompensatory

unless sinoatrial entrance block is present and sinoatrial node is not reset, resulting in either an interpolated beat or a full compensatory pause
- QRS complex similar in morphology to the QRS complex present during sinus rhythm

j. Atrial premature complexes, nonconducted (Fig. 5 and 6)
Suggested by:

- Premature P waves that are abnormal in morphology but not followed by QRS
- P waves that are often hidden in T wave (look for deformed T wave)

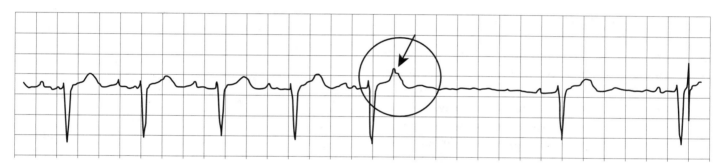

Fig. 5. Nonconducted atrial premature complex (*arrow*) causing a pause.

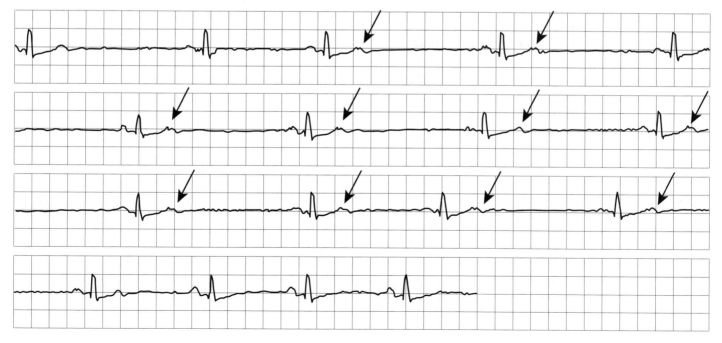

Fig. 6. Nonconducted atrial premature complexes (*arrows*) in bigeminy causing bradycardia; continuous strip.

● The sinus node is usually reset, resulting in RR interval pause

k. Atrial premature complexes with aberrant intraventricular conduction (Fig. 7)
Suggested by:

● P wave that occurs very early
● RBBB pattern is most common, but LBBB or even variable QRS morphology may occur
Note: Also see item **7i**

l. Atrial tachycardia (regular, sustained, 1:1 conduction)
Suggested by:

● Abnormal P waves that are different in morphology from sinus P waves
● Three or more beats in succession
● The atrial rate is generally 100 to 180 beats/min
● Regular rhythm (constant RR interval), except for a warm-up period in the automatic type
● A QRS complex follows each P wave—the QRS complex usually resembles the morphology present during sinus rhythm unless aberrantly conducted
● PR interval may be within normal limits or prolonged
● Secondary ST- and T-wave changes may occur

m. Atrial tachycardia, repetitive (short paroxysms)

● Characterized by recurring short runs of atrial tachycardia interrupted by normal sinus rhythm

Note: Refer to item **21** for definition of atrial tachycardia

n. Atrial tachycardia, multifocal (chaotic atrial tachycardia)
Requires *all* of the following:

● P waves of at least three morphologic patterns
● Absence of one dominant atrial pacemaker (in contradistinction to normal sinus rhythm with multifocal atrial premature complexes)
● Variable PR, RR, and RP intervals
● Atrial rate > 100 beats/min
● Isoelectric baseline between P waves

o. Atrial tachycardia with AV block
Requires *all* of the following:
● Abnormal P waves that are different in morphology from P waves of sinus rhythm
● Atrial rate usually 150 to 240 beats/min
● Isoelectric intervals between P waves in all leads (unlike atrial flutter)
● AV block to a degree beyond simple PR prolongation (second or third degree)
● Rhythm is regular, but ventriculophasic sinus arrhythmia may occur (refer to item **5e** for definition)
Note: Most cases are due to digitalis toxicity. Consider item **14b**

p. Supraventricular tachycardia, unspecified

● Rhythm is regular
● P wave not easily identified

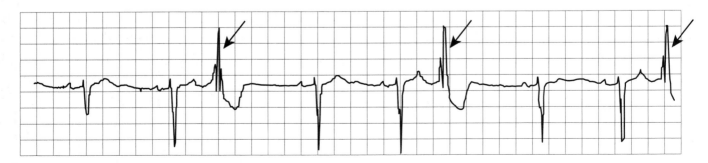

Fig. 7. Atrial premature complexes with aberrant intraventricular conduction (*arrows*).

- QRS complex usually narrow (occasionally aberrant)
Note: If rate is 150 beats/min, rule out atrial flutter with 2:1 block

q. Supraventricular tachycardia, paroxysmal

- Onset and termination sudden
- May have retrograde P wave (see item **2t**)
- Refer to item **2p** for definition of supraventricular tachycardia

r. Atrial flutter

- Rapid regular undulations (F waves), sawtooth pattern usually seen best in leads II, III, aVF, and V_1
- Atrial rate 240 to 340 beats/min. May be faster in children. May be slower in the presence of class 1A, 1C, and 3 antiarrhythmic drugs
- QRS complex may be normal or aberrantly conducted
- Rate and regularity of QRS complexes are variable and depend on the AV conduction sequence
- AV conduction

  - Complete block may occur with or without AV junctional tachycardia (usually digoxin toxicity)
  - May have varying degrees of block (2:1, 4:1, or more)

s. Atrial fibrillation

- P waves are absent. Atrial activity is represented by fibrillatory (f) waves of varying amplitudes, duration, and morphology causing random oscillation of the baseline
- The ventricular rhythm, in the absence of third-degree AV block, is irregularly irregular
- Atrial activity best seen in the right precordial and inferior leads
- Rate is usually 100 to 180 beats/min in the absence of drugs. If rate is < 100 beats/min, conduction system disease is likely to be present. If rate is > 200 beats/min with a QRS complex > 0.12 second in duration, consider Wolff-Parkinson-White syndrome
- Differential diagnoses:

  - Multifocal atrial tachycardia
  - Paroxysmal atrial tachycardia with block
  - Atrial flutter

t. Retrograde atrial activation

- Inverted P waves in leads II, III, and aVF
- Look for retrograde P waves after ventricular premature complexes and other ectopic junctional or ventricular beats

3. AV Junctional Rhythms

a. AV junctional premature complexes
Require *all* of the following:

- Occur early in cycle, in contrast to escape beats
- P wave is inverted in leads II, III, aVF and upright in leads I and aVL
- P wave may precede the QRS by 0.11 second or less, be superimposed on or follow the QRS
- Ventricular complex may show aberration
- Coupling interval is usually constant
- Noncompensatory pause is usually seen
Note: Consider also item **2t**

b. AV junctional escape complexes

- There is decreased sinus impulse formation or conduction from the sinoatrial node, or high-degree AV block at or proximal to the bundle of His. Atrial mechanism may be sinus rhythm, paroxysmal atrial tachycardia, atrial flutter, or atrial fibrillation
- May be seen with post-extrasystolic pause after atrial tachycardia, atrial flutter, or atrial fibrillation

c. AV junctional rhythm, accelerated
Requires *all* of the following:

- Rate > 60 beats/min
- Variable relationship between atrial and ventricular rates. If retrograde block is present, atria remain in sinus rhythm and AV dissociation will be present. If retrograde activation occurs, constant QRS-P interval will be present
- May be seen with atrial fibrillation or atrial

flutter with complete heart block (consider digoxin toxicity)

- Exit block also occurs with digoxin toxicity

Note: Consider items **2t** and **14b**

d. AV junctional rhythm (rate ≤ 60 beats/min)

- RR interval of escape rhythm usually constant (< 0.04-second variation)
- May have isorhythmic AV dissociation (consider item **5d**)
- P wave inverted in leads II, III, aVF and upright in leads I and aVL (consider item **2t**)

4. Ventricular Rhythms

a. Ventricular premature complex(es), uniform, fixed coupling (Fig. 8)
Require *all* of the following:

- Premature with relation to normal cycles, not preceded by P wave (or shorter than expected PR interval, "collapsing PR")
- Coupling interval usually the same for each site or focus (variation usually < 0.08 second)

- Abnormal QRS configuration that is almost always > 0.12 second in duration
- Retrograde capture of atria may occur (consider item **2t**)
- Initial direction of QRS complex is often different from that observed during sinus rhythm
- Usually full compensatory pause is noted
- Compensatory pause requires an undisturbed sinus depolarization due to one of the following:

  - Ventriculoatrial block
  - Sinoatrial entrance block if atrial capture occurs
  - Sinoatrial node discharged before arrival of retrograde wavefront, and thus refractory

b. Ventricular premature complex(es), uniform, non-fixed coupling

- Ventricular premature complexes with variable temporal relationship to regular sinus beats

c. Ventricular premature complex(es), multiform

- Two or more morphologic patterns of ventricular premature complexes present

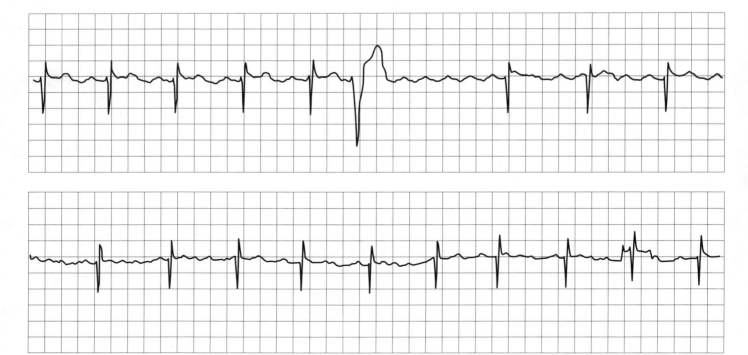

Fig. 8. Ventricular premature complex resulting in concealed retrograde conduction during atrial fibrillation.

d. Ventricular premature complexes, in pairs (2 consecutive)

- Two consecutive ventricular premature complexes of not necessarily the same morphology
  Note: Refer to item **4a** for criteria

e. Ventricular parasystole
An automatic ventricular focus with entrance block and all of the following:

- Rates usually 30 to 56 beats/min
- Varying relationship with the preceding sinus beats
- All interectopic intervals are a multiple of a constant shortest interval
- When fusion beats and lack of fixed coupling are noted, consider parasystole

f. Ventricular tachycardia (≥ 3 consecutive beats)
Rapid succession of three or more beats of ventricular origin (Fig. 9 and 10)

- Abnormal and wide QRS complexes with secondary ST-T changes
  Note: Ventricular tachycardia originating in the septum near the normal conduction system may have a narrow QRS complex
- Rate > 100 beats/min
- Regular or slightly irregular
- Abrupt onset and termination
- AV dissociation is common. On occasion, retrograde conduction and capture of the atria may occur
- Look for ventricular capture and fusion beats as a marker for ventricular tachycardia

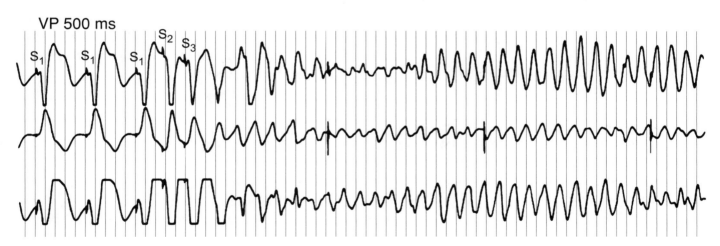

Fig. 9. Torsades de pointes induced at the time of electrophysiologic testing in a patient with congenital Q-T prolongation. A ventricular arrhythmia with a morphology consistent with torsades de pointes was induced after critically timed paired extrastimuli (S_2S_3) were introduced during ventricular pacing (*VP*) at a rate of 120 beats/min (cycle length equals 500 ms). (From Giuliani ER, Gersh BJ, McGoon MD, Hayes DL, Schaff HV [editors]: *Mayo Clinic Practice of Cardiology*. Third edition. Mosby, 1996, p 810. By permission of Mayo Foundation.)

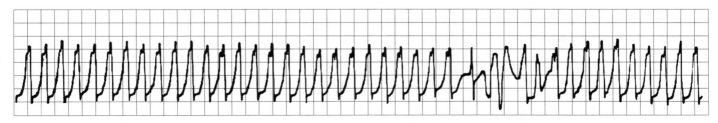

Fig. 10. Monomorphic ventricular tachycardia with fusion complexes. (From Giuliani ER, Gersh BJ, McGoon MD, Hayes DL, Schaff HV [editors]: *Mayo Clinic Practice of Cardiology*. Third edition. Mosby, 1996, p 903. By permission of Mayo Foundation.)

Favors ventricular origin:

- QRS complexes like those of ventricular premature complexes
- Tachyarrhythmia initiated by ventricular premature complexes
- AV dissociation
- Capture or fusion beats
- QRS ≥ 0.14 second if RBBB morphology and ≥ 0.16 second if LBBB morphology when QRS during sinus rhythm < 0.12 second
- Left- or northwest-axis deviation
- All positive or all negative complexes in precordial leads
- In V_1 R > r´ (left rabbit ear taller than right)

Favors supraventricular origin:

- QRS complex like aberrantly conducted atrial premature complexes or QRS in sinus rhythm
- Tachyarrhythmia initiated by atrial premature complexes
- RBBB configuration with rSR´ in V_1

g. Accelerated idioventricular rhythm
Requires *all* of the following:

- Regular rhythm, rate 60 to 110 beats/min
- QRS complexes are abnormal and wide
- Usually AV dissociation
- Capture and fusion beats are common because of slower rate
Note: Also consider items **5a** and **5c**

h. Ventricular escape complexes or rhythm
Requires *all* of the following:

- Rate is usually 30 to 40 beats/min (can be 20 to 50)
- QRS complexes are abnormal and wide
- Occurs when the rate of supraventricular impulse arriving at the ventricle is slower than the inherent rate of the ectopic ventricular pacemaker

i. Ventricular fibrillation

- Chaotic and irregular deflections of varying amplitude and contour
- No P waves, QRS complexes, or T waves

5. Atrioventricular Interactions in Arrhythmias

a. Fusion complexes
Caused by simultaneous activation of the ventricle from two sources. May occur with:

- Ventricular premature complexes
- Wolff-Parkinson-White syndrome
- Ventricular tachycardia
- Ventricular parasystole
- Accelerated idioventricular rhythm
- Paced rhythm

b. Reciprocal (echo) complexes

- The impulse activates a chamber (atrium or ventricle), returns, and reactivates the same chamber

c. Ventricular capture complexes

- Ventricular capture by conducted supraventricular impulses resulting in a fusion beat or a QRS morphology similar to that during sinus rhythm
- Strong but not infallible evidence for rhythm of ventricular origin

d. AV dissociation
Requires *all* of the following:

- Atrial and ventricular activities that are independent
- Ventricular rate is faster than atrial rate
- Always a secondary phenomenon resulting from some other disturbance of cardiac rhythm

e. Ventriculophasic sinus arrhythmia

- PP interval containing a QRS complex is shorter than a PP interval without a QRS
- Common in presence of high-grade AV block

6. AV Conduction Abnormalities

a. AV block, first degree
Requires *all* of the following:

- PR interval ≥ 0.20 second (usually 0.21 to 0.40

second, but may be as long as 0.80 second)
- Each P wave followed by a QRS complex
- Usually constant PR interval (Fig. 11)

b. AV block, second degree-Mobitz type I
(Wenckebach) (Fig. 12 and 13)
Requires *all* of the following:

- Progressive prolongation of PR interval until P

wave fails to conduct to the ventricle
- Progressive shortening of RR interval until P wave is not conducted
- The RR interval containing the nonconducted P wave is shorter than the sum of two PP intervals
- Results in "group" or pattern beating

c. AV block, second degree-Mobitz type II (Fig. 14)

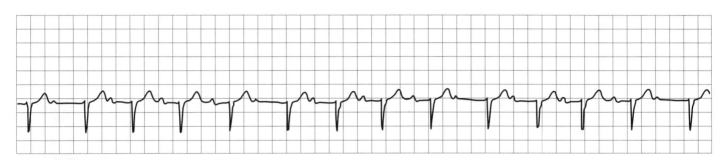

Fig. 11. Changing RP interval affecting the subsequent PR interval during sinus arrhythmia.

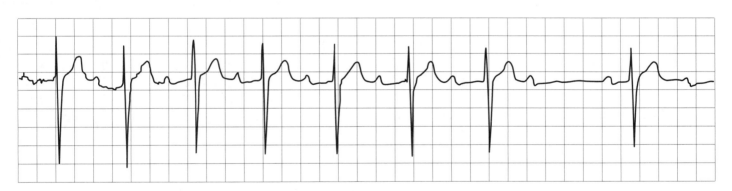

Fig. 12. Atrioventricular block, second degree-Mobitz type I (Wenckebach).

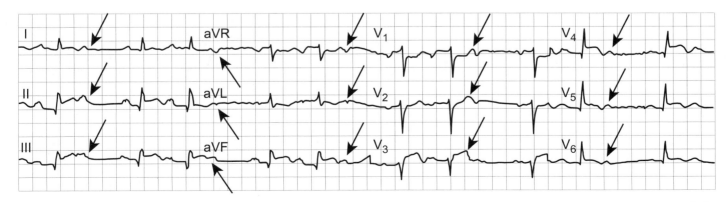

Fig. 13. Acute inferior myocardial infarction with atrioventricular block, second degree-Mobitz type I (Wenckebach), in a 69-year-old man. *Arrows* indicate P waves preceding dropped beats.

Requires *all* of the following:

- There are intermittent nonconducted P waves with no evidence of atrial prematurity
- In conducted beats, PR intervals stay constant
- The RR interval containing the nonconducted P wave is equal to two PP intervals
- 2:1 AV block can be Mobitz type I or II and cannot be distinguished unless:

    - Maneuvers used to increase heart rate and improve AV conduction (atropine and exercise typically will decrease type I block and increase type II block) (Fig. 15), *or*
    - Classic Mobitz type I seen on another part of ECG (then probably type I), *or*
    - If QRS conduction is abnormal with bundle branch block or bifascicular block, then usually Mobitz type II

d. AV block, 2:1

- There are two P waves for each QRS complex

(every other P wave is nonconducted)
Note: Refer to item **6c**

e. AV block, third degree (Fig. 16)
Requires *all* of the following:

- Independent atrial and ventricular activities
- Atrial rate faster than ventricular rate
- Ventricular rhythm maintained by a junctional or idioventricular escape rhythm or ventricular pacemaker
- Ventriculophasic sinus arrhythmia in 30% of cases (consider item **5e**)
- When ventricular rate is *faster* than the atrial rate, AV dissociation is present, not AV block

f. AV block, variable

- Varying degrees of AV block including first-, second- (types I and II), or third-degree block
- Consider this in atrial flutter with variable RR (flutter wave to R wave) intervals after ruling out third-degree AV block

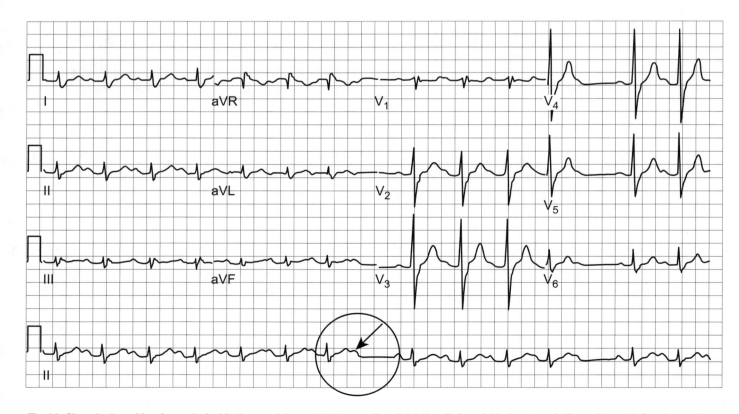

Fig. 14. Sinus rhythm with atrioventricular block, second degree-Mobitz type II, and right bundle branch block. *Arrow* indicates P wave before dropped beat.

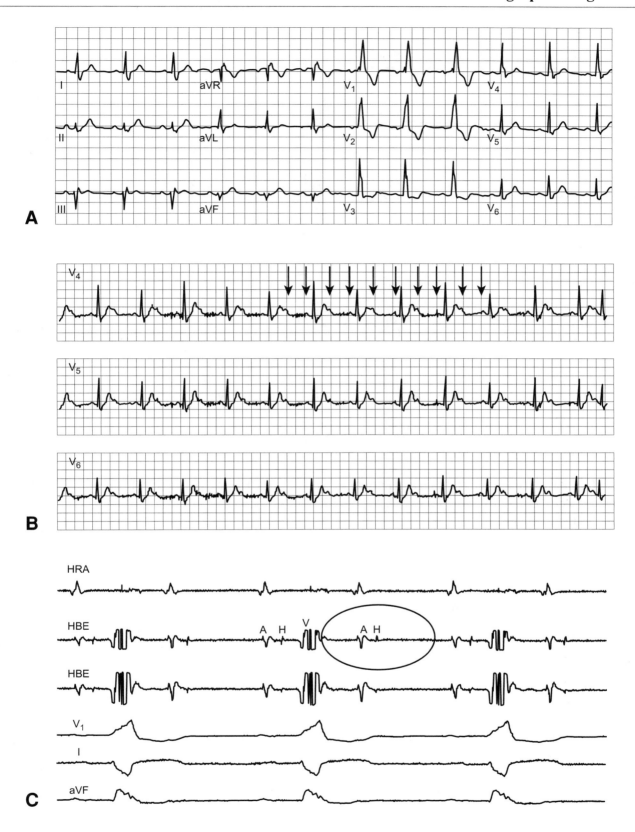

Fig. 15. *A*, Electrocardiograms (ECG) in 59-year-old man. Resting ECG with right bundle branch block. *B*, Exercise ECG with 2:1 atrioventricular block. *Arrows* indicate P waves with conduction of every second beat. *C*, His bundle recording. Right bundle branch block and atrioventricular block distal to His. The highlighted complex shows an atrial (A) followed by a His (H) depolarization but no ventricular (V) depolarization. A, atrial depolarization; H, His bundle depolarization; V, ventricular depolarization; HBE, His bundle electrogram; HRA, high right atrium.

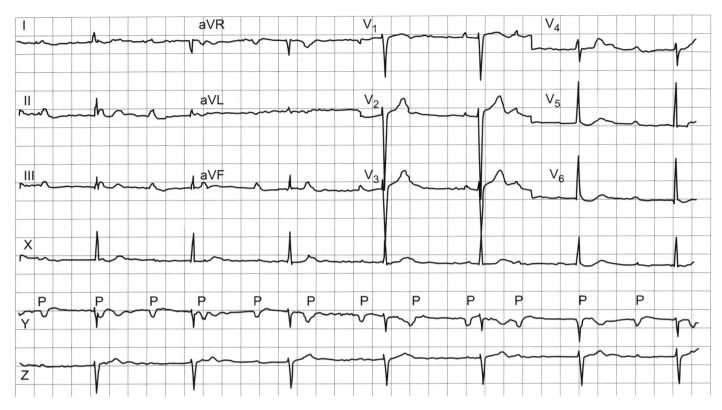

Fig. 16. Complete heart block (third-degree atrioventricular block).

g. Short PR interval (with sinus rhythm and normal QRS duration)
Requires the following:

- Sinus P wave
- PR < 0.12 second

h. Wolff-Parkinson-White pattern (Fig. 17)
Suggested by the following:

- Normal P wave with PR interval < 0.12 second (rarely > 0.12)
- Abnormally wide QRS > 0.10 second
- Initial slurring of QRS (δ wave)
- PJ interval is constant and ≤ 0.26 second

Note: Atrial fibrillation or flutter with QRS that is varying in width (generally wide) and rate > 200 beats/min suggests Wolff-Parkinson-White syndrome

7. Intraventricular Conduction Disturbances

a. RBBB, incomplete

RBBB morphology (rSR´) but QRS duration is 0.09 to 0.11 second (Fig. 18)

b. RBBB, complete
Requires *all* of the following:

- Prolonged QRS ≥ 0.12 second
- Secondary R wave (R´) in right precordial leads, with R´ usually greater than initial R
- Delayed intrinsicoid deflection in right precordial leads > 0.05 second
- Wide S wave in I, V_5, V_6
- Secondary ST-T changes in V_1-V_3
- Axis as determined by initial 0.06 to 0.08 second of QRS should be normal unless concomitant left anterior fascicular block is present

Note: Consider item **12g**

c. Left anterior fascicular block (Fig. 19)
Requires *all* of the following:

- Displacement of mean QRS axis to between -45° and -90°

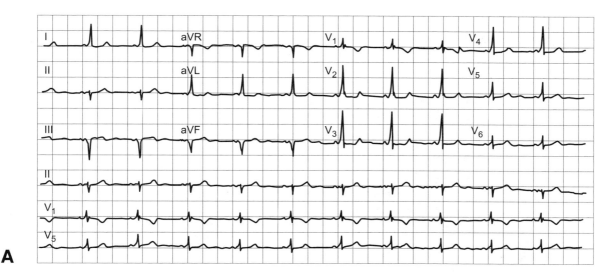

	V$_1$	aVF	aVL
Left lateral	+	+	-
Left posterior/septal	+	-	+
Right posterior/septal	-	-	+
Right lateral/anterior	-	+	+

B

Fig. 17. *A* and *B*, Wolff-Parkinson-White pattern.

- qR complex (or an R wave) in leads I and aVL; rS in lead III
- Normal or slightly prolonged QRS duration (0.08 to 0.10 second)
- No other factors responsible for left-axis deviation, such as:

  - Left ventricular hypertrophy
  - Inferior infarct
  - Emphysema (chronic lung disease)

  Note: Also consider item **9c**

d. Left posterior fascicular block (Fig. 20)

Requires *all* of the following:

- Frontal plane QRS axis of +100° to +180°
- S$_1$ Q$_3$ pattern (deep S wave in lead I, with Q wave in lead III)
- Normal or slightly prolonged QRS duration (0.08 to 0.10 second)
- No other factors responsible for right-axis deviation, such as:

  - Right ventricular hypertrophy
  - Vertical heart
  - Emphysema (chronic lung disease)

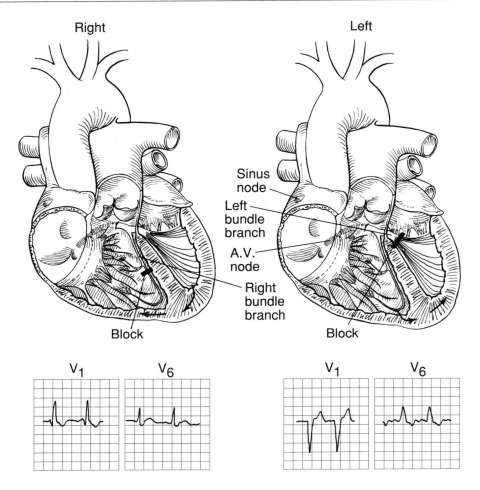

Fig. 18. Drawings of heart show location of right bundle branch block with the characteristic V_1 and V_6, scalar electrocardiographic (ECG) changes RSR´, and terminal sagging of S wave (*left*) and left bundle branch block with the characteristic scalar ECG changes in V_1 and V_6, deep S waves, and broad notched wide QRS (*right*). (From Giuliani ER, Gersh BJ, McGoon MD, Hayes DL, Schaff HV [editors]: *Mayo Clinic Practice of Cardiology.* Third edition. Mosby, 1996, p 94. By permission of Mayo Foundation.)

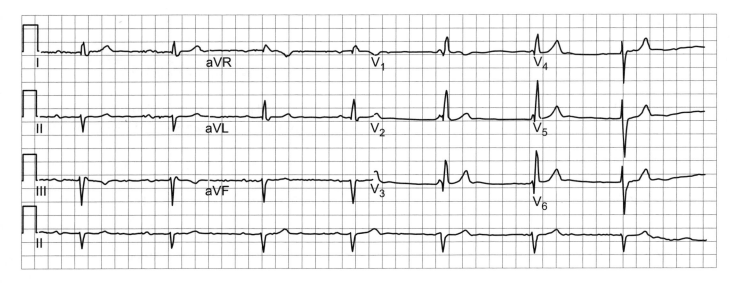

Fig. 19. Complete heart block with right bundle branch block and left anterior fascicular block.

- Lateral wall myocardial infarction
Note: Also consider item **9d**

e. LBBB, complete with ST-T waves suggestive of acute myocardial injury or infarction (Fig. 21, 22, and 23)
Requires the following:

- Fulfills criteria for LBBB (see item **7f**)
- ≥ 1 mm ST elevation concordant with QRS
- ≥ 1 mm ST depression in leads V_1 to V_3
- ≥ 5 mm ST elevation discordant with QRS
- Criteria valid with artificial pacemaker

f. LBBB, complete
Requires *all* of the following:

- Prolonged QRS duration ≥ 0.12 second
- Delayed intrinsicoid deflection in left precordial leads and lead I > 0.05 second
- Broad monophasic R in leads I, V_5, and V_6 which is usually notched or slurred
Note: Also consider items **9c** and **12g**

g. LBBB, intermittent
More common at high rates but also may be bradycardia-dependent

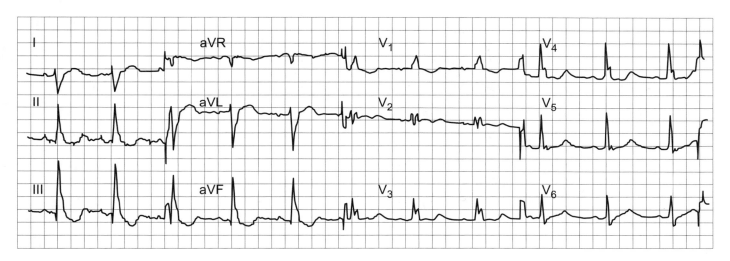

Fig. 20. Left posterior fascicular block and right bundle branch block in a 68-year-old man.

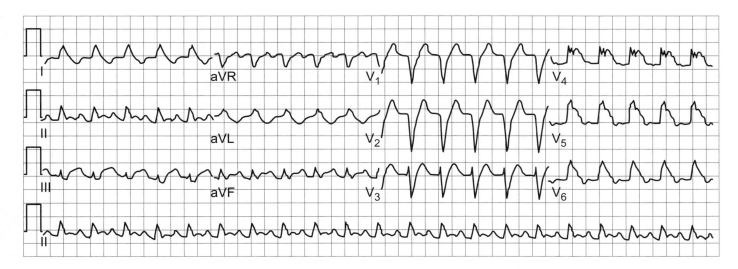

Fig. 21. Left bundle branch block with ST changes of acute anterior injury in a 76-year-old woman presenting with severe dyspnea.

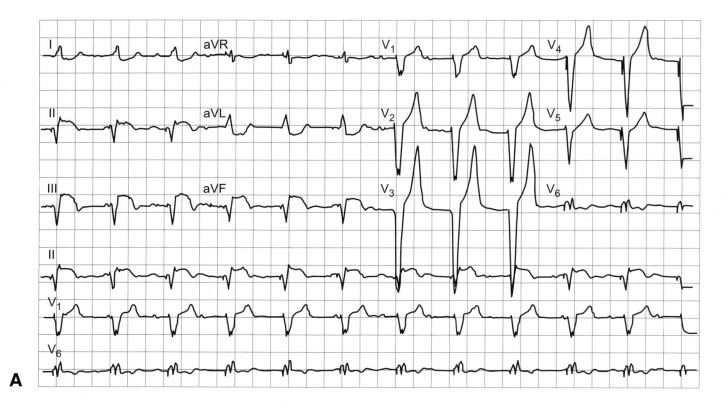

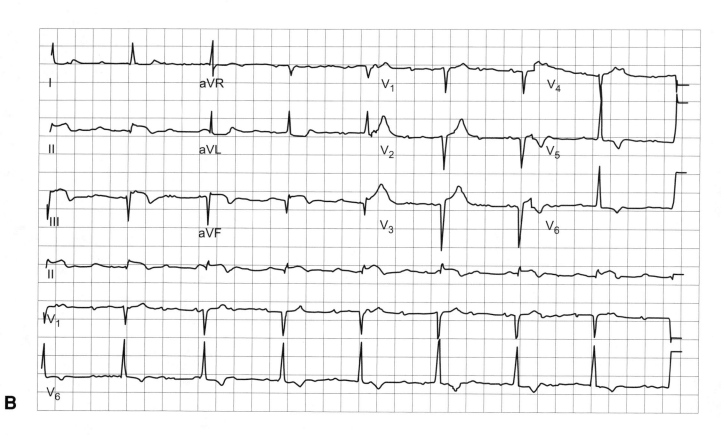

Fig. 22. *A,* Findings in a 78-year-old man presenting with severe chest pain, permanent ventricular pacemaker, and inferior ST elevation. *B,* Acute inferior myocardial infarction with complete heart block; pacemaker is off.

h. Intraventricular conduction disturbance, nonspecific type

- QRS > 0.11 second, but QRS morphology does not satisfy criteria for either LBBB or RBBB
- May also be used when there is abnormal notching of the QRS complex without prolongation
- May occur with antiarrhythmic drug toxicity, hyperkalemia, and hypothermia

Note: Also consider items **12g, 14d,** and **14e**

i. Aberrant intraventricular conduction with supraventricular arrhythmia (specify rhythm)

Note: See item **4f** for criteria of supraventricular vs. ventricular tachycardia

8. P-Wave Abnormalities

a. Right atrial abnormality

- Amplitude > 2.5 mm in leads II, III, or aVF with a normal P-wave duration (P pulmonale), *or*
- Positive amplitude > 1.5 mm in V_1 or V_2, *or*
- P-wave frontal axis 70° or greater (rightward axis)

b. Left atrial abnormality
- Notched P wave with a duration ≥ 0.12 second in leads II, III, or aVF (P mitrale), *or*
- Downward terminal deflection of P wave in V_1 with a negative amplitude of 1 mm and with duration of 0.04 second (Fig. 24)

Biatrial enlargement suggested by any of the following:

- Large biphasic P wave in V_1 with initial positive component 1.5 mm and the P terminal force with a negative amplitude of 1 mm and with a duration of 0.04 second
- Tall, peaked P waves (> 1.5 mm) in right precordial leads (V_1 to V_3) and wide, notched P waves in left precordial leads (V_5 to V_6)

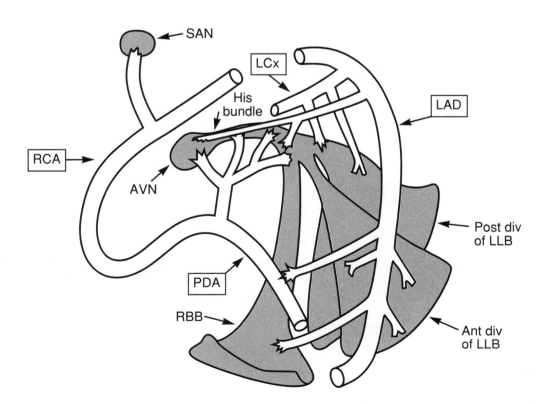

Fig. 23. Diagram of the conduction system and its blood supply. *SAN*, sinoatrial node; *AVN*, atrioventricular node; *LCx*, left circumflex coronary artery; *LAD*, left anterior descending coronary artery; *RCA*, right coronary artery; *PDA*, posterior descending branch of right coronary artery; *RBB*, right bundle branch; *LBB*, left bundle branch. (From *Cardiovasc Clin* 13 No 1:191-207, 1983. By permission of FA Davis Company.)

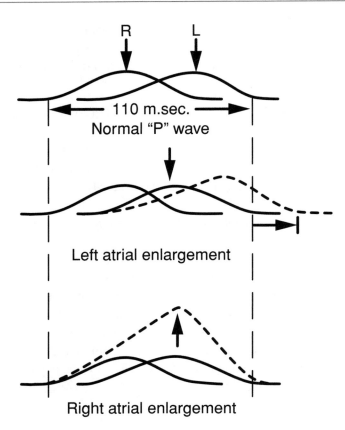

Fig. 24. *Top*, Normal surface P-wave morphology, illustrating right and left atrial activation sequence and normal duration. *Middle*, Left atrial enlargement (*broken line*), illustrating delayed peak and left atrial activation time producing a prolonged P-wave duration and notched P-wave morphology. *Bottom*, Right atrial enlargement (*broken line*), illustrating effective combined right and left atrial voltage peaks occurring at the same time with resulting tall peaked P waves. (From Giuliani ER, Gersh BJ, McGoon MD, Hayes DL, Schaff HV [editors]: *Mayo Clinic Practice of Cardiology*. Third edition. Mosby, 1996, p 83. By permission of Mayo Foundation.)

- P-wave amplitude ≥ 2.5 mm and duration ≥ 0.12 second in limb leads

c. Nonspecific atrial abnormality

- Abnormal P-wave morphology, but not fulfilling criteria for right or left atrial enlargement

9. **Abnormalities of QRS Voltage or Axis**

a. Low voltage, limb leads only

- Amplitude of the entire QRS complex (R + S) is < 5 mm in all limb leads
Note: Consider items **14m, 14o,** and **14t**

b. Low voltage, limb and precordial leads

- Amplitude of the entire QRS complex (R + S) is < 10 mm in each precordial lead
- Amplitude of R + S in limb leads is < 5 mm
- Low voltage can also occur with obesity, pleural effusion, restrictive or infiltrative cardiomyopathies, and diffuse myocardial disease
Note: Consider items **14m, 14o,** and **14t**

c. Left-axis deviation (> -30°)

- Axis -30° to -105°
- Be careful about diagnosing left-axis deviation in presence of inferior infarct
Note: Consider item **7c**

d. Right-axis deviation (> +100°)

- Axis 101° to -106° (+254°)
- Pure right-axis deviation (left posterior fascicular block) should have S_1Q_3 pattern
- Causes:

  - Right ventricular hypertrophy (especially if axis > 100°). Consider item **10c**
  - Vertical heart
  - Chronic lung disease. Consider item **14m**
  - Pulmonary embolus. Consider item **14n**
  - Left posterior fascicular block. Consider item **7d**

e. Electrical alternans (Fig. 25)

- Alternation of amplitude of the P, QRS, or T waves
- Causes:

  - Pericardial effusion causes only a third of cases. But if electrical alternans involves the P wave, QRS complex, and T wave, significant effusion is usually present. Twelve percent of simple pericardial effusions have electrical alternans
  - Severe left ventricular failure
  - Hypertension
  - Coronary artery disease
  - Rheumatic heart disease
  - Supraventricular or ventricular tachycardia

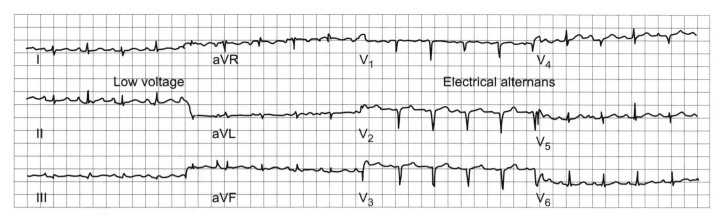

Fig. 25. Electrical alternans in a 51-year-old woman with pericardial tamponade. Note the low QRS voltage in the limb leads and the varying height of the QRS complex on consecutive beats. The RR interval and complex morphology are constant throughout, differentiating electrical alternans from a bigeminal rhythm.

10. Ventricular Hypertrophy

a. Left ventricular hypertrophy by voltage only

- Cornell criteria

  - R wave in lead aVL and S wave in lead V_3
  - > 24 mm in males
  - > 20 mm in females

- Precordial leads

  - The sum of the R wave in lead V_5 or V_6 and the S wave in lead V_1 is > 35 mm in adults older than 30 years (40 mm in those between 20 and 30 years and 60 mm in the 16- to 20-year age group), *or*
  - The sum of the maximal R and the deepest S waves in the precordial leads is > 45 mm, *or*
  - The amplitude of the R wave in lead V_5 is greater than 26 mm, *or*
  - The amplitude of the R wave in lead V_6 is greater than 20 mm

- Limb leads

  - The sum of the R wave in lead I and the S wave in lead II is ≥ 26 mm, *or*
  - The amplitude of the R wave in lead I is 14 mm or more, *or*

  - The amplitude of the S wave in lead aVR is 15 mm or more, *or*
  - The amplitude of the R wave in lead aVF is 21 mm or more, *or*
  - The amplitude of the R wave in lead aVL is 12 mm or more (a highly specific, if insensitive, finding), *or*
  - The R wave in lead V_6 is taller than the R wave in lead V_5, provided there are dominant R waves in both these leads

b. Left ventricular hypertrophy by both voltage and ST-T segment abnormalities

Refer to item **10a** for voltage criteria; the ST-T abnormalities of left ventricular hypertrophy include:

- ST-segment depression in any or all of the following leads: I, aVL, III, aVF, V_4 through V_6
- Subtle ST elevation in V_1 through V_3
- Inverted T waves I, aVL, V_4 through V_6
- Prominent or inverted U waves
- Nonvoltage-related criteria for left ventricular hypertrophy (often with or without prominent voltage and ST-T changes in patients with left ventricular hypertrophy)

  - Left atrial abnormality
  - Left-axis deviation
  - Nonspecific intraventricular conduction delay

- Delayed intrinsicoid deflection
- Low or absent R waves in V_1, V_2, or V_3
- Absent Q waves in left precordial leads
- Abnormal Q waves in inferior leads due to left-axis deviation
- Prominent U waves

● Left ventricular hypertrophy should not be diagnosed in the presence of left-axis deviation when the only criterion for the hypertrophy is in lead aVL (Fig. 26)

c. Right ventricular hypertrophy
   Suggested by one or more of the following:

● Right-axis deviation $\geq +100°$
● R/S ratio in leads V_1 or $V_{3R} > 1$
● R in V_1 + S in V_5 or $V_6 > 10.5$ mm
● Right atrial enlargement
● R wave in $V_1 \geq 7$ mm
● S wave in $V_1 < 2$ mm
● qR in V_1
● R/S ratio in V_5 or $V_6 \leq 1$
● Onset of intrinsicoid deflection in V_1 between 0.35 and 0.55 second

● rSR´ in V_1 with R´ > 10 mm
● Secondary ST-T changes in right precordial leads

To diagnose right ventricular hypertrophy, must exclude:

● Posterior wall myocardial infarction
● Right bundle branch block
● Wolff-Parkinson-White syndrome (type A)
● Dextroposition
● Left posterior fascicular block (lateral wall infarct)
● Normal variant (especially in children)

Criteria to diagnose right ventricular hypertrophy in the presence of RBBB (Fig. 27)

● r´ ≥ 15 mm in lead V_1
● Right-axis deviation of initial vector (unblocked forces)

d. Combined ventricular hypertrophy (Fig. 28)
   Suggested by any of the following:

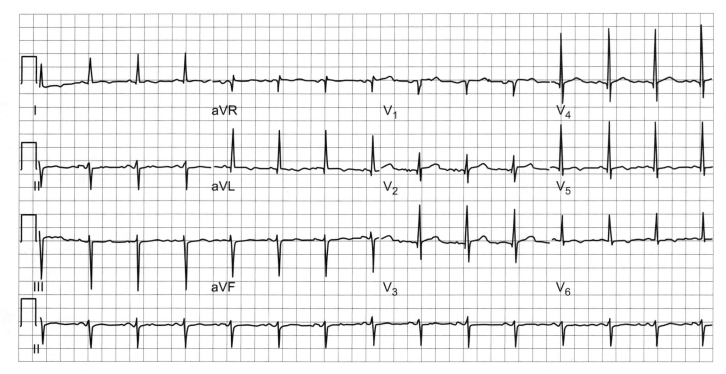

Fig. 26. Left-axis deviation with increased voltage in lead aVL, but not left ventricular hypertrophy.

- ECG meets one or more diagnostic criteria for both isolated left and right ventricular hypertrophy
- Precordial leads show left ventricular hypertro-

phy, but QRS axis in frontal plane > 90°
- R > Q in aVR, S > R in V_5, and T inversion in V_1 in conjunction with signs of left ventricular hypertrophy

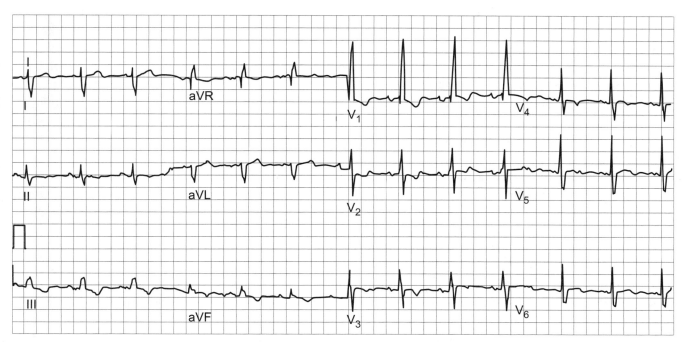

Fig. 27. Right bundle branch block with right ventricular hypertrophy (right-axis deviation, r′ ≥ 15 mm in lead V_1).

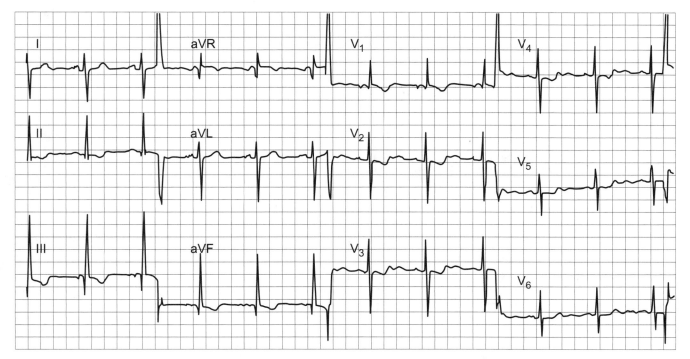

Fig. 28. Combined ventricular hypertrophy: right ventricular hypertrophy (right-axis deviation and amplitude of R wave > wave in lead SV_1) and left ventricular hypertrophy (R wave amplitude > 21 mm in lead aVF).

- Kutz-Wachtel phenomenon—high-voltage equiphasic (R = S) complexes in mid-precordial leads
- Right atrial enlargement with left ventricular hypertrophy pattern in precordial leads

11. Transmural Myocardial Infarction

General considerations:

- Acute myocardial infarction (MI): Q waves, ST elevation with or without reciprocal ST depression
- Recent MI: Q waves, isoelectric ST segments, ischemic T waves
- Old MI: Q waves, isoelectric ST segments, nonspecific T-wave abnormalities, or normal ST and T waves
- "Transmural" MI is defined by *abnormal Q waves* (or R waves in leads V_1 and V_2 in posterior MI). ST-segment elevation without Q waves should be coded under item **12e** (myocardial injury)
- Significant Q waves

  - Duration of Q wave ≥ 0.04 second
  - Amplitude varies according to region of infarct

- ST elevation can persist 48 hours to 4 weeks after MI; longer than 1 month suggests aneurysm
- T-wave inversions may persist indefinitely
- Watch for pseudoinfarctions, such as:

Condition	Pseudoinfarct
Wolff-Parkinson-White (Fig. 29)	Inferior, anteroseptal, posterior
Hypertrophic cardiomyopathy	Inferior, posterior, lateral, anteroseptal
Left bundle branch block	Anteroseptal, anterior, inferior
Left ventricular hypertrophy (Fig. 30)	Anteroseptal, anterior, inferior, lateral
Left anterior fascicular block	Inferior, anterior, lateral
Chronic lung disease or right ventricular hypertrophy	Inferior, posterior, anteroseptal, anterior
Cardiomyopathy	Any
Chest deformity	Any
Normal variant	Posterior, anteroseptal, anterior, lateral

- A Q-wave may be present intermittently in lead aVF in the absence of MI as a result of respiratory effects and low voltage inferiorly (Fig. 31)
- In RBBB, Q-wave criteria apply for all infarcts (Fig. 32)
- Difficult to diagnose any infarct in presence of LBBB (Fig. 21 and 22)

a. Anterolateral infarction, probably acute or recent Requires either of the following:

- Abnormal Q waves in leads V_4, V_5, V_6 having

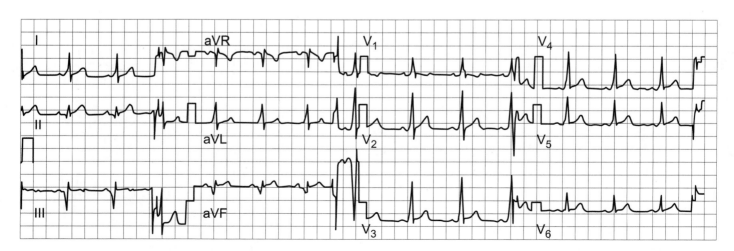

Fig. 29. Pseudo–inferior-posterior myocardial infarction due to Wolff-Parkinson-White pattern.

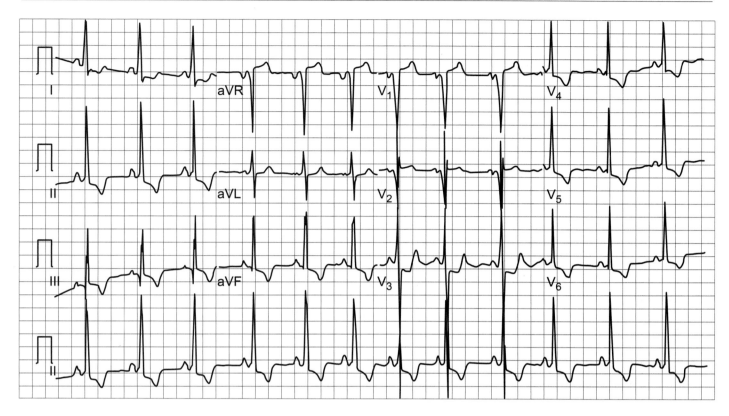

Fig. 30. Left ventricular hypertrophy simulating an anteroseptal myocardial infarction.

amplitude > 15% of total QRS complex
- ST-segment elevation

b. Anterior infarction, probably acute or recent
Requires either of the following:

- rS in V_1 followed by QS or QR in leads V_2 through V_4
- ST-segment elevation

c. Anteroseptal infarction, probably acute or recent (Fig. 32)

- Q or QS deflection in leads V_1 through V_3 and sometimes in V_4 with Q-wave amplitude > 25% of the QRS
- Q in V_1 helps distinguish anteroseptal from anterior infarction
- ST-segment elevation

d. Lateral or high lateral infarction, probably acute

or recent (Fig. 33)
Requires either of the following:

- Q waves in leads I, aVL

  - Q wave in aVL > 50% of the amplitude of QRS, with the Q wave in lead I > 10% of the amplitude of QRS

- ST-segment elevation

e. Inferior (diaphragmatic) infarction, probably acute or recent

- Q waves in leads II, III, aVF, and Q in aVF > 25% amplitude of the R wave
- ST-segment elevation, often with reciprocal ST depression in leads I, aVL, V_1, and V_2

f. Posterior infarction, probably acute or recent (Fig. 34 and 35)

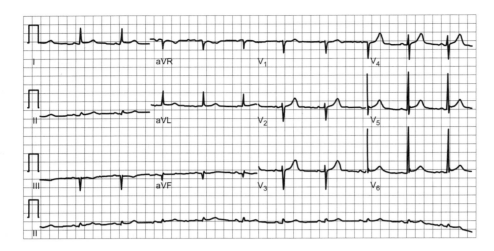

A

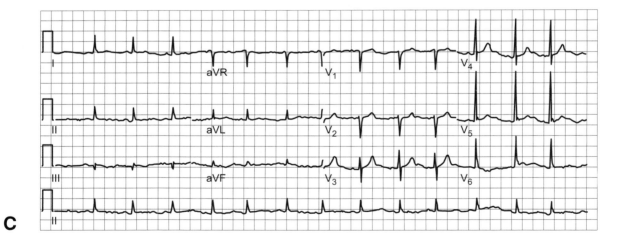

B

C

D

- Disappearance or reduction of Q waves on two consecutive daily ECGs ➔ present day 1, absent day 2

- Occurred in 33% of 167 patients

- Due to respiratory effects on axis shift and low-voltage QRS inferiorly

Fig. 31. *A* through *C*, Electrocardiograms (ECGs) in a 73-year-old man. *A*, Asymptomatic, preoperative ECG on July 9. *B*, Asymptomatic, last prior ECG on January 14, 6 months before noncardiac operation. *C*, Asymptomatic, postoperative ECG on July 10. *D*, Inferior myocardial infarction: Q-wave inconsistency on ECG. (*D*, Data from *Am J Cardiol* 66:1144-1146, 1990.)

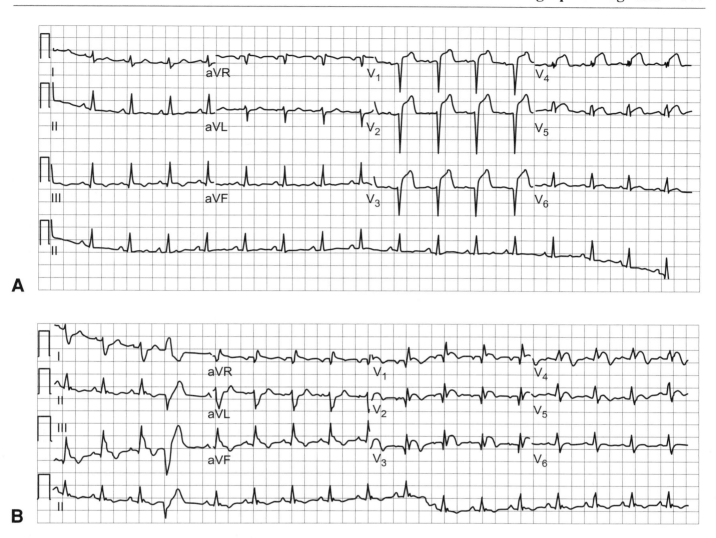

Fig. 32. Electrocardiograms in a 62-year-old man. *A*, Anteroseptal myocardial infarction. *B*, Anteroseptal myocardial infarction in the presence of right bundle branch block.

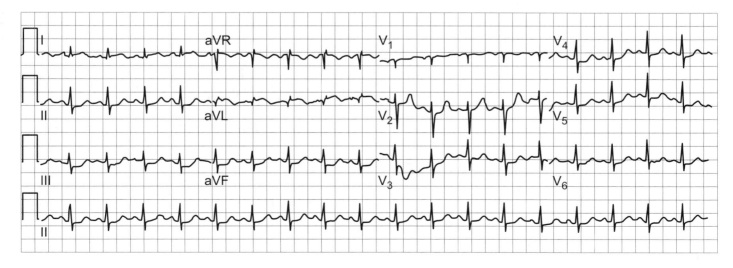

Fig. 33. Acute high lateral wall myocardial infarction in an 80-year-old woman interpreted as normal by computer electrocardiographic reading program.

- Initial R wave in leads V_1 and $V_2 \geq 0.04$ second with $R \geq S$ and ST-segment depression and upright T wave in anterior precordial leads
- Usually associated with inferior MI

g. Anterolateral infarction, probably old or age indeterminate

- See above, no ST elevation

h. Anterior infarction, probably old or age indeterminate

- See above, no ST elevation

i. Anteroseptal infarction, probably old or age indeterminate

- See above, no ST elevation

j. Lateral or high lateral infarction, probably old or age indeterminate

- See above, no ST elevation

k. Inferior (diaphragmatic) infarction, probably old or age indeterminate

- See above, no ST elevation

l. Posterior infarction, probably old or age indeterminate

- See above, no ST changes

m. Probable ventricular aneurysm

- Persistent ST-segment elevation of ≥ 1 mm in one or more leads with associated Q waves. The patient must be ≥ 1 month after infarction to make this diagnosis on basis of electrocardiography

12. ST-, T-, and U-Wave Abnormalities

a. Normal variant, early repolarization

- Some degree of ST elevation is present in most young, healthy individuals, especially in the precordial leads

Suggested by the following:

- Elevated takeoff of ST segment at J junction with QRS
- Distinct notch or slur on downstroke of R wave
- *Upward* concavity of ST segment
- Symmetrically limbed T waves, which are often of large amplitude
- Most commonly involves leads V_2 through V_5, rarely V_6

Sometimes also seen in leads II, III, and aVF

- No reciprocal changes

b. Normal variant, juvenile T waves
Suggested by the following:

- Persistence of negative T wave in leads V_1 through V_3
- Most frequent in young, healthy females
- Usually not symmetrical or deep
- T waves still upright in left precordial leads I, II

c. Nonspecific ST- or T-wave abnormalities
Suggested by any of the following:

- Slight ST depression or elevation
- T wave flat, low, or slightly inverted. T wave normally should be at least 0.5 mm in leads I and II

d. ST- or T-wave abnormalities suggesting myocardial ischemia
Ischemic T-wave changes

- Abnormally tall, symmetrical, upright T waves. QT usually prolonged, and there may be reciprocal changes

Differential diagnosis:

- Hyperkalemia—tall, peaked (tented), symmetrical (QT normal or short)
- Intracranial bleeding—QT long, prominent U waves
- Normal variant

- Symmetrically or deeply inverted T waves

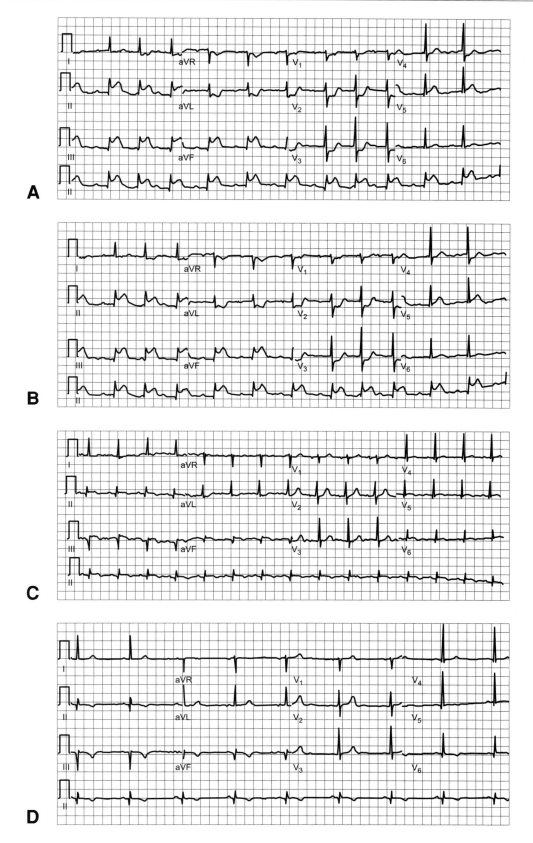

Fig. 34. Electrocardiograms obtained at presentation in 71-year-old man. *A,* With severe chest pain. *B,* Acute inferior-posterior myocardial infarction. ST changes in leads V_1 through V_3 represent posterior injury. *C,* Evolving inferior-posterior myocardial infarction 1 day after presentation. *D,* Inferior-posterior infarction 6 months after presentation.

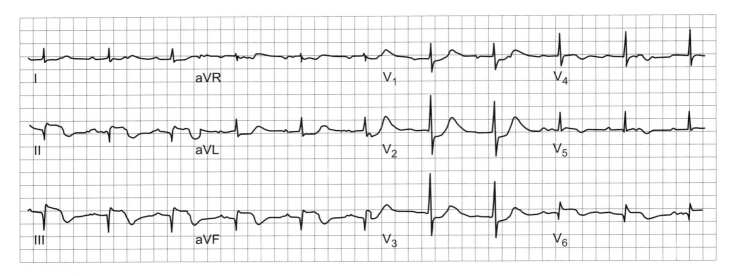

Fig. 35. Acute inferior-posterior-lateral myocardial infarction.

Differential diagnosis:

- Giant T inversion from Stokes-Adams attack
- Post-tachycardia T-wave inversion
- Apical hypertrophic cardiomyopathy
- Post-extrasystolic or pacemaker T-wave inversion
- Central nervous system disease (e.g., intracranial hemorrhage)

● Pseudonormalization of T waves during exercise

Ischemic ST-segment changes

● Horizontal or downsloping ST-segment depression with or without T-wave inversion
● Prinzmetal's angina typically manifests as ST elevation without Q waves

e. ST- or T-wave abnormalities suggesting myocardial injury

● Acute ST-segment elevation with upward convexity in the leads representing the area of infarction
● Reciprocal ST depression in the opposite leads
● Acute posterior injury often has horizontal or downsloping ST-segment depression with upright T waves in leads V_1 through V_3, with or without a prominent R wave in these same leads

f. ST- or T-wave abnormalities suggesting acute pericarditis (Fig. 36)
Four stages:
Stage 1: ST-segment elevation (upwardly concave) in almost all leads except aVR. No reciprocal changes
Stage 2: ST junction (J point) returns to the baseline and the T-wave amplitude begins to decrease
Stage 3: T waves are inverted
Stage 4: Electrocardiographic resolution
Other clues:

● PR depression early
● Low-voltage QRS with pericardial effusion (consider item **14o**)
● Electrical alternans (consider items **9e** and **14o**)
● Sinus tachycardia
● Regional pericarditis after acute MI (Fig. 37 through 39)
  - T waves should normally invert by 48 hours and slowly return to normal over several days to weeks
  - Abnormal T-wave evolution due to regional pericarditis is characterized by either persistently positive T waves or early reversal of normal T-wave inversion
Note: Also consider item **14p**

g. ST-segment or T-wave abnormalities due to intraventricular conduction disturbance or hypertrophy

- *Left ventricular hypertrophy*

  - ST-segment depression with upward convexity and T-wave inversion in left precordial leads
  - Reciprocal changes in right precordial leads
  - In limb leads, ST- and T-wave vectors usually opposite QRS vector

- *Right ventricular hypertrophy:* ST-segment depression and T-wave inversion in right precordial leads (V_1 through V_3) and sometimes in inferior leads (II, III, aVF)

- *LBBB:* ST-segment and T-wave displacement opposite the major QRS deflection

- *RBBB*

  - Uncomplicated RBBB has little ST displacement
  - T-wave vector is opposite terminal slowed portion of QRS. Upright in leads I, V_5, and

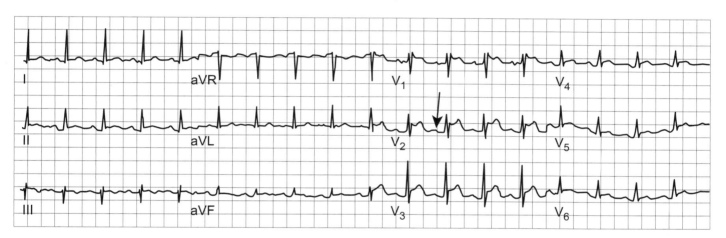

Fig. 36. Acute pericarditis with PR segment depression (*arrow*).

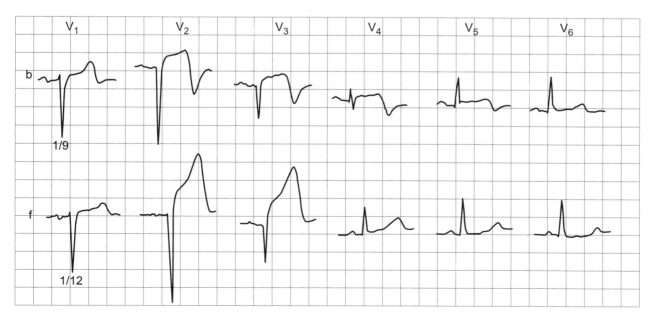

Fig. 37. Regional pericarditis after acute myocardial infarction.

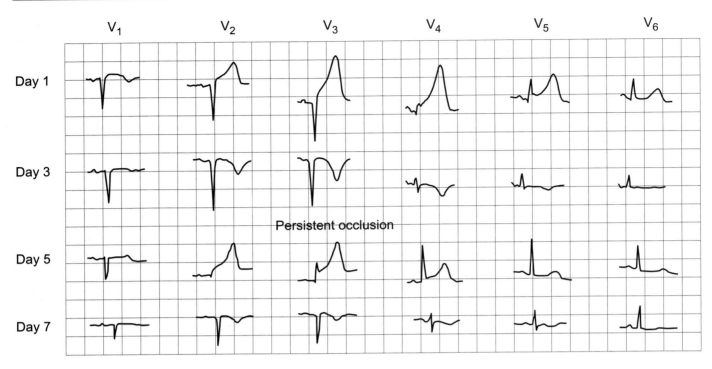

Fig. 38. Normal T-wave evolution after acute myocardial infarction.

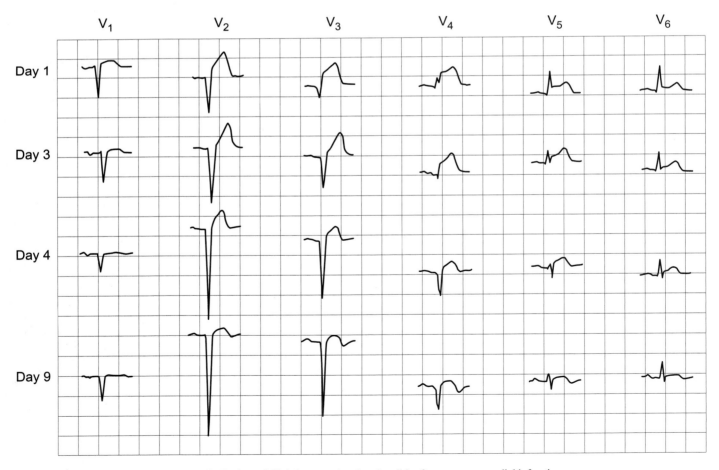

Fig. 39. Persistently positive T waves (leads V_2 through V_6) due to regional pericarditis after acute myocardial infarction.

V_6 and inverted in right precordial leads

h. Post-extrasystolic T-wave abnormality
Any alteration in contour, amplitude, or direction of T wave in sinus beat(s) after ectopic beat(s)

i. Isolated J-point depression

- Most frequent in exercise testing
- In normals, ST segment should be within 1 mm of the isoelectric line by 0.08 second after the J point

j. Peaked T waves
Require either of the following:

- T wave > 6 mm in limb leads
- T wave > 10 mm in precordial leads

Differential diagnosis:

- Acute MI. Also see prolonged QT interval

(item **12k**). Consider item **12e**
- Normal variant. Most commonly mid-precordial leads. May be > 10 mm
- Hyperkalemia. QT normal. Consider item **14e**
- Intracranial bleeding. QT prolonged. Prominent U waves. Consider item **14s**

k. Prolonged QT interval (Fig. 40)

- QT interval varies inversely with heart rate
- Measure lead with a large T wave and distinct termination
- Corrected QT interval = QT_c. $QT_c = QT \div$ the square root of the RR interval (normal, < 0.42 second)

Easier methods:

- Use 0.40 second as the normal QT interval for heart rate of 70 beats/min. For every 10 beats/min change in heart rate from 70 beats/min, adjust by 0.02 second

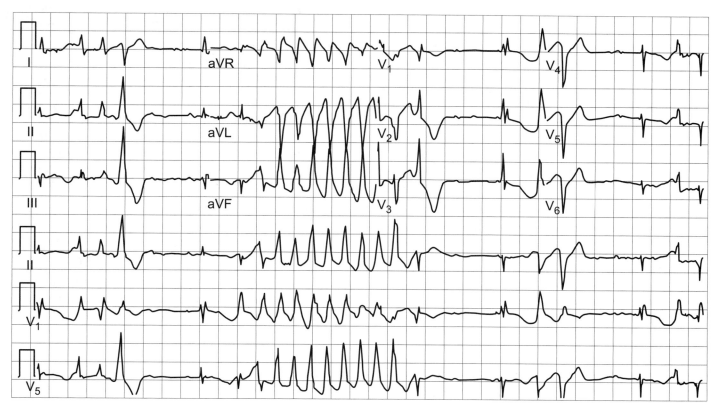

Fig. 40. Complete heart block, right bundle branch block, QT prolongation, and polymorphic ventricular tachycardia in a 76-year-old woman with acute myocardial infarction.

appropriately. Measured value should be within ± 0.07 second of the calculated normal. (Example: For a heart rate of 100 beats/min, the calculated "normal" QT interval would be 0.34; for a heart rate of 50 beats/min, the calculated "normal" QT interval would be 0.44.)
- Should be less than half the RR interval

Note: Also consider items **14c, 14d, 14h, 14s,** and **14u**

l. Prominent U waves

- Largest in leads V_2 and V_3
- Normally 5% to 25% of T wave
- Considered large when amplitude is ≥ 1.5 mm

13. **Pacemaker Function and Rhythm**

a. Atrial or coronary sinus pacing

- Pacemaker stimulus followed by atrial depolarization

b. Ventricular demand pacing

- Pacemaker stimulus followed by a QRS complex of different morphology than intrinsic QRS
- Must demonstrate *inhibition* of pacemaker output in response to intrinsic QRS

c. AV sequential pacing

- Atrial followed by ventricular pacing
- Could be DVI, DDD, DDI, or DOO pacing mode

d. Ventricular pacing, fixed rate (asynchronous)

- Ventricular pacing with no demonstrable output inhibition by intrinsic QRS complexes

e. Dual-chamber, atrial-sensing pacemaker

- DDD and possibly VAT or VDD
- For atrial sensing, need to demonstrate inhibition of atrial output or triggering of ventricular stimulus in response to intrinsic atrial depolarization (Fig. 41)

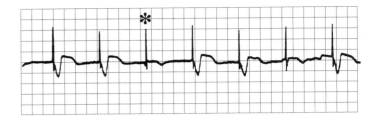

Fig. 41. Rhythm strip demonstrates pseudofusion beat (*asterisk*) and fusion beat (sixth pacing stimulus). (From Giuliani ER, Gersh BJ, McGoon MD, Hayes DL, Schaff HV [editors]: *Mayo Clinic Practice of Cardiology.* Third edition. Mosby, 1996, p 957. By permission of Mayo Foundation.)

f. Pacemaker malfunction, not constantly capturing (atrium or ventricle) (Fig. 42)

- Failure of pacemaker stimulus to be followed by depolarization
- Rule out pseudomalfunction (e.g., pacer stimulus falling into refractory period)

g. Pacemaker malfunction, not constantly sensing (atrium or ventricle) (Fig. 43)

- For pacemakers in inhibited mode, it is failure of pacemaker to be inhibited by an appropriate intrinsic depolarization
- For pacemakers in triggered mode, it is failure of pacemaker to be triggered by an appropriate intrinsic depolarization
- Watch for pseudomalfunction

Premature depolarizations may not be sensed if:

- They fall within the programmed refractory period of the pacemaker
- They have insufficient amplitude at the sensing electrode site

Note: Any stimulus falling within the QRS complex probably does not represent sensing malfunction. Common with right ventricular electrodes in RBBB

h. Pacemaker malfunction, not firing (Fig. 44)

- Failure of appropriate pacemaker output

i. Pacemaker malfunction, slowing

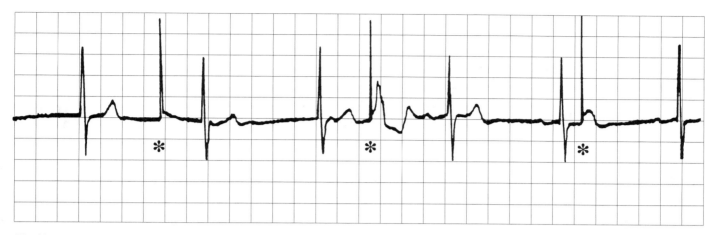

Fig. 42. VVI pacing with failure to capture (*first asterisk*), normal capture (*second asterisk*), and functional noncapture (*third asterisk*) because pacing artifact occurs during ventricular refractoriness. (From Giuliani ER, Gersh BJ, McGoon MD, Hayes DL, Schaff HV [editors]: *Mayo Clinic Practice of Cardiology.* Third edition. Mosby, 1996, p 956. By permission of Mayo Foundation.)

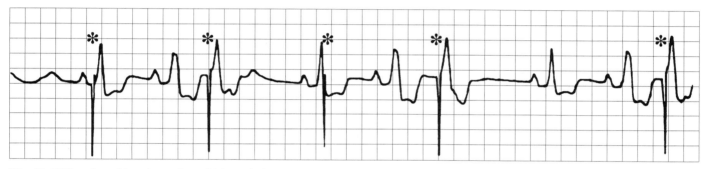

Fig. 43. VVI pacing with undersensing, which results in potentially undesirable competitive ventricular stimulation (*first and fourth asterisks*). (From Giuliani ER, Gersh BJ, McGoon MD, Hayes DL, Schaff HV [editors]: *Mayo Clinic Practice of Cardiology.* Third edition. Mosby, 1996, p 956. By permission of Mayo Foundation.)

- An increase in stimulus intervals over the programmed intervals
- Usually an indicator of end of battery life
- Often noted first during magnet application

14. **Suggested or Probable Clinical Disorders**

   a. Digitalis effect
   Suggested by the following:

- Sagging ST-segment depression with upward concavity
- Decreased T-wave amplitude; T wave may be biphasic
- QT shortening
- Increased U-wave amplitude
- Lengthened PR interval

In left or right ventricular hypertrophy or BBB, ST changes are difficult to interpret, but if typical sagging ST segments are present and QT is shortened, consider digitalis effect

   b. Digitalis toxicity (Fig. 45)

- Almost any type of cardiac arrhythmia resulting from either a disturbance in impulse formation or an impairment of conduction, except BBB
- Typical abnormalities include:

    - Paroxysmal atrial tachycardia with block
    - Atrial fibrillation with complete heart block
    - Bidirectional tachycardia
    - Second- or third-degree AV block with digitalis effect

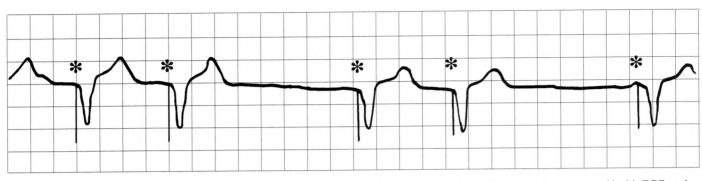

Fig. 44. Oversensing, resulting in an inappropriate, irregular pacemaker bradycardia. It is impossible to tell what is being oversensed in this ECG tracing. (From Giuliani ER, Gersh BJ, McGoon MD, Hayes DL, Schaff HV [editors]: *Mayo Clinic Practice of Cardiology.* Third edition. Mosby, 1996, p 958. By permission of Mayo Foundation.)

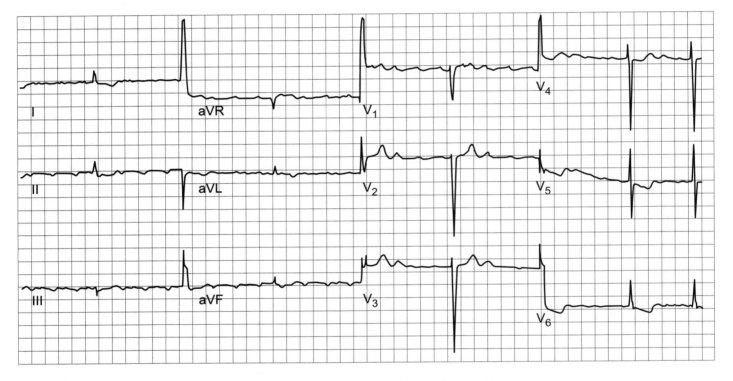

Fig. 45. Paroxysmal atrial tachycardia with atrioventricular block due to digitalis toxicity in a 79-year-old man.

- Complete heart block with accelerated junctional or idioventricular rhythm

c. Antiarrhythmic drug effect
Suggested by the following:

- Decrease in the amplitude of the T wave or T-wave inversion
- ST-segment depression
- Prominent U waves—one of the earliest findings
- Prolongation of the QT_c interval

- Notching and widening of the P waves
- Decrease in the atrial flutter rate

d. Antiarrhythmic drug toxicity
Suggested by the following:

- Widening of the QRS
- Various degrees of AV block
- Ventricular arrhythmias—"torsades de pointes"
- Marked sinus bradycardia, sinus arrest, or sinoatrial block

e. Hyperkalemia (Fig. 46)
Potassium value 5.5-7.5 mEq/L

- Reversible left anterior fascicular block or left posterior fascicular block
- Tall, peaked, narrow-based T waves

Potassium value 7.5-10.0 mEq/L

- First-degree AV block
- Flattening and widening of P waves, later disappearance of P waves ("sinoventricular conduction") or sinus arrest
- ST-segment depression

Potassium value > 10.0 mEq/L

- LBBB, RBBB, markedly widened, diffuse intraventricular conduction delay
- Ventricular tachycardia or fibrillation, idioventricular rhythm

f. Hypokalemia
Suggested by the following:

- Prominent U waves
- ST-segment depression, decreased T-wave amplitude
- Increase in amplitude and duration of the P wave
- Cardiac arrhythmias and AV block may be digitalis-related

g. Hypercalcemia

- Major ECG change is shortened QT_c
- Little effect on QRS, P, and T waves. May see PR interval prolongation

h. Hypocalcemia

- Earliest and most common finding is prolongation of QT_c. Results from ST-segment prolongation

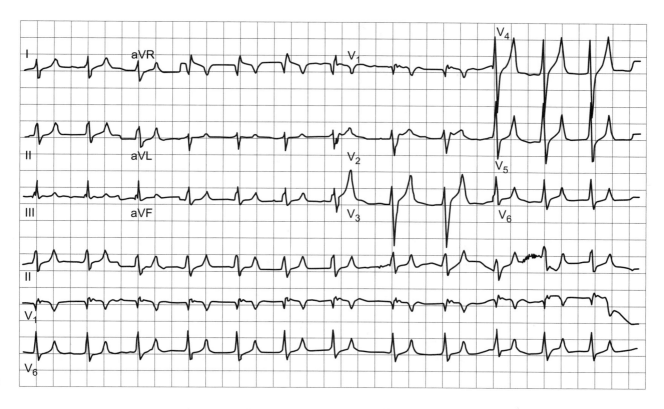

A

Fig. 46. *A*, Unresponsive 35-year-old man with insulin-dependent diabetes and hyperkalemia (potassium, 6.4 mEq/L). *B* and *C*, Asymptomatic 66-year-old man with hyperkalemia (potassium: *B*, 6.0 mEq/L; *C*, 9.2 mEq/L).

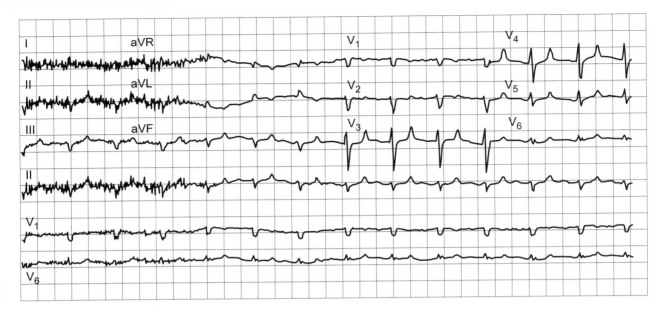

B

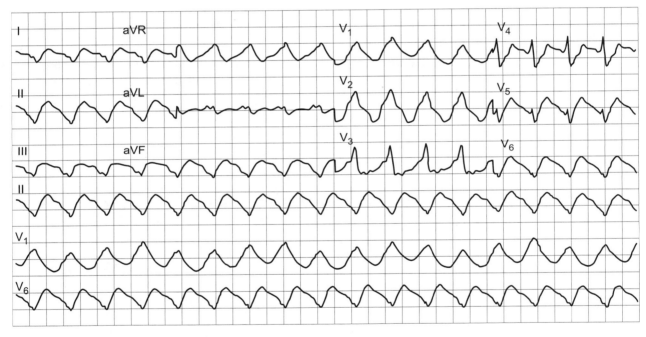

C

- ST-segment prolongation occurs without changing the duration of the T waves. Only hypothermia and hypocalcemia do this
- There can be flattening, peaking, or inversion of T waves

i. Atrial septal defect, secundum (Fig. 47) Suggested by the following:

- Typical RSR´ or rSR´ in V₁ with duration < 0.11 second. Right ventricular conduction

delay in 90%, most are incomplete RBBB
- Right-axis deviation due to right ventricular hypertrophy
- Right atrial enlargement in 36%
- PR interval prolonged in < 20%

j. Atrial septal defect, primum (Fig. 48) Suggested by the following:

- Most have left-axis deviation (in contradistinction to right-axis deviation in secundum atrial

septal defect)
- PR interval prolongation 15% to 40%
- Far-advanced cases have biventricular hypertrophy

k. Dextrocardia, mirror image (Fig. 49)
Suggested by the following:

- Decreasing R-wave amplitude from leads V_1 to V_6
- The P, QRS, and T waves in leads I and aVL are inverted, or "upside down"

- Be wary of lead malposition producing similar findings in leads I and aVL but not in V_1 through V_6

l. Mitral valve disease

- Mitral stenosis

    - No diagnostic findings
    - Combination of right ventricular hypertrophy and left atrial abnormality is suggestive

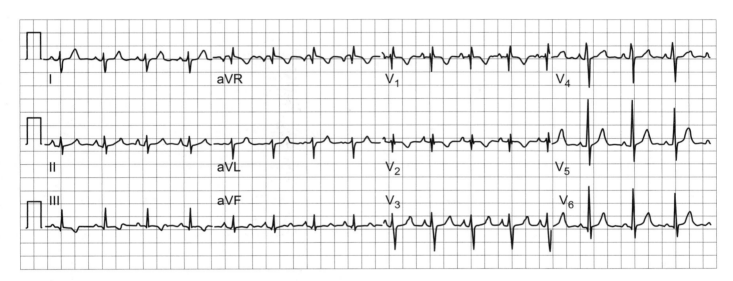

Fig. 47. Right-axis deviation and RSR´ in lead V_1 with duration less than 0.11 second in 6-year-old girl with secundum atrial septal defect.

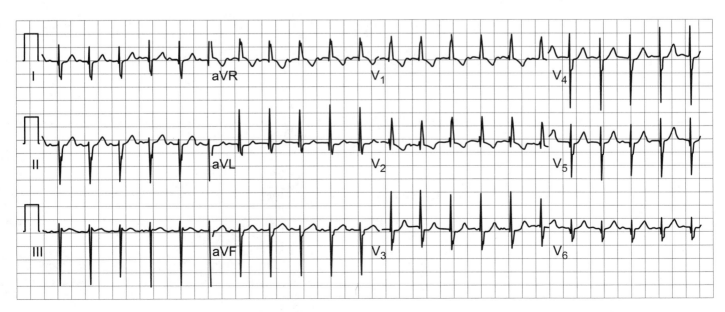

Fig. 48. Left-axis deviation and RSR´ in lead V_1 with duration less than 0.11 second in 1-year-old boy with primum atrial septal defect.

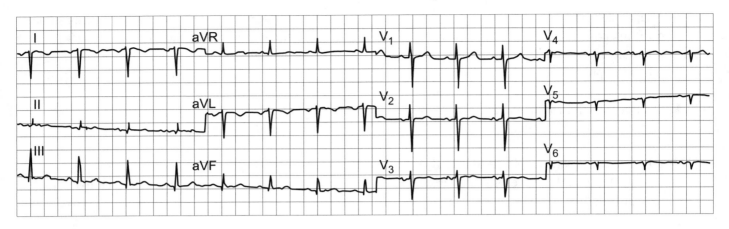

Fig. 49. Dextrocardia.

● Mitral valve prolapse

May see any of the following:

- Flattened or inverted T waves in leads II,
  III, and aVF with or without ST-segment
  depression (sometimes left precordial leads). T-
  wave changes in the right precordial
  leads can be associated with prolapse of leaflets
- Prominent U waves, QT prolongation

m. Chronic lung disease
Suggested by any of the following:

● Right ventricular hypertrophy
● Right-axis deviation
● Right atrial abnormality
● Shift of transitional zone counterclockwise
● Low voltage
● Pseudo-anteroseptal infarct

Right ventricular hypertrophy in the setting of
chronic lung disease:

● Rightward shift of QRS
● T-wave abnormalities in right precordial leads
● ST depression inferiorly
● Transient RBBB
● rSR′ or QR in V_1

n. Acute cor pulmonale, including pulmonary
embolus (Fig. 50)
● ECG abnormalities are frequently transient

● Sinus tachycardia most common
● Findings consistent with right ventricular
pressure overload:

- Right atrial abnormality
- Inverted T waves in leads V_1 through V_3
- Right-axis deviation
- $S_1 Q_3$ and $S_1 Q_3 T_3$ patterns
- Pseudoinfarct pattern in inferior leads
- Transient RBBB
- Various supraventricular tachyarrhythmias

o. Pericardial effusion (Fig. 25)
Suggested by either of the following:

● Low-voltage QRS (consider items **9a** and **9b**)
● Electrical alternans (consider item **9e**)

p. Acute pericarditis
● Refer to item **12f** for criteria

q. Hypertrophic cardiomyopathy (Fig. 51 and 52)
Suggested by the following:

● Left atrial abnormality common
● Majority of cases have abnormal QRS

- Left-axis deviation in 20%
- High-voltage QRS
- Large abnormal Q waves can give pseudoinfarct
  patterns in inferior, lateral, and precordial leads
- Tall R wave in V_1 with inverted T waves
  simulating right ventricular hypertrophy

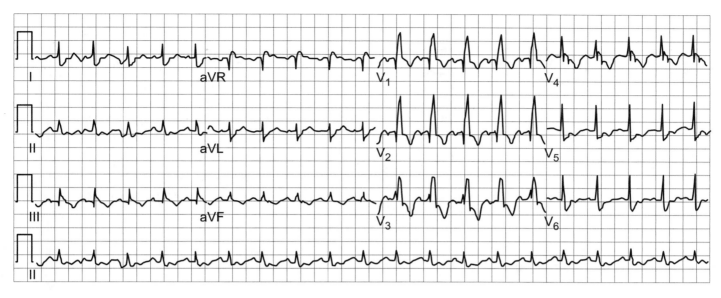

Fig. 50. Electrocardiogram in a 76-year-old man with massive pulmonary embolus.

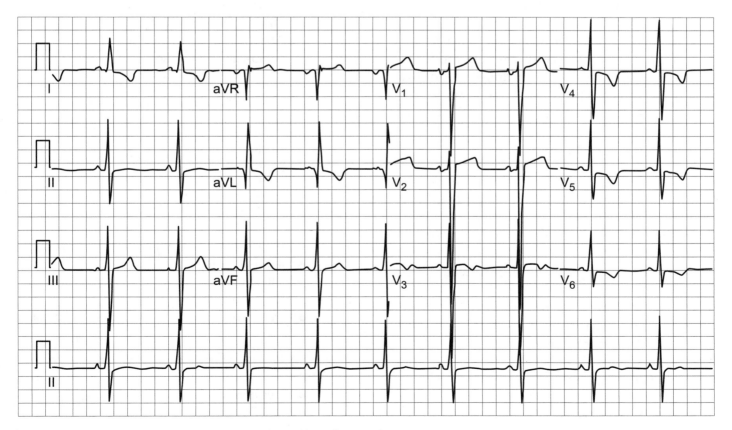

Fig. 51. Electrocardiogram in 21-year-old man with hypertrophic cardiomyopathy.

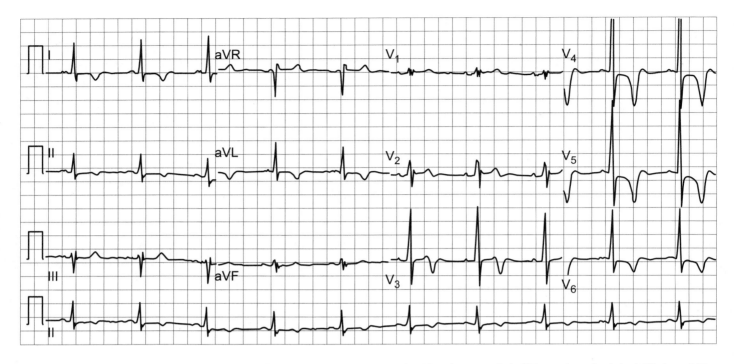

Fig. 52. Electrocardiogram in 72-year-old man with apical hypertrophic cardiomyopathy. Note deep symmetrical T-wave inversion in leads V_3 through V_6.

● ST-T wave abnormalities common

- ST-T wave changes due to ventricular hypertrophy or conduction abnormalities
- Apical variants of hypertrophic obstructive cardiomyopathy have deep lateral, precordial T-wave inversions

r. Coronary artery disease

● Use only when definitive evidence is present (such as acute infarct, diagnostic Q waves)

s. Central nervous system disorder (Fig. 53)

● "Classic changes," usually in precordial leads

- Large upright or deeply inverted T waves
- Prolonged QT interval
- Prominent U waves

● Other changes:

- T-wave notching, loss of amplitude
- Diffuse ST-segment elevation imitating

pericarditis or focal ST-segment elevation imitating acute myocardial injury pattern
- Abnormal Q waves imitating MI
- Almost any rhythm abnormality

Differential diagnosis:

- Acute MI
- Acute pericarditis
- Drug effect

t. Myxedema (Fig. 54)

● Low voltage of all complexes
● Sinus bradycardia
● Flattening or inversion of the T waves
● PR interval may be prolonged
● Frequently associated with pericardial effusion

u. Hypothermia (Fig. 55)

● Sinus bradycardia
● PR, QRS, and QT prolongation
● J waves that may be quite prominent

(Osborne, or "camel-hump" sign)
- 50% to 60% have atrial fibrillation
- Other arrhythmias occur

v. Sick sinus syndrome
Frequently manifests as one or more of the following:

- Sinus bradycardia of marked degree
- Sinus arrest or sinoatrial block
- Bradycardia alternating with tachycardia
- Atrial fibrillation with slow ventricular response preceded or followed by sinus bradycardia,

sinus arrest, sinoatrial block
- Prolonged sinus node recovery time after atrial premature complex or atrial tachyarrhythmias
- AV junctional escape rhythm
- Additional conduction system disease is often present

w. Ebstein's anomaly (Fig. 56)
- Characteristic RBBB with abnormal terminal forces (R' in lead V_1, S in I and aVL)

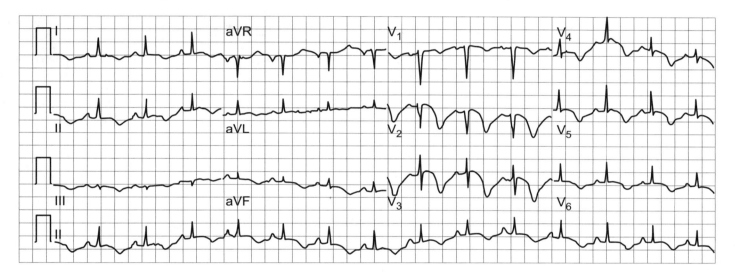

Fig. 53. Electrocardiogram in 65-year-old woman with acute subarachnoid hemorrhage.

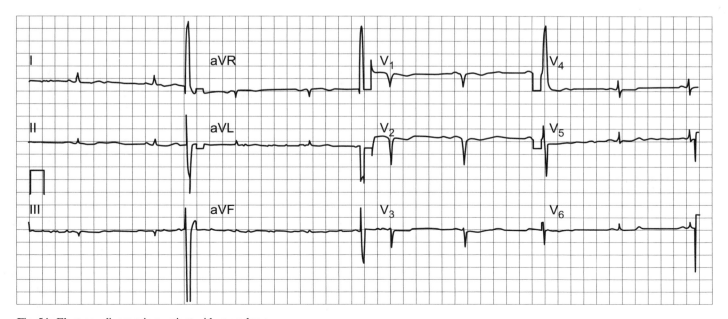

Fig. 54. Electrocardiogram in a patient with myxedema.

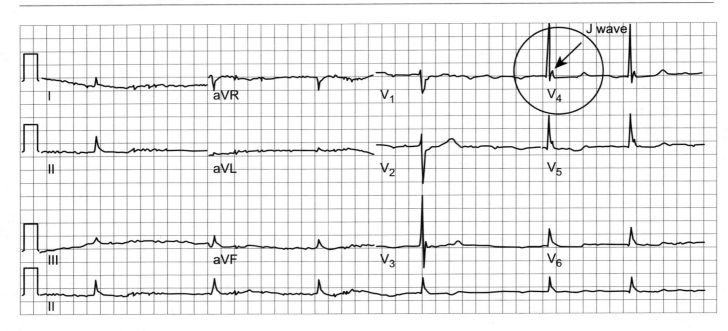

Fig. 55. Electrocardiogram in a 63-year-old woman with hypothermia.

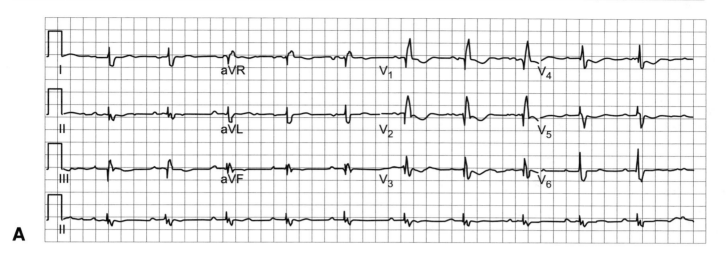

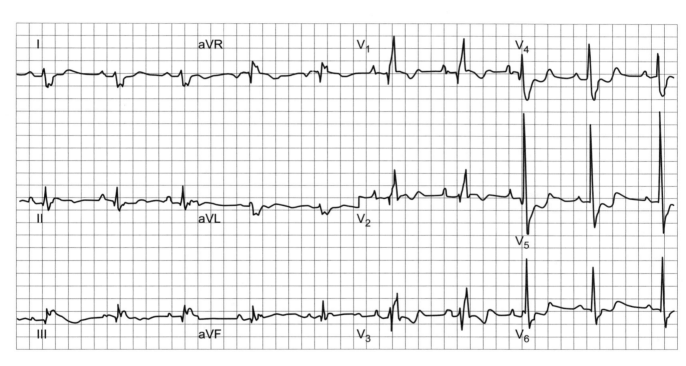

Fig. 56. Electrocardiograms from patients with Ebstein's anomaly. *A*, A 25-year-old man. *B*, A 10-year-old boy.

Notes

Chapter 35

Cardiac Cellular Electrophysiology

Win-Kuang Shen, M.D.

Advancements in molecular biology and cellular electrophysiologic techniques have significantly narrowed the gap in our understanding between single channel electrophysiology and clinical rhythm generation. This chapter reviews the basic cellular mechanisms of action potential generation together with the concepts of impulse formation and propagation.

Important topics for the Cardiology Boards include the mechanisms of clinical arrhythmias, including abnormal automaticity, triggered activity, and reentry. Questions about the effects of antiarrhythmic drugs on action potentials, the electrocardiogram, and rhythms, that is, drug-target interaction, are common. One should be familiar with the recent advancements in cellular electrophysiology and molecular biology of the long QT syndrome.

- The effects of antiarrhythmic drugs on the action potential are an important "examination" subject.
- Cellular electrophysiology and molecular biology of the congenital long QT syndrome are reasonable examination questions.

The Cardiac Action Potential

The cardiac action potential has a characteristic time course that depends on sequential changes in cell membrane permeability, which are due to activation and inactivation of ionic channels. The action potential is divided into five phases (0-4). These phases with their underlying ionic mechanisms are shown in Figure 1 and summarized in Table 1.

Several different types of action potential occur in the heart. The sinoatrial and atrioventricular nodes contain pacemaker cells and have slow upstroke velocity (10 to 15 V/s) and very slow spontaneous depolarization between action potentials (pacemaker depolarization); at the opposite end of the scale are ventricular action potentials that have a fast upstroke (200 to 400 V/s) and no spontaneous depolarization between action potentials. Atrial action potentials are similar to ventricular action potentials but of shorter duration. The action potentials of conducting cells such as Purkinje fibers look similar to ventricular action potentials but may displace spontaneous depolarization.

- The sinoatrial and atrioventricular nodes contain pacemaker cells and have slow upstroke velocity and very slow spontaneous depolarization between action potentials.
- Ventricular action potentials have a fast upstroke and no spontaneous depolarization between action potentials.

Phases of the Action Potential

Phase 0—Rapid membrane depolarization. Phase 0 of the action potential in atrial and ventricular cells is the result of increased sodium permeability, with a rapid inward sodium current (I_{Na}). In nodal cells, phase 0 is the result of increased calcium influx due to activation of calcium channels (I_{Ca}).

Table 1.—Summary of Cardiac Action Potential and Underlying Currents

Action potential phase	SA node	Atrial myocardium	AV node	Purkinje fiber	Ventricular myocardium
0					
Amplitude, mV	50-60	110-120	70-80	120	110-120
V_{max}, V/s	1-10	100-200	5-15	500-700	100-200
Currents	I_{Ca} I_{Na}	I_{Na}	I_{Ca} I_{Na}	I_{Na}	I_{Na}
1					
Overshoot, mV	...	30	...	30	30
Currents	...	I_{to}	...	I_{to} $I_{Cl\,(?)}$	I_{to} $I_{Cl\,(?)}$
2 and 3					
Currents	I_{Ca} I_K	I_{Ca} I_K I_{Kl}	I_{Ca} I_K	I_{Ca} I_K I_{Kl}	I_{Ca} I_K I_{Kl}
Action potential duration, ms	175-250	200-300	100-175	250-400	200-300
Propagation velocity, m/s	< 0.05	0.3-0.4	0.1	2-3	0.3-0.4
4					
Maximal diastolic potential, mV	-50 to -60	-80 to -90	-60 to -70	-90 to -95	-80 to -90
Spontaneous depolarization	+	-	+	+	-
Currents	I_{Ca} I_f*		I_{Ca} I_f*		

AV, atrioventricular; I_{Ca}, calcium current; I_{Cl}, chloride current; I_f, pacemaker current; I_K, delayed rectifier potassium current; I_{Kl}, inward current; I_{Na}, sodium current; I_{to}, transient outward current; SA, sinoatrial.
*Presence or absence depends on maximal diastolic potential.
From Giuliani ER, Gersh BJ, McGoon MD, Hayes DL, Schaff HV (editors): *Mayo Clinic Practice of Cardiology*. Third edition. Mosby, 1996, p 735. By permission of Mayo Foundation.

Phase 1—After the dominant action potential upstroke in atrial and ventricular cells, a brief phase of repolarization due to a transient outward current of potassium ions (I_{to}) temporarily returns the membrane potential toward normal.

Phase 2—Plateau phase. This relatively prolonged phase is the result of a delicate balance between a small outward membrane current and a slow inward current. The outward current is mediated by activation of a potassium-conducting ionic channel (I_K). The inward current is mediated by the slow inward calcium current (I_{Ca}). A striking feature of cardiac electrophysiology is that very few channels open during the plateau. The total conductance during the plateau region of the cardiac action potential is extremely low.

Phase 3—After the end of the plateau zone, repolarization occurs, during which time the membrane potential returns toward the resting level. This phase is due to continued inactivation of the slow inward calcium current and, more importantly, additional activation of outward-going potassium current (I_{Kl}) and the electrogenic sodium-potassium pump (I_p). It is important to note that the duration of the action potential can be influenced greatly by changes in calcium and/or potassium conductance during repolarization. Any factor that promotes potassium current activation will shorten the duration of the action potential. Conversely, the duration of the action potential is prolonged when outward-going potassium currents are inhibited. One of the potassium channels is the ATP-sensitive potassium channel (K_{ATP}), which is important during ischemic conditions. The K_{ATP} channel normally is inactive during physiologic conditions (the channel is inhibited by ATP under physiologic conditions). Under

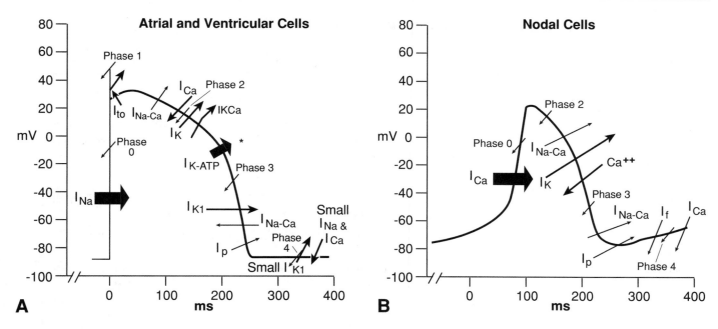

Fig. 1. The various phases of the action potential of, *A*, atrial and ventricular cells and, *B*, nodal cells. The underlying ionic mechanisms of each phase are described in the text. *Activated during ischemia.

conditions such as ischemia or hypoxia, the channel is activated when the intracellular ATP concentration is decreased. This leads to a shortening of action potential duration, presumably decreasing contraction and conserving energy. (A question related to the K_{ATP} channel could be on the Cardiology Boards.)

- The K_{ATP} channel normally is inactive during physiologic conditions (the channel is inhibited by ATP under physiologic conditions). Under conditions such as ischemia or hypoxia, the channel is activated when the intracellular ATP concentration is decreased.

Phase 4—The diastolic portion of the action potential varies. In atrial and ventricular muscle, no spontaneous diastolic depolarization occurs, primarily because of the activation of potassium current (the inward rectifier, I_{Kl}). During this time, the membrane potential is maintained near the equilibrium potential for potassium. In the nodal cells, I_{Kl} is not present. Spontaneous diastolic depolarization occurs as a result of the activation of the pacemaker current (I_f). This forms the basis of automaticity.

- Phase 0—rapid depolarization, the result of increased sodium permeability.
- Phase 1—a brief phase of repolarization due to a transient outward current of potassium ions (I_{to}).

- Phase 2—plateau phase, the result of a delicate balance between a small outward membrane current and a slow inward current.
- Phase 3—repolarization, which is due to inactivation of the slow inward calcium current, activation of the outward-going potassium current (I_{kl}), and the electrogenic sodium-potassium pump (I_p).
- Phase 4—diastolic portion of the action potential.
- Normal automaticity in the nodal cells is a net result of the absence of I_{kl} and the presence of I_f.
- In the nodal cells, I_{kl} is not present.

Mechanisms of Arrhythmias

Arrhythmias arise through three potential mechanisms: 1) disorders of impulse formation, 2) disorders of impulse conduction, and 3) mixed disorders. The classification of arrhythmogenic mechanisms, examples of clinical rhythms, ionic targets, and pharmacology are summarized in Table 2.

Disorders of Impulse Formation

Normal Automaticity
Normal automaticity is defined as spontaneous diastolic depolarization (phase 4 action potential) that occurs in cells with intrinsic automatic mechanisms, that is, normally the

Table 2.—Clinical Arrhythmias, Mechanisms, and Drug Actions

Arrhythmia	Mechanisms	Target mechanisms	Representative drugs
	Automaticity Enhanced normal		
Inappropriate sinus tachycardia		Phase 4 depolarization (decrease)	β-Adrenergic blocking agents
Some idiopathic ventricular tachycardias			Sodium channel blocking agents (block I_f)
	Abnormal		
Ectopic atrial tachycardia		Maximum diastolic potential (hyperpolarization) *or*	M_2 agonists (activate K_{Ach} channel)
		Phase 4 depolarization (decrease)	Calcium or sodium channel blocking agents
Accelerated idioventricular rhythms		Phase 4 depolarization (decrease)	Calcium or sodium channel blocking agents
	Triggered activity EAD		
Torsades de pointes		Action potential duration (shorten) or EAD (suppress)	Pacing, vagolytic agents (increase rate, shorten APD)
			Calcium channel blocking agents, Mg^{2+}, β-adrenergic blockers (suppress EAD)
	DAD		
Digitalis-induced arrhythmias		Calcium overload (unload) or DAD (suppress)	Calcium channel blockers
Certain autonomically mediated ventricular tachycardias		Calcium overload (unload) or DAD (suppress)	β-Adrenergic blockers Calcium channel blockers, adenosine
	Reentry (sodium-channel dependent) Long excitable gap		
Atrial flutter type I		Conduction and excitability (depress)	Atrium: sodium channel blockers (except lidocaine, mexiletine, tocainide)
Circus movement tachycardia in WPW		Conduction and excitability (depress)	Atrium/ventricle: sodium channel blockers
Sustained monomorphic ventricular tachycardia		Conduction and excitability (depress)	Ventricle: sodium channel blockers
	Short excitable gap		
Atrial flutter type II		Refractory period (prolong)	Potassium channel blockers
Atrial fibrillation		Refractory period (prolong)	Potassium channel blockers
Circus movement tachycardia in WPW		Refractory period (prolong)	Class III agents
Polymorphic and sustained monomorphic ventricular tachycardia		Refractory period (prolong)	Class I and III agents
Bundle branch reentry		Refractory period (prolong)	Class I and III agents
Ventricular fibrillation		Refractory period (prolong)	Class I and III agents

Table 2 (continued)

Arrhythmia	Mechanisms	Target mechanisms	Representative drugs
	Reentry (calcium-channel dependent)		
AV nodal reentrant tachycardia		Conduction and excitability (depress)	Calcium channel blockers
Circus movement tachycardia in WPW		Conduction and excitability (depress)	Calcium channel blockers
Verapamil-sensitive ventricular tachycardia		Conduction and excitability (depress)	Calcium channel blockers

APD, action potential duration; AV, atrioventricular; DAD, delayed afterdepolarization; EAD, early afterdepolarization; WPW, Wolff-Parkinson-White syndrome.
Modified from *Circulation* 84:1831-1851, 1991. By permission of the American Heart Association.

sinus node but occasionally in specialized atrial cells, in some regions of the atrioventricular junction, and in Purkinje fibers. These subsidiary pacemaker cells usually are depolarized by impulses propagated from the sinus node before they reach threshold spontaneously, whereas atrial and ventricular cells normally do not demonstrate automaticity.

Intrinsic automaticity is dependent on three major factors: 1) the slope and rate of phase 4 depolarization, which set the rate of impulse formation; 2) the threshold potential—the potential at which an action potential is initiated; and 3) the maximal diastolic potential—the potential from which phase 4 depolarization begins spontaneously. Any factor that slows the rate of phase 4 depolarization, makes the threshold more positive, or makes the maximal diastolic membrane potential more negative will slow the rate of spontaneous pacemaker depolarization. The ionic mechanisms responsible for phase 4 depolarization are discussed above. The many factors capable of influencing the slope and rate of phase 4 depolarization include autonomic mediators, acid-base changes, hypoxia, temperature, extracellular and intracellular ion concentrations, cardioactive medications, and degree of tissue stretch. These factors may act directly on the dominant pacemaker to slow or to accelerate heart rate or they may shift the dominant pacemaker either within the sinus node or to a subsidiary pacemaker.

- Intrinsic automaticity is dependent on three major factors: 1) the slope and rate of phase 4 depolarization, 2) the threshold potential, and 3) the maximal diastolic potential.

Abnormal Automaticity

Abnormal automaticity is defined as an alteration of the normal automatic mechanisms (enhanced automaticity in cells with intrinsic automatic mechanisms) or an occurrence of abnormal automatic mechanisms in cells that do not normally have intrinsic automatic mechanisms. Abnormal automaticity may be present in ischemic or other diseased cardiac tissues. Under experimental conditions, abnormal automaticity can occur by one of three mechanisms: 1) depolarized resting membrane potential (less negative membrane potential), 2) increased slope of diastolic depolarization (phase 4 of the action potential), and 3) more negative threshold membrane potential. Abnormal automaticity occurs most often when the resting membrane potential is partially depolarized, that is, in injured atrial or ventricular cells. When atrial and ventricular resting membrane potentials are decreased to less than - 60 mV, spontaneous depolarization may occur. At this membrane potential in partially depolarized fibers, the fast inward sodium current (I_{Na}) is inactivated, whereas the slow inward calcium current (I_{Ca}) mechanisms remain intact. In this setting, these slow inward currents may result in abnormal automaticity. These cellular mechanisms may also explain why some automatic arrhythmias respond to calcium channel blockers and β-blockers. Approximately 90% of specimens of chronically diseased atrial tissue and 50% of ventricular myocardial specimens obtained at operation may have spontaneous activity. Clinically, it has been shown that some ectopic atrial tachycardias and accelerated idioventricular rhythms are automatic.

- Abnormal automaticity occurs most often when the resting membrane potential is partially depolarized, that is, in injured atrial or ventricular cells.

- Clinically, it has been shown that some ectopic atrial tachycardias and accelerated idioventricular rhythms are automatic.

Triggered Activity/Afterdepolarizations

Another mechanism of arrhythmia generation that has received increasing attention is "triggered activity." This general term is used to describe arrhythmias originating in afterdepolarizations, the genesis of which is critically dependent on previous electrical activity of the heart. These afterdepolarizations, or "oscillatory afterpotentials," are referred to as "early afterdepolarizations" when they occur during phase 2 and phase 3 of the action potential and as "delayed afterdepolarizations" when they occur after complete repolarization (phase 4). The characteristics of each type of afterdepolarization are substantially different from one another.

During the repolarization phases of the action potential (phase 2 and phase 3), delay rectifiers (I_K) and inward rectifiers (I_{K1}) are the major components of outward potassium currents. The inward currents are primarily calcium (I_{Ca}) currents. Theoretically, early afterdepolarization can occur when outward currents are inhibited or inward currents are enhanced (Fig. 2). During phase 2 of the action potential, the membrane potential is reduced, and the calcium current could be responsible for the early afterdepolarization. During phase 3 of the action potential, the membrane potential is more negative than in phase 2, and the sodium current could be responsible for early afterdepolarization.

Because of these different mechanisms responsible for early afterdepolarization, it is not unexpected that the pharmacologic response may vary for triggered arrhythmias caused by early afterdepolarization. Early afterdepolarization may occur with the following (Table 3): hypokalemia, membrane depolarization, hypoxia, acidosis (with or without catecholamines), aconitine, veratridine (induced inward current), cesium (inhibits I_K), and antiarrhythmic agents such as sotalol, N-acetylprocainamide, and quinidine (inhibits I_K). Clinically, torsades de pointes is a form of polymorphic ventricular tachycardia that occurs in the setting of prolonged QT interval (Table 4 and Fig. 2). Early afterdepolarization can be suppressed with the following: increased potassium, acetylcholine (hyperpolarization of transmembrane potential), tetrodotoxin, and antiarrhythmic agents such as lidocaine and procainamide (suppressed sodium current), magnesium, calcium channel blockers, β-blockers (suppressed calcium currents), and potassium channel openers (enhanced potassium currents).

Table 3.—Factors That Influence Early Afterdepolarization

Factor	Increase	Decrease
Autonomic	↑ Sympathetic tone	↓ Sympathetic tone
	↑ Catecholamines	↓ Catecholamines
	↓ Parasympathetic tone	↑ Parasympathetic tone
Metabolic	↑ Hypoxia	↑ O_2
	↑ Acidosis	↓ Acidosis
Electrolytes	Cesium	K^+
	Hypokalemia	Mg^{2+}
Drugs and metabolites	Sotalol	Acetylcholine/adenosine
	N-acetylprocainamide	Lidocaine
	Quinidine	Procainamide
	Aconitine	Ca^{2+} channel blockers
	Veratridine	β-Blockers
		Tetrodotoxin
		K^+ channel openers
Heart rate	Slow	Fast

Delayed afterdepolarization (Fig. 3) may occur with the following: faster heart rate, cardiac glycosides, hypokalemia, hypercalcemia, and catecholamines. All these conditions lead to a final common pathway, namely, an increase in the intracellular concentration of calcium. The fluctuation in the increase in the intracellular calcium concentration has been correlated with activation of an inward ionic current. This current has been named the "transient inward current" (I_t). The ionic channel responsible for this current is thought to be a nonselective cation channel that can conduct either sodium or potassium ions. Under physiologic conditions, this channel predominately conducts sodium ions. The afterpotentials coupled to the oscillatory intracellular calcium concentration may eventually increase in amplitude, reach threshold, and produce a sustained arrhythmia. In contrast to early afterdepolarizations, these oscillating afterpotentials more likely are precipitated by shorter pacing cycle lengths or coupling intervals, producing an increase in the amplitude of the afterdepolarizations and triggered activity when the depolarization threshold is reached.

- Early afterdepolarization may occur with the following: hypokalemia, membrane depolarization, hypoxia, acid-

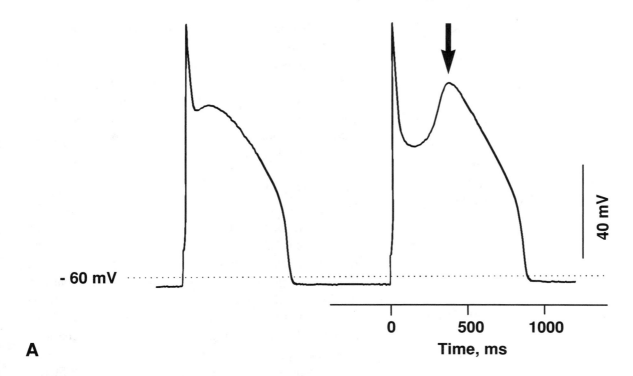

A

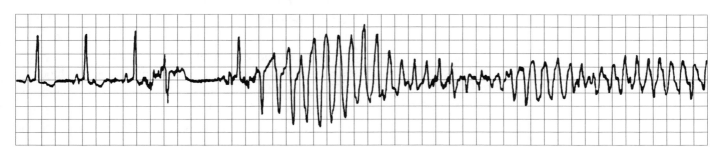

B

Fig. 2. A, Two consecutive action potentials recorded by the current clamp technique in the whole-cell patch configuration from paced single cardiomyocyte isolated from a canine left ventricle. *Arrow*, early afterdepolarization triggered spontaneously during plateau phase of repolarization. *B*, The long-short sequence initiating a run of torsades de pointes in patient with ischemic heart disease. The first beat of tachycardia occurred during repolarization of the cardiac cycle (within the T wave). (From *ACC Current Journal Review* 16-19, 1997. By permission of the American College of Cardiology.)

osis, sotalol, *N*-acetylprocainamide, and quinidine.
- Delayed afterdepolarization may occur with the following: faster heart rate, cardiac glycosides, hypokalemia, hypercalcemia, and catecholamines.

Clinical Significance of Triggered Arrhythmias

Early Afterdepolarizations
It has been proposed that early afterdepolarization may be the mechanism underlying torsades de pointes. In support of this hypothesis is the finding that these potentials are generated by conditions or drugs that are associated with clinical torsades de pointes. Furthermore, torsades de pointes has been reproduced in experimental animals by the administration of cesium, which also decreases outward potassium currents and produces early afterdepolarizations.

- It has been proposed that early afterdepolarization may be the mechanism underlying torsades de pointes.

Delayed Afterdepolarizations
Delayed afterdepolarizations and triggered activity may be

Table 4.—Conditions Associated With Torsades de Pointes

Electrolyte abnormality
  Hypokalemia
  Hypomagnesemia
  Hypocalcemia (rare)
Drug-related
  Antiarrhythmia agents: quinidine, procainamide,
    disopyramide, amiodarone, lidocaine, aprindine
  Psychotropic agents: phenothiazines, tricyclic
    antidepressants
  Organophosphate poisoning
Liquid protein diets
Cardiac disease
  Ischemia
  Myocarditis
  Bradycardia: sinus node disease, atrioventricular block
    with a slow escape rhythm
Central nervous system disease
  Intracranial trauma
  Subarachnoid hemorrhage
  Pneumoencephalography
Congenital syndromes
  Romano-Ward
  Jervell and Lange-Nielsen

From Giuliani ER, Gersh BJ, McGoon MD, Hayes DL, Schaff HV (editors): *Mayo Clinic Practice of Cardiology.* Third edition. Mosby, 1996, p 810. By permission of Mayo Foundation.

the underlying mechanism for arrhythmias that occur during digitalis toxicity, ischemia, increased catecholamines, hypokalemia, and hypercalcemia. Perhaps the most convincing observation that clinical arrhythmias are caused by delayed afterdepolarization is exercise-induced ventricular tachycardia in patients without overt cardiac disease (Fig. 3). This tachycardia is catecholamine-dependent and calcium-sensitive. Exercise-induced ventricular tachycardia frequently responds to adenosine, calcium channel blockers, and β-blockers. These pharmacologic agents decrease the intracellular concentration of calcium and, therefore, inhibit the transient inward current and suppress clinical tachycardia.

● Delayed afterdepolarizations and triggered activity may be the underlying mechanism for arrhythmias that occur during digitalis toxicity, ischemia, increased catecholamines, hypokalemia, and hypercalcemia. All these conditions lead to an increase in intracellular calcium concentration.

Arrhythmias Related to Abnormal Impulse Conduction

Arrhythmias related to reentry are more common than arrhythmias of abnormal automaticity and triggered activity. The mechanism of reentry involves three prerequisite conditions: 1) at least two functionally distinct conduction pathways, 2) unidirectional block in one pathway, and 3) slow conduction down the second pathway.

Two or More Functional Pathways for Conduction
During normal conditions and despite the existence of cross-connections between fibers of the conduction system, the direction of impulse propagation is mostly uniform. Reentry requires an alteration in the uniform propagation of the impulse, so that two or more limbs are present that join proximally and distally to form functional common pathways (Fig. 4). The pathways may be anatomically and/or functionally distinct, as seen in patients with accessory atrioventricular connections or in those with dual atrioventricular node pathways. Pathologic processes such as fibrosis or infarction may result in distinct conduction pathways joining together to form a closed loop.

Unidirectional Block in One Pathway
For reentry to occur, there must be unidirectional block in one pathway. This allows an impulse propagating antegradely down the second pathway to reenter the first pathway and to exit it in a retrograde fashion. Unidirectional block may be due to a structural condition or it may be functional, depending on the disparity in refractoriness in the two limbs.

Slow Conduction Down the Second Pathway
The third prerequisite is slow conduction. Conduction velocity is dependent on the threshold potential, the rate of depolarization of phase 0 of the action potential, the amplitude of the action potential, and the cellular resistance. Slow conduction may be due to decremental conduction, in which the amplitude of the impulse decreases progressively during the passage of the impulse through cardiac tissue. Such slow decremental conduction is seen in areas of the conduction system characterized by slow calcium currents, as in the atrioventricular node. Slow decremental conduction also can be seen in fibers that normally are dependent on fast channel responses but are exposed to ischemia or hypoxia. Slow conduction in one pathway allows recovery of the second pathway, so that retrograde conduction and reentry can occur.

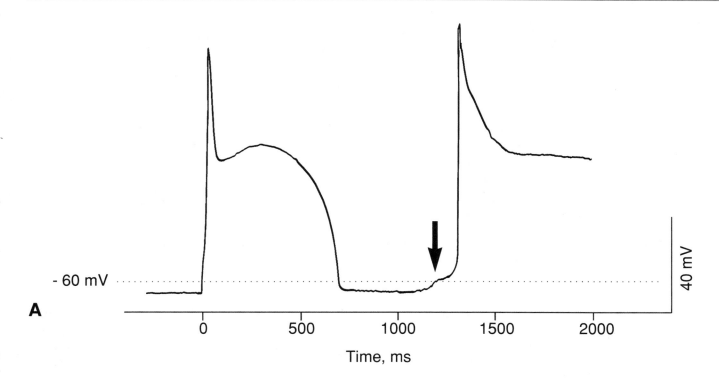

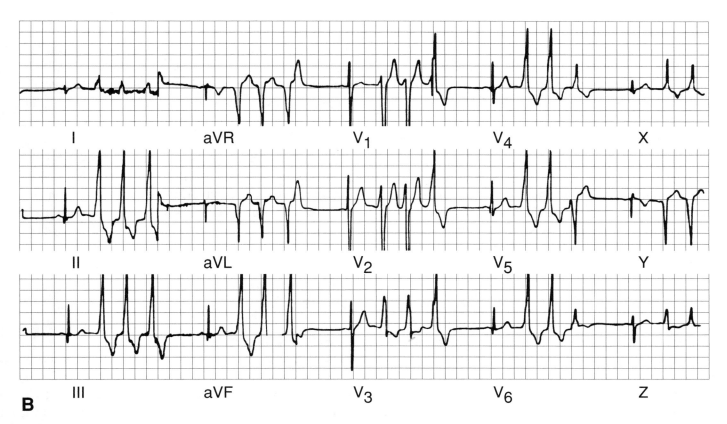

Fig. 3. *A*, With recording techniques similar to those mentioned in Figure 2*A*, a normal action potential is followed by a premature spontaneous depolarization that occurs after depolarization of the preceding action potential. Such a delayed afterdepolarization (arrow) triggered an aberrant action potential. *B*, Exercise-induced nonsustained ventricular tachycardia in a young man without any structural heart disease. The first beat of tachycardia was relatively late (after the T wave) during the cardiac cycle. The morphology (left bundle) and axis (inferior) suggest a right ventricular outflow tract origin. (*A* from *ACC Current Journal Review* 16-19, 1997. By permission of the American College of Cardiology.)

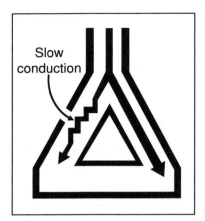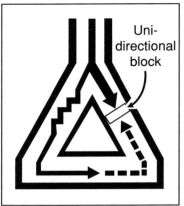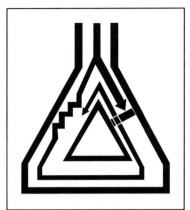

Fig. 4. Arrhythmogenic mechanism of reentry. The conditions for reentry are described in the text. (From Giuliani ER, Gersh BJ, McGoon MD, Hayes DL, Schaff HV [editors]: *Mayo Clinic Practice of Cardiology*. Third edition. Mosby, 1996, p 740. By permission of Mayo Foundation.)

Reentry can occur at any level within the conduction system and can be macroreentry with a large anatomical loop, as in patients with classic preexcitation with accessory atrioventricular pathways. Regardless of the location and size of the pathway, the requisite requirements are the same. In patients with dual atrioventricular node pathways and atrioventricular nodal reentrant tachycardia, the slow conduction pathway usually has a rapid recovery (shorter refractory period). The fast conduction pathway usually has a slower recovery (longer refractory period). Under normal conditions, all conduction is down the fast pathway, and this results in a normal PR interval. However, with an atrial premature contraction, the fast pathway is unexcitable (unidirectional block), but the impulse can propagate, with a delay, down the slow pathway, the result being PR prolongation. With the right circumstances, the impulse then can propagate retrogradely up the fast pathway and give rise to an atrial echo. Sustained reentry results when critical timing exists that allows the impulse to return to the ventricle via the slow pathway.

- Reentry can occur at any level within the conduction system and can be macroreentry with a large anatomical loop, as in patients with classic preexcitation with accessory atrioventricular pathways.

Although reentry around an anatomical obstacle undoubtedly is the mechanism for many arrhythmias, a fixed barrier does need to be present. In these cases, a reentrant arrhythmia may circle an area of functional block that is disseminated in time and space. Such a mechanism has been demonstrated in rabbit atrial myocardium, in which, in the absence of a fixed inexcitable central obstacle, the center of a circuit movement may be invaded by multiple centripetal wavelets converging on and producing block at the center of the circuit. This mechanism, known as "a leading circle" concept, may also be responsible for some clinical rhythm disorders.

Abnormal Impulse Formation and Conduction

Abnormalities of impulse conduction and impulse formation can coexist and lead to clinical arrhythmias. Parasystolic rhythms are thought to result from a focus of myocardial cells that are undergoing cyclic diastolic depolarization and varying rates. These arrhythmias are characterized by abnormal conduction of normal cardiac impulses into the focus ("entrance block") or by abnormal impulses that leave the focus ("exit block") or both. This abnormal conduction may be caused by localized changes in the diastolic potential in the myocardium surrounding the focus and in the focus itself.

Molecular Biology of Cardiac Ion Channels

The Ionic Channel Proteins

Most cardiac channel proteins consist of individual subunits or groups of subunits, with each subunit containing six hydrophobic transmembrane regions (Plate 1). The sodium and calcium channels comprise a single (alpha) subunit containing four internally homologous domains, each composed of six transmembrane segments. The voltage-activated potassium channels are structurally more complex. The genes for the voltage-activated potassium channels encode proteins for only a single subunit containing six transmembrane segments. Four separate subunits are assembled to form a functional voltage-gated potassium channel. The molecular structure of another class of potassium channels, the inward rectifying potassium-selective channels, was recently defined. These channels conduct potassium current much more effectively into the cells than out of the cells. However, the outward current conducted by these channels is physiologically important to maintain the transmembrane potential at rest. Each subunit of the inward rectifying potassium channels contains only two transmembrane-spanning regions. However, a functional inward rectifier is assembled by different combinations of subunits, regulatory proteins (i.e., G proteins), and interactions with other proteins.

- The sodium and calcium channels consist of a single (alpha) subunit.
- Four separate subunits are assembled to form a functional voltage-gated potassium channel.

Inherited "Channelopathies"
Major advances have been made in the molecular biology of the congenital long QT syndromes in recent years. The molecular basis for other potential familial rhythm disorders, including idiopathic ventricular fibrillation and familial atrial fibrillation, is being investigated.

Familial Long QT Syndromes
The phenotypical and genotypical characteristics of familial long QT syndromes are summarized in Table 5. Linkage analysis studies have demonstrated significant genotype heterogeneity in the Romano-Ward long QT syndrome. Currently, at least five gene locations have been linked to the congenital long QT syndrome and more than 40 mutations have been identified.

The first gene linked to the long QT syndrome (LQT1) is located on chromosome 11 and was recently confirmed to be the *KVLQT1* gene. The product of the *KVLQT1* gene is the potassium channel that is a component of I_{Ks}. The second gene, located on chromosome 7 (LQT2), encodes the HERG cardiac potassium channel and is functionally related to the I_{Kr} outward potassium current. The third gene (*SCN5A*) is located on chromosome 3 (LQT3) and encodes the alpha subunit of the cardiac sodium channel (I_{Na}). Functionally, mutations at this gene location appear to impair the inactivation of sodium channels, presumably leading to an enhanced inward current during the repolarization of the cardiac cycle. The fourth gene is located on chromosome 4 (LQT4), but its functional component has not been identified. The fifth gene, located on chromosome 21 (LQT5) encodes the β-subunit (minK of the I_{Ks}). It has been estimated that the first three genetic defects can account for up to 90% of the clinical Romano-Ward long QT syndrome. A recent study reported that homozygous mutation of *KVLQT1*

Table 5.—Familial Long QT Syndromes

Clinical syndrome	Chromosomal location	Ionic channel	Comments
Romano-Ward			Autosomal dominant
LQT1	11p15.5	*KVLQT1* (I_{Ks})	Most common clinical long QT syndrome (30%-50%)
LQT2	7q35-36	*HERG* (I_{Kr})	Symptoms related to stress, catecholamine-sensitive
LQT3	3p21-24	*SCN5A* (I_{Na})	Altered channel inactivation, symptoms are more bradycardia-dependent
LQT4	4q25-27	?	Defect may be a regulatory enzyme for channel function
LQT5	21q22.1-22.2	*KCNE* (1 β-subunit minK of I_{Ks})	Homozygous mutation with *KVLQT1* results in Jervell and Lange-Nielsen syndrome
LQT6 and others	?	?	
Jervell and Lange-Nielsen			Autosomal recessive, deafness
JNL	11p15.5 21q22.1-22.2	*KVLQT1* (I_{Ks}) *KCNE1*(minK)	Homozygous

and the minK causes the Jervell and Lange-Nielsen syndrome.

- At least five gene locations have been linked to the congenital long QT syndrome and more than 40 mutations have been identified.

Attempts have been made to correlate electrocardiographic patterns in patients who have long QT syndrome with a specific genetic defect. Qualitatively, T waves are broad-based and enlarged in amplitude in LQT1 (chromosome 11, I_{Ks} defect), are low in amplitude in LQT2 (chromosome 7, I_{Kr} defect), and have the T-wave late onset but normal duration and amplitude in LQT3 (chromosome 3, a sodium channel defect).

- T waves are broad-based and enlarged in LQT1, have low amplitude in LQT2, and have late onset but normal duration and amplitude in LQT3.

Preliminary observations from pharmacologic interventions targeting the specific genetic defects in long QT syndrome are encouraging. Mexiletine (a sodium channel blocker) increased the heart rate significantly and shortened the QT interval in patients with LQT3 compared with those with LQT2, suggesting that patients with LQT3 may be more likely to benefit from sodium channel blockers and pacing. In patients with LQT2, abnormalities in QT interval and T-wave morphology were corrected after potassium supplementation when serum potassium was increased. These observations support the concept that activation of I_{Kr} is dependent on the extracellular potassium concentration and that potassium supplementation and potassium channel openers may be more beneficial for patients with LQT2.

- Patients with LQT3 may more likely benefit from sodium channel blockers and pacing.
- Potassium supplementation and potassium channel openers may be more beneficial for patients with LQT2.

The relationship between sympathetic activation of clinical arrhythmias and symptoms is complex in patients with long QT syndromes. It has been suggested that clinical events such as syncope and cardiac arrest occur more frequently under conditions of sudden emotional or physical stress in patients with LQT2 and more frequently during sleep or rest in those with LQT3. These differences in clinical presentation may be explained by the inability to shorten the QT interval under sympathetic challenge because of a defect in I_{Kr} in patients with LQT2. It is tempting to suggest that β-adrenergic blocker therapy may be more beneficial for patients with LQT2. Because I_{Kr} is functionally intact in LQT3, shortening of the QT interval in response to a sympathetic activation would be expected.

- Syncope and cardiac arrest occur more frequently under conditions of sudden emotional or physical stress in patients with LQT2 and more frequently during sleep or rest in those with LQT3.

Idiopathic Ventricular Fibrillation

Idiopathic ventricular fibrillation is defined as cardiac arrest in the absence of any structural heart disease or any other identifiable cause of ventricular fibrillation. Recently, a distinct group of patients with idiopathic ventricular fibrillation has been identified. They have electrocardiographic (ECG) features of ST-segment elevation and repolarization abnormalities mimicking an atypical right bundle branch block pattern (Brugada syndrome). Genotypical defects have been located in the *SCN5A* gene encoding the sodium channel. Functionally, more rapid inactivation or nonfunctional sodium channel activities have been characterized (Table 6).

Familial Atrial Fibrillation

Although the clinical entity of familial atrial fibrillation has not been precisely defined, genetic studies have been performed recently in a large family with many members who have lone atrial fibrillation. Gene mutations have been located on chromosome 10. The precise encoded target protein has not been identified (Table 6).

Acquired Cardiovascular Condition and "Electrical Remodeling"

Complex cellular and subcellular changes take place in the setting of acquired cardiovascular disease. "Electrical remodeling" occurs in patients with acquired atrial fibrillation and cardiac diseases, resulting in myocyte hypertrophy and ventricular dilatation (Table 7). Significant intracellular remodeling also has been observed during atrial fibrillation in animal models. The action potential duration is significantly reduced in amplitude in recordings from single atrial cells, corresponding to a decrease in atrial refractoriness, most likely a result of the reduced inward calcium current.

Electrical remodeling also has been observed in cardiovascular conditions leading to ventricular cell hypertrophy

Table 6.—Other Possible Familial "Channelopathies"

Clinical syndrome	Gene/chromosome	Comment
Idiopathic ventricular fibrillation	SCN5A (I_{Na})	ECG abnormalities (RBBB, ST-segment elevation in V_1)
		Cardiac arrest in absence of heart or other abnormalities
Familial atrial fibrillation	10q22-24	Exact gene has not been identified
		Channel regulatory proteins or neurohumoral receptors could be the encoded targets

and ventricular dilatation. Significant reduction of transient outward current (I_{to}) density as well as increases in the calcium-sodium exchange current ($I_{Ca/Na}$) and the inward sodium current (I_{Na}) have been observed. These changes at the ionic channel level could provide explanations for the prolonged duration of the action potential and the increased refractoriness seen in ventricular hypertrophy that could serve as a basis for reentry and triggered types of arrhythmias.

Basic Electrophysiology and Pharmacology

The Action Potential and the Electrocardiogram

The clinical pharmacology of antiarrhythmic drugs is reviewed in the chapter on these drugs. The correlation of ventricular action potentials with the ECG is shown in Figure 5. The rapid depolarization of ventricular cells (phase 0 of the action potential) corresponds to the QRS complex on the surface ECG. During the period of peak ventricular depolarization (phase 1) and the plateau (phase 2), there is little electrical activity that corresponds to the ST segment. The

Table 7.—Acquired Cardiac Diseases and "Electrical Remodeling"

Clinical syndrome	Electrical remodeling
Atrial fibrillation	Shortened action potential duration and atrial refractoriness
	Reduction of I_{to} and I_{Ca}
Hypertrophy and ventricular dilatation	Prolonged action potential duration and ventricular refractoriness
	Reduction of I_{to}
	Increase in $I_{Ca/Na}$ and I_{Na}

acceleration of ventricular repolarization (phase 3) is marked by the appearance of the T wave. With repolarization complete (phase 4), the ECG returns to the isoelectric baseline. The duration of the action potential corresponds to the QT interval on the surface ECG.

The primary approach to the development and administration of antiarrhythmic agents has followed the Vaughan Williams classification (Table 8). Class I antiarrhythmic

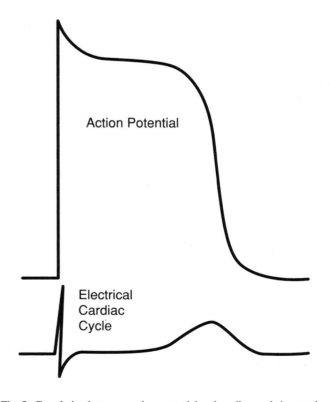

Fig. 5. Correlation between action potential and cardiac cycle in ventricular cells. The QRS duration on the ECG is correlated with phase 0 (sodium channel-dependent) of action potential. The QT interval (repolarization) is correlated with action potential duration (predominantly potassium channel-dependent).

drugs block sodium channels. On the ECG, sodium channel blockade in the ventricular cells is manifested by a prolongation of the QRS duration. However, the action of class I agents is not channel-specific. Particularly, class IA agents (quinidine, procainamide, and disopyramide) can block potassium channels, thus prolonging the QT interval. Class II antiarrhythmic drugs block cardiac β-adrenergic receptors. Inhibition of β-adrenergic activity results in a decrease in sinus rate and atrioventricular nodal conduction. Class III antiarrhythmic drugs characteristically prolong refractoriness. Because most of the drugs in this category have many electrophysiologic effects, it is difficult to attribute their antiarrhythmic action to prolongation of refractoriness alone. Class IV antiarrhythmic drugs are antagonists of calcium channels. These agents are used most commonly to suppress atrioventricular nodal conduction and atrial arrhythmias of an automatic nature. Although this classification system provides a framework

for a large number of antiarrhythmic compounds, it must be emphasized that each drug has unique characteristics that should be considered before one is selected for therapy. As knowledge of electrophysiologic mechanisms (receptors and ion channels) grows, we recognize that many new (adenosine, ATP) and old (digoxin, atropine) drugs do not fit into this classification scheme. The target receptors/channels, basic and clinical electrophysiologic properties, ECG effects, and important proarrhythmic features of the frequently used antiarrhythmic agents are summarized in Table 9.

- Class I antiarrhythmic drugs block sodium channels.
- Class II antiarrhythmic drugs block cardiac β-adrenergic receptors.
- Class III antiarrhythmic drugs characteristically prolong refractoriness.
- Class IV antiarrhythmic drugs are antagonists of calcium channels.

Table 8.—Vaughan Williams Classification of Antiarrhythmic Drugs in Clinical Use

Class I	Class II	Class III	Class IV	Other
IA	Acebutolol	Amiodarone	Diltiazem	Adenosine
Disopyramide	Atenolol	Bretylium	Verapamil	ATP
Procainamide	Esmolol	Sotalol		Digoxin
Quinidine	Metoprolol	Ibutilide		Atropine
	Propranolol			
	Timolol			
IB				
Ethmozine*				
Lidocaine				
Mexiletine				
Phenytoin				
Tocainide*				
IC				
Encainide*				
Flecainide				
Propafenone				

*Discontinued.

Table 9.—Pharmacologic Effects, Electrophysiologic Properties, and Cardiac Side Effects of Antiarrhythmic Drugs

Drug	Relative potency of receptor/channel interaction	Basic electro-physiologic properties	Clinical electro-physiologic properties	ECG effects	Important pro-arrhythmic side effects
Class IA					
Quinidine	Na channel +++ K channel ++ Anticholinergic + α-Adrenergic blockade +	Slow depolarization (phase 0) Prolongs AP duration	Slow His-Purkinje (HV interval) and intra-atrial and intraventricular conduction; prolongs atrial and ventricular refractoriness	Prolongs QRS duration; prolongs QT interval	Torsades de pointes at low heart rate
Procainamide	Na channel +++ K channel ++ α-Adrenergic blockade +	Same as above	Same as above	Same as above	Torsades de pointes, AV blockade
Disopyramide	Na channel +++ K channel + Anticholinergic +++	Same as above	Same as above	Same as above	Torsades de pointes
Class IB					
Lidocaine/ mexiletine	Na channel +	Slows depolarization (phase 0), shortens AP duration	Minimal slowing of His-Purkinje and intraventricular conduction; shortens ventricular refractoriness	Minimal prolongation of QRS duration, shortens QT interval	Minimal delay of AV conduction
Class IC					
Propafenone	Na channel ++++ β-adrenergic blockade + Calcium channel + K channel +	Slows depolarization (phase 0 and phase 4)	Prolongs HV interval, mild prolongation of sinus rate and AH interval	Prolongs QRS duration, minimal reduction of heart rate, and prolongation of PR interval	Proarrhythmia at high heart rate, ventricular tachycardia
Flecainide	Na channel ++++	Slows depolarization (phase 0)	Slows His-Purkinje (HV interval) and intra-atrial and intraventricular conduction	Prolongation of QRS duration	Same as above
Class III					
Sotalol	K channel +++ β-Adrenergic blockade ++	Prolongs AP duration in atrial and ventricular cells, slows depolarization (phase 4 and phase 0) in nodal cells	Prolongs atrial and ventricular refractoriness, slows sinus rate and AV nodal conduction (prolongs AH interval)	Prolongation of QT interval and PR interval, decrease of heart rate	Torsades de pointes at slow heart rate

Table 9 (continued)

Drug	Relative potency of receptor-channel interaction	Basic electro-physiologic properties	Clinical electro-physiologic properties	ECG effects	Important cardiac side effects
Amiodarone	K channel +++ Na channel + α-Adrenergic blockade + β-Adrenergic blockade + Calcium channel +	Prolongation of AP duration, slows depolarization (phase 4 and phase 0) of nodal cells	Same as above	Prolongation of QT interval, slows sinus rate, and prolongs PR interval	Sinus bradycardia, AV blockade
Others					
Adenosine/ ACh	A_1 receptor ++++ M_2 receptor ++++ G-protein-mediated activation of K channel (I_{KACh})	Shortens atrial AP, slows depolarization (phase 4) of nodal cells	Shortens atrial refractoriness, slows sinus rate and AV conduction (prolongs AH interval)	Slows sinus rate and prolongs PR interval	Sinus bradycardia, AV blockade, promotes atrial fibrillation
Atropine	M_2 receptor blockade +++ (anticholinergic)	Negates ACh effects	Increases sinus rate and AV conduction (shortens AH interval)	Increases sinus rate and shortens PR interval	Sinus tachycardia, rapid AV conduction
Digoxin	Na-K pump inhibition +++ Cholinergic +	Decreases resting membrane potential	Slows sinus rate and AV conduction (prolongs AH interval)	Slows sinus rate and prolongs PR interval	Promotes triggered activity

ACh, acetylcholine; AP, action potential; AV, atrioventricular; ECG, electrocardiographic.

Suggested Review Reading

1. Ackerman MJ: The long QT syndrome: ion channel diseases of the heart. *Mayo Clin Proc* 73:250-269, 1998.
A comprehensive review of basic and clinical information on the familial long QT syndrome. Molecular biology information is provided on the various mutations. The clinical diagnostic criteria for long QT syndrome are also discussed.

2. Ackerman MJ, Clapham DE: Ion channels—basic science and clinical disease. *N Engl J Med* 336:1575-1586, 1997.
Review of the basic physiology and structure of ionic channels. Ionic channel abnormalities in diseases such as cystic fibrosis and congenital long QT syndrome are discussed in detail.

3. Brugada R, Tapscott T, Czernuszewicz GZ, et al: Identification of a genetic locus for familial atrial fibrillation. *N Engl J Med* 336:905-911, 1997.
This article confirms that familial atrial fibrillation may be a distinct clinical entity. Mutations on chromosome 10 were identified in a family with numerous members who presumably have lone atrial fibrillation. The precise functional gene has not been identified.

4. Chen Q, Kirsch GE, Zhang D, et al: Genetic basis and molecular mechanism for idiopathic ventricular fibrillation. *Nature* 392:293-296, 1998.

The first article to characterize the mutations on the sodium channel gene in patients with idiopathic ventricular fibrillation.

5. Moss AJ, Zareba W, Benhorin J, et al: ECG T-wave patterns in genetically distinct forms of the hereditary long QT syndrome. *Circulation* 92:2929-2934, 1995.
The authors attempt to correlate T-wave abnormalities with genotypic abnormalities in LQT1, LQT2, and LQT3. This information will be extremely useful in clinical practice if the correlation is confirmed and validated.

6. Peeters HA, Sippensgroenewegen A, Wever EF, et al: Electrocardiographic identification of abnormal ventricular depolarization and repolarization in patients with idiopathic ventricular fibrillation. *J Am Coll Cardiol* 31:1406-1413, 1998.
Electrocardiographic features of patients with idiopathic ventricular fibrillation were analyzed in detail. Evidence of slow conduction and repolarization abnormalities can be identified. The article suggests that the body surface QRST integral mapping is potentially a useful method for identifying patients who may be at increased risk for ventricular fibrillation.

7. Roden DM, Lazzara R, Rosen M, et al: Multiple mechanisms in the long-QT syndrome. Current knowledge, gaps, and future directions. *Circulation* 94:1996-2012, 1996.
The authors discuss the congenital long QT syndrome from molecular biology to clinical cardiology. The various types of familial long QT syndrome are defined by genotypes. A target-specific therapy is suggested.

8. Shen WK, Holmes DR Jr, Packer DL: Cardiac arrhythmias: A. Anatomic and pathophysiologic concepts. In *Mayo Clinic Practice of Cardiology*. Third edition. St Louis, Mosby, 1996, pp 727-747.

Review of the traditional mechanisms of arrhythmogenesis, including automaticity, triggered activity, and reentry, and examples of clinical arrhythmias based on mechanisms.

9. Shen WK, Kurachi Y: Mechanisms of adenosine-mediated actions on cellular and clinical cardiac electrophysiology. *Mayo Clin Proc* 70:274-291, 1995.
Review of adenosine-mediated actions on signal transduction and electrophysiology at the cellular and clinical levels and examples of clinical applications.

10. Task Force of the Working Group on Arrhythmias of the European Society of Cardiology: The Sicilian gambit. A new approach to the classification of antiarrhythmic drugs based on their actions on arrhythmogenic mechanisms. *Circulation* 84:1831-1851, 1991.
Review of the pharmacologic mechanisms of antiarrhythmic agents. In addition to the traditional Vaughan Williams classification, the authors provide information on the properties of antiarrhythmic drugs based on molecular mechanisms.

11. Wit AL, Rosen MR: Afterdepolarizations and triggered activity: distinction from automaticity as an arrhythmogenic mechanism. In *The Heart and Cardiovascular System: Scientific Foundation*. Vol 2. Second edition. New York, Raven Press, 1991, pp 2113-2163.
A comprehensive review of the underlying mechanisms of triggered activity. It provides information to differentiate triggered activity from automaticity on the basis of cellular, pharmacologic, and electrophysiologic properties.

12. Zipes DP, Jalife J: *Cardiac Electrophysiology: From Cell to Bedside*. Second edition. Philadelphia, WB Saunders Company, 1995.
Discussion of molecular biology of ionic channels. Mechanisms of various clinical arrhythmias are also discussed.

Questions

Multiple Choice (choose the one best answer)

1. A 16-year-old girl was admitted to the coronary care unit after an aborted sudden cardiac death. The event occurred early in the morning when she was awakened to answer a telephone call. While she was on the telephone, she suddenly lost consciousness. The paramedics arrived within 5 minutes. She was in ventricular fibrillation. Defibrillation was successful after 3 shocks. The patient was subsequently intubated and transported to the hospital.

   On physical examination, the patient was unresponsive to pain or commands. Her pupils were dilated but reactive to light symmetrically. Her cardiovascular examination was normal. A 12-lead electrocardiogram is shown below. Her past medical history (provided by the mother) was significant for three brief episodes of fainting spells, from which she spontaneously recovered. She was otherwise a healthy teenager. The mother denied any knowledge of substance abuse in the patient's history or any premature death in her family. The family history of the patient's biologic father was unknown.

1A. What is the most likely diagnosis at this time?
   a. Idiopathic ventricular fibrillation
   b. Substance abuse
   c. Anomalous coronary artery
   d. Prolonged QT syndrome
   e. Hypertrophic cardiomyopathy

1B. Within 24 hours, the patient completely recovered neurologically and was extubated. No additional relevant history was obtained from her. During the diagnostic evaluation, which one of the following studies is most likely to further confirm the diagnosis?
   a. Echocardiography
   b. Electrophysiologic testing
   c. Coronary angiography
   d. Isoproterenol infusion
   e. Endomyocardial biopsy

1C. After the diagnosis is established, what is the most appropriate therapy for the patient?
   a. Pacemaker
   b. β-Adrenergic blocker
   c. Defibrillator

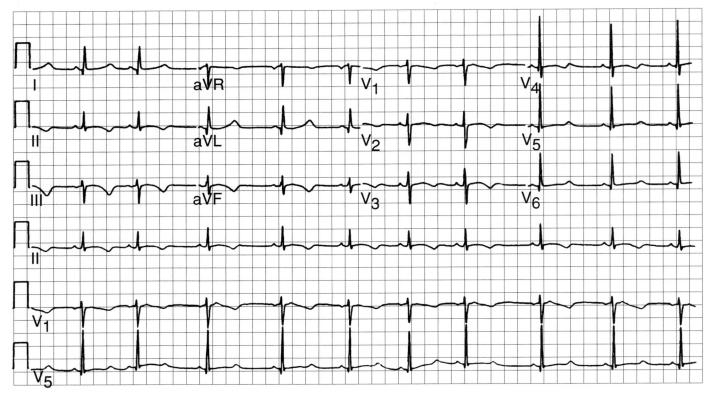

Question 1

d. Gene therapy

e. Cardiac transplantation

2. What is the most common mechanism underlying cardiac tachyarrhythmias?
   a. Triggered activity
   b. Abnormal automaticity
   c. Normal automaticity
   d. Reentry
   e. Parasystole

3. Under ischemic conditions, activation of which one of the following ion channels may provide a myocardial protective mechanism?
   a. Sodium channels (I_{Na})
   b. Calcium channels (I_{Ca})
   c. ATP-sensitive potassium channels (I_{KATP})
   d. The inward rectifier (I_{K1})
   e. Chloride channels (I_{Cl})

4. Which one of the following currents is responsible for maintaining stable resting membrane potential in atrial and ventricular cells?
   a. I_f
   b. I_{Na}
   c. I_{K1}
   d. I_K
   e. I_{Ca}

5. Which one of the following is the most common mechanism underlying abnormal automaticity?
   a. Depolarized resting membrane potential under disease conditions
   b. Increased slope of diastolic depolarization
   c. More negative threshold membrane potential
   d. Prolonged duration of action membrane potential
   e. Decreased slope of phase 0 depolarization

6. A 22-year-old man was referred to the arrhythmia clinic for evaluation of exercise-induced palpitations. He was very athletic and healthy. Noninvasive studies such as 12-lead electrocardiography at baseline, echocardiography, and Holter monitoring were unremarkable. During a treadmill exercise test, tachycardia was induced. The 12-lead electrocardiogram is shown below.

6A. What is the clinical diagnosis?
   a. Supraventricular tachycardia with aberrancy

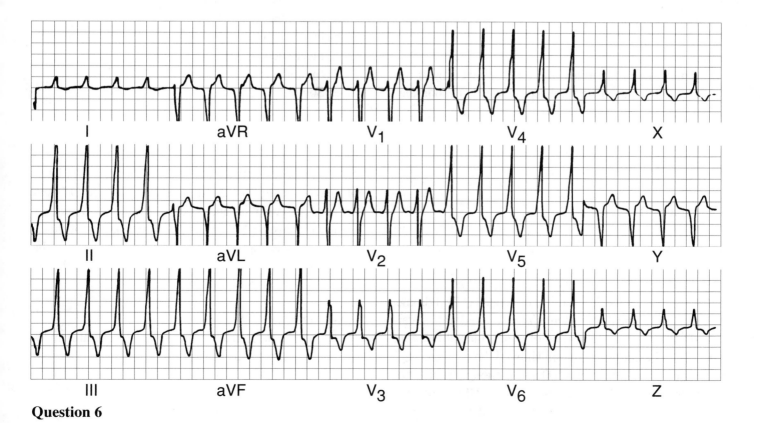

Question 6

b. Fascicular tachycardia
c. Exercise-induced ventricular tachycardia
d. Atrial flutter with 2:1 conduction
e. Wolff-Parkinson-White syndrome

6B. What is the most likely underlying mechanism for this tachyarrhythmia?
   a. Abnormal automaticity
   b. Triggered activity from early afterdepolarization
   c. Triggered activity from delayed afterdepolarization
   d. Reentry
   e. Parasystole

6C. Which one of the following anti-arrhythmic drugs will likely not be effective for this tachyarrhythmia?
   a. Atenolol
   b. Verapamil
   c. Sotalol
   d. Amiodarone
   e. Digoxin

7. Which one of the following antiarrhythmic drugs does *not* prolong the QT interval?
   a. Quinidine
   b. Lidocaine
   c. Sotalol
   d. Procainamide
   e. Ibutilide

8. Which one of the following ion channels is most frequently affected in the familial prolonged QT syndrome?

a. I_{Na}
b. I_{Ks}
c. I_{Kr}
d. I_{Ca}
e. minK

9. Which one of the following antiarrhythmic drugs has the least effect in slowing the conduction via the atrioventricular node?
   a. Calcium channel blockers
   b. β-Adrenergic blockers
   c. Amiodarone
   d. Lidocaine
   e. Sotalol

10. Which one of the following antiarrhythmic drugs may promote atrial fibrillation?
    a. Adenosine
    b. Quinidine
    c. Propafenone
    d. Amiodarone
    e. Atenolol

11. Which one of the following antiarrhythmic drugs is least likely to cause torsades de pointes?
    a. Quinidine
    b. Procainamide
    c. Flecainide
    d. Ibutilide
    e. Sotalol

Answers

1A. Answer d

1B. Answer d

1C. Answer c
  The clinical diagnosis is familial prolonged QT syndrome. The patient's clinical presentation is an aborted sudden cardiac death with documentation of ventricular fibrillation. The 12-lead electrocardiogram showed the corrected QT interval (QTc) is longer than 500 ms. Although the diagnosis in this patient is fairly certain because of the significant prolongation of the QT interval, the isoproterenol infusion challenge can be useful in patients with borderline QT intervals and clinically suspected familial prolonged QT syndrome. The sensitivity and specificity of the isoproterenol infusion test have not been validated. The treatment of choice for this patient is implantation of a defibrillator, because the patient has had a clinical event of sudden cardiac death with documented ventricular fibrillation.

2. Answer d
  It has been estimated that 80% to 90% of clinical arrhythmias are reentry in mechanism.

3. Answer c
  The ATP-sensitive potassium channel is activated under

ischemic conditions, whereas the intracellular ATP level is diminished. Activation of the ATP-sensitive potassium channel shortens action potential duration and decreases calcium influx and energy expenditure. This has been one of the proposed mechanisms of ATP-sensitive potassium channel-mediated myocardial protection.

4. Answer c

I_{K1} (inward rectifier) maintains a stable resting membrane potential in atrial and ventricular cells. I_{K1} is absent in nodal cells.

5. Answer a

The most common mechanism underlying abnormal automaticity is a partially depolarized resting membrane potential under disease conditions. An increased slope of diastolic depolarization is less frequent.

6A. Answer c

6B. Answer c

6C. Answer e

The 12-lead electrocardiogram shows a wide complex tachycardia with a left bundle branch block morphology and inferior axis. The clinical presentation of the patient and the documented arrhythmia are consistent with exercise-induced ventricular tachycardia originating in the right ventricular outflow tract. The proposed underlying mechanism for the exercise-induced ventricular tachycardia is catecholamine-sensitive, calcium-mediated triggered activity from delayed afterdepolarization. Because of the catecholamine sensitivity and calcium-mediated mechanism, β-adrenergic blockers and calcium channel blockers are usually effective in treating this type of ventricular tachycardia. Digoxin increases calcium and potentially promotes delayed afterdepolarization and trigger activity.

7. Answer b

Lidocaine is a weak sodium channel blocker. It does not have a significant potassium channel blockade effect. It does not prolong the QT interval. It is the one antiarrhythmic drug that may shorten the QT interval.

8. Answer b

The most frequently affected ionic channel in the familial prolonged QT syndrome is I_{Ks}, located on chromosome 11 (LQT1).

9. Answer d

Because of its rather specific sodium channel blockade, lidocaine does not have a significant effect on atrioventricular nodal conduction.

10. Answer a

Adenosine activates the $I_{K,Ach}$ channel in atrial tissue. Activation of the $I_{K,Ach}$ channel shortens the action potential duration, thereby shortening the refractoriness of the atrial tissue and promoting the induction of atrial fibrillation.

11. Answer c

Of the choices given, class 1A agents (quinidine and procainamide) and class III agents (ibutilide and sotalol) have a significant potassium channel blocking effect, thus prolonging the QT interval and potentially causing torsades de pointes. Flecainide (a class 1C agent) is a fairly specific sodium channel blocker without a significant potassium channel blocking effect. Prolongation of the QT interval is not associated with flecainide.

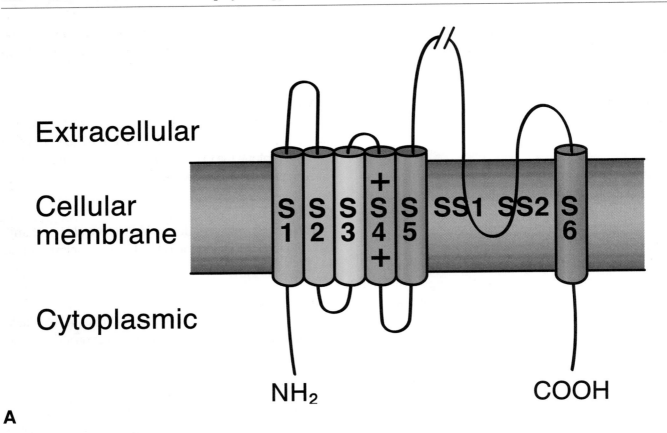

A

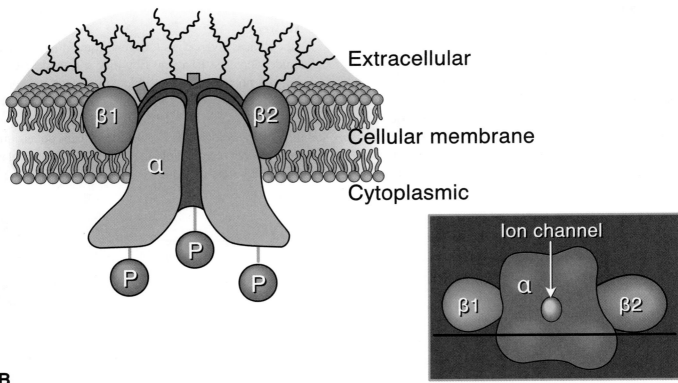

B

Plate 1

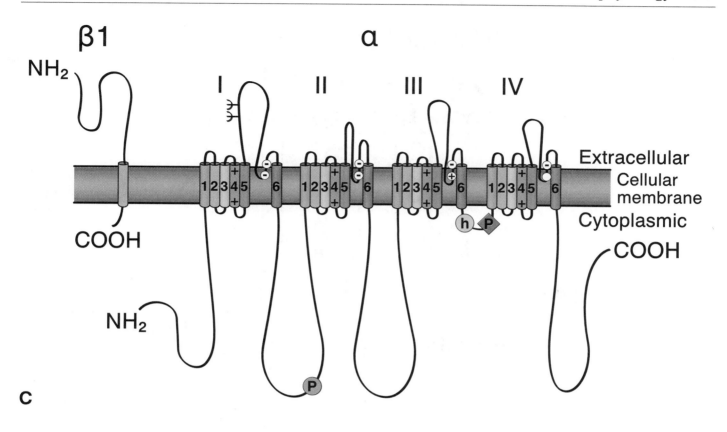

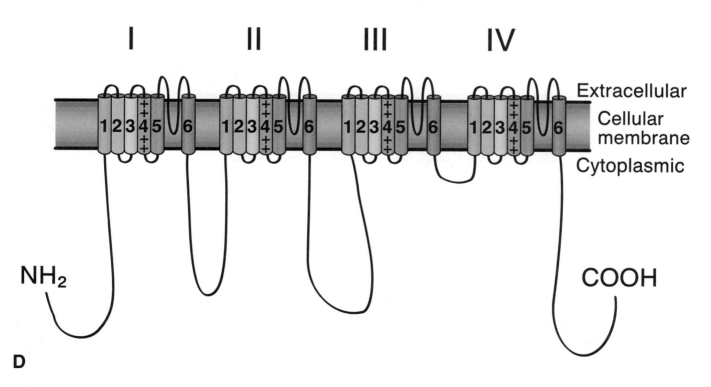

Plate 1 (continued)

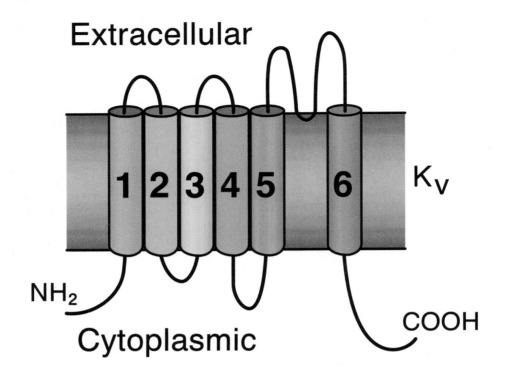

E

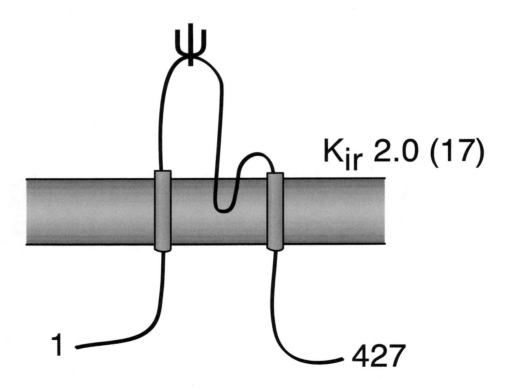

F

Plate 1 (continued). *A*, Diagram of subunit of voltage-gated ionic channel with six transmembrane motifs (S1-S6). It forms the core structure of sodium, calcium, and potassium channels. *B* and *C*, Sodium and, *D*, calcium channels consist of a single α subunit containing four repeats of the six transmembrane segments. Distinct subunits may form specific associations with different α subunits, which may add to the potential diversity of the structure and function of sodium channels. *E*, A single six-transmembrane-segment subunit of a voltage-gated potassium channel. Four separate subunits in combination form the functional voltage-gated potassium channels (K$_V$). *F*, A single subunit of inwardly rectifying potassium channels (K$_{ir}$) contains two transmembrane segments. Various combinations of subunits and interactions with other regulatory proteins modify the functional behavior of inwardly rectifying potassium channels.

Chapter 36

Indications for Electrophysiologic Testing

(Including Tilt Table Testing)

Thomas M. Munger, M.D.

Indications for Electrophysiologic Testing

Electrophysiologic (EP) studies are performed to establish the mechanism for a particular bradycardia or tachycardia rhythm and to guide the selection of treatment, whether it be antiarrhythmic drugs, devices, catheter ablative techniques, or electrosurgery. The indications for EP testing are listed in Table 1. A joint commission's recommendations have been published by the American College of Cardiology/American Heart Association.

Technical Aspects

Catheters

Flexible multipolar, platinum-tipped electrode catheters are introduced into a systemic vein (femoral, internal jugular, subclavian, or brachial) via a percutaneous Seldinger technique. Typical intracardiac electrode recording sites include the high right atrium or atrial appendage, right ventricular apex, and bundle of His area (near the septal leaflet of the tricuspid valve). In studies involving paroxysmal supraventricular tachycardia, a catheter introduced several centimeters into the coronary sinus from the right side of the heart can indirectly provide recordings from the left atrioventricular groove. Catheters can also be introduced into the left atrium and ventricle from the chambers on the right side of the heart through a patent foramen ovale or a transseptal atrial puncture or they can be introduced retrogradely through the femoral artery.

- A catheter introduced several centimeters into the coronary sinus from the right side of the heart can indirectly provide recordings from the left atrioventricular groove.

Definition of EP Conduction Times

Electrical recordings made in sinus rhythm using catheters in the standard position are shown in Figure 1. The His electrogram is marked by "H."

- When reviewing EP tracings on the Cardiology Boards, it is important to review the surface tracings, because these are more familiar to test-takers. Note the paper speed of the recordings; many are recorded at 100 mm/s (four times faster than standard), making *all* rhythms appear "wide-complex" when in fact they are not.

1. *PA interval*: This represents the onset of the earliest atrial event (P wave on atrial electrogram) in any lead (except the His bundle catheter) to the onset of the atrial electrogram in the low right atrial septum (at the His bundle catheter). This represents intra-atrial conduction time.
2. *AH interval*: This is the time from the onset of the atrial electrogram at the His bundle catheter to the onset of the His electrogram at the His bundle catheter. In normal subjects, this interval varies the most, because it is affected by sympathetic and vagal influences.
3. *HV interval*: This is the time from the onset of the His bundle electrogram at the His bundle catheter to the onset of the earliest ventricular event (QRS on ventricular

Table 1.—Indications for Electrophysiologic Study

Definite indications
  Sustained ventricular tachycardia or cardiac arrest
    occurring in the absence of electrolyte imbalance, drug
    toxicity, or acute myocardial infarction
  Syncope of undetermined cause
  Wide QRS tachycardia of undetermined cause
  ICD testing
  Catheter ablation for symptomatic paroxysmal
    supraventricular tachycardia or ventricular tachycardia
  Second-degree atrioventricular block to assess the
    requirement for permanent pacemaker
  Symptomatic hypertrophic cardiomyopathy
  Nonsustained ventricular tachycardia in patient with
    coronary artery disease, ejection fraction $\leq$ 35%, > 3
    weeks post-myocardial infarction (MADIT)
Unestablished indications
  Post-myocardial infarction
  Dilated cardiomyopathy

ICD, implantable cardioverter defibrillator; MADIT, Multicenter Automatic
  Defibrillator Implantation Trial.

electrogram) in any lead (except the His bundle catheter).
4. *ERP*: This is the effective refractory period. For a given
   tissue, it is the longest immediate input interval that fails
   to cause an electrical output; for example, the anterograde
   ERP of the atrioventricular node is defined as the longest
   A_1A_2 (atrial stimuli 1 and 2) interval that fails to cause an
   H_1H_2 interval (His bundle spikes corresponding to A_1A_2).
   At the ERP of the atrioventricular node, the A_2 would fail
   to produce an H_2. An example is shown in Figure 2.
5. *Shortest 1:1 conduction*: This represents the stimulus
   interval below which non-1:1 conduction occurs for a given
   tissue; for example, if the Wenckebach phenomenon of the
   AV node (anterograde) occurred at a 300-ms stimulus interval ($S_1 = 300$ ms) and conduction was 1:1 at 310 ms, then
   the shortest 1:1 conduction would be 310 ms.
6. *Sinus node recovery time*: This provides an assessment
   of intrinsic sinus node function. It can be affected by
   sympathetic/vagal tone and medications. The sensitivity
   of this test for sinus node dysfunction is poor (no better
   than 50%). The corrected sinus node recovery time
   (CSNRT) is "corrected" as follows:

$$CSNRT =$$

Sinus Node Recovery Time (ms) - Sinus Cycle Length
An example of an abnormally long CSNRT is shown in
Figure 3.

Indications

Ventricular Tachycardia/Cardiac Arrest

It is estimated that approximately 35% to 40% of patients
remain at risk for recurrent cardiac arrest after an initial
nonmyocardial infarct-related cardiac arrest when followed
for 2 years after the event. The usual initiating arrhythmia
for cardiac arrest is ventricular tachycardia/ventricular
fibrillation, although more than 10% to 20% of cardiac
arrests are initiated by bradyarrhythmias or supraventricular
arrhythmias. Sustained monomorphic ventricular arrhythmias are inducible at EP testing in a significantly lower
proportion of patients who have spontaneous cardiac arrest
than in those with spontaneous sustained monomorphic
ventricular tachycardia. Arrhythmias induced in survivors
of cardiac arrest have shorter cycle lengths than in patients
without a history of cardiac arrest. After having cardiac
arrest, approximately 35% to 50% of patients have sustained inducible monomorphic ventricular tachycardia. EP
testing in a patient with cardiac arrest can also identify
occult arrhythmia disorders (Wolff-Parkinson-White syndrome, bundle branch reentry ventricular tachycardia) that
are readily treatable with catheter ablation.

The major use of EP testing in patients with cardiac
arrest or sustained ventricular tachycardia is planning
antiarrhythmic drug therapy versus device or ablative
therapy. Early studies demonstrated excellent results
using EP study to identify patients remaining at high risk
for sudden death while receiving drug therapy. Later studies, particularly the Electrophysiologic Study Versus
Electrocardiographic Monitoring (ESVEM) trial, suggested Holter-guided therapy may be as efficacious as EP
study-guided therapy in this regard. In recent years, fewer
drug trials have been used because implantable cardioverter defibrillator nonthoracotomy-lead therapy has
become available.

- More than 10% to 20% of cardiac arrests are initiated by
  bradyarrhythmias or supraventricular arrhythmias.
- After having cardiac arrest, approximately 35% to 50%
  of patients have sustained inducible monomorphic ventricular tachycardia.

Syncope

Syncope is an extremely common clinical problem throughout life, and in many cases it is due to benign mechanisms.
Nonetheless, the potential implications of a syncopal event
are profound concerning independent personal activities

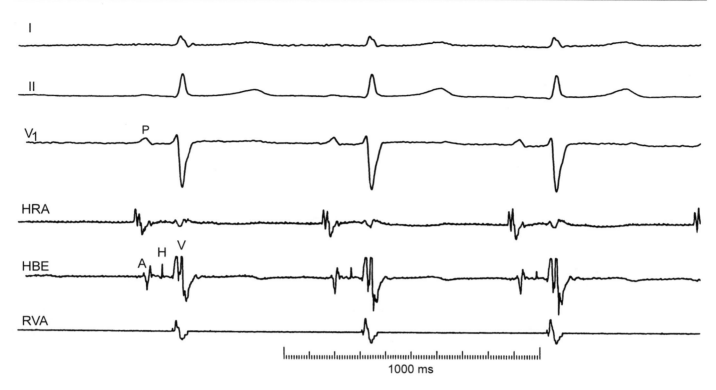

Fig. 1. Electrical recordings made in sinus rhythm using catheters in the standard position. A, atrial electrogram; H, His electrogram; HBE, His bundle electrogram; HRA, high right atrium; RVA, right ventricular apex; V, ventricular electrogram.

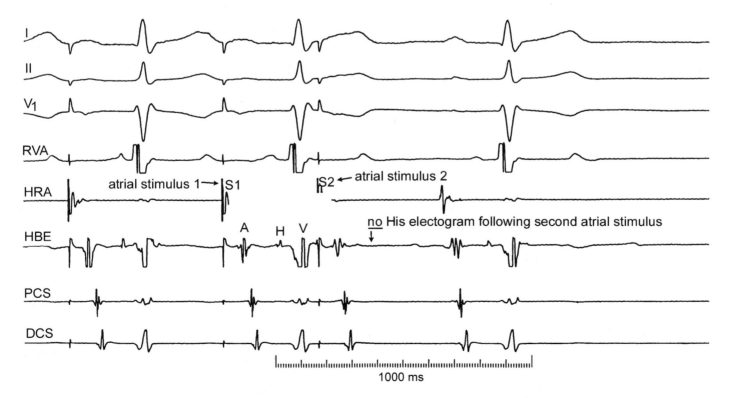

Fig. 2. Effective refractory period of atrioventricular node. DCS, distal coronary sinus; PCS, proximal sinus. Other abbreviations as in Figure 1.

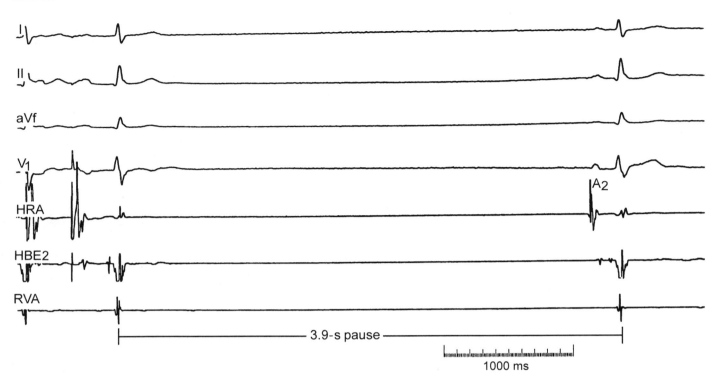

Fig. 3. Example of an abnormally long corrected sinus node recovery time .

(e.g., driving or employment). Also, syncope can be due to potentially life-threatening mechanisms that deserve further clinical evaluation. Syncope due to a cardiac arrhythmia portends a significantly high mortality rate. Diagnostic yields from syncope EP studies vary, ranging between 20% and 90% (Table 2). The probability that an EP study will identify a cause of syncope is greater in those having underlying structural heart disease. In particular, patients with normal resting electrocardiograms (ECGs) and ventricular function have a low diagnostic yield EP study. In this group, paroxysmal supraventricular tachycardia (usually due to atrioventricular nodal reentry tachycardia) and sinus node dysfunction may be found at EP testing, although these entities are still not absolutely ruled out with negative findings on EP study. In patients with cardiovascular disease, the most common findings are inducible sustained ventricular arrhythmias and conduction system disease. Other findings may include carotid sinus hypersensitivity or vasodepressor syncope with the use of head-up tilt testing. EP study should be considered in patients (particularly with cardiac disease) before empiric pacing for recurrent syncope.

● Patients with normal resting ECGs and ventricular function have a low diagnostic yield EP study.

Wide Complex Tachycardia

Between 80% and 95% of all wide complex tachycardias are due to ventricular tachycardia; the rest are due to supraventricular arrhythmias with associated bundle branch aberrancy or accessory pathway conduction. Although atrioventricular dissociation is a useful finding that confirms the presence of ventricular tachycardia, more than 60% of all ventricular tachycardias display 1:1 atrial conduction; thus, the diagnosis of ventricular tachycardia may not be definitely made from the surface ECG. In these cases, EP study is used to determine the cause of wide complex tachycardia. Because most of the supraventricular causes of wide complex tachycardia are amenable to catheter ablation techniques (with a high likelihood of success), it is imperative that these rhythms be diagnosed accurately with EP study.

● Between 80% and 95% of all wide complex tachycardias are due to ventricular tachycardia.

Implantable Cardioverter Defibrillator Testing

Virtually all the newer generation implantable cardioverter defibrillators have the capability of allowing noninvasive programmed ventricular stimulation; thus, reassessment of a patient's arrhythmic substrate can be performed many times noninvasively. Initial assessment of sensing, pacing,

Table 2.—Criteria for Abnormality at Electrophysiologic Study in Patients With Syncope

Variable	Positive	Indeterminate	Negative
CSNRT	> 600 ms	550-600 ms	< 500 ms
SVT	Hypotension	Normotension	No SVT
AV Wenckebach	> 500 ms	< 300 ms	300-500 ms
HV interval	> 100 ms, infra-His block	55-99 ms, < 35 ms	35-55 ms
VT	SMVT	NSMVT, PVT, VF	No VT
CSH	> 5-s pause with symptoms	3- to 5-s pause	< 3-s pause
HUT/VDS	Hypotension/syncope	Asymptomatic hypotension	Normotension

AV, atrioventricular; CSH, carotid sinus hypersensitivity; CSNRT, corrected sinus node recovery time; HUT/VDS, head-up tilt table test in vasodepressor syncope; NSMVT, nonsustained monomorphic ventricular tachycardia; PVT, polymorphic ventricular tachycardia; SMVT, sustained monomorphic ventricular tachycardia; SVT, supraventricular tachycardia; VF, ventricular fibrillation; VT, ventricular tachycardia.

and defibrillation functions is necessary at the time of implantation, during subsequent visits after recurrent shocks, and as part of the routine annual follow-up. Introduction of antiarrhythmic drugs or implantation of a supplemental dual-chamber pacemaker system requires reassessment of implantable cardioverter defibrillator efficacy.

- Virtually all the newer generation implantable cardioverter defibrillators have the capability of allowing noninvasive programmed ventricular stimulation.

Radiofrequency Catheter Ablation

Radiofrequency catheter ablation provides exceptional cure rates for most of the common congenital paroxysmal supraventricular tachycardia syndromes, including Wolff-Parkinson-White syndrome, atrioventricular nodal reentry tachycardia, and paroxysmal junctional reciprocating tachycardia. These rhythms can be ablated with success rates greater than 95%. Radiofrequency ablation of atrial tachycardia, atrial flutter, or ventricular tachycardia is associated with lower success rates (70% to 90%). Catheter ablation should be considered the primary treatment for patients with symptomatic Wolff-Parkinson-White syndrome. An example of radiofrequency energy eliminating the delta wave in a patient with Wolff-Parkinson-White syndrome is shown in Figure 4. Radiofrequency ablation of the slow atrioventricular nodal pathway for atrioventricular nodal reentry tachycardia should also be considered in the early management of this rhythm, usually after failed therapy with β-blockers or calcium-channel blockers.

- Catheter ablation should be considered the primary treatment for symptomatic Wolff-Parkinson-White syndrome.

Second-Degree Atrioventricular Block

EP study should be performed in patients with second-degree atrioventricular block, particularly in the setting of syncope or bundle branch block, to ascertain the level of the block and to determine whether the patient would be a candidate for pacemaker therapy.

Hypertrophic Cardiomyopathy

Investigators at the National Institutes of Health have demonstrated that subsequent events (either cardiac arrest or shocks from implantable cardioverter defibrillators) can be predicted in patients with hypertrophic cardiomyopathy based on either a clinical history of syncope or inducibility of ventricular arrhythmias at EP study. Thus, EP study can be used to provide additional prognostic information for patients with hypertrophic cardiomyopathy.

Emerging and Unestablished Indications

Approximately 3% to 5% of all patients who have a myocardial infarction in the U.S. have cardiac arrest within the following year. Proper risk stratification for the occurrence of cardiac arrest after myocardial infarction has continued to perplex investigators. Certain variables, including depressed left ventricular ejection fraction, congestive heart failure, complex ventricular arrhythmias, and a positive signal-averaged ECG, have identified patient groups at higher risk than normal. Nonetheless, these variables are not specific enough to define all the patient groups that would warrant extremely aggressive, expensive intervention. EP testing appears to provide independent predictive information about fatal electrical events in patients the first year after myocardial infarction, but like the noninvasive variables, specificity is poor.

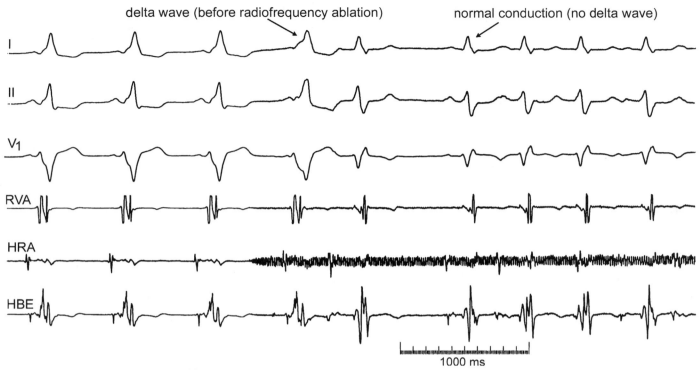

Fig. 4. Elimination of delta wave in Wolff-Parkinson-White syndrome with radiofrequency energy.

Empiric antiarrhythmic drug therapy, when administered to post-myocardial infarction patients, can unfavorably affect mortality. The Cardiac Arrhythmia Suppression Trial (CAST) demonstrated that flecainide, encainide, and moricizine when given in the post-myocardial infarction period to patients at higher risk were proarrhythmic, leading to excess mortality in comparison with placebo. Similar data exist for mexiletine. The data concerning amiodarone have been variable; some studies have shown no effect, and others have demonstrated a beneficial effect in a post-myocardial infarction.

Studies such as the Multicenter Unsustained Tachycardia Trial (MUSTT), the Coronary Artery Bypass Graft (CABG) Patch Trial, and the Multicenter Automatic Defibrillator Implantation Trial (MADIT) have attempted to identify patients at high risk for lethal electrical events and then assess whether antiarrhythmic drugs or implantable cardioverter defibrillator therapy extends survival. MADIT results were released in 1996 and showed favorable effects of implantable cardioverter defibrillators over drug therapy (80% of patients receiving amiodarone) in the management of high-risk patients after myocardial infarction (ejection fraction < 35% and positive EP testing after intravenous procainamide in the setting of complex ventricular ectopy). However, the CABG Patch Trial demonstrated

that a similar high-risk group of patients who were receiving bypass surgery at the time of randomization received no such benefit.

EP testing to predict adverse events in patients with dilated cardiomyopathy is poor and is *not recommended*. A trial called Sudden Cardiac Death in Heart Failure Trial (SCD-HFT) has begun and will examine the possibility that either amiodarone or implantable cardioverter defibrillators may be beneficial if used empirically in these high-risk patients.

- Approximately 3% to 5% of all patients who have a myocardial infarction in the U.S. have cardiac arrest within the following year.
- Empiric antiarrhythmic drug therapy, when administered to post-myocardial infarction patients, can unfavorably affect mortality.

Indications for Head-Up Tilt Testing

Vasodepressor syncope is an extremely common cause of fainting in the general population, accounting for 20% to 40% of all syncopal episodes. Recurrence after the initial event can be expected in 30% of cases. Trigger events for the vasodepressor response vary and can include noxious stimuli, unpleasant sights or smells, anticipated pain, upright posture, heat or dehydration, physical exercise, cough, micturition, sneezing, or coincident medical illness. An initial β-adrenergic stimulus activates cardiac and carotid chemoreceptors/mechanoreceptors that through afferent pathways to the brain release an even greater parasympathetic efferent discharge, causing profound bradycardia and arterial vasodilatation. This sequence of events can be reproduced with isoproterenol head-up tilt testing in approximately 80% of patients who have vasodepressor syncope. The sensitivity and specificity of head-up tilt testing for the vasodepressor response are approximately 80%. Several variations of the tilt protocol exist; in general, it is agreed that the angle for tilting should be between 60° and 80° and at least a 15-minute baseline tilt procedure should be performed. It is not clear whether prolonged tilt procedures on the order of 45 to 60 minutes offer better specificity or sensitivity compared with shorter tilt periods and the addition of isoproterenol or adenosine. The reproducibility of tilt testing is approximately 80%. Thus, using follow-up tilt studies to predict efficacy of therapy generally is not recommended. A positive response to head-up tilt with the development of junctional rhythm and hypotension (as well as clinical syncope) is shown in Figure 5.

- Vasodepressor syncope is an extremely common cause of fainting in the general population, accounting for 20% to 40% of all syncopal episodes.

Complications of Electrophysiologic Study

From a study performed in the 1980s, the most common complications of EP testing included hemorrhage, arterial tear, thrombophlebitis (0.7%); embolic phenomena (0.2%); and cardiac perforation (0.15%). Death, myocardial infarction, and stroke all are exceedingly rare and less common than the rates associated with cardiac angiography. Event rates are higher for patients undergoing catheter ablation because of longer instrumentation times, additional electrode catheters used, and increased number of pharmacologic agents used. The various complications of EP testing are listed in Table 3.

Table 3.—Complications of Electrophysiologic Testing

Death
Myocardial infarction
Stroke
Perforation with tamponade
Arterial tear
Thrombophlebitis
Pulmonary embolism
Pneumothorax
Complete heart block (after radiofrequency ablation)
Plexopathy
Radiation exposure

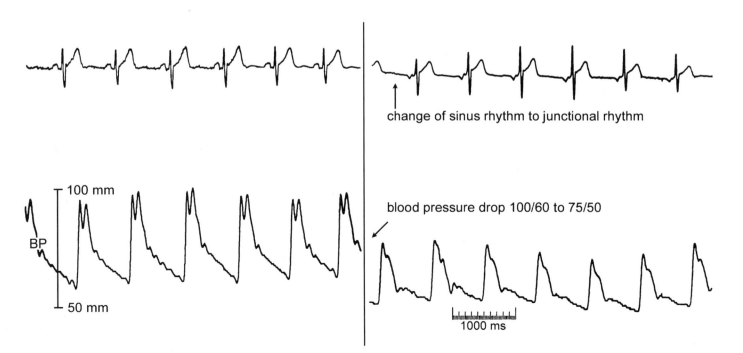

Fig. 5. Head-up tilt test showing development of junctional rhythm and hypotension.

Suggested Review Reading

1. Akhtar M, Williams SV, Achord JL, et al: Clinical competence in invasive cardiac electrophysiological studies. A statement for physicians from the ACP/ACC/AHA Task Force on Clinical Privileges in Cardiology. *Circulation* 89:1917-1920, 1994.

This position-statement paper describes the clinical requirements for cardiologists who want to complete fellowship training in adult clinical cardiac electrophysiology.

2. Bigger JT Jr: Prophylactic use of implanted cardiac defibrillators in patients at high risk for ventricular arrhythmias after coronary-artery bypass graft surgery. *N Engl J Med* 337:1569-1575, 1997.

In this prospective randomized clinical trial, there was no improved survival among coronary artery disease patients who had depressed left ventricular function and an abnormal signal-averaged ECG in whom a defibrillator was implanted prophylactically at the time of elective coronary artery bypass grafting. After an average follow-up of 32 months, the overall mortality in the implanted cardioverter defibrillator group was 23% compared with 21% in the control group (P = 0.6).

3. Brugada P, Brugada J, Mont L, et al: A new approach to the differential diagnosis of a regular tachycardia with a wide QRS complex. *Circulation* 83:1649-1659, 1991.

Four new stepwise criteria that can be applied ensuring a 99% sensitivity and 97% specificity for accurate diagnosis are described in this prospective analysis of 554 wide complex tachycardias. The absence of an RS complex in all precordial leads was highly specific for the diagnosis of ventricular tachycardia. When an RS complex was present in one or more precordial leads, an RS interval greater than 100 ms was specific for ventricular tachycardia.

4. DiMarco JP, Prystowsky EN, Ellenbogen KA, et al: Catheter ablation in patients with cardiac arrhythmias. Circulation 85:390, 1992.

Review article summarizing the technique of arrhythmia catheter ablation.

5. Farrehi PM, Santinga JT, Eagle KA: Syncope: diagnosis of cardiac and noncardiac causes. *Geriatrics* 50:24-30, 1995.

A general review of the cardiac and noncardiac causes of syncope and the pitfalls of some of the common modalities to diagnose this symptom.

6. Gregoratos G, Cheitlin MD, Conill A, et al: ACC/AHA Guidelines for Implantation of Cardiac Pacemakers and Antiarrhythmia Devices: Executive Summary—a report of the American College of Cardiology/American Heart Association Task Force on Practice Guidelines (Committee on Pacemaker Implantation). Circulation 97:1325-1335, 1998.

Consensus guidelines concerning indications for implantation of cardiac pacemakers and implantable cardioverter defibrillators. Excellent overview of class I/II/III indications and strength of data supporting these indications.

7. Moss AJ, Hall WJ, Cannom DS, et al: Improved survival with an implanted defibrillator in patients with coronary disease at high risk for ventricular arrhythmia. *N Engl J Med* 335:1933-1940, 1996.

The MADIT trial was a prospective randomized clinical trial that examined the use of the implantable cardioverter defibrillator (ICD) versus medical therapy in high-risk coronary artery disease patients for the primary prevention of overall and arrhythmic mortality. Entry criteria included left ventricular ejection fraction < 35%, nonsustained ventricular tachycardia on Holter monitoring, and inducible ventricular arrhythmias that were not suppressible with intravenous procainamide. At a mean follow-up of 27 months, 16% of ICD-treated patients versus 39% of medically treated (mostly amiodarone) patients had died (P = 0.009). However, it should be noted that more patients in the ICD group received β-blocker therapy.

8. Munger TM, Packer DL, Hammill SC, et al: A population study of the natural history of Wolff-Parkinson-White syndrome in Olmsted County, Minnesota, 1953-1989. *Circulation* 87:866-873, 1993.

Retrospective, longitudinal analysis of the natural history and epidemiology of a community-based population of patients with Wolff-Parkinson-White (WPW) syndrome in the preablation era. The incidence of sudden death was low and suggested that electrophysiologic testing should not be performed routinely in asymptomatic patients with WPW syndrome.

9. Oribe E, Caro S, Perera R, et al: Syncope: the diagnostic value of head-up tilt testing. Pacing Clin Electrophysiol 20:874-879, 1997.

Prolonged head-up tilt testing had a 93% positive predictive value and a 43% negative predictive value for assessing patients with possible neurocardiogenic syncope.

10. Zipes DP, DiMarco JP, Gillette PC, et al: Guidelines for clinical intracardiac electrophysiological and catheter ablation procedures. A report of the American College of Cardiology/American Heart Association Task Force on Practice Guidelines (Committee on Clinical Intracardiac Electrophysiologic and Catheter Ablation Procedures), developed in collaboration with the North American Society of Pacing and Electrophysiology. *J Am Coll Cardiol* 26:555-573, 1995.
Guidelines, as determined by a joint committee representing the AHA/ACC/NASPE, concerning indications for electrophysiologic procedures and catheter ablation. This is the most recent attempt at creating such a consensus.

Questions

Multiple choice (choose the one best answer)

1. A 54-year-old man has an enlarged cardiac silhouette on a chest radiograph. This was discovered during an employment physical examination. Your physical examination discloses a third heart sound. The electrocardiogram shows left bundle branch block. Echocardiography shows a left ventricular ejection fraction of 25% with mild mitral regurgitation and global dysfunction. Coronary angiography results are normal. Holter monitoring discloses 35,000 premature ventricular contractions, including 1,200 pairs and 85 runs of nonsustained ventricular tachycardia, 3-9 beats in duration. What is the next most appropriate test to request?
   a. Pericardiocentesis
   b. Right ventricular biopsy
   c. Electrophysiologic study
   d. Serum ferritin
   e. Signal-averaged electrocardiogram

2. A 38-year-old man has radiofrequency catheter ablation for atrial tachycardia. On post-procedure day 6, he goes to his local physician with intermittent chest aches over the left precordium which had been present for the previous 24 hours and mild dyspnea. Examination findings are negative, and electrocardiographic/chest radiographic results are unremarkable. What is the next most appropriate test to request?
   a. Echocardiography
   b. Arterial blood gas
   c. Treadmill exercise test
   d. Ventilation perfusion scan
   e. Coronary angiography

3. Which of the following statements about head-up tilt testing is true?
   a. The correct tilt angle can be 45°
   b. The sensitivity of the test is 95% for vasovagal syncope
   c. In a nondifferentiated group of syncope patients, the test would be positive 5% of the time
   d. b + c
   e. None of the above

4. The arrhythmic substrate least likely to be definitely ruled out with a negative electrophysiologic study would be:
   a. Sinus node dysfunction
   b. Severe His-Purkinje disease
   c. Accessory bypass tract
   d. Ventricular tachycardia in a patient with coronary artery disease
   e. Atrioventricular nodal reentry tachycardia

5. An active 68-year-old woman with recurrent syncope has an electrophysiologic study. With atrial pacing at 150 beats/min for 30 seconds, a 7-second atrial pause occurs when pacing ceases. Her baseline examination, electrocardiographic, and echocardiographic findings are all negative. What would be the next appropriate management step?
   a. Implant VVI permanent pacemaker
   b. Implant dual-chamber implantable cardioverter defibrillator
   c. Implant DDDR permanent pacemaker
   d. Implant AAI permanent pacemaker
   e. Atropine

6. Each of the following were entry criteria for patients randomized in the Multicenter Automatic Defibrillator Implantation Trial (MADIT) (which examined drug versus implantable cardioverter defibrillator therapy in high-risk patients for sudden death) *except*:
   a. Left ventricular ejection fraction less than 35%
   b. Inducible electrophysiologic study for sustained ventricular tachycardia
   c. Coronary artery disease
   d. Nonsustained ventricular tachycardia on telemetry
   e. A ventricular tachycardia at electrophysiologic study suppressible with procainamide

7. In a patient with a history of syncope and atrioventricular block, which of the following baseline interval measurements is least likely to be prolonged?
   a. PA
   b. AH
   c. HV
   d. None will be affected
   e. All will be affected

8. In a patient with cardiac arrest, each of the following diagnoses could be identified at electrophysiologic study as a cause of sudden death *except*:
   a. Wolff-Parkinson-White syndrome
   b. Bundle branch reentry ventricular tachycardia

   c. Intramyocardial reentry ventricular tachycardia
   d. Severe His-Purkinje system disease
   e. None of the above

9. Acute success rates for ablation of accessory pathways could be stated as:
   a. 50%-70%
   b. 75%
   c. 85%
   d. 90%-95%
   e. Virtually 100%

10. A 69-year-old woman goes to the emergency department with the following electrocardiogram: Blood pressure is 110/70 mm Hg. She has mild presyncope, palpitations, and no other symptoms. Acutely, and then chronically, she is best treated with:
    a. Adenosine and then radiofrequency ablation
    b. Lidocaine and then coronary angiography/electrophysiologic testing
    c. DC cardioversion and then implantation of a cardioverter defibrillator
    d. Procainamide and then radiofrequency ablation
    e. Lidocaine and then amiodarone

11. The effective refractory period (ERP) of the ventricle would be expected to be prolonged after the administration of each of the following drugs *except*:
    a. Quinidine
    b. Mexiletine
    c. Sotalol
    d. Disopyramide
    e. Amiodarone

12. Overall mortality following myocardial infarction is favorably affected by each of the following *except*:
    a. Sotalol
    b. Simvastatin
    c. Recombinant tissue plasminogen activator
    d. Enalapril
    e. Metoprolol

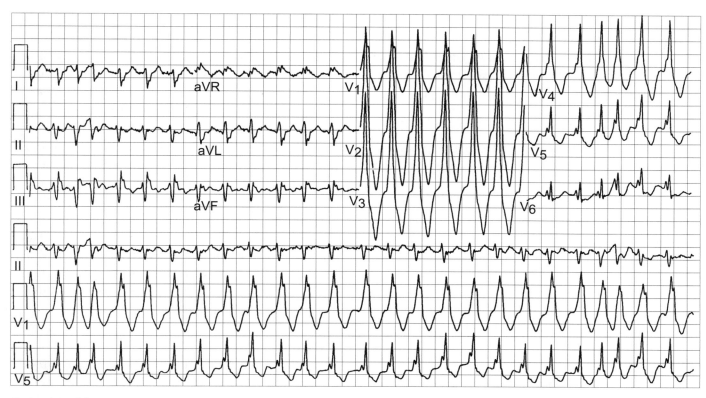

Question 10

Answers

1. Answer d

This patient has the diagnosis of dilated cardiomyopathy. Currently, electrophysiologic testing in such an "asymptomatic" patient is not indicated. Hemochromatosis can cause a secondary cardiomyopathy and should be among several definable causes of dilated cardiomyopathy that should be sought before invasive studies are performed.

2. Answer b

This patient has a presentation compatible with pulmonary embolism, complicating the electrophysiologic study he had 6 days earlier. As such, blood gas is the next appropriate test, followed by an imaging modality like V/Q scanning or cine computed tomography.

3. Answer e

Head-up tilt should be performed at 60° to 80°. The sensitivity and specificity of the test are 80%; approximately 20% to 40% of all syncope patients have vasodepressor as the mechanism of the problem.

4. Answer a

The sensitivity of electrophysiologic testing for sinus node disease is less than 50%. For all the other diagnoses listed, detection rates at electrophysiologic study are greater than 90%.

5. Answer c

There is a pathologic pause following atrial pacing consistent with sinus node dysfunction. The patient should receive pacing with a device that has rate response, in this case the DDDR device.

6. Answer e

For patients to be randomized in the Multicenter Automatic Defibrillator Implantation Trial (MADIT), they had to be nonsuppressible following infusion of procainamide at electrophysiologic study.

7. Answer a

Patients with atrioventricular block can have prolonged AH, HV, or both. PA (intra-atrial conduction time) would not necessarily be expected to be affected in a patient with atrioventricular block.

8. Answer e

All the potentially occult arrhythmia disorders listed—Wolff-Parkinson-White syndrome, bundle branch reentry ventricular tachycardia, intramyocardial reentry ventricular tachycardia, or His-Purkinje disease—could be uncovered at electrophysiologic study in a patient with cardiac arrest.

9. Answer d

Acute success rates for ablation in Wolff-Parkinson-White syndrome are approximately 90% to 95%; right-sided pathways have a lower chance of acute success.

10. Answer d

This patient has preexcited atrial fibrillation due to Wolff-Parkinson-White syndrome and a shortest RR interval during atrial fibrillation of 240 ms; thus, she is at risk for sudden death and should receive radiofrequency ablation to cure the syndrome. Acutely, procainamide is the drug of choice for termination (or DC cardioversion if she becomes hemodynamically unstable). Atrioventricular nodal blocking drugs such as calcium channel blockers and adenosine are contraindicated in this situation.

11. Answer b

The effective refractory period (ERP) of the ventricle will be prolonged in response to antiarrhythmic drugs, which prolong phase III of the action potential, like Vaughan Williams class IA and III drugs. Mexiletine (class IB), if anything, shortens action potential duration.

12. Answer a

Statins, thrombolytics, angiotensin-converting enzyme inhibitors, and β-blockers reduce mortality following myocardial infarction. Empiric use of most antiarrhythmic agents (including D-Sotalol, a class III drug) enhances

Chapter 37

Atrial Fibrillation

Diagnosis, Management, and Stroke Prevention

Paul A. Friedman, M.D.

Epidemiology

Atrial fibrillation is the most common arrhythmia encountered in clinical practice, and its frequency increases with age. Population-based studies have shown its prevalence to be 5% in patients 65 years or older. Common causes and associated conditions include hypertension, cardiomyopathy, valvular heart disease (particularly mitral stenosis), sick sinus syndrome, Wolff-Parkinson-White syndrome (especially in young patients), alcohol use, and thyrotoxicosis. The presence of these conditions should be sought in the history and physical examination of patients with atrial fibrillation.

- Common causes of atrial fibrillation include hypertension, cardiomyopathy, valvular heart disease, sick sinus syndrome, Wolff-Parkinson-White syndrome, thyrotoxicosis, and alcohol use.

History and Physical Examination

Patients with atrial fibrillation may be asymptomatic, or they may present with palpitations, presyncope, dizziness, fatigue, or dyspnea. Frank syncope is less common, and if present, other causes should be considered. These may include pauses in patients with tachycardia-bradycardia syndrome (often with the termination of atrial fibrillation) or ventricular arrhythmias in patients who present with atrial fibrillation in the setting of cardiomyopathy.

Physical examination reveals an irregularly irregular rhythm with variable intensity of the first heart sound. This variability is due to the changing interval between contractions, resulting in changes in filling of the ventricle and variation in the position of the mitral valve leaflets at the initiation of systole. An S_4 is not present because of the lack of a coordinated atrial contraction, and, similarly, an A wave is notably absent. If heart failure is present, the jugular venous pulsations may be increased, an S_3 may be noted, and rales may be present.

- Patients with atrial fibrillation may be asymptomatic or may present with palpitations and dizziness, but less commonly frank syncope.
- The development of overt heart failure suggests the possibility of concomitant cardiac disease (such as cardiomyopathy or valvular heart disease).

Electrocardiographic Differential Diagnosis

Atrial fibrillation is characterized by continuous and irregular activity of the electrocardiographic baseline, caused by swarming electrical currents in the atria. Atrial fibrillation must be distinguished from atrial flutter, which is characterized by repetitive undulations in the baseline which (in typical atrial flutter) yield a sawtooth pattern in the inferior leads (Fig. 1). Multifocal atrial tachycardia (MAT) also can mimic atrial fibrillation. MAT is characterized by premature atrial complexes of at least three different morphologic types; it is distinguished from atrial fibrillation by the presence of an isoelectric baseline between complexes (Fig. 1). Treatments for MAT (calcium channel blockers and control of predisposing conditions) and atrial flutter (medications or catheter ablation) can differ from those for atrial fibrillation.

Even in the absence of a preexisting bundle branch block, intermittent wide QRS complexes are frequent in patients with atrial fibrillation. These can be due to aberrant conduction of the supraventricular impulse (Ashman phenomenon) or ventricular ectopy. In the Ashman phenomenon, after a long RR interval an early impulse from the atria is conducted aberrantly because one bundle branch has not fully recovered from the previous impulse and is still partially refractory. Because the right bundle branch has a longer refractory period than the left, aberrant impulses usually have a right bundle branch block (RBBB) morphology, classically with the right "rabbit ear" taller than the left (rsR´, as seen in "typical" RBBB).

- Atrial fibrillation must be distinguished from atrial flutter (uniform flutter waves) and multifocal atrial tachycardia (isoelectric interval between premature atrial contractions).
- Ashman phenomenon reflects aberrant conduction of atrial impulses and can be characterized by a long-short coupling interval and (usually) RBBB morphology—this will be part of the electrocardiography section of the Cardiology Boards.

Therapy

Therapy for atrial fibrillation can be divided into three broad categories: 1) control of ventricular rate, 2) stroke prophylaxis (for ongoing atrial fibrillation), and 3) maintenance of sinus rhythm (rhythm control). The choice of the approach depends in part on the degree of a patient's symptoms, age and preference, and comorbid conditions. Whether one

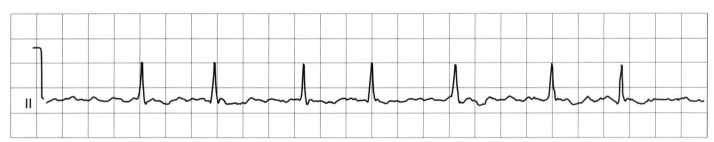

A

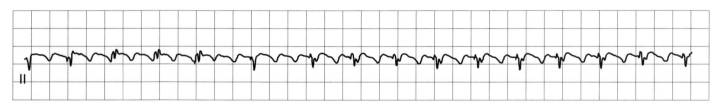

B

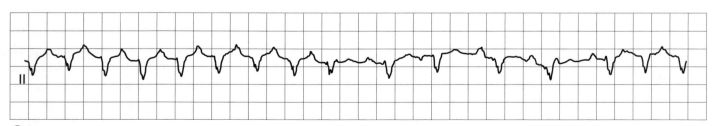

C

Fig. 1. *A*, Atrial fibrillation is characterized by continuous and irregular activity of the electrocardiographic baseline and irregularly irregular ventricular response. *B*, Atrial flutter with repetitive undulations in the baseline, which result in a sawtooth pattern in the inferior leads. *C*, Multifocal atrial tachycardia with premature atrial complexes of at least three different morphologic types and an isoelectric baseline between complexes.

approach is superior to the other is unknown, and this issue is being evaluated in a multicenter trial.

- It is important to know which agents are useful for rate control and which for rhythm control (Table 1).

Rate Control

In the absence of significant conduction disease, atrial fibrillation typically manifests with a rapid and irregular ventricular response. This can result in impairment of systolic and diastolic function due to inadequate filling and can result in ischemia in patients with coronary artery disease. Additionally, in most patients, symptoms are due to the rapid ventricular response.

Importantly, a prolonged rapid ventricular rate can lead to ventricular dysfunction, a *tachycardia-induced cardiomyopathy*. In some patients initially thought to have dilated cardiomyopathy, controlling the ventricular rate has resulted in dramatic improvement in ventricular systolic function. Even in patients with a primary cardiomyopathy and associated atrial fibrillation in whom systolic function fails to improve, rate control remains important for controlling symptoms and preventing deterioration in cardiac function.

- Uncontrolled atrial fibrillation with a rapid ventricular response can lead to a *tachycardia-induced cardiomyopathy*. This is reversible with control of the ventricular rate.

Rate control may alleviate symptoms associated with atrial fibrillation. However, because the atria are persistently fibrillating, stasis and thrombus formation remain possible, and appropriate stroke prophylaxis (discussed below) is still required.

Pharmacologic Control of the Ventricular Rate

Three main categories of drugs are used to blunt the atrioventricular (AV) nodal response in atrial fibrillation: digitalis glycosides, β-adrenergic blocking agents, and calcium channel blockers (Table 1). None of these agents have been shown to be effective for the prevention of recurrent atrial fibrillation. There is one exception: continued use of β-blockers after cardiac operation may prevent recurrence.

Digitalis preparations historically were the first agents available for controlling the ventricular rate in atrial fibrillation. Digoxin primarily has an indirect effect by increasing vagal tone and, thus, slowing AV nodal conduction. Because of its mechanism of action, digoxin is less effective than β-blockers or calcium channel blockers, particularly with exercise, when an increase in sympathetic tone results in more rapid AV nodal conduction. Thus, the optimal role for digoxin in atrial fibrillation is in patients with left ventricular dysfunction (due to its positive inotropy) or as adjunctive therapy in patients being treated with β- or calcium channel blocking agents.

- Digoxin alone is no better than placebo for terminating atrial fibrillation.

Table 1.—Pharmacologic Therapy for Atrial Fibrillation

Agents	Comments
Control of ventricular rate	
β-Adrenergic blockers (e.g., atenolol, metoprolol, propranolol, carvedilol)	Ideal in hyperthyroidism, acute myocardial infarction, chronic congestive heart failure (especially carvedilol), and postoperative patients
Calcium channel blockers (verapamil, diltiazem)	Nifedipine, amlodipine, and felodipine are not useful for slowing atrioventricular conduction
Digoxin	Less effective than β- and calcium channel blockers, especially with exercise. Useful in heart failure
Maintenance of sinus rhythm	
Class IA: quinidine, disopyramide, procainamide	Enhance atrioventricular conduction—rate must be controlled before use. Monitor QTc
Class IC: propafenone, flecainide	Slow atrioventricular conduction. Often first choice in patients with normal heart. Monitor QRS duration
Class III: sotalol, amiodarone	Amiodarone is agent of choice for ventricular dysfunction and after myocardial infarction

- Digoxin is less effective than β- or calcium channel blocking agents for controlling the ventricular rate, and it is best used as an adjunctive agent or for impaired ventricular function.

β-Blocking agents such as propranolol, metoprolol, and atenolol are effective for slowing AV nodal conduction and may be particularly useful when atrial fibrillation complicates hyperthyroidism or myocardial infarction (in which case they reduce the risk of death from infarction). β-Blockers have also been shown to reduce the risk of postoperative myocardial infarction, making them well suited for postoperative atrial fibrillation. Additionally, carvedilol reduces mortality in patients with chronic heart failure and may be a good choice in that setting. Esmolol, because of its intravenous formulation and short half-life, is particularly useful for acute management of atrial fibrillation.

- β-Blocking agents are effective for slowing the ventricular rate in atrial fibrillation, but they do not terminate atrial fibrillation (although they may prevent it postoperatively).
- They are particularly useful in hyperthyroidism, acute myocardial infarction, chronic heart failure, and postoperative situations.

Calcium channel blocking drugs are broadly divided into two groups: dihydropyridines (nifedipine, amlodipine, felodipine) and nondihydropyridines (diltiazem, verapamil). Dihydropyridine agents have little or no effect on AV nodal conduction and have no role in the management of atrial fibrillation. Verapamil and diltiazem are both available in intravenous and oral preparations and are well suited for both acute and chronic rate control. Both diltiazem and verapamil have negative inotropic effects and should be used cautiously in congestive heart failure.

- Diltiazem and verapamil are both effective for rate control in atrial fibrillation; nifedipine, amlodipine, and felodipine are not and have no role in the management of atrial fibrillation.

Although adenosine is very effective for slowing AV nodal conduction, it has no role in the therapy of atrial fibrillation because of its short half-life. It can be useful diagnostically, however, by slowing the ventricular rate transiently, permitting visualization of atrial activity if the diagnosis is in question.

Nonpharmacologic Control of the Ventricular Rate

For patients whose rate cannot be controlled pharmacologically, and for patients in whom medications for rhythm control (discussed below) are either ineffective or not well tolerated, catheter ablation of the AV junction is an alternative therapeutic approach. In this procedure, a catheter is placed percutaneously near the region of the His bundle and radiofrequency energy is delivered, creating complete AV block. For patients with chronic atrial fibrillation, a VVIR pacemaker is implanted, whereas for patients with paroxysmal atrial fibrillation, dual-chamber pacemakers with mode-switching functions are used. These permit the tracking of P waves during sinus rhythm and revert to VVIR (or DDIR) pacing when atrial fibrillation recurs. With this approach, because the fibrillation itself persists in the atria, the risk of thromboembolism is unchanged, and thus appropriate stroke prophylaxis must be prescribed.

Recently, an AV nodal modification procedure has been developed in which radiofrequency energy is used to alter the AV node to slow conduction without the creation of complete heart block, avoiding the need for permanent pacing; however, this technique is newer, has a lower success rate, and has not yet been widely adopted.

Rhythm Control

Rhythm control (maintenance of sinus rhythm) can effectively control symptoms. However, it should be noted that maintaining sinus rhythm has not been shown to decrease the likelihood of thromboembolism, nor has it been shown to prolong survival; in fact, some drugs used to prevent recurrences may actually cause new arrhythmias (proarrhythmias).

Pharmacologic Control of Rhythm

Class IA antiarrhythmic drugs (quinidine, procainamide, and disopyramide) can be used to prevent recurrences, but AV nodal slowing agents must be administered because these drugs enhance AV nodal conduction. A meta-analysis of six randomized controlled trials of quinidine demonstrated that at 1 year, 50% of quinidine-treated patients but only 25% of control patients remained in sinus rhythm ($P < 0.001$). However, deaths were higher in the quinidine-treated group: total mortality 2.9% versus 0.8%, sudden death 0.8% versus 0.0%, respectively. That study highlights the potential problem of proarrhythmia, but given the very small number of patients with sudden death (3 of 413 total patients), the results must be interpreted with caution. Nonetheless, the choice of antiarrhythmic medication is often based on concomitant cardiovascular or other diseases, as summarized in Table 1.

- Class IA agents (quinidine, procainamide, and disopyramide) can be associated with torsades de pointes, particularly at the time of reversion of atrial fibrillation, and their use should be initiated with monitoring to assess QT prolongation.
- These agents also *enhance* AV nodal conduction, so rate control agents should be given before their use.

In patients with structurally normal hearts, type IC agents (flecainide or propafenone) are well tolerated and can safely be started in outpatients. As opposed to IA agents, these slow AV nodal conduction. Close electrocardiographic follow-up to exclude excessive QRS widening (up to 20% beyond baseline is acceptable) and a treadmill test after 3 days to screen for a proarrhythmia are warranted. However, patients who have had a previous myocardial infarction are at increased risk of death with the use of class IC agents, as demonstrated in the Cardiac Arrhythmia Suppression Trial (CAST). After myocardial infarction, amiodarone is well tolerated and has no effect on, or tends to reduce (nonsignificantly), mortality as shown by the European Myocardial Infarction Amiodarone Trial (EMIAT) and the Canadian Amiodarone Myocardial Infarction Trial (CAMIAT). Additionally, patients with systolic dysfunction, especially due to dilated cardiomyopathy, may particularly benefit from amiodarone. In the Grupo de Estudio de la Sobrevida en la Insuficienca Cardiaca en Argentina (GESICA) trial, patients with heart failure treated with amiodarone had improvement in ejection fraction and survival compared with those receiving placebo. Although amiodarone is more effective than other drugs, side effects are more prevalent, resulting in discontinuation of its use in more than 30% of patients in clinical trials. Adverse effects can include pulmonary fibrosis, hepatitis, hypothyroidism, or hyperthyroidism. Patients should be assessed every 3 months during the first year of therapy and every 6 months thereafter to screen for drug toxicity.

- For patients with a normal heart, IC agents (propafenone, flecainide) can usually be used safely in the outpatient setting (with electrocardiography and treadmill testing at 3 days to exclude proarrhythmia).
- Amiodarone has been proved safe after myocardial infarction and in systolic dysfunction

Nonpharmacologic Control of Rhythm

Because of the limitations of pharmacologic therapy, including drug intolerance, proarrhythmia, and recurrence of atrial fibrillation, there has been great interest in non-pharmacologic therapies.

In patients with sick sinus syndrome, atrial pacing reduces thromboembolism, congestive heart failure, and recurrence of atrial fibrillation compared with ventricular demand pacing. Multisite atrial pacing (such as dual-site atrial pacing) and implantable atrial defibrillators have been used to treat patients with atrial fibrillation in small trials, but their role has yet to be determined.

In the surgical maze procedure, linear incisions are made in the atria. These incisions heal to form scars that act as boundaries or corridors that are too narrow to allow atrial reentry to develop, forcing activation down the surgical pathways to the AV node in an orderly manner. In one series, more than 90% of patients were free of arrhythmia without antiarrhythmic agents, and all patients were in sinus rhythm with the use of medical therapy. Patients without a history of thromboembolism were not treated with anticoagulation. Efforts to perform the maze procedure by means of percutaneous catheters (and thus eliminate the need for thoracotomy) are under rapid development, but they currently are not widely available.

Nonpharmacologic Therapy for Atrial Flutter

Unlike atrial fibrillation, which is composed of reentrant wavelets that travel through the atria, typical atrial flutter consists of a single reentrant circuit that follows the tricuspid valve annulus. Radiofrequency catheter ablation of this single circuit has success rates in excess of 90%. This procedure must not be confused with AV node ablation for atrial fibrillation. In atrial flutter ablation, a lesion is placed in the atrium to interrupt the flutter circuit; AV nodal conduction is not impaired, and normal sinus rhythm (with no need for pacing) ensues. In AV node ablation for atrial fibrillation, the AV node (or His bundle) is ablated, preventing atrial impulses from reaching the ventricles, thus controlling the ventricular rate; the atria, however, continue to fibrillate, and a pacemaker is required because of the presence of AV block.

- The surgical maze is effective for controlling atrial fibrillation, but thoracotomy is needed.
- Atrial flutter ablation has a success rate in excess of 90%.

Atrial Fibrillation in Wolff-Parkinson-White Syndrome

Atrial fibrillation in Wolff-Parkinson-White syndrome is of special interest because it is a frequent subject of examination questions, it can be life-threatening, and it requires therapy that is different from the usual treatment for atrial fibrillation. Patients with Wolff-Parkinson-White syndrome have an accessory pathway that can conduct electrical activity from the atrium to the ventricle, bypassing the AV node. Because the accessory pathway does not slow conduction in the same manner as the AV node, the ventricular response to atrial fibrillation can be extraordinarily and dangerously rapid. Because activation down the accessory pathway does not use the normal His-Purkinje system, wide, irregular, and rapid ventricular complexes occur. Use of agents such as calcium channel blockers, β-blockers, or digoxin can result in an even more rapid ventricular response due to blocking of conduction down the AV node (which can limit concealed conduction into the pathway). Therefore, the agent of first choice is procainamide, which will slow accessory pathway and intra-atrial conduction. Should a patient with Wolff-Parkinson-White syndrome and atrial fibrillation become hypotensive, prompt cardioversion should be performed.

- Atrial fibrillation in Wolff-Parkinson-White syndrome should *not* be treated with digoxin or β- or calcium channel blocking agents.
- Atrial fibrillation in Wolff-Parkinson-White syndrome should be treated with procainamide or direct-current cardioversion.

Stroke Prevention

Acute Cardioversion to Normal Sinus Rhythm

Electrical cardioversion from atrial fibrillation is commonly used to control atrial fibrillation. However, up to 7% of patients undergoing cardioversion without anticoagulation experience clinical thromboembolism. This likely results from dislodgment of atrial thrombus with the resumption of atrial systolic activity.

Current guidelines state that patients with atrial fibrillation of more than 48 hours in duration should receive anticoagulation before cardioversion. Several weeks of warfarin therapy before cardioversion can reduce the incidence of cardioversion-associated thromboembolism to about 1%. Additionally, anticoagulation should be continued for 4

weeks after cardioversion because of the increased risk of thromboembolism during that time. Although there are few data on cardioversion in the absence of anticoagulation for atrial fibrillation of recent onset (less than 48 hours), current guidelines do not mandate anticoagulation in this setting. Although historically atrial flutter was thought to confer a low thromboembolic risk, more recent data have questioned this assumption, suggesting that similar anticoagulation guidelines should be followed.

Recently, studies have supported an alternative approach to the management of patients with atrial fibrillation of more than 48 hours. In this approach, intravenous heparin therapy is begun, and then transesophageal echocardiography is performed. In one study of 230 patients, if transesophageal echocardiography showed no evidence of thrombus, cardioversion was safely performed with no thromboembolism. Most patients underwent anticoagulation before, during, and for several weeks after the transesophageal echocardiography and cardioversion, and atrial thrombi were identified in 15% of patients (in whom cardioversion was therefore deferred). A prospective trial is under way to evaluate this approach further.

- Patients with atrial fibrillation of more than 48 hours must receive anticoagulation for 3 weeks before and 4 weeks after cardioversion.
- An alternative approach for patients with atrial fibrillation of more than 48 hours may be transesophageal echocardiography with cardioversion (if no thrombus is found) and 3 to 4 weeks of anticoagulation subsequently, although this approach is less well validated.
- For acute cardioversion, atrial flutter should be treated like atrial fibrillation with regard to anticoagulation.

Chronic Stroke Prevention

Patients with atrial fibrillation due to rheumatic valvular disease have a markedly increased risk of stroke and all should be treated with warfarin, unless there is an absolute contraindication to anticoagulation. Most patients in clinical practice have nonrheumatic atrial fibrillation. A series of landmark studies (listed in Suggested Review Reading) demonstrated that warfarin reduces the incidence of thromboembolism by 68% to 84% in this population. The risk of thromboembolism can be determined by clinical and echocardiographic risk factors, which should be used to guide treatment (Tables 2 and 3). The risk factors for thromboembolism are advanced age, previous transient ischemic attack or stroke, a history of hypertension, diabetes mellitus, and congestive heart failure. Echocardiographic risk factors include depressed left ventricular function and left atrial enlargement. Patients who are younger than 60 years and have no clinical heart disease or hypertension are at extremely low risk and require no treatment, although some physicians recommend aspirin. Thus, a strategy based on age and risk factors has emerged (Table 3). Patients younger than 60 years (65 in some reports) with no risk factors can be given no therapy or aspirin. Patients older than 75, or patients with risk factors, should receive warfarin. In patients treated with warfarin, the International Normalized Ratio (INR) should be maintained in a range of 2.0 to 3.0 (although 2.0-2.5 may be preferable in those > 75 years old). The INR value is preferable to prothrombin time for patient management, because prothrombin time assays vary among laboratories.

Of note, the Stroke Prevention in Atrial Fibrillation (SPAF) III study compared fixed-dose low-intensity warfarin (INR, 1.3-1.5) plus aspirin with dose-adjusted warfarin (mean INR, 2.4) in high-risk patients and found the fixed-dose warfarin plus aspirin treatment insufficient for stroke prevention. Two other warfarin-aspirin–combination studies in other populations (the POST-CABG [Coronary Artery Bypass Grafting] and CARS [Coumadin-Aspirin Reinfarction Study] trials) also found no benefit with low-intensity warfarin combination therapy. These studies support the role for adjusted-dose warfarin for patients with atrial fibrillation at risk for thromboembolism.

- The clinical risk factors for stroke in nonrheumatic atrial fibrillation are age > 75 years, previous transient ischemic attack or stroke, a history of hypertension, diabetes mellitus, and congestive heart failure. (These should be known for the Cardiology Boards.)
- Echocardiographic risk factors are depressed ventricular function and left atrial enlargement.
- Patients < 60 years with structurally normal hearts and no hypertension are at low risk of thromboembolism and require no specific therapy.
- Warfarin should be used to maintain an INR of 2.0 to 3.0 (although 2.0-2.5 is preferable in elderly patients).
- Studies have shown no difference in the risk of stroke between paroxysmal and chronic atrial fibrillation.

> Atrial fibrillation is common and will be included in questions on the Cardiology Boards. Important areas to be familiar with are:

- History and physical examination findings (stressed throughout the Cardiology Boards)
- Agents used for ventricular rate control and agents used for maintenance of sinus rhythm
- Risk factors for thromboembolism in atrial fibrillation
- Atrial fibrillation in Wolff-Parkinson-White syndrome— this is a perennial favorite examination topic
- Stroke prevention trials in atrial fibrillation

Table 2.—Risk Factors for Thromboembolism in Nonrheumatic Atrial Fibrillation

Clinical risk factor	Echocardiographic risk factor
Advanced age	Two-dimensional left ventricular dysfunction
Previous transient ischemic attack or stroke	Left atrial enlargement
Hypertension	
Diabetes (in pooled analysis)	
Heart failure	
Other high-risk clinical settings	
Prosthetic heart valves	
Thyrotoxicosis	

Table 3.—Recommended Management of Nonrheumatic Atrial Fibrillation

Age, yr	Risk factor	Recommendation
< 65	Present	Warfarin, INR 2-3
	No risk factors	Acetylsalicylic acid or nothing
65-75	Present	Warfarin, INR 2-3
	No risk factors	Warfarin or acetylsalicylic acid (based on discussion with patient of relatively low risk of stroke, decrease in risk with warfarin, monitoring needs)
> 75		Warfarin, INR 2-3 (but should be kept closer to 2.0-2.5 because of increased risk of hemorrhage in this age group)

Modified from *Chest* 108 (Suppl):352S-359S, 1995. By permission of the American College of Chest Physicians.

Suggested Review Reading

1. Andersen HR, Nielsen JC, Thomsen PE, et al: Long-term follow-up of patients from a randomised trial of atrial versus ventricular pacing for sick-sinus syndrome. *Lancet* 350:1210-1216, 1997.
Patients with sick sinus syndrome who have atrial pacing have improved survival, less atrial fibrillation, less thromboembolism, and less heart failure than those with ventricular pacing.

2. Anonymous: Risk factors for stroke and efficacy of antithrombotic therapy in atrial fibrillation. Analysis of pooled data from five randomized controlled trials. *Arch Intern Med* 154:1449-1457, 1994.
This article pools original data from five trials to define the risk factors for thromboembolism in nonrheumatic atrial fibrillation.

3. The Boston Area Anticoagulation Trial for Atrial Fibrillation Investigators: The effect of low-dose warfarin on the risk of stroke in patients with nonrheumatic atrial fibrillation. *N Engl J Med* 323:1505-1511, 1990.
Long-term low-dose warfarin therapy (prothrombin time ratio, 1.2-1.5) is highly effective for preventing stroke in patients with nonrheumatic atrial fibrillation.

4. Cox JL, Schuessler RB, Lappas DG, et al: An 8 1/2-year clinical experience with surgery for atrial fibrillation. *Ann Surg* 224:267-273, 1996.
Of 178 patients who had the maze procedure, 93% were arrhythmia free without any antiarrhythmic medication. The remaining patients all had conversion to sinus rhythm with medications. Most patients had echocardiographic atrial transport, and 1 of 107 patients with normal preoperative sinus function required permanent pacing.

5. EAFT (European Atrial Fibrillation Trial) Study Group: Secondary prevention in non-rheumatic atrial fibrillation after transient ischaemic attack or minor stroke. *Lancet* 342:1255-1262, 1993.
Anticoagulation is effective for reducing the risk of recurrent vascular events in patients with nonrheumatic atrial fibrillation and a recent transient ischemic attack or minor ischemic stroke. In absolute terms, 90 vascular events (mainly strokes) are prevented if 1,000 patients are treated with anticoagulation for 1 year. Aspirin is a safe, though less effective, alternative when anticoagulation is contraindicated; it prevents 40 vascular events each year for every 1,000 treated patients.

6. Grogan M, Smith HC, Gersh BJ, et al: Left ventricular dysfunction due to atrial fibrillation in patients initially believed to have idiopathic dilated cardiomyopathy. *Am J Cardiol* 69:1570-1573, 1992.
In this report of tachycardia-induced cardiomyopathy, patients initially thought to have dilated cardiomyopathy and concomitant atrial fibrillation with a rapid ventricular rate had improvement in ejection fraction after rate control or restoration of sinus rhythm.

7. Jensen SM, Bergfeldt L, Rosenqvist M: Long-term follow-up of patients treated by radiofrequency ablation of the atrioventricular junction. *Pacing Clin Electrophysiol* 18:1609-1614, 1995.
Atrioventricular node ablation with permanent pacing is effective for controlling symptoms in patients with difficult to manage atrial fibrillation.

8. Kopecky SL, Gersh BJ, McGoon MD, et al: The natural history of lone atrial fibrillation. A population-based study over three decades. *N Engl J Med* 317:669-674, 1987.
Lone atrial fibrillation (< 60 years old, no overt cardiovascular disease or precipitating illness) is associated with a very low risk of stroke. Routine anticoagulation may not be warranted.

9. Laupacis A, Albers G, Dalen J, et al: Antithrombotic therapy in atrial fibrillation. *Chest* 108 (Suppl 4):352S-359S, 1995.
The report of the fourth American College of Chest Physicians Consensus Conference on Antithrombotic Therapy is an excellent review of the studies of anticoagulation in atrial fibrillation and provides concise recommendations.

10. Manning WJ, Silverman DI, Keighley CS, et al: Transesophageal echocardiographically facilitated early cardioversion from atrial fibrillation using short-term anticoagulation: final results of a prospective 4.5-year study. *J Am Coll Cardiol* 25:1354-1361, 1995.
This prospective trial demonstrated the safety and feasibility of using transesophageal echocardiography to screen for thrombus before cardioversion of atrial fibrillation. Most patients who had anticoagulation (heparin, then warfarin) before and after the echocardiography had cardioversion.

11. Petersen P, Boysen G, Godtfredsen J, et al: Placebo-controlled, randomised trial of warfarin and aspirin for prevention of thromboembolic complications in chronic atrial fibrillation. The Copenhagen AFASAK study. *Lancet* 1:175-179, 1989.
The incidences of thromboembolic complications and vascular mortality were significantly lower in the warfarin group than in the aspirin (75 mg/day) and placebo groups, which did not differ significantly. Thromboembolic complications developed in 5 patients receiving warfarin, 20 receiving aspirin, and 21 receiving placebo. Nonfatal bleeding complications led to withdrawal in 21 patients given warfarin, 2 given aspirin, and none receiving placebo. Thus, anticoagulation therapy with warfarin can be recommended to prevent thromboembolic complications in patients with chronic nonrheumatic atrial fibrillation.

12. Prystowsky EN, Benson DW Jr, Fuster V, et al: Management of patients with atrial fibrillation. A Statement for Healthcare Professionals. From the Subcommittee on Electrocardiography and Electrophysiology, American Heart Association. *Circulation* 93:1262-1277, 1996.
This subcommittee report of the American Heart Association provides an excellent review of the management of atrial fibrillation.

13. Stroke Prevention in Atrial Fibrillation Investigators: Stroke Prevention in Atrial Fibrillation Study. Final results. *Circulation* 84:527-539, 1991.
Aspirin (325 mg/day) reduced the risk of thromboembolism in nonrheumatic atrial fibrillation by 42%, and warfarin (prothrombin time ratio, 1.3-1.8) reduced the risk by 67% compared with placebo. Because of the study design, warfarin was not directly compared with aspirin.

14. Stroke Prevention in Atrial Fibrillation Investigators: Warfarin versus aspirin for prevention of thromboembolism in atrial fibrillation: Stroke Prevention in Atrial Fibrillation II Study. *Lancet* 343:687-691, 1994.
Warfarin may be more effective than aspirin for the prevention of ischemic stroke in patients with atrial fibrillation, but the absolute reduction in stroke rate with warfarin is small. Younger patients without risk factors had a low rate of stroke when treated with aspirin. In older patients, the rate of stroke (ischemic and hemorrhagic) was substantial, irrespective of which agent was given. Patient age and the inherent risk of thromboembolism should be considered in the choice of antithrombotic prophylaxis for patients with atrial fibrillation.

15. Stroke Prevention in Atrial Fibrillation Investigators: Adjusted-dose warfarin versus low-intensity, fixed-dose warfarin plus aspirin for high-risk patients with atrial fibrillation: Stroke Prevention in Atrial Fibrillation III randomised clinical trial. *Lancet* 348:633-638, 1996.
Low-intensity fixed-dose warfarin plus aspirin was insufficient for stroke prevention in patients with nonvalvular atrial fibrillation at high risk for thromboembolism. Adjusted-dose warfarin (target INR, 2.0-3.0) reduced the rate of stroke for high-risk patients.

Questions

Multiple Choice (choose the one best answer)

1. On the electrocardiogram shown below, all of the following are present *except*:
   a. Atrial fibrillation
   b. Premature ventricular contraction
   c. Ashman phenomenon
   d. None of the above

2. A 42-year-old man walks into the emergency room complaining of dizziness and a sensation of racing heartbeats. He takes no medications and has a systolic blood pressure of 100 mm Hg. An electrocardiogram is obtained and is shown below. Which of the following items would be appropriate initial therapy?
   a. Lidocaine
   b. Adenosine
   c. Metoprolol
   d. Procainamide
   e. Diltiazem

3. Hypertension is associated with atrial fibrillation.
   a. True
   b. False

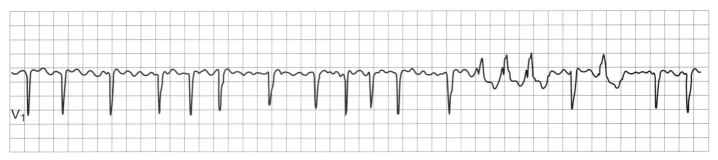

Question 1

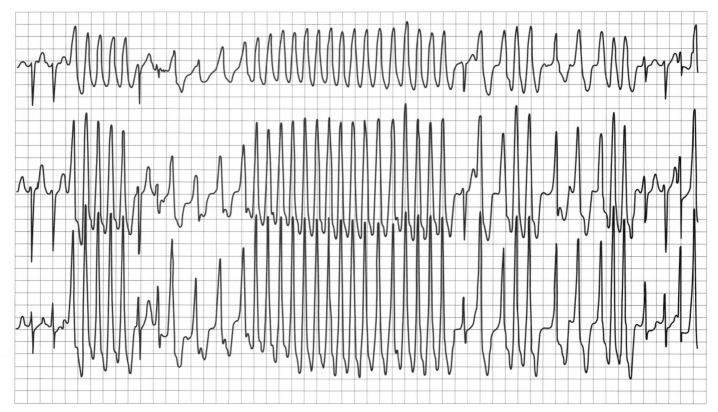

Question 2

4. A 56-year-old man presents complaining of palpitations. An electrocardiogram is obtained and is shown below. Which of the following statements is true?
   a. Adenosine will terminate this rhythm
   b. For successful cardioversion, 200 joules or more is required
   c. Radiofrequency ablation is more than 90% effective
   d. Propafenone has no effect on this rhythm
   e. β-Adrenergic blockers are not effective for controlling the ventricular heart rate

5. A patient with palpitations for 8 days presents to you for evaluation. An electrocardiogram is obtained and is shown on the next page. Which of the following is not a risk factor for stroke in this patient?
   a. Hypertension
   b. Previous cerebrovascular accident
   c. An ejection fraction of 30%
   d. Female patient older than 75 years
   e. All of the above are risk factors

6. For the patient described in question 5, which is *not* an appropriate course of action?
   a. Check electrolyte values and thyroid function
   b. Begin warfarin therapy and plan on cardioversion in 1 month
   c. Begin β-adrenergic blocker therapy
   d. Begin a heparin infusion and perform cardioversion immediately
   e. All of the above are appropriate courses of action

7. For the patient described in question 5, it is appropriate to initiate therapy with all the following medications *except*:
   a. Digoxin
   b. Diltiazem
   c. Procainamide
   d. Metoprolol

8. Paroxysmal atrial fibrillation is associated with an increased risk of stroke compared with chronic atrial fibrillation.
   a. True
   b. False

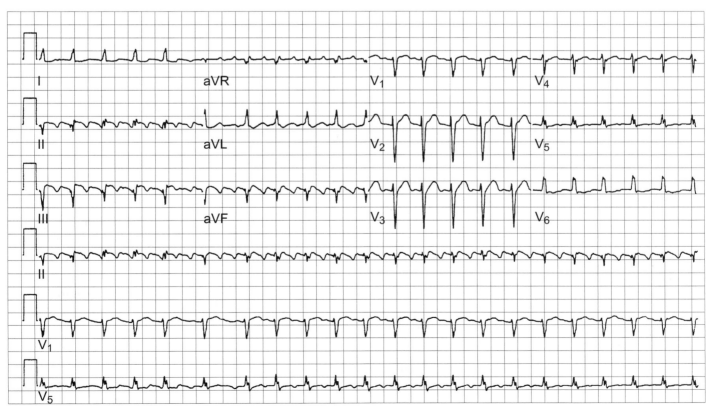

Question 4

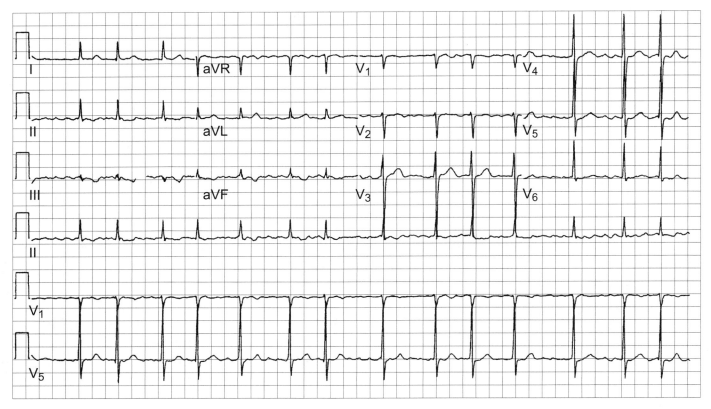

Question 5

Answers

1. Answer b

This tracing demonstrates atrial fibrillation with Ashman phenomenon. The long-short interval and classic right bundle branch morphology with a "right rabbit ear taller than left" demonstrate that this is aberrant conduction. A premature ventricular complex is not present.

2. Answer d

The electrocardiogram shows atrial fibrillation in a patient with Wolff-Parkinson-White syndrome. The widest complexes represent activation down the accessory pathway, whereas narrower ones represent fusion beats in which the ventricles are activated in part by conduction down the atrioventricular node and in part by the accessory pathway. Adenosine shortens the atrial refractory period and causes atrioventricular block and could accelerate the ventricular rate, resulting in degeneration to ventricular fibrillation. Lidocaine has no effect on atrial tissue and is not effective in this setting. Both metoprolol and diltiazem also slow the atrioventricular node, possibly limiting concealed conduction from the node to the accessory pathway and accelerating conduction down the pathway. Procainamide is the agent of choice in this setting. If this fails to control the rhythm, cardioversion is appropriate.

3. Answer a

Hypertension is an etiologic agent in atrial fibrillation. The presence of hypertension also confers increased risk for thromboembolism in patients with atrial fibrillation.

4. Answer c

The rhythm shown is atrial flutter. This rhythm involves intra-atrial reentry in a circuit that is parallel to the tricuspid valve annulus. Administration of adenosine will result in transient atrioventricular node block and clear demonstration of the persistent atrial flutter waves in most cases, but it will not terminate the intra-atrial reentry itself. In some cases, adenosine may cause atrial flutter to degenerate into atrial fibrillation because of its shortening of the atrial effective refractory period. Atrial flutter is a very organized rhythm and can frequently be cardioverted with less than 50 joules.

Atrial flutter ablation is successful in more than 90% of cases. A linear radiofrequency lesion is placed between the tricuspid valve annulus and the inferior vena cava, interrupting the reentrant circuit. Propafenone, a class IC agent, is effective in atrial flutter, although the recurrence rate at 1 year may exceed 50%. Although β-adrenergic blockers do not control the atrial flutter itself, by increasing the degree of atrioventricular block, the ventricular rate is slowed.

5. Answer e

The electrocardiogram shows atrial fibrillation. Atrial fibrillation is characterized by an irregular baseline without clear-cut P waves and an irregularly irregular ventricular response. Several studies have demonstrated that the risk of cerebrovascular accident in patients with nonrheumatic atrial fibrillation is increased with hypertension, previous cerebrovascular accident, and a depressed ejection fraction. It is also increased in women older than 75 years. Patients with structurally normal hearts who are younger than 60 are considered to have "lone atrial fibrillation," which is associated with a very low risk of thromboembolism and requires no specific antithrombotic therapy.

6. Answer d

This patient has atrial fibrillation, which, according to the history, has persisted for 8 days. Patients with atrial fibrillation for more than 24 to 48 hours should have anticoagulation for 3 or 4 weeks before elective cardioversion to diminish the risk of stroke. More recently, emerging evidence suggests that intravenous heparin followed by transesophageal echocardiography and cardioversion if no atrial thrombus is present is an acceptable alternative approach. In this setting, however, continuous anticoagulation for at least 4 weeks after cardioversion is required to prevent postcardioversion thromboembolism.

Beginning a heparin infusion followed by immediate cardioversion is not an appropriate action. Checking electrolyte values and thyroid function to screen for predisposing factors for atrial fibrillation is appropriate. β-Adrenergic blockers are effective for controlling the ventricular rate by limiting the number of atrial signals that can successfully penetrate the atrioventricular node and activate the ventricles. β-Adrenergic blockers or calcium channel blockers, in general, are more effective than digoxin for controlling the ventricular response in atrial fibrillation. β-Adrenergic blockers, calcium channel blockers, and digoxin have not been shown to terminate atrial fibrillation.

7. Answer c

This patient has atrial fibrillation. The digoxin, diltiazem, and metoprolol will slow the atrioventricular node conduction and control the ventricular rate. Although procainamide can be used to restore normal sinus rhythm, it enhances atrioventricular node conduction and could result in an increase in ventricular rate. Therefore, rate control should be achieved before use of procainamide is initiated.

8. Answer b

Randomized studies of nonrheumatic atrial fibrillation in patients with paroxysmal and chronic atrial fibrillation have shown no difference in the rate of stroke between the subgroups. Some authorities believe that patients with infrequent episodes of paroxysmal atrial fibrillation may have a decreased risk of thromboembolism, although this has not been proved.

Notes

Chapter 38

Supraventricular Tachycardia

Marshall S. Stanton, M.D.

> This chapter is a synopsis of all the supraventricular tachycardia subtypes that you are likely to be asked about in Internal Medicine or General Cardiology Examinations, except for atrial fibrillation, which is covered in a separate chapter.

Narrow QRS tachycardias are defined as "abnormal fast rhythms with QRS complexes 100 ms or less in duration." It is improper to use 100 beats/min as the cutoff for tachycardia in this definition because some arrhythmias originating at the atrioventricular (AV) junction are considered tachycardias when they exceed 60 beats/min, the typical upper limit for normal escape rhythms from that region.

It is most useful to divide regular narrow QRS tachycardias into short RP and long RP types (Table 1). This is done by assessing the position of the P wave relative to the QRS (R wave). Short RP tachycardias have the P wave either buried within the QRS or following in the ST segment or T wave; that is, the RP interval is shorter than the PR interval. Conversely, long RP tachycardias have the P wave in front of the QRS; that is, the RP is longer than the PR. **The most important way to begin analyzing any arrhythmia is to identify the atrial activity.** Surface electrocardiographic (ECG) leads II, III, aVF, and V$_1$ usually are the most helpful.

This chapter concentrates on the ECG presentation of regular narrow QRS tachycardias.

- Narrow QRS tachycardias are defined as "abnormal fast rhythms with QRS complexes 100 ms or less in duration."
- It is most useful to divide regular narrow QRS tachycardias into short RP and long RP types.
- To begin the diagnosis of narrow QRS tachycardia:
    Identify the atrial activity.
    Leads II, III, aVF, and V$_1$ are most helpful.
    Determine the relationship of the P waves to the QRS complex.

Short RP Tachycardias

AV Nodal Reentrant Tachycardia

AV nodal reentrant tachycardia is a very common mechanism of paroxysmal tachycardias that occur in young people. In these patients, two pathways exist for conduction of impulses from the atria to the ventricles: the fast pathway (which conducts rapidly) and the slow pathway (which conducts more slowly) (Fig. 1). The typical form of AV nodal reentrant tachycardia is a regular tachycardia with the P wave either not visible (because it is occurring simultaneously with the QRS) or apparent at the end of the QRS or within the ST segment. The reason for this is that the arrhythmia circuit consists of anterograde conduction over the slow pathway and return of the impulse to the atria retrogradely over the fast pathway. This atrial activity may be subtle, but careful comparison with the

Table 1.--Differential Diagnosis of Regular Narrow QRS Tachycardia*†

Short RP (RP < PR)	Long RP (RP > PR)
AV nodal reentrant tachycardia	**Sinus tachycardia**
	Sinus nodal reentrant tachycardia
AV reentrant tachycardia	**Atrial tachycardia**
Nonparoxysmal junctional tachycardia‡	**Nonparoxysmal junctional tachycardia‡**
	Permanent junctional reciprocating tachycardia
	Unusual form of AV node reentry
	Atypical AV reentrant tachycardia

AV, atrioventricular.

*The arrhythmias most important for clinical cardiologists are in boldface type.

†Atrial flutter is often a regular narrow QRS tachycardia, but it is not included in this table because P waves are not present and, thus, it cannot be designated as a short or long RP tachycardia.

‡The RP relation in nonparoxysmal junctional tachycardia is not predictable: there may be retrograde block with resultant AV dissociation or the atria may be captured retrogradely with 1:1 or variable conduction.

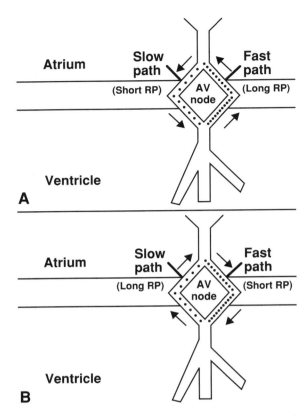

Fig. 1. Mechanisms of supraventricular tachycardia. *A*, Slow-fast form. In this common form of AV nodal reentrant tachycardia, a reentrant circuit is composed of a slow pathway with a short refractory period (*RP*) and a fast pathway with a long refractory period. A premature beat is required to initiate tachycardia, and the tachycardia utilizes the slow pathway for antegrade conduction and the fast pathway for retrograde conduction. *B*, Fast-slow form. In this unusual form of AV nodal reentrant tachycardia, sometimes referred to as "incessant tachycardia," the slow pathway has a long refractory period and the fast pathway has a short refractory period. In contrast to the more common form of AV nodal reentrant tachycardia, a premature beat is not necessary to initiate tachycardia; a normally timed sinus beat may initiate tachycardia. (From Giuliani ER, Gersh BJ, McGoon MD, Hayes DL, Schaff HV [editors]: *Mayo Clinic Practice of Cardiology.* Third edition. Mosby, 1996, p 754. By permission of Mayo Foundation.)

patient's baseline ECG should identify P waves in approximately 50% of patients.

Acutely, this arrhythmia responds well to vagal maneuvers and to adenosine or intravenous calcium channel blockers or β-blockers. Chronic medical therapy is best initiated with AV nodal blocking drugs. Digoxin is tolerated best but is the least effective. Catheter ablation is curative in about 95% of patients and typically involves eliminating the slow pathway; complete AV block can complicate ablation in about 2% of patients.

AV nodal reentrant tachycardia has an abrupt onset and offset, although there may be some slowing of the rate before sudden termination. Rate is not useful in distinguishing this rhythm from others, because it can range from 100 to 280 beats/min.

- AV nodal reentrant tachycardia is a common arrhythmia.
- The circuit involves a fast pathway and a slow pathway.
- The arrhythmia can be terminated with AV nodal blockade.
- Catheter ablation is curative in 95% of patients.

Esophageal Recording

Recording the atrial activity via an esophageal electrode can be helpful because a VA (RP) interval less than 70 ms excludes an accessory pathway from participating in the tachycardia and makes AV nodal reentrant tachycardia likely. The converse is not necessarily true; that is, a VA (RP) interval greater than 70 ms does not exclude AV nodal reentrant tachycardia. The occurrence of functional bundle branch block during AV nodal reentrant tachycardia will not affect the VA interval or the cycle length of the tachycardia, because the bundle branches are not an integral part of the arrhythmia circuit (compare with AV reentrant tachycardia below).

It should be noted that under certain uncommon circumstances, AV block (most often 2:1) can occur, and extremely rarely, retrograde VA block may be seen. Thus, AV dissociation or block does not necessarily rule out AV nodal reentrant tachycardia as the underlying mechanism, but it would be most unusual.

> Esophageal ECG recordings have been shown on the Cardiology Boards, Internal Medicine Boards, and examinations of the Royal College of Physicians.

AV Reentrant Tachycardia

AV reentrant tachycardia involves an accessory pathway in its circuit. Narrow QRS AV reentrant tachycardia uses the AV node as the anterograde limb and an AV accessory pathway as the retrograde limb and is known as "orthodromic reciprocating tachycardia" (Fig. 2). Like AV nodal reentrant tachycardia, AV reentrant tachycardia is typically a short RP tachycardia that has an abrupt onset and offset. One-to-one AV association is a requisite of AV reentrant tachycardia because the atria and ventricles are both integral parts of the arrhythmia circuit. In other words, if AV dissociation occurs, AV reentrant tachycardia can be excluded.

It has been reported that alternation of the amplitude of QRS complexes (QRS alternans) during narrow complex tachycardias strongly suggests orthodromic reciprocating tachycardia. However, in an individual case, this criterion has limited usefulness, and the phenomenon has been seen in other arrhythmias.

Acute treatment of AV reentrant tachycardia usually is aimed at interrupting the circuit in the AV node. Thus, vagal maneuvers, adenosine, and intravenous administration of calcium channel blockers or β-blockers are used. Do not confuse this with the situation of atrial fibrillation in the setting of an accessory pathway, in which digoxin, calcium channel blockers, and β-blockers are contraindicated and the treatment of choice would be intravenous administration of procainamide or cardioversion. For most patients, the treatment of choice for long-term therapy of arrhythmias involving accessory pathways is catheter ablation, which is curative in about 95% of patients.

- AV reentrant tachycardia involves an accessory pathway that may be concealed (i.e., no delta wave) or manifest (i.e., Wolff-Parkinson-White syndrome).
- Acute therapy is aimed at blocking the AV node, which will terminate the arrhythmia.
- Adenosine, verapamil, and other AV nodal blockers are effective in terminating AV reentrant tachycardia but are contraindicated in atrial fibrillation with Wolff-Parkinson-White syndrome.
- Catheter ablation is curative in 95% of patients.

Esophageal Recording

During orthodromic reciprocating tachycardia, esophageal recording shows a VA (RP) interval greater than 70 ms

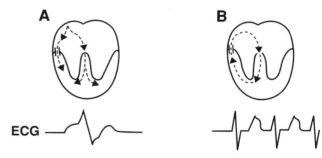

Anterograde conduction present (Wolff-Parkinson-White syndrome)

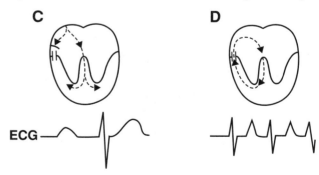

Anterograde conduction absent (concealed Wolff-Parkinson-White syndrome)

Fig. 2. Wolff-Parkinson-White syndrome with manifest (*A* and *B*) and concealed (*C* and *D*) conduction. When anterograde conduction is present down an accessory pathway, the QRS morphology is the product of fusion of input from the atria via the AV node and the accessory pathway producing the typical delta wave. When anterograde conduction down the accessory pathway is absent (*C*), activation of the ventricle proceeds in the normal fashion, and the QRS is normal (hence, concealed bypass tract). The mechanism of tachycardia in both cases is identical: anterograde conduction proceeds down the AV node, and retrograde conduction is via the bypass tract (*C* and *D*). (From Campbell R, Murray A [editors]: *Dynamic Electrocardiography.* Churchill Livingstone, 1985, pp 74-88. By permission of the publisher.)

(Fig. 3). As mentioned above, AV nodal reentrant tachycardia sometimes also has a VA interval greater than 70 ms. Unlike AV nodal reentrant tachycardia, when bundle branch block occurs on the side ipsilateral to the accessory pathway (e.g., left bundle branch block in the presence of a left-sided accessory pathway) the VA interval—and often the cycle length—will be prolonged. This is because the ipsilateral bundle branch is an integral part of the arrhythmia circuit; thus, when block occurs in that bundle, the impulse must travel down the contralateral bundle branch and then traverse the intraventricular septum before reaching the accessory pathway. Therefore, the tachycardia circuit is lengthened.

Nonparoxysmal Junctional Tachycardia

Nonparoxysmal junctional tachycardia is an automatic or triggered rhythm arising in the AV junction and having a relatively slow rate (typically 70 to 130 beats/min), with a gradual onset and offset. The P wave usually occurs simultaneously with or just after the QRS; occasionally, it can precede the QRS or even be dissociated. The P-wave axis is directed superiorly, being negative in the inferior leads. When nonparoxysmal junctional tachycardia is due to digitalis toxicity, there can be alterations in conduction back to the atrium, producing variations such as retrograde Wenckebach phenomenon or complete VA block.

The causes of nonparoxysmal junctional tachycardia include digitalis toxicity, inferior myocardial infarction, myocarditis, and post-mitral valve surgery.

- Suspect nonparoxysmal junctional tachycardia or complete heart block when the ventricular response becomes regular in a patient taking digoxin for atrial fibrillation.

Long RP Tachycardias

Sinus Tachycardia
Although sinus tachycardia would not seem to be a difficult diagnosis to make, at very rapid rates the P wave begins to fuse with the preceding T wave, and this rhythm has been mistaken for other arrhythmias, especially in critically ill patients in whom rates may exceed 180 beats/min. In sinus tachycardia, the P wave precedes the QRS and has a normal morphology, that is, upright in leads I, II, III, and aVF.

Sinus Nodal Reentrant Tachycardia
The P wave precedes the QRS in sinus nodal reentry, and its morphology is identical to that of normal sinus rhythm. The onset and offset are abrupt. Sinus node reentry is easily affected by changes in autonomic tone. Thus, vagal maneuvers slow or terminate the rhythm. Although a wide range of rates may occur, the average rate is about 130 to 140 beats/min. Without the onset or offset being seen, sinus node reentry cannot be distinguished from sinus tachycardia. It is not unusual for this rhythm to be seen on asymptomatic ambulatory ECG recordings.

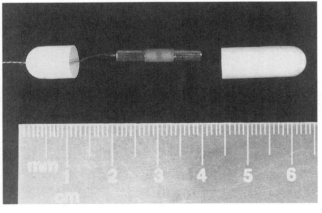

A

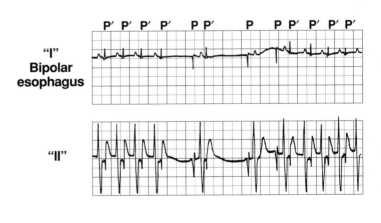

B

Fig. 3. Esophageal recording techniques. *A*, Esophageal pill electrode originally described by Arzbaecher (*Med Instrum* 12:277-281, 1978). *B*, Bipolar esophageal recording from a patient with paroxysmal AV tachycardia that uses a concealed accessory pathway. The bipolar esophageal lead recorded simultaneously with lead II during tachycardia clearly identifies retrograde P waves (P´) with a VA interval of approximately 150 ms. (From Campbell R, Murray A [editors]: *Dynamic Electrocardiography*. Churchill Livingstone, 1985, pp 74-88. By permission of the publisher.)

Atrial Tachycardia

In atrial tachycardia, the impulse comes from a focus in the atrium away from the sinus node. The morphology of the P wave depends on the location of the atrial focus and will differ from the sinus P wave unless the site of origin is near the region of the sinus node. Atrial tachycardia is a long RP tachycardia, because typically the P wave immediately precedes the QRS. Whether 1:1 AV conduction occurs depends on the rate of the tachycardia, presence of AV node blocking drugs or disease, and whether digitalis toxicity is present. Paroxysmal atrial tachycardia with AV block should raise the diagnostic possibility of digitalis toxicity.

The medical treatment of atrial tachycardia is similar to that for atrial flutter and fibrillation. Catheter ablation can eliminate the focus of this arrhythmia, with cure rates of 75% to 90%.

- In atrial tachycardia, the impulse comes from a focus in the atrium away from the sinus node.
- Paroxysmal atrial tachycardia with AV block should raise the diagnostic possibility of digitalis toxicity.

Permanent Junctional Reciprocating Tachycardia

Permanent junctional reciprocating tachycardia represents a specific type of accessory pathway: an AV accessory connection with AV nodal-like properties located in the posteroseptal region. Because of these characteristics, the P wave is seen preceding the QRS and the axis of the P wave is directed superiorly (negative in II, III, and aVF).

Furthermore, although anterograde conduction may occur under special circumstances over the accessory pathway, the QRS is almost always narrow. Permanent junctional reciprocating tachycardia often presents as an incessant arrhythmia, and it may be a cause of tachycardia-induced cardiomyopathy.

- Suspect permanent junctional reciprocating tachycardia in a young patient presenting with cardiomyopathy and an incessant tachycardia that looks like atrial tachycardia.

Unusual Form of AV Nodal Reentrant Tachycardia

As noted above, typical AV nodal reentrant tachycardia is due to an impulse traveling anterogradely down the slow pathway and retrogradely up the fast pathway. In the unusual (atypical) form of AV nodal reentrant tachycardia, the circuit is reversed; that is, anterograde conduction is over the fast pathway and retrograde conduction is over the slow pathway. The P wave will be located in front of the QRS. On the surface ECG, this arrhythmia is identical to permanent junctional reciprocating tachycardia.

Atypical AV Reentrant Tachycardia

Although most accessory pathways conduct rapidly and generate a P wave following the QRS during orthodromic reciprocating tachycardia, a small percentage of accessory pathways conduct slowly, causing a long RP tachycardia.

Suggested Review Reading

1. Calkins H, Langberg J, Sousa J, et al: Radiofrequency catheter ablation of accessory atrioventricular connections in 250 patients. Abbreviated therapeutic approach to Wolff-Parkinson-White syndrome. *Circulation* 85:1337-1346, 1992.

2. Gallagher JJ, Smith WM, Kasell J, et al: Use of the esophageal lead in the diagnosis of mechanisms of reciprocating supraventricular tachycardia. *Pacing Clin Electrophysiol* 3:440-451, 1980.

3. Jackman WM, Beckman KJ, McClelland JH, et al: Treatment of supraventricular tachycardia due to atrioventricular nodal reentry, by radiofrequency catheter ablation of slow-pathway conduction. *N Engl J Med* 327:313-318, 1992.

4. Jackman WM, Wang XZ, Friday KJ, et al: Catheter ablation of accessory atrioventricular pathways (Wolff-Parkinson-White syndrome) by radiofrequency current. *N Engl J Med* 324:1605-1611, 1991.

5. Kalbfleisch SJ, el-Atassi R, Calkins H, et al: Differentiation of paroxysmal narrow QRS complex tachycardias using the 12-lead electrocardiogram. *J Am Coll Cardiol* 21:85-89, 1993.

6. Kastor JA: Multifocal atrial tachycardia. *N Engl J Med* 322:1713-1717, 1990.
Excellent review of multifocal atrial tachycardia.

7. Kerr CR, Gallagher JJ, German LD. Changes in ventriculoatrial intervals with bundle branch block aberration during reciprocating tachycardia in patients with accessory atrioventricular pathways. *Circulation* 66:196-201, 1982.

8. Pieper SJ, Stanton MS: Narrow QRS complex tachycardias. *Mayo Clin Proc* 70:371-375, 1995.

Questions

Multiple Choice (choose the one best answer)

1. Atrioventricular block is not uncommon in:
   a. Sinus tachycardia
   b. Atrial tachycardia
   c. Atrioventricular node reentry
   d. Atrioventricular reentry with an accessory pathway

2. The risk of stroke is increased in patients having:
   a. Sinus tachycardia
   b. Atrial flutter
   c. Atrioventricular node reentry
   d. Wolff-Parkinson-White syndrome
   e. None of the above

3. All the following arrhythmias can be located very near the crista terminalis *except*:
   a. Sinus tachycardia
   b. Sinus node reentry
   c. Atrial tachycardia
   d. Atrioventricular node reentry

4. Intravenous administration of metoprolol may terminate:
   a. Sinus tachycardia
   b. Atrial tachycardia
   c. Atrial flutter
   d. Atrioventricular reentry in Wolff-Parkinson-White syndrome
   e. None of the above

5. Verapamil should never be administered intravenously to a patient with Wolff-Parkinson-White syndrome.
   a. True
   b. False

6. Acceptable therapies for acutely treating atrial fibrillation in a patient with Wolff-Parkinson-White syndrome include all the following *except*:
   a. Procainamide
   b. Ibutilide
   c. Diltiazem
   d. Electrical cardioversion

7. The permanent form of junctional reciprocating tachycardia (PJRT):
   a. Often is an incessant arrhythmia
   b. May present as a cardiomyopathy
   c. Is a type of accessory pathway
   d. Terminates with verapamil
   e. All the above

8. Catheter ablation is well-accepted curative therapy for:
   a. Sinus tachycardia
   b. Atrial fibrillation
   c. Atrioventricular node reentry
   d. Nonparoxysmal junctional tachycardia

9. Long RP tachycardias include:
   a. Atrial tachycardia
   b. Atrioventricular node reentry
   c. Atrioventricular reentry with an accessory pathway
   d. All the above

10. Digoxin toxicity may present with:
    a. Nonparoxysmal junctional tachycardia
    b. Atrial tachycardia
    c. A normal digoxin level
    d. All the above

Answers

1. Answer b
AV block may be associated with atrial tachycardia and suggests the possibility of digitalis toxicity.

2. Answer b
Atrial flutter in addition to atrial fibrillation is associated with an increased risk of stroke that is reduced by anticoagulation therapy with warfarin.

3. Answer d
AV node reentry occurs, as its name implies, within or in proximity to the AV node.

4. Answer d
β-Blockade may slow the heart rate in sinus tachycardia or increase the AV block in atrial tachycardia or flutter. It is unlikely to terminate the arrhythmia.

5. Answer b
Verapamil is contraindicated in atrial fibrillation complicating Wolff-Parkinson-White syndrome, but it may be used cautiously in AV reentry tachycardia complicating Wolff-Parkinson-White syndrome.

6. Answer c
Diltiazem is contraindicated in atrial fibrillation complicating Wolff-Parkinson-White syndrome.

7. Answer e
All these statements are correct.

8. Answer c
Catheter-based therapy is generally ineffective in arrhythmias that are automatic in cause or due to microreentry circuits.

9. Answer a
Atrial tachycardia is a long RP tachycardia.

10. Answer d
Digoxin toxicity is associated with all these statements.

Chapter 39

Ventricular Tachycardia

Thomas M. Munger, M.D.

The anatomical substrate for most cases of ventricular tachycardia (VT) is coronary artery disease with prior myocardial infarction. However, VT may also occur in myocarditis, cardiomyopathy, and, rarely, in structurally normal hearts.

Wide Complex Tachycardia—Differential Diagnosis

In unselected patients presenting with wide complex tachycardias, VT is the diagnosis in 80% of cases. If the patient has underlying structural heart disease, the occurrence of VT as the cause of the rhythm increases to 95%. Features on the surface electrocardiogram (ECG) that favor VT as the diagnosis include fusion beats, capture beats, atrioventricular dissociation (seen in one-third of VT episodes), a wide QRS (> 140 ms), and a northwest axis (Table 1). Figure 1 shows a wide complex tachycardia that has features consistent with VT (QRS duration = 160 ms, AV dissociation [lead II], and ends with fusion beat). Frequently, the cause of wide QRS tachycardia is not readily discerned on the surface ECG (usually VT or supraventricular tachycardia with aberrant conduction), and esophageal recordings or electrophysiologic testing is required to confirm the mechanism of the arrhythmia. Table 2 lists the various arrhythmias that can cause a wide complex tachycardia.

• Features on the surface ECG favoring VT as the diagnosis include fusion beats, capture beats, atrioventricular

dissociation (seen in one-third of VT episodes), a wide QRS complex (> 140 ms), and a northwest axis (Table 1).

Ventricular Tachycardia

Coronary Artery Disease

In the first year after myocardial infarction, clinically detected sustained VT occurs in 2% of patients, but more than 5% of patients experience sudden cardiac death, of which many cases are due to VT/fibrillation. More than 80% of patients in whom post-infarct VT develops also have had other post-infarct complications, including conduction defects, congestive heart failure, primary ventricular fibrillation, and hypotension requiring vasopressors. Patients who present with VT in association with coronary artery disease are more likely to have lower ejection fractions and associated ventricular aneurysms than those who present with ventricular fibrillation. Up to two-thirds of patients with post-infarct VT have an associated left ventricular aneurysm.

Endocardial electrograms are more often abnormal and of longer duration in patients with VT than in those with ventricular fibrillation. The mechanism of VT in most of these patients is myocardial reentry. Several observations support this mechanism, including 1) the ability to initiate and terminate monomorphic VT using programmed ventricular stimulation in more than 95% of patients; 2) the demonstration that VT can be eliminated with either catheter ablation or electrosurgery; 3) the presence of fractionated electrograms during diastole, suggesting an area of slow

Table 1.—Differentiation of Supraventricular Tachycardia With Aberrancy (SVT) From Ventricular Tachycardia (VT) by Means of the Surface Electrocardiogram

Variable	SVT, % of patients	VT, % of patients
Ventricular rate (beats/min)		
100-130	1	13
130-170	27	47
170-200	60	21
> 200	12	19
One-to-one atrial and ventricular relationship	100	33
QRS width, ms		
< 120	76	14
120-140	24	19
> 140	0	67
Mean QRS axis, frontal plane		
-30° or less	7	69
Between -30° and +90°	47	11
More than +90°	43	17
Undetermined	3	3

From Giuliani ER, Gersh BJ, McGoon MD, Hayes DL, Schaff HV (editors): *Mayo Clinic Practice of Cardiology*. Third edition. Mosby, 1996, p 792. By permission of Mayo Foundation.

Table 2.—Differential Diagnosis of Wide Complex Tachycardia

Ventricular tachycardia
Antidromic reciprocating tachycardia
Mahaim fiber tachycardia
Pacemaker-mediated tachycardia
Any supraventricular tachycardia with aberrant conduction (left or right bundle branch block)*
Any supraventricular tachycardia with bystander accessory pathway activation (except junctional tachycardia)*

*Atrial fibrillation, atrial flutter, atrial tachycardia, sinus tachycardia, sinus node reentry tachycardia, typical atrioventricular nodal reentry tachycardia, atypical atrioventricular nodal reentry tachycardia, junctional tachycardia, orthodromic reciprocating tachycardia.

conduction; 4) the high incidence of positive signal-averaged ECGs, indicating an area of slow conduction; and 5) the ability to entrain VT in many patients.

The initial management of patients with VT induced at electrophysiologic study can include antiarrhythmic drug treatment. The probability of an antiarrhythmic drug rendering VT noninducible at subsequent electrophysiologic study decreases as left ventricular ejection fraction or functional class decreases. In the Electrophysiologic Study Versus Electrocardiographic Monitoring (ESVEM) trial, the most effective initial drug tested at electrophysiologic study was sotalol (35% efficacy), as compared with 16% for quinidine and 14% for propafenone. These latter drugs were also associated with twice the clinical recurrence rate of arrhythmia at 1 year compared with sotalol. Amiodarone was not studied in this trial. Our current approach is to test sotalol in patients with an ejection fraction greater than 30%

or to recommend automatic implantable cardioverter-defibrillator (AICD) placement. For patients with an ejection fraction less than 30%, amiodarone therapy or an implantable defibrillator device is advised. For patients with out-of-hospital cardiac arrest, the Antiarrhythmics Versus Implantable Defibrillator (AVID) trial suggested that follow-up results were superior for AICD compared with amiodarone.

Current tiered-therapy implantable defibrillator device systems allow antitachycardia pacing schemes to terminate more than 80% of all spontaneous VTs. After implantation of a defibrillator device, one-third of patients still require antiarrhythmic drug therapy to decrease the frequency of low-energy cardioversion shocks or to suppress atrial arrhythmias that can lead to "inappropriate" shocks.

Electrosurgery is a viable option for patients with discrete left ventricular aneurysms that do not involve the inferior wall/papillary muscle who require other cardiac surgery. Catheter ablation often is a palliative treatment for patients with drug-refractory VT in conjunction with coronary artery disease. Currently, success rates are only about 50% to 75%. Many patients receiving such treatments already have implantable defibrillator devices in place.

- More than 80% of patients in whom VT develops during the first year post-infarct have also had other complications after myocardial infarction.
- The probability of an antiarrhythmic drug rendering VT noninducible at subsequent electrophysiologic study decreases as left ventricular ejection fraction or functional class worsens.

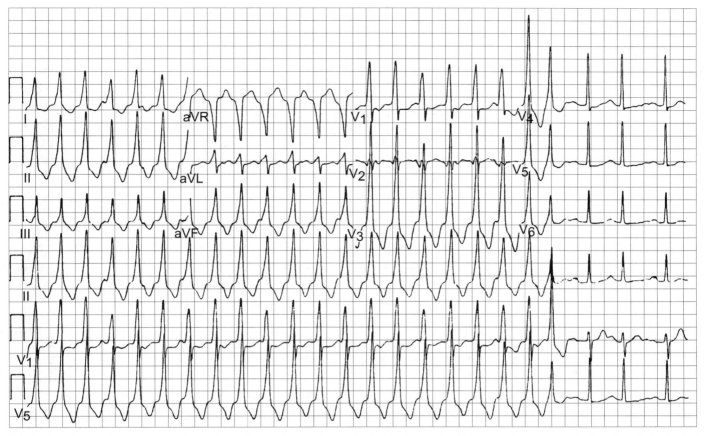

Fig. 1. Ventricular tachycardia with atrioventricular dissociation terminating in sinus rhythm with first-degree atrioventricular block and one fusion beat (*).

- After implantation of a defibrillator device, one-third of patients still require antiarrhythmic drug therapy to decrease the frequency of low-energy cardioversion shocks or to suppress atrial arrhythmias that can lead to "inappropriate" shocks.

Dilated Cardiomyopathy

As in patients with coronary artery disease, the most significant predictor of long-term mortality in patients with dilated cardiomyopathy is left ventricular function. Ventricular arrhythmias occur in more than 90% of patients with dilated cardiomyopathy. More than one-fourth of these patients have nonsustained asymptomatic VT during Holter monitoring for 24-hour periods. The incidence of nonsustained VT increases as the New York Heart Association functional class worsens. The incidence of electrophysiologic-induced monomorphic VT in those with dilated cardiomyopathy who have clinically experienced sustained monomorphic VT is only 50% (much less than for patients with coronary artery disease). Thus, noninducibility of ventricular tachycardia at electrophysiologic testing is much

less predictive for arrhythmia recurrence in patients with dilated cardiomyopathy. There is likely a benefit in treating this group of patients with β-blockers or amiodarone, although there are theoretic reasons why these agents may be detrimental. A recently completed prospective trial using the β-blocker carvedilol demonstrated a significant decrease in overall mortality for patients with congestive heart failure and dilated cardiomyopathy.

Two specific features should be sought in patients with dilated cardiomyopathy and ventricular arrhythmias. The first would be patients with atrial fibrillation and rapid ventricular response or incessant paroxysmal supraventricular tachycardia who present with heart failure. Many of these patients have tachycardia-induced cardiomyopathy, ventricular ectopy, and poor ventricular function—all of which improve with control of the atrial arrhythmias. The second would be left bundle branch block morphology VT due to bundle branch reentry. Many of these patients present with syncope and demonstrate baseline conduction disorders and long HV intervals. This rhythm most often uses the left bundle branch as the retrograde limb of the circuit and the right bundle branch as the anterograde limb, with transseptal conduction completing the loop. This tachycardia is readily diagnosed at electrophysiologic study and can be cured with right bundle branch radiofrequency ablation, with success rates greater than 95%.

- The most significant predictor of long-term mortality in patients with dilated cardiomyopathy is left ventricular function.
- Ventricular arrhythmias occur in more than 90% of patients with dilated cardiomyopathy.

Hypertrophic Cardiomyopathy

A National Institutes of Health prospective study conducted in 1992 involving 230 patients with hypertrophic cardiomyopathy examined the usefulness of electrophysiologic study for predicting subsequent clinical events (cardiac arrests or syncopal implantable defibrillator device shocks). The study examined the relationship of clinical variables, Holter monitoring results, catheterization, and electrophysiologic variables to clinical end points. Only two items were predictive of subsequent clinical events in patients with hypertrophic obstructive cardiomyopathy: a clinical history of syncope or out-of-hospital arrest and inducible ventricular arrhythmias at electrophysiologic testing. Thus, it is reasonable to recommend electrophysiologic testing for patients with symptomatic hypertrophic cardiomyopathy. The role of electrophysiologic study in completely asymptomatic patients with this disease is controversial. The role of electrophysiologic study in patients with hypertrophic obstructive cardiomyopathy who have a significant family history of cardiac arrest but without syncope is unclear.

- Only two items were predictive of cardiac arrest in patients with hypertrophic obstructive cardiomyopathy: a clinical history of syncope or out-of-hospital arrest and inducible ventricular arrhythmias at electrophysiologic testing.

Arrhythmogenic Right Ventricular Dysplasia

"Arrhythmogenic right ventricular dysplasia" (ARVD) is a familial type of right ventricular cardiomyopathy associated with a left bundle branch block type morphology VT. The disease was first described in 1977, and pathologic specimens have disclosed a large degree of fatty infiltration of the right ventricle in patients suddenly dying of this illness. Patients typically were young, often male, and presented with symptoms of hemodynamic compromise. The mechanism of VT in these patients is often myocardial reentry, and VT is frequently inducible at electrophysiologic study. Treatment strategies for these patients have included simple ventriculotomy, disarticulation of the right ventricle, radiofrequency ablation, drug therapy, and implantable defibrillator device. Because patients have been shown to have multiple sites of VT in the right ventricle, success rates for catheter ablation have been similar to those for coronary artery disease. Figure 2 shows VT in a patient with ARVD (note left bundle branch block/left axis deviation, indicating the right ventricular apex as the origin).

- "Arrhythmogenic right ventricular dysplasia" (ARVD) is a familial type of right ventricular cardiomyopathy associated with a left bundle branch type morphology VT.

Ventricular Tachycardia in Patients With a Structurally Normal Heart

Earlier in this century, Parkinson and Papp described an arrhythmia now known as "repetitive monomorphic nonsustained VTs" in patients with normal hearts. Since then, a good prognosis for these patients has been confirmed. These VTs can be divided into those with left bundle branch block morphologies and those with right bundle branch block morphologies.

For patients with left bundle branch block idiopathic VT, initiation by programmed electrical stimulation of the heart is rare (Fig. 2). Frequently, decremental atrial or ventricular pacing is more successful for initiating these rhythms than ventricular extrastimuli. Isoproterenol also can help to initiate this type of VT, which often arises from the right ventricular outflow tract. This type of VT usually is exercise-induced and is often seen in young patients. It has been suggested that an automatic or triggered mechanism underlies this type of VT and explains its response to adenosine, verapamil, β-blockers, and vagal maneuvers. If β-blockers or calcium channel blockers are ineffective in suppressing this arrhythmia, radiofrequency catheter ablation is usually effective.

Right bundle branch block idiopathic VT often is paroxysmal and sustained and is *less* likely to be exercise-induced than left bundle branch block idiopathic VT. It is seen almost exclusively in males. Unlike left bundle branch block VT, this rhythm can be induced with programmed stimulation and isoproterenol in almost 90% of cases. The rhythm classically responds to verapamil given intravenously,

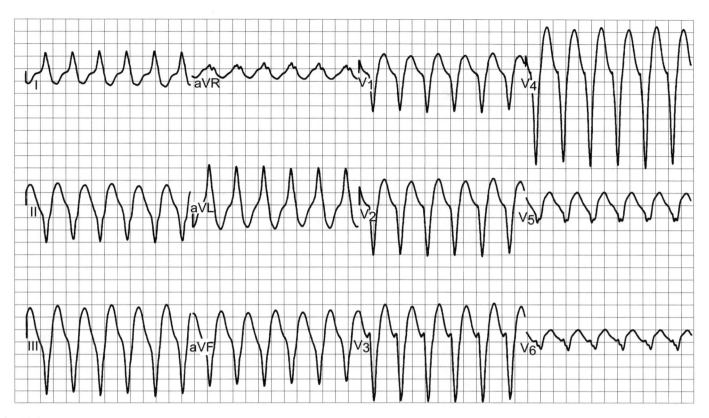

Fig. 2. Ventricular tachycardia.

suggesting a triggered mechanism. The earliest ventricular activation sites are generally in the left ventricular apex or at the mid left ventricular septum. Not uncommonly, discrete electrical potentials can be identified before the ventricular activation at the earliest site, raising the possibility that the Purkinje system participates in the generation of this arrhythmia. If antiarrhythmic drugs are used for right bundle branch block idiopathic VT, class III agents seem to have the best efficacy. Catheter ablation has also been used. The success rate for eradication of this type of VT using catheter ablation is 85% to 90%.

- Right bundle branch block idiopathic VT often is paroxysmal and sustained and is *less* likely to be exercise-induced than left bundle branch block idiopathic VT.

Long QT Syndrome and Polymorphic Ventricular Tachycardia

The long QT syndrome is manifested as triggered ventricular activity and polymorphic ventricular tachycardias, in particular, torsades de pointes. The long QT syndrome can

Table 3.—Genetics of Congenital Long QT Syndrome

Type	Chromosome number	Gene	Exon number	Ion channelopathy
LQT1	11p15.5	*KvLQT1*	16	I_{Ks}
LQT2	7q35-36	*HERG*	16	I_{Kr}
LQT3	3p21-24	*SCN5A*	?	I_{Na}
LQT4	4q25-26	?	?	?
LQT5	21q22	*KCNE1*	?	I_{Ks} (minK)

be either congenital or acquired. Genetic defects in those with the congenital variant have been localized to both potassium and sodium channels, which are encoded on chromosomes 3, 4, 7, 11, and 21 (Table 3).

The long QT syndrome has many secondary causes, including several cardiac and noncardiac drugs, very low calorie diets, cardiac ischemia, and catastrophic events in the central nervous system (Table 4). Treatment for a primary or acquired long QT syndrome in cases of symptomatic polymorphic ventricular tachycardia includes withdrawal of aggravating drugs, magnesium given intravenously, and isoproterenol as well as pacing to increase the ventricular rate and to shorten the QT interval. More chronic therapies include β-blockers, left sympathectomy, mexiletine, and implantable cardioverter defibrillators.

Table 4.—Acquired Causes of Long QT Syndrome

Antiarrhythmic drugs
Astemizole
Bepridil
Central nervous system hemorrhage
Cisapride
Erythromycin
Ischemia
Ketoconazole
Liquid protein diet
Myocarditis
Pentamidine
Phenothiazines
Terfenadine
Tricyclic antidepressants

Suggested Review Reading

1. Ackerman MJ: The long QT syndrome: ion channel diseases of the heart. *Mayo Clin Proc* 73:250-269, 1998.
State-of-the-art review of this rapidly evolving area in the genetic understanding of sudden death and ventricular arrhythmias. The author points out that more than 35 mutations in four cardiac ion channel genes have been identified in the long QT syndrome: KVLQT1 (voltage-gated potassium channel, I_{Ks}, LQT1), HERG (human ether-a-go-go related gene, I_{Kr}, LQT2), SCN5A (incomplete sodium channel inactivation, LQT3), and KCNE1 (minK, a subunit of I_K, LQT5).

2. Akhtar M, Shenasa M, Jazayeri M, et al: Wide QRS complex tachycardia. Reappraisal of a common clinical problem. *Ann Intern Med* 109:905-912, 1988.
One hundred fifty consecutive patients who came to the emergency room with wide QRS tachycardia were evaluated.

Ventricular tachycardia was confirmed in 81%, aberrantly conducted supraventricular tachycardia in 14%, and pre-excited tachycardias in 5%. Ventricular tachycardia was associated with structural heart disease. Criteria implying ventricular tachycardia included atrioventricular dissociation, positive QRS concordance, northwest axis, combination of left bundle branch block and right axis, and QRS duration greater than 140 ms with right bundle branch block and greater than 160 ms with left bundle branch block.

3. Amiodarone Trials Meta-Analysis Investigators: Effect of prophylactic amiodarone on mortality after acute myocardial infarction and in congestive heart failure: meta-analysis of individual data from 6500 patients in randomised trials. *Lancet* 350:1417-1424, 1997.
Trends favoring beneficial effects of amiodarone in post-myocardial infarction patients at risk for sudden cardiac death appeared in trials such as BASIS, CAMIAT, and EMIAT, but overall mortality was little affected. These workers performed meta-analysis on 13 randomized trials of

prophylactic amiodarone in recent post-myocardial infarction patients (n = 8) or in patients with congestive heart failure (n = 5). This included 6,553 patients, 78% who were in post-myocardial infarction trials. Total mortality was reduced by 13% (P = 0.030). Arrhythmic/sudden death was reduced by 29% (P = 0.0003). There was no effect on nonarrhythmic deaths (P = 0.84). The risk of pulmonary toxicity from the drug was 1% per year. The authors concluded that the previous studies, by themselves, were underpowered to examine overall mortality and that in this meta-analysis the drug indeed reduced overall mortality, chiefly having its effect on reducing overall arrhythmic death.

4. Blanck Z, Dhala A, Deshpande S, et al: Bundle branch reentrant ventricular tachycardia: cumulative experience in 48 patients. *J Cardiovasc Electrophysiol* 4:253-262, 1993.

The clinical and electrophysiologic features and follow-up of 48 patients with inducible bundle branch reentrant (BBR) tachycardia. Idiopathic dilated cardiomyopathy and coronary artery disease were present in 19 (39%) and 24 (50%) patients, respectively. All patients had His-Purkinje system disease. BBR tachycardia with left and right bundle branch block morphologies was induced in 46 and 5 patients. During follow-up, congestive heart failure was the most common cause of death.

5. Borggrefe M, Fetsch T, Martinez-Rubio A, et al: Prediction of arrhythmia risk based on signal-averaged ECG in postinfarction patients. *Pacing Clin Electrophysiol* 20:2566-2576, 1997.

This article reviews the method used to record signal-averaged ECGs that can identify slow zones of conduction in post-myocardial infarction patients and its potential clinical usefulness in such patients. It is pointed out that the signal-averaged ECG has been used to predict sudden cardiac death in post-myocardial infarction patients and to screen for inducible ventricular tachycardia in patients with unexplained syncope.

6. Brugada P, Brugada J, Mont L, et al: A new approach to the differential diagnosis of a regular tachycardia with a wide QRS complex. *Circulation* 83:1649-1659, 1991.
The authors used four new ECG criteria and applied them prospectively to 554 cases of tachycardia with widened QRS. When applied in a stepwise fashion, the sensitivity was 99% and the specificity was 97%. Of the criteria, perhaps the easiest remembered is that the absence of an RS

complex in all precordial leads is highly specific for the diagnosis of ventricular tachycardia.

7. Doval HC, Nul DR, Grancelli HO, et al: Nonsustained ventricular tachycardia in severe heart failure. Independent marker of increased mortality due to sudden death. Circulation 94:3198-3203, 1996.
The GESICA trial suggested empiric amiodarone given to patients with congestive heart failure (mostly nonischemic heart failure) would be of benefit. This paper reiterates the importance of nonsustained ventricular tachycardia as a marker for sudden death in patients with congestive heart failure. Such findings have previously been noted in patients with dilated cardiomyopathy.

8. Fananapazir L, Chang AC, Epstein SE, et al: Prognostic determinants in hypertrophic cardiomyopathy. Prospective evaluation of a therapeutic strategy based on clinical, Holter, hemodynamic, and electrophysiological findings. Circulation 86:730-740, 1992.
Clinical, Holter monitoring, cardiac catheterization, and electrophysiologic data were collected on 230 patients with hypertrophic cardiomyopathy and examined by multivariate analysis to predict subsequent life-threatening ventricular arrhythmia events. Ventricular tachycardia on Holter monitoring was present in 115 patients (50%). Sustained ventricular arrhythmia was induced in 82 patients (36%). Two variables were significant independent predictors of subsequent events: sustained ventricular arrhythmia induced at electrophysiologic study (P = 0.002) and a history of cardiac arrest or syncope (P < 0.05). Of interest, this study also showed that Holter monitoring that showed nonsustained ventricular tachycardia or a positive family history of sudden death was predictive of future cardiac events.

9. Fontaine G, Fontaliran F, Frank R: Arrhythmogenic right ventricular cardiomyopathies: clinical forms and main differential diagnoses. Circulation 97:1532-1535, 1998.
An excellent comprehensive state-of-the-art review of this structural heart disease.

10. Grogan M, Smith HC, Gersh BJ, et al: Left ventricular dysfunction due to atrial fibrillation in patients initially believed to have idiopathic dilated cardiomyopathy. Am J Cardiol 69:1570-1573, 1992.
This paper emphasizes the importance of looking for tachycardia-induced cardiomyopathy in patients who present

with unexplained systolic heart failure. Atrial fibrillation with uncontrolled rates and, less commonly, incessant ectopic atrial tachycardia or paroxysmal junctional reciprocating tachycardia can cause this reversible form of heart failure/dilated cardiomyopathy. In this review of 10 patients, the left ventricular ejection fraction increased from a median of 25% to 52% after adequate rhythm management.

11. Julian DG, Camm AJ, Frangin G, et al: Randomised trial of effect of amiodarone on mortality in patients with left-ventricular dysfunction after recent myocardial infarction: EMIAT. *Lancet* 349:667-674, 1997.

The EMIAT trial was a randomized double-blinded placebo-controlled trial designed to assess whether amiodarone would decrease all-cause mortality (primary end point) and arrhythmic death (secondary end point) in survivors of myocardial infarction with a left ventricular ejection fraction of 40% or less. The trial included 1,486 patients (743 in the amiodarone group, 743 in the placebo group). Median follow-up was 21 months. All-cause mortality (103 deaths in the amiodarone group, 102 in the placebo group) and cardiac mortality did not differ; in the amiodarone group, there was a 35% risk reduction (P = 0.05) in arrhythmic deaths. The authors suggested that systematic prophylactic use of amiodarone in all patients with depressed left ventricular function after myocardial infarction was not warranted, because overall mortality was not affected by the presence of the drug.

12. Stevenson WG, Khan H, Sager P, et al: Identification of reentry circuit sites during catheter mapping and radiofrequency ablation of ventricular tachycardia late after myocardial infarction. *Circulation* 88:1647-1670, 1993.

This study developed criteria for distinguishing bystander ventricular tachycardia from actual slow zones of conduction for purposes of mapping and ablating post-infarction reentry ventricular tachycardia (VT). Computer simulation was used to develop the criteria. Endocardial catheter mapping and radiofrequency ablation were then undertaken in 15 patients with 31 drug refractory VTs late after myocardial infarction. Radiofrequency current terminated VT at 24 of 241 sites (10%) in 12 of 15 patients (80%). VT termination was more likely to occur at sites demonstrating entrainment with concealed fusion (odds ratio, 3.4; 95% confidence interval [CI]: 1.4, 8.3), a postpacing interval equal to the VT cycle length (odds ratio, 4.6; 95% CI: 1.6, 12.9), and an S-QRS interval during entrainment of more than 60 ms and less than 70% of the VT cycle length (odds ratio, 4.9; 95% CI: 1.4, 17.1). VT termination was also predicted by the presence of isolated diastolic potentials or continuous electrical activity (odds ratio, 5.2; 95% CI: 1.8, 15.5); however, these types of electrograms were rarely noted (8% of all sites). Taken together, entrainment with concealed fusion, postpacing interval, S-QRS intervals, and isolated diastolic potentials/continuous electrical activity, more than 35% of radiofrequency current applications terminated VT, compared with 4% when none of these criteria were present. Analysis of the postpacing interval and S-QRS interval suggested that 25% of the sites with entrainment with concealed fusion were in bystander areas, not within the reentry circuit.

13. Tsai CF, Chen SA, Tai CT, et al: Idiopathic monomorphic ventricular tachycardia: clinical outcome, electrophysiologic characteristics and long-term results of catheter ablation. *Int J Cardiol* 62:143-150, 1997.

This study assessed the results of radiofrequency catheter ablation therapy in 61 consecutive patients with ventricular tachycardia (VT) in the absence of structural heart disease. Equal numbers of patients had left ventricular or right ventricular VT. Idiopathic left VT was entrained by overdrive ventricular pacing and terminated by verapamil, but not by adenosine (except one case with VT focus at the left ventricular free wall). Most of the successful ablation sites were located at the left ventricular inferior-apical septum. In the right VT group, 20 (67%) of 30 patients had clinically repetitive monomorphic VT. Most of the idiopathic right VT (22/30) required isoproterenol to facilitate induction of VT and originated in the right ventricular outflow tract.

Questions

Multiple Choice (choose the one best answer)

1. A 63-year-old woman comes to the emergency department with palpitations and wide complex tachycardia, as shown below. Blood pressure is 102/65 mm Hg. She has no other complaints. What is a likely therapy the emergency room physician did *not* give in this situation?
   a. Metoprolol
   b. Adenosine
   c. Lidocaine
   d. Carotid sinus massage
   e. Procainamide

2. Which of the following forms of ventricular tachycardia is least likely cured with radiofrequency catheter ablation?
   a. Right ventricular outflow tract ventricular tachycardia
   b. Ventricular tachycardia in the setting of arrhythmogenic right ventricular dysplasia
   c. Bundle branch reentry ventricular tachycardia
   d. Idiopathic left ventricular tachycardia
   e. Quinidine-induced torsades de pointes

3. Which of these arrhythmias is most likely to respond to intravenously administered verapamil?
   a. Right ventricular outflow tract ventricular tachycardia
   b. Ventricular tachycardia in association with arrhythmogenic right ventricular dysplasia
   c. Idiopathic left ventricular tachycardia
   d. Bundle branch reentry ventricular tachycardia
   e. Ventricular tachycardia in association with hypertrophic cardiomyopathy

4. Which of the following features of a wide complex tachycardia most likely rules out supraventricular tachycardia with aberrant conduction?
   a. Atrial ventricular dissociation
   b. Left axis deviation
   c. Blood pressure of 80/50 mm Hg
   d. Ventricular rate of 220 beats/min
   e. QRS duration of 140 ms

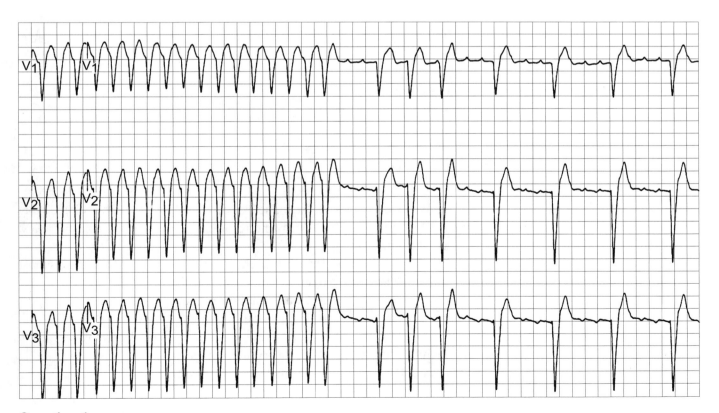

Question 1

5. A 78-year-old woman has syncope. Her electrocardiogram is shown below. Chest radiographic and echocardiographic findings are normal. She is taking an angiotensin-converting enzyme (ACE) inhibitor for hypertension and takes no other medications. Physical examination findings are negative. Serum levels of electrolytes, creatine kinase, and troponin I are normal.

What is the next most appropriate treatment for her in this situation?

a. Temporary pacing
b. Intravenous magnesium
c. Intravenous amiodarone
d. Isoproterenol
e. Atropine

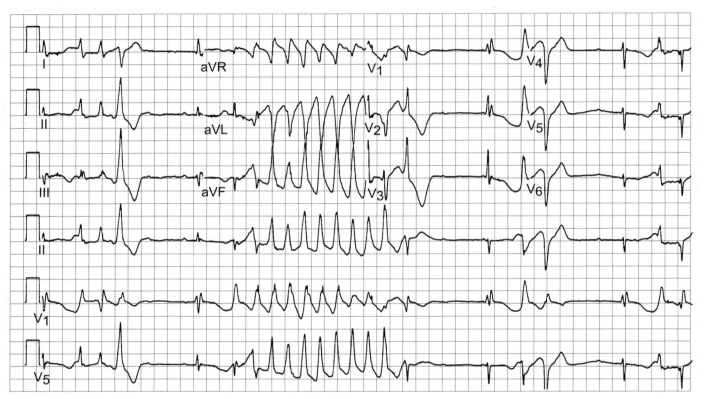

Question 5

6. Each of the following clinical features would favor placement of an implantable cardioverter-defibrillator rather than ablation in a patient with ventricular tachycardia *except*:
   a. Syncope with ventricular tachycardia induction at electrophysiologic study
   b. Right ventricular outflow tract ventricular tachycardia
   c. Multiple morphologies of ventricular tachycardia inducible at electrophysiologic study
   d. No inducible arrhythmias at electrophysiologic study
   e. Arrhythmogenic right ventricular dysplasia

7. Bundle branch reentry ventricular tachycardia is most often seen in patients with:
   a. Dilated cardiomyopathy
   b. Hypertrophic cardiomyopathy
   c. Arrhythmogenic right ventricular dysplasia
   d. Coronary artery disease
   e. Normal structural heart

8. This electrophysiology tracing shows each of the following *except*:
   a. Atrioventricular dissociation
   b. High-to-low atrial activation
   c. Left-sided accessory pathway conduction
   d. Ventricular tachycardia
   e. A tachycardia with right bundle branch morphology

9. The third complex on this electrophysiology tracing is:
   a. Left bundle branch morphology
   b. A premature ventricular contraction
   c. Does not reset the sinus rhythm
   d. B and C
   e. None of the above

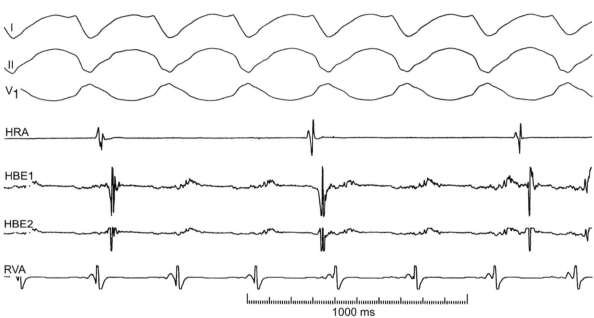

Question 8

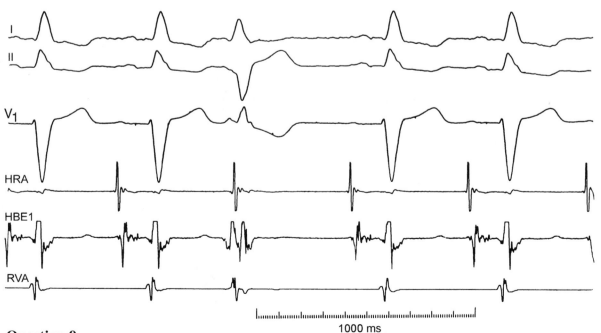

Question 9

10. Each of these antiarrhythmic drugs has Vaughan Williams class I activity *except*:
    a. Amiodarone
    b. Sotalol
    c. Quinidine
    d. Lidocaine
    e. Propafenone

11. This rhythm would respond favorably to each of the following drugs *except*:
    a. Lidocaine
    b. Atenolol
    c. Verapamil
    d. Procainamide

    e. Flecainide

12. An esophageal electrogram recording in a patient with wide complex tachycardia would be most useful:
    a. To identify the location of earliest ventricular activation, thus aiding subsequent ventricular tachycardia mapping
    b. To determine whether intravenous procainamide would terminate the rhythm
    c. To record an accessory pathway potential
    d. To record atrial activity and identify the presence of atrioventricular dissociation
    e. To distinguish ventricular tachycardia due to reentry from ventricular tachycardia due to a triggered mechanism

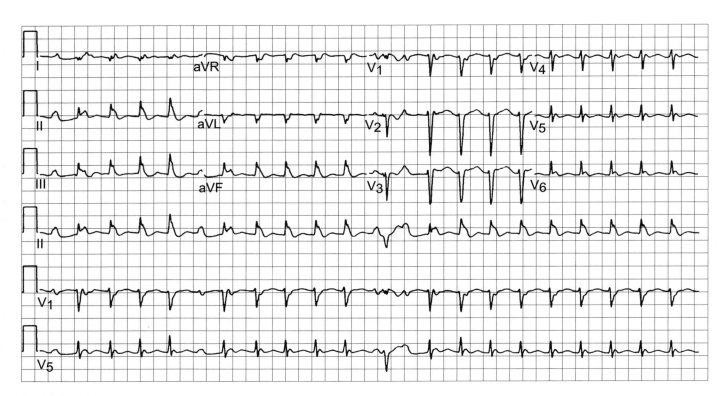

Question 11

Answers

1. Answer c

This patient has a left bundle branch morphology wide complex tachycardia. It appears to be atrial flutter with 1:1 conduction; at the right of the tracing, variable atrioventricular (AV) block occurs with P waves becoming obvious, thus allowing the diagnosis of atrial flutter with aberrant conduction. All the drugs (except lidocaine) and carotid massage could produce enhanced AV nodal block in this situation. Lidocaine has no effect on AV nodal conduction.

2. Answer e

Torsades de pointes (polymorphic ventricular tachycardia) due to QT prolongation is a generalized process involving presumably the entire ventricle. There is no defined focal or slow zone target that can be approached with radiofrequency catheter ablation.

3. Answer c

Reentrant ventricular tachycardia rhythms like those seen in cardiomyopathies would not be expected to respond to verapamil. Idiopathic left ventricular tachycardia is more likely to terminate with a calcium channel blocker than the right ventricular outflow tract type of ventricular tachycardia.

4. Answer a

Patients with supraventricular tachycardia and aberrancy can present with rapid tachycardia (> 200 beats/min) and hypotension. Only northwest axis is highly specific for ventricular tachycardia. QRS duration less than or equal to 140 ms favors supraventricular tachycardia. Atrioventricular dissociation virtually assures that ventricular tachycardia is the cause.

5. Answer e

This patient has bradycardic-dependent polymorphic ventricular tachycardia. There is atrioventricular block on the tracing. The patient is best treated long-term with pacing. However, in the initial acute treatment, atropine would be administered first, followed by temporary pacing.

6. Answer b

Right ventricular outflow tract ventricular tachycardia (presenting in patients with normal hearts) has an excellent long-term prognosis and can be ablated with 85% success.

To allow ablation to be performed in a patient with ventricular tachycardia, one needs a hemodynamically stable ventricular tachycardia that can be induced at electrophysiologic study and mapped. Multiple morphologies of ventricular tachycardia (which are often induced in patients with arrhythmogenic right ventricular dysplasia and coronary artery disease) suggest a lower likelihood that complete ablation and cure can be achieved.

7. Answer a

In patients with dilated cardiomyopathy who present with ventricular tachycardia, the mechanism for the ventricular tachycardia is bundle branch reentry in 50% of cases, as compared with less than 5% of cases of ventricular tachycardia associated with coronary artery disease.

8. Answer c

Atrioventricular dissociation is seen in this electrophysiologic tracing, as is sinus rhythm in the atrium (high-to-low atrial activation sequence) that continues during ventricular tachycardia. There is no evidence for accessory pathway conduction.

9. Answer d

The complex is an interpolated premature ventricular contraction (right bundle branch block morphology) that fails to reset the sinus node.

10. Answer b

Sotalol has β-blocking activity (class II) and potassium channel blocking activity (class III). All the other drugs have sodium channel blocking (class I) activity.

11. Answer a

This rhythm is atrial tachycardia with QRS conduction delay and variable atrioventricular block. Lidocaine has no effect on atrial or atrioventricular nodal tissue and would have no effect on this rhythm.

12. Answer d

Esophageal electrodes allow indirect recording of atrial electrograms and, thus, can identify atrioventricular dissociation and, potentially, ventricular tachycardia. Esophageal electrodes cannot record ventricular or accessory pathway electrograms and cannot determine mechanisms of ventricular tachycardia or its response to therapy.

Notes

Chapter 40

Pacemakers

Margaret A. Lloyd, M.D.
David L. Hayes, M.D.

Indications for Permanent Pacing

Guidelines for implantation of a permanent pacemaker were originally established in 1984 by a joint task force of the American Heart Association and American College of Cardiology, and they were updated in 1991 and 1998.

Indications for permanent pacing are divided into three classes:

- Class I: permanent pacing is acceptable and necessary
- Class II: permanent pacing is acceptable
- Class III: pacing is inappropriate

Class I

Class I indications are those in which pacing is considered necessary, provided the indication is chronic or recurrent and not due to transient underlying causes, such as drugs (commonly antiarrhythmics, β-adrenergic blockers, calcium channel blockers, or digoxin), electrolyte imbalance, or acute myocardial infarction. A single symptomatic episode is sufficient to establish the necessity for pacing, but symptoms must be clearly due to the rhythm disturbance. Indications are as follows:

1. Acquired complete (third-degree) atrioventricular (AV) block. Typical symptoms include syncope, seizures, dizziness, confusion, limited exercise tolerance, and congestive heart failure. Exercise testing may provide evidence of exercise intolerance. Asymptomatic complete AV block is generally an acceptable indication for pacing. Symptoms may be subtle, especially in elderly, inactive patients.

2. Congenital complete (third-degree) AV block with symptomatic bradycardia, exercise intolerance, secondary ventricular ectopy, or congestive heart failure; also, asymptomatic bradycardia with a heart rate less than 50 beats/min in the awake infant.

3. Mobitz I second-degree AV block (Wenckebach) with symptomatic bradycardia.

4. Mobitz II second-degree AV block with symptomatic bradycardia.

5. Symptomatic sinus bradycardia (heart rate < 40 beats/min or documented periods of asystole > 3.0 seconds when awake). Symptoms include syncope or pre-syncope, confusion, seizures, or congestive heart failure, and they must be clearly related to the bradycardia. Pacing in patients with a heart rate more than 40 beats/min may be considered; however, careful documentation of symptoms related to bradycardia is required.

6. Symptomatic sinus bradycardia due to drug treatment for which there is no acceptable alternative (for example, amiodarone or digoxin).

7. Sinus node dysfunction with symptomatic bradycardia. Examples include tachycardia-bradycardia syndrome, episodic sinus arrest, and sinoatrial block.

8. Sinus node dysfunction with life-threatening, bradycardia-dependent arrhythmias. Bradycardia itself need not be symptomatic.

9. Neurocardiogenic syncope. Syncope with more than a 3-second pause with carotid sinus massage.

10. After catheter ablation of the AV junction.

11. Postoperative AV block that is not expected to resolve. Examples include AV block after correction of congenital abnormalities and AV block after valve replacement.

12. Neuromuscular diseases with AV block. Examples include Kearns-Sayre, Erb dystrophy, myotonic muscular dystrophy, and peroneal muscular atrophy.

Class II

Class II indications include those in which permanent pacing may be acceptable, provided that the potential benefit to the patient can be documented. Indications are as follows:

1. Congenital complete (third-degree) AV block with moderate bradycardia.

2. Asymptomatic Mobitz II second-degree AV block.

3. Bifascicular or trifascicular block with syncope that is attributed to transient complete heart block. Other potential causes of syncope must first be excluded.

4. Transient complete (third-degree) or Mobitz II second-degree AV block after acute myocardial infarction.

5. Overdrive pacing in patients with recurrent ventricular tachycardia refractory to other therapy.

6. Syncope and positive tilt-table testing.

7. First-degree AV block with symptoms of pacemaker syndrome, or marked first-degree AV block (PR interval > 300 ms) with left ventricular dysfunction and symptoms of congestive heart failure in which a shorter AV interval results in hemodynamic improvement.

8. Incidental finding at electrophysiologic study of a markedly prolonged HV interval (> 100 ms) or pacing-induced infra-His block.

Class III

Class III indications are those in which permanent pacing is unlikely to be of benefit and therefore is considered inappropriate.

1. Asymptomatic sinus bradycardia.

2. Asymptomatic sinus arrest or sinoatrial block.

3. Bradycardia during sleep.

4. Asymptomatic Mobitz I second-degree AV block (Wenckebach).

5. Transient, asymptomatic ventricular pause with atrial fibrillation.

6. Right bundle branch or left-axis deviation with syncope or pre-syncope.

7. Positive carotid sinus massage (> 3-s pause) without symptoms or with vague symptoms not clearly related to the pause, or recurrent syncope with negative tilt-table testing.

8. AV block expected to resolve and not likely to recur.

Examples include Lyme disease and drug toxicity.

9. Syncope of undetermined cause. Evaluation should include assessment of left ventricular function, neurologic evaluation, Holtor monitoring or an event recorder, exercise testing, and electrophysiologic testing, including tilt-table testing. If the history strongly suggests a cardiogenic cause for the syncope and the evaluation is unrevealing, permanent pacing may be considered. The patient must understand that pacing may not relieve symptoms.

Conduction Disturbances in Acute Myocardial Infarction

Various conduction disturbances may occur during the peri-infarct period, including bradycardia and AV block. Disturbances are usually related to the site of infarction, and they may be transient or permanent. Temporary pacing during the peri-infarct period is not necessarily an indication for permanent pacing.

Inferior Myocardial Infarction

Common conduction disturbances include sinus bradycardia, sinus arrhythmia, sinus arrest, atrial fibrillation or flutter, and AV block. First-degree AV block and Mobitz I second-degree block (Wenckebach) are more common; in a minority of patients, Mobitz II second-degree block or complete (third-degree) AV block develops. Patients who are hemodynamically unstable may require temporary pacing. Conduction defects associated with acute inferior myocardial infarction are usually transient and rarely require permanent pacing.

Anterior Myocardial Infarction

Conduction disturbances are more likely to develop in patients with acute anterior myocardial infarction. Anterior myocardial infarction accompanied by AV block has a poor prognosis and an increased incidence of sudden cardiac death, probably related to the large area of myocardium involved in this type of infarction. Temporary pacing is required for patients who have intermittent or persistent complete heart block, new-onset bifascicular block, or bilateral bundle branch block. Permanent pacing is usually required in these patients.

Other causes of acquired AV block are summarized in Table 1.

- Conduction defects in inferior myocardial infarction are

usually transient and rarely require permanent pacing.

- Conduction disturbances in anterior myocardial infarction may be permanent, and thus permanent pacing is usually required.

Pacing Modes and Nomenclature

The pacemaker code is used to describe pacemaker function. Five positions are used to describe the mode of pacemaker operation (Table 2).

Position I indicates the chamber paced. Five letters are commonly used: "A" for atrium, "V" for ventricle, "D" if both chambers are paced, and "O" if pacing is turned off. "S" is used by some manufacturers to indicate pacing capability in a single-chamber device.

Position II indicates the chamber sensed. Again, five letters are commonly used: "A" for atrium, "V" for ventricle, "D" if both chambers are sensed, and "O" if no sensing is present in any chamber and asynchronous pacing is to occur. "S" is again used by some manufacturers to indicate sensing capability in a single-chamber device.

Position III indicates the response to a sensed signal. "I" indicates that output is inhibited by a sensed event, "T" indicates that a stimulus is triggered by a sensed event, and "D" indicates that a stimulus may be triggered or inhibited by a sensed event. For example, in dual-chamber devices, the atrial output may be inhibited by a sensed atrial event, and the ventricular stimulus triggered by a sensed atrial event (in the absence of a sensed ventricular event). The letter "O" indicates that there is no mode of response, mandating that there be an "O" in the second (sensing) position.

Position IV describes the programmability or rate modulation capability of the device. Five letters are used, in order of complexity: "O" indicates no programmability or rate modulation, "P" indicates simple programmability (usually rate or output) but no rate modulation, "M" indicates multiprogrammability, "C" indicates telemetry capability ("communicating"), and "R" indicates sensor-driven rate responsiveness.

In practice, the "R" designation is the only letter typically used, because most current devices are multiprogrammable with telemetry capability. Rate modulation is achieved by incorporation of a sensor capable of detecting changes in physiologic activity. Various sensors are available, including those that detect changes in activity, body temperature, minute ventilation, and QT interval.

Table 1.—Causes of Acquired Atrioventricular (AV) Block

Idiopathic (senescent) AV block
Coronary artery disease
Calcific valvular disease
Postoperative or traumatic condition
AV node ablation
Therapeutic irradiation of the chest
Infectious
    Syphilis
    Diphtheria
    Chagas disease
    Tuberculosis
    Toxoplasmosis
    Lyme disease*
    Viral myocarditis (Epstein-Barr, varicella, etc.)
    Infective endocarditis
Collagen-vascular
    Rheumatoid arthritis
    Scleroderma
    Dermatomyositis
    Ankylosing spondylitis
    Polyarteritis nodosa
    Systemic lupus erythematosus
    Marfan syndrome
Infiltrative
    Sarcoidosis
    Amyloidosis
    Hemochromatosis
    Malignant disease (lymphomatous or solid tumor)
Neuromuscular
    Progressive external ophthalmoplegia (Kearns-Sayre syndrome)
    Myotonic muscular dystrophy
    Peroneal muscular atrophy (Charcot-Marie-Tooth disease)
    Scapuloperoneal syndrome
    Limb-girdle dystrophy
Drug effect
    Digoxin
    β-Blocking agents
    Calcium-channel–blocking agents
    Amiodarone
    Procainamide
    Class 1C agents: propafenone, encainide, flecainide

*AV block due to Lyme disease does not require permanent pacing.
From Giuliani ER, Gersh BJ, McGoon MD, Hayes DL, Schaff HV (editors): *Mayo Clinic Practice of Cardiology*. Third edition. Mosby, 1996, p 911. By permission of Mayo Foundation.

Table 2.—NASPE/BPEG* Pacemaker Codes

Position	I	II	III	IV	V
Category	Chamber paced	Chamber sensed	Response	Programmability	Antitachycardia functions
	O = None	O = None	O = None	O = None	O = None
	A = Atrium	A = Atrium	T = Triggered	P = Simple programmable	P = Pacing
	V = Ventricle	V = Ventricle	I = Inhibited	M = Multiprogrammable	S = Shock
	D = Dual	D = Dual	D = Dual	C = Communicating	D = Dual
				R = Rate modulation	

*North American Society of Pacing and Electrophysiology and the British Pacing and Electrophysiology Group.
From *Pace* 10:794-799, 1987. By permission of Futura Publishing Company.

Position V indicates the presence of antitachycardia functions and rarely is used. "O" indicates the absence of any such function, "P" indicates a pacing modality (underdrive, burst, and scanning), "S" indicates shocking capability, and "D" indicates both pacing and shocking capabilities. Atrial antitachycardia devices use only pacing, whereas automatic implantable cardioverter-defibrillators typically use both pacing and shocking therapies.

When choosing the appropriate pacing mode for an individual patient, one must consider the underlying rhythm abnormality, chronotropic status (that is, whether the patient can mount an appropriate rate response for a given physiologic activity), and activity level. Table 3 summarizes available pacing modes and appropriate indications.

Permanent Pacing Leads

Pacing leads are either unipolar or bipolar. In a unipolar lead, the distal electrode is the (-) pole and the pulse generator "can" serves as the (+) pole. In a bipolar lead, the distal electrode is the (-) pole and a more proximal electrode on the pacing lead is the (+) pole. Bipolar leads are less susceptible to electromagnetic and electromechanical interference than unipolar leads. (When bipolar leads are used, some pulse generators are capable of being programmed to function in either the unipolar or the bipolar configuration, and some allow designation of pacing and sensing configuration; for example, some pacemakers may allow options of atrial sensing polarity, atrial pacing polarity, ventricular sensing polarity, and ventricular pacing polarity.)

The outer insulation of pacing leads is made of silicone rubber or polyurethane. There are advantages and disadvantages of each type of insulating material.

All pacing leads have some mechanism of fixation to the myocardium and are classified as either active or passive fixation. Active fixation leads usually have a "screw" that is screwed into the endocardium. Passive fixation leads usually have small "tines" that extend from the lead tip. The tines are designed to become entrapped in the endocardial trabeculae and stabilize the lead until scar tissue forms around the lead.

Some leads are designed to maintain a low stimulation or capture threshold. Steroid-eluting leads characteristically have lower acute and chronic thresholds than nonsteroid-eluting leads. In addition to steroid-eluting leads, there are other low-threshold design leads, such as carbon-tipped and platinized electrodes. Low thresholds are desirable in order to maximize the battery life of the device.

Pacemaker Complications

Troubleshooting

Most pacemaker problems result from inappropriate programming, inappropriate mode selection, or lead malfunction. Initial troubleshooting should always include interrogation of the device and evaluation of electrocardiographic tracings. Pacing and sensing thresholds should be evaluated, and lead impedance checked. A chest radiograph should be obtained if lead impedances or electrocardiographic tracings suggest a lead problem (Table 4 and Figure 1).

Failure to sense or capture in the immediate postimplantation period is most likely due to lead micro- or macro-dislodgment or to a poor connection between the lead and the set screw within the pacemaker generator

Table 3.—Indications for Various Pacing Modes*

Mode	Indications Generally agreed on	Indications Controversial	Contraindications
VVI	Atrial fibrillation with symptomatic bradycardia in the CC patient	Symptomatic bradycardia in the patient with associated terminal illness or other medical conditions from which recovery is not anticipated and pacing is life-sustaining only	Known pacemaker syndrome or hemodynamic deterioration with ventricular pacing at the time of implant CI patient who will benefit from rate response Hemodynamic need for dual-chamber pacing
VVIR	Fixed atrial arrhythmias (atrial fibrillation or flutter) with symptomatic bradycardia in the CI patient	As for VVI	As for VVI
AAI	Symptomatic bradycardia as a result of sinus node dysfunction in the otherwise CC patient when AV conduction can be proved normal		Sinus node dysfunction with associated AV block either demonstrated spontaneously or during pre-implant testing Inability to attain adequate atrial sensing
AAIR	Symptomatic bradycardia as a result of sinus node dysfunction in the CI patient when AV conduction can be proved normal		As for AAI
VDD†	Congenital AV block AV block when sinus node function can be proved normal		Sinus node dysfunction AV block accompanied by sinus node dysfunction Inability to attain adequate atrial sensing AV block accompanied by paroxysmal supraventricular tachycardias
VDDR‡			
DDI	Need for dual-chamber pacing in the presence of significant PSVT in the CC patient	Sinus node dysfunction in the absence of AV block and in the presence of significant PSVT in the CC patient	CI patient with a demonstrated need or improvement with rate responsiveness
DDIR§	AV block and sinus node dysfunction in the CI patient in the presence of significant PSVT	Sinus node dysfunction without AV block in the CI patient in the presence of significant PSVT	
DDD	AV block and sinus node dysfunction in the CC patient Need for AV synchrony (to maximize cardiac output) in the CC active patient Previous pacemaker syndrome	For any rhythm disturbance when atrial sensing and capture are possible for the potential purpose of minimizing future atrial fibrillation and improving morbidity and survival	Presence of chronic atrial fibrillation, atrial flutter, giant inexcitable atrium, or other frequent PSVT Inability to attain adequate atrial sensing
DDDR	AV block and sinus node dysfunction in the CI patient	As for DDD	As for DDD

Table 3 (continued)

*DVI as a stand-alone pacing mode (that is, a pacemaker capable of DVI as the only dual-chamber mode of operation) is obsolete. All primary uses of this mode should be considered individually.

†VDD as a stand-alone pacing mode (that is, a pacemaker capable of VDD as the only dual-chamber mode of operation) is currently used primarily as a single-lead VDD system. If a dual-lead system is implanted, then the capability of DDD pacing is desirable.

‡In current single-lead VDDR pacemakers, P-wave tracking occurs as long as the sinus rate is appropriate. However, in the presence of sinus bradycardia or chronotropic incompetence, the pacemaker operates in the VVIR mode.

§DDIR has been supplanted by DDD or DDDR pacemakers with the capability of mode-switching (that is, the pacemaker automatically reprograms to a mode incapable of tracking the atrial rhythm in the presence of an atrial rhythm that the pacemaker classifies as a pathologic rhythm). When the pacemaker recognizes the atrial rhythm as being physiologic, the pacemaker reprograms to the previously programmed mode.

AV, atrioventricular; CC, chronotropically competent (the ability to achieve an appropriate heart rate for a given physiologic activity); CI, chronotropically incompetent (the inability to achieve an appropriate heart rate for a given physiologic activity); PSVT, paroxysmal supraventricular tachyarrhythmia.

(Fig. 2). The most common abnormality in dual-chamber systems is atrial undersensing, due to the technical difficulty in placing the atrial lead in a mechanically stable position.

Failure to output is not synonymous with failure to capture and is usually the result of oversensing (Table 5).

Other pacemaker complications are summarized in Table 6.

- The most common abnormality in dual-chamber systems is atrial undersensing.

Lead Abnormalities

Lead conductor fracture may present with high lead

Table 4.—Interpretation of Radiographic Appearance of the Pacing System

1. Inspect the routine posteroanterior lateral chest radiographs, ignoring the pacing system. Obtain overpenetrated, that is, thoracic, spine films, if necessary
2. Identify the pulse generator location
3. Identify the pulse generator model and polarity
4. Inspect the connector block
5. Determine the lead(s) position:
   a. Transvenous or epimyocardial
   b. Atrial or ventricular, or both
   c. If transvenous, its location within a cardiac chamber of the coronary sinus
6. Determine lead polarity and type of fixation
7. Evaluate lead integrity
8. Look for other specific complications

From Furman S, Hayes DL, Holmes DR Jr: *A Practice of Cardiac Pacing.* Third edition. Futura Publishing Company, 1993, p 400. By permission of the publisher.

impedance, failure to capture, oversensing with inappropriate output inhibition, or muscle stimulation. Lead insulation failure usually presents with low lead impedance, undersensing or oversensing, failure to capture, muscle stimulation, or early battery depletion. Every lead has a characteristic range of normal impedance; generally this range is 300 to 1,000 ohms. Recently introduced high-impedance leads may have significantly higher measured impedance (1,000-1,800 ohms). Steroid-eluting leads characteristically have lower acute and chronic thresholds than nonsteroid-eluting leads (Table 7).

- Lead conductor fracture may present with high lead impedance.
- Lead insulation failure usually presents with low lead impedance.

Crosstalk

Crosstalk develops when an electrical event in one chamber is sensed in the other chamber and inappropriate inhibition of the pacing stimulus occurs in the second chamber. An example is an atrial stimulus that is sensed by the ventricular lead as a ventricular event, with consequent inhibition of ventricular output and ventricular asystole. Crosstalk may occur in several ways. Occasionally, the atrial or the ventricular lead may become dislodged and migrate in the chamber of the other lead. More frequently, crosstalk develops when the stimulus field is large or the stimulus output is high. Although these conditions are more likely to develop when unipolar sensing or pacing is used, crosstalk can occur in bipolar systems. Furthermore, crosstalk may occur within the pacemaker circuitry in some devices (Fig. 3).

Two approaches have been incorporated into the pacemaker circuitry to prevent the occurrence of crosstalk.

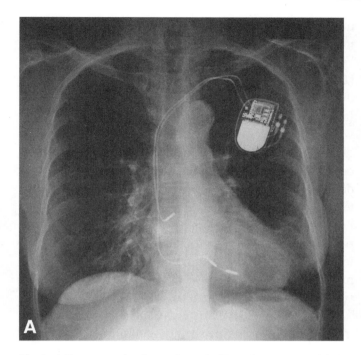

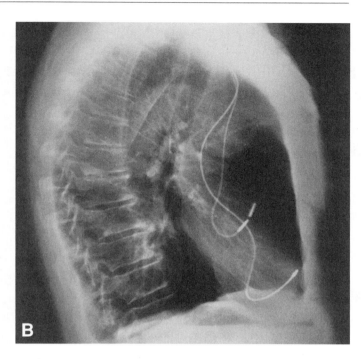

Fig. 1. *A*, Posteroanterior chest radiograph. Normal appearance of dual-chamber pacing system. Pacemaker generator is implanted in the upper left infraclavicular region. One atrial lead is present in right atrial appendage, and one ventricular lead is present in right ventricular apex. Gentle redundancy is present on both leads. Ventricular lead can be clearly visualized as bipolar. *B*, Lateral chest radiograph. Normal appearance of dual-chamber pacing system. Ventricular lead is clearly anterior, therefore in right ventricular apex, and not in coronary sinus (in which case it would be pointing backward toward the spine). Atrial lead is clearly visualized as bipolar.

The first approach is the ventricular blanking period. The blanking period is a period of ventricular insensitivity beginning at the time of the atrial pulse stimulus; during this period, electrical events are not sensed. Depending on the device, the ventricular blanking period may be fixed or programmable. The second approach is safety pacing, in which the sensing of any event during the early portion of the blanking period (12 to 16 ms) is followed by a committed early ventricular stimulus, producing a shortened AV delay (Fig. 4).

There are several ways to treat crosstalk. If the ventricular blanking period is programmable, it can be prolonged. Safety pacing can be programmed "on" if it is not already so programmed. The atrial channel output can be decreased, or the ventricular sensitivity can be programmed to a less sensitive value. Switching from unipolar pacing or sensing to bipolar pacing or sensing may eliminate crosstalk if the pacing system allows this change in lead polarity configuration. If the patient has intact sinus node function, decreasing the pacing rate allows for more native atrial depolarization and less opportunity for crosstalk to occur. Programming the device to a committed AV interval (DVI mode) eliminates crosstalk but may result in competitive

ventricular pacing. Finally, the lead position or the pulse generator may need to be changed.

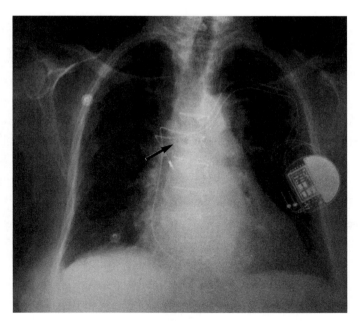

Fig. 2. Posteroanterior chest radiograph, demonstrating dislodgment of the atrial lead (*arrow*) the day after implantation of a permanent dual-chamber pacemaker. Position of the lead does not permit atrial sensing or pacing.

Table 5.—Causes of Pacemaker Malfunction

Failure to capture
    High thresholds with an inadequately programmed output
    Partial conductor coil fracture
    Insulation defect
    Lead dislodgment or perforation
    Impending total battery depletion
    Functional noncapture
    Poor or incompatible connection at connector block
    Circuit failure
    Air in pocket (unipolar pacemaker)
Failure to output
    Circuit failure
    Complete or intermittent conductor coil fracture
    Intermittent or permanently loose set screw
    Incompatible lead or header
    Total battery depletion
    Internal insulation failure (bipolar lead)
    Oversensing any noncardiac activity
    Lack of anodal connector contact*
    Crosstalk
Undersensing
    Morphology of intrinsic event different from that
        measured at implantation
    Lead dislodgment or poor lead positioning
    Lead insulation failure
    Circuit failure
    Magnet application
    Malfunction of reed switch
    Electromagnetic interference
    Battery depletion
    Poor or incompatible connection at connector block
    Circuit failure
    Air in pocket (unipolar pacemaker)

*Examples include unipolar lead in bipolar generator, bipolar lead in pacemaker programmed as unipolar, air in the pocket of a unipolar device, and unipolar pacemaker not in the pocket.

- Crosstalk develops when an electrical event in one chamber is sensed in the other chamber.
- The blanking period is a period of ventricular insensitivity beginning at the time of the atrial pulse stimulus.

Pacemaker Syndrome

Pacemaker syndrome is a hemodynamic abnormality that can result from an inappropriate use of ventricular pacing. It occurs when ventricular pacing is uncoupled from atrial contraction. This syndrome is most common when the VVI mode is used in patients with sinus rhythm, but it can occur in any pacing mode if AV synchrony is lost.

Patients may experience a sensation of fullness in the head and neck, syncope or pre-syncope, hypotension, cough, dyspnea, congestive heart failure, or weakness. Physical findings include cannon A waves and a blood pressure drop when pacing compared with normal sinus rhythm. Levels of atrial natriuretic factor are high. If pacemaker syndrome occurs in a patient with a VVI or VVIR pacemaker, the only definitive treatment is converting to a dual-chamber system. If the patient has only rare episodes of symptomatic bradycardia, it may be possible to alleviate symptoms of pacemaker syndrome by programming the pacemaker to a lower rate limit and programming hysteresis "on." This minimizes pacing and allows the patient to stay in normal sinus rhythm for longer periods.

If single-chamber ventricular pacing is contemplated, a trial of ventricular pacing should be performed at the time of implantation and the blood pressure compared with that during sinus rhythm. If there is a fall in blood pressure with ventricular pacing or if the patient experiences symptoms, dual-chamber pacing should be used; however, an absence of blood pressure drop or symptoms is not a guarantee that pacemaker syndrome will not develop.

- Pacemaker syndrome is a hemodynamic abnormality that can result from inappropriate use of ventricular pacing.
- Levels of atrial natriuretic factor are high in pacemaker syndrome.

Pacemaker-Mediated Tachycardia

Pacemaker-mediated tachycardia can occur only with dual-chamber pacing systems with intact atrial sensing (DDD, DDDR, and VDD systems) (Fig. 5). Types of pacemaker-mediated tachycardia include rapid tracking of atrial fibrillation or flutter and rapid ventricular triggering from electromagnetic interference. Endless-loop tachycardia refers to a specific type of pacemaker-mediated tachycardia in which intact VA conduction results in retrograde "P" waves, which trigger another ventricular stimulation, creating a "loop." The situation can be corrected by lengthening the postventricular atrial refractory period beyond the retrograde "P" wave, so that the "P" wave either is not sensed or does not initiate an AV timing cycle. Many devices offer extension of the postventricular refractory period after a premature ventricular contraction, the most common cause of endless-loop tachycardias, or some other

Table 6.—Pacemaker Complications

Early complications	Late complications	Early or late complications
Pain/ecchymoses	Skin erosion	Lead dislodgment
Pneumothorax	Skin adherence	Pacemaker-related arrhythmias
Hematoma formation	Thrombosis	Twiddler's syndrome
Lead perforation	Radiation damage	Abnormalities induced by medical equipment (MRI, lithotripsy, or surgical cautery)
Intraoperative lead damage	Pacemaker failure	Infection
Subcutaneous emphysema	High thresholds	Pacemaker syndrome
Thoracic duct injury	Lead fracture or insulation defect	Pacemaker allergy
Air embolism		Pulse generator malfunction
Brachial plexus injury		Loose lead/connector block interface
Subclavian artery puncture		

MRI, magnetic resonance imaging.

Modified from Furman S, Hayes DL, Holmes DR Jr: *A Practice of Cardiac Pacing*. Third edition. Futura Publishing Company, 1993, p 538. By permission of the publisher.

algorithm to recognize and terminate pacemaker-mediated tachycardia.

- Endless-loop tachycardia can be corrected by lengthening the postventricular atrial refractory period.

Additional Features

Many dual-chamber devices now have special algorithms to deal with paroxysmal atrial tachyarrhythmias. When a tachyarrhythmia meets the criteria for paroxysmal atrial tachyarrhythmias, the device switches to a non-tracking mode so as *not* to track the tachyarrhythmia and pace the ventricle at an inappropriately high rate. When paroxysmal atrial tachyarrhythmia terminates, the device resumes normal DDD pacing function (Fig. 6).

Additionally, some dual-chamber devices have algorithms that recognize the onset of vasovagal syncope and initiate pacing at a programmable "hysteresis" rate, usually set at 90 to 100 beats/min for optimal treatment of this syndrome (Fig. 7). Some devices have a "sleep" feature, which allows for the lower rate limit to decrease during the night (usually 5-15 beats/min) to conserve battery life.

Finally, most devices have diagnostic features that can provide information such as amount of pacing and sensing in each chamber, number of episodes of paroxysmal atrial tachyarrhythmias, and number of vasovagal episodes. This information is useful to optimize pacing parameters during subsequent programming.

Miscellaneous Causes of Pacemaker Malfunction

Many external conditions can affect pacemaker function and can sometimes be interpreted as intrinsic pacemaker malfunction. A common cause of noncapture is electrolyte disturbance, especially severe hyperkalemia. Toxic levels of procainamide and disopyramide have been shown to increase pacing thresholds; however, no significant problems have occurred at therapeutic levels of these drugs. Class 1C antiarrhythmic agents (flecainide, encainide, and propafenone) have consistently been shown to significantly increase pacing thresholds. This increase is sometimes dramatic, and these agents should be avoided or used with caution in pacemaker-dependent patients.

Systemic steroids can lower pacing thresholds and have been used clinically for this purpose. Pacing thresholds

Table 7.—Intraoperative Evaluation of Pacing System

Defect	Voltage threshold	Current threshold	Lead impedance
Wire fracture	High	High, normal, or low	High
Insulation break	Low	High	Low
Lead dislodgment	High	High	Normal
Exit block	High	High	Normal

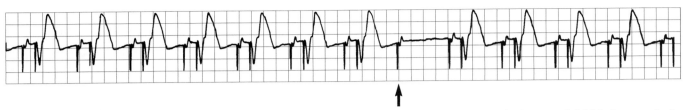

Fig. 3. Electrocardiographic strip demonstrating pacemaker crosstalk. In the eighth complex (*arrow*), the ventricular output is inhibited as a result of sensing of the atrial pacemaker artifact in the ventricular channel.

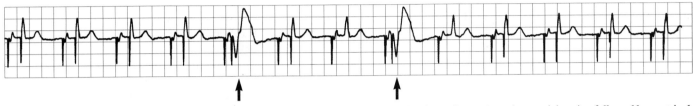

Fig. 4. Electrocardiographic strip demonstrating safety pacing. The fifth (*arrow*) and eighth (*arrow*) complexes have atrial pacing followed by ventricular pacing artifact at a fixed AV interval of 110 ms. At this interval, there is complete depolarization of the ventricle by the pacemaker. The remainder of the complexes on the strip reveal an AV delay of 200 ms and ventricular fusion complexes.

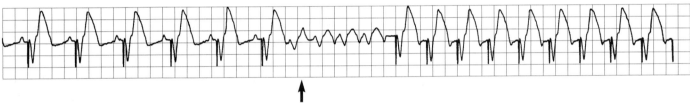

Fig. 5. Electrocardiographic strip demonstrating pacemaker-mediated tachycardia initiated by a ventricular triplet (*arrow*).

usually increase to pretreatment levels when systemic steroid use is discontinued.

- A common cause of noncapture is electrolyte disturbance.
- Toxic levels of procainamide and disopyramide increase pacing thresholds.
- Class 1C antiarrhythmic agents (flecainide, encainide, and propafenone) significantly increase pacing thresholds.

Electromagnetic Interference (EMI) in the Hospital Environment

EMI can affect pacemaker performance. The hospital environment is a frequent source of EMI. Electrocautery can result in inhibition of the pacemaker, and therefore it is desirable to program the pacemaker to an asynchronous mode before starting the surgical procedure, especially in pacemaker-dependent patients. Electrocautery can damage the pacemaker's internal circuitry if used in proximity to the pacemaker, and efforts should be made to keep the cautery electrode at least 6 inches away from the pacemaker during surgical procedures.

- Electrocautery can result in inhibition of the pacemaker.

Magnetic resonance imaging (MRI) uses magnetic and radiofrequency fields that cause all pacemakers to pace asynchronously as a result of closure of the reed switch. Additionally, the radiofrequency field theoretically has the potential to induce rapid, asynchronous pacing. Although patients with pacemakers should avoid MRI, nondependent patients have undergone MRI when the pacemaker output can be lowered below the capture threshold or programmed off. The patient must be carefully monitored throughout the procedure.

- Patients with pacemakers should avoid MRI.

Radiofrequency ablation can result in pacemaker inhibition or reprogramming. The pacemaker programmer should be available during the procedure and the pacemaker interrogated at the end of the procedure to document programmed parameters.

Therapeutic (but not diagnostic) radiation may damage the pacemaker components, resulting in damage to circuits or complete pacemaker failure. Radiation-induced pacemaker failure may present as sudden "no output" or "run-

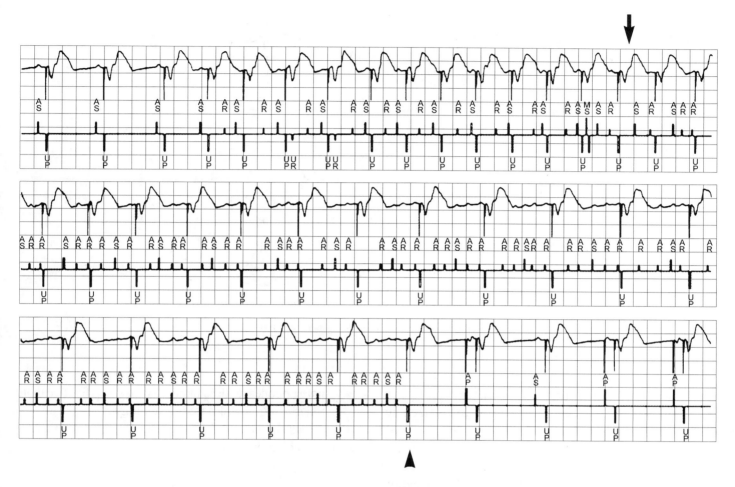

Fig. 6. Electrocardiogram with pacemaker marker channels. Onset of paroxysmal atrial tachycardia, with the device switching from DDD (R) to VVI (R) pacing (*arrow*). At termination of the episode, the device reverts to normal DDD (R) function (*arrowhead*).

away pacemaker." This potential is of special concern in patients receiving therapeutic radiation for breast or chest malignancies. Damage is not related to cumulative dose; but rather it may occur at any time during the course of therapy. If radiation is being used for carcinoma of the breast or lung and the pacemaker is located on the same side as the malignancy, the pacemaker should be moved before initiating radiation. For radiation of any other portion of the body, the generator should be shielded.

- Radiation-induced pacemaker failure may present as sudden "no output" or "runaway" pacemaker.

Electroshock therapy for depressive disorders does not result in pacemaker malfunction but it may cause significant electrocardiographic artifact and could potentially reprogram the pacemaker.

Extracorporeal shock-wave lithotripsy may interfere with

pacemaker function. The lithotriptor is usually synchronized to the ventricular output or the pacemaker ventricular stimulus, so programming the pacemaker to fixed rate ventricular pacing is safe. If the lithotriptor is synchronized to the atrial stimulus, loss of ventricular output may result and should be avoided. Therefore, before lithotripsy, the pacemaker should be programmed to the VOO, VVI, or DOO mode. The focal point of the lithotriptor should be at least 6 inches away from the pulse generator to avoid damage to the device.

- Extracorporeal shock-wave lithotripsy may interfere with pacemaker function.
- Before lithotripsy, the pacemaker should be programmed to the VOO, VVI, or DOO mode.

All pacemakers should be interrogated before and after the aforementioned procedures to ensure that inadvertent reprogramming or damage to the pacemaker has not occurred.

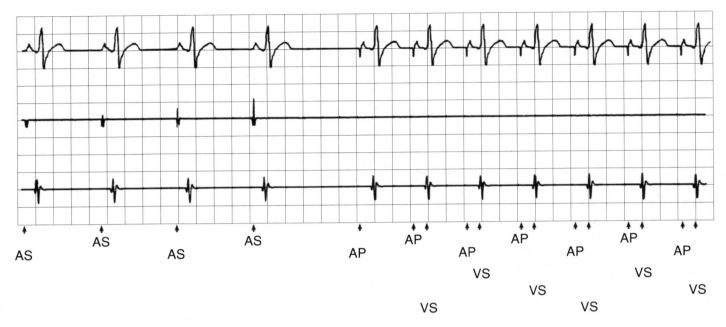

Fig. 7. Electrocardiogram showing onset of vasovagal symptoms, treated with pacing therapy at 100 beats/min.

EMI in the Nonhospital Environment

Permanent damage to pacing systems by electrical equipment outside the hospital environment is unlikely; however, temporary interference may occur with exposure to certain devices and electromagnetic fields. Potential sources of exposure include heavy electric motors and arc welding. Devices such as airport security detectors and ham radios may cause single-beat inhibition, but they should not cause significant clinical sequelae. Microwave ovens do not interfere with pacemaker function.

● Microwave ovens do not interfere with pacemaker function.

Currently, there is a great deal of interest in potential EMI from cellular phones and from antitheft devices or electronic article surveillance equipment. At this time, the advice for patients with pacemakers who use cellular phones is as follows: analog phones are less likely to cause interference than phones using digital-based technology; for most non–pacemaker-dependent patients, cellular phones available in the United States are safe; and all patients should avoid carrying an activated phone in a pocket directly over the pacemaker.

Antitheft devices appear capable of pacemaker interference. However, at this time, information is very limited and definitive clinical advice is not available.

● Analog phones are less likely to cause interference than phones using digital-based technology.

● Patients should avoid carrying an activated phone in a pocket directly over the pacemaker.

Expanding Indications for Pacing

Protocols are in progress to evaluate dual-chamber pacing to optimize cardiac output and minimize the outflow tract gradient in patients with hypertrophic obstructive cardiomyopathy. Additionally, some patients with dilated cardiomyopathies and reduced left ventricular function may benefit from dual-chamber pacing, with echocardiographic optimization of the AV delay to maximize cardiac output. Dual-site atrial pacing to prevent atrial fibrillation is being evaluated.

Temporary Pacing

Temporary ventricular or atrial pacing can be used in patients with symptomatic bradycardia, either transiently if the cause is reversible or as a bridge to permanent pacing. Common transvenous approaches include the internal jugular vein, the subclavian vein, the femoral vein, and, less often, the external jugular vein.

There are two major types of temporary ventricular pacing catheters: a rigid, firm catheter, and a more flexible, balloon-tipped catheter. Although the balloon-tipped catheter may be easier to advance into the right ventricular apex, the firmer catheter usually provides a more stable position for the catheter. Pulmonary artery catheters are available which have an extra port through which a temporary pacing wire can be placed. These are advantageous in that they can be placed quickly without fluoroscopic guidance; however, the pacing wire is relatively unstable. Atrial "J" catheters are available for cases in which atrial pacing is required, for example, atrial overdrive pacing or dual-chamber temporary pacing for patients who hemodynamically do not tolerate single-chamber ventricular pacing.

Potential complications of temporary pacing include those complications that occur with permanent pacing: bleeding, infection, lead dislodgment, and pneumothorax (Fig. 8). The risk of cardiac perforation is higher with temporary pacing catheters because of the stiffness of the catheters.

External pacing systems are available and can be used in patients with intermittent conduction disturbances or to maintain rhythm until a transvenous pacing catheter can be placed. Disadvantages of external pacing include occasional difficulty maintaining capture and potentially significant discomfort from the pacing stimulus for some patients.

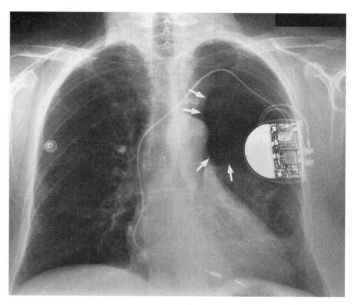

Fig. 8. Posteroanterior chest radiograph revealing pneumothorax the day after pacemaker implantation.

- Potential complications of temporary pacing include those complications that occur with permanent pacing: bleeding, infection, lead dislodgment, and pneumothorax.

Suggested Review Reading

1. Ellenbogen KA: *Cardiac Pacing.* Second edition. Cambridge, MA, Blackwell Science, 1996.

2. Ellenbogen KA, Kay GN, Wilkoff BL: *Clinical Cardiac Pacing.* Philadelphia, WB Saunders Company, 1995.

3. Furman S, Hayes DL, Holmes DR Jr: *A Practice of Cardiac Pacing.* Third edition. Mt. Kisco, NY, Futura Publishing Company, 1993.

4. Gregoratos G, Cheitlin MD, Conill A, et al: ACC/AHA guidelines for implantation of cardiac pacemakers and antiarrhythmia devices: a report of the American College of Cardiology-American Heart Association Task Force on Practice Guidelines (Committee on Pacemaker Implantation). *J Am Coll Cardiol* 31:1175-1209, 1998.

5. Hayes DL, Wang PJ, Reynolds DW, et al: Interference with cardiac pacemakers by cellular telephones. *N Engl J Med* 336:1473-1479, 1997.

6. Kusumoto F, Goldschlager N: Cardiac pacing. N Engl J Med 334:89-97, 1996.

7. Lamas GA, Orav EJ, Stambler BS, et al: Quality of life and clinical outcomes in elderly patients treated with ventricular pacing as compared with dual-chamber pacing. *N Engl J Med* 338:1097-1104, 1998.

8. Mason JW, Hlatky MA: Do patients prefer physiologic pacing? (Editorial.) *N Engl J Med* 338:1147-1148, 1998.

9. Roelke M, Bernstein AD: Cardiac pacemakers and cellular telephones (editorial). *N Engl J Med* 336:1518-1519, 1997.

Questions

Multiple Choice (choose the one best answer)

1. All of the following statements regarding temporary pacing after inferior myocardial infarction are true *except*:
   a. Transient sinus bradycardia is common and rarely necessitates temporary pacing
   b. Patients who are hemodynamically unstable may require temporary pacing
   c. Patients who require temporary pacing in the peri-infarct period usually require subsequent permanent pacing
   d. Patients rarely develop permanent high-grade atrioventricular block after inferior wall myocardial infarction

2. Which of the following regarding anterior myocardial infarction is *true*?
   a. Conduction disturbances are usually transient
   b. Progressively higher grades of atrioventricular block in the absence of hemodynamic instability are an indication for temporary pacing
   c. Atrioventricular block during the peri-infarct period has a favorable prognosis
   d. Anterior myocardial infarction accompanied by atrioventricular block has a lower incidence of sudden cardiac death than inferior infarction

3. The abnormality present in the pacing strip below is:
   a. Consistent atrial undersensing
   b. Consistent ventricular undersensing
   c. Intermittent ventricular undersensing
   d. Intermittent atrial undersensing

4. All of the following pacing system abnormalities can be detected on the chest radiograph *except*:
   a. Insulation break
   b. Fracture of the pacing lead coil
   c. Macro-dislodgment of the pacing lead
   d. Migration of the pulse generator

5. Which of the following regarding the intraoperative evaluation of the pacing system is *false*?
   a. Wire fracture usually presents with a low impedance
   b. Insulation break usually presents with a low impedance
   c. Lead dislodgment typically presents with a high-voltage threshold
   d. Exit block typically presents with a high-voltage threshold

6. Which of the following regarding pacemaker-mediated tachycardia is *false*?
   a. A dual-chamber system must be present
   b. Intact atrial sensing is required
   c. Premature ventricular contractions frequently initiate

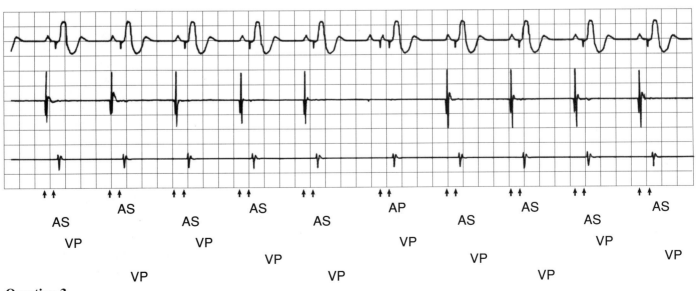

Question 3

pacemaker-mediated tachycardia

   d. Shortening the postventricular atrial refractory period will correct the problem

7. All of the following devices or procedures may cause electromagnetic interference *except*:

   a. Electrocautery

   b. Magnetic resonance imaging

   c. Microwave ovens

   d. Arc welding

8. In the electrocardiographic strip shown below, the pacing mode may be all of the following *except*:

   a. DDD

   b. DDDR

   c. DVI

   d. VDD

9. Which of the following is *not* an AHA/ACC class I indication for pacing?

   a. Congenital complete heart block with symptomatic bradycardia

   b. Sinus node dysfunction with symptomatic bradycardia

   c. Mobitz I second-degree atrioventricular block (Wenckebach) with symptomatic bradycardia

   d. Atrial fibrillation with a 4-second pause during sleep

10. The most common site of pacing lead fracture is:

   a. Between the first rib and clavicle

   b. As the ventricular lead crosses the tricuspid valve

   c. In the pulse-generator pocket

   d. Within the superior vena cava as a result of friction between the two leads

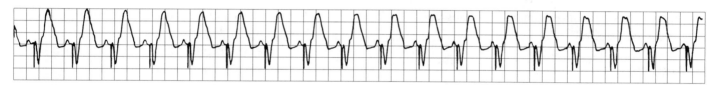

Question 8

Answers

1. Answer c

Conduction abnormalities in the peri-infarct period in patients with inferior myocardial infarction are almost always transient and rarely require permanent pacing.

2. Answer b

Temporary pacing is required in progressive block because complete heart block may develop suddenly. The other statements are false.

3. Answer d

The sixth complex has an intrinsic "p" wave that is not sensed; this is followed by an atrial pacemaker artifact and another "p" wave and subsequent ventricular pacing.

4. Answer a

The lead insulation is not visible radiographically, and breaks typically cannot be seen on the radiograph. All the others can be detected.

5. Answer a

Wire fracture usually presents with a high impedance. The rest of the statements are true.

6. Answer d

Lengthening, not shortening, the PVARP can correct pacemaker-mediated tachycardia. The other statements are true.

7. Answer c

Microwave ovens do not interfere with pacemaker function. All of the other devices listed may cause electromagnetic interference.

8. Answer c

The "p" waves are clearly sensed in this example; in the DVI mode, only the ventricle is sensed. The three other choices are all possible.

9. Answer d

In the absence of symptoms, a 4-second pause during sleep is not a class I indication.

10. Answer a

Although fracture of the coil or the insulation can occur anywhere along the lead, the most common site is where the lead passes between the rib and clavicle. Also known as subclavian crush syndrome, it can be avoided by placing the insertion of the lead into the subclavian vein as lateral as possible, or using an extrathoracic approach.

Chapter 41

Overview of Implantable Cardioverter-Defibrillators

Marshall S. Stanton, M.D.

> The key study points for the Cardiology Boards are the following:
> - Accepted indications for implantation of implantable cardioverter-defibrillators (ICDs)
> - General results of randomized trials involving ICDs
> - Key features of devices approved by the Food and Drug Administration. (Note: Questions about investigational devices should not be included in the Cardiology Boards)
> - Contraindications and warnings for patients with an ICD

Ventricular tachyarrhythmias present a difficult management problem for the physician. Although many drugs are available for controlling abnormal rhythms, their success rates are less than 50% for control of either supraventricular or ventricular arrhythmias. Concern also exists about whether drugs remain effective as a disease progresses and whether the arrhythmogenic substrate changes. Further, each drug has its own side effect profile, including the potential for proarrhythmia.

Various ICDs have been developed to aid in the management of lethal ventricular arrhythmias. They all have in common the need for one or more ventricular myocardial leads to sense the cardiac rate, pace, and deliver cardioversion-defibrillation shocks. Today, in almost all patients, a cardioverter-defibrillator can be implanted without performing a thoracotomy (that is, transvenous lead[s] and, if necessary, in rare circumstances, a subcutaneous lead [patch or array]).

ICDs function by continuously monitoring the cardiac rate and delivering therapy when the rate exceeds the programmed rate cutoff. If a device is programmed to deliver shocks for treatment of tachyarrhythmias with a rate cutoff of 175 beats per minute, then shortly after the heart rate exceeds 175 beats per minute the device charges and delivers a shock directly to the heart.

- Today, in almost all patients, a cardioverter-defibrillator can be implanted without performing a thoracotomy.

Features

Today, all ICDs have the capacity to provide backup ventricular demand (VVI) pacing in addition to delivering shocks. This feature is very useful for patients with intermittent heart block or other bradyarrhythmias. Placement of a separate pacemaker into a patient who has a defibrillator has the potential to cause serious pacemaker-defibrillator interactions. If it becomes necessary to insert a pacemaker in a patient who already has a defibrillator, it is mandatory to assess for pacemaker-defibrillator interactions at the time of implantation. This assessment should be performed only by someone with experience in this type of evaluation. ICDs with backup bradycardia pacing but without antitachycardia pacing (ATP) capability are not used frequently, but they are a cost-saving option for patients in whom ATP will not be needed (such as patients with ventricular fibrillation only). ICDs that can perform dual-chamber or rate-responsive pacing are available in certain models.

- Placement of a separate pacemaker into a patient who has a defibrillator has the potential to cause serious pacemaker-defibrillator interactions.

The most commonly implanted defibrillators have the additional ability to attempt termination of ventricular tachycardia with ATP. The obvious advantage of this feature is that an arrhythmia can be terminated painlessly without delivery of a shock. These ICDs are multiprogrammable, allowing the physician to adjust many aspects of tachycardia detection and therapy and thereby to customize the device to an individual patient. To begin with, different zones can be programmed for detection of ventricular tachyarrhythmias such that slower arrhythmias can be treated with ATP before progressing to shocks, whereas faster tachycardias can be treated more aggressively (Table 1). For example, slow ventricular tachycardia (126 to 160 beats per minute) is managed with the therapies programmed into tachycardia zone 1. The patient first receives the ATP formatted for ATP_1. If that series of ATP sequences is unsuccessful, the device then delivers the ATP programmed as ATP_2. Shocks then are delivered if the arrhythmia persists after delivery of these ATP sequences: 1-J and 5-J shocks are attempted before progressing to high-energy 34-J shocks. A faster ventricular tachycardia (161 to 200 beats per minute) is treated with a different series of therapies that the physician chooses. Still faster ventricular tachycardia (more than 200 beats per minute) or ventricular fibrillation is treated with only high-energy shocks. If the patient's heart rate slows to less than 50 beats per minute, the ICD provides rate support with backup demand ventricular pacing (VVI). The number of zones, the detection rates of the different zones, and specifics of the different therapies are all programmable. This feature is of critical importance because most patients present with various types of rhythm problems necessitating different detection and therapy schemes.

Indications for Placement

As with any treatment, a patient's other underlying diseases may alter the choice of ICD therapy. For example, if a

Table 1.—Implantable Cardioverter-Defibrillator, Example of Function

Zone	Heart rate, bpm	Therapy
Tachycardia zone 3	> 200	34-J shocks
Tachycardia zone 2	161-200	ATP_1/1-J shock/5-J shock/34-J shock
Tachycardia zone 1	126-160	ATP_1/ATP_2/1-J shock/5-J shock
Normal rhythm zone	50-125	
Bradycardia zone	< 50	VVI pacing

Abbreviations: ATP, antitachycardia pacing; VVI, ventricular demand.

patient has metastatic cancer and a predicted survival of less than 1 year, ICD therapy may not be appropriate. ICDs are indicated in the following circumstances:
- Cardiac arrest due to ventricular fibrillation or ventricular tachycardia not due to a transient or reversible cause
- Spontaneous sustained ventricular tachycardia
- Syncope of undetermined origin with clinically relevant, hemodynamically significant sustained ventricular tachycardia or ventricular fibrillation induced at electrophysiologic study when drug therapy is not effective, not tolerated, or not preferred
- Nonsustained ventricular tachycardia with coronary artery disease, prior myocardial infarction, left ventricular dysfunction, and inducible ventricular fibrillation or sustained ventricular tachycardia at electrophysiologic study that is not suppressible by a class I antiarrhythmic drug

It is *not* appropriate to implant a defibrillator in the following cases:
- Syncope of unknown cause without inducible ventricular arrhythmias at electrophysiologic study
- Ventricular arrhythmias due to reversible causes (proarrhythmia, severe electrolyte disturbance, ischemia)
- Incessant ventricular tachycardia

Some patients have indications that are between the extremes of definitely indicated and not indicated. These are patients thought to be at high risk for sudden death but who have not yet had lethal ventricular arrhythmias, such as patients with familial dilated cardiomyopathy, long QT syndrome, or hypertrophic cardiomyopathy whose family members have died suddenly.

Nonthoracotomy Lead Systems

Advances have been made such that the leads required for pacing, sensing, and defibrillation can all be placed without the need for a thoracotomy. Different configurations have been used, but all have in common a lead in the right ventricle which acts as one of the poles for defibrillation and also provides pacing and sensing. The second "lead" for defibrillation often is the pulse generator metallic can itself. A third lead can be added in the subcutaneous region of the left lateral chest wall, and this is needed in approximately 5% of cases. This subcutaneous lead may be a patch or an array of three separate wires linked together. In some nonthoracotomy systems, the third lead can be placed in the coronary sinus, but this placement is done infrequently because of increased lead dislodgment from this position.

Shock Waveforms

Studies have shown that biphasic shocks are more efficient (require lower energies) than monophasic shocks. All currently marketed ICDs use biphasic shock waveforms, although there are differences between those used by different manufacturers.

Size

Newer ICDs are small. Available ICDs can be consistently implanted in the pectoral region, analogous to how pacemakers are implanted.

Diagnostic Features

When a patient returns for follow-up, it sometimes is difficult to determine what type of rhythm caused the ICD to deliver therapy. All devices can give information about the cycle length (that is, rate) of the rhythm. Many also can provide visual information in the form of a stored electrogram. This gives the physician the opportunity to review an intracardiac version of an electrocardiogram, which can aid in determining whether device therapy was appropriate. Despite this advanced feature, in some instances it is still not possible to be certain whether a ventricular or supraventricular arrhythmia caused the ICD to deliver therapy.

Complications

Operative mortality with nonthoracotomy ICDs is less than 1%. This is an improvement over the 1% to 4% mortality reported when epicardial patches were used. Infection of the pulse generator or lead(s) occurs in approximately 2% of cases, and this necessitates removal of the entire system. Other complications include lead fracture or dislodgment, inappropriate delivery of therapy because of overdetection of sinus tachycardia or atrial arrhythmias, initiation of ventricular arrhythmias by inappropriate device therapy, hemothorax, pneumothorax, hematoma of the pulse generator pocket, undersensing, arrhythmia exacerbation early after implantation, and early battery depletion.

- Operative mortality with nonthoracotomy ICDs is less than 1%.

Efficacy

Patients who have cardiac arrest unrelated to acute myocardial infarction have approximately a 35% chance of recurrent lethal ventricular arrhythmia within the first 6 to 12 months after their event. Considering the severe cardiac disease and generally poor prognosis of most patients who receive ICDs (mean ejection fraction in most series is about 35%), survival in patients with such devices is excellent. A database of almost 10,000 patients with implantable defibrillators showed a 5-year survival free of sudden death of more than 95% and a total 5-year survival of 79%. Other, separate studies have shown excellent survival rates. Whether ICDs prolong survival in patients with severe left ventricular dysfunction has been questioned. Some authors argue that such patients die of progressive heart failure regardless of the presence of ICDs and perhaps do not benefit from these devices. Other studies present data arguing that these patients do benefit. The issue remains unresolved because no randomized trials have addressed this question. Although the topic remains debated, it is this author's opinion that the low risk associated with implantation of ICDs today is far outweighed by the benefit obtained, as evidenced by the impressive survival in many published studies. Currently, the option of ICD therapy should not be withheld from anyone with life-threatening ventricular arrhythmias in whom drug therapy cannot be proved to be effective.

Additional benefits not measured by survival are realized in patients with ICDs. Hospitalizations are reduced because single episodes of device-treated arrhythmias need not require admission to the hospital. Recurrence of ventricular tachycardia or ventricular fibrillation in a patient without an ICD certainly would prompt hospitalization if the individual were to survive. Additionally, patients often have a sense of security in knowing that they have a device continuously monitoring their heart rhythm which can resuscitate them within seconds of a recurrence.

- Patients who have cardiac arrest unrelated to acute myocardial infarction have approximately a 35% chance of recurrent lethal ventricular arrhythmia within the first 6 to 12 months.

Contraindications and Warnings

Patients with ICDs or pacemakers should not undergo magnetic resonance imaging. Lithotripsy is contraindicated if the pulse generator is in the field. Although arc welding is listed as a contraindication, we have published data showing that some patients can be allowed to do this activity if they are evaluated in their work environment. Cautery that is used during operation potentially can cause oversensing, and thus ICDs should be inactivated before cautery is used. As mentioned above, special testing must be performed to assess for pacemaker-ICD interactions when one device is placed in the setting of the other. There are no official guidelines for the follow-up of patients with ICDs. Table 2 outlines the author's recommendations. These are suggestions, and they should be tailored to the individual patient. The importance of follow-up is to ensure that the ICD system (pulse generator and lead[s]) continues to function normally with time.

- Magnetic resonance imaging is contraindicated in patients with ICDs.
- Lithotripsy is contraindicated if the pulse generator is in the field.

Clinical Trials Involving ICDs

Primary Prevention Studies

MADIT

The Multicenter Automatic Defibrillator Implantation Trial (MADIT) assessed the best way to treat patients with

Table 2.—Follow-Up Schedule of Patients With Implantable Cardioverter-Defibrillators

Time	Place	Procedure[*]
One month after implantation	Outpatient clinic	Interrogation Assessment of battery Pacing threshold Sensing
Three months and 1 year after implantation, then yearly, plus as needed[†]	Outpatient hospital	Interrogation Assessment of battery Pacing threshold Sensing VT induction VF induction Chest roentgenography[‡]
Six months, then 6 months between the yearly VT/VF induction visits	Outpatient clinic	Interrogation Assessment of battery Pacing threshold Sensing Chest roentgenography[‡]

[*]Re-formation of the capacitors occurs automatically in most devices. If not, this should be performed as specified by the device's manufacturer.
[†]Additional full testing of the device with arrhythmia induction should be performed when there is a significant change in the patient's status (such as after a myocardial infarction) or after addition or removal of antiarrhythmic drug therapy.
[‡]The chest roentgenogram must be reviewed carefully for any evidence of lead dislodgment or fracture.
Abbreviations: VF, ventricular fibrillation; VT, ventricular tachycardia.

coronary artery disease and nonsustained ventricular tachycardia. Results were released in March 1996, when the trial was stopped prematurely by its Safety and Data Monitoring Board. For inclusion, the left ventricular ejection fraction had to be less than 35%, patients had to be in New York Heart Association class I or II, and they must have had inducible ventricular tachycardia at baseline electrophysiologic study and after administration of intravenous procainamide. Patients were then randomized for immediate placement of an ICD or serial electrophysiologic testing to identify a successful drug. The total number of randomized patients was 196. Fifteen deaths occurred in the ICD group and 39 deaths in the electrophysiologic group. The hazard ratio was 0.46 (54% mortality reduction; $P = 0.009$). Survival was 96% at 1 year and 86% at 2 years in the ICD group and 76% and 68%, respectively, in the electrophysiologic group. One potential criticism of the study is that there was no control group. Thus, it is not known whether the patients in the ICD group received a benefit or merely avoided the deleterious effect that could have occurred from the drug therapy in the electrophysiologic group. This argument can be somewhat rebutted by the finding that 80% of the patients in the electrophysiologic group were treated with amiodarone, a drug that, in other studies, has not increased mortality in similar populations. Because of this study, the Food and Drug Administration has granted one defibrillator manufacturer labeling for the use of ICDs in patients who meet the MADIT criteria.

CABG-Patch

Winning the "best acronym award," the CABG-Patch trial enrolled 900 patients who were undergoing coronary artery bypass grafting (CABG) and who had a left ventricular ejection fraction less than 35% and a positive signal-averaged electrocardiogram. Half the patients were randomized to receive an ICD with epicardial patches, and the other half received no antiarrhythmic therapy. There was no significant difference in overall survival between the two groups; 2-year survival was approximately 84%. Thus, prophylactic use of ICDs is not indicated in patients undergoing CABG.

SCD-HeFT

Whether ICDs can improve survival when used prophylactically in patients with congestive heart failure is the aim of the Sudden Cardiac Death-Heart Failure Trial (SCD-HeFT). Patients with a left ventricular ejection fraction less than 35% due to any cause and New York Heart Association functional class II or III are eligible for entry. Patients are randomized to standard therapy for congestive heart failure, standard therapy plus amiodarone, or standard therapy plus ICD placement. The trial is still ongoing.

MUSTT

The Multicenter UnSustained Tachycardia Trial (MUSTT) addressed the problem of the appropriate management of patients with nonsustained ventricular tachycardia associated with known coronary disease and ventricular dysfunction (ejection fraction less than 40%). This study compared conservative medical management with antiarrhythmic therapy. All patients underwent a baseline risk stratification by electrophysiologic study. Seven hundred four patients had inducible sustained ventricular tachycardia and were randomized to either standard medical management (angiotensin-converting enzyme inhibitors or β-adrenergic blockers) or electrophysiologically guided antiarrhythmic drug therapy and

ICD placement in patients in whom drug therapy failed. If monomorphic ventricular tachycardia was not inducible at electrophysiologic study, the patients received no antiarrhythmic therapy. All patients in the antiarrhythmic therapy group initially received an antiarrhythmic drug, but after failure of at least one drug they were eligible to receive an ICD. The number of patients who received an ICD was approximately equal to the number who finished the study receiving antiarrhythmic drug therapy. The cardiac death rate was significantly reduced at 2 years (12% versus 18%) and at 5 years (5% versus 32%) in the patients who had electrophysiologically guided treatment compared with the patients who had standard medical therapy alone. Patients who received antiarrhythmic drugs did no better than patients assigned to usual medical treatment, and all the beneficial effects in the aggressive treatment arm occurred in patients who received ICDs.

Secondary Prevention Studies

AVID

The Antiarrhythmics Versus Implantable Defibrillator (AVID) trial compared medical and device therapies for patients who had sudden death or hemodynamically significant sustained ventricular tachycardia. Those enrolled were randomized either to receive an ICD or to be treated with amiodarone or sotalol. The trial was stopped prematurely in April 1997 when just more than 1,000 patients (of an anticipated 1,200) were enrolled. Patients randomized to receive an ICD had significantly improved survival compared with those treated with amiodarone or sotalol. Risk reduction for death was reduced 38% at 1 year and 30% at 3 years. More than 80% of patients in the drug arm of the study received amiodarone. This study provides compelling evidence of the improved survival in patients with lethal ventricular arrhythmias who are treated with ICDs and argues for use of such devices as first-line therapy in these patients.

CIDS

The Canadian Implantable Defibrillator Study is testing the therapeutic benefit of amiodarone compared with ICD implantation in patients who have: 1) cardiac arrest, 2) ventricular tachycardia with syncope, or 3) inducible ventricular tachycardia or fibrillation and have an ejection fraction of 35% or less. More than 600 patients were randomized to either immediate ICD placement or amiodarone drug therapy. After 3 years of follow-up, patients in the ICD group had a 20% risk reduction ($P = 0.07$) compared with those in the amiodarone group. Pulmonary complications occurred in 12% of the ICD group and 20% of the amiodarone group.

CASH

The Cardiac Arrest Study Hamburg (CASH) is a German study whose primary objective is to compare the incidence of sudden death, cardiac mortality, and total mortality in survivors of cardiac arrest randomized to one of four treatments: ICD, amiodarone, metoprolol, and propafenone.

The propafenone limb was discontinued from the study in March 1992 because of an increase in mortality (total mortality 29.3% in patients randomized to propafenone versus 11.5% in the ICD group, $P = 0.01$). At completion of the study, there was no difference in mortality between patients randomized to metoprolol and those in the amiodarone group. Overall mortality was reduced 37% ($P = 0.047$) in patients assigned to ICD compared with those in the metoprolol and amiodarone groups.

Suggested Review Reading

1. The Antiarrhythmics Versus Implantable Defibrillators (AVID) Investigators: A comparison of antiarrhythmic-drug therapy with implantable defibrillators in patients resuscitated from near-fatal ventricular arrhythmias. *N Engl J Med* 337:1576-1583, 1997.

2. Bardy GH, Troutman C, Poole JE, et al: Clinical experience with a tiered-therapy, multiprogrammable antiarrhythmia device. *Circulation* 85:1689-1698, 1992.

3. Bigger JT Jr: Prophylactic use of implanted cardiac defibrillators in patients at high risk for ventricular arrhythmias after coronary-artery bypass graft surgery. *N Engl J Med* 337:1569-1575, 1997.

4. Calkins H, Brinker J, Veltri EP, et al: Clinical interactions between pacemakers and automatic implantable cardioverter-defibrillators. *J Am Coll Cardiol* 16:666-673, 1990.

5. Fetter JG, Benditt DG, Stanton MS: Electromagnetic interference from welding and motors on implantable cardioverter-defibrillators as tested in the electrically hostile work site. *J Am Coll Cardiol* 28:423-427, 1996.

6. Gregoratos G, Cheitlin MD, Conill A, et al: ACC/AHA guidelines for implantation of cardiac pacemakers and antiarrhythmia devices: a report of the American College of Cardiology/American Heart Association Task Force on Practice Guidelines (Committee on Pacemaker Implantation). *J Am Coll Cardiol* 31:1175-1209, 1998.

7. Moss AJ, Hall WJ, Cannom DS, et al: Improved survival with an implanted defibrillator in patients with coronary disease at high risk for ventricular arrhythmia. *N Engl J Med* 335:1933-1940, 1996.

8. Wietholt D, Block M, Isbruch F, et al: Clinical experience with antitachycardia pacing and improved detection algorithms in a new implantable cardioverter-defibrillator. *J Am Coll Cardiol* 21:885-894, 1993.

Questions

Multiple Choice (choose the one best answer)

1. The AVID Trial showed that patients with which of the following had improved survival when treated with an implantable cardioverter-defibrillator compared with amiodarone or sotalol?
   a. Ventricular fibrillation
   b. Nonsustained ventricular tachycardia and a low ejection fraction
   c. Hypertrophic cardiomyopathy
   d. Both a and b
   e. All of the above

2. An accepted indication for placing an implantable cardioverter-defibrillator in a patient with nonsustained ventricular tachycardia and a low ejection fraction after myocardial infarction is sustained ventricular tachycardia inducible at electrophysiologic study.
   a. True
   b. False

3. A 65-year-old man with idiopathic dilated cardiomyopathy has a sudden syncopal spell while sitting in a chair. Physical examination shows no orthostasis and a soft S_3 gallop, but it is otherwise unremarkable. Electrocardiography reveals sinus rhythm and left bundle branch block. Ejection fraction is 25% by echocardiography. Electrophysiologic study shows normal sinus node recovery time, normal AH and HV intervals, no infra-His block, and no inducible supraventricular or ventricular arrhythmias. Result of the tilt test is normal. What is the next most appropriate action?
   a. No further evaluation or treatment
   b. External or insertable loop recorder
   c. Amiodarone
   d. Permanent pacemaker
   e. Implantable defibrillator

4. Implantable defibrillators are available that can do each of the following *except*:
   a. Sense the atrium to aid in discrimination of supraventricular from ventricular arrhythmias
   b. Pace AV sequentially
   c. Store an intracardiac electrogram
   d. Store hemodynamic data
   e. Painlessly terminate ventricular tachycardia

Answers

1. Answer a

2. Answer a

3. Answer b

4. Answer d

Notes

Chapter 42

Sudden Cardiac Death

Joseph G. Murphy, M.D.
Thomas M. Munger, M.D.

Sudden death that is not due to trauma or other accidental cause is due predominantly to cardiac causes (Table 1). Sudden cardiac death results in about 350,000 deaths annually in the U.S. Sudden death occurs in elderly patients with known heart disease, in asymptomatic middle-aged patients without known cardiac disease, and in a small number of apparently healthy young athletes.

Definition of Sudden Cardiac Death

Sudden cardiac death is nonaccidental, unexpected death due to a cardiac cause within 1 hour after the onset of acute symptoms. Although many of these patients have a previous diagnosis of cardiac disease, the time and mode of death are unexpected.

Epidemiology of Sudden Cardiac Death

Prospective studies have reported that about 50% of all deaths due to coronary heart disease are sudden and occur either as the presenting symptom or within 1 hour after the onset of other new cardiac symptoms. In comparison with the general population, the risk of sudden cardiac death is highest in patients who have already had a significant cardiac event such as an out-of-hospital cardiac arrest or new onset of heart failure or unstable angina or who are in one of the high-risk subgroups after recovery

from acute myocardial infarction.

- 350,000 sudden cardiac deaths occur in the U.S. annually.
- 50% of all cardiac deaths in the U.S. are sudden.
- 80% to 90% of sudden nontraumatic deaths have a cardiac cause.

Cardiac Diseases Associated With Sudden Cardiac Death

Ischemic Heart Disease

Ischemic heart disease is the primary cause of sudden cardiac death. Most of these patients have two- or three-vessel coronary artery disease (defined as > 75% stenosis). Sudden death is the first clinical manifestation of coronary heart disease in 25% of patients with coronary artery disease (Table 2). Although myocardial infarction does not evolve in most patients resuscitated from sudden death, many (> 75%) of them have evidence of previous infarcts. Risk factors for sudden death include ventricular dysfunction (ejection fraction < 40%) and more than 10 ventricular ectopic beats per minute.

The Cardiac Arrhythmia Suppression Trial (CAST) tested the hypothesis that suppression of premature ventricular contractions with class IC antiarrhythmic drugs would decrease the risk of sudden death after myocardial infarction. The treated group had excess mortality because of a proarrhythmic effect by class IC agents.

Table 1.—Cardiovascular Disease States Associated With Sudden Death

Coronary artery disease
 Atherosclerosis
 Infectious disease (syphilis)
 Inflammatory disorder (rheumatic vasculitis)
 Congenital anomaly
 Coronary artery embolism
 Coronary artery aneurysm
Valvular heart disease
 Mitral valve prolapse
 Aortic stenosis
Cardiomyopathy or myocarditis
 Idiopathic disorder
 Hypertrophic cardiomyopathy
 Infectious disease
 Sarcoidosis
 Amyloidosis
 Muscular dystrophy
 Arrhythmogenic ventricular dysplasia
Prolonged QT interval
 Idiopathic disorder
 Congenital anomaly
 Medication-related disorder
 Liquid protein diet
Metabolic abnormalities
 Hyperkalemia or hypokalemia
 Hypercalcemia or hypocalcemia
 Hypomagnesemia
 Increased levels of catecholamines
Congenital heart disease
 Primary pulmonary hypertension
 Tetralogy of Fallot
 Congenital heart block
 Ebstein anomaly of the heart
Medication
 Antiarrhythmic agents
 Antidepressant drugs
 Major tranquilizers
Intracardiac tumor
 Primary
 Metastatic
Cardiac ganglionitis
Wolff-Parkinson-White syndrome
No apparent underlying cardiac disease

From Giuliani ER, Gersh BJ, McGoon MD, Hayes DL, Schaff HV (editors): *Mayo Clinic Practice of Cardiology*. Third edition. Mosby, 1996, p 867. By permission of Mayo Foundation.

Table 2.—Survival in Patients With Out-of-Hospital Cardiac Arrest

Chances of survival are increased if:
 Initial rhythm is ventricular tachycardia or fibrillation rather than bradycardia-asystole
 Cardiopulmonary resuscitation is initiated quickly
 Defibrillation is implemented immediately
 Heart rate after initial defibrillation is more than 100 beats/min
 Postresuscitation rhythm is sinus, paced, or atrial fibrillation

From Giuliani ER, Gersh BJ, McGoon MD, Hayes DL, Schaff HV (editors): *Mayo Clinic Practice of Cardiology*. Third edition. Mosby, 1996, p 874. By permission of Mayo Foundation.

Valvular Heart Disease

Untreated critical aortic stenosis is frequently associated with sudden death. Even after successful aortic valve replacement surgery, an excess risk of sudden death still exists (possibly because of residual left ventricular hypertrophy), although it is less than that of patients without surgical treatment. Stenotic lesions of other cardiac valves are associated with a much lower risk of sudden death than aortic stenosis. Regurgitant valve lesions (chronic aortic regurgitation and acute mitral regurgitation) may also cause sudden death, but the risk is much less than that associated with aortic stenosis.

Mitral valve prolapse, a common condition, may be epidemiologically associated with a small excess risk of sudden death, but overall the prevalence and clinical outcome of mitral valve prolapse are more favorable than previously thought (*N Engl J Med* 341:1-7, 1999; *N Engl J Med* 341:8-13, 1999).

Congenital Heart Disease

The congenital heart lesions most commonly associated with sudden cardiac death are aortic stenosis and conditions with right-to-left intracardiac shunts with Eisenmenger physiology. Other causes of pulmonary hypertension, including primary pulmonary hypertension, are also associated with an excess risk of sudden death. Sudden cardiac death is reported as a late complication after surgical repair of complex congenital lesions, including tetralogy of Fallot, transposition of the great arteries, and atrioventricular canal. Ebstein anomaly is associated with Wolff-Parkinson-White syndrome.

Wolff-Parkinson-White Syndrome

The risk of sudden death in Wolff-Parkinson-White syndrome is about 0.1 per year and is usually due to the onset of atrial fibrillation with rapid ventricular conduction. This syndrome is amenable to cure with radiofrequency ablation at the time of electrophysiology study.

Long QT Syndromes

The long QT syndromes, either congenital or acquired, are associated with a significant risk of sudden death. The hereditary congenital long QT syndrome has been reported in two forms: that associated with deafness (Jervell and Lange-Nielsen syndrome) and that without deafness (Romano-Ward syndrome).

Patients with long QT syndrome are highly susceptible to fatal ventricular arrhythmias, particularly the torsades de pointes form of ventricular tachycardia. Predictors of high risk are associated deafness, female sex, syncope, and documented torsades de pointes or previous ventricular fibrillation.

The acquired form of prolonged QT interval is associated with the use of specific drugs, including antiarrhythmic, antipsychotic, and psychotropic drugs, terfenadine (Seldane), and lithium. It is also associated with electrolyte abnormalities, hypothermia, and central nervous system injury.

Dilated Cardiomyopathy and Heart Failure

Up to 50% of deaths in patients with heart failure are categorized as sudden cardiac deaths. The risk of sudden death is proportional to the extent of ventricular dysfunction as measured by the ejection fraction. Although many patients with heart failure have underlying severe coronary artery disease, nonischemic dilated cardiomyopathy from any cause is also associated with a significant risk of sudden death. All causes of acute cardiac failure may result in sudden death, either because of the circulatory failure itself or secondary to arrhythmias. Electrophysiologic testing is of limited value for risk stratification in patients with dilated cardiomyopathy, and noninducibility of ventricular tachycardia is not predictive of a low risk of sudden death.

Hypertrophic Cardiomyopathy

Hypertrophic cardiomyopathy (HCM) is associated with a substantial risk of sudden death, estimated at 2% to 4% annually in adults and 4% to 6% in children and adolescents. No good predictors of sudden death in HCM are available, but certain high-risk groups can be identified, including young age at symptom onset, strong family history of either HCM or unexplained sudden death, and

worsening symptoms. However, in most studies, more than 50% of sudden deaths occurred in patients without any functional limitations. The mechanism of sudden cardiac death in patients with HCM was initially thought to be outflow tract obstruction, possibly as a consequence of exercise or catecholamine stimulation, but the current view is that most sudden deaths in HCM are primarily arrhythmogenic rather than hemodynamic in cause. Many patients with HCM have a high prevalence of premature ventricular contractions and nonsustained ventricular tachycardia on ambulatory monitoring. Rapid or polymorphic symptomatic nonsustained tachycardias (or both) have better predictive power than stable and asymptomatic nonsustained ventricular tachycardia, which has poor predictive power for sudden cardiac death in patients with HCM. Patients with nonobstructive HCM also have a high risk of ventricular arrhythmias and are at increased risk for sudden death. The apical variant of HCM, seen more commonly in Japanese patients, probably has a lower risk of sudden death than the nonapical variants, suggesting that an electrophysiologic mechanism secondary to the hypertrophied muscle itself has a role.

The question of whether the pathogenesis of the arrhythmias represents an interaction between electrophysiologic and hemodynamic abnormalities or is a consequence of electrophysiologic derangement of hypertrophied muscle has not been answered.

Inflammatory and Infiltrative Heart Disease

Almost all inflammatory and infiltrative heart diseases are associated with sudden cardiac death, with or without concomitant cardiac failure. Acute viral myocarditis with left ventricular dysfunction is commonly associated with cardiac arrhythmias, including malignant ventricular lethal arrhythmias.

Idiopathic Ventricular Fibrillation

Idiopathic ventricular fibrillation is a diagnosis of exclusion and accounts for 2% to 3% of sudden cardiac deaths. This condition is characterized by the occurrence of ventricular fibrillation in the absence of any clinically identifiable structural or functional cardiac abnormality. An important aspect of this condition is that ventricular fibrillation recurs in about 33% of patients within 4 years. Most patients are younger than other patients with sudden death due to underlying cardiac disease. The role of electrophysiologic testing in this condition is controversial, and nonspecific findings, including polymorphic ventricular tachycardia and ventricular fibrillation, are frequently induced. Noninducibility of ventricular fibrillation at electrophysiologic testing is not a reliable predictor of future prognosis, and an automatic implantable cardioverter defibrillator should be considered in all cases.

A specific variation of unexplained nocturnal sudden death, which has many names (Bangungut in Filipino males, Pokkuri in Japanese males, and Nonlaitai in Laotian males), has been documented in young Southeast Asians. Death usually occurs during sleep and is due to ventricular fibrillation. In many cases, pathologic examinations have revealed subtle cardiac abnormalities. Brugada syndrome is characterized by right bundle branch block, persistent ST-segment elevation, and sudden death due to ventricular fibrillation.

Sudden Death

Sudden Cardiac Death in Athletes

Sudden cardiac death in athletes is rare but attracts considerable public attention (the annual incidence is about 4 deaths/1 million athletes). The commonest cause in those 35 years or younger is HCM, followed by coronary artery anomalies, aortic rupture in those with Marfan syndrome, coronary artery disease, and cocaine abuse. Although the left ventricle is enlarged in many competitive athletes, left ventricular wall thickness should not exceed 13 mm and diastolic filling abnormalities should be absent. In those older than 35 years, coronary artery disease is the predominant cause of death, followed by valvular heart disease (usually aortic stenosis) and HCM. Rarely, the congenital long QT syndromes or Wolff-Parkinson-White syndrome may be the cause of death.

Treatment of Aborted Sudden Death

An underlying pathophysiologic cause should always be sought in all patients who have had an aborted sudden death, and the cause should be corrected if possible (e.g., aortic valve replacement in critical aortic stenosis) and ameliorated if full correction is not possible (e.g., β-blockers for patients with severe nonrevascularizable coronary artery disease). In many patients, an invasive electrophysiology study is performed to determine the risk of a future arrhythmogenic event. Implantable defibrillator placement and/or amiodarone therapy can decrease the risk of sudden death, as evidenced by the MADIT and AVID studies (discussed in Chapter 73). Some patients with aborted sudden death will have severe anoxic brain injury, in which case conservative management of their cardiac disease is more appropriate.

Prevention of Sudden Death in Patients With Left Ventricular Dysfunction

Sudden death occurs in about 3% of patients soon after dismissal from the hospital after myocardial infarction. This is approximately 60,000 deaths annually in the U.S. Sudden death due to ventricular arrhythmias is also an important cause of death in patients with heart failure due to any cause. In patients with dilated cardiomyopathy, sudden death accounts for up to 50% of the total number of deaths.

Patients with nonsustained ventricular tachycardia are at risk for sudden death, as are those with impaired left ventricular function (ejection fraction < 40%), clinical heart failure, or conduction block. Beginning in the 1960s, it became clear that patients with nonsustained ventricular tachycardia on telemetry after myocardial infarction were at high risk for sudden death compared with those without ventricular ectopy. It was suggested that suppression of complex ventricular ectopy in patients at high risk after myocardial infarction would have a beneficial effect on mortality. The Cardiac Arrhythmia Suppression Trial (CAST) demonstrated clearly that this "premature ventricular contraction hypothesis" about patients who had had myocardial infarction was wrong and that suppression of premature ventricular contractions with class IC antiarrhythmic agents increased mortality in this group of patients.

- Sudden death occurs in about 3% of patients soon after hospital dismissal.
- High-risk patients are patients who have had myocardial infarction and have nonsustained ventricular tachycardia, ventricular dysfunction, clinical heart failure, or conduction block

Several antiarrhythmic drugs (including mexiletine, flecainide, encainide, and sotalol) have been shown in clinical trials to adversely affect mortality (despite suppressing nonsustained ventricular tachycardia salvos) when given prophylactically after myocardial infarction to patients at higher risk for sudden death. In contrast, amiodarone has not been shown to have an adverse effect after myocardial infarction, and in some trials has shown benefit. The European Post-MI Amiodarone Trial (EMIAT) was a randomized, double-blinded, placebo-controlled trial designed to test whether amiodarone would reduce all-cause mortality (primary end point) and arrhythmic death (secondary end point) in survivors of myocardial infarction with a left ventricular ejection fraction of 40% or less. All-cause mortality and cardiac mortality were not significantly reduced overall, but amiodarone decreased the risk of arrhythmic death by 35% ($P = 0.05$). The Canadian Amiodarone Trial (CAMIAT) reported a similar finding. The conclusion of these trials was that routine use of amiodarone prophylactically in all patients with depressed left ventricular function after myocardial infarction was not warranted, because overall mortality was not affected by the drug. However, meta-analysis has been performed of 13 randomized trials of prophylactic amiodarone in patients who recently had myocardial infarction (8 trials) or patients who had congestive heart failure (5 trials). This included 6,553 patients, 78% of whom were in post-myocardial infarction trials. Total mortality was decreased by 13% ($P = 0.03$). Arrhythmic/sudden death was decreased by 29% ($P = 0.0003$). The conclusion of the meta-analysis study was that the individual amiodarone studies by themselves were underpowered to detect an overall mortality effect, but amiodarone reduced overall mortality, chiefly because of its effect on reducing overall arrhythmic death.

Multicenter Automatic Defibrillator and Multicenter Unsustained Tachycardia Trials

For patients with coronary artery disease, the role of the implantable defibrillator (ICD) has been clarified by two recent excellent trials.

Multicenter Automatic Defibrillator Implantation Trial (MADIT)

MADIT, published in 1996, demonstrated that the ICD improves overall survival in comparison with antiarrhythmic therapy when used as a primary preventive tool in high-risk patients after myocardial infarction. MADIT included patients who had ejection fractions less than 35%, asymptomatic nonsustained ventricular tachycardia, and myocardial infarction at least 3 weeks before entry into the study. Patients were also required to have inducible ventricular tachycardia at electrophysiologic testing that was not suppressible with intravenous procainamide. Patients were randomly assigned to ICD or antiarrhythmic therapy (mainly amiodarone). At follow-up, patients receiving ICDs had a 54% reduction in overall mortality compared with those receiving antiarrhythmic therapy.

- ICD improves overall survival when compared to antiarrhythmic therapy in high-risk patients after myocardial infarction.

Multicenter Unsustained Tachycardia Trial (MUSTT)

MUSTT was reported at the American College of Cardiology meeting in March 1999. Inclusion criteria for this trial included coronary artery disease, an ejection fraction less than 40%, nonsustained ventricular tachycardia, and positive electrophysiologic study for inducible monomorphic ventricular tachycardia. A total of 351 patients were randomly assigned to electrophysiologic study-guided therapy, which included at least one evaluation of the effectiveness of antiarrhythmic therapy (the criteria for initial success being suppression of inducible ventricular tachycardia at electrophysiologic testing by antiarrhythmic drug) and 353 patients to no antiarrhythmic therapy. For total mortality, there was a significant trend favoring electrophysiologic study-guided therapy, with a risk reduction of 10% at 5 years compared with no antiarrhythmic therapy. The 5-year mortality was 52% in the electrophysiologic study-guided group and 58% in the nontreatment group ($P = 0.06$). Of greater importance was the finding of additional mortality benefit in patients who received ICD therapy ($n = 167$) compared with those who received exclusively antiarrhythmic drug therapy in the electrophysiologic study-guided therapy group. When examined as separate groups, the patients who received electrophysiologic study-guided antiarrhythmic drug therapy did worse than those who received no therapy, mimicking the results of CAST. The 5-year survival for patients in MUSTT who received an ICD was 75%, compared with 52% for the no treatment group and 45% for those who received electrophysiologic study-guided antiarrhythmic drug therapy. The difference was significant ($P < 0.001$). Thus, MUSTT confirmed the MADIT approach to patients with coronary artery disease who are at risk after myocardial infarction.

The 5-year survival for patients in MUSTT was as follows:
- Patients who received an ICD, 75%
- Patients who received no antiarrhythmic therapy, 52%
- Patients who received electrophysiology study-guided antiarrhythmic drug therapy, 45%.

Recommendations for Monitoring Patients After Myocardial Infarction

Telemetry or Holter monitoring should be performed on all patients who had myocardial infarction and have depressed left ventricular function (ejection fraction < 40%). If nonsustained ventricular tachycardia is present (at least one triplet per 24 hours), invasive electrophysiologic testing should be scheduled. If inducible monomorphic ventricular tachycardia is elicited during electrophysiologic testing, prophylactic ICD placement is recommended to achieve an overall survival benefit as well as prevention of sudden death.

ICD in Patients With Nonischemic Heart Disease

In patients with congestive heart failure without coronary artery disease (dilated cardiomyopathy, valvular heart disease, congenital heart disease), the role of prophylactic ICD placement is unproven. An NIH-sponsored trial, Sudden Cardiac Death in Heart Failure Trial (SCD-HeFT), is addressing this issue. This trial enrolls patients with an ejection fraction less than 35% who have New York Heart Association class II or III heart failure. Patients are randomly assigned to conventional heart failure therapy, amiodarone therapy,

or ICD implantation. Of interest is that no documented ventricular arrhythmia is required for entry, nor is electrophysiologic testing required (because this testing has been shown to be a poor predictor of fatal arrhythmias in patients with noncoronary left ventricular dysfunction). It is anticipated that SCD-HeFT enrollment will be completed by the year 2000.

Our understanding of the benefits of prophylactic treatment of patients who are at high risk for arrhythmic death has evolved considerably during the last 30 years. In the 1960s and 1970s, the predictors for poor outcomes were identified, and for many years drug therapy was the mainstay of treatment. However, trials such as CAST and MUSTT have shown that both empiric and electrophysiologic study-guided drug therapy are inferior to ICD therapy, which is now the mainstay of preventive therapy for patients at high risk for sudden death.

Suggested Review Reading

Amiodarone Trials

1. Amiodarone Trials Meta-Analysis Investigators: Effect of prophylactic amiodarone on mortality after acute myocardial infarction and in congestive heart failure: meta-analysis of individual data from 6500 patients in randomised trials. *Lancet* 350:1417-1424, 1997.

MADIT Trial

2. Moss AJ, Hall WJ, Cannom DS, et al: Improved survival with an implanted defibrillator in patients with coronary disease at high risk for ventricular arrhythmia. *N Engl J Med* 335:1933-1940, 1996.

MUSTT Trial

3. Buxton AE, et al: Survival results from the MUSTT trial. Presented at the general sessions at the American College of Cardiology, New Orleans, Louisiana, 1999.

Chapter 43

Normal and Abnormal Cardiac Electrophysiology

Douglas L. Packer, M.D.

The Heart's Electrical System

Sinus Node

The sinus node is a tapered cylindrical structure that lies subepicardially at the junction between the right atrium and the superior vena cava. Histologically, the sinus node consists of several cell types that are embedded within a connective tissue stroma. Round or ovoid P cells are probably the site of impulse formation, and transitional cells, which are considerably greater in number, serve as the link between the P cells and the remaining atrial tissue (Fig. 1).

Atrioventricular (AV) Node

The AV node is a dense structure positioned in the subendocardium of the low right atrium at the apex of the triangle of Koch (formed by the ostium of the coronary sinus, the tendon of Todaro, and the septal attachment of the tricuspid valve leaflet). Several cell types are present within the AV node, including P cells similar to those found in the sinoatrial node, N (or nodal) cells comprising the compact node, and transitional cells between atrial and nodal tissue (Fig. 2).

● The P cells within the sinoatrial node are probably the site of formation of normal cardiac impulse.

Intra-Atrial Pathways

There is evidence for the preferential spread of atrial activation between the sinus and AV nodes via intranodal pathways, but whether these are true tracts or simply preferential pathways of conduction remains unclear. These tracts are the anterior internodal tract, which curves leftward and anteriorly around the superior vena cava; the middle internodal tract, which crosses toward the interatrial septum to join the anterior internodal tract; and the posterior pathway, which exits posteriorly from the sinus node and courses toward the inferior vena cava. Bachmann's bundle may represent an alternative specialized tract for impulse propagation between atria (Fig. 3).

● Intra-atrial pathways are less well defined tracts than the His-Purkinje system.

His-Purkinje System

The His bundle begins from the inferior portion of the AV node, penetrates the fibrous portion of the interventricular septum, and travels down across the muscular septum to the remainder of the ventricles. The right bundle branch is more discrete than the left bundle branch. Activation of the right ventricle spreads peripherally through specialized Purkinje fibers. Alternatively, the left bundle branch, which may be described in terms of the left anterior and left posterior hemifascicles, is less discrete, particularly proximally, where the left bundle proper is a sheet of specialized conducting tissue rather than a discrete bundle. Purkinje cells of the bundle and peripheral branches are large: 15 to 30 μm in diameter and 20 to 100 μm in length. These cells, in turn, arborize with actual myocardial cells to facilitate

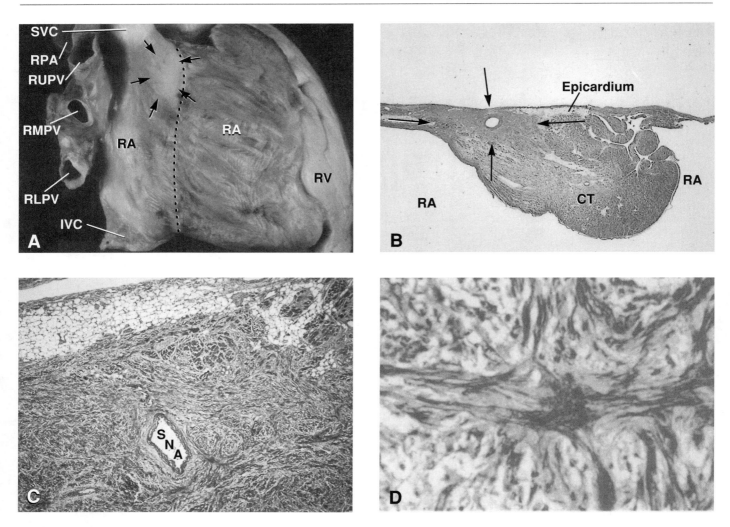

Fig. 1. Sinus node. *A*, The sinus node (*arrows*) lies in the sulcus terminalis (*dotted line*) near the cavoatrial junction. (Right lateral view from 32-year-old man.) *B*, The sinus node (*arrows*) is a subepicardial structure that overlies the superolateral portion of the crista terminalis. (Trichrome x5; from 61-year-old man.) *C*, The sinus nodal artery courses through the center of the sinus node. (Trichrome x20; from 20-year-old man.) *D*, The specialized myocardial cells of the sinus node form an interlacing pattern. (Trichrome x100; from 20-year-old man.) CT, Crista terminalis; IVC, inferior vena cava; RA, right atrium; RLPV, right lower pulmonary vein; RMPV, right middle pulmonary vein; RPA, right pulmonary artery; RUPV, right upper pulmonary vein; RV, right ventricle; SNA, sinus node artery; SVC, superior vena cava. (From Giuliani ER, Gersh BJ, McGoon MD, Hayes DL, Schaff HV [editors]: *Mayo Clinic Practice of Cardiology*. Third edition. Mosby, 1996, p 481. By permission of Mayo Foundation.)

local ventricular activation. The vascular supply of the conduction system is shown in Figure 4.

Tissue Electrophysiologic Properties

Fast Action Potentials

Atrial, ventricular, and His-Purkinje tissues show characteristic action potentials with rapid upstrokes (phase 0), as described by V_{max} (most rapid rate of increase of the upstroke of the action potential), the values of which range up to 300 V/s in atrial and ventricular tissue and up to 900 V/s in Purkinje tissue (Fig. 5). In these tissues, the upstrokes of the action potential are generated by inward sodium current. The action potential durations are shortest in atrial cells, intermediate in ventricular myocytes, and longer in Purkinje cells. The duration of the action potential and the characteristic contours of repolarization are determined largely by outgoing potassium currents, although inward calcium currents contribute to a lesser degree (Fig. 6). The latter currents are more responsible for phase 2 of the action potential. Resting membrane potentials typically range from -80 to -90 mV, and activation thresholds from -60 to -70 mV. The action potential amplitudes are large, ranging from 90 to 130 mV.

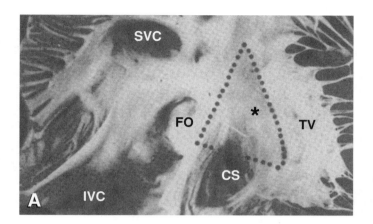

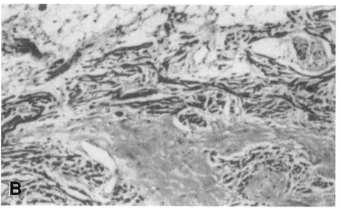

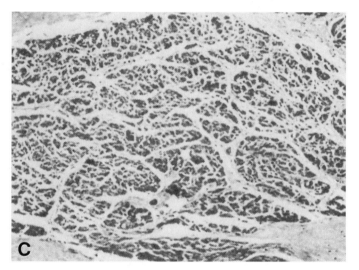

Fig. 2. Atrioventricular conduction system. *A*, The atrioventricular (AV) node (*) lies within the triangle of Koch (*dotted lines*), along the right atrial aspect of the AV septum. (Opened right atrium from 32-year-old man.) *B*, The node is characterized by an interlacing pattern of specialized myocardial cells. (Trichrome x50; from 20-year-old man.) *C*, The AV bundle consists of parallel bundles of specialized myocardial cells. (Trichrome x50; from 20-year-old man.) CS, coronary sinus; FO, fossa ovalis; IVC, inferior vena cava; SVC, superior vena cava; TV, tricuspid valve. (From Giuliani ER, Gersh BJ, McGoon MD, Hayes DL, Schaff HV [editors]: *Mayo Clinic Practice of Cardiology*. Third edition. Mosby, 1996, p 483. By permission of Mayo Foundation.)

- Upstrokes of the action potential are generated by inward sodium current.
- Action potential durations are shortest in atrial cells, intermediate in ventricular myocytes, and longer in Purkinje cells.

Slow Action Potentials

In contrast, the sinoatrial nodal and AV nodal cells are activated by slow inward calcium-carried currents. As such, the rates of activation and inactivation are slower, membrane potentials range from -40 to -70 mV, activation thresholds range from -30 to -40 mV, and the V_{max} of the upstroke of action potentials is typically slow, less than 15 V/s (Fig. 7). In addition, cells of the sinus and AV nodal regions demonstrate phase 4 depolarization, in which there is a gradual reduction in the negativity of the membrane potential during the diastolic interval. These cells also are highly influenced by both sympathetic and

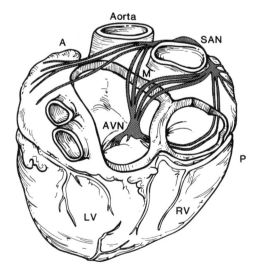

Fig. 3. Posterior schematic of the heart with internodal pathways connecting the sinoatrial node (SAN) and atrioventricular node (AVN). The anterior internodal tract (A) curves leftward and anteriorly around the superior vena cava. The middle internodal tract (M) crosses toward the interatrial system to join the anterior internodal tract. The posterior pathway (P) exits posteriorly and courses toward the inferior vena cava. LV, left ventricle; RV, right ventricle. (From Giuliani ER, Gersh BJ, McGoon MD, Hayes DL, Schaff HV [editors]: *Mayo Clinic Practice of Cardiology*. Third edition. Mosby, 1996, p 730. By permission of Mayo Foundation.)

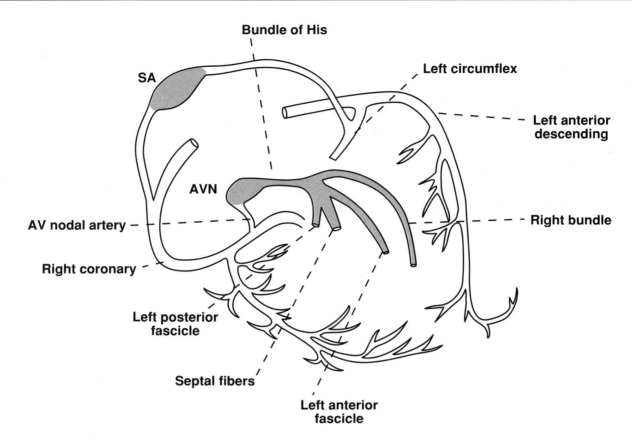

Fig. 4. Schematic of the vascular supply to the cardiac conduction system. The sinus node artery may arise from the right coronary artery (55% to 65%) or as a branch of the left circumflex (35% to 45%). The atrioventricular node (AVN) artery arises from the right coronary artery in 90% of patients. The right coronary artery also supplies the common His bundle and portions of the right bundle. The left anterior descending coronary artery also supplies blood to the His bundle via septal perforators and the "left anterior fascicle." The left posterior fascicle usually receives a blood supply from both the right coronary artery (posterior descending) and the left anterior descending artery. SA, sinoatrial node. (From Giuliani ER, Gersh BJ, McGoon MD, Hayes DL, Schaff HV [editors]: *Mayo Clinic Practice of Cardiology*. Third edition. Mosby, 1996, p 731. By permission of Mayo Foundation.)

parasympathetic nerve input, which increases or decreases the rate of phase 4 depolarization. Similarly, these cells may be modulated by catecholamines or acetylcholine. Because conduction is driven by the slow inward current, conduction velocities are more on the order of 0.01 to 0.1 m/s. In contrast, velocities in fast current tissue range from 0.5 to 3.0 m/s.

Table 1 lists the features of fast and slow inward currents of the action potential.

- Sinoatrial nodal and AV nodal cells are activated by slow inward calcium-carried currents.

Tissue Refractoriness

In addition to the action potential durations, all cardiac cells show refractoriness, which is the fundamental resistance to reexcitation after a previous electrical activation.

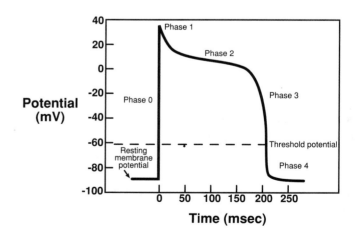

Fig. 5. Action potential with five phases. The resting membrane potential is -90 mV. In spontaneously active cells, there is slow diastolic depolarization during phase 4, which returns the fiber toward the threshold potential. (From Giuliani ER, Gersh BJ, McGoon MD, Hayes DL, Schaff HV [editors]: *Mayo Clinic Practice of Cardiology*. Third edition. Mosby, 1996, p 734. By permission of Mayo Foundation.)

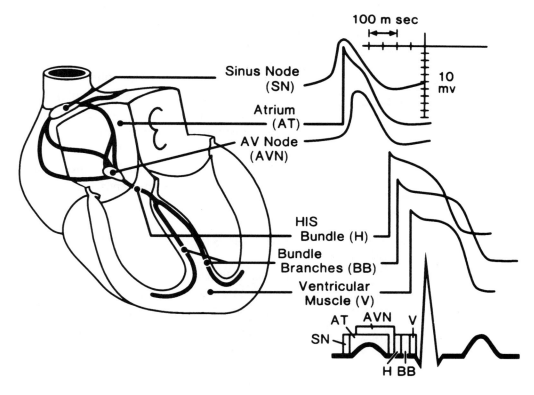

Fig. 6. Action potentials recorded from different regions of the heart. Action potentials from the sinus and certain cells in the atrioventricular (AV) node are similar and distinct from those from the rest of the heart. (From Giuliani ER, Gersh BJ, McGoon MD, Hayes DL, Schaff HV [editors]: *Mayo Clinic Practice of Cardiology*. Third edition. Mosby, 1996, p 734. By permission of Mayo Foundation.)

Table 1.—Distinguishing Features of Fast and Slow Inward Currents of the Action Potential

Characteristic	Fast current	Slow current
Main ion	Na^+	Ca^{2+}
Rates of activation and inactivation	Rapid	Slow
Activation threshold, mV	-60 to -70	-30 to -40
Resting membrane potential, mV	-80 to -90	-40 to -70
Conduction velocity, m/s	0.5 to 3.0	0.01 to 0.1
Action potential amplitude, mV	100 to 130	35 to 75
Recovery	Prompt	Delayed, outlasts full repolarization
Current decreased by	Tetrodotoxin	Manganese, verapamil, D600,
	Decreased resting membrane potential	nifedipine, diltiazem, perhexiline, acetylcholine
	Local anesthetics	
Current enhanced by	Veratridine	Catecholamines, cAMP
Role in nodal automaticity	Doubtful	Probable
Role in toxic or ischemic arrhythmias	?	Possible

From Giuliani ER, Gersh BJ, McGoon MD, Hayes DL, Schaff HV (editors): *Mayo Clinic Practice of Cardiology*. Third edition. Mosby, 1996, p 736. By permission of Mayo Foundation.

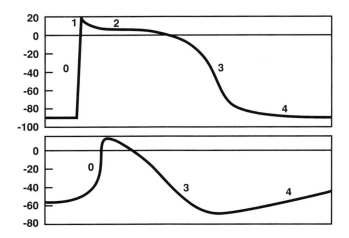

Fig. 7. Action potentials recorded by intracellular electrodes from two types of cardiac cells. *Top*, Action potential recorded from a cell that is dependent mainly on a rapid-current, fast-channel response. *Bottom*, Action potential recorded from a sinus node cell that is dependent on a slow inward current. The latter current is characterized by lower resting and activation potentials and slower conduction velocity. Numbers 0-4 refer to the phases shown in Figure 5. (From Giuliani ER, Gersh BJ, McGoon MD, Hayes DL, Schaff HV [editors]: *Mayo Clinic Practice of Cardiology*. Third edition. Mosby, 1996, p 736. By permission of Mayo Foundation.)

This resistance can be described in terms of effective refractoriness, which can be measured by the introduction of an extrastimulus. In such testing, the effective refractory period is the longest paired S_1-S_2 impulse coupling interval that does not activate the cell when introduced at twice the diastolic threshold during the diastolic interval.

- Effective refractory period is the longest paired S_1-S_2 impulse coupling interval that does not activate the cell.

Tissue Innervation

All cardiac tissue is innervated by both sympathetic and parasympathetic nerves. In atrial tissue, parasympathetic nerve stimulation produces shortening of the duration of the action potential and slowing of conduction. Sympathetic nerve activation also may shorten the duration of the action potential, but it accelerates conduction. In AV nodal tissue, parasympathetic nerve stimulation, as mediated by acetylcholine release, results in the slowing of conduction and prolongation of refractoriness, whereas the opposite reaction occurs with sympathetic nerve stimulation. In contrast, refractoriness of ventricular tissue typically is decreased by sympathetic nerve activation but increased by parasympathetic nerve activation. Interestingly, both sympathetic and parasympathetic nerve stimulation have

relatively little effect on ventricular conduction. These nerves follow a characteristic course to the individual myocardial cells. Both sets of fibers typically enter the ventricles in the region of the AV groove. Although sympathetic fibers may initially course in a subendocardial location, they penetrate the ventricular wall location to course along the epicardial surface. The opposite occurs with parasympathetic nerve fibers.

- Sympathetic and parasympathetic nerve stimulation have relatively little effect on ventricular conduction.

Normal Rhythm Generation

Cardiac cells demonstrate the ability for spontaneous action potential formation (automaticity). This manifests itself in a hierarchical pattern: sinus nodal tissue tends to be more automatic than atrial tissue, which is, in turn, more automatic than AV nodal, His-Purkinje, or ventricular cells. This hierarchy is due to differences in the intrinsic automaticity of the cells, which is dependent on 1) the slope and rate of phase 4 depolarization, which sets the rate of impulse formation; 2) the threshold potential, at which the action potential is initiated; and 3) the maximal diastolic potential, from which phase 4 spontaneous depolarization begins. Typically, normal sinus node rates range between 60 and 100 bpm. In contrast, junctional tissue produces rates in the range of 50 to 60 bpm, and ventricular automaticity, when observed in the absence of higher pacemakers, usually produces rates of only 30 to 45 bpm.

- Sinus nodal tissue tends to be more automatic than atrial tissue, which is, in turn, more automatic than AV nodal, His-Purkinje, or ventricular cells.

Sinus Node Recovery Time

Sinus node function can be assessed in terms of sinus node recovery time or the time required for repeat sinus node activation after prolonged overdrive suppression of the node by pacing the atria at rates of 100 to 175 bpm. Normal values of sinus node recovery times are usually less than 1,500 ms. The corrected sinus node recovery time provides a more accurate description of sinus node "normalcy." This is calculated by subtracting the baseline sinus rate from the sinus node recovery time. Normal values of the corrected sinus node recovery time are typically < 550 to 600 ms. Because of sinus node automaticity, it is significantly more difficult to assess recovery times from overdrive suppression of AV nodal or junctional tissue. Nevertheless, in the absence of a functioning sinus node or after the creation of AV conduction system block, lower-level pacemakers can emerge, at the above-mentioned rates.

Abnormal Rhythm Generation

Abnormal Automaticity
Abnormal automaticity may create impulse formation in regions other than the sinus node. Such automaticity may occur in ischemic or other diseased cardiac tissues. Spontaneous depolarization of affected cardiac fibers occurs, particularly when atrial or ventricular resting membrane potentials are reduced to values less than -60 mV. Abnormal atrial automatic rhythms typically arise from the region of the crista terminalis, around pulmonary veins, or in the pericoronary sinus orifice region. Some ventricular tachycardias, which also may be automatic in mechanism, are usually catecholamine-dependent.

Triggered Automaticity
An additional mechanism of abnormal arrhythmia generation is that of triggered automaticity. This term is used to describe arrhythmias originating from afterdepolarizations or oscillatory afterpotentials occurring during diastole which reach threshold and generate subsequent action potentials. These afterdepolarizations are typically dependent on prior activation of the heart and can be further classified as early afterdepolarizations if they occur during phase 2 or 3 of the action potential or as delayed afterdepolarizations if they occur after complete repolarization. The early afterdepolarizations are typically pause-dependent. Such a pause may be set up by a prior premature depolarization. Early afterdepolarizations are facilitated by low potassium level, low magnesium level, or potassium channel block with agents such as quinidine, N-acetylprocainamide, sotalol, or other class I or III antiarrhythmic agents (Table 2). Various other drugs may similarly prolong the action potential duration by modulation of constituent ionic currents. Some of these include erythromycin, pentamidine, and terfenadine. Early afterdepolarizations are probably responsible for torsades de pointes, which is polymorphic ventricular tachycardia with QRS morphologies that appear to twist around an isoelectric baseline, occurring in the setting of a prolonged QT interval. Similar

Table 2.—Factors That Influence Early Afterdepolarization

	Increase	Decrease
Autonomic	↑ sympathetic tone	↓ sympathetic tone
	↑ catecholamines	↓ catecholamines
	↓ parasympathetic tone	↑ parasympathetic tone
Metabolic	↑ hypoxia	↑ O_2
	↑ acidosis	↓ acidosis
Electrolytes	C_s^+	K^+
	Hypokalemia	Mg^{2+}
Drugs and metabolites	Sotalol	Acetylcholine/ adenosine
	N-acetylprocainamide	Lidocaine
	Quinidine	Procainamide
	Aconitine	Ca^{2+} channel blockers
	Veratridine	β-Blockers
		Tetrodotoxin
		K^+ channel openers
Heart rate	Slow	Fast

From Giuliani ER, Gersh BJ, McGoon MD, Hayes DL, Schaff HV (editors): *Mayo Clinic Practice of Cardiology*. Third edition. Mosby, 1996, p 738. By permission of Mayo Foundation.

abnormalities may occur in patients with the congenital long QT syndromes.

In contrast, delayed afterdepolarizations, which occur during phase 4 of diastole, are more likely to occur after rapid, repetitive pacing. These are thought to be related to accumulation of intracellular calcium and activation of a nonspecific cation channel. The most common cause of the delayed afterdepolarization type of arrhythmia is digitalis toxicity. With digitalis, the sodium-potassium pump is inhibited, producing an increase in intracellular sodium and subsequent acceleration of sodium for calcium exchange. Both abnormal atrial and ventricular arrhythmias may have triggered automaticity as an underlying mechanism. A potential clue to the presence of such a mechanism is the termination of arrhythmias with calcium channel blockers or adenosine, although reentrant arrhythmias under certain circumstances may be interrupted by these agents.

- Early afterdepolarizations are probably responsible for torsades de pointes.
- The most common cause of the delayed afterdepolarization type of arrhythmia is digitalis toxicity.

Arrhythmias Related to Abnormal Impulse Conduction

AV Conduction

Electrical impulse propagation through atrial, ventricular, or specialized tissues occurs with each cardiac activation. Purkinje tissue may have conduction velocities of 1 to 3 m/s, but conduction velocity in atrial or ventricular tissue is significantly slower, about 0.3 m/s. On the scale of the intact heart, conduction through the atrium can be expressed as the PA interval, taken as the onset of the surface P wave to the activation of the atrial tissue in the region of the AV node, as recorded on the His bundle electrogram. The normal PA interval is 20 to 50 ms.

In addition, conduction through the AV node is reflected by the AH interval, or the point of earliest rapid upstroke of the atrial deflection on the His bundle electrogram to the similar rapid onset of the deflection recorded from the His bundle. Under normal conditions, the AH interval ranges between 60 and 120 ms. In some patients, enhanced AV nodal physiology may be observed, in which the AH interval may be less than 60 ms, prolongation of the AH interval which typically occurs with faster pacing is limited, and propagation via the AV node persists with atrial pacing rates in excess of 200 bpm (Fig. 8).

Conduction through the His-Purkinje system is reflected in the HV interval, which is taken as the onset of the His bundle deflection to the onset of the ventricular deflection recorded on the His bundle electrogram or the onset of the QRS. Normal HV intervals range between 35 and 60 ms. In patients with diseased His-Purkinje conduction, HV intervals are longer than 60 ms. The exact implication of HV intervals in the range of 60 to 80 ms is unclear. In patients with syncope, bifascicular conduction block on the surface electrocardiogram, and an HV interval longer than 70 ms, infra-His block is the likely cause of the syncopal episode. AV block below the His bundle during rapid atrial pacing also suggests significant conduction system disease, which should be treated with permanent ventricular pacing.

In 0.1% of patients, normal activation of the ventricles via the AV conduction system can be short-circuited. This may result from the presence of an accessory pathway that bridges atrial and ventricular tissue. Because a portion of the ventricle may be activated before the onset of activation of the His-Purkinje system, ventricular tissue is said to be preexcited. This phenomenon is accompanied by the appearance of slurred upstrokes of surface QRS complexes (delta waves) and a very short or negative HV interval.

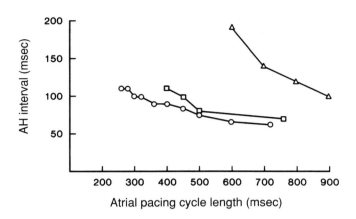

Fig. 8. Response of atrioventricular (AV) node to atrial pacing. Most common response is a gradual increase in the AH interval and then AV node block at less than 200 beats/min. This is seen in patient □, in whom the resting AH is 70 ms at 80 bpm and increases to 110 ms at 150 bpm and then AV node Wenckebach periodicity. Patient ○ had accelerated AV node conduction with an initial AH of 60 ms, which increased to 110 ms with atrial pacing at 250 bpm (240 ms). Patient △ had abnormal AV node conduction and an initial AH of 100 ms, which increased to 190 ms with pacing at 100 bpm (600 ms). AV node Wenckebach periodicity then developed. (From Giuliani ER, Gersh BJ, McGoon MD, Hayes DL, Schaff HV [editors]: *Mayo Clinic Practice of Cardiology*. Third edition. Mosby, 1996, p 832. By permission of Mayo Foundation.)

- Conduction through the atrium can be expressed as the PA interval.
- The normal PA interval is 20 to 50 ms.
- Conduction through the AV node is reflected by the AH interval.
- Under normal conditions, the AH interval ranges between 60 and 120 ms.
- Conduction through the His-Purkinje system is reflected in the HV interval.
- Normal HV intervals range between 35 and 60 ms.

Reentry Arrhythmias

Conduction abnormalities in cardiac tissue may contribute to reentrant arrhythmias. The mechanisms of reentry involve three requisite conditions: 1) at least two functionally distinct conducting pathways, 2) unidirectional block in one pathway, and 3) slower conduction down a second conduction pathway, with return via the second pathway (Fig. 9). Initially, these mechanisms of reentry were observed in the setting of an anatomical obstacle around which a circulating impulse could propagate. Subsequent studies have clearly demonstrated that reentry also may occur in the absence of such an obstacle, strictly because of the properties of conduction and refractoriness in atrial or ventricular tissue. One form of

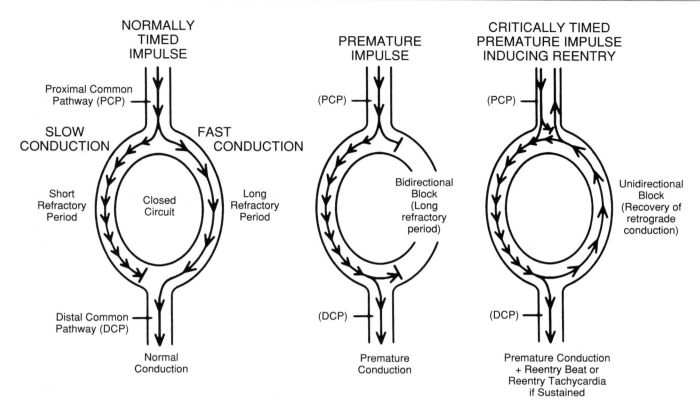

Fig. 9. Description of a reentrant circuit as a mechanism in initiating and sustaining tachycardia. (From Giuliani ER, Gersh BJ, McGoon MD, Hayes DL, Schaff HV [editors]: *Mayo Clinic Practice of Cardiology*. Third edition. Mosby, 1996, p 781. By permission of Mayo Foundation.)

such reentry is referred to as "functional." In this type of reentry, a circulating impulse travels around an area of tissue rendered refractory by centripetal activation of the center of circuit. Although the anatomical obstacle form of reentry may be more likely to occur in the presence of atrial flutter or ventricular tachycardia in patients with islands of infarcted myocardium, functional reentry is undoubtedly operative in other forms of atypical atrial flutter or atrial fibrillation.

For understanding of the reentrant arrhythmias, it is often useful to consider the wavelength of a tachycardia, which is the minimal tachycardia circuit length that is necessary for the perpetuation of a reentrant arrhythmia, given the electrical properties of that circuit. The wavelength is the product of the functional refractory period and the conduction velocity. If conduction velocity is slowed or refractoriness is decreased, the minimal potential circuit length is similarly decreased, leading to an increased likelihood of an arrhythmia. However, when tissue refractoriness is significantly prolonged, as may be the case with an antiarrhythmic drug, the wavelength needed to perpetuate a reentrant arrhythmia may increase. If the available circuits are of only limited size, that increase in refractoriness could

produce a favorable elimination of the reentrant arrhythmia. In the case of atrial fibrillation, such an increase in refractoriness due to a drug results in the need for progressively larger tissue circuits for perpetuation of arrhythmia. Because the atria are of finite size in patients with atrial fibrillation, the five to seven circulating wavelets that typically comprise atrial fibrillation increase in size and undergo coalescence to progressively fewer circuits and subsequent elimination of atrial fibrillation.

The mechanisms of reentry involve three requisite conditions:

- At least two functionally distinct conducting pathways.
- Unidirectional block in one pathway.
- Slower conduction down a second conduction pathway.

Arrhythmias Associated With Preexcitation

Orthodromic Reciprocating Tachycardia

An additional form of macro-reentry is that of orthodromic reciprocating tachycardia in patients with accessory pathways. In these patients, an electrical impulse propagates down the normal AV conduction system, inscribing a normal QRS complex on a surface electrocardiogram during tachycardia. The electrical impulse then propagates to an accessory pathway bridging between ventricular and atrial tissue, leading to retrograde atrial activation via the pathway (Fig. 10A). If the accessory pathway is well removed from the region of the interventricular or atrial septum, atrial activation as recorded on catheters positioned along the free-wall regions of the AV groove may show earlier atrial activation than that present in the septum. This is clearly distinctive from retrograde atrial activation via the normal VA conduction system. With return of the electrical impulse through the atria back down the normal AV conduction system, the cycle repeats itself.

Antidromic Tachycardia

In some patients, the pattern of excitation may reverse, yielding an "antidromic tachycardia" (Fig. 10B). In such patients, activation of the ventricle proceeds via the accessory pathway, inscribing a maximally preexcited QRS complex on the surface electrocardiogram during tachycardia. Subsequent activation of the atria occurs via the normal VA conduction system, yielding activation of the atria in the center of the atrial septum and subsequent reactivation of the ventricles via the accessory pathway.

Dual AV Nodal Physiology

Some patients with dual AV nodal physiology may have AV nodal reentrant tachycardia. These patients may be viewed conceptually as having dual AV nodal pathways in which the electrical impulses activating the ventricle proceed via a fast pathway with a long refractory period or via a slow pathway with shorter refractoriness. In these patients, an atrial premature complex may produce block in the fast pathway, resulting in delayed AV nodal propagation through the "slow" pathway. If this conduction is sufficiently slow to allow recovery of the fast pathway, retrograde return activation via the fast structure may lead to repeat atrial activation and subsequent conduction through the slow AV nodal pathway. Because an electrical impulse conducts through the His-Purkinje system into the ventricles with each circulating impulse, a tachycardia with a narrow QRS complex is observed.

Ventricular Tachycardia

In a similar but more microscopic fashion, ventricular tachycardia may occur in patients with diseased ventricular myocardium, such as that caused by a prior myocardial infarction. In these patients, the islands of infarcted tissue surrounded by some strands of continuing functional tissue may provide the requisite two or more potential conduction

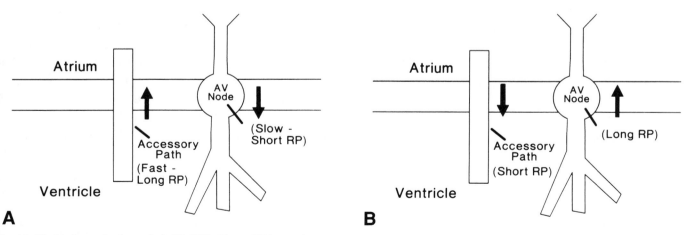

Fig. 10. Mechanisms of tachycardia in Wolff-Parkinson-White syndrome. *A*, Reciprocating tachycardia (also called orthodromic tachycardia). This is the most common mechanism of tachycardia observed in Wolff-Parkinson-White syndrome. In this form, tachycardia is often initiated by a premature atrial beat that blocks in the accessory pathway and then is conducted antegrade down the atrioventricular (AV) node. The impulse then is conducted retrograde to the atrium over the accessory pathway and returns to the ventricle over the AV node. In this manner, a reciprocating tachycardia is sustained. Unless functional bundle branch block is present, the QRS complex will be narrow, going to its antegrade conduction down normal AV conduction tissues. *B*, More unusual form of reciprocating tachycardia (sometimes called antidromic tachycardia) observed in Wolff-Parkinson-White syndrome in which the antegrade limb of the reentry circuit is the accessory pathway and the retrograde limb is the AV node. In this circumstance, the QRS complex is wide. RP, refractory period. (From Giuliani ER, Gersh BJ, McGoon MD, Hayes DL, Schaff HV [editors]: *Mayo Clinic Practice of Cardiology*. Third edition. Mosby, 1996, p 772. By permission of Mayo Foundation.)

pathways. With a ventricular premature complex, block may occur in one pathway, with subsequent propagation occurring via a second conducting pathway. If this conduction is sufficiently slow, the impulse may return via the first pathway, leading to completion of the reentrant circuit.

- Orthodromic reciprocating tachycardia occurs when an electrical impulse propagates down the normal AV conduction system, inscribing a normal QRS complex on a surface electrocardiogram during tachycardia.

- Antidromic tachycardia occurs when activation of the ventricle proceeds via the accessory pathway, inscribing a maximally preexcited QRS complex on the surface electrocardiogram during tachycardia.

Questions

Multiple Choice (choose the one best answer)

1. All of the following statements regarding the atrioventricular node are true *except*:
   a. Conduction through the node displays decremental behavior
   b. It is positioned in the subendocardium at the base of the triangle of Koch
   c. It is composed of nodal cells and transitional cells
   d. It is a right atrial structure

2. In which of the following tissues is the upstroke of the action potential generated by ingoing calcium currents?
   a. Atrial
   b. Atrioventricular nodal
   c. His-Purkinje
   d. Ventricular

3. Conduction velocity is most rapid in:
   a. Atrial tissue
   b. Atrioventricular nodal tissue
   c. His-Purkinje tissue
   d. Ventricular tissue

4. Repolarization of myocardial cells is determined mostly by:
   a. Outgoing sodium current
   b. Ingoing calcium current
   c. Outgoing potassium current
   d. Ingoing chloride current

5. All of the following statements regarding atrioventricular nodal cells are true *except*:
   a. The resting membrane potential is typically -80 to -90 mV
   b. The activation threshold ranges between -30 and -40 mV
   c. The upstroke of the action potential is carried by the inward calcium current
   d. Conduction in the atrioventricular node proceeds at a velocity of 0.01 to 0.1 m/s

6. Vagal stimulation in each of the following tissue types changes the action potential duration *except* in the:
   a. Atrioventricular node
   b. His-Purkinje system
   c. Ventricular myocardium
   d. Atrial myocardium

7. Early afterdepolarizations are favored by:
   a. High potassium concentrations
   b. Type III antiarrhythmic drugs
   c. Fast underlying heart rates
   d. Increased magnesium concentrations

8. The underlying arrhythmia mechanism most likely present in digitalis toxicity is:
   a. Reentry
   b. Delayed afterdepolarizations
   c. Enhanced automaticity
   d. Early afterdepolarizations

9. A normal HV interval is:
   a. 25 to 50 ms
   b. 35 to 60 ms
   c. 50 to 80 ms
   d. 60 to 100 ms

10. Patients with the Wolff-Parkinson-White syndrome typically show each of the following features *except*:
    a. A wide QRS complex during normal sinus rhythm
    b. A narrow complex supraventricular tachycardia
    c. A delta wave on the surface QRS
    d. A normal HV interval on the His-bundle recording

11. Prerequisite conditions for a reentrant arrhythmia include all of the following *except*:
    a. Two functionally distinct conducting pathways
    b. An anatomical obstacle around which the impulse reenters
    c. Unidirectional block in one pathway
    d. Slow conduction via one pathway with return via the second

12. Atrial fibrillation is most often caused by:
    a. Three or four repetitively firing automatic or triggered foci
    b. Reentry around multiple anatomical obstacles
    c. Four to seven circulating wavelets of functional reentry
    d. A combination of early and delayed afterdepolarizations

13. Antidromic reciprocating tachycardia in a patient with Wolff-Parkinson-White syndrome refers to:
    a. Atrioventricular conduction proceeding via the normal atrioventricular conduction system with return via the accessory pathway
    b. Atrioventricular conduction via the accessory pathway with return via the normal ventriculoatrial conduction system
    c. Atrioventricular nodal reentrant tachycardia with additional conduction via the accessory pathway
    d. None of the above

14. Patients with atrioventricular nodal reentrant tachycardia usually have:
    a. Dual atrioventricular nodal physiology
    b. A concealed accessory pathway
    c. Retrograde atrial activation spreading from the free wall of the atrioventricular groove to the septum
    d. A wide QRS complex during tachycardia

15. The most common mechanism of arrhythmias in sustained ventricular tachycardia is:
    a. Sympathetically facilitated enhanced automaticity
    b. Reentry involving ventricular myocardium
    c. Triggered automaticity arising from early afterdepolarizations
    d. Reflection of propagated impulses

Answers

1. Answer b

The atrioventricular node is positioned in the low right atrium at the apex of the triangle of Koch (ostium of the coronary sinus, tendon of Todaro, and septal attachment of tricuspid valve leaflet). It is composed of nodal and transitional cells.

2. Answer b

The sinoatrial and atrioventricular nodal cells are activated via slow inward calcium-carrying currents, in contrast to atrial, ventricular, and His-Purkinje cells, which are activated by the inward sodium current.

3. Answer c

Conduction velocity is most rapid in His-Purkinje tissue.

4. Answer c

The outgoing potassium current is the principal determinant of repolarization of myocardial cells.

5. Answer a

The resting membrane potential of atrioventricular nodal cells is -40 to -70 mV.

6. Answer c

Vagal stimulation has little effect on the ventricular myocardial action potential, increases it in the atrioventricular node, and reduces it in the atrial myocardium.

7. Answer b

Early afterdepolarizations are facilitated by a low potassium level, low magnesium level, and class I or III antiarrhythmic drugs and are typically pause-dependent.

8. Answer b

Delayed afterdepolarizations are characteristic of digitalis toxicity.

9. Answer b

The normal HV interval is 35 to 60 ms.

10. Answer d

The HV interval in Wolff-Parkinson-White syndrome is either negative or very short.

11. Answer b

Anatomical block is not necessary for a reentrant arrhythmia.

12. Answer c

Atrial fibrillation typically is associated with four to seven circulating wavelets of functional reentry, although reentry around fixed anatomical obstacles undoubtedly plays a role. Single or multiple repetitively firing foci can lead to atrial fibrillation, but this is a less common mechanism than reentry.

13. Answer b

Antidromic reciprocating tachycardia in a patient with Wolff-Parkinson-White syndrome is atrioventricular conduction via the accessory pathway with return via the normal ventriculoatrial conduction system.

14. Answer a

Patients with atrioventricular nodal reentrant tachycardia usually have dual nodal physiology.

15. Answer b

The most common mechanism of arrhythmias in sustained ventricular tachycardia is reentry involving ventricular myocardium.

Notes

Chapter 44

Atlas of Electrophysiology Tracings

Douglas L. Packer, M.D.

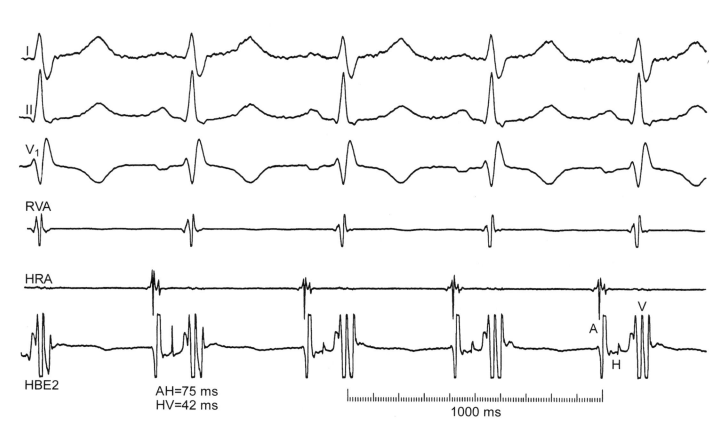

Fig. 1. *Normal sinus rhythm with normal conduction intervals*. Despite the presence of right bundle branch block, the AH interval of 75 ms and HV interval of 42 ms shown on the electrogram labeled HBE2 are normal. The AH interval is measured from the first discrete, rapid atrial deflection to the first deflection of the His bundle. The HV interval is taken from the first discrete, rapid His deflection to the onset of the surface QRS or ventricular deflection on the HBE2 channel, as indicated by the straight line. HBE, His bundle electrogram; HRA, high right atrium; RVA, right ventricular apex.

713

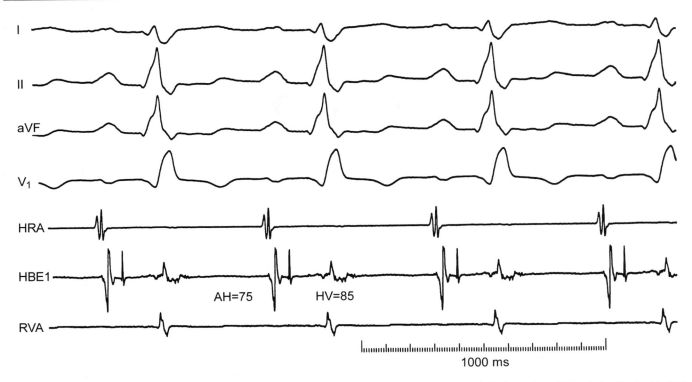

Fig. 2. *Normal sinus rhythm with infra-His conduction delay*. Here, the HV interval is grossly prolonged. In the setting of bifascicular block, this finding is accompanied by a 12% risk of progression to complete heart block. The HV interval is 85 ms in duration. A normal HV interval is less than 60 ms. See Figure 1 for explanation of abbreviations.

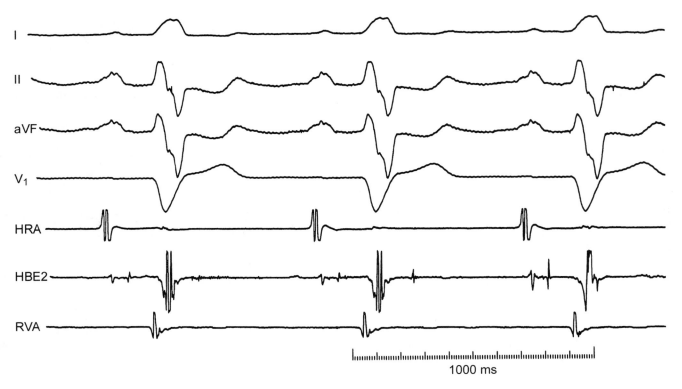

Fig. 3. *Normal sinus rhythm with left bundle branch block QRS morphology (negative deflection in V₁ lead) and a prolonged HV interval*. The infra-His conduction time is grossly prolonged at 100 ms. In a patient with a history of syncope, this interval would be a sufficient indication for pacemaker implantation. See Figure 1 for explanation of abbreviations.

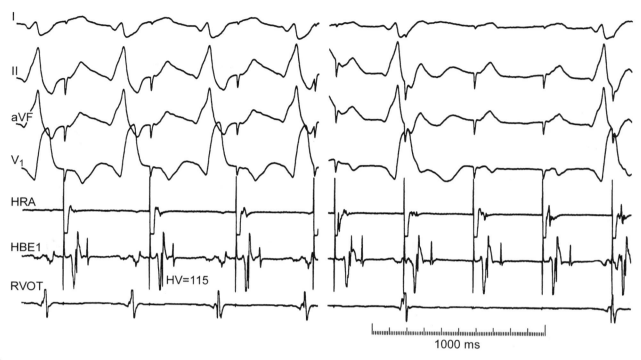

Fig. 4. *Atrial pacing with infra-His block.* The left panel shows atrial pacing (note sharp pacing spikes) at a rate of 100 bpm. The HV interval is 115 ms. The right panel shows faster pacing at 150 bpm, which produced infra-His block (after the sharp His spike on the HBE1 tracing). Only two ventricular complexes are seen on the right ventricular outflow tract (RVOT) tracing. See Figure 1 for explanation of other abbreviations.

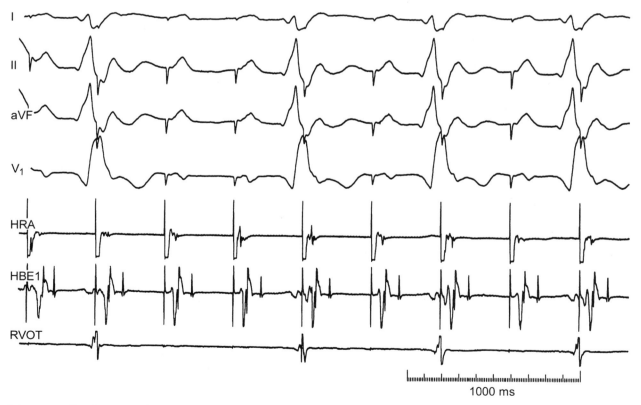

Fig. 5. *Longer recording during atrial pacing demonstrating block within or below the His bundle.* With atrial pacing at a rate of 150 bpm, recurrent conduction interruption at a level within or below the His bundle is noted. This is a type 1 indication for pacemaker implantation. Note that only four ventricular complexes are seen on the right ventricular outflow tract (RVOT) tracing. See Figure 1 for explanation of other abbreviations.

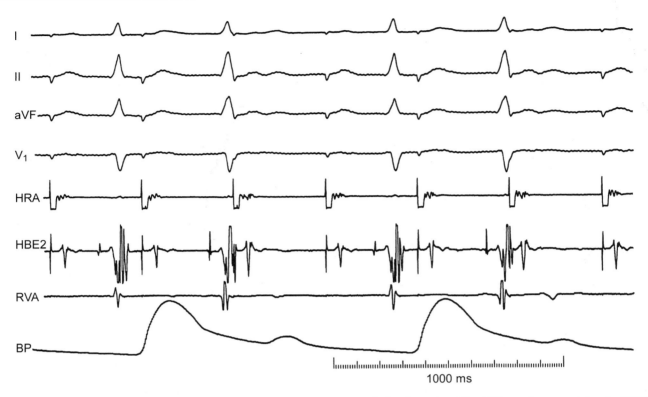

Fig. 6. *Atrial pacing with Wenckebach block in the atrioventricular node.* Note the gradual prolongation of the AH interval, as recorded on the HBE2 electrogram during atrial pacing at a rate of 150 bpm. BP, blood pressure. See Figure 1 for explanation of other abbreviations.

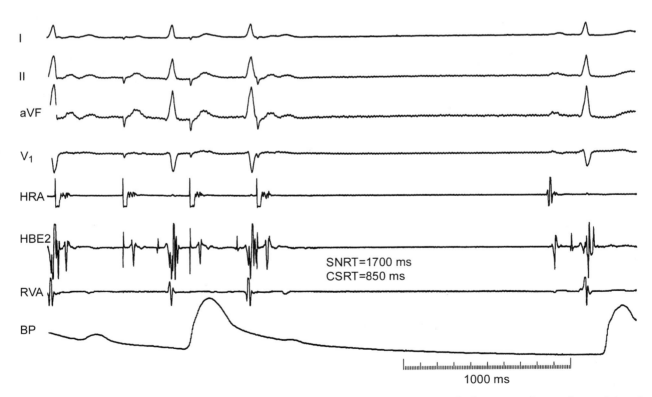

Fig. 7. *Abnormal sinus node recovery time (SNRT) after atrial pacing (150 bpm).* Here, 1,700 ms was required to generate the next sinus node impulse. The corrected sinus node recovery time (CSRT), which equals the SNRT - sinus cycle length, also was prolonged at 850. A value more than 600 is abnormal. BP, blood pressure. See Figure 1 for explanation of other abbreviations.

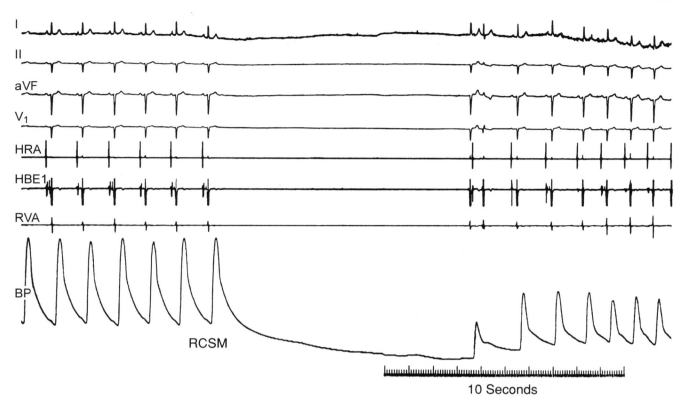

Fig. 8. *Response to right carotid sinus massage (RCSM) in the setting of carotid sinus hypersensitivity.* Note the 10-s pause precipitated by RCSM. BP, blood pressure. See Figure 1 for explanation of other abbreviations.

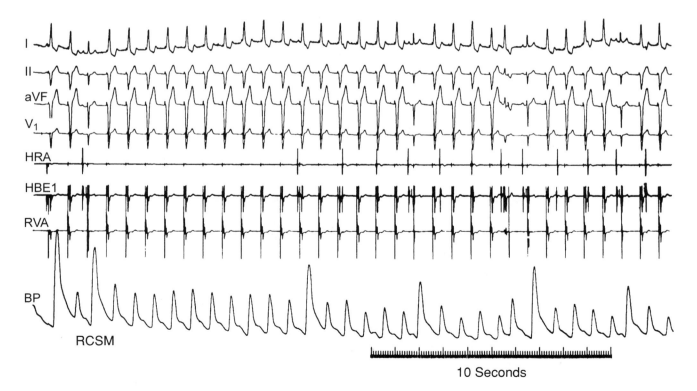

Fig. 9. *Partial recovery of blood pressure (BP) with ventricular pacing during right carotid sinus massage (RCSM).* Note the absence of atrial activity on the high right atrium (HRA) channel in the left half of the figure. BP recovers to a less than normal value during ventricular pacing. This suggests the presence of both cardioinhibitory and vasodepressor components of the carotid hypersensitivity. See Figure 1 for explanation of other abbreviations.

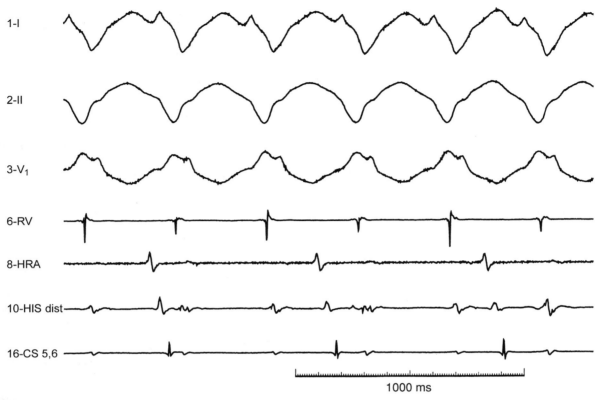

Fig. 10. *Wide complex tachycardia with right bundle branch block morphology.* Note the presence of a ventricular deflection on the right ventricular (RV) channel accompanying each QRS complex. In contrast, the presence of ventriculoatrial dissociation is indicated by the presence of only three atrial deflections on the high right atrium (HRA) or coronary sinus (CS) 5,6 tracings. This is consistent with the diagnosis of ventricular tachycardia. dist, distal electrode.

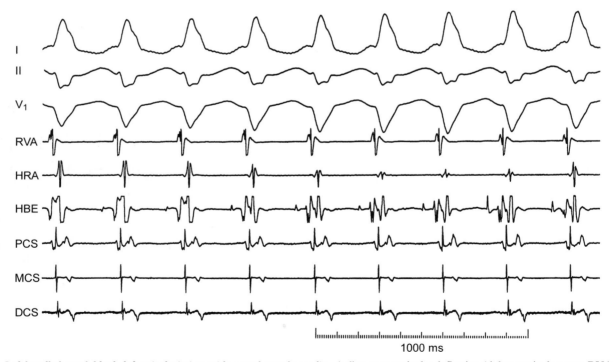

Fig. 11. *Left bundle branch block, left-axis deviation, wide complex tachycardia.* A discrete ventricular deflection (right ventricular apex, RVA, channel) is seen with each QRS complex. There is also an atrial deflection on the high right atrium (HRA) channel indicating a 1:1 atrioventricular relationship. Each ventricular deflection on the His-bundle electrogram (HBE) channel, however, shows a discrete high-frequency His-bundle deflection, indicating that this is a supraventricular tachycardia. DCS, distal coronary sinus; MCS, mid-coronary sinus; PCS, proximal coronary sinus.

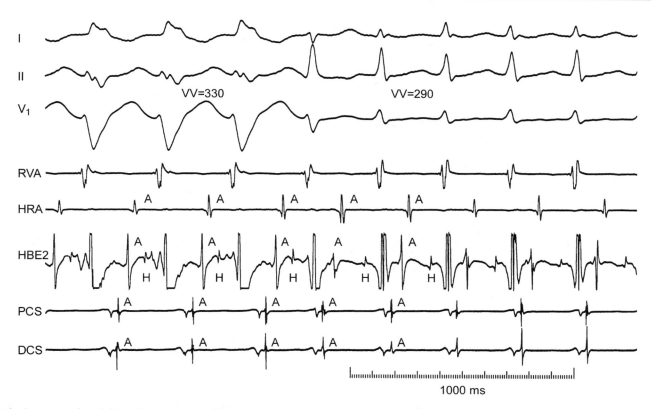

Fig. 12. *Conversion from left bundle branch block during atrioventricular reentrant tachycardia to normal QRS morphology tachycardia* in a patient with a left freewall accessory pathway. Importantly, the VV intervals shorten from 330 to 290 ms with the loss of bundle branch aberrancy. This is diagnostic for a freewall accessory pathway on the same side as the bundle branch block. The atrial and ventricular deflections are clearly marked. DCS, distal coronary sinus; PCS, proximal coronary sinus. See Figure 1 for explanation of other abbreviations.

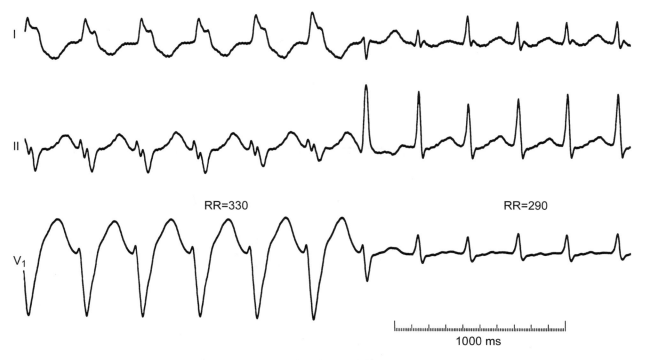

Fig. 13. *Surface electrocardiogram demonstrating conversion of left bundle branch block aberrancy during atrioventricular reentrant tachycardia to a normal QRS tachycardia.* The RR interval of 330 ms during the left bundle branch block aberrant supraventricular tachycardia is longer than that during the narrow QRS complex. This provides sufficient information for making the diagnosis of a left freewall accessory pathway-mediated tachycardia.

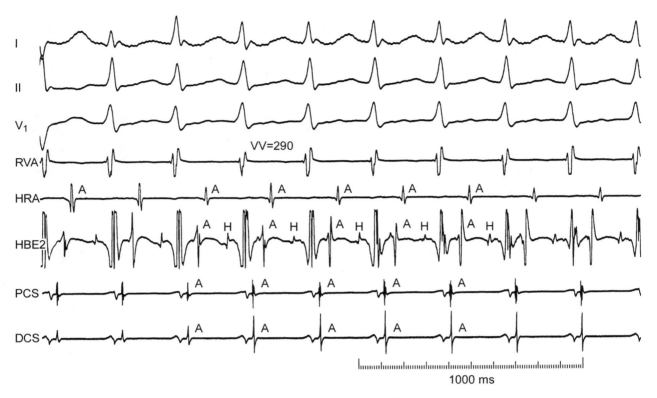

Fig. 14. *Atrioventricular reentrant tachycardia using a left freewall accessory pathway.* Note that the earliest retrograde atrial activation on the proximal (PCS) and distal (DCS) coronary sinus channels occurs before the atrial deflection on the His-bundle electrogram (HBE2) or high right atrium (HRA) channels. The distance from the onset of the surface QRS to the earliest retrograde atrial deflection is 75 ms, which is also consistent with this diagnosis. RVA, right ventricular apex.

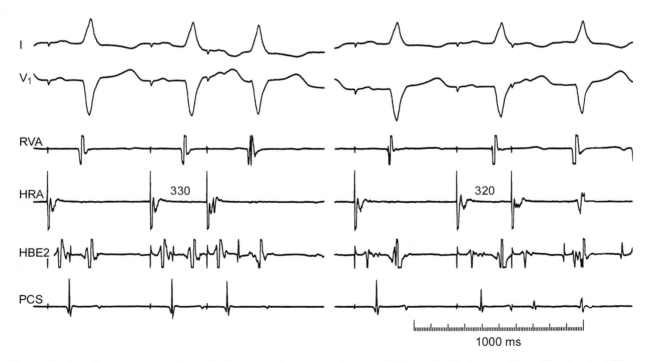

Fig. 15. *Introduction of a premature atrial complex during atrial pacing.* It is introduced 330 ms after the last paced beat. Note that the AH interval generated is relatively short at 130 ms. The right panel shows a premature atrial complex introduced 10 ms earlier, at 320 ms after the last paced atrial beat. Note the significant prolongation of the AH interval out to 230 ms. PCS, proximal coronary sinus. See Figure 1 for explanation of other abbreviations.

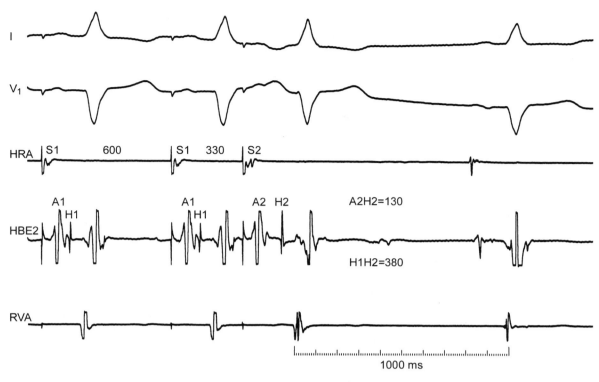

Fig. 16. *Expanded view of the impact of the timing of a premature atrial complex on the A2H2 interval.* The interval is 130 ms. In this patient with dual atrioventricular nodal physiology and atrioventricular nodal reentrant tachycardia, the impulse is proceeding down the fast pathway. See Figure 1 for explanation of abbreviations.

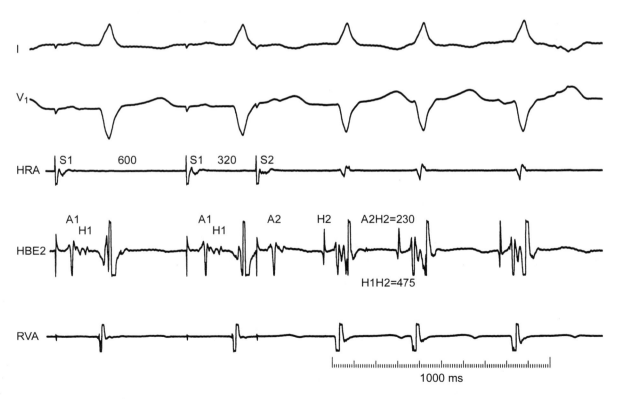

Fig. 17. *Jump in the A2H2 interval with introduction of a premature atrial complex.* A 10-ms decrease in the S1S2 coupling interval to 320 ms results in a dramatic prolongation of the A2H2 interval to 230 ms. This indicates that the premature atrial complex produced block in the fast pathway but conducted to the ventricle via the slow pathway. Note also the onset of atrioventricular nodal reentrant tachycardia. See Figure 1 for explanation of abbreviations.

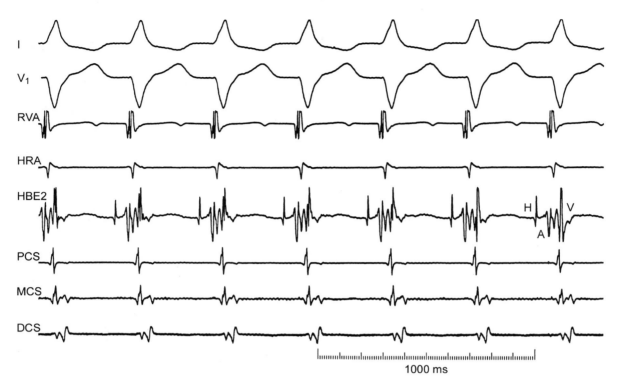

Fig. 18. *Intracardiac tracings of atrioventricular nodal reentrant tachycardia.* The QRS complex is narrow, and atrial deflections are seen with each QRS complex. This 1:1 atrioventricular relationship, with a sharp His-bundle deflection preceding the surface QRS, is consistent with a supraventricular tachycardia dependent on atrioventricular nodal conduction. The final complex shows the His-bundle deflection followed by a surface QRS complex and a normal HV interval. The retrograde atrial deflection, however, times with the onset of the surface QRS, giving a ventriculoatrial interval of zero. Usually, this interval is 10 to 55 ms. In this case, it took an equal amount of time for the reentrant impulse to return back to the atrium as it did for one to proceed down the His-Purkinje system to yield a QRS complex. DCS, distal coronary sinus; MCS, mid-coronary sinus; PCS, proximal coronary sinus. See Figure 1 for explanation of other abbreviations.

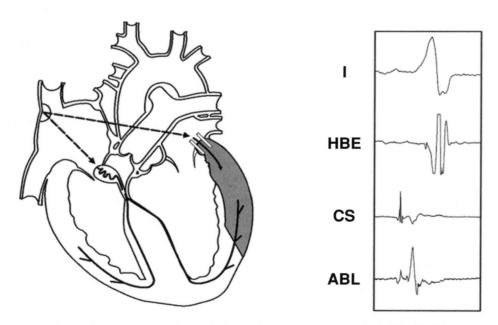

Fig. 19. *Ventricular preexcitation via an accessory pathway.* A characteristic delta wave is seen in limb lead I. This occurs well before the first sharp, discrete deflection on the His-bundle electrogram (HBE) channel, which is the "His deflection." An ablation catheter (ABL) placed near the accessory pathway shows that the local ventricular deflection actually occurs before the onset of the surface QRS. A line is drawn to reflect the timing from the onset of the surface QRS. Note that much of the ventricular deflection on the ablation (ABL) lead and a small Kent potential occur before the onset of the surface lead. The His-bundle spike on the HBE lead, however, is well after the onset of the surface QRS. CS, coronary sinus.

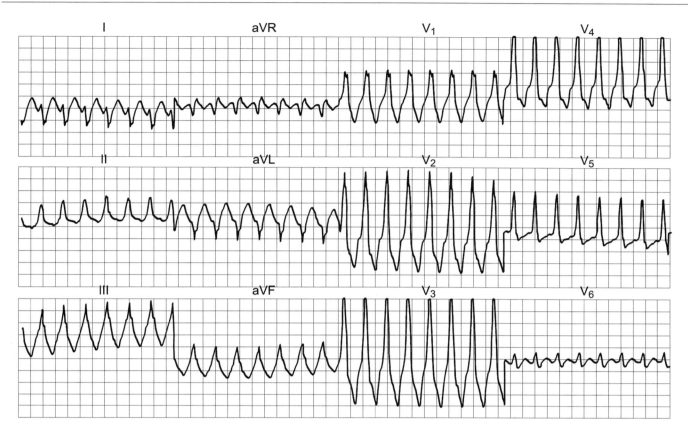

Fig. 20. *Electrocardiograms show antidromic reciprocating tachycardia.* Ventricular activation is via the accessory pathway. As a result, all of the QRS complexes show maximal preexcitation, with characteristic delta waves. Retrograde atrial activation occurs via the atrioventricular node.

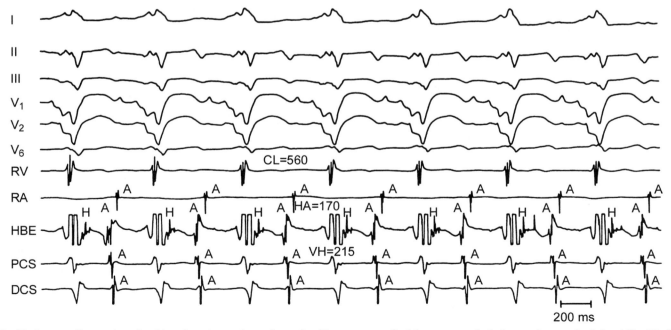

Fig. 21. *Intracardiac tracing of antidromic reciprocating tachycardia.* Note presence of a delta wave, particularly prominent on leads I and V_1. The His-bundle deflection occurs well after the local ventricular activation on the HBE lead. This is followed by retrograde atrial activation via the atrioventricular conduction system. Note that the atrial deflection (A) on the HBE channel precedes any of the other atrial depolarizations. DCS, distal coronary sinus; HBE, His-bundle electrogram; PCS, proximal coronary sinus; RA, right atrium; RV, right ventricle.

Notes

Chapter 45

Noncardiac Surgery in Patients With Heart Disease

André C. Lapeyre III, M.D.
Clarence Shub, M.D.

The American College of Cardiology and the American Heart Association (ACC/AHA) have published guidelines for the perioperative evaluation and management of patients with heart disease who are to have noncardiac operations. The guidelines recommend a conservative approach. Expensive testing, invasive strategies, and revascularization are rarely, if ever, warranted just to "get the patient through an operation." Rather, the indications for extensive perioperative testing or revascularization are generally similar to those in a nonoperative setting.

- Testing or revascularization is *not* indicated just to "get the patient through an operation."

Impact of Coronary Artery Disease

The risk of a perioperative myocardial infarction in patients without clinical evidence of heart disease is approximately 0.15%. In patients with clinical heart disease, the risk of a perioperative myocardial infarction can be stratified according to the cardiovascular profile of the patient (major, intermediate, minor, or no clinical predictors of increased risk) and according to the cardiac stress of the operation (high, medium, or low stress or risk).

- Patients without clinical evidence of heart disease are at low risk (about 0.15%) of perioperative myocardial infarction.

The rate of mortality in association with perioperative myocardial infarction is significantly higher than that with an infarct unrelated to operation. Previously, the significance of perioperative myocardial infarction was less well recognized and the antemortem diagnosis was more difficult. Increased awareness of the problem, better patient selection, improved anesthetic and operative techniques, improved perioperative monitoring and management, and improved diagnostic techniques (including the newer enzymatic tests) have all contributed to a significant reduction in mortality from perioperative myocardial infarction.

The risk of perioperative reinfarction is highest in the first 6 months after an index myocardial infarction. This risk decreases with increasing time between the index infarction and the planned operation. According to the ACC/AHA guidelines, an elective surgical procedure can be performed before the 6 months has elapsed as long as the patient underwent postinfarction risk stratification. Absence of postinfarction ischemia, a negative postinfarction stress test, and complete myocardial revascularization after infarction suggest a reduced risk of reinfarction with an elective operation. The ACC/AHA guidelines still suggest that it is prudent to wait at least 4 to 6 weeks before proceeding with an elective operation.

- Risk of perioperative reinfarction varies inversely with the time between the index infarction and the operation.
- Patients with negative postinfarction risk stratification or complete postinfarction myocardial revascularization

can proceed with elective operation at 4 to 6 weeks after infarction.

The risk of perioperative reinfarction is *not* significantly different between patients who have had a Q-wave infarction and those who have had a non–Q-wave infarction.

- Recent Q-wave and non–Q-wave myocardial infarctions are associated with the same risk of perioperative reinfarction.

Preoperative Cardiac Risk Indices

Risk factors in patients undergoing noncardiac operation include 1) the type of operation (intrathoracic and intra-abdominal procedures have a higher risk than limb operations); 2) the presence and severity of coronary artery disease, especially if unstable (heart failure or unstable angina); 3) status of left ventricular function (ejection fraction); 4) age of patient; 5) severe valvular heart disease, especially aortic stenosis; 6) serious cardiac arrhythmias; 7) associated medical conditions, for example, chronic obstructive pulmonary disease, hypoxemia, diabetes mellitus, and renal insufficiency; and 8) overall functional status.

The benefit of using a risk factor approach to cardiac risk estimation was first demonstrated by Goldman et al. and later modified by Detsky et al. By multivariate analysis of 39 variables in 1,001 patients, 9 variables were statistically significant and had independent predictive value for perioperative cardiac events. A point score was derived statistically, and a cardiac risk index calculated (Table 1). The cardiac risk index is strongly predictive of perioperative risk (Table 2).

Perioperative risks can be stratified further into major-, intermediate-, and low- (minor) risk categories (Table 3). Active conditions are more important than dormant ones, and the degree of abnormality is also important. The presence of major risk predictors warrants further evaluation and (usually) treatment that may delay or cancel the elective operation. The urgency of a noncardiac operation may dictate patient management. Thus, a patient with a recent myocardial infarction and an acute abdominal crisis generally requires laparotomy without delay. The presence of intermediate predictors of increased perioperative risk warrants careful clinical assessment and, when appropriate, use of additional cardiac testing. Minor predictors have

Table 1.--Preoperative Cardiac Risk Index, Derived by Goldman and Colleagues

Variable	Point score
History	
Age > 70 yr	5
Preoperative myocardial infarction	
within preceding 6 mo	10
Physical examination	
S_3 gallop or elevated JVP (> 12 cm H_2O)	11
Significant valvular aortic stenosis	3
Electrocardiogram	
Rhythm other than sinus or atrial ectopy	7
Documentation of > 5 VPC/min at any time	7
General medical status	
PaO_2 < 60 or $PaCO_2$ > 50 torr	
K^+ < 3.0 or HCO_3 < 20 mEq/L	3
BUN > 50 or creatinine > 3.0 mg/dL	
Chronic liver disease or debilitated patient	
Operation	
Intraperitoneal, intrathoracic, or aortic	3
Emergency	4
Total possible points	53

BUN, blood urea nitrogen; JVP, jugular venous pressure; VPC, ventricular premature complex.
Modified from *N Engl J Med* 297:845-850, 1977. By permission of the Massachusetts Medical Society.

relatively less clinical importance.

High-risk operation (Table 4) includes 1) major intrathoracic procedures, 2) abdominal (intraperitoneal) operations, 3) aortic surgical procedures (e.g., aortic aneurysmectomy), and 4) peripheral vascular operation.

High-risk operation has been associated with a higher incidence of postoperative congestive heart failure and a threefold greater incidence of myocardial infarction in comparison with other general surgical procedures. A major operation is often associated with large extravascular and intravascular fluid shifts or blood loss and postoperative hypoxemia. The magnitude and duration of the procedure are also important. Patients undergoing peripheral vascular operations are at high risk, primarily because of the increased incidence of associated coronary artery disease. Emergency major operations, especially in the elderly, are considered high-risk.

Intermediate-risk operation includes 1) carotid endarterectomy, 2) head and neck procedures, 3) orthopedic and

Table 2.--Perioperative Outcome Stratified by Cardiac Risk Index

Risk class	Patients, no.	Total points	Life-threatening complications,* no. (%)	Cardiac deaths, no. (%)
I	537	0–5	4 (0.7)	1 (0.2)
II	316	6–12	16 (5)	5 (2)
III	130	13–25	15 (11)	3 (2)
IV	18	≥ 26	4 (22)	10 (56)
			—	—
			39	19

*Perioperative myocardial infarction, pulmonary edema, or ventricular tachycardia without cardiac death.
From *N Engl J Med* 297:845-850, 1977. By permission of the Massachusetts Medical Society.

prostate operations, and 4) less extensive intraperitoneal and intrathoracic procedures.

Low-risk operation includes 1) ophthalmologic procedures, 2) endoscopic surgery, 3) breast surgery, and 4) uncomplicated herniorrhaphy.

- High-risk operation includes major intrathoracic, abdominal (intraperitoneal), and aortic surgical procedures (e.g., aortic aneurysmectomy).
- Patients undergoing peripheral vascular operations are also at high risk, primarily because of the increased incidence of associated coronary artery disease.

Nonvascular Versus Vascular Surgery

Overall, perioperative cardiac event rates recently have decreased markedly, especially for patients undergoing *nonvascular* operations, partly because of improved patient selection, anesthetic techniques, and perioperative management. Most studies have focused on patients having *vascular* procedures, because they are at higher risk.

Routine coronary angiography performed before a vascular operation has demonstrated that more than one-half of patients with clinically suspected coronary artery disease have severe multivessel or inoperable coronary artery disease. Even patients with peripheral vascular disease and no previous history of heart disease may have severe coronary artery disease, especially those with diabetes mellitus.

- Even patients with peripheral vascular disease and no previous history of heart disease may have severe coronary artery disease, especially those with diabetes mellitus.

Valvular Heart Disease

In patients with valvular heart disease, the risk of noncardiac operation depends on 1) the type, anatomical location, and severity of the valve lesion; 2) left ventricular systolic function; and 3) New York Heart Association (NYHA) functional class.

Patients with severe symptomatic aortic stenosis pose the greatest risk and, ideally, should undergo corrective aortic valve operation or, in selected cases, balloon valvuloplasty before having a noncardiac operation. However, aortic balloon valvuloplasty has inherent risks, including significant vascular access complications, especially in the elderly. A selected, small group of patients from the Mayo Clinic who had critical aortic stenosis and who were not candidates for (or refused) aortic valve operation or valvuloplasty had noncardiac operations without having major complications; nonetheless, most patients with aortic stenosis should be considered high risk and aortic valve replacement is generally warranted. Patients with severe mitral stenosis are at increased risk for the development of perioperative congestive heart failure, especially if tachycardia occurs. Patients with milder degrees of aortic or mitral stenosis have a lower risk.

Generally, patients with aortic or mitral regurgitation, especially if they have only mild symptoms, seem to be at lower risk than those with stenotic lesions. Patients with advanced symptoms (NYHA class III-IV) of congestive heart failure and those with severe valvular regurgitation and left ventricular systolic dysfunction are at greater risk (regardless of the mechanism) and should undergo further evaluation and treatment before having a noncardiac operation, especially if it includes a high-risk surgical procedure (Table 4).

Table 3.--Clinical Predictors of Increased Perioperative Cardiovascular Risk (Myocardial Infarction, Congestive Heart Failure, Death)

Major risk
    Unstable coronary syndromes
        Recent myocardial infarction[*] with evidence of important ischemic risk by clinical symptoms or noninvasive study
        Unstable or severe[†] angina (Canadian class III or IV)
    Decompensated congestive heart failure
    Significant arrhythmias
        High-grade atrioventricular block
        Symptomatic ventricular arrhythmias in the presence of underlying heart disease
        Supraventricular arrhythmias with uncontrolled ventricular rate
    Severe valvular disease
Intermediate risk
    Mild angina pectoris (Canadian class I or II)
    Prior myocardial infarction by history of pathologic Q waves
    Compensated or prior congestive heart failure
    Diabetes mellitus
Minor risk
    Advanced age
    Abnormal ECG (left ventricular hypertrophy, left bundle branch block, ST-T abnormalities)
    Rhythm other than sinus (e.g., atrial fibrillation)
    Low functional capacity (e.g., inability to climb one flight of stairs with a bag of groceries)
    History of stroke
    Uncontrolled systemic hypertension

ECG, electrocardiogram.
[*]The American College of Cardiology National Database Library defines recent myocardial infarction as more than 7 days but 1 month or less (30 days).
[†]May include "stable" angina in patients who are unusually sedentary.
From *Circulation* 93:1278-1317, 1996 and *J Am Coll Cardiol* 27:910-948, 1996. By permission of the American Heart Association and the American College of Cardiology.

- Patients with severe symptomatic aortic stenosis pose the greatest risk and, ideally, should undergo corrective aortic valve operation before having a noncardiac operation.
- Patients with severe mitral stenosis are at increased risk for the development of perioperative congestive heart failure, especially if tachycardia occurs.
- Patients with advanced symptoms (NYHA class III-IV) of congestive heart failure and those with severe valvular regurgitation and left ventricular systolic dysfunction

Table 4.--Cardiac Risk[*] Stratification for Noncardiac Surgical Procedures

High (reported cardiac risk often > 5%)
    Emergency major operations, particularly in the elderly
    Aortic and other major vascular
    Peripheral vascular
    Anticipated prolonged surgical procedures associated with large fluid shifts or blood loss
Intermediate (reported cardiac risk generally < 5%)
    Carotid endarterectomy
    Head and neck
    Intraperitoneal and intrathoracic
    Orthopedic
    Prostate
Low[†] (reported cardiac risk generally < 1%)
    Endoscopic procedures
    Superficial procedures
    Cataract
    Breast

[*]Combined incidence of cardiac death and nonfatal myocardial infarction.
[†]Do not generally require further preoperative cardiac testing.
From *Circulation* 93:1278-1317, 1996 and *J Am Coll Cardiol* 27:910-948, 1996. By permission of the American Heart Association and the American College of Cardiology.

are at greater risk (regardless of the mechanism) and should undergo further evaluation and treatment before having a noncardiac operation, especially if it includes a high-risk surgical procedure.

Hypertrophic Obstructive Cardiomyopathy

In general, patients with hypertrophic obstructive cardiomyopathy tolerate noncardiac operations reasonably well. However, some of them are at increased risk. Hemodynamic changes associated with an anesthetic-related decrease in peripheral resistance, hypovolemia, or adrenergic stimulation may increase the left ventricular outflow tract gradient and lead to hemodynamic deterioration.

- In patients with hypertrophic obstructive cardiomyopathy, hemodynamic changes associated with an anesthetic-related decrease in peripheral resistance, hypovolemia, or adrenergic stimulation may increase the left ventricular outflow tract gradient and lead to hemodynamic deterioration.

Preoperative Cardiovascular Functional Assessment

The ability of a patient to exercise is an important indicator of how well he or she will tolerate noncardiac operation. If a patient is able to exercise moderately (4–5 metabolic equivalents [METs]) without symptoms, the risk is relatively low. Preoperative exercise stress testing is an important objective means of functional assessment before a noncardiac operation (Table 5) and is especially important when the functional status of the patient is unclear.

Postoperative cardiac risk is increased in patients with abnormal findings on a preoperative exercise stress test and in those who are unable to exercise to a moderate workload (e.g., 4–5 METs). In one study of patients undergoing symptom-limited exercise radionuclide angiography before a peripheral vascular operation, perioperative cardiac events occurred only in those unable to exercise at a relatively low workload of 400 kg-m/min (4.5 METs for a 70-kg patient). Activities such as digging in the garden, shovelling light earth, and walking at a brisk pace (3.5-4 mph) are associated with energy costs in the 5-MET range. Climbing a flight of stairs, scrubbing floors, and playing golf generally exceed 4 METs. Strenuous sports (swimming or tennis) exceed 10 METs (Table 6).

- If a patient is able to exercise moderately (4-5 METs) without symptoms, the perioperative risk is relatively low.
- In general, postoperative cardiac events occur more frequently in patients with abnormal findings on a preoperative exercise stress test and in those who are unable to exercise to a moderate workload (e.g., 4–5 METs).
- Activities such as digging in the garden, shovelling light earth, and walking at a brisk pace (3.5-4 mph) are associated with energy costs in the 5-MET range. Climbing a flight of stairs, scrubbing floors, and playing golf generally exceed 4 METs.

Preoperative Functional Assessment of Patients Unable to Exercise

In patients unable to exercise adequately, pharmacologic stress testing (intravenous dipyridamole [or adenosine] thallium [or sestamibi] imaging or dobutamine stress echocardiography) has been used as an alternative means of stress testing. The data are most valuable if the test results are negative (high *negative* predictive value). Patients with

Table 5.--Prognostic Gradient of Ischemic Responses During an ECG-Monitored Exercise Test

Patients with suspected or proven CAD

High risk
    Ischemia induced by low-level exercise* (< 4 METs or heart rate < 100 bpm or < 70% age predicted) manifested by one or more of the following:
        Horizontal or downsloping ST depression > 0.1 mV
        ST-segment elevation > 0.1 mV in noninfarct lead
        Five or more abnormal leads
        Persistent ischemic response > 3 min after exertion
        Typical angina

Intermediate risk
    Ischemia induced by moderate-level exercise (4-6 METs or heart rate 100-130 bpm [70%-85% age predicted]) manifested by one or more of the following:
        Horizontal or downsloping ST depression > 0.1 mV
        Typical angina
        Persistent ischemic response > 1-3 min after exertion
        Three or four abnormal leads

Low risk
    No ischemia or ischemia induced at high-level exercise (> 7 METs or heart rate > 130 bpm [> 85% age predicted]) manifested by:
        Horizontal or downsloping ST depression > 0.1 mV
        Typical angina
        One or two abnormal leads

Inadequate test
    Inability to reach adequate target workload or heart rate response for age without an ischemic response. For patients undergoing noncardiac operation, ability to exercise to at least the intermediate-risk level without ischemia should be considered a low risk for perioperative ischemic events

CAD, coronary artery disease; ECG, electrocardiographically; MET, metabolic equivalent; bpm, beats per minute.

*Workload and heart rate estimates for risk severity require adjustment for patient age. Maximal target heart rates for 40- and 80-year-old subjects taking no cardioactive medication are 180 and 140 bpm, respectively.

From *Circulation* 93:1278-1317, 1996 and *J Am Coll Cardiol* 27:910-948, 1996. By permission of the American Heart Association and the American College of Cardiology.

normal scans are at very low risk. The opposite is not true, however, and positive stress tests continue to have a low *positive* predictive value for perioperative events. The incorporation of clinical factors improves the specificity and predictive value of a positive dipyridamole thallium scan. Demonstration of a thallium redistribution defect in the presence of one or more *clinical* risk factors has been associated with a higher incidence of perioperative cardiac

Table 6.--Estimated Energy Requirements for Various Activities

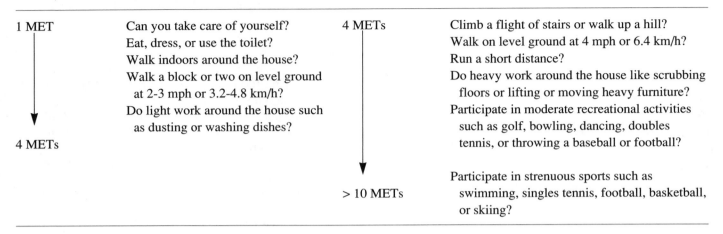

MET, metabolic equivalent.
From *Circulation* 93:1278-1317, 1996 and *J Am Coll Cardiol* 27:910-948, 1996. By permission of the American Heart Association and the American College of Cardiology.

complications than in patients with a reversible thallium defect but without such clinical risk factors. Severe ischemia has greater predictive value than mild ischemia, but the total area of ischemia is more predictive than the severity in any single ventricular segment. In addition to thallium redistribution, ischemic electrocardiographic changes during the test are predictive of perioperative events.

Clinical Approach to Preoperative Assessment and Management

Generally, the perioperative risk for nonvascular non–high-risk operations is low, in any case limiting the predictive value of stress testing. Standard clinical evaluation should suffice in most of these low-risk patients.

Functionally active patients without major or intermediate risk factors in whom there is no clinical suspicion of coronary artery disease do not need to undergo *routine* stress testing before a noncardiac operation, especially for a low-risk procedure. Patients with chronic stable angina who are active and able to perform activities of daily living (4–5 METs) probably will be able to tolerate the stress of most types of noncardiac operations. This group of patients routinely would not require preoperative stress testing. For optimal use of resources, the ACC/AHA guidelines recommend that if a patient has had coronary revascularization within the past 5 years and if the clinical status has remained stable without recurrent symptoms or signs of

ischemia, additional cardiac testing generally is not needed. For patients with ischemic heart disease who have not had coronary revascularization but who have undergone coronary evaluation in the past 2 years (assuming adequate testing and favorable outcome of testing), it usually is unnecessary to repeat testing unless there has been an acceleration of angina or new symptoms of ischemia have appeared during the interim. For patients at intermediate risk, consideration of both the functional capacity and the level of operation-specific risk is necessary. Further noninvasive testing should be considered for patients with poor functional capacity or moderate functional capacity before a high-risk procedure is performed. Patients about to undergo a high-risk operation, especially if they have significant clinical risk factors, should be considered for preoperative stress testing. In selected patients with known coronary artery disease and significant (class III or IV) symptomatic limitation or accelerating angina, preoperative coronary angiography is often indicated, as it would be even if a noncardiac operation were not being contemplated.

Coronary revascularization before noncardiac operation can decrease perioperative cardiac mortality to approximately 1% or less, compared with 2.4% for patients with similar coronary artery disease treated medically. However, the potential risks (morbidity and mortality) of coronary artery bypass grafting itself, especially in patients older than 70 years, must also be considered before a noncardiac operation is performed. A multicenter study of percutaneous transluminal coronary angioplasty has demonstrated an overall mortality of 1% (2.8% in the presence of triple-vessel disease), a 4.3% incidence of nonfatal myocardial infarction, and a need for emergency coronary artery bypass grafting in 3.4% of patients. The strategy of performing coronary angiography and percutaneous transluminal coronary angioplasty before noncardiac operation in order to reduce the risk of a noncardiac procedure depends on individual circumstances and has not yet been proved beneficial by controlled clinical trials.

In most ambulatory patients who are active enough to perform adequate stress testing, the exercise electrocardiographic treadmill test is usually preferred because it provides an estimate of both functional capacity and ischemic response. In patients with an abnormal resting electrocardiogram (e.g., left ventricular hypertrophy, left bundle branch block, digitalis effect, and nonspecific ST-T abnormalities), a cardiac imaging exercise test such as exercise echocardiography or myocardial perfusion imaging should be considered. The choice of the specific test depends on various factors, especially local expertise with a specific technique.

Interventional procedures rarely are needed just to lower the risk of noncardiac operation, unless the intervention is thought to be indicated anyway, that is, if the patient were not undergoing a noncardiac operation. Thus, the strategy of performing coronary revascularization just to avoid perioperative cardiac complications should be reserved for only a small subset of very high-risk patients.

According to ACC/AHA guidelines, class I indications for preoperative coronary angiography for patients with suspected or proven coronary artery disease (Table 7) include the following:

1) High-risk results of noninvasive testing
2) Severe (class III-IV) angina unresponsive to medical therapy
3) Unstable angina
4) Nondiagnostic or equivocal noninvasive test results in a high-risk patient, for example, multiple clinical risk factors in a patient undergoing high-risk operation (see above)

Coronary angiography generally is not indicated in low-risk patients or in those who are asymptomatic after coronary revascularization and have good exercise capacity.

- Generally, the perioperative risk for nonvascular non–high-risk operations is low, limiting the predictive value of cardiac stress testing. Standard clinical evaluation should suffice in most of these low-risk patients.
- Patients with chronic stable angina who are active and able to perform activities of daily living (4–5 METs) probably will be able to tolerate the stress of most types of noncardiac operations.
- If a patient has undergone coronary revascularization within the past 5 years and if the clinical status has remained stable without recurrent symptoms or signs of ischemia, additional cardiac testing generally is not needed.
- For patients with ischemic heart disease who have not had coronary revascularization but who have undergone coronary evaluation in the past 2 years (assuming adequate testing and favorable outcome of testing), it usually is unnecessary to repeat testing unless there has been an acceleration of angina or new symptoms of ischemia have appeared during the interim.
- In selected patients with known coronary artery disease and significant (class III or IV) symptomatic limitation or accelerating angina, preoperative coronary angiography is often indicated, as it would be even if a noncardiac operation were not being contemplated.
- The strategy of performing coronary angiography and "preventive" percutaneous transluminal coronary angioplasty before operation in order to reduce the risk of noncardiac surgery, although logical, has not been proved in controlled clinical trials.

Preoperative Hemodynamic Assessment and Intraoperative Hemodynamic Monitoring

If overt congestive heart failure is present, medical therapy should be optimized preoperatively, but dehydration and hypotension from overly aggressive diuretic and vasodilator therapy must be avoided. In patients with overt congestive heart failure, preoperative or intraoperative monitoring with Swan-Ganz catheters may be useful, especially with high-risk procedures, so that intravenous fluid and drug therapy can be guided optimally. Monitoring should be continued into the postoperative period, when major extravascular fluid mobilization could precipitate pulmonary edema in patients with severe valvular heart disease or left ventricular dysfunction. The risks of invasive hemodynamic monitoring have to be balanced against the potential benefits. Many patients can be managed adequately on a clinical basis without the need for invasive hemodynamic monitoring. Randomized trials have not proved a major benefit from invasive hemodynamic monitoring with regard to decreasing perioperative cardiac morbidity.

Table 7.--Indications for Coronary Angiography* in Perioperative Evaluation Before (or After) Noncardiac Operation

Class I†--Patients with suspected or proven CAD
    High-risk results during noninvasive testing
    Angina pectoris unresponsive to adequate medical therapy
    Most patients with unstable angina pectoris
    Nondiagnostic or equivocal noninvasive test in a high-risk patient undergoing a high-risk noncardiac surgical procedure

Class II‡
    Intermediate-risk results during noninvasive testing
    Nondiagnostic or equivocal noninvasive test in a lower risk patient undergoing a high-risk noncardiac surgical procedure
    Urgent noncardiac operation in a patient convalescing from acute MI
    Perioperative MI

Class III§
    Low-risk noncardiac operation in a patient with known CAD and low-risk results on noninvasive testing
    Screening for CAD without appropriate noninvasive testing
    Asymptomatic after coronary revascularization, with excellent exercise capacity ($\geq$ 7 METs)
    Mild stable angina in patients with good LV function, low-risk noninvasive test results
    Patient is not a candidate for coronary revascularization because of concomitant medical illness
    Prior technically adequate normal coronary angiogram within 5 years
    Severe LV dysfunction (e.g., ejection fraction < 20%) and patient not considered candidate for revascularization procedure
    Patient unwilling to consider coronary revascularization procedure

CAD, coronary artery disease; MI, myocardial infarction; MET, metabolic equivalent; LV, left ventricular.
*If results will affect management.
†Class I: conditions for which there is evidence for or general agreement that a procedure be performed or a treatment is of benefit.
‡Class II: conditions for which there is a divergence of evidence or opinion about the treatment.
§Class III: conditions for which there is evidence or general agreement that the procedure is not necessary.
From *Circulation* 93:1278-1317, 1996 and *J Am Coll Cardiol* 27:910-948, 1996. By permission of the American Heart Association and the American College of Cardiology.

- If overt congestive heart failure is present, medical therapy should be optimized preoperatively.
- In patients with overt congestive heart failure, preoperative or intraoperative monitoring with Swan-Ganz catheters may be useful, especially with high-risk procedures, so that intravenous fluid and drug therapy can be guided optimally.
- Randomized trials have not proved a major benefit from invasive hemodynamic monitoring with regard to decreasing perioperative cardiac morbidity.

Assessment of Preoperative Medications

Patients should continue to take their cardiovascular medications up to the time of the operation and should resume taking them as soon after the operation as possible. Treatment with β-adrenergic blockers, which reduce postoperative ischemia and improve perioperative outcomes, should remain uninterrupted as long as possible, especially in patients with coronary artery disease. Postoperative sinus tachycardia should be prevented in these patients, especially if ischemia developed on preoperative stress testing. In selected patients, treatment with β-blockers, and other cardiac medications if need be, can be continued until the morning of the operation. Patients taking β-blockers who have an operation may experience involuntary "drug withdrawal" if the medication is not administered early in the postoperative period. This problem has been prevented in recent years by temporary intravenous administration of β-blockers, such as esmolol, until the patient is able to resume taking medications orally. Although calcium entry blockers and anesthetics have additive vasodilator and negative inotropic effects, most patients who take these agents can be anesthetized safely.

Although mild or moderate hypertension usually does not warrant delaying the operation, severe (stage III or IV) hypertension (i.e., systolic pressure > 180 mm Hg and diastolic pressure > 110 mm Hg) should be controlled before the operation is performed. Patients with hypertension whose blood pressure is controlled with medication usually tolerate anesthesia better than those with poorly controlled blood pressure. The decision to delay the operation to achieve improved blood pressure control should take into account the urgency of the operation. Significant perioperative hypertension occurs in approximately 25% of patients with hypertension, appears unrelated to preoperative control, and occurs frequently in patients undergoing abdominal aortic aneurysm repair and other peripheral vascular procedures, including carotid endarterectomy. If oral intake of antihypertensive medications must be interrupted, parenteral therapy may be needed perioperatively. Various antihypertensive medications can be used, including intravenous β-blockers, vasodilators, calcium entry blockers, and angiotensin converting enzyme inhibitors. For patients taking clonidine orally, it may be helpful to switch to a long-acting clonidine cutaneous patch preoperatively to avoid "rebound hypertension" perioperatively.

- Treatment with β-blockers improves perioperative outcomes and should remain uninterrupted as long as possible, especially in patients with coronary artery disease. Postoperative sinus tachycardia should be prevented in these patients.
- Although calcium entry blockers and anesthetics have additive vasodilator and negative inotropic effects, most patients who take these agents can be anesthetized safely.
- Although mild or moderate hypertension usually does not warrant delaying the operation, severe hypertension should be controlled before the operation is performed.

Arrhythmias and Conduction Disturbances

Clinical evaluation should seek to uncover any underlying heart or pulmonary disease, drug toxicity, and electrolyte or metabolic abnormality that might be causing arrhythmias or conduction disturbances. Symptomatic or hemodynamically significant arrhythmias should be treated before the patient undergoes a noncardiac operation; the indications for treatment are similar to those for the nonoperative setting. It is important to correct even mild degrees of preoperative hypokalemia in patients taking digitalis. The respiratory alkalosis that is normally produced during general anesthesia may cause a decrease in extracellular potassium concentration and provoke arrhythmias. Asymptomatic conduction system disease such as bundle branch block, bifascicular block, or even

trifascicular block does not predict high-grade or complete heart block during a noncardiac operation and does not by itself mandate prophylactic temporary pacing.

- Symptomatic or hemodynamically significant arrhythmias should be treated before the patient undergoes a noncardiac operation.
- It is important to correct even mild degrees of preoperative hypokalemia in patients taking digitalis.
- Asymptomatic conduction system disease such as bundle branch block, bifascicular block, or even trifascicular block does not predict high-grade or complete heart block during a noncardiac operation and does not by itself mandate prophylactic temporary pacing.

Approach to Patients Requiring Chronic Oral Anticoagulation

The issue of discontinuation of oral anticoagulation in the perioperative setting requires balancing the thromboembolic potential of the patient's cardiovascular disease with the hemorrhagic risk of the operation. For most cardiovascular problems, including bioprosthetic valves, the acute thromboembolic potential is low to moderate. Mechanical prosthetic valves, especially those in the tricuspid or mitral position, or patients with recent embolic episodes from, for example, cardiomyopathies, atrial fibrillation, ventricular aneurysms, or acute infarctions, have high thromboembolic potential. Unfortunately, there are no large randomized trials studying the risk of thromboembolism versus the risk of hemorrhage in various conditions and types of operation. The lack of solid data is reflected in the vague wording of the recommendation in both the ACC/AHA guidelines and the Fourth Consensus Conference on Anticoagulation (*Chest* 1992;102 [Suppl]:445S-455S):

> For patients who require minimal invasive procedures (dental work, superficial biopsies), we recommend briefly reducing the INR to the low or subtherapeutic range, and resuming the normal dose of oral anticoagulation immediately following the procedure. Perioperative heparin therapy is recommended for patients in whom the risk of bleeding on oral anticoagulation is high and the risk of thromboembolism off anticoagulation is also high (major surgery in the setting of mitral valve prosthesis). For patients between these two extremes, physicians must assess the risk and benefit of reduced anticoagulation versus perioperative heparin therapy.

Several small studies have suggested that patients with low or moderate risk can have an international normalized ratio (INR) less than 2.0 for 5 to 7 days with relative safety. A reasonable approach to these patients would be to discontinue the use of warfarin several days in advance of the operation, which should be performed as soon as the INR is 1.5 or less. Oral anticoagulation is resumed as soon as possible postoperatively, and heparin is reserved for patients whose INR is less than 2.0 for 5 days or more. In patients at high risk of thromboembolic complications, intravenous heparin coverage can be instituted until 6 hours before the operation and then resumed as soon as possible postoperatively. The use of heparin can be discontinued once the INR is therapeutic for at least 24 hours.

Although the use of subcutaneous low-molecular-weight heparin seems attractive, there have been no studies showing either safety or efficacy in this setting. The use of low-molecular-weight heparin for this indication should await data from good clinical trials.

- Five days of subtherapeutic INR for patients with low to moderate thromboembolic risk is probably reasonable.
- Perioperative heparin coverage should be used in patients with a high thromboembolic risk.
- Perioperative use of subcutaneous low-molecular-weight heparin as an alternative to standard anticoagulation should await good clinical trials.

Suggested Review Reading

1. Eagle KA, Brundage BH, Chaitman BR, et al: Guidelines for perioperative cardiovascular evaluation for noncardiac surgery: an abridged version of the report of the American College of Cardiology/American Heart Association Task Force on Practice Guidelines. *Mayo Clin Proc* 72:524-531, 1997.
This is the condensed version of the full guidelines (reference 2). Although not the "reference" work or full work that cardiologists should read and understand, it provides a quick update.

2. Eagle KA, Brundage BH, Chaitman BR, et al: Guidelines for perioperative cardiovascular evaluation for noncardiac surgery. Report of the American College of Cardiology/American Heart Association Task Force on Practice Guidelines (Committee on Perioperative Cardiovascular Evaluation for Noncardiac Surgery). *J Am Coll Cardiol* 27:910-948, 1996, and *Circulation* 93:1278-1317, 1996.
This is the "definitive" evidence-based review of the literature, up to the date of publication of the article, done by

the joint committee of the ACC and AHA. The practice guidelines in this article are certain to be the major basis for any board questions about this topic. This article contains 229 references.

3. Goldman L, Caldera DL, Nussbaum SR, et al: Multifactorial index of cardiac risk in noncardiac surgical procedures. *N Engl J Med* 297:845-850, 1977.
The authors prospectively collected clinical and laboratory data on patients about to undergo noncardiac operation. From the resulting prospective data, they developed a multivariate model of the risk factors predicting perioperative myocardial ischemic events. This is a classic article presenting some of the most often-cited data.

4. L'Italien GJ, Paul SD, Hendel RC, et al: Development and validation of a Bayesian model for perioperative cardiac risk assessment in a cohort of 1,081 vascular surgical candidates. *J Am Coll Cardiol* 27:779-786, 1996.
This study presents data showing the accuracy of simple clinical markers for predicting a perioperative myocardial event even before high-risk vascular procedures. The

predictive accuracy was reliable using a separate valida-tion set of patients.

5. Mangano DT, Layug EL, Wallace A, et al: Effect of atenolol on mortality and cardiovascular morbidity after noncardiac surgery. *N Engl J Med* 335:1713-1720, 1996.
This study was a double-blind, randomized assessment of atenolol perioperatively. The authors demonstrated a long-term benefit of 7 days of perioperative therapy with atenolol.

6. Mason JJ, Owens DK, Harris RA, et al: The role of coronary angiography and coronary revascularization before noncardiac vascular surgery. *JAMA* 273:1919-1925, 1995.
The authors show by decision analysis that the use of routine preoperative coronary arteriography in even very high-risk vascular operation is associated with worse outcomes than very selective use of angiography.

7. Pasternack PF, Imparato AM, Baumann FG, et al: The hemodynamics of β-blockade in patients undergoing abdominal aortic aneurysm repair. *Circulation* 76 (Suppl 3):III-1-III-7, 1987.
This study shows a significant benefit of β-adrenergic block-ers for preventing perioperative myocardial infarction in patients undergoing repair of an abdominal aortic aneurysm.

8. Tiede DJ, Nishimura RA, Gastineau DA, et al: Modern management of prosthetic valve anticoagulation. *Mayo Clin Proc* 73:665-680, 1998.
This is an excellent state-of-the-art review of anticoagu-lation for prosthetic valve, including the perioperative management of patients with prosthetic valves who are to undergo noncardiac operations.

9. Mangano DT, Hollenberg M, Fegert G, et al: Perioperative myocardial ischemia in patients under-going noncardiac surgery. I. Incidence and severity during the 4 day perioperative period. *J Am Coll Cardiol* 17:843-850, 1991.

10. Mangano DT, Wong MG, London MJ, et al: Perioperative myocardial ischemia in patients under-going noncardiac surgery. II. Incidence and severity during the 1st week after surgery. *J Am Coll Cardiol* 17:851-857, 1991.
The authors studied 100 patients at significant risk for

perioperative ischemia. They found that anesthesia and operation were not associated with increased ischemia during the postoperative period (especially the first 3 days). Immediate preoperative ischemia also was not increased. Ischemia at both times was associated with persistent increased heart rates. Perioperative ischemia was usual-ly silent and associated with a worse long-term outcome. This finding suggests a role for preoperative anxiety relief, postoperative pain relief, and perioperative β-adrenergic blockade.

11. Katholi RE, Nolan SP, McGuire LB: The management of anticoagulation during noncardiac operations in patients with prosthetic heart valves. A prospective study. *Am Heart J* 96:163-165, 1978.

12. Tinker JH, Tarhan S: Discontinuing anticoagulant ther-apy in surgical patients with cardiac valve prostheses. Observations in 180 operations. *JAMA* 239:738-739, 1978.
The authors of references 11 and 12 report that there is minimal risk associated with discontinuing prosthetic valve anticoagulation for a short period to allow elective non-cardiac operation. Different methods of discontinuing and resuming the anticoagulation are suggested.

13. O'Keefe JH Jr, Shub C, Rettke SR: Risk of noncar-diac surgical procedures in patients with aortic steno-sis. *Mayo Clin Proc* 64:400-405, 1989.

14. Torsher LC, Shub C, Rettke SR, et al: Risk of patients with severe aortic stenosis undergoing noncardiac surgery. *Am J Cardiol* 81:448-452, 1998.
The authors of references 13 and 14 report that patients with severe aortic stenosis can undergo necessary non-cardiac operation without first having the aortic valve replaced. This is very important information, especially for patients with aortic stenosis who require either urgent operation or operation in which the surgical findings have an impact on expected prognosis (most often malignancy resection).

15. Detsky AS, Abrams HB, Forbath N, et al: Cardiac assessment for patients undergoing noncardiac surgery. A multifactorial clinical risk index. *Arch Intern Med* 146:2131-2134, 1986.
This article describes an important multifactorial clinical risk index for patients undergoing noncardiac surgery.

Examination Strategy

For the purposes of the Cardiology Boards, the *most important* information to remember about evaluating patients with heart disease before noncardiac operation includes all of the following:

 a. The clinical indicators of high, intermediate, and low risk for a cardiac event in the perioperative period
 b. The surgical procedures associated with high, intermediate, and low risk for precipitating perioperative myocardial infarction and cardiac complications
 c. Patients with peripheral vascular disease are at a very high risk of a perioperative cardiac event, and these patients should have some type of stress test before an elective vascular operation
 d. The indications for preoperative testing and revascularization are similar to those in the nonoperative setting and not based on getting the patient through the planned operation
 e. Goldman's risk stratification nomogram

Do not sacrifice the questions on the risks of noncardiac operation because there will likely be many direct and indirect "core" questions regarding this topic. This is an important enough topic for the American College of Cardiology and American Heart Association to develop a task force and practice guidelines. The article and nomogram of Goldman et al. provide very useful information, but they are only part of the full strategy. Not all patients with peripheral vascular disease need preoperative stress tests (examples: active, asymptomatic patients having carotid endarterectomy; active, asymptomatic patients having abdominal aortic aneurysm repair; patients who had complete coronary revascularization less than 5 years earlier and who remain moderately active and asymptomatic). Patients can generally be "gotten through" the operation itself even in the presence of significant cardiac disease, and so the indications for preoperative testing and revascularization are similar to those in the nonoperative setting and based on a patient's long-term cardiac requirements.

Questions

Multiple Choice (choose the one best answer)

 1. A 65-year-old man is referred for cardiovascular evaluation before planned repair of an asymptomatic 6-cm abdominal aortic aneurysm. His prior medical history includes moderate hypertension, now controlled with hydrochlorothiazide and enalapril, and hypercholesterolemia, for which he follows a low-fat diet and takes niacin. He smoked for 5 years in his 20s and then stopped. His heaviest physical activity is bowling in a league 3 evenings per week, which causes no symptoms. His examination reveals the following: pulse, 60 beats/min; respirations, 14/min; jugular venous pressure, 6 cm H_2O; blood pressure, 130/70 mm Hg; clear lungs; normal cardiac sounds except for a soft S_4; and a palpable, nontender abdominal aortic aneurysm with a bruit along the aneurysm. Laboratory evaluation shows normal values for sodium, potassium, hemoglobin, and fasting glucose. Your recommendation would be:

 a. Preoperative treadmill exercise testing and clearance for operation if results are negative
 b. Preoperative testing to include electrocardiography, exercise stress with sestamibi or echocardiographic imaging, and lipid profile. If these tests are negative, proceed with aneurysm repair and postoperative risk factor modification
 c. Clearance for operation with perioperative β-adrenergic blocker coverage
 d. Preoperative electrocardiography only; if results are normal, then clearance for aneurysm repair with postoperative risk stratification and risk factor modification
 e. Advise the patient to have the aneurysm repaired with an endovascular catheter-based technique
 f. Advise the patient to have coronary angiography and carotid ultrasonography before surgical repair

2. A 35-year-old woman is referred for cardiovascular evaluation of a heart murmur before elective vaginal hysterectomy. She relates that she has known about the murmur since childhood. She does not know whether she ever had rheumatic fever. She denies any other medical problems and takes no medications. There is no family history of heart disease. On examination, she appears healthy and not overweight. Her blood pressure is 110/58 mm Hg. The jugular venous pressure and waves are normal. Her lungs are clear to auscultation. Her apical impulse is strong and not displaced, and the rest of the precordium is normal. There is a grade 2/6 systolic murmur along the left sternal border without radiation, which increases with standing and Valsalva maneuver. There is no associated thrill. All pulses feel full, and there are no bruits or radiated murmurs. The first and second sounds are normal, and there are no extra sounds. She frequently plays doubles tennis and "lasts" as well as her partner or the opponents. Your recommendation would be:
   a. Proceed with operation after bacterial endocarditis prophylaxis
   b. Tell the patient to delay her operation until she has had a full evaluation, including chest radiography, electrocardiography, and echocardiography
   c. The anesthesiologist should be alerted to avoid volume depletion and hypotension. The patient can proceed to operation with bacterial endocarditis prophylaxis
   d. The patient should not proceed to elective noncardiac operation until she has had the murmur corrected
   e. The anesthesiologist should be alerted to the patient's condition and should have β-adrenergic blockers available. She can then proceed to operation with bacterial endocarditis prophylaxis

3. A 65-year-old man is referred for evaluation before planned total hip replacement. He has had progressive disability due to pain in the hip and can now walk only across the room. The patient uses a wheelchair to go any longer distance. Three years ago the patient had 5-vessel coronary artery bypass for unstable angina and was following a good walking program until his hip limited him 9 months ago. He remains asymptomatic and is taking metoprolol (100 mg twice a day), aspirin (325 mg a day), and a multivitamin. On examination, the patient's blood pressure is 120/60 mm Hg, and his

cardiopulmonary examination is normal. His electrocardiogram is normal. You would recommend:
   a. The patient should proceed with operation without additional cardiovascular evaluation
   b. Dipyridamole thallium scanning should be done, and if no reversible abnormality is found, then proceed with hip replacement
   c. The patient should have dobutamine echocardiography and proceed with hip replacement if no inducible ischemia is identified
   d. The patient should avoid hip operation unless coronary angiography demonstrates patent grafts
   e. The patient should undergo arm ergometry stress testing and proceed to hip operation if he is asymptomatic and has a negative electrocardiogram at a workload of 150 kg/m per minute

4. An 85-year-old man is referred for evaluation before carotid endarterectomy. He had a transient ischemic attack 3 weeks ago, initially treated with heparin and aspirin. He has never had a myocardial infarction and has a normal electrocardiogram. He occasionally gets angina when polka dancing. He denies angina while doing light gardening at his home. You would recommend:
   a. He should have an exercise treadmill test, and if he completes stage II, then proceed with endarterectomy
   b. He should have coronary angiography before undergoing endarterectomy
   c. He should be advised to take warfarin for 3 to 6 months and then switch to 1 aspirin per day in an attempt to avoid carotid endarterectomy because of his cardiac risk
   d. He should proceed to endarterectomy and be taking aspirin
   e. He should be given β-adrenergic blockers, aspirin, and nitrates. If a stress test on medications is negative, he can proceed with endarterectomy

5. A 60-year-old woman is referred for evaluation before cholecystectomy for cholelithiasis. She has been paraplegic since age 45 years as a result of a spinal cord injury that occurred while skiing. With her enforced sedentary lifestyle, she has gained weight and has had hypercholesterolemia and hyperglycemia, both treated with medication. She denies angina. She is taking diltiazem for blood pressure control. On examination, her blood pressure is 150/85 mm Hg. She is very overweight. The heart sounds and pulses are normal.

Her electrocardiogram shows left-axis deviation but no other abnormalities. Which of the following statements is correct?

a. She is asymptomatic and has a normal electrocardiogram and so can proceed to cholecystectomy

b. She has multiple risk factors and is referred for a high-risk operation and so should have preoperative dobutamine echocardiography

c. She has multiple risk factors and is referred for an intermediate-risk operation and so should have preoperative adenosine sestamibi scanning

d. She is asymptomatic. Therefore, because she has only minor clinical predictors and is not having a high-risk operation, she can proceed to cholecystectomy without additional cardiac testing

e. She should have stone dissolution therapy to avoid the cardiac risk of operation

6. You are called to the emergency room to evaluate a patient who has fallen and broken a hip. The orthopedist wants to do an open reduction and internal fixation. The orthopedist believes that the patient will recover faster this way but that she can be treated with traction if necessary. The emergency room physician heard a loud murmur and noted that the electrocardiogram showed left ventricular hypertrophy. The patient is a 70-year-old woman. She states that she occasionally gets light-headed while doing her housework and gardening. On examination, she has a grade 4/6 crescendo-decrescendo harsh murmur along the left upper sternal border. The second heart sound is single. There is a loud fourth heart sound. Your recommendation would be:

a. Proceed to hip operation from the emergency room but have 72 hours of monitoring in the intensive care unit postoperatively

b. Start the patient on a β-adrenergic blocker in the emergency room and then proceed to hip operation with intravenous β-blocker coverage

c. Advise that the patient undergo cardiac catheterization and coronary angiography preoperatively

d. Advise that the patient have a dipyridamole stress test and proceed to operation if the stress test is normal

e. Advise the patient to consider traction until she can have operation to fix the murmur

7. You are called by a family physician who regularly refers patients to you. The requested telephone consultation is clearance for a 75-year-old woman to have a cataract

operation. She had a myocardial infarction 3 years ago and was treated with thrombolysis. She has since done well and is without anginal symptoms. During the past 3 years, her activity level has decreased because of increasing difficulty with her vision and with exertional dyspnea. The physician wants to know if she can proceed with the cataract operation or whether she should be referred to you first. Your advice would be:

a. Perform echocardiography. If normal, proceed to cataract operation

b. The patient's exercise tolerance and prior cardiac history put her into a high-risk population, and she should have a full evaluation with you as soon as possible

c. A treadmill exercise test should be performed by the family physician, and the patient should be referred to you if it shows an ischemic response to exercise

d. The patient should be sent to you for risk stratification either before or after the cataract procedure. This is low-risk and need not be delayed

e. The patient should be referred to you only if examination or chest radiography shows evidence of poorly compensated congestive heart failure from her previous infarction

8. A 55-year-old man, whom you treated for an acute myocardial infarction in the coronary care unit 2 months ago, presents with severely symptomatic cholelithiasis. There is no evidence of infarction of the gallbladder or of infection. The surgeon is strongly recommending operation very soon because several gallstones appear to be small enough to become impacted in the bile ducts. At the time of the infarction, the patient presented in congestive failure, but this resolved promptly in the first 24 hours and has not recurred. His current cardiovascular examination is normal. He completed phase I and II cardiac rehabilitation without recurrent symptoms or any dysrhythmias. He had a low-level treadmill test without symptoms or electrocardiographic changes before hospital dismissal after his myocardial infarction. He is scheduled for a high-level stress test in 3 weeks. Because he had no myocardial ischemia on his first stress test, he did not have coronary angiography. You would advise:

a. He should have immediate angiography with revascularization of any culprit lesions before proceeding to cholecystectomy

b. He should undergo a risk stratification stress test

immediately. Unless this shows that he is in the high-risk category, he should proceed with urgent cholecystectomy

c. He should have echocardiography. If his left ventricular ejection fraction is less than 30%, he should undergo anesthesia with Swan-Ganz monitoring and be in the intensive care unit postoperatively for at least 72 hours

d. Because the cholecystectomy is urgent, he should proceed with the operation immediately without further cardiac testing, especially because he has been asymptomatic in cardiac rehabilitation. He should have the cholecystectomy done laparoscopically

e. He should avoid the operation for 4 to 6 months after infarction, unless his condition becomes an absolute emergency

9. You are asked to advise about the perioperative management of anticoagulation for a 69-year-old woman. As a child, she had rheumatic fever. Subsequently, she had mitral valve replacement with a Starr-Edwards valve for severe mitral stenosis complicated by pulmonary hypertension, right heart failure, and tricuspid insufficiency. She initially did well, and then recurrent problems developed which necessitated a second operation for aortic valve replacement with a Starr-Edwards valve. She again did well until 3 years ago, when she had progressive right heart failure due to tricuspid insufficiency and had a St. Jude tricuspid valve replacement. She now needs major elective noncardiac operation. At her last valve replacement, coronary angiography revealed normal coronary arteries. She is maintained on warfarin with an international normalized ratio (INR) of 3 to 3.5. In addition to bacterial endocarditis prophylaxis, your recommendation would be:

a. Discontinue use of warfarin and admit her to the hospital for intravenous administration of heparin as soon as her INR is subtherapeutic (< 2.5). Once her INR while receiving full heparin coverage is less than 1.5, she can proceed with operation. Use of heparin should be started as soon as possible postoperatively, as should warfarin therapy. Heparin therapy can be discontinued as soon as her INR has been more than 2.5 for 24 hours

b. Discontinue her use of warfarin as an outpatient. Admit her to the hospital and perform the operation as soon as her INR is 1.5 or less. Restart warfarin therapy early postoperatively and use heparin only if

her INR will be less than 2 for more than 5 days

c. Discontinue her use of warfarin as an outpatient and begin subcutaneous therapy with low-molecular-weight heparin. Admit her to the hospital once the INR is less than 1.5 and proceed with the operation. Restart the warfarin therapy as soon as possible postoperatively. Use intravenous heparin or subcutaneous low-molecular-weight heparin if her INR will be less than 2 for more than 5 days

d. Admit her to the hospital and give her heparin as soon as the INR is less than 2. Continue heparin therapy through the operation because of her very high risk with three prosthetic valves. Stop the use of heparin postoperatively once the INR is more than 2 for 24 hours or if absolutely necessary to control major bleeding

e. Reverse her anticoagulation with fresh frozen plasma on the way to the operating room to minimize the time that her valves are at risk. Heparin therapy should be started as soon as possible postoperatively, as well as warfarin therapy. Use of heparin can be discontinued as soon as her INR has been more than 2 to 2.5 for 24 hours

10. A 68-year-old man who is a patient of your partner's is admitted for you to evaluate during the weekend because of multiple episodes of new left hemisphere transient neurologic symptoms. Computed tomography of the head is normal. While taking heparin and aspirin, the patient has no further episodes of neurologic symptoms. Your partner performed coronary angiography on the patient 3 weeks ago for stable class III angina despite optimized β-adrenergic blockers, nitrates, aspirin, lipid concentrations, blood pressure, and glucose value. The patient was scheduled for coronary artery bypass operation in another week. The arch aortogram and cerebral angiogram that you obtain now show a 70% to 80% plaque in the left carotid bulb and minimal disease in the right carotid artery. Your review of the coronary angiogram shows the following lesions: 60% left main coronary artery, 50% proximal left anterior descending, 70% middle left anterior descending, 60% first diagonal, 70% distal circumflex, 50% second obtuse marginal, and 80% distal right coronary. The neurovascular surgeon states that the patient needs carotid endarterectomy. The cardiac surgeon states that the patient needs a coronary procedure. In the hospital, while receiving intravenous heparin and aspirin, the patient is asymptomatic.

The surgeons refuse to do a combined, simultaneous procedure because of the documented increased perioperative risk of performing combined procedures, but each is reluctant to do the first procedure for fear of a major event in the other circulation. Your partner is on vacation for 2 weeks. The surgeons and the patient turn to you for recommendation. You would recommend:

a. The patient should be given warfarin for 6 months and the surgical options reconsidered then

b. The patient should have the carotid endarterectomy first, and the coronary bypass can be done as soon as surgically cleared by the neurosurgeon

c. The patient should have the coronary bypass first, and the carotid endarterectomy can be done as soon as surgically cleared by the cardiac surgeon

d. The patient should have percutaneous transluminal coronary angioplasty or stenting of the 80% coronary lesion and then have the carotid endarterectomy 2 or 3 days later. After the endarterectomy, the patient should take aspirin and full-dose β-adrenergic blockers and have a repeat stress test. If the stress test is positive, the patient should then proceed to coronary artery bypass procedure

e. The surgeons need to reconsider doing a combined procedure

11. A 55-year-old woman is referred to you for preoperative evaluation because of a heart murmur. She denies any previous history of cardiac disease and denies any cardiovascular symptoms. She is active taking care of a two-story home but does no specific exercise. She does not smoke and takes no medications except a multivitamin and calcium. On examination, her blood pressure is 110/60 mm Hg, pulse is 64 beats/min and regular, respirations are 16/min, and the jugular venous waves are normal. The carotid pulses are normal. The lungs are clear, and there is a grade 2 to 3/6 systolic murmur that radiates widely over the left chest. The murmur decreases with the held phase of the Valsalva maneuver and returns to its previous level after 7 or 8 beats. Her creatinine, electrolyte, and fasting glucose values and lipid panel are normal. Chest radiography shows prominence of the upper left heart border, but the cardiothoracic ratio is normal and the lungs are clear. Electrocardiography shows prominent voltage that does not meet the criteria for left ventricular hypertrophy. In addition to endocarditis prophylaxis, you would advise:

a. She is cleared for operation with perioperative β-adrenergic blockade and preoperative hydration to avoid hypovolemia

b. She needs a preoperative stress test

c. She needs preoperative echocardiography

d. She needs preoperative left ventriculography and coronary angiography

e. She is cleared for operation with a recommendation to avoid overhydration and hypertension

Answers

1. Answer d

Although abdominal aortic aneurysm repair is a high-risk surgical procedure and is highly associated with coronary atherosclerosis, this patient's risk profile is low. With a normal electrocardiogram, he has no clinical predictors of a perioperative event, and so further preoperative testing is unnecessary. He does have risk factors, and these should be stratified postoperatively (especially his lipid status) and modified as appropriate.

2. Answer c

Her murmur is that of mild to, at most, moderate hypertrophic cardiomyopathy. She is asymptomatic at good exercise levels. There is no family history of heart disease, which includes no history of sudden death. She can safely undergo operation as long as volume depletion (which might increase her gradient) and hypotension are avoided. She will need bacterial endocarditis prophylaxis for a transvaginal procedure.

3. Answer a

The patient had symptoms of angina before his bypass and has remained asymptomatic since that procedure. Although he has recently become sedentary, he was active without symptoms until relatively recently, and he is within 5 years of complete surgical revascularization. Therefore, he does not need additional cardiovascular testing before his hip replacement. Any risk factors should be addressed postoperatively.

4. Answer d

Polka dancing is moderately high exertion of 6 to 8 METs. The patient is at moderately low risk because of his exercise capacity and asymptomatic status with light gardening (4.5 to 5 METs). Carotid endarterectomy is an intermediate-risk procedure. He can proceed to endarterectomy without formal cardiac testing. Aspirin is reasonable for both his cardiac and carotid disease. He does not need to have a negative stress test, just an adequate exercise capacity. Postoperatively, he should have risk stratification and risk factor modification appropriate to any patient with evidence of cardiac disease.

5. Answer c

Hyperglycemia in a patient who is taking an oral agent is an intermediate clinical predictor. Cholecystectomy is a moderate-risk operation. The patient is very sedentary and has an exercise capacity of 2 METs, at best. She cannot exercise because of her paraplegia. She needs pharmacologic stress testing for risk stratification preoperatively.

6. Answer e

For the purposes of the Cardiology Boards, the patient has significant symptomatic aortic stenosis and should have this corrected before undergoing anything but an emergency operation. For your practice, you should be aware of the newer data showing that selected patients can safely undergo an orthopedic operation if you, the anesthesiologist, and the surgeon are careful to avoid volume depletion, volume overload, and hypotension.

7. Answer d

A cataract operation is very low-risk, and the patient can proceed without preoperative specialized cardiac tests. However, she has coronary artery disease, prior myocardial infarction, and progressive exertional dyspnea at probably a very low level of exertion. She needs risk stratification, regardless of the operation. If her stratification shows that she is at high cardiac risk, this should be addressed irrespective of her cataract procedure.

8. Answer b

The patient's major cardiac risk is reinfarction, and neither Swan-Ganz monitoring nor monitoring in the intensive care unit has been shown to affect this. Although the risk of reinfarction decreases with time from the initial infarction, operation can be done with reasonable safety much earlier if appropriate risk stratification has been done and shows a low risk. Although it would be important for the patient's long-term prognosis to know his ejection fraction, the critical issue for the upcoming operation is exercise capacity and inducible ischemia. If his exercise capacity is good, then his left ventricular function will be adequate for the operation. The urge to push for revascularization before cholecystectomy must be tempered by the very high mortality associated with an infarcted or infected gallbladder or with pancreatitis precipitated by an impacted gallstone if either of these occurs in the immediate period after coronary artery bypass. Thus, a risk-stratifying stress test and, if the result shows a low risk, proceeding to cholecystectomy is the best course in this patient. Perioperative β-adrenergic blockade would also be very reasonable.

9. Answer a

Aortic mechanical valves have a moderate to high thromboembolic potential. Mitral mechanical valves have a high thromboembolic potential. Tricuspid mechanical valves have a very high thromboembolic potential. Thus, this patient needs an aggressive approach to protection of her valves perioperatively. Protection with heparin both pre-operatively and as soon as possible postoperatively while waiting for the INR to become therapeutic is best in a high-risk situation such as this. In lower-risk settings, using heparin only if the INR is less than 2 for more than 5 days is a reasonable approach. The use of low-molecular-weight heparin in this setting is unproved. Trials are under way, but at least one has been put on hold by the Food and Drug Administration for safety concerns. Until there are data on this method, it should be reserved for clinical investigation studies and not used clinically, especially in high-risk settings. The operation is elective, and so the fresh frozen plasma approach is unwarranted, although in an emergency setting this would be the approach. Vitamin K should not be used because of the possible procoagulant phase and the need for re-anticoagulation postoperatively.

10. Answer b

The surgeons are correct that morbidity and mortality are higher with a combined procedure than with two-staged operations. Coronary revascularization by operation or catheter intervention is rarely indicated to "get a patient through" a noncardiac operation. Rather, revascularization is for the long-term. This patient's angina is stable and your partner and the surgeon are willing to wait weeks for an elective coronary artery bypass. The carotid lesion is currently the more symptomatic and unstable lesion and should be corrected first. In addition, carotid endarterectomy is not a high cardiac-risk procedure, especially with ongoing β-adrenergic blockade in combination with adequate pain and anxiety relief. Both the neurosurgeon and the anesthesiologist should be alerted to the increased cardiac risk with carotid surgery in this patient.

11. Answer e

The patient's findings are most consistent with asymptomatic mitral regurgitation. The chest radiograph confirms slight left atrial enlargement, but the patient is in sinus rhythm. Regurgitant lesions rarely cause difficulty with operation unless there is evidence of heart failure from the regurgitation. Because the patient has mitral regurgitation, the primary cardiac risk is pulmonary edema, which can be precipitated by either overhydration or hypertension. Hypertension can significantly increase the regurgitant fraction across the mitral valve, thus causing pulmonary edema. This is not hypertrophic cardiomyopathy, in which the murmur should increase with the Valsalva maneuver.

Chapter 46

Magnetic Resonance Imaging and Computed Tomography of the Heart and Great Vessels

John A. Rumberger, Ph.D., M.D.
Jerome F. Breen, M.D.
Donald L. Johnston, M.D.

Magnetic resonance imaging (MRI) and electron beam x-ray computed tomography (EBCT) provide information regarding the structure, function, and perfusion of the heart which is not possible with other imaging methods.

The standard imaging views for CT and MRI are as follows: the tomographic view along the transverse cardiac axis perpendicular to the long axis of the left ventricle is called the "short-axis" view; images comprising long-axis images generated by slicing in the vertical plane through the short-axis perspective represent the "vertical long-axis" view; the other long-axis view, generated by slicing along the horizontal plane through the short-axis perspective, is the "horizontal long-axis" view (Fig. 1).

Magnetic Resonance Imaging

Basic Principles of MRI

Magnetic resonance is a result of the magnetic properties of certain nuclei (mobile hydrogen nuclei or protons) that, when placed in an external magnetic field, act similarly to small bar magnets and temporarily align themselves with the field. The spinning nuclei also possess angular momentum, resulting in vibration at a precise frequency (Lamour frequency) about the major axis of the external field. When additional radio-frequency energies (pulse sequences) are applied at the Lamour (resonance) frequency, the nuclei absorb the radio-frequency energy and become "excited," and the magnetic moment deviates from alignment with the

external magnetic field. The fluctuating magnetic moment can be detected by an external coil, and this constitutes the MRI signal.

The MRI signal depends on the number of nuclei present, the time for them to relax (T1, T2), and the time at which the signal is measured. T1 is a measure of the longitudinal return to alignment with the static magnetic field. T2 is a measure of the time it takes for the transverse magnetization to diminish. T1 and T2 relaxation times are affected by the local biochemical and magnetic environments. Thus, the MR signal is dependent on inherent properties of the various tissues interrogated (hydrogen, T1, T2) and variables that can be manipulated by the imager. The difference in MR signal between tissues (MR contrast) can be enhanced by varying the pulse sequences and with the addition of paramagnetic contrast agents.

- The MR phenomenon is a result of magnetic properties of certain nuclei (mobile hydrogen nuclei or protons in standard MRI).
- MR signal difference between tissues (MR contrast) can be enhanced by varying the pulse sequences and with the addition of paramagnetic contrast agents.

Technique of MRI

A standard spin-echo MR image results from many repetitions of the MR phenomenon and is not simply a "snapshot." Acquisition of the signal data must therefore be gated to the electrocardiogram. An irregular rhythm can seriously

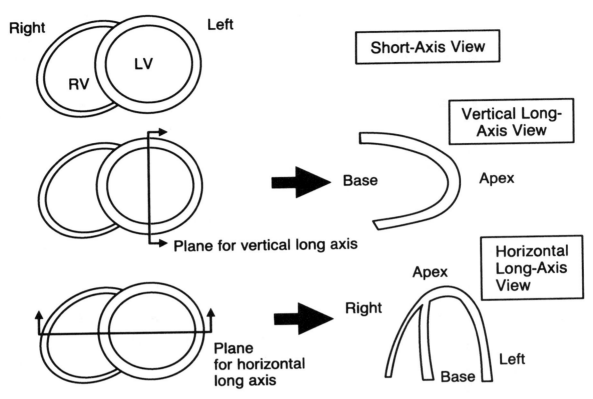

Fig. 1. Standardization of imaging planes for presentation of clinical data with magnetic resonance imaging, computed tomography, and positron emission tomography. LV, left ventricle; RV, right ventricle.

degrade image quality in standard MRI techniques. Even with regular cardiac rhythms, an adequate QRS complex may be difficult to obtain because of induced electrical potentials in the leads produced by the changing magnetic gradients, the radio-frequency pulses, and the beating heart in the strong external magnetic field. Similarly, because of induced voltages, pacemaker function can be seriously degraded by the MR signal; thus, the presence of a pacemaker typically is a contraindication to MRI.

Imaging time with standard spin-echo techniques is relatively long. Although multiple levels spanning the entire heart can be obtained simultaneously, the need for many separate signal acquisitions for adequate spatial resolution and adequate signal-to-noise ratio results in a scan time of about 5 minutes for a patient with an average heart rate.

Although spin-echo technique is the mainstay of anatomic cardiac imaging by providing high spatial resolution, physiologic imaging is provided by "fast" MR techniques. One of these techniques, known as "cine MRI," uses very rapid excitations and signal measurement sequences, which markedly increase the number of images that can be obtained at a given anatomical location during a single acquisition.

Standard spin-echo imaging results in only one cardiac phase per tomographic level, with each level being at a different phase in the cardiac cycle. Cine MRI can yield up to 64 images per level, which can be reviewed in real-time. The time to image the entire heart with this method depends on the spatial and temporal resolution desired.

- The presence of a pacemaker or pacemaker leads is a contraindication to MRI.

Clinical Applications of MRI
MRI has multiple applications in cardiology.

1. Because of the tomographic imaging capabilities of MRI, quantitation of left and right ventricular volumes, left ventricular muscle mass, and regional and global systolic and diastolic function is possible. MRI (along with ultrafast or electron beam CT) is superior to echocardiography for defining these parameters.

2. Additionally, the pericardium, central pulmonary emboli, and intracardiac thrombi and tumors can be visualized (Fig. 2 through 6). Pericardial thickness can be measured and adhesions demonstrated.

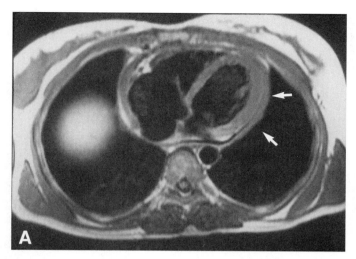

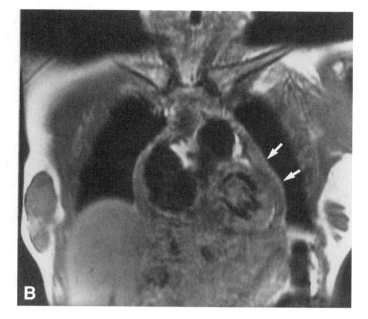

Fig. 2. Axial (*A*) and coronal (*B*) spin-echo images demonstrate thickened pericardium surrounding the heart (*arrows*), consistent with constrictive pericarditis.

MRI can accurately detect extracardiac extension of intracardiac masses and cardiac involvement by lymphomas, mediastinal tumors, and breast and lung carcinomas. MRI is the method of choice for visualization of right ventricular dysplasia, which is characterized by wall thinning and fatty infiltration of the right ventricular apex.

3. One of the most common applications of cardiac

MRI is to assess congenital heart disease. MRI provides excellent anatomic imaging in patients with anomalous connections between the aorta, pulmonary artery, and venous circulation. Pulmonary artery branch stenosis, pulmonary atresia, persistent left superior vena cava, and patent ductus arteriosus are well seen (Fig. 7 through 10).

4. Several imaging methods, including MRI, have been

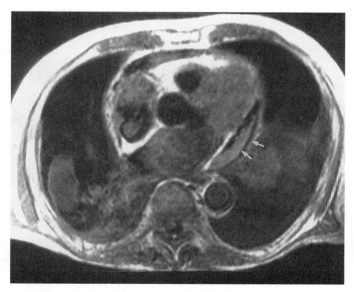

Fig. 3. Spin-echo image in a 45-year-old man with symptoms of constrictive pericarditis demonstrates areas of low and medium signal intensity within the pericardial space, consistent with an organizing pericardial effusion (*arrows*). (From Giuliani ER, Gersh BJ, McGoon MD, Hayes DL, Schaff HV [editors]: *Mayo Clinic Practice of Cardiology*. Third edition. Mosby, 1996, p 298. By permission of Mayo Foundation.)

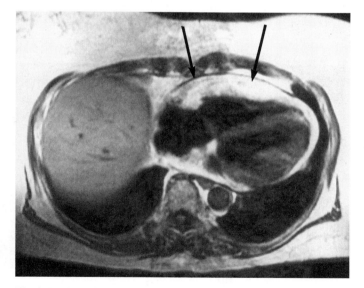

Fig. 4. Marked thickening of the pericardium was suspected on the basis of echocardiographic examination. Magnetic resonance imaging shows a normal-thickness pericardium (*arrows*) and a large amount of epicardial fat mimicking pericardial thickening. Note the identical high-intensity signal from subcutaneous fat and epicardial fat.

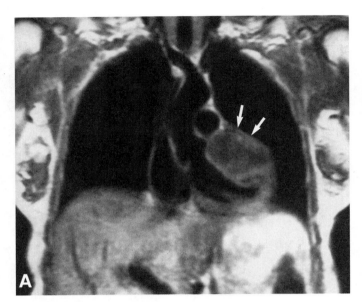
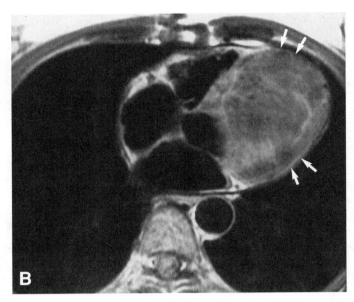

Fig. 5. Coronal (*A*) and transverse (*B*) images demonstrate a large left ventricular tumor (*arrows*). (From Giuliani ER, Gersh BJ, McGoon MD, Hayes DL, Schaff HV [editors]: *Mayo Clinic Practice of Cardiology.* Third edition. Mosby, 1996, p 290. By permission of Mayo Foundation.)

shown to be effective for the diagnosis of aortic dissection. MRI can demonstrate ostial involvement of the coronary arteries by the aortic dissection and thrombus and blood flow in the false lumen. MRI can also localize the communication between the true and false aortic lumina and show the anatomical extent of the dissection and whether the arch vessels or visceral vessels are involved. Rupture into the mediastinum and pleural cavity also is well seen. MRI is

comparable, or superior, to transesophageal echocardiography and conventional x-ray CT; its sensitivity is about 95%, and its specificity is up to 98% (Fig. 11).

MRI is an excellent imaging method in aortic disease, especially for aortic aneurysm, coarctation of the aorta, and the aortic root dilatation characteristic of Marfan disease.

5. MRI can detect the location and patency of coronary artery bypass grafts and anomalous coronary arteries

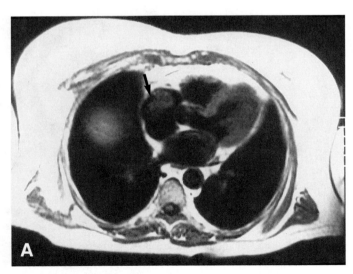
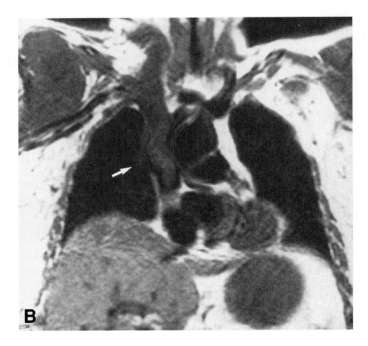

Fig. 6. Axial image (*A*) demonstrates a soft tissue mass in the right atrium (*arrow*). Coronal image (*B*) shows that this mass extends from the superior vena cava. The patient had a history of renal cell carcinoma. The tumor extended from a shoulder metastasis into the right atrium.

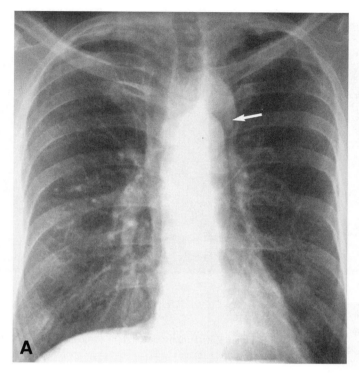

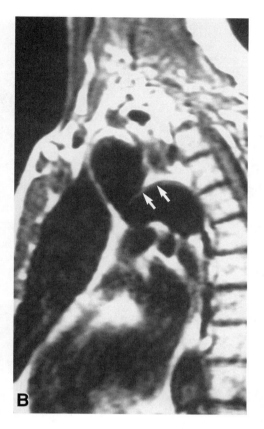

Fig. 7. *A*, Plain film demonstrates an abnormal "3" contour to the aortic arch (*arrow*). Oblique magnetic resonance image (*B*) demonstrates an aortic coarctation with shelf-like narrowing (*arrows*).

(especially an anomalous circumflex artery that arises from the right coronary artery or right coronary sinus and traverses between the aorta and pulmonary artery, which may be associated with sudden cardiac death).

6. Recently, development of three-dimensional MRI techniques that image a small bolus of gadolinium has provided high-quality images of the aorta and its major branches. The technique and image projections are very similar to those of conventional catheter aortography (Fig. 12 through 14).

7. MR angiography of peripheral arteries and veins can be readily performed. The examination time is approximately 60 minutes, longer than with conventional peripheral angiography, but it can be done noninvasively in an outpatient setting without exposure to radiation or use of conventional iodinated contrast media. Additionally, information can be obtained about resting flow velocity in peripheral vessels.

8. MR angiography of the coronary arteries has been reported but has so far shown limited application. With images oriented perpendicular to the coronary artery, the presence of a bright signal from moving blood indicates patency. Projection-type images of the proximal coronary arteries have provided convincing evidence that

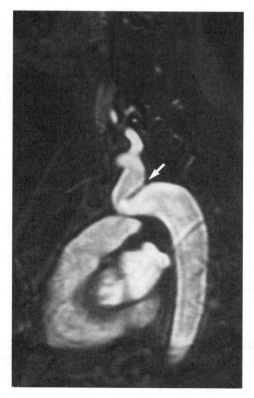

Fig. 8. Breath-hold gadolinium-enhanced magnetic resonance angiogram demonstrates an aortic coarctation (*arrow*).

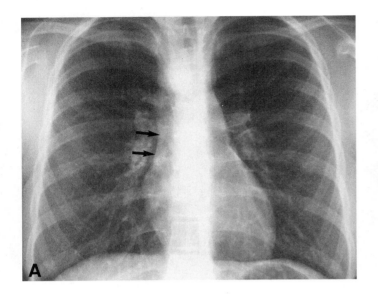

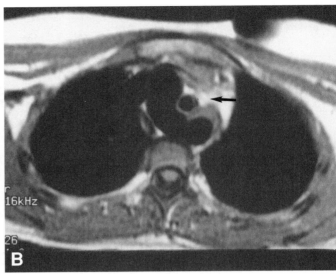

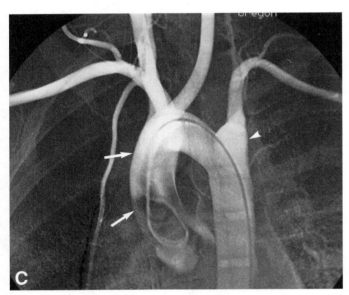

Fig. 9. *A*, Plain film demonstrates a right aortic arch (*arrows*). *B*, Axial magnetic resonance image at the level of the arch demonstrates the takeoff of an aberrant left subclavian artery (*arrow*). *C*, Conventional contrast angiogram confirms the presence of a right aortic arch (*arrows*) with aberrant left subclavian artery (*arrowhead*).

non–flow-limiting disease can be detected. Complications of coronary artery disease, such as ventricular aneurysms, are well demonstrated by MRI (Fig. 15 through 17).

9. Velocity-encoded cine MRI is a useful method of evaluating and quantitating large-vessel flow rates within the cardiovascular system. Velocities up to 6 m/s can be mapped, including those associated with extracardiac ventriculopulmonary conduits and mitral and aortic stenosis. In some studies, a close correlation has been shown between MRI and Doppler echocardiography in the assessment of pressure gradients and single-valve regurgitation. Applications of MRI to quantitation of myocardial perfusion, using intravenous injection of paramagnetic contrast agents, have shown promising early results, but the clinical utility of such methods remains to be substantiated (Fig. 18).

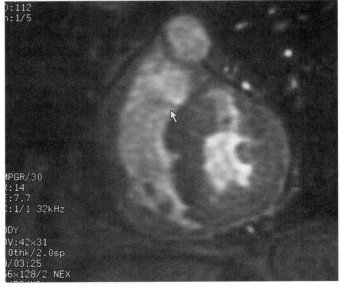

Fig. 10. Single frame from a cine acquisition in the short-axis plane demonstrates a muscular ventricular septal defect. There is a tiny shunt seen as a turbulent jet entering the outflow region of the right ventricle (*arrow*).

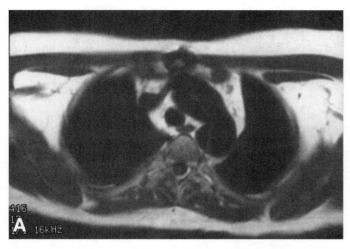 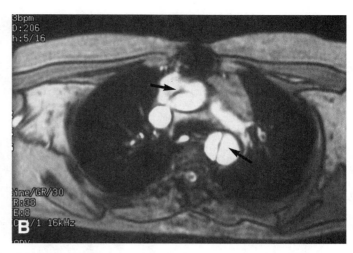

Fig. 11. Intimal flaps seen in this type A dissection by both "black blood" (*A*) and "white blood" (*B*) (*arrows*) magnetic resonance imaging techniques. *B* is a single frame from a cine acquisition.

- MRI has been shown to be effective for the diagnosis of aortic dissection.

Limitations of MRI

A patient's claustrophobia and irregular cardiac rhythm are the two most common causes for a nondiagnostic MRI examination. Morbidly obese patients may not fit within the MRI magnets.

No known biologic ill effects have been shown to occur with current MR techniques.

Metal agents are attracted by the strong magnetic field associated with MRI scanning. MRI is contraindicated in patients

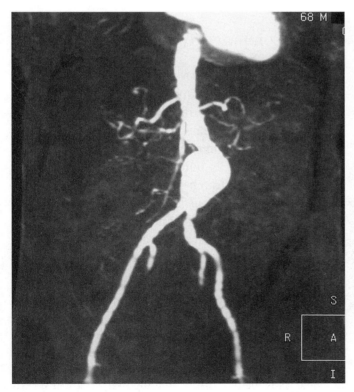

Fig. 12. Gadolinium-enhanced magnetic resonance angiogram of the abdominal aorta demonstrates an infrarenal aortic aneurysm. The patient also has renal failure and dilated cardiomyopathy (note the massive left ventricle).

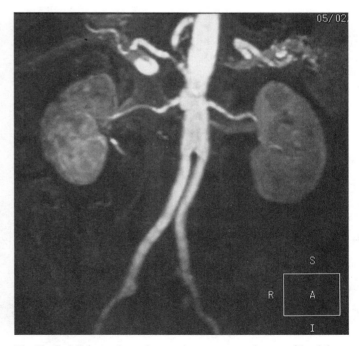

Fig. 13. Gadolinium-enhanced magnetic resonance angiogram of the abdominal aorta demonstrates a widely patent bifurcated aortic graft and widely patent renal arteries.

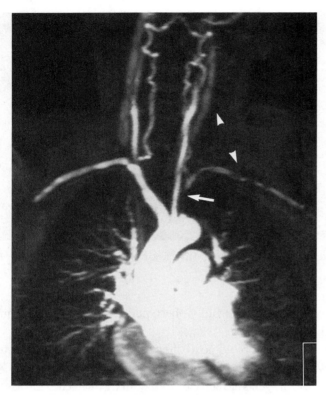

Fig. 14. Gadolinium-enhanced magnetic resonance angiogram of the aortic arch and great vessels demonstrates an occluded left subclavian artery origin (*arrow*) and a left vertebral steal (*arrowheads*).

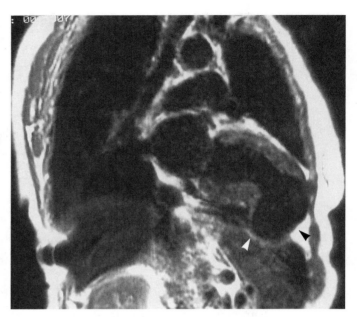

Fig. 15. Oblique image through the left ventricle demonstrates a large true apical aneurysm (*arrowheads*).

with pacemakers, old nonfunctional pacemaker leads, temporary epicardial leads placed at the time of cardiac operation, internal cardiac defibrillators, or certain ferromagnetic cerebral aneurysm clips. The presence of surgical clips, vascular coils, sternotomy wires, and metallic orthopedic implants is not a contraindication; however, all may produce image artifacts. Coronary stents may be imaged 4 to 6 weeks after implantation. Several prosthetic heart valves experience some attractive force when placed in the bore of an MR imager; however, the force generated is small compared with that experienced by valves during the normal cardiac contraction. With the exception of patients with an older Starr-Edwards (pre-6000) valve and suspected dehiscence of that valve, MRI can be accomplished safely in all patients with prosthetic valves. Hemodynamically unstable patients are unsuitable for MRI because of the difficulty with clinical monitoring within the scanner and the imaging time needed (about 30 minutes).

- Claustrophobia and an irregular rhythm are the two most common causes for a nondiagnostic MRI examination.
- MRI is contraindicated in patients with pacemakers, internal cardiac defibrillators, or certain ferromagnetic cerebral aneurysm clips.

X-Ray Computed Tomography

The major limitation of conventional CT for cardiac imaging is the prolonged scan times (2 to 5 seconds per image), which result in image blurring.

In 1979, a fast CT scanner designed specifically to image the beating heart was introduced. This scanner (called by various names, such as "ultrafast CT," "cine CT," and the now-preferred "electron beam CT") uses a conventional parallel tomographic acquisition system coupled to unique electron beam scanning technology. This technology acquires images from an electrocardiographic "trigger." Up to 8 cm of the myocardium can be scanned nearly simultaneously. Individual scan times for EBCT are about 50 ms, which provides sufficient temporal resolution to define cardiac anatomy, function, and flow.

Recently, a method known as "spiral" (also called "helical") CT was introduced by several manufacturers and has replaced conventional x-ray CT during the past several years. This method offers imaging of the body at speeds as fast as 600 ms, continuous volume scanning, and rapid (1-4 seconds) image reconstruction. Unlike EBCT, it cannot provide detailed images of the heart and myocardium

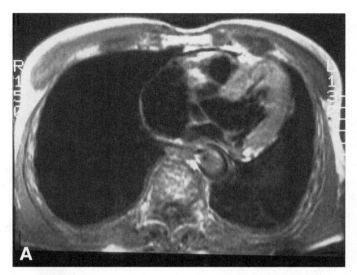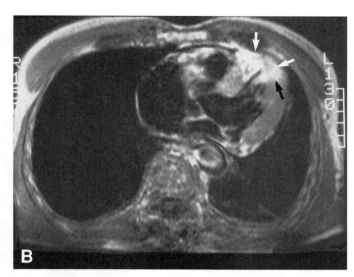

Fig. 16. Magnetic resonance images in a 58-year-old man 7 days after anterior infarction. *A*, Spin-echo image without contrast enhancement is unremarkable. *B*, After gadolinium administration, image shows marked enhancement (*arrows*) in the anterior wall and anterior septum. (From Giuliani ER, Gersh BJ, McGoon MD, Hayes DL, Schaff HV [editors]: *Mayo Clinic Practice of Cardiology*. Third edition. Mosby, 1996, p 295. By permission of Mayo Foundation.)

because of motion artifact, but it is of value for examination of great vessel abnormalities.

Method of CT Scanning

Regardless of the scanning instrument, CT often involves intravenous injection of iodinated contrast media to allow for selective opacification of vascular structures. This is needed because the x-ray densities of tissue and flowing blood are similar.

Current electron beam scanning options include an electrocardiographic-triggered, rapid sequence, polytomo-graphic (2 to 12 levels), 50 ms/scan acquisition for studies requiring information from temporal sequences (such as cardiac function and flow) and a single-slice, 100 ms/scan acquisition for studies requiring improved density and spatial resolution from static images (such as coronary artery calcium).

Applications of CT Imaging

EBCT has multiple applications in cardiology.

EBCT has been extensively validated by several laboratories for quantitation of left and right ventricular volumes and remains the most accurate in vivo method for

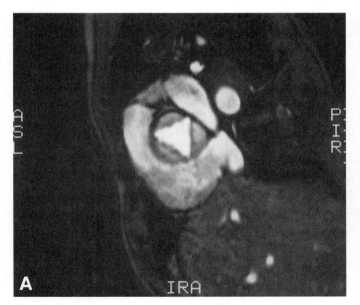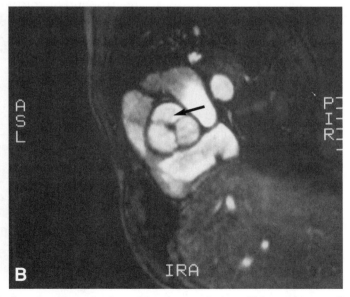

Fig. 17. Short-axis views through the level of the aortic valve demonstrate a trileaflet valve. The patient has mild aortic regurgitation, which results in a small area of signal void caused by a central jet of turbulent flow in diastole (*arrow*).

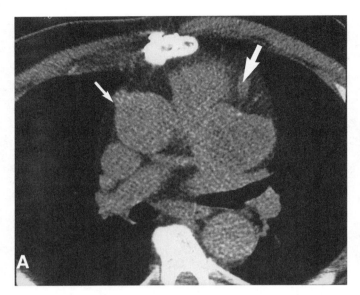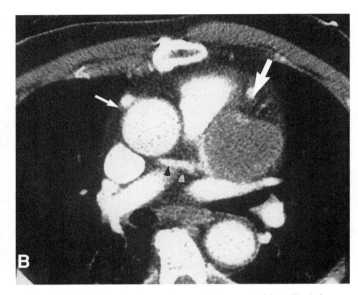

Fig. 18. Computed tomography imaging studies in a 60-year-old man with recurrent angina after three-vessel coronary artery bypass grafting. The left anterior descending coronary artery (*large arrows*) and right coronary grafts (*small arrows*) are patent, as shown by contrast enhancement on computed tomography images (*A* and *B*). The graft to an obtuse marginal vessel (*arrowheads*) is patent proximally but leads to a mass. The high signal centrally in the mass establishes the diagnosis of thrombus, likely in a pseudoaneurysm. (From Giuliani ER, Gersh BJ, McGoon MD, Hayes DL, Schaff HV [editors]: *Mayo Clinic Practice of Cardiology*. Third edition. Mosby, 1996, p 294. By permission of Mayo Foundation.)

measurement of left and right ventricular muscle masses. Additionally, regional and global systolic and diastolic function can be determined. Applications of changes in global and regional systolic wall thickening and ejection fraction during exercise have been reported. As with MRI, congenital heart disease, aortic disease (including aneurysms and dissections), abnormalities of the pericardium (including constriction and effusion), and intracardiac and extracardiac masses, tumors, and thrombi can be visualized. The abilities to identify and quantify discrete calcified coronary artery plaque were recently demonstrated for EBCT using thin high-spatial-resolution tomograms, and this method is of value for diagnosing asymptomatic coronary artery plaque. By quantification of the extent of calcification (calcium score), EBCT recently was shown to offer prognostic information regarding future cardiac events. Increased calcium scores correlate with overall plaque burden and future cardiac events in patients younger than 70 years. Calcium scores are not predictive of individual stenosis severity or anatomical location. This unique application for EBCT does not require the use of contrast media and thus can be done in virtually all subjects. Although coronary calcium can be seen on conventional and spiral CT examinations of the heart, these two methods, because of lack of electrocardiographic gating, are not able to adequately quantify the extent of calcified plaque.

Both EBCT and spiral CT are excellent for identifying proximal pulmonary artery emboli, and EBCT also may allow for evaluation of pulmonary blood flow in a manner analogous to measurement of myocardial and renal blood flow.

In preliminary studies, EBCT and spiral CT have been shown to facilitate, with appropriate three-dimensional reconstruction methods, the production of great vessel, peripheral, and coronary CT angiograms. EBCT can accurately assess the patency of bypass grafts.

Conventional CT, spiral CT, and EBCT all have clear clinical applications for diagnosing and following acute and chronic aortic dissections or aneurysms. These methods offer complete definition of other potentially involved vessels, such as the brachiocephalic trunk and the renal and splanchnic arteries (Fig. 19 through 28).

- The abilities to identify and quantify discrete calcified coronary artery plaque were recently demonstrated for EBCT using thin high-spatial-resolution tomograms. This method is of value for diagnosing asymptomatic coronary artery plaque and for identifying patients at risk for future cardiac events, especially patients with diabetes.

Limitations of CT Scanning

The major limitations of CT are the necessity for radiation exposure and, in most circumstances, the need for intravascular contrast media. Thus, the method is relatively

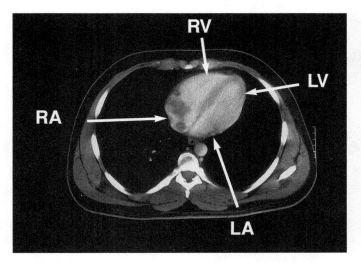

Fig. 19. Horizontal long-axis x-ray computed tomography image demonstrates a filling defect in the right atrium (RA). This filling defect is a right atrial myxoma. LA, left atrium posteriorly; LV, left ventricle laterally; RV, right ventricle anteriorly.

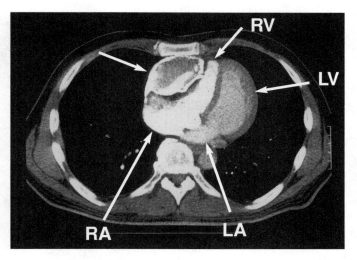

Fig. 20. Horizontal long-axis computed tomography image demonstrates a heavily calcified mass (*arrows*) compressing the right ventricle (RV). This mass resulted in obstruction to right ventricular outflow. The mass is a large, calcified pericardial cyst. LA, left atrium; LV, left ventricle; RA, right atrium.

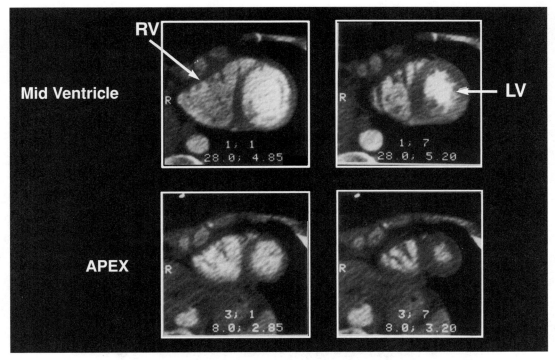

Fig. 21. Multilevel short-axis electron beam computed tomography images at end-diastole (left) and end-systole (right) in a 21-year-old woman with arrhythmogenic right ventricular dysplasia. The left ventricle (LV) is normal in size and function. The right ventricle (RV) is dilated and distorted and has prominent trabeculations consistent with fatty infiltration.

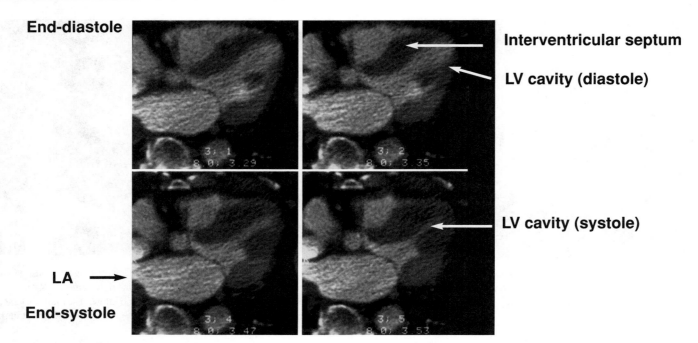

Fig. 22. Sequential vertical long-axis images using electron beam computed tomography at end-diastole and end-systole in a patient with hypertrophic cardiomyopathy. Note that the interventricular septum is hypertrophied and the overall left ventricular (LV) cavity is small and nearly obliterates (hyper-ejection fraction) with contraction. LA, left atrium.

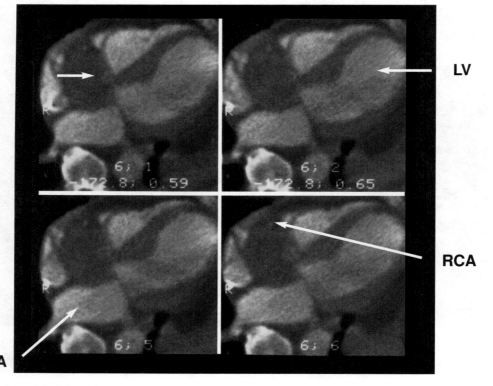

Fig. 23. Long-axis images at base of the left ventricle (LV) demonstrate a mass (*arrow*) compressing the area of the left ventricular outflow tract. This non-contrast-enhancing (and thus nonvascular) structure is an aortic root abscess. It is shown encroaching on the mid-portion of the right coronary artery (RCA). LA, left atrium.

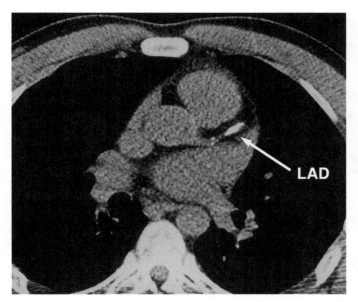

Fig. 24. Noncontrast, thin-slice electron beam computed tomography scan at base of the heart demonstrates dense coronary artery calcification in the proximal portion of the left anterior descending (LAD) coronary artery. There also is some moderate calcification in the distal portion of the left main coronary artery. This relatively extensive coronary calcification was associated with advanced coronary disease at coronary arteriography.

in particular, for pediatric applications does not require sedation, as is necessary with MRI and conventional CT.

Examination Strategy

MRI and CT images have all been shown in the Cardiology Boards. The clinical applications and limitations of the imaging techniques are stressed in the examination. MRI and CT images of aortic dissections, pericardial disease, cardiac tumors, and thrombi should be reviewed. Advanced images of complex congenital heart disease are unlikely to be shown. An important examination issue is knowledge of metallic devices that render MRI an unsafe procedure. The role of detection of coronary calcium by EBCT is controversial but may be included on the examination.

Images of CT and MRI studies that would be reasonable to use for Cardiology Board questions are included in the following pages. These studies include 1) pericardial disease (constrictive pericarditis, pericardial cyst, pericardial effusion), 2) cardiac tumors (intramural or intracavitary), 3) aortic disease (coarctation or dissection), 4) non-complex congenital heart disease (ventricular septal defect), 5) vascular disease (abdominal aortic aneurysm, renal artery disease, cerebrovascular disease), 6) myocardial disease (aneurysms, infarction, right ventricular dysplasia, hypertrophic obstructive cardiomyopathy), 7) coronary calcification, and 8) bypass graft patency.

contraindicated in most patients with a significantly increased creatinine level or in patients with allergy to contrast media. The advantages, especially with EBCT, are that image quality is almost uniformly excellent and scanning can be accomplished rapidly. Thus, scanning in patients who are ill or,

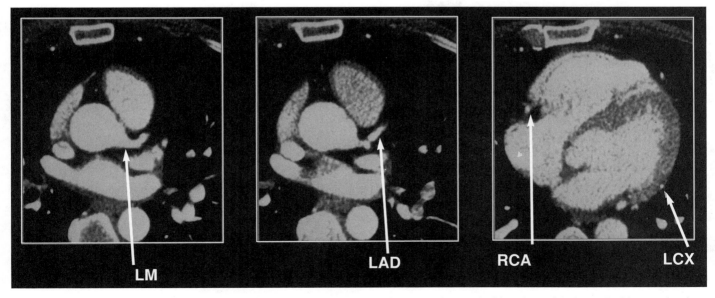

Fig. 25. Serial, contrast-enhanced, thin-section electron beam computed tomography scans at base and mid-portions of the heart. In this normal patient, patency of all major epicardial coronary arteries is noted. LM, left main coronary artery; LAD, left anterior descending coronary artery; RCA, mid-right coronary artery; LCX, mid-left circumflex coronary artery.

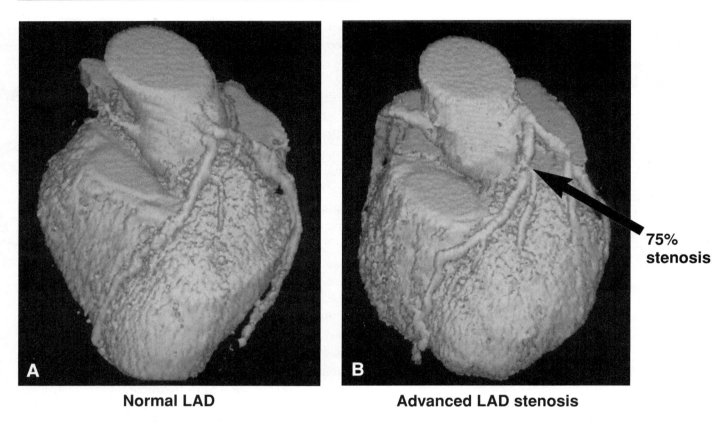

Normal LAD   **Advanced LAD stenosis**

Fig. 26. Three-dimensional coronary arteriography performed with a shaded surface projection method from intravenous contrast-enhanced, thin-section imaging using electron beam computed tomography. *A*, Normal coronary arteriogram. *B*, Stenosis of left anterior descending (LAD) coronary artery.

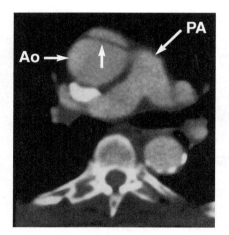

Fig. 27. Contrast-enhanced x-ray computed tomography scan at base of the aorta (Ao). There is a large dissection (*arrow*) of the proximal aorta (aortic type A dissection). PA, pulmonary artery.

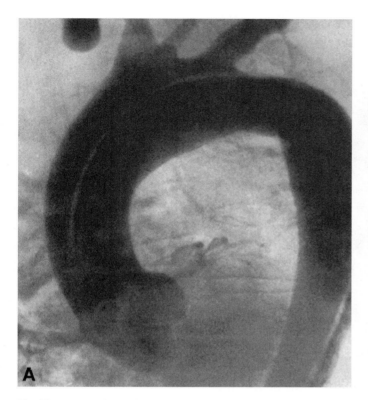
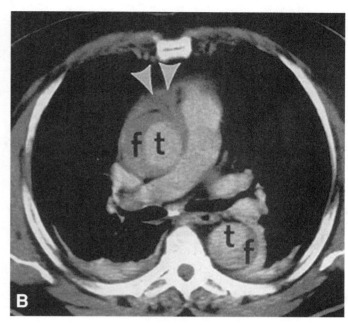

Fig. 28. *A*, A nondiagnostic aortogram in a patient with a dissection. *B*, Computed tomography shows the dissection. Note the presence of the dissection in both the ascending and the descending aortic sections, which is not appreciated on the single-view aortogram. *Arrowheads* show a small mediastinal hematoma. f, false lumen; t, true lumen. (From Lindsay J Jr [editor]: *Diseases of the Aorta.* Lea & Febiger, 1994, p 213. By permission of Williams & Wilkins.)

Suggested Review Reading

1. Globits S, Higgins CB: Assessment of valvular heart disease by magnetic resonance imaging. *Am Heart J* 129:369-381, 1995.
Discusses the "natural" contrast of MRI for assessing both regurgitant and stenotic valves and the developing method of measuring blood flow velocities, similar to what is done with Doppler echocardiography.

2. Greaves SM, Hart EM, Aberle DR: CT of pulmonary thromboembolism. *Semin Ultrasound CT MR* 18:323-337, 1997.
Discusses applications of spiral and EBCT for evaluation of pulmonary embolism, citing advantages over ventilation-perfusion scanning as a means to augment or supplant pulmonary angiography.

3. Hartiala J, Knuuti J: Imaging of the heart by MRI and PET. *Ann Med* 27:35-45, 1995.
Discusses the role of MRI as an adjunct to currently available heart tests. Also comments on the evolving role of PET in cardiac studies.

4. Reichek N: Magnetic resonance imaging for assessment of myocardial function. *Magn Reson Q* 7:255-274, 1991.
Discusses in some detail the premise that MRI can be used to perform all manner of studies for ventricular function. It provides an excellent background. Be aware, however, that many of these studies still remain difficult to do with MRI, although there is promise that this will change in the future.

5. Rumberger JA: Quantifying left ventricular regional and global systolic function using ultrafast computed tomography. *Am J Card Imaging* 5:29-37, 1991.
Review of the applications of ultrafast (now called electron beam) CT for evaluation of left and right ventricular volumes, muscle mass, and function.

6. Rumberger JA, Sheedy PF II, Breen JF, Fitzpatrick LA, Schwartz RS: Electron beam computed tomography and coronary artery disease: scanning for coronary artery calcification. *Mayo Clin Proc* 71:369-377, 1996.
Review of literature on clinical applications of EBCT scanning for calcium.

7. Rumberger JA, Simons DB, Fitzpatrick LA, Sheedy PF, Schwartz RS: Coronary artery calcium area by electron-beam computed tomography and coronary atherosclerotic plaque area. A histopathologic correlative study. *Circulation* 92:2157-2162, 1995.
Report evaluating the measurement of coronary calcium area by EBCT with histologic plaque areas. Key points are that not all plaque has calcium, but that calcium provides a surrogate estimation for total coronary atherosclerotic plaque burden.

8. Schmermund A, Bell MR, Lerman LO, Ritman EL, Rumberger JA: Quantitative evaluation of regional myocardial perfusion using fast X-ray computed tomography. *Herz* 22:29-39, 1997.
Reviews applications of EBCT for assessment of regional myocardial perfusion.

9. Shapiro EP: Magnetic resonance imaging of the heart: a cardiologist's viewpoint. *Top Magn Reson Imaging* 2:1-12, 1990.
Early review of MRI and its potential for the future.

10. Tempany CM, Zerhouni EA: Clinical magnetic resonance imaging of the vascular system. *Top Magn Reson Imaging* 2:13-30, 1990.
Expands on the concepts presented in the article by Shapiro with regard to imaging of the blood vessels. Peripheral MRI vascular imaging (called MRA) has assumed a leading role for evaluation of the carotid arteries, cerebrovascular system, and peripheral vascular system.

11. Wexler L, Higgins CB, Herfkens RJ: Magnetic resonance imaging in adult congenital heart disease. *J Thorac Imaging* 9:219-229, 1994.
One area that MRI has excelled in, mainly because of the difficulties with at least transthoracic echocardiography, has been in the assessment of complex congenital heart disease.

Questions

Multiple Choice (choose the one best answer)

1. These magnetic resonance imaging (MRI) scans (top, transverse cardiac; bottom left, sagittal; bottom right, coronal) show the following abnormality:
   a. Metastatic tumor to the pericardium
   b. Left atrial myxoma
   c. Right atrial myxoma
   d. Cor triatriatum

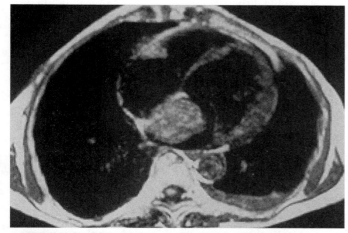

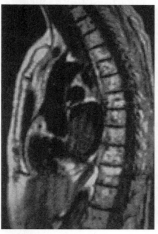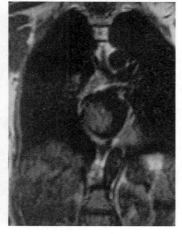

Question 1

2. MRI of the heart is contraindicated in which of the following clinical situations?
   a. Presence of a Björk-Shiley mitral valve prosthesis
   b. Presence of a Carpentier-Edwards mitral valve prosthesis
   c. Intracoronary stent
   d. Prior cerebral aneurysm operation with residual clips
   e. Atrioventricular sequential pacemaker

3. A 75-year-old man with long-standing hypertension and cigarette usage is brought to the emergency department after a motor vehicle accident. There is a question of possible cervical spine trauma, and he is wearing a cervical collar. He has abdominal pain and nausea. Although his oxygenation is adequate, the patient is confused and thrashing about. Sedation is necessary, an orotracheal tube is inserted for airway protection, and the patient is mechanically ventilated. The blood pressure is 190/100 mm Hg, the heart rate is 95 beats/min, and the pulse is bounding in the right brachial artery but less prominent in the left brachial artery. His complexion is ruddy, but the femoral and peripheral pulses are not palpable and the extremities are cool. A portable chest radiograph shows hyperlucent lung fields that are generally clear, proper placement of the orotracheal tube, and an enlarged aorta and mediastinum. He has an increased anterior-posterior chest dimension, and the heart sounds are soft and best appreciated in the subxiphoid area. There are no murmurs. An electrocardiogram shows left ventricular hypertrophy and diffuse T-wave inversion but no ST-segment elevation. You make a presumptive diagnosis of aortic dissection and decide to order an additional test to confirm the diagnosis. The patient has no known allergies. Baseline serum chemistry values are normal. The imaging method of choice is:
   a. A transthoracic two-dimensional echocardiographic examination
   b. A transesophageal two-dimensional echocardiographic examination
   c. MRI of the thorax and abdomen
   d. Computed axial (x-ray) tomography (CT) examination of the chest and abdomen with and without contrast

4. A 43-year-old black woman is referred for consultation. She has sharp, nonradiating central chest pain at variable times during the day. It can come on at rest and may be relieved with food, but she also has had it when climbing stairs. She has moderate dyspnea on exertion, which is also new. The chest pain has been present for the past 6 months and has had some increase in frequency, especially within the past 2 weeks. She smokes about 10 cigarettes per day and has done so for 15 years. She is an accountant and has had significant job-related mental stress recently. Her mother has diabetes and high blood pressure at age 65 years. Her father died of a "coronary" at age 58. She has one brother, age 35, who has hypertension. Her total cholesterol value is 235

mg/dL, triglyceride value is 200 mg/dL, and high-density lipoprotein is 33 mg/dL. Her serum chemistry values are otherwise normal. Electrocardiography (ECG) shows an incomplete left bundle branch block with normal sinus rhythm. She has never had a prior ECG. A chest radiograph had shown a borderline enlarged heart and a question of some fullness in the upper mediastinum, and her internist ordered an electron beam computed tomography (EBCT) chest examination. The patient is referred for further evaluation. The mediastinum and lungs were normal by EBCT, and a tomogram from the base of the heart is shown in the figure below. On physical examination she is obese (weight, 90 kg). She has a large anteroposterior diameter and large breasts, but the lungs are clear. There are no abnormalities in jugular venous pulsations. The heart sounds are distant, but there are no murmurs or gallops. All peripheral pulses are intact and normal. After review of the history, physical examination, CT, ECG, and laboratory data, you would do which of the following?

a. Perform a routine treadmill exercise examination
b. Advise the patient that coronary angiography is necessary
c. Perform a stress thallium test
d. Advise on a weight-reduction, low-cholesterol diet. Reassure the patient that the pain is not cardiac in origin

5. A 65-year-old man with no known history of cardiac or vascular disease has been hospitalized for a moderate-sized left hemispheric cerebrovascular accident. You are called for consultation regarding a possible cardiac source for embolism. Carotid ultrasonography showed only minimal plaque in both carotid arteries. The referring doctor had requested a transthoracic echocardiogram, which showed a normal-appearing proximal aorta, an enlarged left ventricle, moderate left atrial enlargement, no right-to-left shunting, and no apparent cardiac thrombosis. The sonographer noted, however, that the examination was difficult and that the left ventricular apex was not well seen. You order an EBCT examination with contrast. The tomographic images confirm the enlarged left and right ventricles. All four pulmonary veins are well seen, as is the left atrium, and there is no apparent thrombosis. The image shown below is from a mid-ventricular tomographic level with imaging done in the neutral (transverse cardiac) plane. You recommend the following:

a. No further testing and no additional medications
b. Further testing with biplane transesophageal echocardiography
c. No further testing, but you request that aspirin be added to the patient's medications and that a stress test be performed
d. Initial warfarin therapy and further cardiac workup as an outpatient

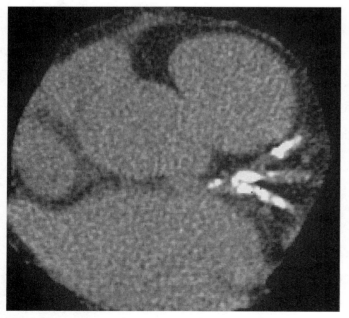

Question 4

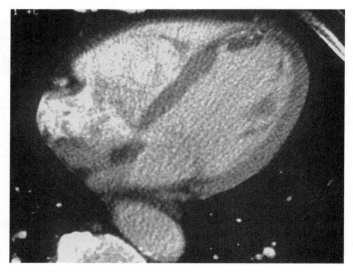

Question 5

6. A 60-year-old Hispanic man is referred for cardiac consultation because of progressive exertional dyspnea and peripheral edema during the past 3 months. He has a past history of crescendo angina, coronary angiography, and coronary bypass grafting performed 6 months previously. Preoperatively, he had a left ventricular ejection fraction of 60% and no regional wall motion abnormalities as assessed by echocardiography. He had a brief episode of atrial fibrillation after operation but has not had angina since. He is currently taking a β-adrenergic blocker and aspirin on a daily basis. Rehabilitation has been slow, and he has been able to perform only 1 to 2 minutes on a treadmill in the cardiovascular health clinic before he stops because of dyspnea. He denies orthopnea and paroxysmal nocturnal dyspnea. His major concern is the development of some ankle edema, worse on the leg from which the saphenous vein was harvested. On physical examination, he has soft heart sounds with an S_4 and a mid-systolic murmur with radiation to the axilla. His lungs show scattered crackles, mostly at the bases, and he has 15 cm H_2O jugular venous pressure at a 45° angle with a slight increase in venous pressure with deep inspiration. The liver span is increased, and there is some right upper quadrant tenderness. It is difficult to assess whether there is a hepatojugular reflux due to the increased jugular venous pressure. You obtain a spiral CT examination of the chest. The figure shows non-contrast CTs at several midcardiac levels. You decide that left and right heart catheterization is necessary. Which of the following hemodynamic factors would be most consistent with the clinical history and the CT images?

a. LVEF 45%; LVEDP 30 mm Hg; RVEDP 25 mm Hg; RAP 23 mm Hg
b. LVEF 65%; LVEDP 12 mm Hg; RVEDP 12 mm Hg; RAP 12 mm Hg
c. LVEF 45%; LVEDP 20 mm Hg; RVEDP 30 mm Hg; RAP 32 mm Hg
d. LVEF 65%; LVEDP 28 mm Hg; RVEDP 28 mm Hg; RAP 29 mm Hg
(LVEF, left ventricular ejection fraction; LVEDP, left ventricular end-diastolic pressure; RVEDP, right ventricular end-diastolic pressure; RAP, right atrial pressure)

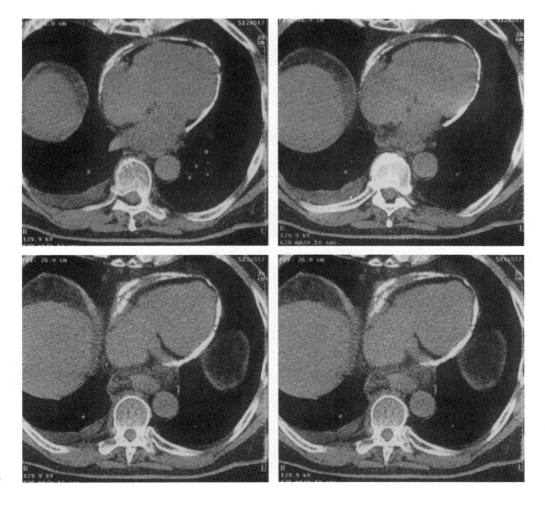

Question 6

7. A 47-year-old white male accountant is referred to the cardiovascular health clinic for advice on an exercise program. He has not done regular exercise for the past 10 years and now wants to lose weight and "get in shape." He has an extensive family history of coronary artery disease; his 50-year-old brother recently had a coronary artery bypass procedure, and his father died after a myocardial infarction at age 49. The patient himself has no known cardiac history and was a competitive athlete in high school and college. He is a vegetarian and avoids animal fats of any kind. He does not smoke. On examination his weight is 91 kg and his height is 5 feet 9 inches. There are no abnormalities on cardiac or pulmonary examination. Baseline laboratory testing shows normal serum chemistry values: total cholesterol, 210 mg/dL; triglycerides, 120 mg/dL; high-density lipoprotein, 38 mg/dL; and low-density lipoprotein, 169 mg/dL. You perform a monitored, graded stress test to assess his cardiovascular performance before designing an exercise program. He exercises to 7 METs with a total time of 11 minutes and stage III on a modified protocol. ECG is normal at rest and normal at peak stress with a maximal heart rate of 155 beats/min and a systolic blood pressure of 120 mm Hg at rest and 175 mm Hg at peak exercise. The testing is stopped because of fatigue. A chest radiograph previously ordered by his referring internist had shown a vague, solitary, 1-cm nodule in the left lung field, and an EBCT examination was ordered to assess the nodule. You have all examinations for review. The lung nodule is not seen on the EBCT, and the remainder of the lungs and mediastinum are normal. The figure shows a representative image from the EBCT examination at the base of the heart. You recommend which of the following?

a. Reassurance, an exercise program with aim of weight loss, continue a low-fat diet

b. Reassurance, an exercise program with aim of weight loss. Prescribe an HmG Co-A reductase inhibitor with aim of achieving a low-density lipoprotein value less than 120 mg/dL. Recheck the lipid values in 1 to 2 months

c. Advise him not to start an exercise program at this time and refer him for stress/perfusion imaging

d. Refer him for coronary angiography

8. Some metallic medical devices may dislocate or heat in the magnetic field of MRI. Which of the following metallic devices is generally regarded as a contraindication to MRI scanning of the heart?

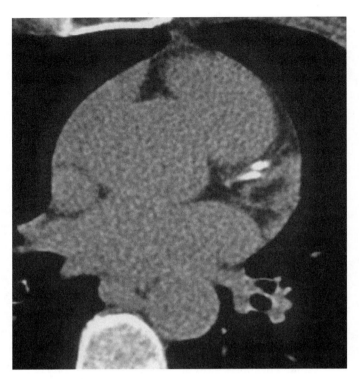

Question 7

a. Prosthetic hip
b. St. Jude heart valve
c. Cerebral aneurysm clip
d. Ureteric stent

9. Which one of the following heart valves is considered more ferromagnetic than the others and therefore presents a hypothetical risk of dislocation or heating during MRI of the heart in a patient with suspected valve dehiscence?

a. Starr-Edwards pre-6000 series (caged ball)
b. St. Jude (bileaflet valve)
c. Björk-Shiley (tilting disk valve)
d. Medtronic-Hall (tilting disk valve)

10. You placed a metallic Palmaz-Schatz stent in the proximal left anterior descending coronary artery in a patient 1 month ago. Now you are asked by a colleague in neurology whether the patient can undergo non-emergency MRI of the head, scheduled for today. You should answer:

a. Only if the MRI scanning is an emergency procedure
b. Ideally, never perform MRI for this patient
c. Imaging can be done in 6 months, when the stent is completely endothelialized
d. Yes, go ahead and image today

11. A 54-year-old woman presents to the outpatient clinic after referral from her internist for evaluation of "congestive heart failure." She has had progressive dyspnea since age 52. Before that date, she had no significant history of cardiac or pulmonary disease. She is postmenopausal and has had estrogen replacement for several years. She has an increased jugular venous pressure with a v wave and no respiratory variation. The lungs show distant breath sounds but are generally clear. There is an S₃ gallop at the sternal border, a holosystolic murmur at the base of the heart, and a parasternal heave. She has 3+ bilateral pitting edema to the thighs, and they are tender. On careful examination you believe you feel a venous "cord" in the left thigh, which is moderately greater in circumference than in the right thigh. She has a pectus deformity and is claustrophobic. The serum creatinine value is mildly increased at 1.1 mg/dL. You order an EBCT examination of the left and right ventricles. Shown below is a single image taken at the mid-heart. C, coronary sinus; IVC, inferior vena cava; LV, left ventricle; RA, right atrium; RV, right ventricle. What is the likely diagnosis?
    a. Idiopathic dilated cardiomyopathy
    b. Isolated right ventricular failure due to severe tricuspid valve incompetence
    c. Chronic pulmonary embolism syndrome with right heart failure and pulmonary hypertension
    d. Myocardial infarction with predominant right ventricular involvement and failure

12. A coronary calcification score of 100 Hounsfield units on an Imatron-computed tomography (CT) scan in an asymptomatic 50-year-old man indicates all of the following *except*:
    a. The calcification is likely located in the proximal coronary arteries
    b. The patient is in the 75th percentile (more calcium than 75% of men his age) for coronary calcification
    c. Occlusion of at least one coronary artery is likely
    d. Risk factor modification might slow progression of coronary calcification

13. A patient with which of the following pacing devices can be safely placed in an MRI scanner?
    a. DDD, not pacemaker-dependent
    b. VVI, not pacemaker-dependent
    c. Implantable cardioverter-difibrillator
    d. None of the above
    e. All of the above

14. A patient with renal failure (creatinine, 3.4 mg/dL) and thrombocytopenia (platelet count, 35,000 mm³) presents with a pericardial effusion. You are concerned about a paracardiac malignancy and would like to characterize the pericardial effusion further. What would be the best method of evaluating this possibility?
    a. Transesophageal echocardiography (TEE)
    b. Electron beam computed tomography (EBCT)
    c. Magnetic resonance imaging (MRI)
    d. Pericardial tap

15. Which of the following imaging methods has a clinically acceptable sensitivity in the diagnosis of proximal pulmonary emboli?
    a. EBCT
    b. "Breath-hold" MRI
    c. Transesophageal echocardiography (TEE)
    d. Contrast transthoracic echocardiography
    e. All of the above

16. Compared with EBCT, radioisotope perfusion-ventilation scanning performed for the diagnosis of pulmonary embolus:
    a. Has low specificity for pulmonary emboli
    b. Readily detects right heart thrombus
    c. Is more likely to be of intermediate probability in chronic obstructive pulmonary disease
    d. Is hazardous in a patient with renal failure

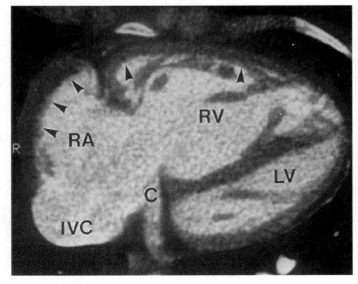

Question 11

17. A 65-year-old man with a known ascending thoracic aortic aneurysm (5 cm) and a bicuspid aortic valve is being followed on a yearly basis by a referring physician. The most recent transthoracic echocardiogram shows an increase in the diameter of the aneurysm to 5.8 cm. The patient is referred to you for further evaluation. You want to confirm the results of the echocardiogram. You should consider ordering:
    a. CT
    b. MRI with contrast (Magnevist)
    c. Transesophageal echocardiography (TEE)
    d. Any of the above

18. Which statement about cardiac MRI is true?
    a. Prosthetic heart valves heat excessively from radio-frequency exposure during MRI
    b. Prosthetic valves cause image artifact that prevents adequate visualization of most other cardiac structures
    c. Placed in the wrong position, ECG electrodes often burn the patient's skin during MRI scanning
    d. Pacemaker wires may heat excessively in an MRI scanner

19. A 40-year-old woman presents with progressive dyspnea, initially with effort and now at rest. There is some mild cyanosis, a pansystolic murmur, and a loud P_2. Refer to the accompanying MRI scans (see below) from the mid-ventricular level (top) and at the level of the root of the pulmonary artery (bottom). Ao, aorta; LV, left ventricle; PA, pulmonary artery; RA, right atrium; RV, right ventricle. What is the diagnosis?
    a. Chronic pulmonary embolism and right ventricular hypertrophy
    b. Ventricular septal defect with right ventricular hypertrophy
    c. Hypertrophic cardiomyopathy
    d. Obliterative cardiomyopathy

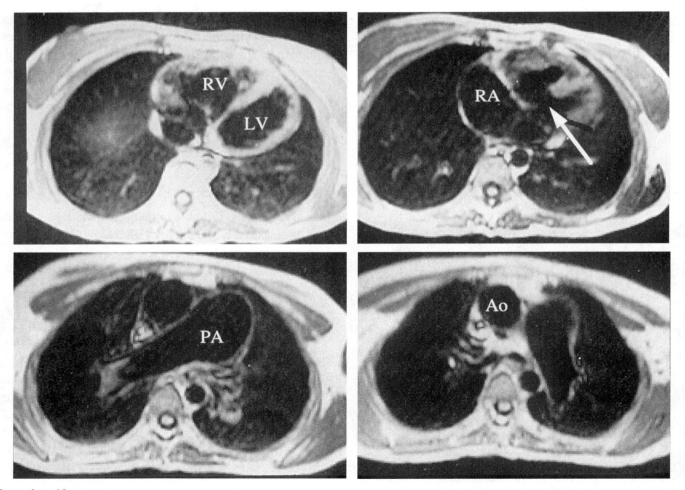

Question 19. (From Duerinckx AJ, Higgins CB, Pettigrew RI [editors]: *MRI of the Cardiovascular System*. Raven Press, 1994, pp 170-171. By permission of the publisher.)

Answers

1. Answer b

The transverse cardiac image for MRI, as with CT, is viewed as if from the patient's feet. Thus, left-sided structures appear on the right side of the image. The left and right ventricular and both atrial chambers are well seen. This is a left atrial myxoma that is attached at the interventricular septum.

2. Answer e

Mechanical cardiac valves, the C-ring support structures for tissue valves, coronary stents, and modern-day aneurysm clips are made of nonferrous material and are not contraindications to MRI. However, if there is a question of valve dehiscence, then MRI is relatively contraindicated. Permanent and temporary pacemakers and implantable defibrillator devices are contraindications.

3. Answer d

A transthoracic echocardiographic examination, especially in a patient with chronic obstructive pulmonary disease, is inadequate to examine the aorta. A transesophageal echocardiographic examination is contraindicated if there is a possibility of cervical damage or unknown esophageal or gastric conditions. MRI is not possible in acutely ill patients or patients requiring mechanical ventilation. The most rapid means to assess the entire aorta in a patient with no allergy to contrast media is x-ray CT.

4. Answer b

This young woman has coronary atherosclerosis with extensive calcification of the proximal left anterior descending coronary artery, as seen on the EBCT examination and according to symptoms consistent with angina. Although its presence may not necessarily correspond to the extent of coronary stenoses, this amount of calcium is consistent with advanced disease. A treadmill test would not be best because she already has an abnormal ECG. Thallium/stress imaging may not improve the diagnostic yield because left bundle branch block can be associated with false-positive abnormalities in the interventricular septum. An adenosine or dipyridamole thallium test would be a viable alternative, but these are not listed as choices. The patient requires further evaluation. From the constellation of findings, coronary angiography would be the most efficient and probably cost-effective means to make the diagnosis.

5. Answer d

The mid-ventricular EBCT examination shows an area of calcification at the apex of the heart and a large, nonenhancing, low-density object within the chamber of the left ventricle, at the apex. This represents a left ventricular apical thrombosis. The presence of calcium indicates that the patient may well have had a prior infarction at the apex with potential for aneurysm formation. Unless absolutely contraindicated, this patient requires initiation of warfarin with an international normalized ratio (INR) of approximately 3.0. Because there was no prior diagnosis of heart disease, further cardiac workup as an outpatient for occult ischemic disease is needed after recovery from the acute stroke.

6. Answer d

This patient has some features consistent with congestive heart failure, pulmonary venous hypertension, and possibly right-sided failure. However, the CT examination shows nondilated left and right ventricles with extensive calcification and thickening of the entire pericardium. Given that his ventricular function was normal preoperatively and there have been no additional ischemic events, it is likely that his left ventricular ejection fraction has remained normal. This patient has clinical and CT features that are consistent with constrictive pericardial disease, normal left ventricular ejection fraction, and increased pressures of the right and left ventricles that equilibrate at end-diastole. In this patient, constrictive pericarditis has developed as a complication of prior cardiac operation.

7. Answer b

This man has a significant family history of premature coronary artery disease but has relatively average lipid values. The presence of moderate amounts of coronary calcification in the left anterior descending coronary artery by EBCT confirms that he has coronary atherosclerosis. However, despite the presence of coronary calcium, he has no symptoms and the physiologic testing suggests that there is no associated ischemia; thus, he should be allowed to enter an exercise program. With a low-density lipoprotein value of 160 mg/dL, given his spartan eating habits, it is unlikely that it can be decreased sufficiently by altering an already healthful diet. In the face of proven heart disease, a low-density lipoprotein value less than 100 is recommended. In the absence of cardiac symptoms, the additional expense of a stress/perfusion scan is not warranted. Likewise, in the absence of any evidence for stress-induced ischemia, coronary angiography is not indicated.

8. Answer c

A prosthetic hip is made of titanium or cobalt-chromium alloy and has no significant ferromagnetic properties. It does not heat and is not significantly magnetic. It may create a large image artifact in the hip on MRI. The St. Jude valve and ureteric stent are also made of nonferromagnetic materials and can be scanned with MRI. They may produce a small image artifact. Although most likely safe, cerebral aneurysm clips should be tested in a magnet before implantation. Made of nonferromagnetic materials, shaping during manufacture can induce some magnetism, and the clip may torque in an MRI scanner. Also, because displacement of an aneurysm clip could be fatal, it is imperative to confirm that the metal used is indeed nonmagnetic, as indicated on the device package insert. A patient's operative record also should confirm that the aneurysm clip used is rated nonferromagnetic.

9. Answer a

The risk of displacement of the Starr-Edwards pre-6000 series valve is hypothetical. This valve shows more magnetism than any other implanted valve, but it is still quite small. All other bioprosthetic and mechanical valves can be imaged in an MRI system. Artifact occurs around the valve, making it impossible to assess the structure of the valve with MRI.

10. Answer d

Patients with coronary artery stents can be safely imaged in an MRI scanner. A small artifact occurs in the coronary artery. There is no evidence of significant heating. Some manufacturers recommend that MRI be withheld in patients with stents for varying periods of time. Practically, these recommendations are unneeded, and MRI is safe immediately after stent placement.

11. Answer c

This woman has been dyspneic since estrogen replacement therapy was started. She has physical examination findings that could suggest deep venous thrombosis. Results of her cardiac examination could represent various problems, including tricuspid regurgitation and other causes of pulmonary hypertension. The EBCT image, however, demonstrates a small left ventricular cavity, a D-shaped interventricular septum, a dilated and hypertrophied right ventricle and right atrium, and a dilated inferior vena cava. The constellation of these findings strongly suggests a chronic pulmonary embolism syndrome with severe pulmonary hypertension.

12. Answer c

Often the calcium is located in the proximal coronary arteries. Normal calcium scores have been established at Mayo Clinic for sex and age. This patient has more calcium than 75% of men his age. A significant (50% diameter narrowing) stenosis is likely (sensitivity and specificity 85%), but severe coronary artery disease occurs with higher scores (> 400). Although further research is required, the calcium score likely can be modified by aggressive risk factor modification.

13. Answer d

It is generally accepted that, ideally, no patient with a pacemaker should be placed in an MRI scanner. However, in an emergency, MRI may be possible in a patient with a pacemaker, especially if the patient is not pacemaker-dependent. After the pacemaker is turned off, an assistant located in the magnet room with the patient should monitor the patient's pulse. This monitoring is necessary because the radio-frequency signal applied during imaging distorts the electrocardiographic signal. The pacemaker should be checked when the patient comes out of the magnet. For a pacemaker-dependent patient, it might be possible to switch the pacemaker to the asynchronous mode above the patient's usual heart rate before imaging. By doing this, inhibition and triggering of the pacemaker by the radio-frequency pulse can be averted.

14. Answer c

TEE does not completely visualize structures around the heart, where one might expect to see a malignancy. EBCT requires a contrast agent, and this may worsen the patient's renal function. Like EBCT, MRI has a wide window of view and is useful for the detection of paracardiac masses but does not require nephrotoxic contrast. Bleeding may occur with pericardial tap in this patient.

15. Answer a

Breath-hold MRI is not sufficiently reliable to be recommended for routine clinical use. TEE does not adequately visualize all of the proximal pulmonary arteries. An exogenously administered echocardiographic contrast agent enhances visualization of pulmonary arteries, but the acoustical window is frequently inadequate in this region.

16. Answer c

A report indicating a high probability for the presence or absence of pulmonary embolus on perfusion-ventilation lung scanning is about as reliable as EBCT. However, EBCT is not significantly affected by lung disease, and therefore a report of intermediate probability for pulmonary embolus is much less likely by EBCT. Unfortunately, EBCT requires a contrast agent, which is toxic in patients with renal failure.

17. Answer d

All the tests listed provide good visualization of the ascending aorta. TEE may overall be the least reliable, although in experienced hands it should be as good as CT and MRI. An MRI study should include contrast images for visualization of the lumen and standard spin-echo images to visualize the wall of the aorta.

18. Answer d

Prosthetic heart valves are not known to heat excessively during MRI. Although valves cause image artifact, it is generally localized around a valve, and the chambers of the heart and the ascending aorta can be readily seen. Although it is possible to burn a patient with an electrocardiography electrode, this is rare. Pacemaker wires have been shown to heat in in vitro studies. Because pacemakers are considered a contraindication to MRI, whether this is clinically significant is unclear. Temporary pacemaker wires placed at cardiac operation should be removed before MRI is performed.

19. Answer b

The left ventricle is not dilated. The right ventricle is hypertrophied. There is marked dilatation of the main pulmonary artery and right and left main pulmonary arteries. The interventricular septum appears to be intact in the mid-ventricular tomogram at top left, but the top right tomogram, representing a level immediately caudad, has a clear signal void in the region of the interventricular septum. This represents a large membranous ventricular septal defect that resulted in right ventricular pressure overload and likely pulmonary hypertension and pulmonary artery dilatation.

Notes

Chapter 47

Echocardiography for Boards

Sharonne N. Hayes, M.D.
Fletcher A. Miller, Jr., M.D.

This chapter addresses aspects of echocardiography that are important for the Cardiology Examinations. Intravascular echocardiography is reviewed in the chapter on coronary artery physiology. Knowledge of echocardiography is tested in several ways in the Cardiology Examinations. You will be asked to identify two-dimensional or Doppler still frame images and/or to use the image to guide clinical decision making. Be aware of the relative strengths, weaknesses, and incremental value of information obtained by different echocardiographic methods in order to best answer questions involving choices of optimal diagnostic evaluations.

The American College of Cardiology, American Heart Association, and the American Society of Echocardiography have developed and published practice guidelines for the use of echocardiography. These guidelines make recommendations about the appropriate (indicated) and inappropriate use of echocardiography. Familiarity with these guidelines is recommended. The inappropriate use of echocardiography for "screening" in patients in whom the information will be redundant (ejection fraction previously measured by left ventriculography) or will not change management ("ruling out" mitral valve prolapse in a patient without signs or symptoms of mitral valve prolapse) is not only cost-ineffective, it will negatively affect your board score. The guidelines divide indications into categories (I, generally indicated; IIa, conflicting evidence but in favor of usefulness; IIb, conflicting evidence, less well-established indications; and III, generally thought not to be useful or contraindicated). Some of the class III indications are listed in Table 1.

Transthoracic Echocardiography

Anatomical and functional assessment of cardiac valves, myocardium, and pericardium as well as quantitation of cardiac chamber dimensions, areas, and volumes are important aspects of the echocardiographic examination.

Doppler echocardiography uses the Doppler effect; that is, the frequency of sound waves increases or decreases as the sound source moves toward or away from the observer (Equation 1).

Equation 1.—Frequency Shift (Δf)

$$\Delta f = \frac{2 f_t\, v \cos\theta}{c}$$

Δf = Doppler frequency shift
f_t = transmitted frequency
$\cos\theta$ = (angle theta), angle between the vector of the moving object and interrogating beam
c = (constant), velocity of sound in tissue or water (1,560 m/s)
v = velocity of the moving object

This Doppler frequency shift is detected and translated into a blood flow velocity (Equation 2) by the Doppler transducer and instrument.

Equation 2.—Velocity (v) (m/s)

$$v = \frac{c}{2\cos\theta} \cdot \frac{\Delta f}{f_t}$$

(Definitions as in Equation 1)

The velocity of blood can be used to determine gradients, intracardiac pressures, volumetric flow, and valve areas.

Pulsed-wave and continuous-wave Doppler are the two most commonly used spectral Doppler modalities (Table 2). Pulsed-wave Doppler is "site-specific" and allows the measurement of blood velocities at a particular region of interest. The disadvantage of pulsed-wave Doppler is aliasing of the signal when velocities reach one-half of the pulse repetition frequency, or the Nyquist limit (Fig. 1). This property limits the maximal velocity that can be measured with pulsed-wave Doppler.

Continuous-wave Doppler measures all velocities in the path of the ultrasound beam, is not site-specific, and is not limited by aliasing. The disadvantage of continuous-wave Doppler is that although very high velocities can be recorded, the anatomical site cannot be localized accurately. Continuous-wave Doppler is typically used to measure high-velocity jets and gradients.

Color flow imaging is computer-enhanced pulsed-wave Doppler that displays the velocity and directional information of blood flow. Red depicts blood flow toward the transducer and blue, away from the transducer. Color flow imaging, like pulsed-wave Doppler, has a Nyquist limit and displays aliasing. Color flow imaging is used to detect, localize, and semiquantitate abnormal flow, such as valvular regurgitation, shunts, or intracavitary obstruction.

Transesophageal Echocardiography

Transesophageal echocardiography (TEE) is used intraoperatively, when transthoracic images are poor, or when detailed evaluation of a structure not well seen on transthoracic studies is required, including the left atrial appendage, thoracic aorta, prosthetic valves, pulmonary veins, mitral valve lesions, and congenital heart disease. TEE transducers are generally biplane or multiplane and allow visualization of the heart from the base to the apex and the thoracic aorta from the diaphragm to the aortic valve, depending on the location and plane of the transducer in the esophagus or stomach.

Complications with TEE occur in fewer than 1.0% of patients and include arrhythmias, hypoxia, laryngeal spasm, esophageal tears, and provocation of heart failure. Rare fatalities have been reported. TEE should be performed where resuscitative equipment is available and with continuous electrocardiography, blood pressure, and pulse oxymetric monitoring.

The major abnormalities to identify on TEE examination questions are the following (Fig. 2 to 8):
Left atrial myxoma
Left atrial thrombus
Patent foramen ovale
Spontaneous echo contrast
Ruptured mitral valve chordae/papillary muscle
Aortic dissection
Aortic debris

Stress Echocardiography

Stress echocardiography is based on the concept that left ventricular wall motion (myocardial thickening) is impaired by ischemia. Echocardiography accurately detects both resting and ischemia-induced wall motion abnormalities. Ischemia is induced by exercise or, pharmacologically, by dobutamine, dipyridamole, or adenosine or, at the time of TEE, by atrial pacing. Baseline images and hemodynamic measurements are obtained and repeated immediately

Table 1.—ACC/AHA Guidelines for the Clinical Application of Echocardiography: Conditions for Which Echocardiography Is Usually Not Indicated*

Patients in whom results of echocardiography will have no impact on diagnosis or clinical decision making because of comorbid conditions, patient preferences, etc.

Routine reevaluation of asymptomatic or clinically stable adults with stable signs and symptoms with

    Mild aortic stenosis

    Mild-to-moderate mitral stenosis

    Mild valvular regurgitation

    Mitral valve prolapse with mild mitral regurgitation

    Valve replacements

    Recent myocardial infarction

    Small pericardial effusion

    Right ventricular function and COPD

    Insignificant congenital heart disease (ASD, small VSDs, etc.)

Asymptomatic heart murmur in adult that is thought to be functional by an experienced clinician

"Rule out" mitral valve prolapse in patients with ill-defined symptoms and no history of or physical signs of mitral valve prolapse

"Rule out" endocarditis in patients with fever, a nonpathologic or no murmur, and no bacteremia

"Rule out" prosthetic valve endocarditis in patients with transient fever and no bacteremia

Evaluation of chest pain when a noncardiac cause is apparent

Diagnosis of chest pain/acute myocardial infarction in patients with an electrocardiogram "diagnostic" of myocardial infarction

Patients with edema, normal venous pressure, and no evidence of heart disease

Evaluation of left ventricular ejection fraction in patients with recent contrast or radionuclide determination of ejection fraction

Pericardial friction rub early after uncomplicated myocardial infarction or cardiac surgery

Reevaluation in hypertensive patients to guide antihypertensive therapy based on left ventricular mass regression or to assess left ventricular function in asymptomatic patients

Palpitations without documented arrhythmia or isolated premature ventricular contractions for which there is no clinical suspicion of heart disease

Pre-cardioversion transesophageal echocardiogram

    When cardioversion is required emergently

    Patients receiving long-term therapeutic anticoagulation without mitral valve disease or hypertrophic cardiomyopathy

    Previous negative transesophageal echocardiogram with no clinical suspicion of change

Syncope with no clinical suspicion for heart disease, classic neurogenic syncope, or recurrent syncope with a previously documented cause

Screening for cardiovascular disease in unselected populations or competitive athletes without clinical evidence of heart disease

"Rule out" myocardial contusion in hemodynamically stable patients with a normal electrocardiogram

ACC, American College of Cardiology; AHA, American Heart Association; ASD, atrial septal defect; COPD, chronic obstructive pulmonary disease; VSD, ventricular septal defect.

*It is important to understand the clinical situations in which echocardiography is very helpful and in which it is either not helpful or a poor use of resources. Data from *Circulation* 95:1686-1744, 1997. By permission of the American Heart Association.

after exercise or after each dose of the pharmacologic agent.

Images from several cardiac cycles are digitized and stored, and the best images from multiple views are displayed and compared in quad-screen format. The normal response to exercise is improved (hyperdynamic) left ventricular function and decreased ventricular cavity size (end-systolic volume) (Table 3). The development of a new or the worsening of a preexisting regional wall motion abnormality indicates ischemia, whereas no change in a preexisting wall motion abnormality indicates infarction. If there is improvement in contractility in a preexisting wall motion abnormality, viable myocardium is present. Normal resting myocardial wall motion that does not improve reflects inadequate workload, beta blockade, or global ischemia.

Pharmacologic stress is useful in patients unable to

Table 2.—Optimal Utilization of Doppler Modalities

Pulsed-wave	Continuous wave
Flow volume	Valvular and other stenotic
Diastolic filling variables	gradients
Pulmonary/hepatic vein	Intracardiac pressure
flow	Mitral regurgitant velocities
Localizing site of flow	Pressure half-time measurements
disturbance	Intracavitary gradients

exercise. Graded dobutamine infusion (5 to 40 µg/kg per minute in 3-minute stages) increases myocardial oxygen demand by increasing contractility, heart rate, and systolic blood pressure. Patients who have an inadequate response to dobutamine may be given atropine (0.25 to 0.5 mg/60 s) until target heart rate is achieved.

Stress echocardiography may allow hibernating myocardium to be differentiated from infarction, using a low dose of dobutamine as stimulation. Viable myocardium reacts by increased thickening in response to a low dose of dobutamine, then function deteriorates as ischemia develops at higher doses. Early results have correlated well with rest redistribution thallium imaging.

Doppler stress echocardiography is used to evaluate patients with valvular heart disease. Supine bicycle ergometry is particularly well suited to Doppler evaluation of mitral, tricuspid, and aortic valve flow during exercise. Changes in valve gradients and areas, the degree of regurgitation, and changes in pulmonary artery pressure with stress provide important insight into the physiologic significance of many valvular, myocardial, and pulmonary conditions. These examinations should be tailored to the specific clinical question and are particularly useful in evaluating patients with symptoms out of proportion to resting valvular abnormalities, mitral stenosis with moderate gradients, and aortic stenosis with decreased left ventricular function. The American Society of Echocardiography has outlined a general approach to the utility of standard stress electrocardiographic and stress echocardiographic techniques for various clinical situations (Table 4).

The sensitivity and specificity and prognostic power of stress echocardiography are comparable to those of stress thallium or sestamibi nuclear studies. The technique requires accurate and rapid poststress image acquisition, because ischemia-induced wall motion abnormalities may resolve quickly, and close attention to image quality, systolic

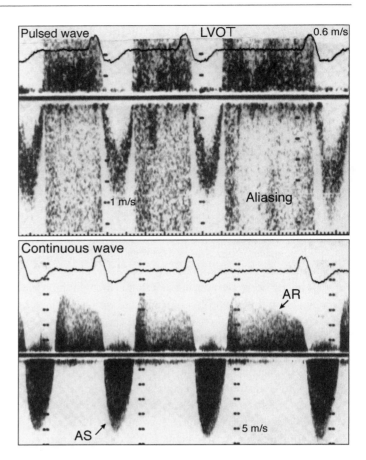

Fig. 1. Pulsed-wave and continuous-wave Doppler spectra from a patient with aortic stenosis (*AS*) and regurgitation. The pulsed-wave sample volume is in the left ventricular outflow tract (*LVOT*) and demonstrates aliasing and "wrapping around" the baseline of the high velocity aortic regurgitation signal (*AR*). The continuous-wave signal displays the entire AS and AR signals. (From Oh JK, Seward JB, Tajik AJ: *The Echo Manual*. Little, Brown and Company, 1994. By permission of Mayo Foundation.)

thickening, and ancillary signs of ischemia, such as left ventricular dilatation.

Contrast Echocardiography

For many years, hand-agitated saline ultrasound contrast administration has been performed to enhance echocardiographic studies. Peripheral venous injection of agitated saline is useful for the detection and semiquantitation of congenital or acquired intracardiac or intrapulmonary shunts and enhances regurgitant jets such as tricuspid regurgitant profiles. The size and instability of these bubbles and their inability to cross the pulmonary vascular bed have precluded opacification of left-sided chambers without intracardiac injection. Several gas-filled sonicated contrast agents have been developed that are injected intravenously and are able to

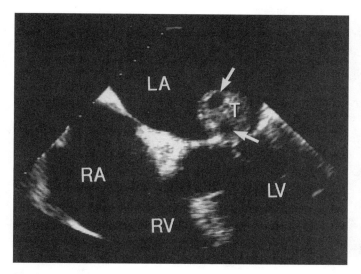

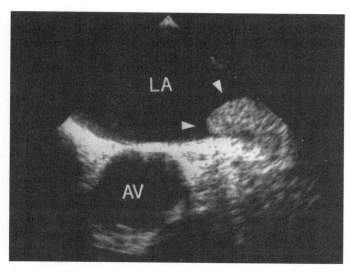

Fig. 2. Left atrial (*LA*) myxoma; transverse four-chamber transesophageal echocardiographic plane. Cystic echolucencies (*arrows*) are clearly seen within this myxoma (*T*); they were not evident on transthoracic examination. The myxoma appears to be attached to the mitral valve but was found to be attached to the mitral annulus on off-axis imaging. *LV*, left ventricle; *RA*, right atrium; *RV*, right ventricle. (From Freeman WK, Seward JB, Khandheria BK, Tajik AJ: *Transesophageal Echocardiography*. Little, Brown and Company, 1994, p 345. By permission of Mayo Foundation.)

Fig. 3. Left atrial (*LA*) appendage thrombus; transverse transesophageal echocardiographic plane, basal short-axis view. A protruding thrombus (*arrowheads*) fills the appendage of the left atrium. This thrombus was slightly mobile on real-time evaluation. *AV*, aortic valve. (From Freeman WK, Seward JB, Khandheria BK, Tajik AJ: *Transesophageal Echocardiography*. Little, Brown and Company, 1994, p 374. By permission of Mayo Foundation.)

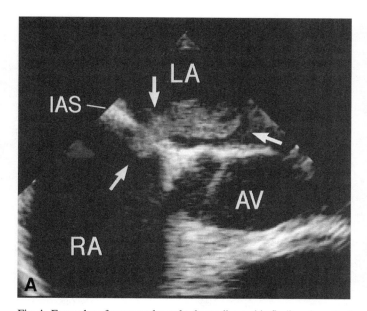

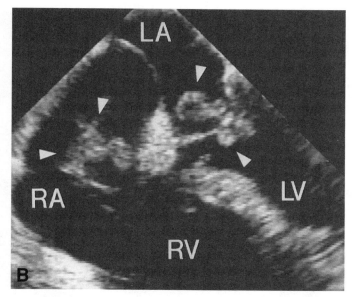

Fig. 4. Examples of transesophageal echocardiographic findings in patients with paradoxical embolism. In each case, a thrombus (*arrows* or *arrowheads*) is crossing through a patent foramen ovale. *IAS*, interatrial septum. Other abbreviations as in Figure 2. (From Freeman WK, Seward JB, Khandheria BK, Tajik AJ: *Transesophageal Echocardiography*. Little, Brown and Company, 1994, p 487. By permission of Mayo Foundation.)

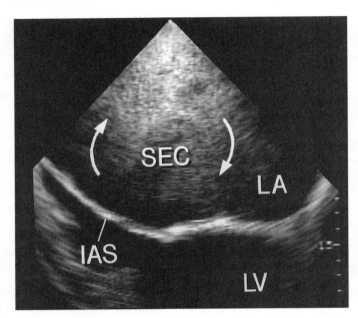

Fig. 5. Dense spontaneous echocardiographic contrast swirling (*arrows*) in the left atrium. *SEC*, spontaneous echocardiographic contrast. Other abbreviations as in Figures 2 and 4. (From Freeman WK, Seward JB, Khandheria BK, Tajik AJ: *Transesophageal Echocardiography*. Little, Brown and Company, 1994, p 478. By permission of Mayo Foundation.)

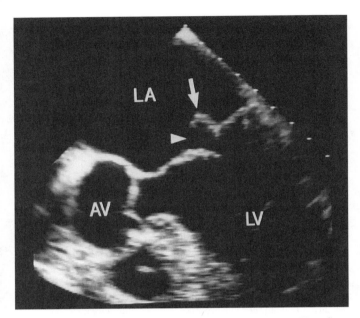

Fig. 6. Mitral valve prolapse with flail leaflet; left ventricular (*LV*) outflow view in the transverse plane. There is prolapse of the posterior mitral leaflet, with a flail leaflet segment (*arrow*) producing a large deficiency in coaptation (*arrowhead*) with the anterior leaflet. Other abbreviations as in Figures 2 and 3. (From Freeman WK, Seward JB, Khandheria BK, Tajik AJ: *Transesophageal Echocardiography*. Little, Brown and Company, 1994, p 507. By permission of Mayo Foundation.)

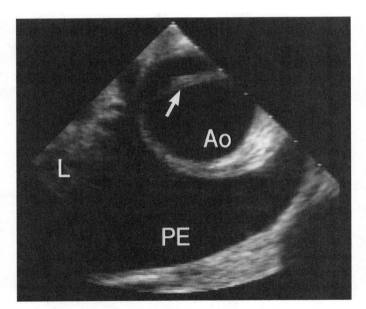

Fig. 7. Acute aortic dissection complicated by pleural effusion. A left pleural effusion within the posteromedial costophrenic angle highlights the dissected (*arrow*) descending thoracic aorta (*Ao*); a portion of the left lung (*L*) is also noted within the effusion. *PE*, pleural effusion. (From Freeman WK, Seward JB, Khandheria BK, Tajik AJ: *Transesophageal Echocardiography*. Little, Brown and Company, 1994, p 440. By permission of Mayo Foundation.)

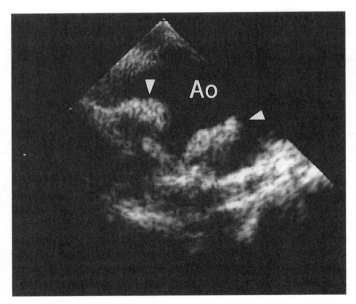

Fig. 8. Extensive atherosclerotic debris within the descending thoracic aorta; transverse transesophageal echocardiographic plane. A "shaggy" appearance of the lumen of the aorta (*Ao*) is produced by several partially mobile lesions (*arrowheads*) projecting far into the aortic lumen. This patient presented with diffuse atheroembolic cutanous infarcts of the feet and "blue toe" syndrome. (From Freeman WK, Seward JB, Khandheria BK, Tajik AJ: *Transesophageal Echocardiography*. Little, Brown and Company, 1994, p 454. By permission of Mayo Foundation.)

Table 3.—Interpretation by Regional Wall Motion (WM) Analysis

Rest	Stress	Interpretation
Normal WM and contractility	→ Hyperdynamic	Normal
Normal WM	→ New WM abnormality or	Ischemia
	→ Lack of hyperdynamic WM	Ischemia
WM abnormality	→ Worsening (hypokinesis → akinesis, akinesis → dyskinesis)	Ischemia
WM abnormality	→ Unchanged	Infarct
Akinetic WM	→ Improved to hypokinetic or to normal WM	Viable myocardium

→ Stress induces.

Table 4.—Clinical Situations and Recommended Echocardiographic Techniques

| | Typical chest pain | | | | | | | |
	Normal ECG, can exercise	Abnormal ECG, can exercise	Cannot exercise	Atypical symptoms	Preoperative risk	Myocardial viability	Pulmonary hypertension	Valvular disease
Exercise ECG	+++	-	-	-	+	-	-	-
Exercise echo	+	+++	-	+++	+	-	+++	+++
Pharmacologic stress echo	-	-	+++	+	+++	+++	+	+
Stress Doppler	-	-	-	-	-	-	+++	+++

ECG, electrocardiography (-gram); echo, echocardiography.
Symbols: -, not recommended; +++, preferred; +, acceptable alternative.
Modified from J Am Soc Echocardiogr 11:97-104, 1998. By permission of the American Society of Echocardiography.

traverse the pulmonary circulation and produce myocardial contrast and enhance visualization of the left ventricular endocardial border. These agents help identify myocardial infarction, ischemia, and viability. The use of contrast-enhanced exercise and pharmacologic stress studies may aid in the detection and quantitation of myocardium at risk. These agents also enhance Doppler signals, allowing more accurate assessment of valvular abnormalities.

Assessment of Ventricular Function (Systolic, Diastolic, Global, and Regional)

Left ventricular systolic global function can be evaluated with several echocardiographic techniques. These include two-dimensional (2-D) volumes derived from two-chamber and four-chamber area and length measurements (modified Simpson's method or summation of disks), left ventricular mass, left ventricular ejection fraction from 2-D volumes (Equation 3) or 2-D-directed M-mode (Equation 4), and fractional shortening (Equation 5).

Equation 3.—Ejection Fraction (EF) (%)

$$EF = \frac{LVED_V - LVES_V}{LVED_V} \times 100$$

$LVED_V$ = left ventricular end-*diastolic* volume
$LVES_V$ = left ventricular end-*systolic* volume

(Formula can be applied to any contracting cavity; volumes are measured by modified Simpson's method with on-line software)

Equation 4.—Ejection Fraction (EF) (%)

$$EF = \frac{LVED_D^2 - LVES_D^2}{LVED_D^2} \times 100$$

$LVED_D$ = averaged left ventricular
    end-*diastolic* diameter
$LVES_D$ = averaged left ventricular
    end-*systolic* diameter

Equation 5.—Fractional Shortening (FS) (%)

$$FS = \frac{LVED_D - LVES_D}{LVED_D} \times 100$$

$LVED_D$ = left ventricular end-*diastolic* diameter
$LVES_D$ = left ventricular end-*systolic* diameter

(This formula can be applied to any contracting cavity or muscle)

Cardiac output can be derived from 2-D volumes or by using Doppler echocardiographic techniques (Equations 6, 7, 8, and 9).

Equation 6.—Stroke Volume (SV) (mL)

$$SV = LVED_V - LVES_V$$
(Definitions as in Equation 3)

Equation 7.—Stroke Volume (SV) (mL)

$$SV = Area \times TVI$$

Area = (πr^2) (i.e., the cross-sectional area [cm^2] through which velocity is recorded)

$$\pi r^2 = \pi \left(\frac{d}{2}\right)^2 = 0.785d^2$$

d = diameter
r = radius
TVI = time velocity integral = stroke distance (cm). The distance over which blood travels in one cardiac cycle (the cycle velocity [cm/s] divided by time [s]).

Equation 8.—Cardiac Output (CO) (L/min)

$$CO = Stroke\ Volume \times Heart\ Rate$$

Equation 9.—Cardiac Index (CI) (L/min per m^2)

$$CI = \frac{Cardiac\ Output}{Body\ Surface\ Area}$$

Regional left ventricular function is based on the 2-D assessment of the contractility of 16 left ventricular wall segments (6 segments at the base and mid-ventricle and 4 at the apical level) (Fig. 9). A numerical score is given to each segment depending on contractility: 1 = normal, 2 = hypokinesis, 3 = akinesis, 4 = dyskinesis, and 5 = aneurysm. A wall motion score index can then be derived (Equation 10). Several studies have demonstrated adverse prognostic significance from high wall motion scores.

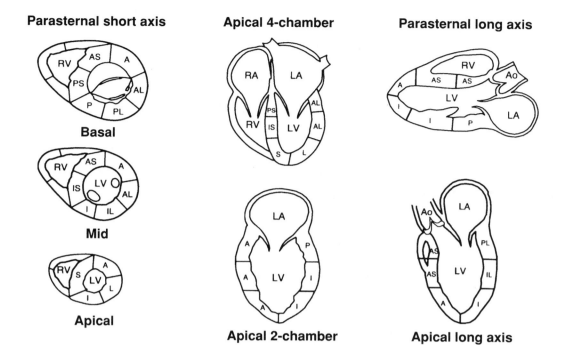

Fig. 9. Schema of the 16 left ventricular wall segments used to assess regional systolic function and wall motion score index.

Equation 10.—Wall Motion Score Index

Sum of Wall Scores ÷ Number of Segments Visualized

Scoring of segmental contraction
1 = normal
2 = hypokinetic
3 = akinetic
4 = dyskinetic
5 = aneurysm

(Note: *hyper*dynamic walls are considered normal and = 1)

Diastolic functional variables measured during an echocardiographic examination include isovolumic relaxation time (the period from atrioventricular valve closure to mitral valve opening), E- and A-wave velocities, E/A ratio, and deceleration time (Fig. 10). Because numerous factors, including heart rate and rhythm, loading conditions, age, and contractility, can affect mitral inflow patterns, pulmonary and hepatic venous tracings are also assessed as an adjunct to the mitral inflow pattern findings (Fig. 11).

Three general categories of diastolic filling abnormalities include the following (Fig. 10 and 11):

1. Relaxation Abnormality—characterized by prolonged isovolumic relaxation time (> 110 ms) and deceleration time (> 240 ms) and predominant A-wave velocity, with low E-wave velocity (E/A ratio < 1.0). Pulmonary and hepatic venous systolic forward flow predominate. Slow myocardial relaxation due to hypertrophy or other factors prolongs early filling, making the atrial contribution to filling more prominent.

2. Restrictive Physiology—characterized by short isovolumic relaxation time (< 60 ms) and deceleration time (< 150 ms) and high E-wave and low A-wave velocity (E/A ratio > 2.0). This pattern occurs when the ventricle is stiff (i.e., poor compliance). There is a rapid increase in left ventricular pressure during the early filling phase, resulting in the short deceleration time. The high left ventricular end-diastolic pressure diminishes the atrial contribution to filling. Pulmonary venous forward flow occurs predominately during diastole. The velocity and flow duration of the atrial reversal are increased. Hepatic venous systolic flow is decreased. This pattern can be seen in conditions in which left atrial pressure is high and there is a rapid increase in left ventricular diastolic pressure, as in patients with decompensated heart failure and restrictive cardiomyopathy.

3. Pseudonormal Physiology—a transitional phase

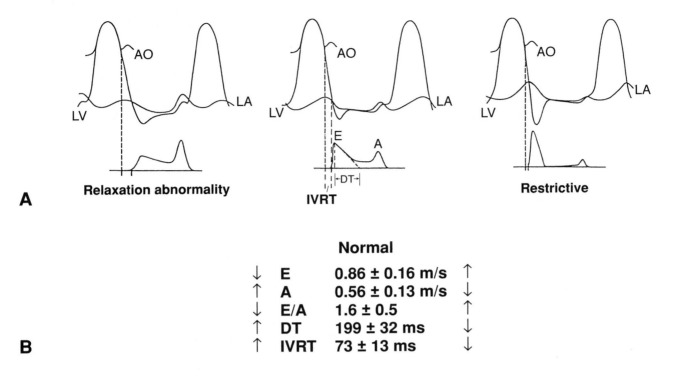

A Relaxation abnormality   IVRT   Restrictive

Normal

↓	E	0.86 ± 0.16 m/s	↑
↑	A	0.56 ± 0.13 m/s	↓
↓	E/A	1.6 ± 0.5	↑
↑	DT	199 ± 32 ms	↓
↑	IVRT	73 ± 13 ms	↓

B

Fig. 10. *A*, Schematic left ventricular (LV), aortic (AO), and left atrial (LA) pressure tracings and corresponding mitral inflow Doppler spectrum. *B*, Range of normal values and direction of change with diastolic dysfunction. A, atrial contraction; DT, deceleration time; E, early filling phase; IVRT, isovolumic relaxation time. (From Oh JK, Seward JB, Tajik AJ: *The Echo Manual*. Little, Brown and Company, 1994. By permission of Mayo Foundation.)

between abnormal relaxation and restriction; that is, relaxation is delayed and left atrial pressure is increased. The mitral inflow pattern appears "normal." The pulmonary venous flow profile is useful in differentiating this pattern from true normal. Pulmonary venous systolic forward flow is decreased, diastolic forward flow is increased, and atrial reversals are of high velocity and longer duration.

Hemodynamic Assessment

The following is a list of commonly used echocardiographic hemodynamic variables and their clinical usefulness:

   1. Pressure Gradients (maximal instantaneous and mean)—valvular stenosis, prosthetic valve, left and right ventricular outflow tract obstruction, and coarctation.

   2. Intracardiac Pressures—right ventricular, pulmonary artery, and left ventricular systolic and end-diastolic pressures.

   3. Volumetric Flow—stroke volume, cardiac output, regurgitant volume and fraction, and shunt fraction (Qp/Qs).

   4. Valve Areas—continuity equation and pressure half-time.

   5. dP/dt.

   6. Diastolic Filling Variables.

To make these measurements, it is essential to understand and to use the modified Bernoulli equation (Equation 11 and Fig. 12), in which the pressure drop across a stenosis is equal to $4v^2$, and the concept of the time velocity integral (TVI or stroke distance) (Fig. 13).

Equation 11.—Gradient (ΔP) (mm Hg)

$$\Delta P = 4(v_2^2 - v_1^2)$$

or

$$\Delta P = 4v^2$$

P = pressure
v_2 = accelerated velocity across a stenosis
v_1 = velocity proximal to a stenosis
Note: Normally v_1 is much smaller than v_2 and can usually be omitted. Therefore, the equation can be simplified to $4v^2$
v = velocity across any vessel, chamber, or valve

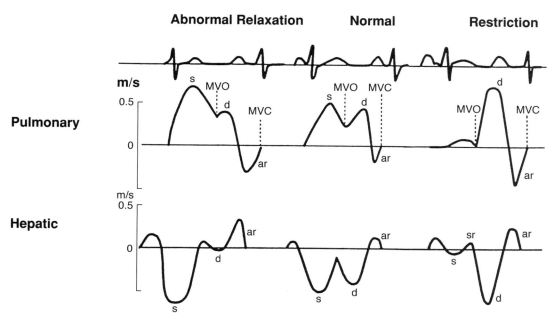

Fig. 11. Schema of pulmonary and hepatic vein flow velocities in normal and abnormal diastolic filling. ar, atrial reversal; d, diastolic; MVC, mitral valve closure; MVO, mitral valve opening; s, systolic; sr, systolic reversal. (From Oh JK, Seward JB, Tajik AJ: *The Echo Manual*. Little, Brown and Company, 1994. By permission of Mayo Foundation.)

When comparing Doppler-derived gradients with those measured invasively, it is important to remember that the maximal instantaneous gradient measured by Doppler is not equal to the peak-to-peak gradient measured at catheterization (Fig. 14). The maximal instantaneous gradient is always higher than the "nonphysiologic" (i.e., nonsimultaneous) peak-to-peak gradient. Doppler- and catheter-derived mean pressure gradients are comparable.

By using the modified Bernoulli equation (Equation 11) and the measured Doppler velocity of a regurgitant or restrictive flow jet, the pressure difference between the two chambers can be calculated. If the pressure in one of the chambers can be measured accurately or estimated noninvasively, the pressure in the other chamber can be derived.

For example,

RV or PA systolic pressure = 4 (TR systolic velocity)^2 + RA pressure

PA diastolic pressure = 4 (PR end-diastolic velocity)^2 + RA pressure

LA pressure = Systolic BP - 4 (MR systolic velocity)^2

RV systolic pressure = Systolic BP - 4 (VSD velocity)^2

where RV = right ventricle, PA = pulmonary artery, TR = tricuspid regurgitation, RA = right atrium, PR = pulmonary regurgitation, LA = left atrium, BP = blood pressure, MR = mitral regurgitation, and VSD = ventricular septal defect.

Right atrial pressure can be estimated by any one or a combination of techniques, including clinical estimate of central venous pressure, nomograms derived from Doppler catheter correlation studies, or echocardiographic estimates based on right atrial and inferior vena cava size and inferior vena caval reactivity to inspiratory effort. In practice, if the right atrium and inferior vena cava appear normal, 5 mm

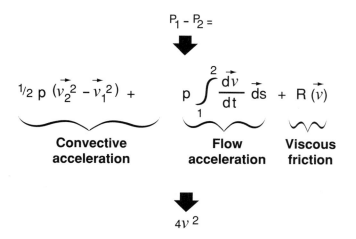

$$P_1 - P_2 =$$

$$\frac{1}{2}\,p\,(\vec{v_2}^2 - \vec{v_1}^2) + \quad p\int_1^2 \frac{\vec{dv}}{dt}\,\vec{ds} + R\,(\vec{v})$$

Convective acceleration — **Flow acceleration** — **Viscous friction**

$$4v^2$$

Fig. 12. Derivation of the modified Bernoulli equation that measures the pressure difference ($P_1 - P_2$) across a restrictive orifice. In most clinical situations, the viscous friction and flow acceleration components are negligible and can be ignored. If the proximal velocity (v_1) is very small compared with the distal velocity (v_2), as in severe aortic stenosis, then the proximal velocity term can be omitted, resulting in the simplified equation $\Delta P = 4v^2$.

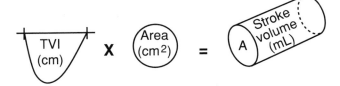

Fig. 13. The time velocity integral (TVI) is the calculated area under the Doppler spectrum over time. It is also known as "stroke distance," because it represents the distance (cm) that blood travels with each stroke or beat. The stroke volume (mL) is the volume of the cylinder formed by the product of the cross-sectional areas (cm^2) of the blood vessel or orifice and the distance (TVI) that the blood moves in a specified time period (i.e., systole, diastole).

Hg is used for right atrial pressure estimates. If the patient is elderly and/or the inferior vena cava is mildly dilated or has blunted inspiratory collapse, 10 to 14 mm Hg is assumed. If the inferior vena cava is plethoric, has little or no inspiratory motion, or the clinical examination findings are consistent with marked increase of central venous pressure, then 20 mm Hg or more is added to the pressure difference measured by Doppler echocardiography.

Regurgitant volume and fraction (Equations 12 and 13) and Qp/Qs (Equation 14) are obtained by comparing the flow through a nonregurgitant reference valve with flow through the affected valve or chamber (Plate 1).

Equation 12.—Regurgitant Volume (mL)

$$\text{Regurgitant Volume} = SV_{valve} - SV_{systemic}$$

SV_{valve} = flow volume (Area x TVI) across the regurgitant valve (forward plus regurgitant flow)

$SV_{systemic}$ = systemic flow measured elsewhere in an unaffected area of the heart (Area x TVI)

Equation 13.—Regurgitant Fraction (%)

$$\text{Regurgitant Fraction} = \frac{SV_{valve} - SV_{systemic}}{SV_{valve}}$$

(Definitions as in Equation 12)

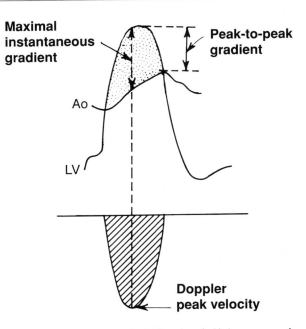

Fig. 14. Schema of left ventricular (LV) and aortic (Ao) pressure tracings and the corresponding Doppler velocity spectrum demonstrating the difference between peak-to-peak and maximal instantaneous gradients. The mean gradient (hatched area) is the area under the curve of the Doppler spectrum and is closely correlated with the mean gradient measured invasively (stippled area). (From Oh JK, Seward JB, Tajik AJ: *The Echo Manual*. Little, Brown and Company, 1994. By permission of Mayo Foundation.)

Equation 14.—Pulmonary-to-Systemic Flow Ratio (Qp/Qs)

$$\frac{Qp}{Qs} = \frac{Area_{PV} \times TVI_{PV}}{Area_{LVOT} \times TVI_{LVOT}}$$

Qp = pulmonary stroke volume (usually measured at pulmonary valve annulus [PV])

Qs = systemic stroke volume (usually measured at left ventricular outflow tract [LVOT])

The continuity equation, which is based on the principle of conservation of mass ("what goes in must come out"), states that flow proximal and distal to an orifice must be equal in a closed system (Equation 15). Rearrangement of the continuity equation allows calculation of stenotic and regurgitant orifice areas by measuring three variables and solving for the fourth (Equation 16).

Equation 15.—Continuity Equation

$$Flow_{proximal} = Flow_{distal}$$
$$A_1 \times TVI_1 = A_2 \times TVI_2$$

$$A_1 \times TVI_1 = \text{proximal flow}$$
$$A_2 \times TVI_2 = \text{flow across valve}$$

Equation 16.—Valve Area (cm^2)

(Rearrangement of Continuity Equation [Equation 15])

$$A_2 = A_1 \times \frac{TVI_1}{TVI_2}$$
$$A_2 = \text{area of the stenotic valve } (cm^2)$$

Mitral valve area can be measured with the continuity equation or the pressure half-time method (Equations 17 and 18).

Equation 17.—Pressure Half-Time (PHT) (ms)

$$PHT = DT \times 0.29$$

PHT = time required for the peak gradient
     to decrease by one-half
DT = deceleration time (time [ms] it takes
     the maximal velocity to decrease to zero)
0.29 = an algebraic constant that converts
     velocity to gradient

Equation 18.—Mitral Valve Area (MVA) by
Half-Time Measurement (cm^2)

$$MVA = \frac{220}{PHT} \quad \text{or} \quad \frac{759}{DT}$$

220 and 759 = empiric time constants equating to a
     mitral valve area of approximately 1 cm^2

(Definitions as in Equation 17)

The proximal isovelocity surface area (PISA) method is a variation of the continuity equation and uses the property of flow convergence of fluid as it approaches a restrictive orifice. Blood forms multiple concentric "shells," or hemispheres, of isovelocity. As the surface area decreases, the velocity increases. The velocity at a given distance from the orifice (v_r) can be measured by altering the aliasing velocity of the color flow Doppler signal. The flow rate through the orifice can be calculated (Equation 19). The effective regurgitant orifice (ERO), also referred to as "regurgitant orifice area" (ROA), and regurgitant volume can be calculated using the continuity equation

and the peak velocity and TVI of the continuous-wave mitral regurgitant signal (Equations 20 and 21). Variations of the PISA technique also allow calculation of flow rate and volume and orifice area of stenotic mitral valves, atrial and ventricular septal defects, and aortic coarctation (Plate 2).

Equation 19.—PISA Flow Rate (mL/s)

$$Flow = 2 \pi r^2 \times v_r$$

Flow = instantaneous flow rate (mL/s)
r = radial distance of isovelocity shell
     from orifice (cm)
v_r = flow velocity radius "r" (cm/s)

Equation 20.—Effective Regurgitant Orifice (ERO) (cm^2)

$$ERO = \frac{Flow \text{ (mL/s)}}{v_{MR} \text{ (cm/s)}}$$

v_{MR} = peak velocity of continuous-wave mitral
     regurgitant signal

Equation 21.—Regurgitant Volume (mL)

$$\text{Regurgitant volume} = ERO \ (cm^2) \times TVI_{MR} \ (cm)$$

ERO = effective regurgitant orifice
TVI_{MR} = time velocity integral of
     continuous-wave mitral
     regurgitant signal

The following examples are frequently given on Cardiology Examinations. You should be able to identify the Doppler signals and the hemodynamic significance of the following:

Aortic stenosis—transvalvular velocity, gradient, and aortic valve area by the continuity equation (Plate 3)

Aortic regurgitation—pressure half-time, diastolic flow reversals in aorta

Mitral stenosis—transvalvular gradient, pressure half-time, and mitral valve area

Mitral regurgitation—regurgitant volume, fraction, systolic flow reversals in pulmonary veins

Pulmonary artery pressure—tricuspid regurgitant velocity

Hypertrophic cardiomyopathy—left ventricular intra-cavity gradient

Tricuspid regurgitation—systolic flow reversals in hepatic veins and marked dilated inferior vena cava and hepatic veins

Evaluation of Specific Disorders

Aortic Stenosis

1. M-Mode/2-D—valve morphology (unicuspid, bicuspid, or tricuspid), and calcification.

2. Doppler—peak aortic velocity, TVI, mean gradient (Plate 3), and aortic valve area by the continuity equation (Equation 16).

Severe aortic stenosis is usually present if the peak aortic velocity is 4.5 m/s or greater, the mean pressure gradient is 50 mm Hg or greater, the valve area is 0.75 cm^2 or smaller, or the LVOT-to-aortic valve TVI ratio is ≤ 0.25. A small aortic valve area associated with a low gradient and a low cardiac output state requires careful evaluation to differentiate decreased left ventricular function due to severe aortic stenosis from milder aortic stenosis with unrelated myocardial dysfunction. Dobutamine echocardiography has been used to increase contractility and to increase cardiac output to differentiate anatomical from "relative" aortic stenosis.

The major pitfall in assessment of aortic stenosis is underestimation of the gradient and overestimation of the valve area when the highest velocity Doppler signal is not obtained because of technical or anatomical factors.

Mitral Stenosis

1. M-Mode/2-D—valve morphology, doming or "hockey stick" (long axis) (Fig. 15), "fish mouth" (short axis), leaflet and subvalvular thickening, calcification and mobility (echocardiographic score), commissural anatomy, and left atrial size.

2. Doppler—mean gradient, mitral valve area by continuity equation, pressure half-time, and planimetry methods (Equations 16 to 18), pulmonary artery pressure, and degree of mitral regurgitation. All three methods of assessment of mitral valve area by echocardiography correlate well with invasive measures, but each has unique features that render it more or less accurate in a given patient (Table 5). Therefore, all three methods should be performed to achieve an integrated approach to the severity of mitral stenosis.

A high transvalvular gradient with normal pressure half-time may reflect severe mitral regurgitation rather than mitral stenosis. Severe mitral stenosis is usually present if the mitral valve area is 1.0 cm^2 or less, the mean resting pressure gradient is 10 mm Hg or greater, or the pressure half-time is 220 ms or longer. Exercise Doppler echocardiography can be very useful to assess stress-induced changes in gradient, mitral valve area, and pulmonary artery pressures.

TEE is essential before percutaneous mitral balloon valvuloplasty and can help define further the presence or absence of commissural fusion and calcification. The presence of heavy calcification at both commissures, significant subvalvular disease, and marked leaflet thickening and immobility predict suboptimal results for valvuloplasty. Left atrial thrombus must be excluded to avoid embolic complications.

Aortic Regurgitation

1. M-Mode/2-D—valve morphology, left ventricular size and function, premature mitral valve closure, diastolic opening of the aortic valve (severe aortic regurgitation), fluttering of the mitral valve, and etiology: Marfan syndrome, bicuspid aortic valve, endocarditis, and dissection.

2. Color Flow Imaging—ratio of jet width or area to left ventricular outflow tract width or area (mild, < 30%; severe, > 60%).

3. Pulsed-Wave Doppler—holodiastolic flow reversals in the descending or abdominal aorta are indicative of significant regurgitation.

4. Continuous-Wave—pressure half-time (mild, ≥ 400 ms; severe, ≤ 250 ms). High left ventricular end-diastolic pressure can shorten pressure half-time, causing overestimation of the severity of regurgitation.

5. Quantitative Methods—regurgitant volume and fraction. Regurgitant fraction (mild < 30%; severe > 55%) or regurgitant volume ≥ 60 mL; effective regurgitant orifice (mild, < 0.10 cm^2; severe, ≥ 0.30 cm^2); left ventricular diastolic dimension in chronic aortic regurgitation (mild, < 6.0 cm; severe, ≥ 7.5 cm).

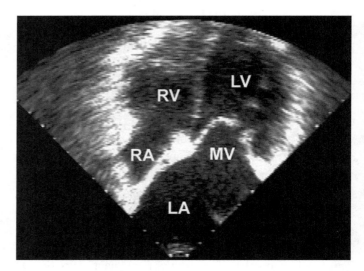

Fig. 15. Rheumatic mitral stenosis with left atrial (*LA*) enlargement and obvious doming of the anterior mitral leaflet. *LV*, left ventricle; *MV*, mitral valve; *RA*, right atrium; *RV*, right ventricle.

Table 5.—Limitations and Pitfalls in Assessing Mitral Valve Area

2-D planimetry

    Dependent on 2-D image quality, gain-setting, and ability to visualize the minimal orifice area

    Less accurate when extensive calcification is present

    Difficult after commissurotomy because of irregular orifice

Doppler pressure half-time

    Tachycardia

    Nonlinear pressure decay

    Significant or acute aortic regurgitation increases the rate of left ventricular pressure rise and shortens pressure half-time
      (mitral valve area overestimated)

    Immediately after percutaneous mitral valvuloplasty when hemodynamics are not stable (mitral valve area overestimated)

Continuity equation

    Cumbersome to perform, multiple measurements are subject to error

    Mitral valve area underestimated when significant mitral regurgitation is present

An integrated approach using these quantitative and semi-quantitative methods of evaluation should be used because all the above can be influenced by factors other than the degree of aortic regurgitation (Plate 4).

A restrictive mitral inflow pattern may be seen in acute severe aortic regurgitation.

Mitral Regurgitation

1. M-Mode/2-D—valve morphology, left ventricular size and function, and etiology: mitral valve prolapse, flail leaflet, mitral annular calcification, papillary muscle dysfunction or rupture, and endocarditis.

2. Color Flow Imaging—jet size and jet/left atrial area ratio. Color flow imaging jet size is influenced by instrument settings (pulse repetition frequency, depth, etc.), loading conditions, and jet direction. A jet that runs adjacent to the left atrial wall carries more regurgitant volume than a similarly sized "free jet."

3. Pulsed-Wave Doppler—systolic reversals in the pulmonary vein indicate severe mitral regurgitation.

4. Quantitative Methods—regurgitant volume and fraction. The PISA method allows assessment of regurgitant volume and effective regurgitant orifice area using the concept of the continuity equation and flow convergence.

5. TEE—useful in assessing mitral valve morphology and in visualizing the color flow jet and pulmonary veins and useful intraoperatively before and after mitral valve repair.

Tricuspid Regurgitation

M-mode/2-D–valve morphology and right ventricular size and function to determine cause of tricuspid regurgitation

(rheumatic valve, prolapse, Ebstein anomaly, carcinoid valve, right ventricular infarct, secondary to pulmonary hypertension or tricuspid valve injury). Severe tricuspid regurgitation is suggested by color-flow regurgitant jet area ≥ 30% of right atrium, annular dilatation ≥ 4 cm, increased tricuspid inflow velocity > 1.0 m/s, or systolic flow reversal in the hepatic vein.

Prosthetic Valves

The range of "normal" hemodynamic variables (gradient, effective orifice area, etc.) for a given prosthetic valve type and location is broad. The best approach for assessing an individual patient is to perform a baseline transthoracic 2-D and hemodynamic evaluation early postoperatively to establish the patient's own "normal values" for later comparison.

"Normal" regurgitation is present in virtually all prosthetic valves and has been well characterized in vitro and in vivo. This "physiologic" regurgitation is usually of low volume and velocity and appears as a nonaliased jet and should be differentiated from pathologic regurgitation. Normal prosthetic valves are inherently "stenotic," with higher transvalvular gradients than native valves.

Prosthetic valve dysfunction includes valvular and perivalvular regurgitation, obstruction, endocarditis, abscess, dehiscence, and thromboembolism. A complete transthoracic 2-D evaluation may be limited by acoustical shadowing by the prosthesis. Doppler echocardiography usually can assess valve gradients and effective orifice areas accurately, detect and quantitate regurgitation, and provide ancillary information about pulmonary pressure and left ventricular systolic and diastolic function.

Unexpectedly high transvalvular gradients or small effective orifice areas should be assessed further to exclude valve dysfunction. If available, comparison with a previous echocardiographic study is invaluable. If no change has occurred and the patient is clinically stable, it is likely that the hemodynamics are "normal" for that patient and valve or that a prosthesis-patient mismatch is present; that is, the valve is relatively undersized for the patient's body size and hemodynamics. High gradients may also occur in the presence of increased transvalvular flow such as anemia or other high output states, but effective orifice areas should remain relatively normal in these conditions. High velocities present in otherwise normal valves may be due to localized high-velocity jets and distal pressure recovery, which may lead to Doppler gradients that are higher than those measured by catheter. This has been observed most commonly in smaller Starr-Edwards and St. Jude prosthetic valves.

TEE is an invaluable complementary examination, especially in mitral and tricuspid prostheses, to visualize valve motion, ring abscess, thrombus, or endocarditis and to assess the degree of regurgitation.

Chest Pain/Acute Myocardial Infarction

Echocardiography is useful in excluding other causes of chest pain (pericarditis, large pulmonary embolus, aortic dissection, etc.), to assess global and regional left ventricular function, to localize myocardial infarction, to identify patients who may benefit from revascularization, and to document the effect of therapy (thrombolysis or percutaneous transluminal coronary angioplasty). The absence of regional wall motion abnormalities during chest pain virtually excludes ischemia and can be a useful study to aid in triage of patients who come to the emergency room. A restrictive pattern of left ventricular diastolic filling or a high wall motion score index may predict a poor prognosis. Infarct-related complications may be readily assessed with echocardiography (Table 6).

Hypertrophic Cardiomyopathy

M-mode and 2-D echocardiography are useful in establishing the diagnosis of hypertrophic cardiomyopathy, evaluating the degree and morphology (asymmetric, symmetric, apical, etc.) of the hypertrophy, and assessing left ventricular function. Typical M-mode features of hypertrophic cardiomyopathy include mid-systolic aortic valve notching and systolic anterior motion of the mitral apparatus. Also, 2-D echocardiography can demonstrate systolic anterior motion and mitral valve morphology.

Table 6.—Echocardiographic Detection of Complications of Acute Myocardial Infarction and Associated Features

Right ventricular infarction
    Dilated right atrium and right ventricle with regional wall motion abnormalities
    Significant tricuspid regurgitation
    Inferior vena cava, dilation or plethora
Pericardial effusion/tamponade
Mitral regurgitation
    Ischemic—papillary muscle dysfunction or annular dilatation
    Ruptured papillary muscle
Ventricular septal defect
    Color flow localization
    Right ventricular dilatation
    Elevated right ventricular pressure
    Inferior vena cava plethora
Left ventricular free wall rupture
    Pericardial effusion/tamponade
    Pericardial thrombus
    Extracardiac flow
Pseudoaneurysm (contained rupture)
    Narrow neck, thin-walled
Aneurysm
    Myocardial thinning, 90% located at apex
Left ventricular thrombus

Pulsed-wave Doppler and color flow imaging are useful in localizing the presence and site of left ventricular outflow tract or mid-ventricular obstruction. The degree of obstruction (pressure gradient) is defined by a characteristic continuous-wave Doppler late-peaking, dagger-shaped signal. The peak gradient is calculated with the modified Bernoulli equation ($4v^2$). Measurement of the gradient during the Valsalva maneuver, administration of amyl nitrite, or exercise can demonstrate the dynamic nature of the obstruction.

Diastolic abnormalities in hypertrophic cardiomyopathy are strongly associated with symptoms of dyspnea and exercise intolerance and should be carefully assessed. Isovolumic relaxation period flow is present occasionally and is due to asynchronous ventricular relaxation. Normally, there is little or no flow during the isovolumic relaxation period when both the mitral and aortic valves are closed. It is important not to confuse this flow with the mitral E wave.

Infective Endocarditis

Echocardiography is the diagnostic procedure of choice for detecting valvular vegetations (Plate 5). It has the additional benefit of being able to detect abscesses, valve perforation, rupture or aneurysm, fistula, dehiscence of a prosthetic valve, and hemodynamic consequences (shunt or regurgitation). The combination of transthoracic echocardiography and TEE has a sensitivity for vegetations in the range of 90% to 95% of native valves and 85% to 90% of prosthetic valves. Patients with suspected infective endocarditis should have a baseline transthoracic study and, in most cases, a transesophageal study. TEE is superior to transthoracic echocardiography in diagnosing valve ring abscess. Serial echocardiographic examinations may be helpful, especially in patients with congestive heart failure, fever, or persistently positive blood cultures.

Whether echocardiographic characteristics of vegetations provide prognostic information about mortality or complications is controversial. The false-negative rate for detection of vegetations is low (< 5%), but in patients with clinical features consistent with infective endocarditis and negative initial TEE findings, it may be reasonable to repeat the study in 1 or 2 weeks.

Pericardial Disease

1. Effusion—Echocardiography is the diagnostic procedure of choice for detecting and evaluating pericardial effusion. An effusion is defined as "an echo-free space present throughout the cardiac cycle." Large effusions may be associated with a "swinging heart."

2. Tamponade—2-D and M-mode features of tamponade are not sensitive but can be quite specific; they include diastolic collapse of the right atrium or right ventricle and inferior vena cava plethora with blunted inspiratory collapse. Doppler findings of cardiac tamponade are more sensitive and are based on ventricular interdependence due to the relatively fixed cardiac volume and reduced response of intrapericardial pressures to changes in intrathoracic pressures. With inspiration, left ventricular filling is impaired, whereas right ventricular filling is favored. Doppler findings include an inspiratory increase in isovolumic relaxation time and decreased mitral E-wave velocity, with reciprocal changes in tricuspid valve inflow tracings. Pulmonary venous, hepatic venous, and left ventricular outflow tract tracings show similar respiratory flow changes. Echocardiographically guided pericardiocentesis with or without catheter drainage is the initial therapy of choice for most patients with tamponade (aortic dissection with tamponade excepted).

3. Constrictive Pericarditis—2-D and M-mode features of constrictive pericarditis include thickened or hyperechoic pericardium, abnormal "jerky" septal motion, respiratory variation in ventricular size, and a dilated inferior vena cava. Doppler features of constriction are similar to those of tamponade, with an inspiratory decrease in left-sided flow (Fig. 16). Expiratory hepatic vein diastolic flow reversals are often prominent. Restrictive cardiomyopathy usually shows no significant respiratory changes in mitral inflow; therefore, Doppler echocardiography is useful in differentiating constriction from restriction.

The Thoracic Aorta

Although transthoracic echocardiography often can visualize the aortic root and arch, most of the aorta cannot be evaluated. With TEE, the entire thoracic aorta can be seen in most patients with a biplane or multiplane examination. Dissection can be evaluated with TEE (Fig. 17) as well as or better than with CT or aortography. Because time is often critical in suspected dissection, TEE has additional advantages: 1) it can be brought rapidly to the bedside of patients whose condition is unstable and 2) it allows assessment of cardiac function and associated conditions (aortic regurgitation, pericardial effusion). Aortic aneurysm, rupture, ulcer, debris, abscess, and coarctation are all easily evaluated with TEE.

Source of Embolus

Cardiovascular sources of emboli may account for 20% to 40% of all strokes. Potential sources of emboli detectable with transthoracic echocardiography or TEE include intracardiac thrombus or mass, valvular vegetation, thoracic aortic debris, atrial septal aneurysm, and patent foramen ovale. In the absence of overt cardiac disease on the basis of history, physical examination, or electrocardiographic findings, the yield from a transthoracic echocardiogram for identification of a cardiac source of embolus is less than 1% and is not routinely recommended. The transthoracic examination, if performed, should focus on left ventricular function and on excluding abnormalities such as valvular heart disease and tumors. Several studies have concluded that proceeding directly to TEE is a clinically useful and cost-effective strategy for evaluation of stroke, especially in younger patients and those in sinus rhythm. TEE is particularly well suited for excluding left atrial and left atrial appendage thrombus, spontaneous echo contrast, patent foramen ovale, and lesions in the thoracic aorta.

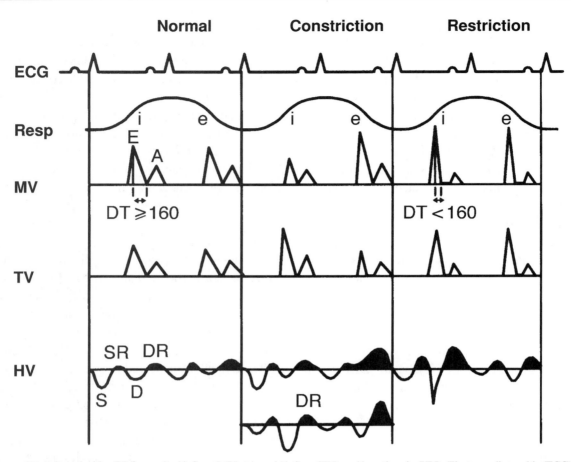

Fig. 16. Schema of Doppler velocities (V) from mitral inflow (MV), tricuspid inflow (TV), and hepatic vein (HV). Electrocardiographic (ECG) and respirometer recordings (Resp) with inspiration (i) and expiration (e) are also represented. The relative changes from normal caused by restrictive or constrictive pericarditis are represented. Both restriction and constriction are characterized by short deceleration time (DT), but patients with constriction demonstrate reciprocal changes in filling of the left and right sides of the heart with respiration, whereas patients with restriction do not. D, diastolic; DR, diastolic reversal; S, systolic; SR, systolic reversal.

Atrial Fibrillation and Cardioversion

Transthoracic echocardiography is usually performed in patients who present with an initial episode of atrial fibrillation. An assessment of left ventricular function is particularly useful for diagnostic purposes and management because several antiarrhythmic and rate-controlling agents are relatively contraindicated in patients with significant left ventricular systolic dysfunction or heart failure. Associated disorders such as hypertensive heart disease and valvular lesions can be assessed, and low-risk persons with "lone atrial fibrillation" can be identified.

Currently, TEE is being used to exclude intracardiac, especially left atrial appendage, thrombus to allow safe and early cardioversion to sinus rhythm and to avoid the traditional 3- to 6-week period of pre-cardioversion anticoagulation. The sensitivity and specificity of TEE for the detection of thrombus are high (95% to 100%), and

early return of sinus rhythm has several potential physiologic advantages. Early small studies that compared conventional therapy (4 weeks of anticoagulation with warfarin before and after cardioversion) with a TEE-guided strategy of early cardioversion while the patient received anticoagulation treatment with heparin followed by 4 weeks of warfarin reported similar safety profiles and lower costs if transthoracic echocardiography was not performed. Larger studies are under way. Approximately 10% to 20% of patients with atrial fibrillation lasting longer than 48 hours have been found, on TEE, to have atrial thrombi. Patients with identified atrial thrombi or in whom thrombus cannot be excluded for technical reasons should not undergo early cardioversion. When a thrombus is identified at the initial study, many advocate follow-up TEE after 4 weeks of anticoagulation before reconsideration of cardioversion (Plate 6).

Intraoperative Transesophageal Echocardiography

Intraoperative TEE is ideally suited to assist surgeons in planning and evaluating the results of surgical procedures (Table 7). The transesophageal probe generally is placed after endotracheal intubation and, ideally, the transesophageal examination is performed before surgery begins, to minimize interference from personnel and electrocautery. The postoperative study provides on-line real-time evaluation of the surgical intervention, allowing the surgeon to determine, before the chest is closed, whether the treatment is adequate. The collaboration of surgeons, echocardiologists, and anesthesiologists is critical for optimal use of the technique.

Table 7.—Indications for Intraoperative Transesophageal Echocardiography

Plan optimal surgical approach
    Mitral valve repair versus replacement
    Sizing of aortic homograft and valve prosthesis
    Congenital heart surgery
    Recognize associated abnormalities requiring intervention
      (e.g., patent foramen ovale)
    Location and extent of septal myectomy
    Extent of repair for aortic dissection
Verify achievement of optimal surgical result
    Determine adequacy of valve repair—residual
      regurgitation/stenosis
    Residual left ventricular outflow tract obstruction after
      myectomy
    Prosthetic valve function
Recognize and/or manage early surgical complications
    Ventricular septal defect
    Dynamic left ventricular outflow tract obstruction after
      aortic valve replacement
    Intracardiac air
    Pericardial effusion or tamponade
    Left or right ventricular dysfunction/ischemia
    Cause of hypotension or difficulty weaning from
      cardiopulmonary bypass
Emergency assessment of hemodynamic instability in the
    operating room during noncardiac surgery

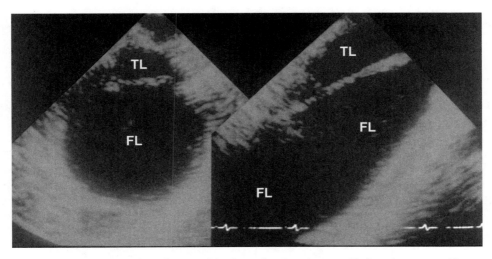

Fig. 17. Transesophageal echocardiogram of the descending thoracic aorta with dissection present. *TL*, true lumen; *FL*, false lumen.

It is important to be able to identify the M-mode and/or 2-D features of the following in a still frame photograph:

Left ventricular aneurysm—most are apical (or less frequently, inferobasal), thin-walled, absent endocardium (Fig. 18)

Left ventricular pseudoaneurysm—narrow neck, discontinuity of endocardium

Left ventricular thrombus—usually adjacent to area of akinesis, dyskinesis, scar

Dilated cardiomyopathy

Hypereosinophilic syndrome—right ventricular and left ventricular endocardial thickening (deposition of eosinophilic clot) at apices up to the mitral valve

Amyloid heart disease—thick left ventricular and right ventricular walls, valve leaflet thickening, biatrial enlargement, "granular, sparkling" myocardium

Carcinoid heart disease—thickened, tethered, immobile tricuspid and pulmonary valves with significant regurgitation with or without stenosis, right ventricular volume overload

Hypertrophic cardiomyopathy—systolic anterior motion of the mitral valve, apical hypertrophic cardiomyopathy, aortic valve mid-systolic closure

Cor pulmonale—right ventricular enlargement, hypertrophy, "D-shaped" left ventricle

Pericardial effusion/tamponade—right atrial/right ventricular diastolic collapse

Mitral valve prolapse—thickened, redundant leaflets that break the plane of the mitral annulus in systole; look for flail segment, ruptured chordae

Mitral stenosis—leaflet thickening, "hockey stick" deformity, commissural fusion, left atrial enlargement

Bicuspid aortic valve—eccentric closure, "doming"

Aortic regurgitation—diastolic flutter of the mitral valve, root dilatation, premature mitral closure, flail leaflet, left ventricular dilatation

Aortic aneurysm—associated Marfan syndrome

Sinus of Valsalva aneurysm—dilated sinus of Valsalva with shunt into right atrium, right ventricle, or other chamber after rupture

Atrial septal defect—secundum, primum, sinus venosus

Ventricular septal defect—infarct, membranous, ventricular septal aneurysm

Dilated coronary sinus—usually caused by persistent left superior vena cava

Ebstein anomaly—downward displacement and fusion of tricuspid leaflets, associated atrial septal defect

Infective endocarditis—vegetation, ring abscess, valve disruption (Fig. 19)

Left atrial myxoma—mass in the left atrium; most common attachment is the interatrial septum

Transplanted heart—elongated atria with prominent suture lines (Fig. 20)

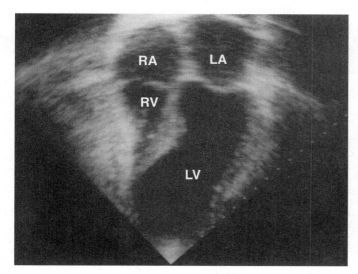

Fig. 18. Large left ventricular (*LV*) apical aneurysm due to old anteroapical transmural infarction. *LA*, left atrium; *RA*, right atrium; *RV*, right ventricle.

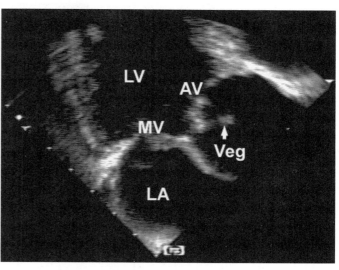

Fig. 19. Transesophageal echocardiogram of a patient with a valvular vegetation (*Veg*) on the aortic surface of a native aortic valve (*AV*). *LA*, left atrium; *LV*, left ventricle; *MV*, mitral valve.

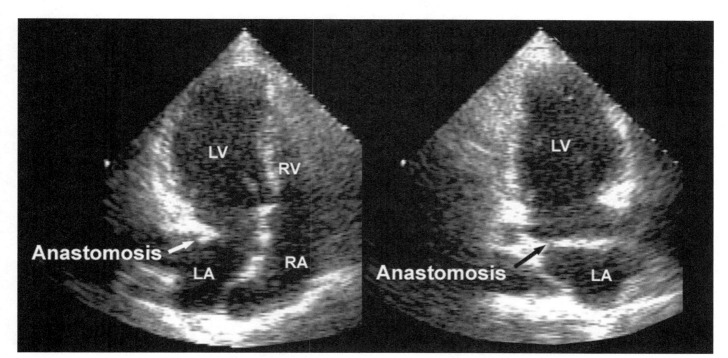

Fig. 20. Status after cardiac transplantation. The left atrial anastomotic site is clearly visible (*arrow*). *LA*, left atrium; *LV*, left ventricle; *RA*, right atrium; *RV*, right ventricle.

Suggested Review Reading

1. Armstrong WF, Pellikka PA, Ryan T, et al: Stress echocardiography: recommendations for performance and interpretation of stress echocardiography. Stress Echocardiography Task Force of the Nomenclature and Standards Committee of the American Society of Echocardiography. *J Am Soc Echocardiogr* 11:97-104, 1998.

A position paper on the clinical usefulness of stress echocardiography, with a review of accuracy and prognostic studies.

2. Basnight MA, Gonzalez MS, Kershenovich SC, Appleton CP: Pulmonary venous flow velocity: relation to hemodynamics, mitral flow velocity and left atrial volume, and ejection fraction. *J Am Soc Echocardiogr* 4:547-558, 1991.

3. Cheitlin MD, Alpert JS, Armstrong WF, et al: ACC/AHA guidelines for the clinical application of echocardiography: executive summary. A report of the American College of Cardiology/American Heart Association Task Force on Practice Guidelines (Committee on Clinical Application of Echocardiography). Developed in collaboration with the American Society of Echocardiography. *J Am Coll Cardiol* 29:862-879, 1997.

Guidelines and recommendations for optimal clinical use of echocardiography by a panel of experts. Class III indications ("procedure is not useful/effective") should be particularly noted.

4. Chuah SC, Pellikka PA, Roger VL, et al: Role of dobutamine stress echocardiography in predicting outcome in 860 patients with known or suspected coronary artery disease. *Circulation* 97:1474-1480, 1998.

5. Fleischmann KE, Hunink MG, Kuntz KM, Douglas PS: Exercise echocardiography or exercise SPECT imaging? A meta-analysis of diagnostic test performance. *JAMA* 280:913-920, 1998.

A meta-analysis of 44 studies comparing exercise echocardiography and nuclear perfusion imaging found similar sensitivities for the detection of coronary artery disease but somewhat better specificity for exercise echocardiography.

6. Kaul S, Senior R, Dittrich H, et al: Detection of coronary artery disease with myocardial contrast echocardiography: comparison with ^{99m}Tc-sestamibi single-photon emission computed tomography. *Circulation* 96:785-792, 1997.

7. Klein AL, Tajik AJ: Doppler assessment of pulmonary venous flow in healthy subjects and in patients with heart disease. *J Am Soc Echocardiogr* 4:379-392, 1991.

8. McCully RB, Roger VL, Mahoney DW, et al: Outcome after normal exercise echocardiography and predictors of subsequent cardiac events: follow-up of 1,325 patients. *J Am Coll Cardiol* 31:144-149, 1998.

Patients who have normal findings on exercise echocardiography and who achieve an adequate workload (men, > 7 METs; women, > 5 METs) have an excellent prognosis, even if they have an intermediate or high pre-test probability of having coronary artery disease. Additional clinical variables identified patients at higher risk (age, workload, angina during exercise test, echocardiographic left ventricular hypertrophy).

9. Nishimura RA, Tajik AJ: Quantitative hemodynamics by Doppler echocardiography: a noninvasive alternative to cardiac catheterization. *Prog Cardiovasc Dis* 36:309-342, 1994.

Summary of noninvasive quantitative hemodynamic assessment in the echocardiographic lab, with excellent graphics and examples.

10. Oh JK, Seward JB, Tajik AJ: *The Echo Manual.* Second edition. Philadelphia, Lippincott-Raven Publishers, 1999.

Excellent resource for nearly all board-pertinent echocardiography. Hundreds of figures and still frames to review.

11. Pellikka PA, Roger VL, Oh JK, et al: Stress echocardiography. II. Dobutamine stress echocardiography: techniques, implementation, clinical applications, and correlations. *Mayo Clin Proc* 70:16-27, 1995.

A "how-to" article on performing dobutamine stress echocardiographic studies, with indications, pitfalls, and limitations of the technique described.

12. Popp R, Agatston A, Armstrong W, et al: Recommendations for training in performance and interpretation of stress echocardiography. Committee on Physician Training and Education of the American Society of Echocardiography. *J Am Soc Echocardiogr* 11:95-96, 1998.

The authors stress the need for specific training in the technique in order to achieve and to maintain accuracy.

13. Quinones MA, Waggoner AD, Reduto LA, et al: A new, simplified and accurate method for determining ejection fraction with two-dimensional echocardiography. *Circulation* 64:744-753, 1981.
Validation studies of the method most commonly used to determine left ventricular ejection fraction (Equation 4).

14. Roger VL, Pellikka PA, Oh JK, et al: Stress echocardiography. I. Exercise echocardiography: techniques, implementation, clinical applications, and correlations. *Mayo Clin Proc* 70:5-15, 1995.

15. Schiller NB, Shah PM, Crawford M, et al: Recommendations for quantitation of the left ventricle by two-dimensional echocardiography. American Society of Echocardiography Committee on Standards, Subcommittee on Quantitation of Two-Dimensional Echocardiograms. *J Am Soc Echocardiogr* 2:358-367, 1989.
Rationale for and technical aspects of echocardiographic quantitation of left ventricular dimensions, volumes, mass, and segmental wall motion analysis.

16. Seward JB, Khandheria BK, Freeman WK, et al: Multiplane transesophageal echocardiography: image orientation, examination technique, anatomic correlations, and clinical applications. *Mayo Clin Proc* 68:523-551, 1993.

17. Tajik AJ, Seward JB, Hagler DJ, et al: Two-dimensional real-time ultrasonic imaging of the heart and great vessels. Technique, image orientation, structure identification, and validation. *Mayo Clin Proc* 53:271-303, 1978.
Step-by-step 2-D examination with anatomical correlation of images.

18. Appleton CP, Jensen JL, Hatle LK, et al: Doppler evaluation of left and right ventricular diastolic function: a technical guide for obtaining optimal flow velocity recordings. *J Am Soc Echocardiogr* 10:271-292, 1997.

19. Nishimura RA, Abel MD, Hatle LK, et al: Assessment of diastolic function of the heart: background and current applications of Doppler echocardiography. II. Clinical studies. *Mayo Clin Proc* 64:181-204, 1989.

20. Nishimura RA, Housmans PR, Hatle LK, et al: Assessment of diastolic function of the heart: background and current applications of Doppler echocardiography. I. Physiologic and pathophysiologic features. *Mayo Clin Proc* 64:71-81, 1989.

21. Oh JK, Appleton CP, Hatle LK, et al: The noninvasive assessment of left ventricular diastolic function with two-dimensional and Doppler echocardiography. *J Am Soc Echocardiogr* 10:246-270, 1997.
References 18-21: Diastolic function as assessed by echocardiography. Practical tips on measuring and interpreting Doppler signals and clinical correlations. Factors influencing diastolic function and individual measurements as well as pitfalls are discussed.

Questions

Multiple Choice (choose the one best answer)

1. A 68-year-old woman had an uncomplicated myocardial infarction 4 days ago. She has stopped smoking and is taking aspirin, β-blockers, and atorvastatin for hyperlipidemia. Before dismissal, a symptom-limited stress test was planned. Shortly before this test was performed, she had a brief syncopal episode and now has mild chest pain. Her heart rate is 80 beats/min and blood pressure is 90/60 mm Hg. Her echocardiogram is shown. What is the next step in management?
   a. Urgent coronary angiography
   b. Thrombolytic therapy
   c. Cardiac surgical consultation
   d. Emergency pericardiocentesis
   e. Aortic root angiography

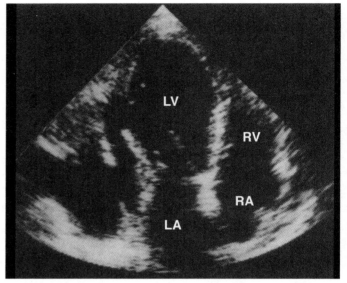

Question 1

2. The following echocardiogram is most consistent with:
   a. A restrictive pattern of left ventricular diastolic filling
   b. Amyloid heart disease
   c. Anteroseptal myocardial infarction
   d. Tricuspid regurgitant velocity of 3.9 m/s

3. The following 2-D echocardiogram would be most consistent with:

   a. Exertional angina and recent ischemic stroke
   b. Peripheral edema and ascites
   c. Diastolic heart murmur
   d. Chest pain and syncope

4. A 58-year-old man undergoes stress echocardiography. He has several risk factors for ischemic heart disease, a history of paroxysmal atrial fibrillation, and atypical chest pain. His medications are digoxin, aspirin, and niacin.

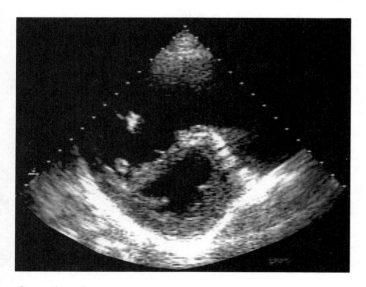

Question 2

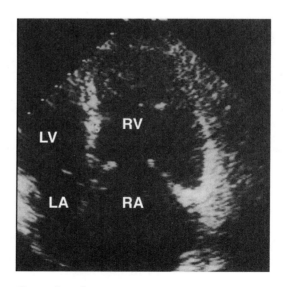

Question 3

He exercises 8 minutes on the Bruce protocol, and heart rate increases from 72 to 126 beats/min and blood pressure from 120/70 to 152/60 mm Hg. He stops because of fatigue and has no chest pain. The exercise ECG is nondiagnostic because of the digoxin effect.

The echocardiographic images were interpreted as follows:

Wall segment	Rest	Stress
Anterior	Normal	Hypokinetic
Septum	Normal	No change
Inferior	Hypokinetic	Hypokinetic
Lateral	Normal	Hyperdynamic
Ejection fraction	55%	55%

The most likely coronary artery anatomy at angiography is which of the following?
a. LAD, 100% occluded; RCA, 100% occluded
b. LAD, 70% occluded; RCA, 70% occluded
c. LAD, 100% occluded; RCA, 70% occluded
d. LAD, 70% occluded; RCA, 100% occluded
e. The exercise test results are nondiagnostic

Note: LAD, left anterior descending coronary artery; RCA, right coronary artery.

5. A 75-year-old woman with chronic obstructive pulmonary disease complains of dyspnea on exertion. Her cardiac silhouette is enlarged on a chest radiograph. The ECG demonstrates sinus rhythm with left bundle branch block.

The accompanying pulmonary vein pulsed-wave Doppler recording is most consistent with which of the following?
a. Severe pulmonary hypertension (cor pulmonale)
b. Aortic stenosis with a mean gradient of 62 mm Hg
c. Mitral regurgitant volume of 122 mL
d. Severe mitral stenosis with a valve area of 1.0 cm^2
e. Aortic regurgitant volume of 80 mL

6. A 65-year-old woman with iron deficiency anemia (hemoglobin, 10.2 g/dL) complains of fatigue. She has no cardiac symptoms. She has a grade III/VI systolic ejection murmur. An echocardiogram shows normal left ventricular size and function and an ejection fraction of 70%. The aortic valve is calcified, and there is very mild aortic regurgitation. The following hemodynamic data were obtained:

Heart rate	70 beats/min
Blood pressure	140/90 mm Hg
Left ventricular outflow tract diameter	2.2 cm
Left ventricular outflow tract velocity	1.4 m/s
Left ventricular outflow tract TVI	30 cm

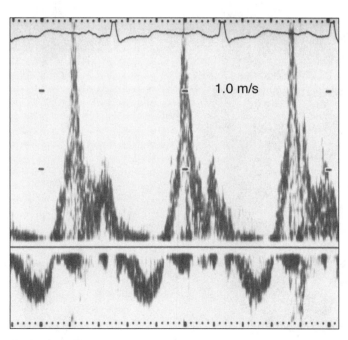

1.0 m/s

Question 5

Aortic velocity   3.5 m/s
Aortic TVI   75 cm
Tricuspid regurgitant velocity   2.4 m/s

Your next recommendation to the patient is which of the following?

a. Consultation with a cardiac surgeon
b. Catheterization of the right and left sides of the heart, with coronary angiography
c. Endocarditis prophylaxis and repeat echocardiography in 6 to 12 months
d. Exercise thallium stress test

7. You care for two patients (A and B) with idiopathic dilated cardiomyopathy. The following clinical and echocardiographic data are provided.

	Patient A	Patient B
Age	50 yr	30 yr
Ejection fraction	15%	25%
End-diastolic diameter	86 mm	72 mm
Left atrial size	36 mm	48 mm
Pulmonary artery systolic pressure	45 mm Hg	60 mm Hg

Which patient has a worse long-term prognosis and is more likely to be symptomatic?

a. "A," because the ejection fraction is lower
b. "B," because the E/A ratio is 4.5
c. "A," because left ventricular dilatation is more profound
d. "B," because pulmonary hypertension is more severe
e. "A," because the patient is older

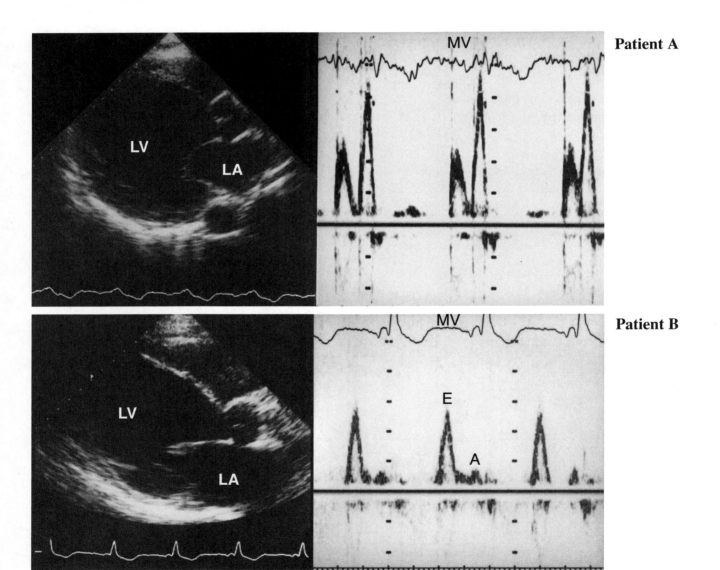

Patient A

Patient B

Question 7. (From Oh JK, Seward JB, Tajik AJ: *The Echo Manual.* Little, Brown and Company, 1994. By permission of Mayo Foundation.)

8. A 55-year-old woman presents with this echocardiogram. Most likely accompanying signs or symptoms include:

a. Blood cultures positive for *S. aureus*
b. Bone pain, anorexia, and hepatic mass
c. Dyspnea, fatigue, transmitral mean gradient 5 mm Hg
d. "Life-long" cardiac murmur

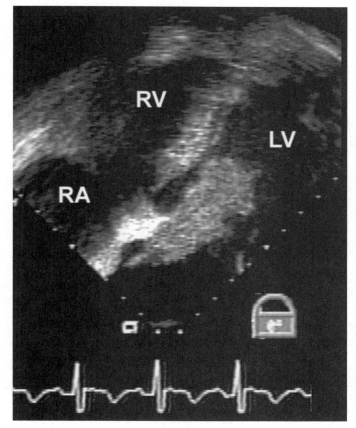

Question 8

Answers

1. Answer c

The 2-D image demonstrates left ventricular free wall rupture near the lateral apex, resulting in pseudoaneurysm formation after myocardial infarction. Echocardiography is an invaluable tool for evaluating recurrent chest pain or new murmurs after myocardial infarction. Patients with impending left ventricular rupture often have chest pain due to localized pericarditis, which may be associated with characteristic ECG changes. Frequently, the patient has a premonitory syncopal or near syncopal episode several hours or days before catastrophic hemodynamic collapse. Other patients, such as this one, have a "contained rupture," as indicated by the large echo-free space adjacent to the left ventricle. Pseudoaneurysms are at high risk for rupture and should be repaired surgically.

2. Answer d

The still frame is an example of right ventricular enlargement due to pressure or volume overload. The left ventricle is small and the interventricular septum is flattened (D-shaped ventricle). The right ventricle is enlarged and pulmonary artery systolic pressure is elevated.

Pulmonary artery systolic
$$\text{pressure} = 4v^2_{TR} + RAP$$
$$= 4 \times (3.9)^2 + 10 \text{ mm Hg}$$
$$= 61 + 10$$
$$= 71 \text{ mm Hg}$$

If volume overload due to severe tricuspid regurgitation or left-to-right shunting is the primary pathophysiology, then right ventricular enlargement occurs, but pulmonary hypertension and right ventricular failure are often late occurrences. In primary pulmonary hypertension, the right ventricle

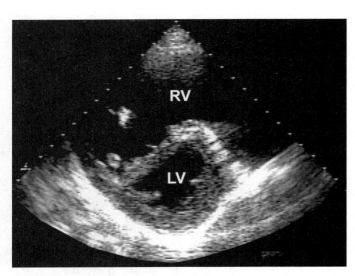

Answer 2

responds initially with hypertrophy, but late in the course of the disease right ventricular dilatation and failure often develop. A similar 2-D appearance may be seen in isolated right ventricular infarction.

3. Answer b

The tricuspid valve has the classic appearance of carcinoid heart disease. The leaflets are thickened, retracted, and immobile and do not coapt, resulting in severe tricuspid regurgitation and, ultimately, signs of right-sided heart failure. Carcinoid heart disease is usually manifested by fibrosis of the endocardium and valve tissue in the chambers of the right side of the heart because of release of vasoactive substances from liver metastases.

4. Answer d

The patient's exercise performance was adequate for diagnostic purposes. A stress test in combination with an imaging modality was necessary because of the effect of digoxin on the ECG. The anterior wall and septum corresponding to the LAD coronary artery distribution had an "ischemic" response to exercise. The normal resting myocardium did not improve or become hypokinetic. The inferior wall response is consistent with infarction in the territory of the right coronary artery. Only the lateral wall had a normal response to stress.

5. Answer c

The pulmonary vein tracing is most consistent with severe mitral regurgitation. Normally in sinus rhythm, systolic forward flow in the pulmonary vein is more prominent than

diastolic forward flow. As mitral regurgitation worsens, pulmonary venous systolic forward flow gradually diminishes and diastolic flow predominates. When mitral regurgitation becomes severe, blood refluxes into the pulmonary veins during systole, causing reversal of flow (below the baseline).

6. Answer c

The echocardiographic data are consistent with mild to moderate aortic stenosis, with aortic valve area (calculated using the continuity equation) of 1.3 cm^2.

$$AVA\ (cm^2) = \pi\,r^2_{LVOT}\ \times\ \frac{TVI_{LVOT}}{TVI_{AV}}$$

$$= 0.785\ (Diameter_{LVOT})^2 \times \frac{TVI_{LVOT}}{TVI_{AV}}$$

$$= 0.785 \times (2.2)^2 \times \frac{30}{85}$$

$$= 1.3\ cm^2$$

Pulmonary artery pressure is normal.

$$Pressure_{PA}\ (mm\ Hg) = 4v^2_{TR} + Pressure_{RA}\ (assumed)$$

$$= 4\ (2.4)^2 + 5$$
$$= 28\ mm\ Hg$$

Stroke volume and cardiac output are in the upper normal range (114 mL and 8.0 L/min, respectively), most likely because of the excellent systolic function and anemia.

$$Stroke\ Volume\ (mL) = Area_{LVOT} \times TVI_{LVOT}$$
$$= 0.785 \times (2.2)^2 \times 30$$
$$= 114\ mL$$

$$Cardiac\ Output\ (L/min) = SV\ (mL) \times HR\ (beats/min)$$
$$= 114 \times 70$$
$$= 7,980\ mL/min$$
$$= 8.0\ L/min$$

The patient should be advised to use appropriate antibiotic prophylaxis for infective endocarditis. The degree of aortic stenosis tends to progress, often at an unpredictable rate. Follow-up clinical examination and echocardiography should be recommended.

In this patient, there is no current indication for aortic valve surgery, because she has no symptoms. Invasive hemodynamic assessment of aortic stenosis is rarely indicated and is usually reserved for those cases in which the echocardiogram is technically inadequate or there is a major discrepancy between the clinical and echocardiographic impressions.

7. Answer b

Several investigators have shown that a restrictive pattern of left ventricular diastolic filling (E/A ratio > 2.5; deceleration time <150-160 ms) is one of the strongest independent predictors of symptoms and increased mortality in patients with dilated cardiomyopathy. The Doppler pattern of restriction indicates high left ventricular end-diastolic pressure, resulting in more dyspnea and a worse New York Heart Association functional class.

Ejection fraction, atrial and ventricular size, pulmonary pressure, and age all contribute to the overall prognosis of patients with dilated cardiomyopathy. The differences in these variables, however, have not been shown to reliably identify those with a poorer prognosis who may benefit from more aggressive medical management or earlier cardiac transplantation. Aggressive medical management of heart failure can improve the diastolic variables, and this change has been associated with improvement in symptoms and prognosis.

Restrictive physiology has also been associated with worse symptoms and prognosis in patients with acute myocardial infarction and amyloid heart disease.

8. Answer c

Myxomas are the most common primary cardiac tumors. Although myxomas may arise from any endocardial surface, over 75% originate in the left atrium and 15% to 20% in the right atrium. Of atrial tumors, 85% originate from the atrial septum, often near the fossa ovalis membrane. These large tumors often prolapse into the mitral valve during diastole, causing obstructive hemodynamics and symptoms of mitral stenosis. This myxoma is large and is attached near the fossa ovalis membrane (arrow). Diastolic (a) and systolic (b) still frames are shown. Although cardiac myxomas can mimic many clinical entities, over 50% present with signs and symptoms of mitral valve disease. Over one-third have embolic phenomena and approximately 15% are asymptomatic. While fever, elevated sedimentation rate, and weight loss may be present in 25% to 50% of cases, blood cultures are not positive. Secondary or metastatic tumors of the heart do not typically attach to the atrial septum. Hepatomas usually affect the heart by direct extension up the inferior vena cava into the right atrium.

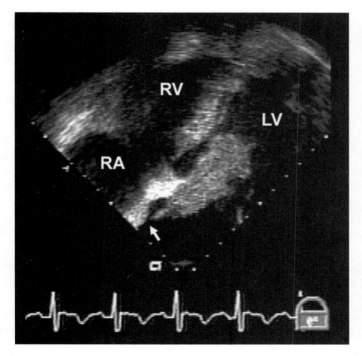

a

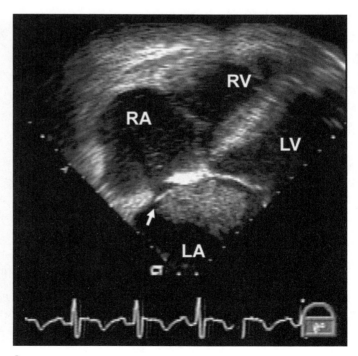

b

Answer 8

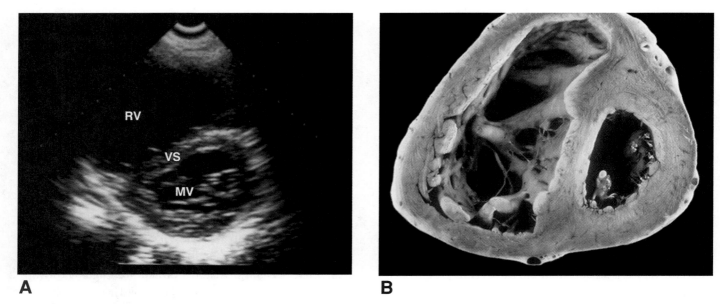

A B

Plate 1. *A*, Parasternal short-axis view demonstrating the D-shaped left ventricular cavity and enlarged right ventricular (*RV*) cavity in pulmonary hypertension. Similar appearances are present in RV volume overload; however, flattening of the ventricular septum (*VS*) persists during the entire cardiac cycle in RV and pulmonary artery pressure overload, whereas it disappears during systole in RV volume overload. *MV*, mitral valve. *B*, Corresponding pathology specimen. (From Oh JK, Seward JB, Tajik AJ: *The Echo Manual*. Second edition. Lippincott-Raven Publishers, 1999, p 217. By permission of Mayo Foundation.)

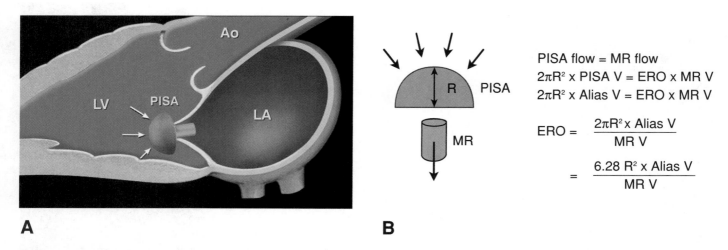

A B

Plate 2. *A*, Diagram of proximal isovelocity surface area (PISA) (*arrows*) of mitral regurgitation. As blood flow converges toward the mitral regurgitant orifice, blood-flow velocity increases gradually and forms multiple isovelocity hemispheric shells. The flow rate calculated at the surface of the hemisphere is equal to the flow rate going through the mitral regurgitant orifice. Ao, aorta. *B*, Calculation and derivation of effective regurgitant orifice (ERO) area of mitral regurgitation (MR) using the PISA method. R, PISA radius; V, velocity. (From Oh JK, Seward JB, Tajik AJ: *The Echo Manual*. Second edition. Lippincott-

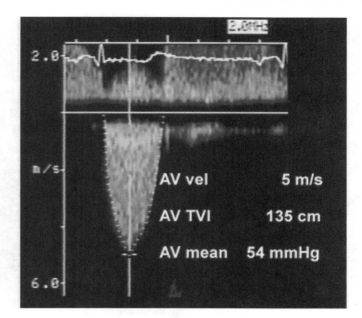

Plate 3. Doppler signal obtained from the apical window in a patient with severe, symptomatic calcific aortic stenosis. LVOT vel = 1 m/s; LVOT TVI = 20 cm; LVOT diameter = 2.0 cm. By continuity equation, aortic valve area = 0.47 cm^2. AV vel = 5 m/s; AV TVI = 135 cm; mean gradient across the aortic valve = 54 mm Hg. AV, aortic valve; LVOT, left ventricular outflow tract; vel, velocity; TVI, time velocity integral.

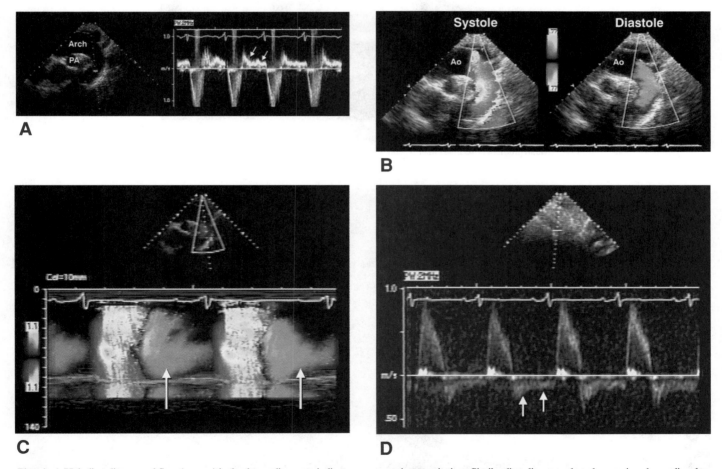

Plate 4. *A*, Holodiastolic reversal flow (*arrows*) in the descending aorta indicates severe aortic regurgitation. Similar diastolic reversal can be seen in a descending thoracic aneurysm or shunt into the aorta during diastole (as in Blalock-Taussig shunt). The sample volume usually is located just distal to the takeoff of the left subclavian artery. *PA*, pulmonary artery. *B*, Two-dimensional color-flow imaging of the descending thoracic aorta during diastole. The orange-red flow in the descending aorta during diastole indicates flow toward the transducer, that is, reversal flow due to severe aortic regurgitation. *Ao*, aorta. *C*, Color M-mode from the descending thoracic aorta shows holodiastolic reversal flow (*arrows*). *D*, Pulsed-wave Doppler recording of abdominal aorta showing diastolic flow reversal (*arrows*) in severe aortic regurgitation. (From Oh JK, Seward JB, Tajik AJ: *The Echo Manual.* Second edition. Lippincott-Raven Publishers, 1999, p 121. By permission of Mayo Foundation.)

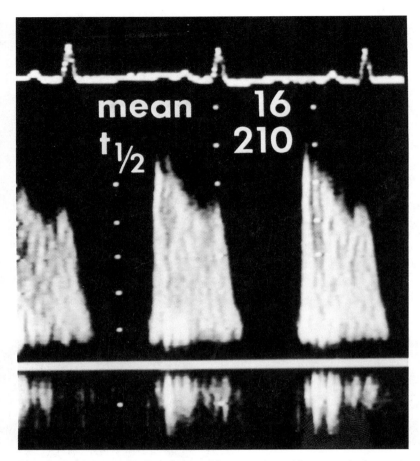

Plate 5. Continuous-wave Doppler signal from a patient with severe mitral stenosis. Mean gradient is 16 mm Hg. Pressure half-time (t $_{1/2}$) is 210 ms. Mitral valve area by pressure half-time method is 1.0 cm^2.

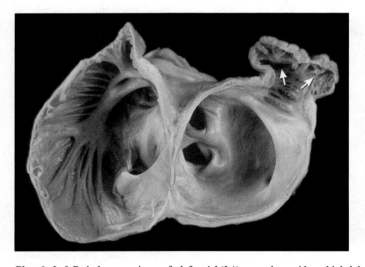
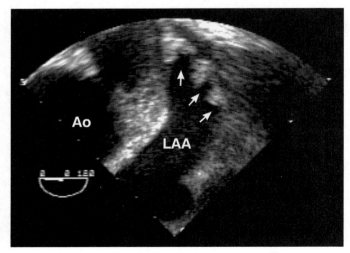

Plate 6. *Left*, Pathology specimen of a left atrial (*LA*) appendage with multiple lobes (*arrows*). *Right*, Transesophageal view of multilobed (*arrows*) LA appendage (*LAA*). *Ao*, aorta. (From Oh JK, Seward JB, Tajik AJ: *The Echo Manual*. Second edition. Lippincott-Raven Publishers, 1999, p 255. By permission of Mayo Foundation.)

Chapter 48

Nuclear Cardiology

Thomas Behrenbeck, M.D., Ph.D.
Timothy F. Christian, M.D.
Brian P. Mullan, M.D.

> Important examination topics in nuclear cardiology include the assessment of myocardial viability, preoperative assessment of cardiac risk for noncardiac surgery, and pharmacologic stress testing.

Nuclear cardiology imaging techniques are most useful for the assessment of left ventricular function and measurement of coronary blood flow in both acute and chronic coronary syndromes (Table 1). Nuclear studies are used less commonly in the diagnosis of valvular and congenital heart disease, primary myocardial disorders, intracardiac thrombi, and autonomic nervous system disorders.

Basics of Radionuclide Imaging

Radionuclide imaging uses a special camera that images photons generated by radioisotopes. Photons are emitted in all directions from the point of origin. Ideally, the photon leaves the patient in a straight line and is captured by the detector. What is more likely is that the photon will be scattered by intervening tissue between the radiation source and the detector. The scattering, or "Compton effect," is the most common event after photon emanation and poses a significant problem for the detection and localization of the original position of the photon. A second possibility is the absorption of the photon by tissue attenuation, making it "invisible" to detection. Photon absorption (photoelectric

Table 1.—Application of Nuclear Cardiology Imaging Procedures

Coronary artery disease
    Acute—assessment of myocardial salvage by reperfusion therapy and prognosis
    Chronic—diagnosis, assessment of therapy, viability, and prognosis
Cardiomyopathy—left and right function, serial assessment, and prognosis
Valvular heart disease—left and right ventricular function, regurgitant fraction, timing of intervention, and assessment of therapy
Congenital heart disease—shunt quantification and ventricular function
Other conditions
    Preoperative cardiac risk assessment before noncardiac surgery
    Chronic obstructive pulmonary disease—left and right ventricular function
    Left ventricular dysfunction after chemotherapy

absorption) is more prevalent in "dense tissues" (with high atomic numbers) such as calcium and depends on the energy of the photon (the less photon energy, the more absorption in the body). Both thallium and technetium, the two most common cardiac radionuclide isotopes, have enough energy to render absorption unimportant in clinical imaging.

- Photons are units of energy measured in kiloelectron volts (keV).
- Gamma radiation is the form of energy in nuclear imaging.
- Photons are scattered, detected, or absorbed by tissue.

Tissue attenuation has an important role during image acquisition. The higher the energy of the original isotope, the greater the likelihood that the photon will leave the body (i.e., the lower the attenuation).

- The higher the isotope energy, the less chance for scatter or absorption.
- The closer to the detector the photon originates (anterior vs. posterior), the greater the chance for detection.
- The larger the patient, the fewer photons that reach the detector.

Isotopes and Detector Equipment

The two most commonly used isotopes are technetium-99m (^{99m}Tc) and thallium-201 (^{201}Tl). Technetium (half-life, 6 hours) is used in both myocardial perfusion studies and radionuclide angiography and is formed on site from molybdenum-99 (^{99}Mo). The parent compound ^{99}Mo has a half-life of 66 hours and is easily transported. From this generator, the metastable ^{99m}Tc is constantly formed and eluted. During the decay of ^{99m}Tc to Tc-99, photons are emitted with a characteristic 140-keV photopeak. In contrast, ^{201}Tl is generated in a cyclotron facility and transported as a finished product; it has a half-life of 73 hours.

The thallium isotope radiodecay process is more complex, with most (93%) photons (x-rays) in the 80-keV range (69-83 keV). The physical properties of technetium make it the more desirable imaging agent. Its higher, more uniform energy profile provides better tissue transmission (less absorption) and less scattering; its shorter half-life and physical characteristics allow use of significantly higher radioactive doses without patient risk, all of which contribute to better image quality with ^{99m}Tc compared with ^{201}Tl. A typical myocardial perfusion or radionuclide angiographic dose of 30 mCi ^{99m}Tc is approximately equivalent in total body radiation dose to a 2-mCi dose of ^{201}Tl. The biologic properties of thallium provide some unique, important applications in cardiology, especially in the area of myocardial viability.

- ^{201}Tl and ^{99m}Tc are the two most commonly used isotopes in nuclear cardiology.

- ^{201}Tl has a lower energy spectrum (80-keV electron signature), has a longer half-life (73 hours), and is more expensive than ^{99m}Tc.
- ^{99m}Tc emits a 140-keV photon and has a short half-life (6 hours).

Photon Detection (Imaging Chain)

The quality of image acquisition depends on the number of nonscattered photons detected by the camera. There is constant radioactive decay with radiation of photons. A sufficient number of photons need to be detected to form a high-quality image.

Imaging Equipment

The photon detector in nuclear studies is a sodium iodide crystal that converts gamma rays into visible light. This signal is then piped through a photocathode into a photomultiplier tube, converting light into an electrical signal that generates the study images. There are two principal detector configurations. The more common is the single crystal camera, which consists of a large sodium iodide crystal connected to an array of photomultiplier tubes. Less commonly, multicrystal gamma cameras are used for first-pass ejection fraction studies. Elimination of scattered photons is achieved by using a lead collimator with cylindrical holes. Energy windows set around the expected energy peak (e.g., 140 keV for ^{99m}Tc) further help reduce unwanted scatter. The need for gamma camera collimation to ensure satisfactory spatial resolution creates a significant limitation in nuclear studies.

Imaging Techniques

Radionuclide Angiography

The two principal imaging methods in clinical nuclear cardiology are radionuclide angiography (RNA) and perfusion imaging. In RNA, an isotope, usually ^{99m}Tc, is tagged to a biologic carrier (albumin or, more commonly, red blood cells). The biologic half-life of the labeled blood cells thus prepared is about 20 hours, and the usable blood pool activity of ^{99m}Tc is approximately 6 hours. Resting images are obtained in the anterior, lateral, and left anterior oblique (LAO) projections. Images are electrocardiographically (ECG)-gated throughout the cardiac cycle. A satisfactory image is based on sufficient photon capture, so many cardiac cycles (200-300) need to be sampled. Ideally, heart rate should be constant because any significant variation in the rate or arrhythmia may degrade the image. Exercise RNA using a supine or semi-recumbent bicycle exercise reduces motion artifacts during imaging. Because it takes approximately 40 seconds to reach a heart rate plateau and the camera acquisition lasts 2 minutes, each exercise stage lasts 3 minutes. This usually precludes imaging for more than one view. Conventionally, the LAO view is obtained throughout exercise. This yields a left ventricular image that is subdivided into five segments (Fig. 1). These segments roughly correspond to the three coronary artery territories as follows: the two septal segments are perfused by the left anterior descending artery, the inferior apical segment is perfused by the right coronary artery, and the circumflex artery supplies the two lateral segments. Quantitative or qualitative regional wall motion analysis is performed. Count-based nuclear angiography does not require any assumptions regarding the geometry of the ventricle and it is well suited for an accurate, operator-independent assessment of left ventricular dysfunction and ejection fraction. Several approaches have been developed to quantitate ventricular volumes. Variation in body size, chest wall attenuations, and the distance of the left ventricle to the detector pose significant limitations for interindividual comparison. However, serial measurements in a patient are reliable because imaging conditions remain essentially unchanged and are sensitive to small changes in cardiac function. Other clinical variables assessed are size and function of the right ventricle and the size of the atrial chambers and great vessels. Aside from systolic function variables, diastolic function can also be analyzed. First half filling fraction (the proportion of early diastolic filling), rate of peak filling, and time to peak filling are clinical variables that distinguish delayed ventricular relaxation from restrictive filling patterns.

- RNA requires ECG gating. Cardiac rhythms with little beat-to-beat variation are essential.
- RNA does not require geometric assumptions regarding ventricular shape.
- Ejection fraction determination by RNA is excellent, with little intraindividual and interindividual variation, particularly in patients with a low ejection fraction (< 30%).
- Volume determination is dependent on several complex variables (such as heart-to-detector distance and chest wall thickness).
- Stress RNA is performed in one view only (usually LAO).

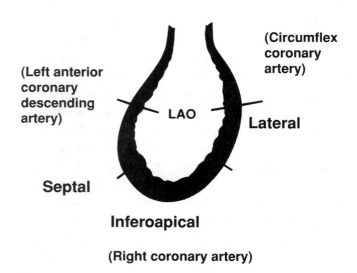

Fig. 1. The left anterior oblique (LAO) view is commonly used in exercise radionuclide angiography. The five segments are roughly attributable to the three coronary artery territories. Note the relative underrepresentation of the right coronary artery and overrepresentation of the circumflex coronary artery.

^{201}Tl and Sestamibi Imaging

Thallium-201

^{201}Tl is a potassium analogue and is avidly taken up by myocardial cells. Uptake of the isotope into the myocardium is related directly to coronary blood flow. After the initial injection, usually following pharmacologic stress or exercise, a complex distribution and redistribution process occurs. Initially, the hypoperfused ischemic myocardium shows less isotope uptake. However, over time (about 7 hours), the thallium equilibrates with the blood pool. Myocardial washout after the initial active uptake phase also occurs. The net results of the redistribution process lead to further thallium uptake in the hypoperfused ischemic myocardium. Thus, the initially hypoperfused or ischemic myocardium shows an initially reduced uptake that is visible as a "defect," which normalizes with time. A more recent technique speeds up this process by "enriching" the blood pool with an additional 1 mCi of isotope before acquisition of redistribution images, the so-called reinjection technique. This significantly increases the sensitivity and specificity of the technique. In thallium imaging, 3 mCi is usually injected during peak exercise or pharmacologic stress, with an additional dose of 1 mCi approximately 30 minutes before the resting images (usually 4 hours after stress).

Images are acquired in one of two ways: the older method

is planar imaging, in which a camera is placed in three fixed positions, not unlike RNA imaging. In single photon emission computed tomographic (SPECT) imaging, a camera rotates 180° around the patient and 30 images are acquired in a "stop-and-shoot" fashion, with each image taking about 30 to 40 seconds for acquisition. The images are then reconstructed by computer to form a three-dimensional representation of the myocardium, which is superior to planar imaging in the detection of a previous myocardial infarction, diagnosis of milder forms of coronary artery disease, and detection of multivessel coronary disease.

Another feature of thallium imaging is the recognition of increased lung uptake immediately after exercise, which indicates heart failure and is strongly associated with left main coronary artery disease, three-vessel disease, and significant left ventricular dysfunction. It is available in both planar and SPECT imaging.

^{99m}Tc (Sestamibi)

Because ^{201}Tl has less than ideal photon energy and a long half-life, technetium compounds have been developed to facilitate higher quality scans and to reduce artifacts. Three agents have been approved using ^{99m}Tc isotopes: teboroxime, tetrafosmin, and sestamibi, the last of which is the one most widely used.

As with thallium, Tc-sestamibi is distributed in relation to coronary blood flow and requires an intact cell membrane for uptake. After entering the myocardial cell, Tc-sestamibi is transported through the cytoplasm and bound to the mitochondria. Unlike thallium, Tc-sestamibi uptake from a clinical point of view is irreversible, with no significant late tissue washout. Thus, Tc-sestamibi is ideally suited for imaging acute myocardial infarction and unstable angina. Because of its higher photon energy, it is also preferred in large patients (> 100 kg) and in women to reduce breast artifacts (soft tissue attenuation). Compared with ^{201}Tl, Tc-sestamibi imaging is superior in the detection of single-vessel coronary artery disease and may be used with a first-pass study to assess global left ventricular function. In the rest/stress protocol, the exercise or stress portion is usually performed 24 hours after initial imaging to avoid high-background isotope counts. It also can be performed as a two-dose study (low dose/high dose) in a 1-day stress/rest study. More recently, SPECT ^{99m}Tc-sestamibi images have been gated for left ventricular function and regional wall motion assessment.

- Thallium is a potassium analogue that requires active membrane transport.

- Unlike thallium, sestamibi is actively taken up and bound "irreversibly" to intracellular mitochondria.
- Sestamibi is the preferred imaging agent in large (> 100 kg) patients and women with large breasts.

Positron Emission Tomography

Positron emission tomography (PET) imaging agents emit two high-energy photons (511 keV) simultaneously in opposite directions. A PET scanner consists of a circular array of detectors that allow these photon pairs to be detected (coincidence detection). This type of imaging leads to better spatial resolution, as compared with conventional isotope SPECT, and with attenuation correction, it is possible to calculate absolute myocardial blood flow and metabolic activity (previously impossible with SPECT). Imaging is relatively fast compared with SPECT, yielding high temporal resolution.

Two different groups of imaging agents are used in PET scanning. The first group measures myocardial perfusion; the agents most commonly used are rubidium-82 (half-life, 75 seconds), nitrogen-13 ammonia (half-life, 10 minutes), and oxygen-15 water (half-life, 2 minutes). The second group measures metabolic processes and includes carbon-11-labeled fatty acids (half-life, 20 minutes) and fluorine-18 fluorodeoxyglucose (FDG) (half-life, 110 minutes). Oxidative metabolism and oxygen consumption can be assessed with C-11 acetate. With this variety of tracers, PET can help in the evaluation of regional myocardial blood flow, metabolic processes, oxygen consumption, receptor activity, and membrane function. To date, two cardiac clinical applications have emerged: 1) the noninvasive detection of coronary artery disease and the assessment of its severity and 2) the assessment of myocardial viability. The initial "head-to-head" comparison indicated a higher diagnostic accuracy of PET scanning over SPECT thallium, particularly in the inferior-posterior region of the heart, an area where SPECT is subject to a greater error rate, attributed partly to diaphragmatic attenuation. Detection of single-coronary artery disease also appears improved, but selection bias may favor PET imaging. As yet, no conclusive evidence indicates that PET imaging provides additional diagnostic accuracy to justify its higher cost. PET imaging has become the reference standard for the detection of viable myocardium, particularly using the intrinsic capability of perfusion *and* metabolic imaging to detect areas of decreased perfusion (with rubidium-82 or N-13 ammonia) but preserved metabolism (F-18 FDG). This perfusion-metabolism mismatch indicates ischemic or hibernating myocardium and allows it to be differentiated from myocardial fibrosis, which can be difficult for SPECT imaging.

- PET scanning is based on coincidence detection.
- Higher energy and technical principle allow better spatial resolution and faster image acquisition than conventional SPECT.
- PET is the reference standard for detection of viable myocardium.
- PET is the only clinical technique to calculate absolute myocardial blood flow.

Stress Techniques

Stress imaging requires two perfusion studies: one representing basal coronary artery blood flow and the other, coronary blood flow during stress. Typically with maximal exercise, blood flow is increased up to fivefold over that of the resting condition. A significant fixed coronary artery stenosis does not permit a maximal increase in regional blood flow in the territory of the stenosed vessel, thus creating a flow differential and inhomogeneous distribution of the radioisotope (Fig. 2 and Plate 1). In patients who are unable to exercise, pharmacologic stress may be preferred (Plate 2). The following pharmacologic agents are widely used.

Dipyridamole (0.56 mg/kg body weight) or adenosine (140 µg/kg per minute over 6 minutes)—These agents are able to increase coronary blood flow up to 400% (adenosine, which blocks adenosine reuptake, increases blood flow slightly more than dipyridamole). In the presence of a fixed coronary artery stenosis, blood is preferentially diverted to the epicardium because of its higher capacitance. This does not represent a "true" steal effect, although this may occur in very severe stenoses. Side effects are common with both drugs and usually are more pronounced—but also shorter-lived—with adenosine. Common side effects are light-headedness, flushing, headache, and nausea. More serious side effects are hypotension (usually counteracted by administration of fluid), chest pain (most often nonspecific and not associated with perfusion defects), respiratory arrest (usually reversible by either discontinuation of adenosine or administration of aminophylline), and ECG changes (usually indicating severe multivessel disease). Absolute contraindications for both drugs include unstable angina, severe asthma, and allergy to dipyridamole/adenosine or aminophylline, which reverses the effects of dipyridamole. Relative contraindications are resting hypotension, severe mitral and aortic stenosis, carotid artery stenosis, and bronchospasm (can be avoided by pretreatment with

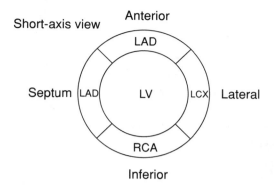

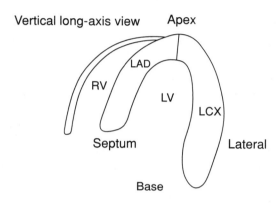

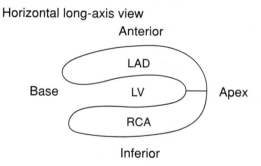

Fig. 2. Cardiac nuclear imaging planes and coronary artery distribution. LAD, left anterior descending coronary artery; LCX, left circumflex coronary artery; LV, left ventricle; RCA, right coronary artery; RV, right ventricle.

β-agonists). Stress testing with adenosine or dipyridamole (not dobutamine) is the preferred method in patients with baseline or exercise-induced left bundle branch block.

Dobutamine—This agent acts through the catecholamine system by increasing heart rate, ventricular contractility, and systolic blood pressure. Coronary blood flow is maximally increased 1.5- to 2.5-fold. Dobutamine is administered by titrating the dose stepwise (up to 40 µg/kg per minute) to a target heart rate of 85% of the maximal predicted heart rate. In patients receiving β-blocker therapy, this goal may require additional administration of 0.5 to 1.0 mg of atropine.

- Pharmacologic stress tests are more sensitive for the detection of myocardial ischemia in patients with symptom-limiting claudication.
- Adenosine is more potent than dipyridamole for increasing coronary artery blood flow.
- Dipyridamole or adenosine, *not* dobutamine, is the preferred agent for patients with left bundle branch block.
- Dobutamine is helpful in low doses for the detection of viable myocardium.

Infarct Pyrophosphate Imaging

Pyrophosphate tagged with ^{99m}Tc accumulates in necrotic cardiac tissue, producing a "hot spot." Imaging is performed 3 hours after the injection of 10 to 15 mCi of ^{99m}Tc-phosphate. Imaging cannot be performed before 4 hours after myocardial infarction; peak uptake occurs 2 to 3 days after infarction and declines at 1 week. Pyrophosphate infarct scanning is now rarely used.

Sensitivity and Specificity of Nuclear Cardiac Imaging

The power of any diagnostic test (its ability to detect disease) depends on the incidence or prevalence of disease in the population studied. If a test result is positive in a patient with a very low probability of disease, the result likely is false-positive. Conversely, in patients with a high likelihood of disease, a negative result is likely false-negative. To define the pretest likelihood of significant coronary artery disease, it is necessary to consider sex, age, and clinical symptoms. Four levels of pretest probability are recommended by the American College of Cardiology/American Hospital Association guidelines: high (> 90%), intermediate (10%-90%), low (< 10%), and very low (< 5%). Stress testing is not helpful in the high, low, or very low incidence groups, because the chance that the patients will have (low, very low groups) or will not have (high group) disease is small. A test result in the "opposite direction" (i.e., a negative result in a group of patients with a high likelihood of disease, e.g., a 65-year-old man with typical angina who smokes) does not exclude disease.

If 1,000 people are considered, with a prevalence of disease of 1%, the number of people who have the disease is only 10. If a test has an 80% sensitivity and a 90% specificity, only 8 patients will have a true-positive result; however, 99 patients will have a false-positive result.

The sensitivity of a test indicates the number of people who have the disease and in whom the test is positive, and specificity indicates the number of people who do not have

the disease and in whom the test is negative. Thus, nuclear imaging studies work best (provided sensitivity and specificity are equally strong) when the pretest likelihood is in the intermediate range. The sensitivity and specificity of several radionuclide imaging methods are listed in Table 2.

Prognosis in Coronary Artery Disease

Exercise duration, peak heart rate achieved, rate response during exercise, peak blood pressure achieved, blood pressure response, and presence and severity of ST-segment depression or elevation in relation to exercise stage achieved are important predictors of prognosis and probability of significant coronary artery disease. The workload achieved is expressed in METs (metabolic equivalents) or rate pressure products. One MET is the expression for baseline oxygen consumption (estimated to be 3.5 mL oxygen, by body weight/min). Various exercise protocols increase this oxygen requirement by multiples over baseline. The most commonly applied exercise protocol in the United States, the Bruce protocol, is the equivalent of 5 METs after completion of stage I.

Patients who are able to achieve high MET levels and those who achieve peak heart rates exceeding 120 beats/min have a good prognosis. Various underlying conditions (anemia, hyperthyroidism, chronic obstructive pulmonary disease, valvular disease, deconditioning) increase oxygen demand at any given level of exercise; conversely, β-blockade will reduce oxygen consumption for a similar workload. Failure

Table 2.—Sensitivity and Specificity of Radionuclide Imaging Methods

Test	Sensitivity, %	Specificity, %
Exercise		
Planar thallium	82	88
Planar sestamibi	84	83
SPECT thallium	90	80
SPECT sestamibi	90	93
Adenosine/dipyridamole		
Planar thallium	82	75
SPECT thallium	89	78
Dobutamine		
SPECT thallium	82	73

SPECT, single photon emission computed tomography.

to increase blood pressure during exercise is an important predictor of left ventricular dysfunction and left main coronary artery or three-vessel disease.

Exercise-induced ST-segment depression is the cardinal indicator in ECG tracings of the presence of disease. The degree of ST-segment depression is correlated with a higher probability of significant coronary artery disease, independent of other risk factors (e.g., diabetes mellitus). ST-segment depression is not helpful in localizing the myocardial segment or the coronary artery stenosis. In contrast, ST-segment elevation is accurate in localizing the myocardium in jeopardy.

- Never view cardiac nuclear scans in isolation, but always evaluate in conjunction with the exercise variables.
- There may be important information in nonimaging variables:

  Exercise duration (in relation to age)
  Peak heart rate (left ventricular dysfunction, medication)
  Peak blood pressure (a decrease is pathologic)
  Onset of ST-segment changes (in minutes and heart rate)
  Time to recovery of ST-segment changes to baseline

Imaging Variables

Radionuclide Angiography
The main prognostic variables in exercise RNA are the changes in ejection fraction from rest to exercise and the resting and stress regional wall motion abnormalities. A decrease by 5 ejection fraction points from rest is pathologic; however, the absolute peak exercise ejection fraction is a more powerful prognostic indicator by itself than the change in ejection fraction. Other imaging variables are the changes in left and right ventricular size from rest to exercise and the development of new exercise-induced regional wall motion abnormalities. A normal response is a decrease in end-systolic and increase in end-diastolic left ventricular volume with increased stroke volume. A decrease in end-diastolic volume is abnormal.

Myocardial Perfusion Imaging
In perfusion imaging, the main indicators of disease are the presence or absence of redistribution or reperfusion abnormalities and presence or absence of fixed myocardial defects (Plate 3). Post-exercise left ventricular dilatation

is an important indicator of exercise-induced left ventricular dysfunction, particularly if isotope uptake does not suggest severe coronary artery disease. In thallium imaging, increased lung uptake, assessed in the anteroposterior position, is a poor prognostic sign, suggestive of left ventricular dysfunction and heart failure (Plate 4).

Clinical Disease Entities

Myocardial Infarction
^{99m}Tc-sestamibi is useful in assessing the extent of infarct severity, future prognosis for cardiac events, and myocardium at risk. After injection, the isotope binds irreversibly with the myocardial cells, reflecting the state of coronary blood flow at time of injection. In patients with acute coronary syndrome, the isotope can be injected during the symptomatic phase and imaging can be delayed for several hours. Measurement of the myocardium at risk is important because it is highly predictive of final infarct size, even if reperfusion is successful. Final infarct size is a major determinant of long-term patient survival. Because the amount of scarring is inversely correlated with the "residual" ejection fraction in the absence of myocardial stunning or hibernation, measurements of resting ejection fraction are also helpful for prognosis.

In patients who have had a myocardial infarction, assessment of residual stress-induced ischemia with either RNA or myocardial perfusion imaging is predictive of future cardiac events. This is independent of the stress method used (exercise or dipyridamole/adenosine). Recent studies have examined the safety of stress testing within 48 to 72 hours after infarction. The data are not yet conclusive. A current problem is the application of prethrombolytic historical data to post-infarction risk stratification. Since the introduction of aggressive revascularization strategies, final infarct size has decreased substantially, improving long-term survival and decreasing the likelihood of future adverse cardiac events. Predismissal exercise testing in the thrombolytic/interventional era addresses an entirely different population, one with a lower incidence of severe residual coronary artery disease. Additional studies are necessary to test the validity of previously established post-infarction risk stratification algorithms in the current clinical environment.

Since the advent of echocardiography for the assessment of mechanical complications in acute myocardial infarction (papillary muscle rupture with subsequent mitral regurgitation, septal infarction with intracardiac shunt, formation of left ventricular aneurysm and pseudoaneurysm), radionuclide tests are reserved for patients in whom echocardiography is not feasible or yields nondiagnostic images.

Assessment of therapeutic success by either thrombolysis or primary percutaneous transluminal coronary angioplasty is an important clinical issue, with two primary aspects: the determination of early reperfusion and the verification of myocardial salvage. Early (18-48 hours) imaging with ^{99m}Tc-sestamibi can identify patients with both coronary artery patency and myocardial salvage; however, it cannot distinguish between patients with persistent occlusion and those who have had vessel patency restored too late for myocardial salvage.

Unstable Angina

Patients with unstable angina should be considered for radionuclide tests only if the medical history or ECG changes are absent or inconclusive. Patients with stuttering symptoms but pain-free intervals may benefit from rest sestamibi imaging, with injection of the isotope during episodes of angina. Once injected, aggressive pharmacotherapy can be used without compromise of the "anginal" image. In patients with known coronary artery disease and unstable angina who are not suitable for complete revascularization or surgical intervention, ^{99m}Tc-sestamibi imaging may identify the culprit lesion to facilitate focused intervention. After being stabilized, patients can undergo myocardial perfusion imaging to determine the risk of future cardiac events. The size of the perfusion defect (the number of segments with reduced uptake) is a more powerful predictor of future events than the severity of underperfused myocardium. Patients who have undergone partial revascularization can be assessed for the completeness of myocardial perfusion or the functional significance of the unrevascularized stenoses.

- RNA does not have a routine value in the acute setting of myocardial infarction apart from measurement of the ejection fraction.
- Perfusion imaging (sestamibi) aids in determination of post-infarction prognosis by evaluating both the myocardium at risk and the ultimate defect size.
- Patients with unstable angina can benefit from SPECT sestamibi to determine the extent and severity of resting ischemia.
- Extensive moderate perfusion defects have a worse prognosis than localized severe perfusion defects.

Chronic Ischemic Disease

Radionuclide imaging has a central role in the diagnosis and prognosis of chronic ischemic disease. Both ^{201}Tl- and ^{99m}Tc-based radiopharmaceuticals yield similar results. Theoretic considerations would favor ^{99m}Tc-sestamibi in patients with significant tissue attenuation (obesity, breast attenuation), resulting in a better specificity (Plate 5). In patients without a history of myocardial infarction but severely reduced resting coronary blood flow, ^{99m}Tc-sestamibi may show a defect with only minimal uptake, suggestive of myocardial infarction. Because of the absence of redistribution, comparison with a resting study may not distinguish between these two entities. ^{201}Tl may provide additional viability information in this setting. PET imaging would be the reference standard. ^{99m}Tc-sestamibi first-pass assessment of left ventricular function (ejection fraction) provides important additional information for risk stratification.

SPECT imaging is more accurate than planar imaging in the diagnosis of coronary artery disease, particularly in localization of the hypoperfused territory. Radionuclide imaging is at least as powerful as coronary angiography in predicting future cardiac events and performs even better in patients with previous myocardial infarction. SPECT perfusion imaging is least sensitive in the lateral wall (circumflex artery territory), and exercise RNA may be more appropriate if clinical questions concern the circumflex coronary artery or its obtuse marginal branches.

In patients receiving antianginal therapy (β-blockers, calcium antagonists, and nitrates), the ischemic threshold may not be reached despite the presence of significant coronary artery stenoses. Imaging in such a situation may be useful to assess the efficacy of therapy; however, it may obfuscate the diagnosis of coronary artery disease. Tapering and discontinuing the drug treatment (β-blockers and calcium antagonists 48 hours and nitrates 12 hours before testing) are recommended whenever possible to improve diagnostic accuracy if exercise stress testing is considered. Pharmacologic stress testing (dipyridamole or adenosine, *not* dobutamine) does not appear to be affected because of the different mechanisms of coronary flow enhancement and, thus, may be preferable if the antianginal therapy cannot be discontinued temporarily.

Women have a higher likelihood (up to 45%) of false-positive treadmill exercise results. Myocardial perfusion imaging is a useful adjunct to evaluate such cases, and breast attenuation makes ^{99m}Tc-sestamibi the isotope of choice. Elderly patients may be a diagnostic problem because of their inability to achieve adequate exercise levels; thus, pharmacologic testing is preferable, particularly in the setting of preoperative risk assessment. When exercised, patients with resting, exercise-induced, or pacemaker-dependent left bundle branch block often exhibit myocardial perfusion defects in the septum in the absence of coronary artery stenoses. These defects usually are not present with pharmacologic testing (dipyridamole or adenosine), which is the stress method of choice in this patient group. Patients with known significant hypertensive blood pressure response during exercise may also benefit from pharmacologic stress testing, because hypertension-induced myocardial ischemia may be indistinguishable from coronary stenosis-induced ischemia.

Noninvasive testing usually is not indicated for predicting future cardiac events in asymptomatic patients because of the low positive predictive value in this group. An exception may be patients without symptoms but positive stress ECG findings, because the presence or absence of sizable perfusion defects has important prognostic implications. The absence of perfusion defects even in the presence of symptoms indicates an excellent prognosis, with an event rate of 0.9% per year, which is comparable to that of the general population. A normal study is also an important predictor of favorable outcome, even in the presence of known coronary artery disease.

- Screening asymptomatic patients with nuclear stress testing is not efficient.
- Severe hypertension can cause ischemia without coronary artery disease.
- A negative test is a powerful predictor of an excellent prognosis, even in the presence of known coronary artery disease.

Preoperative Risk Assessment

Patients undergoing noncardiac vascular surgery have a high incidence of concomitant coronary artery disease. Pharmacologic stress testing has been studied extensively, because most of these patients cannot achieve a satisfactory exercise level. Patients with a normal resting ECG and normal cardiac history and cardiac examination findings have a low perioperative risk. A normal pharmacologic stress myocardial perfusion scan is associated with a low incidence of perioperative cardiac events. An abnormal test has a positive predictive value between 15% and 30% for perioperative cardiac events. Patients undergoing noncardiac, nonvascular surgery

should not routinely be stressed unless coronary artery disease is documented or suspected.

Assessment of Cardiac Risk and Prognosis

RNA is useful in assessing the risk and success of revascularization and medical treatments. Resting ejection fraction provides important information regarding long-term prognosis and for decision making regarding surgical, medical, or interventional therapy; appropriate levels of exercise activity; rehabilitation; and work status. A decrease in the ejection fraction during exercise or a poor peak exercise ejection fraction is associated with a poor long-term prognosis for survival.

In myocardial perfusion imaging, the presence of increased lung uptake on thallium imaging is also associated with a poor prognosis. This, together with marked post-stress dilatation of the left ventricle and multiple perfusion defects, is suggestive of either left main coronary artery or severe three-vessel coronary artery disease. Patients with left main coronary artery disease may not have regionally reduced uptake in the septum, anterior, and lateral walls but rather have a more general pattern of perfusion abnormalities and increased lung uptake (lung/heart ratio $\geq 50\%$). With use of all three criteria, 86% of all patients in this high-risk category can be identified. The number of affected myocardial segments is more important than the severity of hypoperfusion and more predictive for long-term survival than the number of angiographically documented diseased vessels. Peripheral coronary artery lesions are usually associated with smaller perfusion defects, which are associated with a better prognosis. Patients with stable chronic angina or asymptomatic patients with coronary artery disease should not undergo serial nuclear exercise testing unless their pattern of symptoms or exercise capacity changes. Similarly, patients who have successfully undergone catheter-based intervention or bypass surgery and are symptom-free do not benefit from serial stress testing unless the clinical variables have changed.

Assessment of Myocardial Viability

Patients with severe coronary artery disease may have impairment of their resting flow in several coronary arteries, with subsequent severe left ventricular dysfunction and congestive heart failure. It is important to assess whether revascularization, that is, restoration of normal resting flow, would result in improvement of left ventricular function and, thus, prognosis. This situation, labeled "hibernating myocardium," needs to be distinguished from "myocardial stunning," in which temporary cessation or critical reduction of coronary blood flow has resulted in loss of myocardial contractility. Even though the clinical substrate is similar (i.e., loss of systolic function), myocardial stunning is usually self-reversing and contractility returns when coronary blood flow resumes. Stunning should be suspected if there is normal or near-normal isotope uptake in the presence of severe regional left ventricular dysfunction. A cardiomyopathic process or severe valvular heart disease may simulate stunning.

To remain viable, the cell has to retain its membrane integrity and its ability to generate high-energy phosphate compounds crucial for contraction. This requires adequate blood flow and supply of nutrients. Because thallium and sestamibi are dependent on active uptake by the cell, these tracers are well suited to assessing viability. It is helpful to consider the myocardial cell as a "dual-purpose unit" capable of discontinuing contraction while maintaining cell integrity. Because thallium is first distributed according to blood flow, later images (after at least 3-4 hours and, preferably, 24 hours) are indicative of myocardial viability.

Rest thallium protocols have been developed to improve diagnostic accuracy for myocardial viability and consist of immediate, 4-hour, and 24-hour images. An alternative is injection of another small amount of thallium (usually 1-2 mCi) before the rest images, which has excellent positive (85%) and negative (90%) predictive accuracy for improvement of regional wall function with revascularization. Recent data suggest that thallium may not be as specific as dobutamine echocardiography for predicting recovery of left ventricular function. This difference may be due to the inability of dobutamine to detect viable cells without contractile reserve, which would be detected by thallium. Myocardial segments with markedly improved thallium uptake in the delayed images have an excellent chance for functional recovery, whereas segments with minimal uptake and minimal redistribution in late images do not recover, possibly because of cellular dedifferentiation. ^{99m}Tc-sestamibi has also been used to assess cell viability, but because of its lack of late redistribution it may underestimate viability in segments with severely impaired resting flow. PET scanning is the reference method for assessment of myocardial viability by evaluating independently the absolute coronary (regional) blood flow and the residual metabolic activity using rubidium-82 or nitrogen-13 ammonia for the assessment of coronary artery blood flow and fluorine-18 FDG to assess metabolic activity. Cost considerations and PET availability have prevented broad clinical application of PET assessment of viability.

- PET scanning is the only method for detection of viable myocardium using both flow and metabolic variables.
- Not all myocardial cells that show thallium uptake recover contractility.
- Resting/reinjection thallium protocols enhance accuracy for the detection of myocardial viability.

Other Conditions

Myocarditis is usually diagnosed on the basis of the medical history and the physical examination, ECG, and chest radiographic results. Radionuclide studies are not used routinely to demonstrate an inflammatory process, although cell necrosis in this setting has been documented with gallium-67 citrate, ^{99m}Tc-pyrophosphate, and, more recently, indium-111-labeled antimyosin antibodies. Although myocardial perfusion imaging is not helpful, serial assessment of resting right and left ventricular function is useful in documenting the course of disease.

Similar considerations pertain to dilated cardiomyopathies. Here, the additional assessment of diastolic function variables can help to further define cardiac risk and prognosis. Exercise RNA is not useful in cardiomyopathy. A special case is doxorubicin cardiotoxicity associated with cancer chemotherapy, particularly in patients with preexisting left ventricular dysfunction, because they are at greater risk for congestive heart failure. Currently, it is recommended that treatment with doxorubicin be discontinued if serial assessment indicates left ventricular function is below normal.

Hypertrophic Cardiomyopathy

In patients with poor echocardiographic windows, RNA may be helpful in assessing systolic and diastolic function. Myocardial perfusion imaging is *not* helpful in diagnosing accompanying coronary artery disease, but it can detect exercise-induced ischemia, which is associated with a high risk for subsequent cardiac events, including sudden cardiac death. An abnormal thallium perfusion study in hypertrophic cardiomyopathy is associated with a significant adverse prognosis.

Restrictive Cardiomyopathies

RNA may be helpful in assessing ventricular function, left ventricular volume, and diastolic function in patients with suspected restrictive cardiomyopathy. ^{99m}Tc-pyrophosphate or gallium-67 imaging is abnormal in restrictive cardiomyopathy but is not discriminatory for restrictive cardiomyopathy, because it is also abnormal in other infiltrative conditions, including amyloidosis, sarcoidosis, progressive systemic sclerosis (scleroderma), and cardiac tumors.

Congenital Heart Disease in Adults

RNA may be used to assess left-to-right shunting by documenting persistent high levels of activities in the lung or right ventricle because of early recirculation. Time activity curves from various cardiac chambers and extracardiac compartments can be used to differentiate intracardiac from extracardiac shunts. Right-to-left shunts can be detected by early passage through the left chambers or the aorta. Quantification has been performed using pulmonary-to-systemic flow ratios from time activity curves over the right lung in left-to-right shunting. Secondary variables, including left and right ventricular function, can be assessed with RNA.

In patients with known congenital coronary abnormalities, perfusion imaging is helpful in assessing the possible hemodynamic severity of the anatomical abnormality.

Post-transplantation Cardiac Disease

The most common causes of death in the perioperative period after cardiac transplantation are ventricular dysfunction and allograft rejection. Radionuclide imaging is useful in assessing abnormal left or right ventricular function or both. It should be noted that during the first few days after transplantation, myocardial dysfunction most likely is not due to rejection. Subsequently, left ventricular dysfunction in the absence of other causes is suggestive of rejection. There is evidence that serial assessment of left ventricular function may detect moderate rejection by detecting only a small decrease in the ejection fraction (e.g., 63% from 67%). Compared with normal hearts, donor hearts usually show increased cardiac mobility, paradoxical septal motion, and leftward rotation with posterior-axis displacement.

Increased antimyosin antibody uptake correlates with biopsy findings of rejection. Transplant-related coronary artery disease preferentially involves the mid and distal coronary vessels. Clinical symptoms are unreliable because chest pain does not occur in a denervated heart. Thus, the initial presentation of severe coronary artery disease in a transplanted heart may be sudden cardiac death, myocardial infarction, or congestive heart failure. Exercise stress and SPECT ^{201}Tl and sestamibi have been shown to have a sensitivity and specificity comparable to those of the native heart.

Valvular Heart Disease

RNA can reliably and serially assess left and right ventricular ejection fraction. In the absence of valvular incompetence on both sides of the heart, the difference between right- and left-sided ejection fractions can be used to calculate regurgitant volumes of mitral or aortic regurgitation. Additional variables such as increased end-systolic and end-diastolic volumes are useful because they imply a poor prognosis.

In mitral valve prolapse, nonspecific myocardial perfusion defects, particularly in the inferior septum, may occur. RNA is not useful in assessing concomitant coronary artery disease because in patients with valvular heart disease nonspecific regional wall motion abnormalities are common.

Questions

Multiple Choice (choose the one best answer)

1. Which of the following statements regarding technetium is correct?
   a. Technetium has a higher energy than thallium
   b. Technetium poses a higher radiation risk to the patient at a dose equivalent to thallium
   c. Technetium is generated in a cyclotron
   d. The half-life of technetium is longer than that of thallium
   e. Technetium has a less uniform energy profile than thallium

2. Which of the following statements is correct regarding radionuclide angiography?
   a. Diastolic function cannot be assessed because electrocardiographic gating is required
   b. Heparin can interfere with radionuclide imaging
   c. In patients with left bundle branch block, pharmacologic stress testing combined with radionuclide angiography is preferred over perfusion imaging
   d. The presence of a pacemaker precludes the use of radionuclide angiography
   e. Exercise radionuclide angiography presents all coronary artery territories equally

3. A 45-year-old woman (156 cm, 82 kg) undergoes radionuclide testing. She reports chest pain lasting for 45 to 80 minutes, constant and nonradiating. She is uncertain about the relationship of her symptoms to exercise but has experienced similar episodes at rest. All the following statements are incorrect *except*:
   a. A positive test would not establish the diagnosis of coronary artery disease
   b. Thallium is preferred over technetium because of its superior imaging characteristics
   c. A pharmacologic stress test would make the test more specific
   d. The test should be terminated when the patient has exercised to 85% of maximal predicted heart rate
   e. The test should be terminated if electrocardiography shows 2 mm or more of ST depression in the absence of symptoms

4. An exercise test with single photon emission computed tomography (SPECT) thallium imaging is performed (shown below) on the patient described in question 3. She exercised for 11 minutes on a Bruce protocol to a peak heart rate of 178 beats per minute and a blood pressure of 180/80 mm Hg. The following statements are correct *except*:
   a. There is a reversible defect in the apex/anterior wall suggestive of coronary artery disease
   b. The finding on the SPECT thallium probably is a breast artifact
   c. The excellent double product (peak heart rate times peak systolic blood pressure) further reduces the likelihood of coronary artery disease
   d. Technetium would have been the preferred imaging agent
   e. A subsequent coronary angiogram will most likely be negative

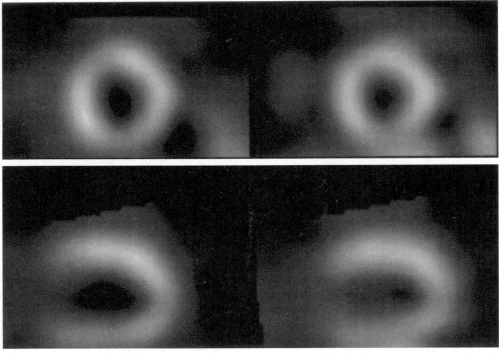

Stress   **Rest**

Question 4

5. Which of the following statements regarding pharma-cologic stress testing is correct?
   a. Dipyridamole causes more side effects than adeno-sine
   b. High-level dobutamine radionuclide angiography (20-40 µg/kg per minute) is useful to assess viabil-ity in patients with known left ventricular dysfunc-tion
   c. Side effects caused by adenosine but not dipyrid-amole can be reversed with theophylline
   d. Adenosine results in a larger increase of blood flow than dipyridamole or dobutamine
   e. Dobutamine radionuclide angiography is useful to assess coronary artery disease in patients with left bundle branch block

6. A 65-year-old man is referred to you for preoperative assessment of cardiac risk. The patient is scheduled for laminectomy at level T10-11. He has several coronary risk factors, including diabetes, smoking, hypertension, and significant peripheral vascular disease. You elect to perform an adenosine thallium test. The patient does not indicate any symptoms. The blood pressure drops by 20 mm Hg from baseline but returns to normal with-in 1 minute after the cessation of the adenosine infu-sion. Representative planar and long-axis images in both the horizontal and vertical orientations are shown below. Which of the following statements is correct?
   a. The drop in blood pressure is clinically important
   b. The absence of symptoms is reassuring
   c. The absence of markedly reversible defects is reas-suring
   d. The post-stress left ventricular dilatation is worri-some for significant coronary artery disease
   e. A coronary angiogram would have better defined the functional significance of the coronary artery lesions

7. A patient with known idiopathic cardiomyopathy is referred to you for assessment of left ventricular func-tion. Echocardiography and a radionuclide angiography at rest had been performed. The ejection fraction was 17% by echocardiography and 20% by radionuclide

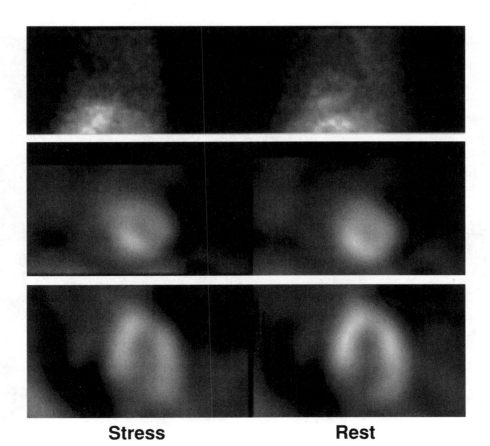

Stress   **Rest**

Question 6

angiography. A year later, repeat echocardiography and radionuclide angiography were done on follow-up. Ejection fraction was 25% by echocardiography and 15% by radionuclide angiography. You are asked to comment on these findings. What is the correct conclusion?

a. There is significant improvement in left ventricular function

b. The left ventricular function is about the same

c. Further deterioration of left ventricular function has occurred

d. The presence of regional wall motion abnormalities refutes the diagnosis of idiopathic dilated cardiomyopathy

e. Additional factors would not be helpful in further risk stratification

8. A patient with known coronary artery disease (preoperative coronary angiogram showed a 30% left main, 100% proximal left anterior descending, 100% proximal circumflex, 90% first marginal, 70% right coronary artery disease) who had subsequent coronary artery bypass grafting (CABG, left internal mammary artery to left anterior descending, right internal mammary artery to right posterior descending artery [PDA], saphenous vein graft to circumflex and saphenous vein graft to obtuse marginal) 1 year ago returns to you with new-onset angina. You perform an exercise single photon emission computed tomography (SPECT) thallium test (shown below) and compare his current results with the preoperative results. Which of the following conclusions is correct?

a. The patient probably underwent incomplete revascularization

b. An angioplasty of the PDA graft should be considered if medical therapy fails

c. Percutaneous transluminal coronary angioplasty of the native right coronary artery should be considered

d. Medical therapy should be considered

e. The patient is a candidate for another CABG

9. A 52-year-old patient (168 cm, 131 kg) is referred with symptoms of class III dyspnea. The patient is a smoker, is sedentary, and has significant chronic obstructive pulmonary disease (COPD) and hyperlipidemia. You want to assess the left ventricular function to distinguish a possible respiratory or cardiac reason for his dyspnea. Which

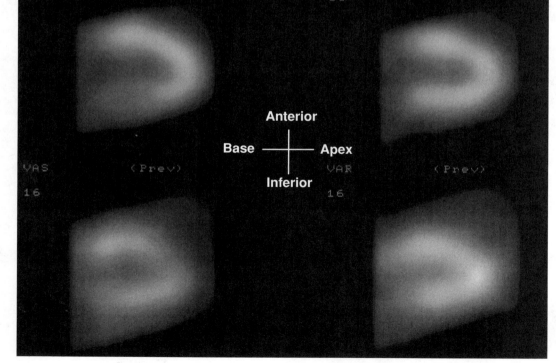

Stress   **Rest**

Question 8   **Vertical long-axis views**

of the following statements is *incorrect* in this setting?

a. Transthoracic echocardiography will probably yield unsatisfactory images

b. First-pass sestamibi is helpful, especially if 30 mCi is used to improve photon statistics

c. The heart volumes measured and images by radionuclide angiography are affected by body habitus and are likely to be smaller than in a normal-weight person

d. Radionuclide angiography is challenging because of the patient's COPD

e. Electron beam computed tomography is the imaging method of choice in this patient

10. Select the best statement regarding radionuclide angiography.

a. Exercise radionuclide angiography is performed with a camera in the anteroposterior or lateral position

b. The left anterior oblique position is always at 45°, similar to coronary angiography

c. Determination of ejection fraction by radionuclide angiography requires a regular rhythm and is best with a low-energy all-purpose (LEAP) collimator

d. There is little interindividual variation in the determination of ventricular volumes

e. Determination of ejection fraction by radionuclide angiography is very discriminate in hyperdynamic ventricles

11. A 56-year-old woman (160 cm, 88 kg) is referred to your practice for cardiac evaluation. She is a non-smoker, has increased lipid values and a family history of coronary artery disease, has no diabetes, has borderline hypertension, is 10 years postmenopausal, and is taking hormone replacement therapy. She achieves 96% of her functional aerobic capacity. The test is stopped because of general fatigue; mild dyspnea is also noted. She underwent resting single photon emission computed tomography sestamibi imaging the day before. As part of your quality assurance, you notice the increased liver uptake (see figure below) after the exercise test and you request reimaging after a light meal. Following reimaging after stress, a short-axis tomogram, correctly aligned, is shown in the right lower corner. Which statement is correct?

a. This represents single-vessel disease

b. This most likely represents an artifact from juxtaposed splanchnic activity or diaphragmatic attenuation

c. Adenosine would have been the preferred stress method in this patient

d. A coronary angiogram should be ordered with the intention of catheter-based intervention

e. The patient can be treated medically with an antianginal regimen

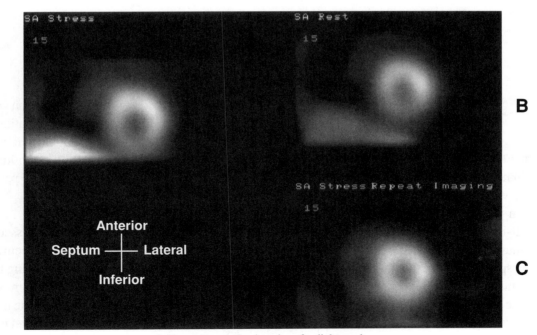

A, Stress; *B*, rest; *C*, reimaging after light meal.

Question 11

12. All the following conditions can produce an artifactual defect in the inferior segments *except*:
    a. Partial volume effect
    b. Diaphragmatic attenuation
    c. Motion artifact
    d. Obesity
    e. Adjacent tissue uptake (liver/loop of bowel)

13. Which of the following is true when myocardial perfusion imaging using thallium-201 is compared with positron emission computed tomography (PET)?
    a. They provide images of similar quality in all patients
    b. They provide for quantification of absolute regional myocardial blood flow
    c. They have similar applicability in defining myocardial viability
    d. Imaging can be done without the need for an on-site cyclotron

14. A 45-year-old patient with diabetes who weighs 250 pounds and has an ejection fraction of 24% and known three-vessel coronary artery disease by coronary angiography presents complaining of shortness of breath despite intensive medical treatment. The cardiac surgeon is skeptical that left ventricular function would improve after coronary artery bypass grafting because a non-exercise 24-hour thallium study showed predominantly fixed perfusion defects. Which of the following studies would you order to pursue the possibility of myocardial viability further?
    a. Low-dose dobutamine echocardiography
    b. Positron emission computed tomography (PET) with ^{18}F fluorodeoxyglucose (FDG)
    c. PET with FDG and nitrogen-13–labeled ammonia
    d. PET with carbon-11-palmitate
    e. None of the above; if 24-hour thallium imaging does not demonstrate myocardial viability, none of these tests will likely be helpful

15. Which test is appropriate for assessing left ventricular viability and the likelihood of functional recovery with revascularization in a patient with systolic ventricular dysfunction?
    a. Positron emission computed tomography with ^{18}F fluorodeoxyglucose (FDG) and nitrogen-13–labeled ammonia
    b. Rest, 24-hour thallium study
    c. Low-dose dobutamine echocardiography
    d. All of the above

Answers

1. Answer a

Thallium and technetium are the two most commonly used isotopes in nuclear cardiology tests. Technetium has a higher energy, with a characteristic 140 keV photon peak. It is eluted from the stable molybdenum-99 compound, which has a half-life of 66 hours and is easily transported. In contrast, thallium-201 is generated from a cyclotron facility and then transported as a finished product. The energy profile of technetium is not only higher but also more homogeneous because the thallium radio-decay process has a marked variability in photon energy, the majority ranging from 69 to 83 keV, but other, particularly lower, energy peaks are also present. The higher energy signature in technetium also allows better penetration and transmission through tissue; thus, the residual radiation in a patient is markedly less for technetium than it is for thallium. Therefore, larger doses can be used to improve imaging characteristic, without endangering the patient.

2. Answer b

Diastolic function can be well assessed with radionuclide angiography. For enhancing accuracy, a different mode of gating has been used, increasing the gating cycle to 64 rather than the conventional 32 frames for better cycle resolution. This, of course, enhances the time necessary to obtain the images to achieve the required photon statistics, but diastolic function analysis has been established as a valid tool with radionuclide angiography. Pharmacologic stress testing is indeed the preferred choice in patients undergoing radionuclide testing for the diagnosis of coronary artery disease. However, the problem with left bundle branch block is a significant change in contraction pattern, which can unpredictably change with additional exercise. Radionuclide angiography is based on the assessment of regional wall motion and thus is not the optimal test for assessing patients with left bundle branch block. The presence of a paced rhythm does not preclude the use of radionuclide angiography, particularly if the patient is paced at a stable rhythm and is capable of achieving a heart rate plateau after adjustment during the various stages of exercise. Pacemakers are often programmed to emulate this physiologic response to exercise while increasing the heart rate according to breathing or motion pattern.

Exercise radionuclide angiography is usually performed with a camera in a modified left anterior oblique position for maximal separation of the right and left ventricles. This projection overrepresents the circumflex coronary artery with two segments, the left anterior descending also with only two segments, and the right coronary artery with one segment (inferoapical), thus constituting a skewed pattern for assessment of the coronary artery territories.

Heparin has been shown to interfere with the labeling of red blood cells with technetium. It is fairly rare but occurs in approximately 5% of patients, requiring retagging of the red blood cells under special precautions.

3. Answer a

The patient described presents a clinical dilemma. As a 45-year-old woman, she has a low pretest likelihood of coronary artery disease. Thus, she is not a good candidate for exercise testing or imaging. The chance is that a positive result would be false-positive rather than true-positive. In women of this age, a pharmacologic stress test would increase the sensitivity but would not increase the specificity. Thus, the predictive accuracy of a negative test result is similar for exercise or pharmacologic testing. The test should not be terminated when the patient has exercised to 85% of her maximal predicted heart rate because of the significant variability in heart rate response in individual patients, and also it should not be terminated if electrocardiography shows more than 2 mm of ST depression, unless it is accompanied by other clinical criteria (signs of reduced perfusion, hemodynamic compromise, hemodynamically significant arrhythmia). In a woman of her size (moderately obese given her height), sestamibi should be chosen because of its superior imaging characteristics.

4. Answer a

This question shows the importance of incorporating nonimaging findings into the exercise test as well as the importance of recognition of imaging artifacts. This patient exercises to an excellent double product and functional aerobic capacity. From the previous question, it is evident that the patient is in a "low pretest likelihood of disease" group. The reversible defect in the apex and anterior wall is thus not suggestive of coronary artery disease, but other reasons should be considered. The finding most likely is a breast artifact. Considering the nonimaging factors, the patient exercised well to a good functional aerobic capacity at 11 minutes on a Bruce protocol with an excellent double product. In most female patients, a technetium perfusion tracer is the preferred imaging agent because of its superior imaging characteristics. This would also obviate coronary angiography, which will most likely be negative in this clinical setting.

5. Answer d

Pharmacologic stress testing is an important adjunct to imaging for the assessment of coronary artery disease. Adenosine results in a larger increase of coronary blood flow than dipyridamole or dobutamine. Dipyridamole, with its slower onset and slower cessation, is usually better tolerated than adenosine. The side effects of both agents can be reversed with theophylline, although because adenosine has a very short half-life, stopping the infusion is usually sufficient if adverse reactions develop.

High-dose dobutamine (20-40 µg/kg per minute) is useful to establish the diagnosis of coronary artery disease. In contrast, low-dose dobutamine (5-10 µg/kg per minute) is used to assess viability in patients with left ventricular dysfunction. Left bundle branch block creates a dyssynergic contraction pattern, and the use of dobutamine stress would only exacerbate these abnormalities, often unpredictably. Thus, it is not helpful for distinguishing a coronary origin for the regional wall motion abnormality.

6. Answer d

Adenosine stress testing is helpful in patients whose exercise capacity is limited by orthopedic, neurologic, or peripheral vascular problems. Symptoms can be misleading, because many patients complain about headaches, flushing, dyspnea, and chest discomfort, which is most likely noncardiac. Also, the absence of symptoms does not indicate the absence of disease. A drop in blood pressure is common with adenosine because of peripheral vasodilatation and usually can be ameliorated, if necessary, with a small amount of saline or Ringer lactate infusion. The key feature in the scan is the marked post-stress dilatation. As emphasized in this chapter, the clinical background always needs to be considered in the interpretation of scans. In a patient with marked cardiovascular risk factors, the likelihood of disease is high, and the absence of a markedly reversible defect in the presence of significant post-stress dilatation is worrisome for significant, equally distributed disease in which the extent of reversibility underestimates the true extent of coronary artery disease. Coronary angiography is helpful for delineating the coronary anatomy but does not assess the functional significance of coronary artery lesions.

7. Answer c

The key to this question lies in the imaging characteristic of each technique. Assessment of left ventricular function by echocardiography is based on the inward motion of the myocardium and wall thickening. In a large, hypocontractile ventricle, the inward motion is minimal and significant variance in the determination of left ventricular function can easily occur. In contrast, radionuclide angiography is based on count statistics. In a large ventricle with poor function, the end-diastolic and end-systolic counts are very high. Thus, high-quality determination of left ventricular function can be obtained in patients who are in stable sinus rhythm. In hyperdynamic ventricles, the markedly exaggerated inward motion allows excellent wall motion discrimination and assessment of left ventricular function by echocardiography. In contrast, the low count density in end-systole in the hyperdynamic ventricle may lead to a slight exaggeration in the assessment of left ventricular function by radionuclide angiography. A decrease in ejection fraction of 5% by radionuclide angiography at this level is a significant change in left ventricular function. Even in patients with known idiopathic cardiomyopathy and absent coronary artery disease, segmental wall motion is not homogeneous. The inferior and inferolateral segments, possibly due to the diaphragmatic buttressing, appear to contract better than the remaining segments. This does not indicate coronary artery disease but is a common finding in this disease state. Additional factors such as stroke volume by echocardiography, diastolic function by both echocardiography and radionuclide angiography, and shape dimensions by echocardiography are useful to further aid in risk stratification.

8. Answer d

This is a complex medical situation, which is more frequently encountered with successful bypass surgery. This patient had significant coronary artery disease preoperatively. He had successful and complete revascularization with bypasses bridging all significant lesions. The postoperative SPECT thallium images (vertical long-axis representation) show a reversible basal inferior defect with otherwise normal uptake. This is most compatible with progression of the lesion in the native right coronary artery or even possible occlusion. Because this represents one-vessel disease, medical therapy is indicated, and angioplasty of the right coronary artery could be considered at a later point only if intractable angina resolves. Angioplasty of the graft to the PDA is not warranted because it is most likely patent given the normal uptake in the remainder of the inferior wall. Thus, the patient is not a candidate for another CABG.

9. Answer e

This question pertains to the choice of optimal test in a challenging patient who is severely obese with significant COPD. Transthoracic echocardiography will most likely be hampered by both the body size and the significant COPD, which of course is not a problem for isotope transmission. The tissue attenuation in this markedly obese patient, however, would make the heart appear smaller because of both distance to the detector and tissue attenuation. A first-pass sestamibi is potentially helpful. However, if significant left ventricular dysfunction or right ventricular dysfunction is present, the bolus may be of inferior quality and thus result in erroneous measurements. Electron beam computed tomography is not readily available and would also suffer from attenuation given the patient's size.

10. Answer c

Full resting radionuclide angiography is performed in three positions, the anteroposterior, a left anterior oblique equivalent, and a lateral position. The left anterior oblique position is always adjusted for optimal alignment of the septum orthogonal to the imaging plane to best discriminate right from left ventricular function. Cranial tilt is sometimes needed and thus a standard left anterior oblique projection is usually not used. Radionuclide angiography is strictly based on count statistics and does not rely on the presumption of a certain contraction pattern or volumetric determinations. Even though there is little intraindividual variation in the ventricular volumes, body habitus, weight, position of the heart in the thoracic cavity, and thus distance to the detector are critical variables that are difficult to account for in the clinical setting. Thus, there is significant interindividual variation. An accurate assessment of left ventricular function is possible only if the patient is in regular rhythm. Use of a LEAP collimator provides optimal counts; improved resolution from a high-resolution collimator is not critical. Determination of left ventricular ejection fraction by radionuclide angiography is very accurate in patients with poor ventricular function because the high count density at both end-diastole and end-systole results in superior quality images, unlike a hyperdynamic ventricle, which has low counts at end-systole.

11. Answer b

On the initial scan, increased liver uptake adjacent to the inferior segment is noted. Because of the filtered back-projection reconstruction algorithm, artificially low isotope uptake is noted. A light snack or meal can sometimes help in reducing the increased uptake in the liver or adjacent bowel. In this case, reimaging indicates a normal uptake throughout the myocardium. The rest image shows an inferior defect similar to that present in the original stress views and likely represents artifact. If this were a thallium-201 study, this would represent "reverse" distribution. Most likely this represents diaphragmatic attenuation and not coronary artery disease.

12. Answer a

Several conditions can cause reduced uptake in the inferior wall. The most notable is diaphragmatic attenuation due to body habitus, such as obesity. A motion artifact also can contribute to reduced inferior uptake, although this is most likely accompanied by reduced uptake, in the contralateral wall. Adjacent tissue uptake, most notably in the liver and bowel, is also responsible for reduced uptake in the inferior segments and needs to be carefully recognized. Partial volume effects occur when reduced myocardial mass is present, which is common at the ventricular apex with its cone shape. This does not play a significant role in the inferior portions, particularly at the base and mid-ventricular level, where diaphragmatic attenuation is usually noted.

13. Answer d

Thallium-201 is a weak radioactive compound, and image quality is not universally excellent, especially in obese patients. Additionally, thallium "scatters," and positrons do not. Thus, imaging with PET is superior for obese patients. Thallium cannot be used to define absolute myocardial perfusion, although it can be used to define relative differences in perfusion between regions. Although some data suggest that thallium can be used to define myocardial viability using reinjection/scanning methods, it is generally accepted that PET, if available, is more applicable for defining myocardial viability using fluorodeoxyglucose. Because rubidium-82 can be generated with a portable device, all PET scanning need not require an on-site cyclotron. Because thallium has a sufficiently long half-life, it can be stored locally for several days before its use.

14. Answer c

PET may show myocardial viability where the rest thallium study does not. Viability detected at rest indicates resting ischemia (hibernation) and suggests that revascularization would improve left ventricular function. Low-dose dobutamine infusion may recruit additional myocardial contraction despite resting ischemia and also suggests that left ventricular function will improve with revascularization. However, in this obese patient with very poor left ventricular function, PET is the better viability test. Because a mismatch in perfusion and glucose metabolism indicates hibernation, both FDG and nitrogen-13–labeled ammonia images must be obtained.

15. Answer d

All of the tests can show hibernation and serve as useful guides for revascularization in patients with left ventricular dysfunction. FDG uptake in an area of reduced perfusion on the ammonia image, redistribution of thallium at 24 hours after injection at rest, and contraction of a hypokinetic segment with low-dose dobutamine (5 to 10 μg/kg per minute) all indicate probable myocardial hibernation.

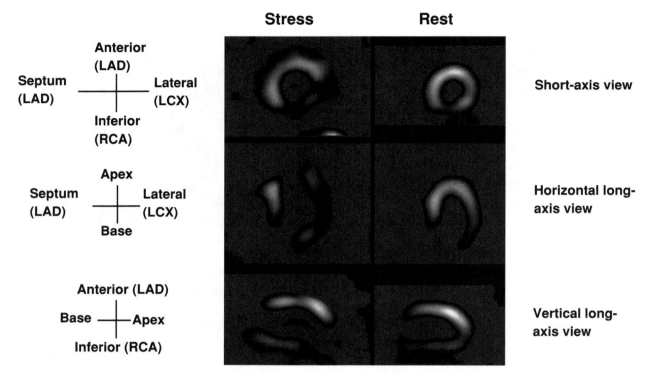

Plate 1. Stress-induced left ventricular dilatation with marked ischemia due to three-vessel coronary artery disease. LAD, left anterior descending coronary artery territory; LCX, left circumflex coronary artery territory; RCA, right coronary artery territory.

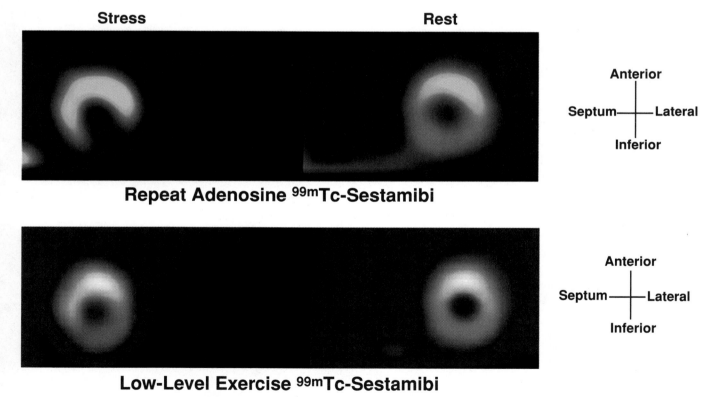

Plate 2. Short-axis images from a patient with significant coronary artery disease (left anterior descending and right coronary arteries) and peripheral vascular disease. The first study represents an adenosine stress ^{99m}Tc-sestamibi (*upper panels*); the second study (*lower panels*) is a symptoms-limited treadmill exercise test. The exercise was stopped because of claudication. Note that symptoms in the second test prevented the patient from reaching the same ischemic threshold as in the first study. The inferior/inferolateral defect is more severe on the stress adenosine study.

Short-axis

Stress   **Rest**

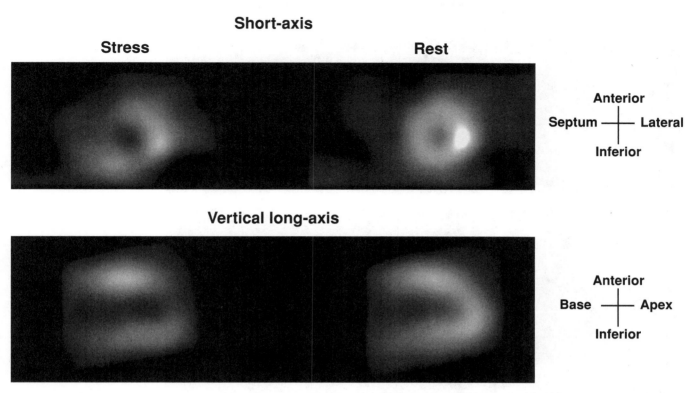

Anterior

Septum ┼ Lateral

Inferior

Vertical long-axis

Anterior

Base ┼ Apex

Inferior

Plate 3. Short-axis (*upper panels*) and vertical long-axis (*lower panels*) views in a patient with significant disease of the left anterior descending and right coronary arteries. Note severely decreased uptake in the apex, septal, and inferior regions, with marked redistribution in all affected territories. There is transient left ventricular dilatation with stress-induced myocardial ischemia.

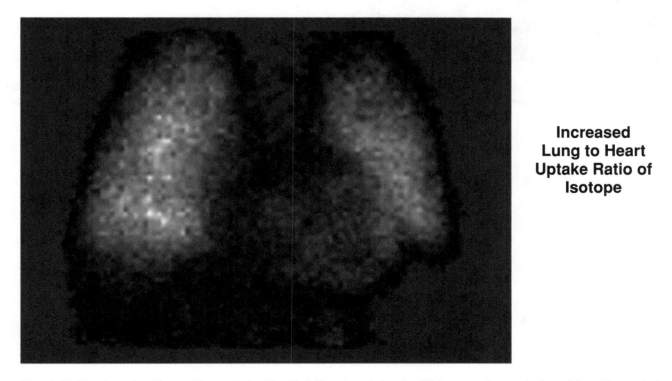

**Increased
Lung to Heart
Uptake Ratio of
Isotope**

Plate 4. Thallium image in a 67-year-old man who has New York Heart Association class IV dyspnea and congestive heart failure. Note markedly increased pulmonary uptake on the anteroposterior image and cardiac enlargement. The left ventricular ejection fraction was 18%.

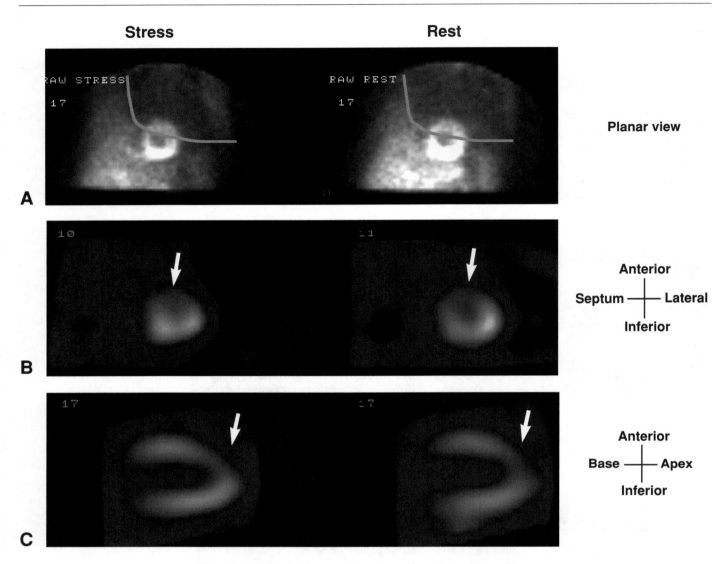

Stress   **Rest**

Planar view

Anterior

Septum —|— Lateral

Inferior

Anterior

Base —|— Apex

Inferior

Plate 5. Planar (*A*) and anteroposterior short-axis (*B*) and long-axis (*C*) views in a markedly overweight patient. Note the defect across the anteroseptal, anterior, and anterolateral segments (*arrow*). The defect is unchanged from stress to rest images. This is consistent with breast artifact. Coronary arteriograms showed normal coronary arteries.

Chapter 49

Exercise Stress Testing

Joseph G. Murphy, M.D.
Thomas Behrenbeck, M.D, Ph.D.

Questions about exercise testing (treadmill exercise test [TMET]) are frequent in both cardiology and internal medicine examinations. The principal areas to understand are the indications for exercise testing, the risks associated with TMET, criteria for a positive test result, and the limitations of the test in various patient populations.

TMET has the advantage over other stress testing modalities because it is widely available at relatively low cost, provides an excellent assessment of the functional capacity of the patient, and has reasonable sensitivity and specificity for the diagnosis of flow-limiting coronary artery disease in patient populations at intermediate risk of coronary artery disease. The disadvantages of TMET are that it has a lower sensitivity and specificity for the diagnosis of myocardial ischemia than imaging-based stress tests and it cannot be used to diagnose myocardial ischemia in patients with other significant noncardiac limitations to TMET, including orthopedic conditions and respiratory disease.

Safety of Exercise Testing

Overall, exercise testing is a safe procedure, but myocardial infarction, stroke, cardiac arrest, and death are all well-recognized complications (Table 1). The risk of death is about 1 per 10,000 patients, and the risk of cardiac arrest is about 2 per 10,000 patients. Absolute and relative contraindications to exercise testing are summarized in Table 2. Exercise testing after myocardial infarction is safe. Submaximal testing can be performed as early as 3 to 7 days after an uncomplicated myocardial infarction and a symptom-limited TMET, 3 to 6 weeks later.

Table 1.—Complications of Exercise Testing

Minor complications
    Supraventricular tachycardia
    Chronotropic incompetence
    Inotropic incompetence
    Excessive chronotropic response
    Excessive inotropic response
    Ventricular ectopic activity
    Congestive heart failure
    Focal or global cerebrovascular ischemia
Major complications
    Supraventricular tachycardia
    Ventricular tachycardia-fibrillation
    Stroke
    Myocardial infarction
    Death

From Giuliani ER, Gersh BJ, McGoon MD, Hayes DL, Schaff HV (editors): *Mayo Clinic Practice of Cardiology*. Third edition. Mosby, 1996, p 140. By permission of Mayo Foundation.

Table 2.—Contraindications to Exercise Testing

Acute phase of an unstable coronary syndrome
Severe heart failure
Active myocarditis or pericarditis
High-grade atrioventricular block
Severe aortic stenosis
Uncontrolled hypertension
ECG abnormalities that preclude ECG interpretation (LBBB, WPW syndrome, etc.)
Unable to exercise for any reason
Uncontrolled arrhythmias
Other uncontrolled severe illnesses, active endocarditis, recent pulmonary embolus

ECG, electrocardiographic; LBBB, left bundle branch block; WPW, Wolff-Parkinson-White.

Indications and Contraindications to TMET

Diagnosis of Coronary Artery Disease

The primary indication for exercise testing is to diagnose flow-limiting coronary artery disease and myocardial ischemia in patients considered to have an intermediate pretest probability of coronary artery disease on the basis of symptoms and risk factors. The mean sensitivity and specificity of TMET in this population is about 70%. TMET is less useful in patients with vasospastic angina and those with either a high or low pretest probability of coronary artery disease on the basis of age, symptoms, and sex. In a patient with a high pretest probability of coronary artery disease (e.g., a 60-year-old male smoker with typical angina), a negative TMET result does not reliably exclude significant coronary artery disease and is likely to be a false-negative result, whereas in a patient with a low probability (e.g., a 30-year-old female nonsmoker with atypical chest pain), a positive TMET result is probably a false-positive result (Table 3). In both cases, the diagnostic accuracy of TMET would be low, and alternative diagnostic strategies should be considered. Predictive variables for the presence of coronary artery disease are shown in Table 4.

Unless a patient presents with an acute coronary syndrome (sudden death, myocardial infarction, unstable angina), when coronary angiography may be the most appropriate initial diagnostic investigation, most patients with suspected significant coronary artery disease or myocardial ischemia (or both) should undergo exercise testing to assess cardiac risk.

The choice of the initial stress-test modality should be

Table 3.—Noncoronary Causes of ST-Segment Depression

Ischemic
    Increased impedance due to
        Aortic stenosis
        Muscular obstruction, as in hypertrophic cardiomyopathy
        Hypertension
    Increased wall stress due to left ventricular dilatation, including
        Volume overload states of aortic insufficiency
        Mitral insufficiency
        Left-to-right shunts
        Arteriovenous fistulas
    Decreased oxygen supply, as in
        Anemia
        Abnormal oxygen-binding affinity of hemoglobin, e.g., hemoglobin Malmö, left shift of oxygen-hemoglobin dissociation curve
        Competitive binding to hemoglobin of nonoxygen compounds such as carbon monoxide
        Low-output states, such as mitral stenosis
        Desaturation of hemoglobin due to chronic obstructive pulmonary disease, right-to-left shunts
Membrane repolarization abnormalities due to
    Digitalis
    Glucose-potassium shifts after meals
    Hypokalemia and electrolyte disorders
    Toxic states and drugs, including diazepam
    Hyperadrenergic syndrome
    Abnormal depolarization with left bundle branch block, pacemaker, right bundle branch block, preexcitation
    Cardiomyopathies
    Left ventricular hypertrophy
    Hyperventilation
Idiopathic mechanisms—mitral prolapse
Miscellaneous—artifact from inadequate recording equipment

From Giuliani ER, Gersh BJ, McGoon MD, Hayes DL, Schaff HV (editors): *Mayo Clinic Practice of Cardiology*. Third edition. Mosby, 1996, p 134. By permission of Mayo Foundation.

based on an evaluation of the patient's resting electrocardiogram (ECG) and physical ability to exercise. For risk assessment, the exercise test should be the standard initial mode of stress testing used in patients with a normal ECG who are not taking digoxin. Patients unable to exercise because of physical limitations (e.g., arthritis, amputation, severe peripheral vascular disease, severe chronic obstructive pulmonary

Table 4.—Predictive Variables for Coronary Artery Disease on the Treadmill Exercise Test by Multivariate Analysis

Males	Females
Test duration	ST depression at rest, in mm
R-wave change, in mm	
Age	Presence or absence of downsloping ST segment
% maximal heart rate achieved	
Maximal heart rate achieved	R-wave change, in mm
Presence or absence of abnormal ECG at rest	Age
	Use of estrogen (yes/no)
ST depression with exercise, in mm	ST depression with exercise, in mm
Presence or absence of angina during test	Test duration
	Presence or absence of angina during test

From Giuliani ER, Gersh BJ, McGoon MD, Hayes DL, Schaff HV (editors): *Mayo Clinic Practice of Cardiology*. Third edition. Mosby, 1996, p 137. By permission of Mayo Foundation.

disease, or general debility) should undergo pharmacologic stress testing in combination with myocardial imaging.

In patients with a well-documented myocardial infarction or previous abnormal coronary angiographic findings, a diagnostic TMET is redundant, but TMET can be used to evaluate the ischemic threshold and overall cardiac risk.

Exercise Testing Before Revascularization

Patients scheduled for myocardial revascularization should have objective evidence of ischemic myocardium, especially if typical angina is not present. The limitation of the exercise ECG in this setting is that exercise-induced ST-segment depression poorly localizes the culprit epicardial coronary stenosis, and exercise imaging studies may be more appropriate. The exception to this rule is when the patient has multivessel disease and the culprit vessel does not need to be accurately defined or when exercise-induced ST-segment elevation accurately localizes the culprit vessel. Ischemia in the territory of the circumflex coronary artery presents a special difficulty because TMET has significantly lower sensitivity and specificity for posterior wall myocardial ischemia.

Exercise Testing After Revascularization

After coronary revascularization (percutaneous transluminal coronary angioplasty [PTCA] or coronary artery bypass grafting [CABG]), exercise testing may be used in symptomatic

patients to distinguish between cardiac and noncardiac causes of recurrent chest pain. If a medical management decision is to be based on the presence or absence of exercise-induced ischemia, the exercise ECG is generally adequate. A stress imaging study is preferred if the site and extent of ischemia or left ventricular function (or both) must be assessed.

In symptomatic patients after PTCA, a positive exercise test is predictive of restenosis. A negative exercise test in this setting has a lower accuracy for the exclusion of restenosis than TMET has for the exclusion of de novo myocardial ischemia. The use of surveillance exercise tests in asymptomatic patients after myocardial revascularization to look for PTCA restenosis after PTCA or graft disease after CABG is controversial. A reasonable strategy advocated by the American College of Cardiology/American Heart Association task force is "to perform exercise testing in selected patients considered to be at particularly high risk, including those with decreased left ventricular function, multivessel CAD [coronary artery disease], proximal left anterior descending disease, previous sudden death, diabetes mellitus, hazardous occupations, and suboptimal PTCA results." The sensitivity of exercise ECG is in the range of 40% to 55% for post-PTCA restenosis, reflecting the high prevalence of one-vessel disease in this population.

The predictive accuracy of exercise ECG for detecting graft disease after CABG in symptomatic patients is not well established, and stress imaging is preferred in this group of patients.

TMET in Patients With Baseline ECG Changes

In patients with less than 1 mm of ST-segment depression on the baseline ECG because of digoxin use or left ventricular hypertrophy, TMET is an acceptable stress test, but the specificity is lower than when the baseline ECG is normal. In patients with more than 1 mm of ST-segment depression on the baseline ECG, TMET is of little diagnostic value. In patients with baseline ECG abnormalities, a negative stress test is more helpful clinically than a positive test.

Patients with the following baseline ECG abnormalities are unsuitable for diagnostic TMET: preexcitation (Wolff-Parkinson-White) syndrome, electronically paced ventricular rhythm, more than 1 mm of resting ST-segment depression, or complete left bundle branch block. Note that right bundle branch block is not a contraindication to TMET.

Diagnostic Criteria for a Positive Stress Test

The classic criteria for a positive TMET is new 1 mm or greater horizontal or downsloping ST-segment depression persisting for 80 ms beyond the J point on any ECG lead, as compared with the baseline ECG. Upsloping ST-segment depression should be considered nondiagnostic for myocardial ischemia or negative. Although specificity is lowered somewhat by resting ST-segment depression, TMET is still a reasonable first option for patients with less than 1 mm of baseline ST-segment depression because of digoxin or left ventricular hypertrophy who otherwise have an intermediate pretest probability of obstructive coronary artery disease. Exercise-induced ST-segment depression reflects subendocardial ischemia, which is often circumferential in location and does not well localize the ischemic zone of the heart. Exercise-induced ST-segment elevation generally reflects transmural ischemia, but it may also be seen over the site of a ventricular aneurysm or in the setting of exercise-induced coronary artery spasm.

Other ECG markers of myocardial ischemia include an increase in R-wave amplitude (also a marker of left ventricular dysfunction) and widening of the QRS complex.

One of the best predictors of future cardiac events on exercise testing is maximal exercise capacity as measured by maximal exercise duration, maximal metabolic equivalent (MET) level achieved, maximal heart rate, and heart rate-blood pressure product. When interpreting exercise test results, it is important to consider the level of exercise at which ECG changes of ischemia occurred and the presence of other ancillary clinical markers of ischemia, including hypotension (or lack of augmentation of systolic blood pressure during exercise) and the onset of anginal pain, exercise-induced arrhythmias, and the recovery time needed to reverse ST-segment changes or angina.

The indications for stopping TMET are listed in Table 5.

The Duke treadmill score incorporates both groups of prognostic markers (exercise capacity and exercise-induced ischemia).

Treadmill Score = Exercise Duration (in minutes)
− 5 x (ST depression in mm)
− 4 (severity of angina [0-2 scale])

TMET in Unstable Angina

Patients with unstable angina should be classified as "low," "moderate," or "high risk" on the basis of their history, physical examination findings, and initial resting ECG. In low-risk patients with unstable angina who are evaluated as outpatients, exercise or pharmacologic stress testing generally should be performed within 72 hours after presentation. In low- or moderate-risk patients with unstable angina who

have been hospitalized for evaluation, exercise or pharmacologic stress testing generally should be performed unless cardiac catheterization is otherwise indicated. Testing can be safely performed when patients have been free of active ischemic or heart failure symptoms for a minimum of 48 hours. In general, as with patients with stable angina, TMET should be the standard stress test for patients with a normal resting ECG who are not taking digoxin. High-risk patients should have angiography.

TMET After Myocardial Infarction

TMET is used in three settings after myocardial infarction. 1) A submaximal TMET before hospital dismissal after myocardial infarction to assess overall prognosis, to select patients who require coronary angiography and possible myocardial revascularization, and to objectively evaluate the response to medical therapy and activity prescription. 2) A symptom-limited TMET is performed 2 to 6 weeks after dismissal after myocardial infarction for prognostic assessment, activity prescription, and evaluation of medical therapy and cardiac rehabilitation if predismissal exercise testing was not performed. 3) TMET is performed late after discharge for prognostic assessment, activity prescription, and evaluation of medical therapy and cardiac rehabilitation if the early exercise test was submaximal. Routine TMET following coronary angiography is not required, but the assessment of ischemia

Table 5.—Indications for Stopping an Exercise Test

1. Clearly positive stress test response (>2-mm horizontal ST-segment depression)
2. New ST-segment elevation >2 mm in leads without a preexisting Q wave
3. Achievement of target heart rate
4. Progressive angina
5. Limiting symptoms (dyspnea, claudication, etc.) or patient's request to stop
6. New onset supraventricular tachycardia, atrial fibrillation, or atrial flutter
7. Sustained or nonsustained ventricular tachycardia
8. Second- or third-degree atrioventricular block
9. New left bundle branch block
10. A decrease in systolic blood pressure of 10 mm Hg or more
11. Severe hypertension
12. A decrease in heart rate with continued exercise

in the distribution of a coronary lesion of borderline severity may be useful. TMET is also an important adjunct in designing an exercise program as part of comprehensive cardiac rehabilitation.

In general, patients who are unable to perform an exercise test have a much higher adverse event rate than those who are able to exercise. Symptomatic ischemic ST-segment depression on exercise testing after thrombolytic therapy increases the risk of cardiac mortality twofold.

Adjunctive Use of Ventilatory Gas Analysis With TMET

Metabolic exercise testing using ventilatory gas analysis is used to assess the response to therapy in patients with heart failure, especially those who are being considered for heart transplantation, and to differentiate cardiac from pulmonary limitations as a cause of exercise-induced dyspnea. The variables measured include oxygen uptake ($\dot{V}O_2$), carbon dioxide output ($\dot{V}CO_2$), minute ventilation, and ventilatory/anaerobic threshold. $\dot{V}O_2$ at maximal exercise is considered the best index of aerobic capacity and cardiorespiratory function. Equations for predicting maximal aerobic capacity during TMET are given in Table 6.

Treadmill Exercise Testing in Special Situations

Diagnosis of Coronary Artery Disease in Women

Despite the consensus that TMET has a lower sensitivity and probably a lower specificity in women than in men, the routine use of stress imaging studies as the initial test for the diagnosis of coronary artery disease in symptomatic women is not justified. The reasons for these differences between men and women are poorly understood but may reflect the lower prevalence of flow-limiting coronary disease in women than in men of the same age, estrogen effects, and the inability of many older women to exercise to maximal aerobic capacity.

Diagnosis of Coronary Artery Disease in the Elderly

Pharmacologic imaging stress testing is required more often in the elderly than in the young because of their frequent inability to exercise adequately. TMET has a lower specificity in elderly patients than in younger patients because of resting ECG abnormalities, but it has a higher sensitivity because of the greater prevalence of obstructive coronary

Table 6.—Equations* for Predicting Maximal Aerobic Capacity During Treadmill Testing

Subjects	$\dot{V}O_2$, mL/(kg • min)
Active men[†]	69.7 - (0.612 x age)
Sedentary men	57.8 - (0.445 x age)
Active women[†]	44.4 - (0.343 x age)
Sedentary women	41.2 - (0.343 x age)

*Age is in years.
† "Active" means frequent aerobic exercise or sufficient exertion at least once a week to cause perspiring.
From Giuliani ER, Gersh BJ, McGoon MD, Hayes DL, Schaff HV (editors): *Mayo Clinic Practice of Cardiology*. Third edition. Mosby, 1996, p 132. By permission of Mayo Foundation.

artery disease. The result is that the application of standard ST-segment response criteria to elderly subjects has an overall accuracy similar to that of younger patients.

Coronary artery disease is highly prevalent in symptomatic elderly patients.

Exercise Testing in Asymptomatic Persons Without Known Coronary Artery Disease

Routine screening of asymptomatic men or women by TMET is not recommended except for asymptomatic men older than 40 years and women older than 50 years who plan to start vigorous exercise or those in occupations in which impairment might affect public safety (e.g., commercial pilots) or those who are at high risk for coronary artery disease because of other diseases (e.g., chronic renal failure).

The rationale for this position is that although the relative risk of a subsequent cardiac event is increased in asymptomatic patients with a positive exercise test result, the absolute risk of a cardiac event (death or myocardial infarction) is still low (about 1% annually).

Valvular Heart Disease

The primary value of exercise testing in valvular heart disease is to assess the exercise capacity of the patient. Many patients with chronic valvular heart disease decrease their exercise capacity gradually over many years and, thus, are not fully aware of the true extent of their disability.

TMET in Aortic Stenosis

TMET can be very useful in patients with moderate aortic

stenosis who have nonspecific symptoms and in those with severe aortic stenosis who have minimal symptoms. Great care should be taken with these patients, because the risk of an adverse event during TMET is increased, and exercise should be terminated for exercise-induced bradycardia, lack of the expected increase in systolic pressure, or increasing ventricular ectopy.

TMET in Mitral Stenosis

Because the major indication for surgery in mitral stenosis is symptom status, exercise testing is of most value when a patient is thought to be asymptomatic because of inactivity or when a discrepancy exists between the patient's symptoms and the valve area.

TMET is not accurate for diagnosing coronary artery disease in patients with significant valvular heart disease, because of false-positive responses due to left ventricular hypertrophy and baseline ECG changes.

Investigation of Heart Rhythm Disorders

TMET generally has a limited role in the investigation of most heart rhythm disorders. It may be used in the evaluation of patients with known or suspected exercise-induced arrhythmias and the response of patients to treatment with medical or ablative therapy for exercise-induced arrhythmias. TMET may also be used as an aid in pacemaker programming in patients with rate-adaptive pacemakers, and it may be used to assess control of the ventricular response to exercise in patients with atrial fibrillation.

Questions

Multiple Choice (choose the one best answer)

1. A 33-year-old woman has recurrent chest pain. The episodes last several hours and are constant in severity, with no radiation of the pain. They occur with and without exercise and are unrelated to posture or meals. She does not have hypertension, does not smoke, has a normal lipid profile, and does not have diabetes mellitus. A stress test is performed. The patient exercises for 12 minutes on a Bruce protocol, achieving more than 100% of her predicted functional aerobic capacity at a peak heart rate of 156 beats/min. She does not experience any angina or dyspnea on exertion. The electrocardiographic tracing shows 1 mm of horizontal ST-segment depression beginning at 4 minutes into the exercise and at a heart rate of 96 beats/min. At peak exercise, the ST segments in leads V_2-V_6 are horizontally depressed 3 mm from the isoelectric line. Which of the following statements is true?

   a. A positive test result is a good predictor of hemodynamically significant coronary artery disease in this patient

   b. There is a higher chance for a false-positive result than a true-positive result in this patient

   c. The test would be a good predictor of coronary artery disease in this patient if its specificity were 90%

   d. There is a higher chance for a false-negative result than a false-positive result in this patient

   e. For safety reasons, the test should have been stopped at 1 mm of ST-segment depression in the fourth minute of exercise

2. A 50-year-old patient is referred for a general cardiac evaluation. He does not complain of any angina; however, he is physically inactive and deconditioned. His cardiac risk factors include a strong family history of coronary artery disease at an age younger than 60 years. He is a current smoker at a low level (5 cigarettes a day), he has stage 1 hypertension, and he has moderately increased lipid levels (low-density lipoprotein, 160 mg/dL). You elect to perform a stress test in which the patient achieves 4.5 minutes on a Bruce protocol (approximately 60% of his predicted functional aerobic capacity). The peak heart rate increases to 110 beats/min, and there is a hypertensive blood pressure response of 220/100 mm Hg. The patient does not experience angina; however, the test was stopped because of general fatigue and dyspnea on exertion. The electrocardiographic tracings indicate no evidence of ischemia. In your experience, the electrocardiographic stress test has a sensitivity of 70% and a specificity of 50% for hemodynamically significant coronary artery disease. You will accept a 90% level of certainty of the presence or absence of disease. You also assume a likelihood of 50% that the patient has significant coronary artery disease (pretest probability). You can thus conclude:

   a. Given the current sensitivity and specificity, a negative test result will confirm the absence of disease
   b. There is a greater probability of a false-negative than a false-positive result in the patient
   c. Increasing the test specificity to 90% would reduce the risk of a false-positive result
   d. There are more false-positive than true-negative results
   e. Increasing the specificity to 90% would markedly reduce the probability of a true-negative test

3. A 70-year-old man comes for evaluation of recurrent chest pain. He is very active, walks 2 miles a day, but has noticed early chest pain within 6 minutes, which he is able to "walk through." He stopped smoking 10 years ago after a 100-pack-year history. His family history cannot be elicited because he was adopted. He does not have hypertension, but his cholesterol level is increased at 230 mg/dL (low-density lipoprotein, 140 mg/dL). You perform a stress test, in which the patient achieves 130% of his predicted functional aerobic capacity. The test is stopped because of 3 mm of ST-segment depression at peak exercise. The patient notices angina at

approximately 4 minutes into the test; however, the symptoms subside with continued exercise. His peak heart rate is 105 beats/min and his blood pressure response is normal. The ST-segment depression starts in the inferior and lateral leads at 2.5 minutes into the exercise. According to your epidemiologic data, the pretest likelihood of disease in men of this age with angina is approximately 95%. Assuming a test sensitivity of 70% and a test specificity of 50%, you conclude with a certainty level of 90% or more:

   a. A negative test would have been helpful to rule out coronary artery disease
   b. The chance that the patient has no disease if the test had been negative is approximately 20%
   c. There is a greater chance of a false-positive than a false-negative test result in this patient
   d. The patient should have been sent directly for coronary angiography
   e. A positive test result is useful to confirm coronary artery disease

4. A patient is referred for review of a treadmill exercise test. On review of the resting exercise, you notice that left ventricular hypertrophy by voltage criteria is present. You then evaluate the stress electrocardiogram (ECG) that has been performed. Which of the following statements is *not* correct?

   a. The stress ECG is positive for ischemia if 2 mm or more of horizontal or downsloping ST-segment depression is present at 0.08 second after the J point
   b. The stress ECG is positive for ischemia if 1 to 2 mm of additional horizontal or downsloping ST-segment depression is present 0.08 second after the J point
   c. The stress ECG is negative for ischemia if less than 1 mm of additional ST-segment depression is noted
   d. The stress ECG is negative for ischemia if there is pseudonormalization of an inverted T wave which occurs without ST-segment depression
   e. The stress ECG is nondiagnostic for ischemia if 1 mm or more of ST-segment elevation occurs in a lead in which preexisting pathologic Q waves are present

5. The following new findings on stress electrocardiograms (ECGs) are considered nondiagnostic for myocardial ischemia *except*:

   a. > 1 mm of ST-segment elevation in the presence of existing Q wave

b. ≥ 2 mm of ST-segment depression in the presence of left ventricular hypertrophy by Sokoloff (voltage) criteria

c. ≥ 1 mm of ST-segment depression in leads V_1-V_3 in the presence of right bundle branch block

d. ≥ 1 mm of ST-segment depression in the presence of digitalis

e. ≥ 1 mm of ST-segment depression in the presence of Wolff-Parkinson-White syndrome

6. In regard to the end points of an exercise test, the following statements are correct *except*:
   a. The test should be stopped when 85% of the maximal predicted heart rate is reached
   b. The perceived exertion scale (Borg scale) is helpful in the pediatric population
   c. β-Adrenergic blockers prevent achievement of an adequate exercise capacity
   d. A decrease in blood pressure should always result in termination of the test
   e. The perceived exertion scale (Borg scale) is helpful for assessing functional aerobic capacity

7. The following criteria are contraindications for exercise testing *except*:
   a. Serum potassium of 3.0 mEq/L
   b. Symptomatic aortic stenosis
   c. Severe arterial hypertension (resting blood pressure, 200/110 mm Hg)
   d. Bradyarrhythmias
   e. Hypertrophic obstructive cardiomyopathy

8. The following criteria are absolute indications for termination of an exercise test *except*:
   a. Moderate to severe angina, typical
   b. Increase in nervous symptoms (ataxia, dizziness, near syncope)
   c. Cyanosis or pallor
   d. Chest pain
   e. Subject's desire to stop

9. In the diagnosis of coronary artery disease, the usefulness of exercise testing is less well established (class IIB) in all of the following patient groups *except*:
   a. Patients with a high pretest probability of disease
   b. Patients with a low pretest probability of disease

c. Patients with less than 1 mm of baseline ST-segment depression and patients taking digoxin

d. Patients with left ventricular hypertrophy of less than 1 mm of ST-segment depression

e. Patients with preexcitation

10. A false-positive exercise stress test is more likely in the following patient groups *except*:
    a. Patients with left ventricular hypertrophy by both Estes and Sokoloff criteria
    b. Patients with resting ST-segment depression
    c. Patients taking digitalis
    d. Women undergoing pharmacologic stress testing

11. A 60-year-old man is referred because of new weight loss. You diagnose a gastric ulcer on endoscopy, which persists despite adequate medical treatment. Gastric surgery is recommended. The patient also has a history of coronary artery disease, treated with coronary artery bypass grafting approximately 3 years ago. The patient still smokes, but he exercises on a daily basis, walking approximately 3 miles a day in a little less than an hour. He denies any shortness of breath or angina. Before approving him for operation, from a cardiac perspective you would recommend the following:
    a. A symptom-limited exercise test
    b. Resting echocardiography
    c. Exercise thallium test
    d. Send patient directly to operation
    e. Coronary angiography

12. A patient with known coronary artery disease reports worsening of his dyspnea on exertion. There is a history of a bipolar psychiatric disorder, and the patient has had many evaluations because of similar complaints, all of which have been negative. You would like to quantitate the patient's exercise tolerance and order a stress test. On the day of the test, you receive a call from the stress laboratory, indicating that the patient has left bundle branch block. You would do which of the following?
    a. Cancel the test because you cannot interpret the electrocardiogram
    b. Proceed with the test
    c. Change the test to dobutamine echocardiography
    d. Change the test to adenosine thallium test
    e. Perform coronary angiography

Answers

1. Answer b

This situation represents the classic problem of combining the power of a test with the incidence of disease in the population. On the basis of the patient's age and sex and the absence of strong risk factors, she has a low risk of hemodynamically significant coronary artery disease. Because the incidence of coronary artery disease is expected to be very low in this patient, a true-positive test is less likely than a false-positive test. Thus, a positive test result would not be a good indicator for coronary artery disease. Increasing the test specificity to 80% would only modestly increase its positive predictive value, still not sufficient to make it a reliable diagnostic test. Diagnostic stress testing should, in general, be a symptom-limited test, and modest changes in electrocardiographic tracings should not lead to termination of the test.

2. Answer c

The problem of test sensitivity and specificity is common, regardless of the evaluating test chosen for a specific diagnosis. One always needs to be aware of the pretest likelihood of disease, which in this case is approximately 50%. This means that half of the test population will have true disease and half will not. Thus, you can easily calculate the proportions of test subjects, given the power of your test, that would be in each category (false-positive and negative, true-positive and negative). From these calculations, it is apparent that the probability of disease despite a negative stress test is 38%, given the specificity indicated initially. Increasing the specificity of the test to 90% would reduce the false-negative rate to 25%, still below the acceptable certainty level of 90%.

3. Answer d

This patient probably should have been sent directly for coronary angiography. The fact that the patient is able to exercise after the initial onset of ischemia is not helpful diagnostically. The pretest likelihood of significant coronary disease of 95% makes the probability that no significant disease is present, even if there was a negative stress test (true negative ÷ true negative + false negative), extremely low (8%). The probability of disease even with a negative test is still 92%, indicating that a negative test would not be helpful in this case. The incidence of disease in this patient group is the predominant factor in the diagnostic strategy. The high workload achieved indicates a good prognosis but not the absence of disease.

4. Answer b

A joint commission of the ACC/AHA (J Am Coll Cardiol, July 1997) developed new guidelines for the interpretation of stress ECGs. Review of the literature indicated that stress ECGs that show left ventricular hypertrophy by voltage criteria only (not fulfilling Estes criteria for the diagnosis of hypertrophy) can be interpreted like a regular stress ECG, with the caveat that horizontal or downsloping ST-segment depression of 1 to 2 mm is considered nondiagnostic but suggestive of ischemia. Horizontal or downsloping ST-segment depression of 2 mm or more indicates that the stress ECG is positive. Conversely, ST-segment depression of less than 1 mm or pseudonormalization of an inverted T wave is still considered negative for ischemia. ST-segment elevation in the presence of existing Q waves is a special case in which the ECG has to be interpreted as nondiagnostic.

5. Answer b

The label "nondiagnostic ECGs" has been redefined according to the recently published guidelines of a joint commission of the ACC/AHA. ST-segment elevation in the presence of existing Q waves cannot be interpreted as indicating ischemia, particularly in the presence of voltage criteria for left ventricular hypertrophy. In contrast, ST-segment depression 2 mm or more in the presence of left ventricular hypertrophy by voltage criteria alone is interpretable as a positive exercise test. Answers c, d, and e are similar to the previously published guidelines, in which the ST-segment changes in patients taking digoxin, the anteroseptal leads in patients with concomitant right bundle branch block, and the ECG of patients with Wolff-Parkinson-White syndrome cannot be accurately interpreted in respect to myocardial ischemia.

6. Answer b

This question deals with the desired end points of a stress test and an indication for termination. Even though exercise tests are often stopped at 85% of the patient's maximal predicted heart rate, this is not the optimal way to perform stress tests. This should occur only if the diagnosis of coronary artery disease is known and the goal of the exercise test is to assess the risk or degree of ischemia in a patient who wants to commence an exercise regimen. For the diagnosis of coronary artery disease, the threshold of 85% of the maximal predicted heart rate is very often inaccurate because of the marked variability present in heart rate response.

The Borg perceived exertion scale is helpful for assessing functional aerobic capacity and is often used in adults to gauge the level of fatigue. This is particularly important in radioisotope imaging. In contrast, the perceived exertion scale is not very helpful in young (pediatric and juvenile) patients because their onset of exhaustion can be very rapid and factors such as anxiety and apprehension play an important role.

β-Adrenergic blockers blunt the heart rate response; however, even in their presence, a good exercise capacity as estimated in metabolic equivalents should be achieved. A decrease in blood pressure should be carefully monitored by the physician and generally should lead to termination of the test only if it is accompanied by other significant clinical symptoms such as pallor, ischemia, significant dyspnea on exertion, or rhythm disturbances. If the blood pressure becomes lower than the resting blood pressure, termination of the test is recommended. At peak exercise in the otherwise asymptomatic patient, blood pressure readings can often be misjudged because of the interference of treadmill noise and patient motion with Korotkoff sounds.

7. Answer d

There are many contraindications for exercise testing, some of which are listed above. Significant electrolyte abnormalities are a cause of concern because affected patients are at risk for ventricular dysrhythmias to stress testing. Severe arterial hypertension is another contraindication. The blood pressure value of 200/110 mm Hg was somewhat arbitrarily suggested by the recent exercise guidelines of a joint commission of the ACC/AHA. The accuracy of the stress test is reduced in the presence of hypertension, particularly because hypertension itself can cause an ischemic response. Often, hypertensive patients with increased baseline blood pressure measurements show no further increase in blood pressure if some peripheral vascular relaxation mechanisms are still preserved.

Bradyarrhythmias and tachyarrhythmias also present problems. Often, bradyarrhythmias are alleviated if the conduction system is partially preserved and still responsive to catecholamines. Hypertrophic obstructive cardiomyopathy and asymptomatic, moderate aortic stenosis are relative contraindications to exercise testing. In affected patients, exercise testing is often used to objectify their exercise capacity. Severe symptomatic aortic stenosis, however, is an absolute contraindication, and an exercise test should not be performed in affected patients.

8. Answer d

Moderate to severe angina, an increase in nervous system symptoms, signs of poor perfusion, and a subject's desire

to stop are all absolute indications for terminating the exercise test. Increasing chest pain, however, is only a relative indication and needs to be judged in the presence of other accompanying factors, such as electrocardiographic changes, changes in the hemodynamic response to exercise, and increasing dysrhythmia.

9. Answer e

Guidelines have been established to assess the usefulness of exercise testing in patients with the diagnosis of obstructive coronary artery disease. The classification used is based on the following criteria:

1. Class I includes conditions in which there is objective evidence of, or general agreement by clinicians in the specialty on, the usefulness and effectiveness of a given procedure, treatment, or test.
2. Class II is subdivided into two groups. Class IIA indicates conditions in which there is evidence or opinion favoring the usefulness or efficacy. Class IIB "turns the corner" by indicating conditions in which the usefulness and efficacy are less well established. In class III, there is evidence or general agreement that a test is not useful or is even harmful. On the basis of these classifications, answers a, b, c, and d are categorized as class IIB, indicating that there is less established evidence for the usefulness or efficacy of exercise testing in this setting. It is important to know these criteria when considering exercise testing for the diagnosis of coronary artery disease. The last option, preexcitation, is a class III option, together with electronically paced ventricular rhythms with more than 1 mm of ST-segment depression at rest or left bundle branch block. This classification pertains to the diagnosis of obstructive coronary artery disease, *not* the assessment of functional aerobic capacity in patients with various underlying diseases. The only established indication for considering exercise testing in the diagnosis of obstructive coronary artery disease (class I) is an intermediate pretest probability of coronary artery disease in an adult on the basis of sex, age, and symptoms and less than 1 mm of resting ST-segment depression. Patients with complete right bundle branch block may be included if one considers that only leads V_3-V_6 can be interpreted. A more marginal but class IIA indication is vasospastic angina.

10. Answer d

All the patient groups listed have a higher proportion of false-positive tests when undergoing exercise testing, particularly women undergoing stress testing. There is still some debate about whether exercise testing becomes more sensitive and specific in women at an advanced age, but data are still pending. However, there is evidence that use of pharmacologic stress testing, particularly coupled with an imaging method, may improve the accuracy of the test significantly.

11. Answer d

This question relates to preoperative exercise testing. You are asked to assess the risk of a perioperative cardiac event in this patient. Certain key features help make the decision. This patient has stable, asymptomatic coronary artery disease. Despite his persistent risk factors, he is able to exercise well without symptoms. His bypass procedure was only 3 years ago, which is in favor of patency of the coronary grafts, although his smoking is worrisome. In the absence of angina or heart failure, the patient's perioperative risk is low and largely determined by the risk of the gastric procedure and not his coronary artery disease per se.

12. Answer b

This question addresses the exercise tolerance of the patient, *not* the diagnosis of coronary artery disease, which has been established. Optimally, you would like to know whether the left bundle branch block is new in onset, but this information is not available. Because the diagnosis has been established, you do not necessarily need to rely on the electrocardiographic information. Dobutamine echocardiography would be similar to an exercise thallium test, in that it would also be subject to false-positive regional wall motion abnormalities. An adenosine thallium test would aid in establishment of the diagnosis, but this is not the goal of the test. Coronary angiography does not assess the functional significance of a lesion. In this situation, assessment of the exercise tolerance and the hemodynamic factors (heart rate and blood pressure response) provides valuable information to objectify the symptoms in this patient. Another good choice would have been a stress test, including the assessment of oxygen uptake, but this is not a listed option for the question.

Notes

Chapter 50

Invasive Hemodynamics

Rick A. Nishimura, M.D.

Cardiac Output

Measurement of volumetric flow rate (i.e., stroke volume or cardiac output) is an important variable for evaluating systolic performance of the heart. Stroke volume is the amount of blood that the heart is able to eject during systole and occurs during the systolic ejection period from aortic valve opening to aortic valve closure. This ejection phase index depends on the loading conditions of the heart (afterload and preload) and on the intrinsic contractility of heart muscle. It provides an overall measurement of the ability of the heart to meet the metabolic demands of the body.

Volumetric flow can be measured by several methods. These include the Fick method, the indicator dilution method, and the Doppler flow velocity method. Cardiac catheterization methods are based on the principle outlined by Fick in 1870: for any circulation, the amount of an indicator substance in the blood leaving the circulation must equal the amount of the substance entering plus any amount added to the circulation during transit. The total amount of substance passing any point in the circulation per unit of time is the product of its concentration (which is measured) and the flow rate (which is the unknown value). The Doppler method is based on the hydrodynamic principle of flow through a rigid tube, in which the velocity of flow times the area through which the flow occurs equals the flow rate.

Each method has inherent advantages and limitations. The Fick measurement of cardiac output is the most accurate measurement for low output states. The indicator dilution method is the most accurate method for high output states. In a properly performed Doppler examination, Doppler-derived cardiac output may be the most accurate and reproducible method overall for determination of volumetric flow rates.

Methods used to measure cardiac output:
- Fick method
- Indicator dilution method
- Dopper flow velocity method

- The Fick measurement of cardiac output is the most accurate measurement for low output states.
- The indicator dilution method is the most accurate method for high output states.

It is important to understand the limitations of cardiac output calculation in both low and high cardiac output states.

Fick Method

The Fick method, a time-honored technique, uses the amount of oxygen extracted by the body, as measured by the arterial-venous oxygen difference, to calculate cardiac output. This difference is divided into the oxygen consumption of the body, which is usually measured through a gas exchange method or, less accurately, by estimation from a patient's body weight. Knowledge of the oxygen-carrying capacity of the blood is required; thus, it is necessary to measure the concentration of hemoglobin in the blood. A properly performed Fick method requires a tight-fitting gas exchange mask at equilibrium (no movement of the patient or movement of catheters inside the patient). Simultaneous measurement of oxygen saturation in the arterial system and in the mixed venous system (main pulmonary artery) is required. The formula for calculating cardiac output is

$$\text{Cardiac Output} = \frac{O_2 \text{ Consumption}}{(A\text{-}V)O_2 \times \text{Hemoglobin Concentration} \times (\text{Vol \%}) \times 10}$$

Where $(A\text{-}V)O_2$ is the arterial-venous oxygen difference, and Vol % is calculated by multiplying the product of hemoglobin by a factor of 1.36.

The advantage of the Fick method over the other methods is that the variables are measured during steady state. The Fick method of calculating cardiac output is the most accurate method if the heart rate or rhythm is irregular, as in atrial fibrillation. Because lower cardiac output results in a higher arterial-venous oxygen difference, the Fick cardiac output method is most accurate for low output states. The total error in determining cardiac output is 10% to 15%.

The disadvantage of the Fick cardiac output method is that it requires simultaneous measurement of oxygen consumption by the body, and this may be difficult to do because of the logistic problem of obtaining a tight gas exchange coupling. It is not of use in patients undergoing cardiac interventions (e.g., valvuloplasty), because it cannot detect rapid changes in cardiac output.

- The Fick method of calculating cardiac output is the most accurate method if the heart rate or rhythm is irregular, as in atrial fibrillation.

> Common errors in calculating cardiac output by the Fick method include forgetting to multiply the volume percent by 10 and omitting the constant (1.36) for the oxygen-carrying capacity per gram of hemoglobin.

Indicator Dilution Method

The indicator dilution method of calculating cardiac output

is the method used most commonly by cardiologists. Originally, the indicator dilution method was performed by injecting indocyanine green into one cardiac chamber and sampling the concentration of dye downstream. Although a continuous infusion of dye would be the most accurate method, the use of bolus injections has evolved for logistic reasons. Although the green dye injection method is still used in some laboratories, the thermodilution cardiac output method is more popular. This consists of injecting a bolus of cold liquid in a proximal portion of the heart and sampling the changes in temperature as the solution mixes distally with warm blood.

The measurement of cardiac output is based on a time intensity (or temperature) curve, with concentration on the y-axis and time on the x-axis (Fig. 1). The area underneath the time intensity curve is related inversely to cardiac output if the dye dissipates immediately after measurement. Because of recirculation of dye through the body, extrapolation of the descending limb of the curve is necessary. The disappearance of dye from the human circulation is exponential; thus, the area under the curve can be determined by assuming a monoexponential decrease of the curve to baseline:

$$\text{Cardiac Output} = \frac{I}{\int_0^\infty c(t)dt}$$

where I = amount of indicator injected and c(t) = concentration as a function of time.

The use of an indicator dye method requires that adequate mixing of the dye (or cold saline) be complete before sampling occurs. Therefore, the optimal method requires that a mixing chamber be interposed between the injection site and the sampling site. The best sampling site is the chamber or great vessel closest to the mixing chamber. The indicator dye solution can be injected into the pulmonary artery or left atrium and the concentration can be sampled in the ascending aorta. For the thermodilution method, the cold solution is injected into the right atrium, and the changes in temperature are sampled in the pulmonary artery.

The indicator dilution method is most accurate in patients with high output states. It is less accurate as cardiac output decreases. This method is inaccurate in the presence of irregular heart rates or rhythms and when coexistent regurgitation of a valve between the ejection site and sampling site is significant. Under the best conditions, the

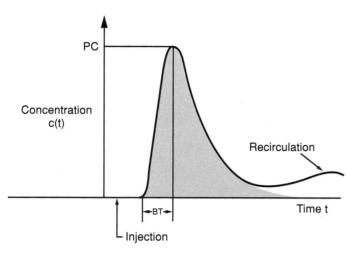

Fig. 1. Indicator time-concentration curve for circulation without shunts. The shaded area is produced by "first-pass" dye. The unshaded area results from recirculation of indicator and is ignored for calculations of cardiac output. *PC*, peak concentration of initial deflection; *BT*, buildup time for initial peak. (From Brandenburg RO, Fuster V, Giuliani ER, et al: *Cardiology: Fundamentals and Practice*. Vol. 1. Year Book Medical Publishers, 1987, p 423. By permission of Mayo Foundation.)

variability in thermodilution cardiac output can be as much as 15% to 20%.

- The indicator dilution method is inaccurate in the presence of irregular heart rates or rhythms and when coexistent regurgitation of a valve between the ejection site and sampling site is significant.

Doppler Cardiac Output

Volumetric flow rate also can be measured by Doppler echocardiography. This method incorporates the hydraulic principle of flow through a rigid tube. If the area of the tube and the velocity of the flow are known, the product of velocity times area provides a measure of volumetric flow rate. In the pulsatile model, the time velocity integral of the measured Doppler velocity times the area through which the flow occurs provides a measurement of stroke volume, and stroke volume multiplied by heart rate equals cardiac output.

There are limitations to using Doppler echocardiography for measurement of volumetric flow. The orifice through which the flow is measured must be a fixed circular orifice. The velocity profile is assumed to be flat, but in humans, flow profiles are usually parabolic. Changes in the position of the sample volume in relation to the heart with respiration also may cause erroneous measurements.

Various sites in the heart and great vessels have been used for measurement of volumetric flow rate by Doppler echocardiography, including the ascending aorta, descending aorta, mitral annulus, mitral valve, tricuspid annulus, tricuspid valve, aortic valve, and right ventricular outflow tract. The sampling site that is most accurate is the left ventricular outflow tract, because the area is relatively constant and the velocity profile is most laminar.

Of all the methods, Doppler measurement of cardiac output potentially is the most accurate on a beat-to-beat basis, but it is also the most operator-dependent method. Care must be taken to obtain an accurate measurement of the diameter of the left ventricular outflow tract, because an error in the diameter measurement is squared when it is converted to area. The velocity profile changes within the left ventricular outflow tract, and different positions of the sample volume may result in different velocity measurements. Also, care must be taken to ensure that the Doppler beam is parallel to the outflow tract velocity.

- Of the three methods commonly used to calculate cardiac output, Doppler echocardiography is the one most susceptible to operator error.

Pressures and Resistance

Pressures
Measurement of intracardiac pressure and pressure in the great vessels is achieved most accurately with cardiac catheterization. Indirect noninvasive measurements have been used, including sphygmomanometry and Doppler velocities; however, they rely on several assumptions. Thus, cardiac catheterization is required for the most accurate measurement of absolute pressures.

Fluid-filled catheter systems are most widely used by cardiologists. The pressure waveforms generated in the cardiac chambers or great vessels are transmitted through the fluid column in the catheter lumen to a pressure transducer. Most pressure transducers are the strain-gauge type, with a diaphragm in direct contact with the fluid column in the catheter. Changes of pressure in the fluid deform this diaphragm and induce a change in electrical potential that is proportional to the pressure change. This potential is calibrated, amplified, and displayed as intracardiac pressure. Zeroing and calibration of the pressure transducers are required before each procedure.

Pressure waves are always distorted with fluid-filled

catheters, primarily because of the oscillatory and dampening characteristics of the catheter-fluid column. These distortions may be minimized by 1) minimizing the number and length of stopcocks and connectors between the catheter and the transducer, 2) flushing out all microbubbles in the system, 3) avoiding making measurements after injection of contrast agent or withdrawal of blood, 4) using continuous flushing with heparin, and 5) using catheters of the largest practical size, preferably with a side hole in the ventricles. Artifacts may occur because of incomplete seals between the catheter and the connectors, inadequate initial calibration, and inaccurate zero balance.

The most accurate way of measuring intracardiac pressures is to use high-fidelity manometer-tipped catheters, in which an electronic manometer transducer is placed on the end of the catheter and inserted directly into the cardiac chamber. The electronic pressures need to be balanced and calibrated to the absolute fluid-filled pressures.

- The most accurate way of measuring intracardiac pressures is to use high-fidelity manometer-tipped catheters.

Normal values for heart pressures are shown in Table 1. Right and left atrial pressures normally have three distinct positive waves and two negative descents. The "a" wave is the pressure increase at atrial contraction. The "c" wave is the pressure increase during isovolumic contraction of the ventricle as the atrioventricular valve bulges back into the atrium. The x descent occurs after the "a" and "c" waves and is related to atrial relaxation, descent of the annulus toward the apex, and the compliance of the atrium itself. The "v" wave is the increase in atrial pressure when the atrioventricular valve is closed as blood comes in from either the vena cava or the pulmonary veins. At the peak of the "v" wave, the atrioventricular valve opens and blood rushes from the atria into the ventricles, causing a y descent. On the right side of the heart, the "a" wave usually is slightly larger than the "v" wave, but on the left side, the "v" wave usually is slightly larger than the "a" wave. The z point on the atrial pressure trace is the pressure of the atria just before the onset of ventricular contraction. The mean right and left atrial pressures are the standard measurements used for clinical assessment.

The left and right ventricular pressures are usually measured at maximal systolic pressure, minimal early diastolic pressure, and ventricular end-diastolic pressure. End-diastolic pressure is defined as the ventricular pressure just before the onset of ventricular contraction after atrial contraction. The first derivative of the ventricular pressure

Table 1.—Normal Values for Heart Pressures

	Pressure, mm Hg*	
Chamber	Average	Range
Right atrium	5	±2
Right ventricle	25/5	±5/±2
Pulmonary artery	25/10	±5/±2
Left atrium	10	±2
Left ventricle	120/15	±20/±5

*The easiest way to remember the normal intracardiac pressures is as multiples of 5.

curves during isovolumic contraction is used as a measurement of systolic contractility, that is, peak positive dp/dt. The peak positive dp/dt may be divided by the absolute pressure at which it occurs to normalize for pressure. The first derivative of the ventricular pressure curve during isovolumic relaxation provides a measurement of the rate of ventricular relaxation, that is, the peak negative dp/dt. The peak positive and negative dp/dt are dependent on the load imposed on the left ventricle.

The time constant of relaxation, or Tau, has been used to measure the rate of relaxation and is less dependent on loading conditions. Various methods have been proposed for measuring the time constant of relaxation. In the most commonly used method (the method of Weiss et al.), the ventricular pressure from aortic valve closure to mitral valve opening is fitted to a monoexponential equation and allowed to decay to 0 mm Hg. The following equation is used to calculate Tau (T) by this method:

$$P(t) = P_0 \times e^{-t/T}$$

Other methods of measuring Tau include using a nonzero asymptote and a biexponential fit. Other diastolic variables of ventricular pressure include measurement of the height of the rapid filling wave and the pressure just before the onset of atrial contraction—the "pre-a wave."

Aortic and pulmonary pressures are measured in terms of peak systolic pressure, end-diastolic pressure, and mean pressure. For the aorta, the mean pressure can be assumed to be one-third the difference between the maximal and minimal aortic pressures. For the pulmonary circulation with normal pulmonary pressures, the mean pressure can be assumed to be one-half the difference between the maximal and minimal pulmonary pressures.

Resistance

The great vessels impose an afterload on the ventricles, and this is related to both flow and absolute pressure. Because the cardiovascular system is pulsatile, the ideal measurement of this afterload would be arterial impedance. However, this measurement is difficult to obtain in humans, and its use has been restricted to laboratory investigations. Although arterial resistance is less accurate as a measurement of afterload, it is the clinically used parameter obtained at the time of cardiac catheterization. Resistance is derived from a hydrodynamic model of continuous flow. The resistance of flow through a rigid tube is defined as follows:

$$\text{Resistance} = \frac{\text{Pressure Difference}}{\text{Cardiac Output}}$$

Systemic arterial resistance is mean systemic aortic pressure divided by cardiac output. Pulmonary artery resistance is mean pulmonary artery pressure divided by cardiac output. A measurement of pulmonary arteriolar resistance is mean pulmonary artery pressure minus mean left atrial pressure divided by cardiac output.

Several types of units have been used to describe arterial resistance. A Wood unit is millimeters of mercury times minute divided by liters, with no conversion factor used. Wood units can be indexed to body surface area. Another unit of arterial resistance is "dynes $\cdot$ s $\cdot$ cm^{-5}," which is the same as a Wood unit multiplied by a constant of 80. Normal values for arterial resistance are listed in Table 2.

- Wood units $\cdot$ 80 = dynes $\cdot$ s $\cdot$ cm^{-5}

Intracardiac Shunts

Intracardiac shunting of blood may be due to either congenital or acquired lesions. Shunting may occur because oxygenated blood from the left heart passes into the systemic venous blood ("left-to-right shunt") or because unoxygenated venous blood passes directly into the arterial circulation ("right-to-left shunt"). In the presence of complex congenital heart disease, it may be confusing to think in terms of left-to-right or right-to-left shunts. The following terms are helpful in describing shunts in complex cases and in calculating shunts:

1. Effective flow (EF)—Quantity of systemically mixed venous blood that circulates through the lungs, is oxygenated,

Table 2.—Normal Values for Arterial Resistance

Type	Resistance	
	Wood units	Dynes$\cdot$s$\cdot$cm^{-5}
Pulmonary arteriolar resistance	0.84 ± 0.29	67 ± 23
Pulmonary arteriolar resistance index (per m^2)	1.54 ± 0.68	123 ± 54
Total pulmonary resistance	2.56 ± 0.64	205 ± 51
Systemic resistance	14.4 ± 2.2	1,130 ± 178

and then circulates through systemic capillaries.

2. Recirculated systemic flow (RSF)—Amount of relatively desaturated, systemically mixed venous blood that recirculates directly to the aorta without being oxygenated by the lungs.

3. Recirculated pulmonary flow (RPF)—The quantity of fully saturated pulmonary venous blood that recirculates to the pulmonary artery without passing through the systemic capillaries.

4. Total pulmonary flow (PF)—Effective flow plus recirculated pulmonary flow.

5. Systemic flow (SF)—Effective flow plus recirculated systemic flow.

In most cases, the question of the presence of intracardiac shunting is raised before cardiac catheterization is initiated. However, there may be instances in which a shunt is suspected only at the time of cardiac catheterization, by finding a "step-up" on a routine measurement of right heart oxygen saturation or finding desaturation when arterial blood gases are measured. When this is present, it is necessary to perform a complete cardiac catheterization study for shunt determination. This consists of 1) performing a complete measurement of saturation, 2) measuring oxygen consumption, 3) considering administration of 100% oxygen, and 4) obtaining dye curves.

Two Methods of Intracardiac Shunt Detection

Traditionally, the detection and quantitation of intracardiac shunts have been performed in a cardiac catheterization laboratory. With the advent of two-dimensional and transesophageal echocardiography, the clinical need for invasive evaluation of intracardiac shunts has virtually disappeared. However, for the Cardiology Boards, it is important to understand the methods used for the detection and measurement of intracardiac shunts at the time of cardiac catheterization. Intracardiac shunts can be detected and quantitated with two separate methods: oximetry and dye curves. The advantage of oximetry is its availability in all laboratories. However, it is a relatively insensitive technique and may miss small shunts. Also, many times, it is difficult to localize the position of the intracardiac shunt by oximetry alone. Dye curves, especially double-sampling dye curves, overcome these limitations of oximetry. However, dye curves are more difficult to perform and their use is limited to a few medical centers in the United States. Nonetheless, for the Cardiology Boards, it is important to understand the concepts of both oximetry and double-sampling dye curves.

Saturations—Left-to-Right

A properly performed saturation measurement should include sampling the saturation at the following sites: the inferior vena cava at the level of the renal arteries, the inferior vena cava below the diaphragm, the inferior vena cava at the diaphragm, the lower right atrium, the mid-right atrium, the high right atrium, the low superior vena cava, the high superior vena cava, the right ventricle, the pulmonary artery, and a systemic arterial location. Hemoglobin and blood gas concentrations should be measured simultaneously at the arterial site. Technical points about catheter position include 1) turning the catheter away from the hepatic vein when sampling from the inferior vena cava, 2) turning the catheter away from the tricuspid valve when sampling from the right atrium, and 3) aspirating all the static blood within the catheter before withdrawing a blood sample in each location for determining oxygen saturation. Normally, the blood in the superior vena cava is less saturated than the blood in the inferior vena cava because of a higher degree of oxygen extraction from the vessels in the head and upper extremity. Therefore, a mixed venous saturation is calculated from the inferior vena cava (IVC) and superior vena cava (SVC):

$$\text{Mixed Venous Saturation} = \frac{3\,\text{SVC} + 1\,\text{IVC}}{4}$$

An oxygen "step-up," which indicates a left-to-right shunt, is significant when there is a step-up of more than 7% at the atrial level, a 5% step-up at the ventricular level, and a 5% step-up at the pulmonary artery level (Table 3).

For measuring shunt flow with oximetry, it is easiest to use the concept of the Fick equation applied to the different circulations. According to this equation (as described above), flow is proportional to oxygen consumption divided by arteriovenous oxygen difference from the most proximal site to the most distal site. Thus, different flows can be determined, as follows:

$$\text{Effective Flow} = \frac{O_2\ \text{Consumption}}{PV\,O_2 - MV\,O_2}$$

$$\text{Total Pulmonary Flow} = \frac{O_2\ \text{Consumption}}{PV\,O_2 - PA\,O_2}$$

$$\text{Total Systemic Flow} = \frac{O_2\ \text{Consumption}}{FA\,O_2 - MV\,O_2}$$

where FA = femoral artery, MV = mixed venous, PA = pulmonary artery, and PV = pulmonary vein.

Recirculated Pulmonary Flow = Total Pulmonary Flow - Effective Flow

Recirculated Systemic Flow = Total Systemic Flow - Effective Flow

The degree of shunt is reported in two ways: Qp/Qs and percentage shunt.

$$\text{Qp/Qs} = \frac{\text{Total Pulmonary Flow}}{\text{Total Systemic Flow}}$$

$$\%\ \text{Left-to-Right Shunt} = \frac{\text{Recirculated Pulmonary Flow}}{\text{Total Pulmonary Flow}}$$

$$\%\ \text{Right-to-Left Shunt} = \frac{\text{Recirculated Systemic Flow}}{\text{Total Systemic Flow}}$$

Dye Curves—Left-to-Right Shunt

Dye curves are a more sensitive and more accurate method for the detection and quantitation of intracardiac shunts.

Table 3.—Oximetry for Shunts

Location	Step-up, $O_2\%$ saturated		Shunt detection, Qp/Qs
	Maximum	Mean	
SVC-IVC/RA	> 11	> 7	1.5-1.9
RA/RV	> 10	> 5	1.3-1.5
RV/PA	> 5	> 5	1.3

IVC, inferior vena cava; PA, pulmonary artery; RA, right atrium; RV, right ventricle; SVC, superior vena cava.

Single-sampling dye curves consist of injecting dye proximal to an intracardiac shunt and sampling distally to a shunt. Double-sampling dye curves consist of injecting dye proximal to the shunt and sampling both distally to the shunt in the arterial circulation and proximally to the recirculation of the shunt on the venous side (Fig. 2).

A single-sampling dye curve usually is performed by injecting dye into the pulmonary artery and sampling in the ascending aorta or femoral artery. If a left-to-right

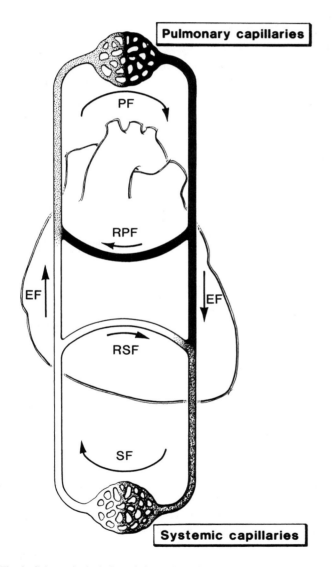

Fig. 2. Schematic depiction of circulation with intracardiac shunting. *EF*, effective flow; *PF*, pulmonary flow; *RPF*, recirculated pulmonary flow; *RSF*, recirculated systemic flow; *SF*, systemic flow. (From Brandenburg RO, Fuster V, Giuliani ER, et al: *Cardiology: Fundamentals and Practice.* Vol. 1. Year Book Medical Publishers, 1987, p 423. By permission of Mayo Foundation.)

shunt is present, the descending limb of the dye curve has a secondary bump. Because it may be difficult to determine whether an extra bump is present, double-sampling dye curves have become standard for diagnosing left-to-right shunts. A complete dye curve measurement should consist of injecting dye first into the pulmonary trunk and simultaneously sampling in the ascending aorta and right ventricle. In the absence of a shunt, sampling in the ascending aorta should produce a normal dye curve. Dye should not appear in the right ventricle until after the blood has fully recirculated through the body. In the presence of a left-to-right shunt, dye appears early in the right ventricle, concomitant with the appearance of dye in the ascending aorta. The magnitude of the shunt can be calculated by comparing the area underneath the two curves, using a forward triangle method.

After an intracardiac shunt has been diagnosed, further evaluation by double-sampling dye curves can provide information about shunt localization. This should be done by injecting dye into the right pulmonary artery and sampling the left pulmonary artery and ascending aorta. Next, the dye should be injected into the left pulmonary artery, with sampling in the right pulmonary artery and ascending aorta. In the presence of anomalous pulmonary venous drainage, the dye will appear early after it is injected into one pulmonary artery but not the other. In the presence of an intracardiac shunt, the dye will appear early after it is injected into either pulmonary artery.

After the question of a partial anomalous pulmonary venous drainage has been answered, injections should be made into the main pulmonary artery, with simultaneous sampling in the ascending aorta and in the right side of the heart. The second sampling site should be made in the right ventricle, then in the right atrium, superior vena cava, and inferior vena cava. The early appearance of dye in the right ventricle alone indicates a shunt at the ventricular level. The appearance of dye in the atrium and ventricle indicates a shunt at the atrial level, and the early appearance of dye in the superior vena cava or inferior vena cava indicates the presence of an anomalous pulmonary venous connection with these venous sites (Fig. 3 and 4).

Evaluation of Arterial Desaturation

Whenever arterial desaturation (arterial saturation < 95%) occurs, an effort must be made to determine whether it is due to a right-to-left shunt, an intrapulmonary shunt, or a pulmonary parenchymal abnormality. The simplest method to determine this is to inject a saline contrast into the right

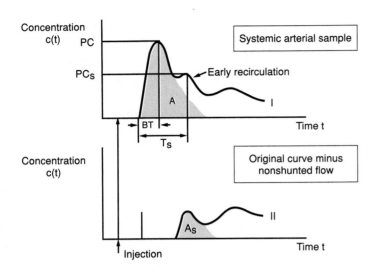

Fig. 3. Pulmonary recirculation, or left-to-right shunt. *Curve I*, Time-indicator concentration relationship from a typical systemic arterial sample. Total pulmonary flow is proportional to shaded area A. *Curve II*, Generated by subtracting, point-by-point, from curve I the portion of the curve bounding area A. Shunt flow is then proportional to the shaded area A_S. An approximate formula uses: *PC*, peak indicator concentration of initial deflection; PC_S, peak indicator concentration of early recirculation from the shunt; *BT*, buildup time for PC; and T_S, time from initial appearance of dye until PC_S. (From Brandenburg RO, Fuster V, Giuliani ER, et al: *Cardiology: Fundamentals and Practice.* Vol. 1. Year Book Medical Publishers, 1987, p 425. By permission of Mayo Foundation.)

side of the heart under two-dimensional echocardiographic guidance. If no shunt is present, saline contrast will not appear in the left side of the heart. If there is an intracardiac shunt, saline contrast will appear immediately. If there is intrapulmonary shunting, saline contrast will appear after six to seven beats. In orthodeoxia platypnea, intrapulmonary shunting occurs only when the person is standing and not when supine.

If an echocardiographic contrast agent is not available, 100% oxygen can be given over 15 minutes to achieve equilibration, and then saturation can be measured. In the presence of pulmonary abnormalities, arterial saturation increases. If there is an intracardiac shunt, the administration of oxygen does not affect desaturation. If the left atrium can be entered through either an atrial septal defect or a patent foramen ovale, sampling of pulmonary vein saturation also can be used to determine the cause of arterial desaturation.

Single sampling dye curves also can be used to detect right-to-left shunts. In the presence of a right-to-left shunt, the ascending limb of the dye curve has an early rise, reflecting the direct shunting of blood through the cardiac chambers.

Stenotic Valvular Lesions

Hemodynamic Assessment of Mitral Stenosis

Mitral stenosis now can be diagnosed readily with two-dimensional and Doppler echocardiography. Many physicians consider Doppler echocardiography to be the standard for determining mitral stenosis hemodynamics. However, for the Cardiology Boards, it is necessary to know what information can be obtained at the time of cardiac catheterization.

In mitral stenosis, a gradient occurs between the left atrium and left ventricle during diastole. This can be measured directly from catheters placed in the left ventricle and left atrium (this requires transseptal cardiac catheterization). In many laboratories, pulmonary artery wedge pressure has been used as an indirect measurement of left atrial pressure in patients with mitral stenosis, but this has inherent problems for determining mean mitral gradient. A properly performed pulmonary artery wedge pressure assessment requires an end-hole catheter and confirmation of a saturation more than 97%. Even when a properly obtained pulmonary artery wedge pressure assessment is used, the mean mitral gradient can still be

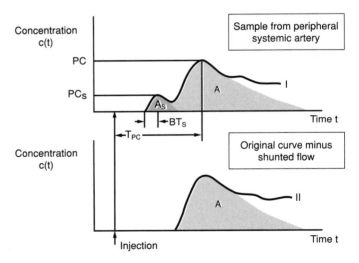

Fig. 4. Time-indicator concentration curves for systemic recirculation, or right-to-left shunt. The magnitude of shunt flow is proportional to the area A_S under *curve I*. After extrapolation of the downslope of the initial deflection toward zero, the portion of the curve bounding A_S is subtracted from curve I point-by-point to produce *curve II*. The area A is proportional to systemic flow. An approximate formula using the forward-triangle technique makes use of: PC_S, peak concentration of initial (shunt flow) deflection; *PC*, peak concentration of the second (systemic flow) deflection; BT_S, buildup time to PC_S; and T_{pc}, time from injection to PC. (From Brandenburg RO, Fuster V, Giuliani ER, et al: *Cardiology: Fundamentals and Practice.* Vol. 1. Year Book Medical Publishers, 1987, p 426. By permission of Mayo Foundation.)

overestimated by up to 50% to 70%. This is due to a delay in the time for transmission of the pulmonary artery wedge pressure and a dampening of the y descent that is normally present in a true left atrial pressure. The pulmonary artery wedge pressure should be "time-shifted" so that the peak of the "v" wave coincides with decreasing left ventricular pressure at the time of mitral valve opening. However, even with this, the gradient may still be overestimated.

The mean mitral valve gradient depends not only on the degree of obstruction across the mitral valve but also on cardiac output and diastolic filling period. Therefore, the Gorlin equation has been used to derive a calculated mitral valve area, which theoretically takes into consideration flow and duration of flow across the mitral valve:

$$\text{Area} = \frac{\text{Flow}}{44.3 \times C \times \sqrt{\Delta P}}$$

where $C = 0.85$ and ΔP = pressure gradient.

$$\text{Mitral Flow} = \frac{1{,}000 \times \text{Cardiac Output (L/min)}}{\text{Heart Rate (beats/min)} \times \text{DFP (s/beat)}}$$

where DFP = diastolic filling period.

Accurate measurement of mitral valve area by cardiac catheterization requires accurate measurement of mean mitral valve gradient and cardiac output. The limitations of both of these have been discussed. In addition, the mitral valve area is erroneous at both low and high heart rates. Also, it is not accurate with concomitant significant mitral regurgitation because of a higher flow across the mitral valve than is reflected in the measurement of cardiac output.

Because of problems with the calculated mitral valve area, another indirect measurement of the severity of mitral stenosis is used—diastolic half-time. This is the time it takes for the peak left atrial/left ventricular pressure gradient to decrease by 50%. It is more accurate than the Gorlin equation for mitral valve area in cases of atrial fibrillation with variable RR intervals and concomitant mitral regurgitation. The original investigations concerning diastolic half-time proposed that a half-time of 100 ms = mild mitral stenosis, of 200 ms = moderate mitral stenosis, and of 300 ms = severe mitral stenosis.

Diastolic half-time depends on the relative compliance between the left ventricle and left atrium and will be erroneous when there is a marked abnormality of compliance.

This occurs in patients with ventricular compliance abnormalities, such as restriction to filling or severe abnormal relaxation, and in those with acute changes in atrial compliance, for example, immediately after balloon valvuloplasty or after mitral valve surgery.

Hemodynamic Assessment of Aortic Stenosis

In a patient with aortic stenosis, the diagnosis and measurement of the severity of stenosis can be made in most cases by Doppler echocardiography, by obtaining both the mean aortic valve gradient and the calculated valve area. However, in contrast to mitral stenosis, the Doppler examination in a patient with aortic stenosis is highly operator-dependent, and the severity of stenosis can be grossly underestimated if there is a large theta angle between the Doppler beam and the aortic stenotic jet. Thus, cardiac catheterization may be needed to determine the severity of the stenosis if there is a discrepancy between the clinical impression and the echocardiographic results.

The aortic valve gradient is an important variable to measure in a patient with aortic stenosis. Several types of gradients are reported. The peak-to-peak gradient, the one most commonly used in cardiac catheterization laboratories, is the difference between the peak left ventricular and peak aortic pressure. This is a nonphysiologic measurement because it is obtained from nonsimultaneous recordings. Doppler echocardiographic assessment of the aortic valve gradient provides instantaneous gradients between the left ventricle and aorta. The peak aortic velocity is converted to gradient, resulting in a maximal instantaneous gradient. This maximal instantaneous gradient is usually 30% to 40% greater than the peak-to-peak gradient. The mean aortic valve gradient provides the most information about the severity of obstruction and should be the gradient used by both Doppler and cardiac catheterization methods.

There are several ways the aortic valve gradient can be measured in a cardiac catheterization laboratory. The most common one is the "pull-back" method, in which a catheter is placed in the left ventricle and quickly pulled back into the aorta while the peak pressure is recorded in both places. The difference between the two peak pressures is the gradient across the aortic valve. In most circumstances, this "peak-to-peak" gradient approximates the true mean aortic valve gradient, especially at very high pressure gradients (> 50 mm Hg). However, it will not provide an accurate transaortic gradient in cases of low-output states or irregular rhythms, as with atrial fibrillation or multiple ectopic beats.

The optimal method for obtaining an aortic valve gradient is simultaneously to use two different catheters—one in the left ventricle and one in the aorta—to measure a mean aortic valve gradient. This can be accomplished by a transseptal approach or by using two different arterial accesses. A simultaneous femoral pressure from the sidearm of a sheath has been used to obtain an aortic valve gradient. However, the discrepancy between the femoral artery pressure and the ascending aorta pressure may be significant because of transmission delay and compliance of the peripheral arterial tree, and this may lead to overestimation or underestimation of the mean gradient.

The aortic valve gradient depends on flow and severity of obstruction. Therefore, an equation for aortic valve area has been described by Gorlin et al. that incorporates pressure and flow for measurement of the severity of stenosis. For this measurement, mean aortic valve gradient, systolic ejection period, heart rate, and cardiac output are needed.

$$\text{Area} = \frac{\text{Flow}}{44.3 \times C \times \sqrt{\Delta P}}$$

$$\text{Aortic Flow} = \frac{1{,}000 \times \text{Cardiac Output (L/min)}}{\text{Heart Rate (beats/min)} \times \text{SEP (s/beat)}}$$

$$C = 1.0$$

where SEP = systolic ejection period.

A modified Hakke equation can be used for aortic stenosis.

$$\text{Area} = \frac{\text{Cardiac Output}}{\sqrt{\Delta P}}$$

There are limitations to calculation of aortic valve area. Measurement of flow through the aortic valve needs to be accurate. In a patient with severe concomitant aortic regurgitation, neither the Fick method nor the thermodilution method can be used, because they will underestimate aortic flow. Aortic valve areas are inaccurate at low and high heart rates, at low and high cardiac outputs, and in the presence of irregular rhythms.

Regurgitant Valvular Lesions

Regurgitant valvular lesions often are assessed in a cardiac catheterization laboratory by injecting contrast into a cardiac chamber or great vessel and visually estimating the amount of contrast that leaks backward into a more proximal chamber. This approach is only semiquantitative, and it has many limitations. Regurgitant fractions have been used in some cardiac catheterization laboratories, but they are cumbersome and have many sources of error. Doppler echocardiographic techniques that provide a more quantitative assessment of the severity of a regurgitant lesion (i.e., volumetric regurgitant fractions, proximal isovelocity surface area, conservation of momentum) will probably be incorporated into clinical practice during the next decade. However, for the Cardiology Boards, it is necessary to know the two cardiac catheterization techniques.

Injections of Contrast Media

For many years, left ventriculography has been the standard for semiquantitation of mitral regurgitation It consists of injecting 45 to 50 mL of contrast medium at a rate of 12 to 14 mL/s into the left ventricle during cineangiography and examining the appearance of the contrast medium in the left atrium. This requires that a large-bore catheter with side holes be well positioned in the left ventricle. Sellars criteria have been established for a semiquantitative estimate of the degree of mitral regurgitation (Table 4).

Left ventriculography has many well-known limitations. The degree to which the contrast medium opacifies the left atrium depends on many factors, including the size and compliance of the left atrium, the size of the left ventricle, the function of the left ventricle, the amount of contrast medium injected, and the rate of injection. Also, catheter entrapment of the mitral apparatus or movement of the

Table 4.—Sellars Criteria for Estimating Degree of Mitral Regurgitation

Grade	Criterion
1+	Contrast medium does not completely fill left atrium
2+	Contrast medium completely opacifies left atrium but does not reach intensity of that in left ventricle
3+	Contrast medium completely opacifies left atrium and reaches intensity of that in left ventricle after 4 or 5 beats
4+	Contrast medium completely opacifies left atrium and reaches intensity of that in left ventricle within first 2 or 3 beats

catheter into the left atrium can produce erroneous results. Premature beats caused by the catheter or jet of contrast medium also result in erroneous interpretations.

The same concept and grading system are used for determining the severity of aortic regurgitation by aortic root angiography. At least 50 to 60 mL of contrast medium is injected into the aortic root at a rate of 20 mL/s, and the severity of aortic regurgitation is evaluated by the amount of contrast medium visualized in the left ventricle. As with left ventriculography, the visual estimate of the degree of aortic regurgitation depends on several factors, including the position of the catheter, the amount of contrast medium injected, rate of injection, the size of the aortic root, and the size and function of the left ventricle.

Regurgitant Fractions

Regurgitant fractions are calculated routinely in cardiac catheterization laboratories. Although this method was once considered the standard by early investigators, it has been shown to be prone to a large degree of error; thus, it is not routinely used in most clinical laboratories. Nonetheless, for the Cardiology Boards, it is important to understand the concept.

For mitral regurgitation, the regurgitant fraction (RF) is the percentage of the total amount of blood ejected by the left ventricle which goes back into the left atrium. The RF is the regurgitant volume (RV) divided by the total amount of blood the ventricle ejects in one beat (total volume [TV]). TV is derived from the left ventriculogram by subtracting the end-systolic volume (ESV) from the end-diastolic volume (EDV). The forward flow volume (FFV) is the amount of blood the ventricle ejects out the aortic valve and is equal to the systemic flow. Thus, this FFV is obtained from the Fick equation. The regurgitant volume is the TV - FFV.

$$TV = EDV - ESV \text{ (from left ventriculography)}$$

$$FFV = \frac{\text{Cardiac Output}}{\text{Heart Rate (from the Fick equation)}}$$

$$RV = TV - FFV$$

$$RF = RV/TV$$

- Regurgitant Fraction $= \dfrac{\text{Regurgitant Volume}}{\text{Total Ventricular Volume}}$

The major limitation of this technique is the inability to obtain accurate measurements of angiographic stroke volumes. Various methods have been proposed for making such measurements, including monoplane vs. biplane approaches, planimetrically determined area vs. videodensitometry measurements, and various geometric assumptions of left ventricular size. Each of these methods has inherent limitations. A similar approach can be used for patients with aortic regurgitation.

Pressure Contours

The severity of regurgitant lesions is assessed indirectly by examining various pressure curves. In patients with severe mitral regurgitation, there usually is a large "v" wave on the left atrial or pulmonary capillary wedge pressure. However, the height of the "v" wave also depends on the left atrial compliance and on cardiac output and, thus, in itself is an insensitive and nonspecific finding. In patients with severe aortic regurgitation, there usually is a rapid increase in left ventricular diastolic pressure as well as a rapid decrease in aortic diastolic pressure; however, these pressure contours are related to other factors, such as the intrinsic compliance of the left ventricle and the impedance of the aorta.

Questions

Multiple Choice (choose the one best answer)

A 64-year-old man comes to the cardiac catheterization laboratory for evaluation of "a hole in his heart." He has had progressive dyspnea on exertion for 5 years and has no prior documented cardiac or medical history. An echocardiogram reveals mild right-sided chamber enlargement, but no atrial septal defect is seen on either transthoracic or transesophageal echocardiography.

The following data are obtained:

Intracardiac location	% Saturation
Inferior vena cava below diaphragm	71
Inferior vena cava at diaphragm	70
Low right atrium	74
Mid right atrium	79
High right atrium	80
Low superior vena cava	79
High superior vena cava	64
Right ventricle	77
Pulmonary artery	78
Left ventricle	98

Intracardiac location	Pressure, mm Hg
Right ventricle	70/15
Pulmonary artery	70/40
Left ventricle	190/90

1A. What is the first step in assessment in the catheterization laboratory?
   a. Perform left ventriculography and coronary angiography
   b. Perform right ventriculography
   c. Determine intracardiac saturations and pressures
   d. Perform double-sampling dye curves
   e. Administer 100% O_2

1B. What is his Qp/Qs ratio?
   a. 1:1
   b. 1.5:1.0
   c. 2.0:1.0
   d. 2.5:1.0
   e. 3.0:1.0

1C. What is the tentative diagnosis?
   a. Right-to-left shunt at atrial level
   b. Left-to-right shunt at atrial level
   c. Left-to-right shunt at ventricular level
   d. Right-to-left shunt at ventricular level
   e. Other

1D. What else should be done at this time?
   a. Send patient for operation
   b. Medical observation
   c. Infusion of nitroprusside
   d. Exercise
   e. Attempt to cross a patent foramen ovale

2. A patient is brought to the cardiac catheterization laboratory for evaluation of the severity of mitral regurgitation. A left ventriculogram shows an end-diastolic volume of 150 mL and end-systolic volume of 50 mL. At a heart rate of 80 beats/min, the cardiac output by the Fick method is 6.4 L/min. The calculated regurgitant fraction is:
   a. 20%
   b. 40%
   c. 60%
   d. 80%
   e. 100%

3. A patient is brought to the cardiac catheterization laboratory for evaluation of the severity of mitral stenosis. Calculated using simultaneous measurements of pulmonary artery wedge pressure and left ventricular pressure, the mean transmitral gradient is 9 mm Hg at a heart rate of 90 beats/min and a diastolic filling period of 0.450 s. The cardiac output by the Fick method is 3.0 L/min. The calculated mitral valve area is approximately:
   a. 0.5 cm^2
   b. 1.0 cm^2
   c. 1.5 cm^2
   d. 2.0 cm^2
   e. Insufficient data to calculate the mitral valve area

4. At the time of cardiac catheterization, a patient has a mean aortic valve gradient of 64 mm Hg and a cardiac output by the Fick method of 4 L/min. Severe aortic regurgitation is also present. Which of the following is true?
   a. Cardiac output determined with thermodilution would

give a more accurate aortic valve area

b. The calculated aortic valve area is lower than the actual aortic valve area

c. Doppler aortic valve area by continuity equation is less accurate than catheterization

d. The aortic regurgitation should not affect the calculated aortic valve area

e. The calculated aortic valve area is 2.0 cm^2

5. A patient with mitral stenosis has a mean transmitral gradient of 5 mm Hg at a heart rate of 70 beats/min and a pressure half-time of 160 ms by Doppler. At cardiac catheterization, calculated using simultaneous measurements of pulmonary artery wedge pressure and left ventricular pressure (confirmed saturation of 98%), the mean transmitral gradient is 11 mm Hg at a heart rate of 75 beats/min and a mitral valve area of 0.9 cm^2. The severity of mitral stenosis is:
   a. Mild
   b. Moderate
   c. Severe
   d. Indeterminate

6. For assessing the cause of arterial desaturation, which of the following is *not* useful?
   a. Double-sampling dye curves
   b. Repeat determination of the saturation after administration of 100% O_2.
   c. Pulmonary vein saturation
   d. Single-sampling dye curve: right atrium to femoral artery
   e. Saline contrast injection under two-dimensional echocardiography

7. A patient has the following baseline values: blood pressure, 120/70 mm Hg; percentage saturation pulmonary artery, 75%; percentage saturation femoral artery, 98%. After a drug is given, the values are as follows: blood pressure, 110/50 mm Hg; percentage saturation pulmonary artery, 85%; and percentage saturation femoral artery, 98%. Which drug is the most likely to be infused?
   a. Isoproterenol
   b. Norepinephrine
   c. Propranolol
   d. Metoprolol
   e. Phenylephrine

8. A patient has the pattern shown on the next page in the right ventricular and left ventricular pressure curves with elevation and end-diastolic equalization of the pressures in the left and right ventricles. Which of the following may be present?
   a. Constrictive pericarditis
   b. Amyloid heart disease
   c. Right ventricular infarction
   d. Severe tricuspid regurgitation
   e. Restrictive cardiomyopathy
   f. All of the above

9. A left ventricular pressure volume curve is displayed on the next page. Which of the following best demonstrates the effect of infusion of nitroprusside?
   a. Line a to b
   b. Point c to d
   c. Point c to e
   d. Point f to g
   e. None of the above

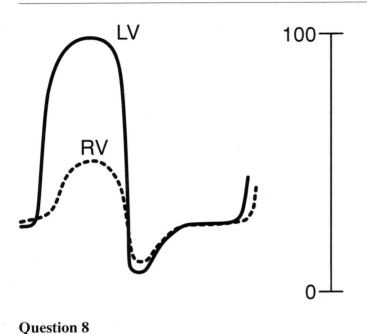

Question 8

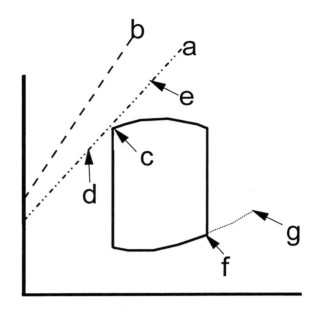

Question 9

Answers

1A. Answer c
1B. Answer b
1C. Answer e
1D. Answer c

Intracardiac saturations should be initially measured to locate the approximate level of the intracardiac shunt before dye curves or contrast injection is done. The most significant step-up in oxygen saturation is between the high superior vena cava (SVC) and low SVC, suggesting a left-to-right shunt into the SVC, probably from an anomalous pulmonary venous connection. Pulmonary arteriolar resistance should be measured and the effect of nitroprusside estimated if resistance is increased.

2. Answer a

Total cardiac output equals stroke volume (150 mL - 50 mL) times heart rate (80) and is 8.0 L/min. The difference between Fick cardiac output and total cardiac output is the regurgitant volume: 1.6 L/min = 20% regurgitant fraction.

3. Answer b

4. Answer b

The Fick method of cardiac output estimates pulmonary blood flow, which equals systemic blood flow in the absence

of a cardiac shunt. In the presence of severe valvular regurgitation, blood flow across the aortic valve is much higher than Fick cardiac output, leading to an understimation of valve area.

5. Answer a

6. Answer a

Double-sampling dye curves are used to localize left-to-right shunts only. Single-sampling dye curves may be used to assess both right-to-left and left-to-right cardiac shunts.

7. Answer a

Cardiac output increased, as evidenced by an increase in pulmonary artery saturation but without an increase in blood pressure. The most likely drug was isoproterenol.

8. Answer f

This tracing shows a dip-and-plateau pattern compatible with all the suggested diagnoses.

9. Answer b

Point C occurs at aortic valve closure when aortic pressure is greater than left ventricular pressure. If arterial resistance is decreased by nitroprusside, cardiac output will increase and end-diastolic volume will decrease with a lower ventricular pressure.

Chapter 51

Atlas of Hemodynamic Tracings

Naeem K. Tahirkheli, M.D.
Rick A. Nishimura, M.D.

Arterial Pulses

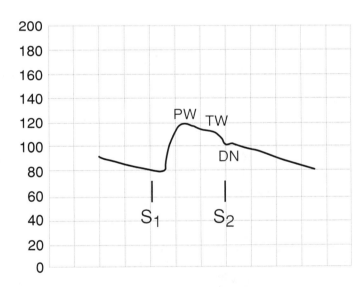

Fig. 1. Normal carotid arterial pulse. It consists of two systolic waves. The initial rise is called the "percussion wave" (PW), and the subsequent wave is called the "tidal wave" (TW), which is due to reflected energy from the aorta. The dicrotic notch (DN) signifies aortic closure. S_1, first heart sound; S_2, second heart sound.

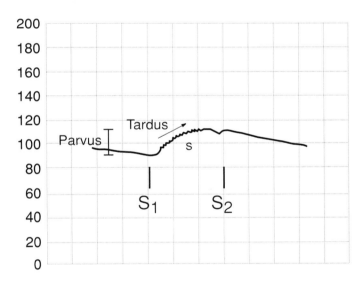

Fig. 2. The parvus (low amplitude) and tardus (slow uprising, arrow) pulse of severe calcified aortic stenosis. The irregularity in the slowly uprising pulse is from the turbulence created by the stenotic aortic valve and, on palpation, is often felt as a shudder (S) in the carotid pulse. Note that the degree to which a pulse is parvus and tardus is correlated with the severity of aortic stenosis. S_1, first heart sound; S_2, second heart sound.

Double arterial pulses can be divided into two main categories. In the first category, the double pulses span different cardiac cycles and include pulsus alternans and pulsus bigeminus (not illustrated). Pulsus alternans is frequently associated with heart failure, with one cardiac cycle having a higher pulse pressure while the preceding and following pulses have lower pulse pressure. Pulsus bigeminus is secondary to a bigeminal rhythm, in which fixed-interval premature ventricular contractions occur after every sinus beat. Therefore, a small-amplitude pulse due to the premature ventricular contraction follows every sinus-mediated larger amplitude pulse.

The second category of double pulses includes bifid, bisferiens, and dicrotic pulses (see below). The split in the pulse in this category is within one cardiac cycle. In the case of dicrotic pulse, a diastolic component is added to the systolic pulsation. The terms "bifid" and "bisferiens" are sometimes used interchangeably; however, bisferiens (twice-beating pulse) refers to two distinct pulsations and is more appropriate for the pulse character in hypertrophic cardiomyopathy. A bifid pulse is a double impulse pulse frequently observed in combined aortic stenosis and aortic regurgitation or severe aortic regurgitation alone.

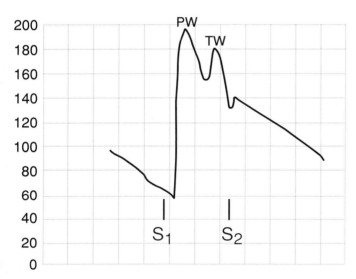

Fig. 3. A bifid pulse in combined aortic regurgitation and stenosis. Note the increased pulse pressure resulting from the lower diastolic blood pressure combined with the increased systolic pressure (blood pressure 200/60 mm Hg). The first peak is the percussion wave (PW) and the second peak is the tidal wave (TW). Note that no specific features of this pulse are related to the severity of the aortic regurgitation. S_1, first heart sound; S_2, second heart sound.

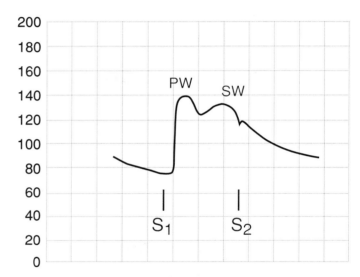

Fig. 4. Spike-and-dome pattern of hypertrophic obstructive cardiomyopathy. After the initial percussion wave (PW), a late systolic sustained secondary wave (SW) can easily be palpated because the two pulsations are frequently distinct. This may also be referred to as a "bisferiens pulse." Note, however, that not all patients with hypertrophic obstructive cardiomyopathy have such a pulse. S_1, first heart sound; S_2, second heart sound.

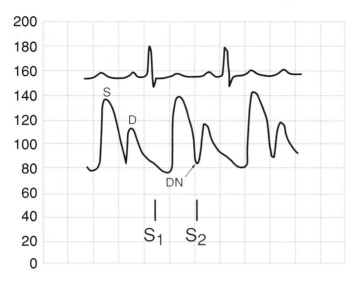

Fig. 5. Dicrotic pulse. This pulse may be seen in significant left ventricular dysfunction and increased peripheral arterial resistance. A systolic wave (S) and a large diastolic wave (D) follow aortic valve closure (dicrotic notch, DN). S_1, first heart sound; S_2, second heart sound.

Right Heart Catheterization

Considerable controversy surrounds the use of pulmonary artery flotation catheters to monitor critically ill patients. Connors et al. (*JAMA* 276:889-897, 1996) reported that after adjustment for treatment selection bias, the use of pulmonary artery flotation catheters was associated with increased mortality and poor use of resources. The American College of Cardiology published an Expert Consensus Document (*J Am Coll Cardiol* 32:840-864, 1998) on the appropriate use and indications for the use of right heart catheters. It should be noted that the original Connors paper included patients primarily with multiorgan and respiratory disease rather than cardiac disease.

Technical Considerations When Interpreting Pulmonary Artery Wedge Tracings

Pulmonary artery balloon catheters primarily yield three important hemodynamic measures: pulmonary artery pressure, pulmonary artery wedge pressure, and cardiac output, from which pulmonary arteriolar resistance can be calculated. Pulmonary artery wedge pressure approximates left atrial pressure, which in turn approximates left ventricular end-diastolic pressure.

A fundamental question is, "When in the respiratory cycle should the pulmonary artery wedge pressure be measured?" Measurement at end-expiration is common in intensive care

units, whereas most cardiac catheterization laboratories record the mean wedge pressures averaged throughout the respiratory cycle.

Pulmonary artery occlusion pressure accurately reflects pulmonary venous pressure only when pulmonary venous and pulmonary artery pressures exceed pulmonary alveolar pressure. In mechanically ventilated patients on positive end-expiratory pressure, alveolar pressure may exceed pulmonary artery and venous pressures, thus making measurements of pulmonary wedge pressure inaccurate

True pulmonary capillary pressure normally exceeds wedge pressure by a few millimeters of mercury, but in septicemia and inflammatory disorders, this discrepancy can be much higher. Left atrial pressure reflects left ventricular end-diastolic pressure only in the absence of significant mitral valve disease (stenosis or regurgitation). Other discrepancies may occur because of changes in left ventricular compliance which may be present in critically ill patients. Thermodilution cardiac output may be inaccurate in the presence of arrhythmias, tricuspid regurgitation, intracardiac shunting, or low cardiac output states.

Indications for the Use of Bedside Right Heart Catheterization

- To differentiate between cardiac (hemodynamic) and noncardiac (abnormal capillary permeability) pulmonary edema
- In patients with coexisting cardiac and pulmonary disease who have not had a response to conventional heart failure therapy
- Differentiation of cardiogenic from noncardiogenic shock (hypotension); this occurs particularly when a trial of intravascular volume expansion has failed to correct hypotension
- To guide the use of inotropic or mechanical cardiac support
- Guidance of therapy in patients with concomitant forward (hypotension, oliguria or azotemia) and backward (dyspnea and/or hypoxemia) heart failure
- Determination of whether pericardial tamponade is present when echocardiography is inadequate
- Guidance of perioperative management in selected patients with decompensated heart failure undergoing intermediate- or high-risk noncardiac surgery
- Detection of the presence of pulmonary vasoconstriction and its reversibility in patients being considered for heart transplantation

Contraindications to Pulmonary Artery Catheter Placement

Absolute Contraindications

- Right-sided endocarditis, mechanical tricuspid or pulmonic valve prosthesis, right-sided thrombus or tumor
- Patients who are terminally ill, for whom aggressive management would be considered futile, are not candidates for pulmonary catheter placement

Relative Contraindications

- Coagulopathy, including recent thrombolytic therapy, recent implantation of permanent pacemaker, left bundle branch block, bioprosthetic tricuspid valve

Acute Myocardial Infarction

Indications in acute myocardial infarction include

- Differentiation between cardiogenic and hypovolemic shock when the initial therapy with intravascular volume expansion and low-dose inotropic drugs has failed
- Guidance of management of cardiogenic shock with pharmacologic and/or mechanical support in patients with or without coronary reperfusion therapy
- Short-term guidance of pharmacologic and/or mechanical management of acute mitral regurgitation before surgical correction
- Establishment of severity of left or right shunting and short-term guidance of pharmacologic and/or mechanical management of ventricular septal rupture for surgical correction
- Guidance for management of complicated right ventricular infarction
- Guidance for management of acute pulmonary edema not responding to the standard treatment
  A relative contraindication in acute myocardial infarction is thrombolytic and/or anticoagulant therapy.

Perioperative Use in Cardiac Surgery

- Differentiation between causes of low cardiac output when clinical and/or echocardiographic assessment is inconclusive

- Differentiation between right and left ventricular dysfunction and pericardial tamponade when clinical and/or echocardiographic assessment is inconclusive
- Guidance of management of severe low cardiac output syndromes
- Diagnosis and guidance of management of pulmonary hypertension in patients with systemic hypotension and evidence of inadequate organ perfusion

Primary Pulmonary Hypertension

- Exclusion of postcapillary (increased pulmonary artery occlusion pressure) causes of pulmonary hypertension
- Establishment of diagnosis and assessment of severity of precapillary pulmonary hypertension
- Selection and establishment of safety and efficacy of long-term vasodilatory therapy based on acute hemodynamic responses
- Assessment of hemodynamic variables before lung transplantation

Complications of Right Heart Catheterization

Central Venous Access Problems

These include arterial puncture, bleeding at the site of insertion, nerve injury, pneumothorax, and air embolism.

Arrhythmias

Transient arrhythmias frequently occur as the catheter is passed through the pulmonary outflow tract. Sustained ventricle arrhythmias are quite rare and seen primarily in patients with myocardial ischemia or a history of ventricle arrhythmias. Rarely, right bundle branch block may be precipitated or, in patients with preexisting left bundle branch block, complete heart block may occur.

Catheter Problems

These complications are related to the catheter residing in the pulmonary artery and include pulmonary artery rupture, thrombophlebitis, venous or intracardiac thrombus formation, pulmonary infarction, and endocarditis.

Venous Pulses

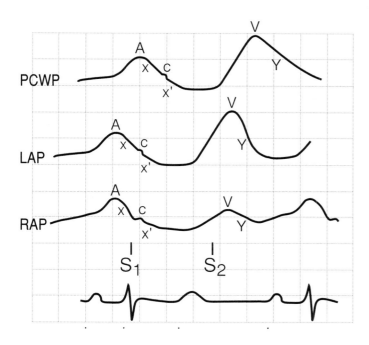

Fig. 6. Top to bottom, tracings of normal pulmonary capillary wedge pressure (PCWP), left atrial pressure (LAP), and right atrial pressure (RAP). The A wave is due to atrial contraction and the downward X descent, to atrial relaxation. The brief outward C wave is caused by a cephalad motion of the closing atrioventricular valve. The downward X' descent is a continuation of the original X descent after atrioventricular valve closure. The V wave occurs with passive atrial filling. The Y descent denotes atrial emptying into the ventricle after opening of the atrioventricular valve. This figure shows important differences in the three pressure tracings. The A wave is the first upward deflection on the hemodynamic tracing after the start of the P wave in the ECG and is within the PR segment of the ECG tracing for the right and left atrial pressure tracings. Because of the reflection of the left atrial pressure across the pulmonary vasculature, there is a time delay in PCWP tracings. Therefore, the A wave of PCWP is toward the end of the PR segment, as shown here. Similarly, the V wave is located in the TP segment of the ECG for the LAP and RAP tracings. In PCWP, the V wave may be in the latter half of the TP segment, occasionally extending into the PR segment. Another difference between the right- and left-sided pressures is that the A wave is the dominant wave of the LAP tracing, whereas the V wave is the larger of the two upward waves in the LAP and PCWP tracings. Finally, the major difference between the LAP and PCWP is the rapidity of the Y descent. The LAP tracing usually has a distinct sharp Y descent, whereas that of the PCWP tracing is more gentle. This difference can be important clinically when estimating the pressure gradient across the mitral valve (mitral stenosis), in which the use of PCWP as a surrogate for LAP may tend to overestimate the pressure gradient. S_1, first heart sound; S_2, second heart sound.

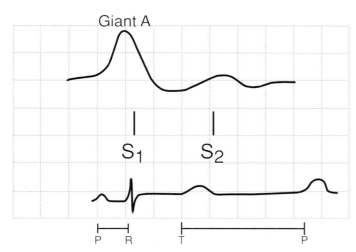

Fig. 7. Right atrial pressure tracing showing a giant A wave. This is usually associated with a poorly compliant ventricle. Note: the *giant* A wave is different from the *cannon* A wave, which refers to the pressure generated when the right atrium contracts against a closed tricuspid valve (not shown here) and is usually seen in patients with complete heart block. Cannon A waves are an intermittent phenomenon, whereas giant A waves are seen with every sinus beat. S_1, first heart sound; S_2, second heart sound.

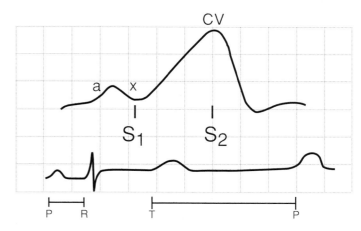

Fig. 8. A CV wave in a pulmonary capillary wedge pressure tracing. This is frequently seen in patients with significant mitral regurgitation. Note that although the A wave is characteristically delayed (end of the PR segment) for a pulmonary capillary wedge pressure tracing, the upward deflection of the CV wave is much earlier (beginning or slightly before the TP segment) than would be expected. Because of the incompetent valve, the CV wave is not only larger, it also starts early in systole. S_1, first heart sound; S_2, second heart sound.

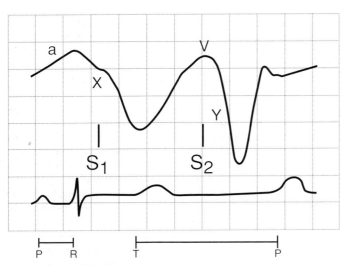

Fig. 9. Right atrial pressure tracing in constrictive pericarditis. Note the sharp X and Y descents. S_1, first heart sound; S_2, second heart sound.

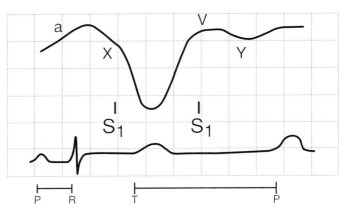

Fig. 10. Right atrial pressure tracing in pericardial tamponade. Note the sharp X descent, but a minimal or absent Y descent, consistent with minimal passive atrial emptying. S_1, first heart sound; S_2, second heart sound.

Apex Impulses in Disease

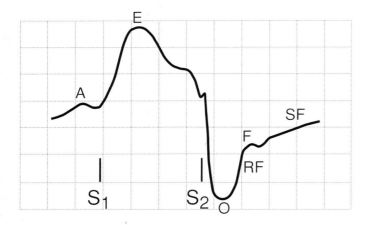

Fig. 11. Normal apex pulse (apex beat cardiogram). The normal apex pulse has several waves. The initial A wave is the outward expansion, "upward deflection on the apex cardiogram," of the apical area due to left atrial contraction. E represents maximal ejection. Note that the upward deflection has occurred entirely in the first half of systole; therefore, a normal apical impulse should be palpable only during the first half of systole. The notch in the downward slope coincides with the second heart sound (S_2) and the closure of the aortic valve, signifying the end of systole. As systole ends, the left ventricle relaxes, accelerating its retraction from the chest wall (downward slope on the apex cardiogram), which ends at O. The O point marks mitral valve opening. As the left ventricle dilates because of blood flowing through the open mitral valve, an upward deflection is noted, the rapid filling wave (RF). The F point is the peak of this rapid filling and is synchronous with the timing of the third heart sound. The slow filling wave (SF) signifies slow ventricular filling during mid-diastole, before atrial contraction. Note: in a normal heart, only the E point during the early part of systole is palpable. S_1, first heart sound.

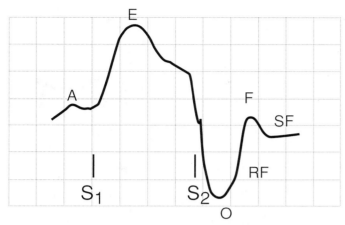

Fig. 12. In conditions in which the the rapid filling wave (RF) is steep and tall (e.g., increased filling due to severe mitral regurgitation or restrictive filling pattern), the F point is more pronounced. This may be appreciated as an audible or palpable third heart sound.

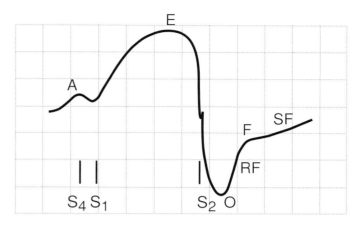

Fig. 13. In aortic stenosis with normal left ventricular function, the apex impulse is strong, prolonged, and reaches a sustained peak, E, in late systole. Contrast this with a normal apex in which peak E is reached in early systole. Also, the amplitude of the A wave may be increased, thereby making it palpable. This would coincide with the fourth heart sound (S_4). S_1, first heart sound; S_2, second heart sound.

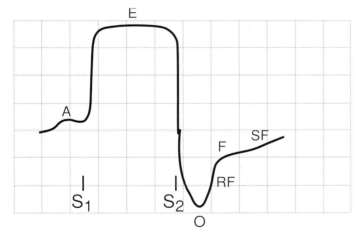

Fig. 14. There is significant dyskinesis of the apical impulse in patients with a left ventricular aneurysm. In contrast to left ventricular hypertrophy, the peak is reached early in systole and, in contrast to the normal impulse, remains sustained throughout systole. Additionally, the apical impulse extends over a wider area corresponding to the ventricular aneurysm. S_1, first heart sound; S_2, second heart sound.

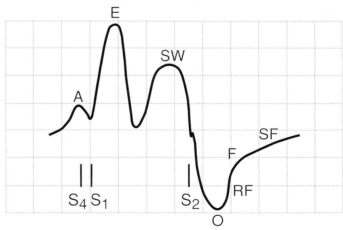

Fig. 15. The classic "triple-ripple" apical impulse of hypertrophic obstructive cardiomyopathy. There is a rapid and early rise to the E point, after which there is sudden cessation and even withdrawal of the apical impulse (corresponds to dynamic outflow obstruction, which peaks in mid-systole) until mid-systole, when a more sustained secondary wave (SW) may be palpable. Additionally, the A wave amplitude may also be increased and, thus, palpable. This corresponds to an audible fourth heart sound (S_4) from the left ventricle. These three peaks are frequently referred to as the "triple-ripple apical impulse of hypertrophic obstructive cardiomyopathy." Note, however, that this classic representation is not universally found in hypertrophic obstructive cardiomyopathy.

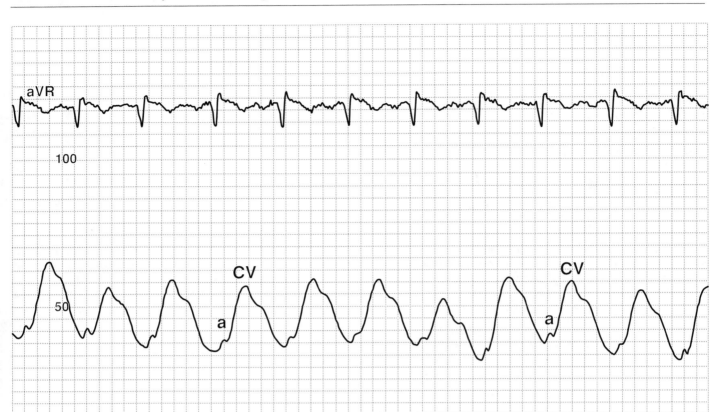

Fig. 16. Pulmonary capillary wedge pressure tracing in a patient with severe mitral regurgitation due to ruptured capillary muscle in association with acute myocardial infarction. The large CV waves measured on this tracing averaged 60 mm Hg. Note that the start of the CV wave in this tracing (before the TP segment of the ECG) is earlier than would be expected in a normal V wave.

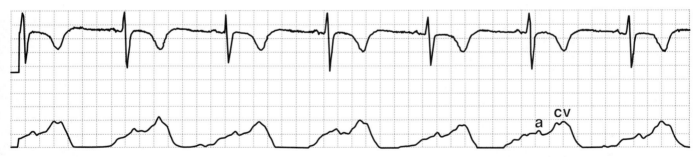

Fig. 17. Pulmonary capillary wedge pressure tracing of a patient with severe mitral regurgitation. Note that the CV waves are not as prominent as the previous tracing (Fig. 16). Also note the early start of the CV wave in relation to the ECG.

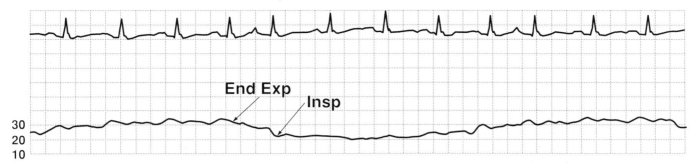

Fig. 18. Variations of pulmonary capillary wedge pressure during spontaneous breathing. The negative intrathoracic pressure generated during the inspiratory phase (Insp) of spontaneous respiration results in an artificial lowering of the pulmonary capillary wedge pressure. During the end-expiratory phase (End Exp). there is relative apnea and the pulmonary capillary wedge pressure here best approximates the left ventricular end-diastolic pressure. As shown in the figure, this point occurs just before the negative dip in the pulmonary capillary wedge pressure. During positive pressure ventilation, end expiration remains the optimal time to measure pulmonary capillary wedge pressure. However, because of positive pressure ventilation, pulmonary capillary wedge pressure is artificially increased during the inspiratory phase and end-expiration occurs just before the upward (positive) shift in the pressure. Therefore, it is important to remember respiratory variations/modes when measuring pulmonary capillary wedge pressure. Note that in most catheterization laboratories, multiple cardiac cycles across respiratory phases are averaged to obtain the mean wedge pressure.

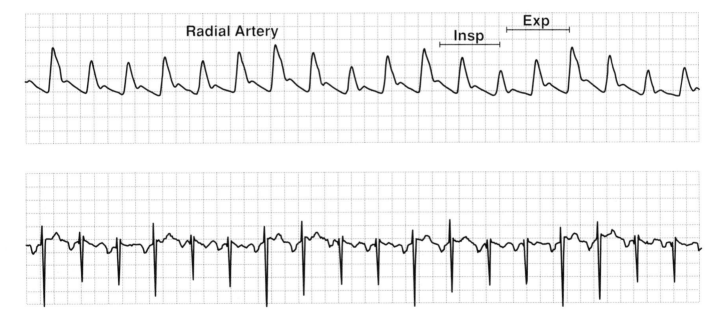

Fig. 19. Pulsus paradoxus and electrical alternans in pericardial tamponade. Radial artery pressure tracing showing a significant decrease in systolic blood pressure with inspiration consistent with pulsus paradoxus. Electrical alternans is also noted: the changing height of the QRS complexes. Exp, expiration; Insp, inspiration.

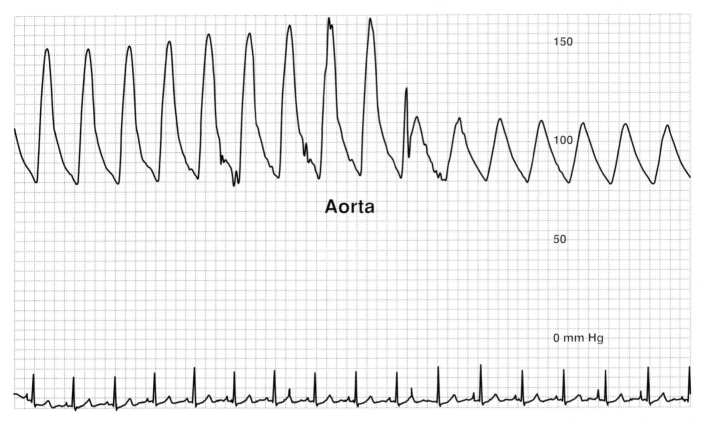

Fig. 20. Coarctation of the aorta. Pullback from the ascending aorta to below the subclavian artery, showing the pressure difference across the coarctation.

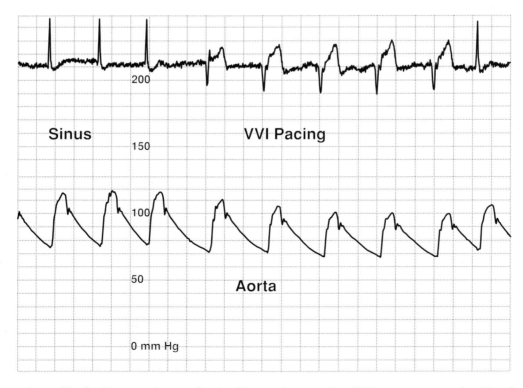

Fig. 21. Pacemaker syndrome. The first 3 beats are sinus-mediated and the next 4 are paced by a VVI permanent pacemaker. Note the decrease in systolic blood pressure while being paced.

Valvular Heart Disease

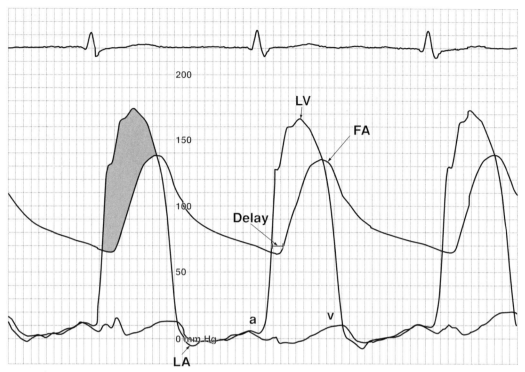

Fig. 22. Aortic stenosis. Pressure tracings from the left ventricle (LV), femoral artery (FA), and left atrium (LA). The shaded area represents the gradient between the LV and FA. Because of the transmission of pressure to a peripheral artery, there is a delay (*arrow*) in the upstroke of the FA. If this is not taken into account, the gradient across the aortic valve can be over- or underestimated.

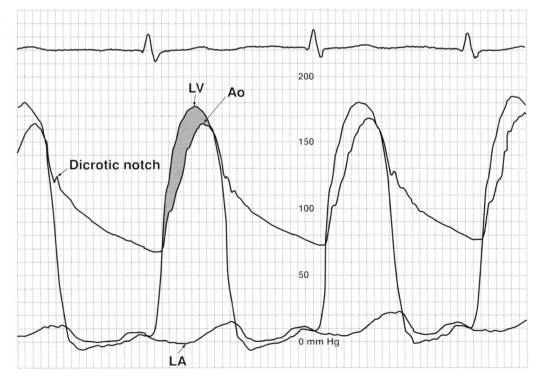

Fig. 23. Aortic stenosis. This is from the same patient as in Figure 22; however, instead of the femoral artery, aortic pressure (Ao) is used to measure the gradient (shaded area) across the aortic valve. Compare this figure with Figure 22, and note the obvious difference in measured gradients.

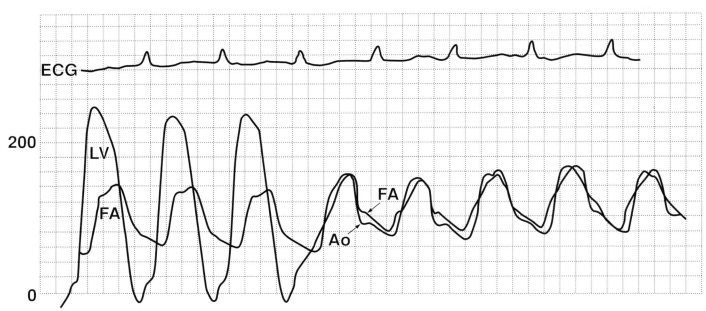

Fig. 24. Carabello sign. Pullback of the left ventricular catheter into the femoral artery (FA). The FA pressure increases when the catheter is withdrawn from across the critically stenosed aortic valve (Ao).

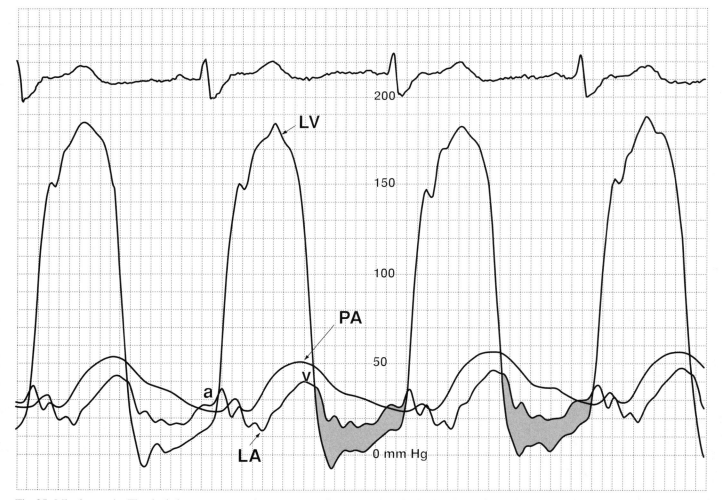

Fig. 25. Mitral stenosis. The shaded area represents the pressure gradient across the mitral valve. LV, left ventricular pressure; PA, pulmonary artery pressure; LA, left atrial pressure; a, left atrial A wave; v, left atrial V wave.

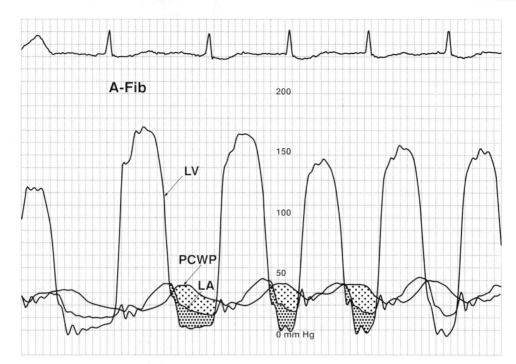

Fig. 26. Severe mitral stenosis. Simultaneous left ventricular (LV), pulmonary capillary wedge pressure (PCWP), and left atrial (LA) pressure tracings. This case illustrates the possibility of overestimating the mitral valve gradient if the PCWP rather than the true LA pressure is measured. Large stiple, gradient between PCWP and LV (false gradient across the mitral valve); small stiple, gradient between LA and LV (true gradient across the mitral valve).

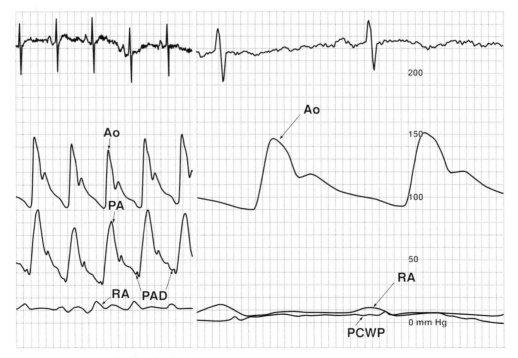

Fig. 27. Pulmonary hypertension. Right heart catheterization is frequently used to identify the cause of pulmonary hypertension, that is, cardiac vs. pulmonary cause. This can be readily appreciated while assessing the relationship of pulmonary artery diastolic pressure (PAD) and pulmonary capillary wedge pressure (PCWP). Normally, and in cases in which pulmonary hypertension is due to a cardiac cause (e.g., left ventricular dysfunction, mitral stenosis), PWCP is 2 to 3 mm less than PAD. However, when the hypertension has a pulmonary cause (e.g., primary pulmonary hypertension, secondary pulmonary hypertension from thromboemboli, pulmonary fibrosis), the PAD may be significantly higher, while the pulmonary artery wedge pressure remains normal, producing a significant difference between these two pressures. In this figure, the patient had primary pulmonary hypertension with a mean PAD of 35 mm Hg and a PCWP of only 7 mm Hg. Note that the right atrial pressure, RA, is slightly higher than the PCWP. Ao, aorta.

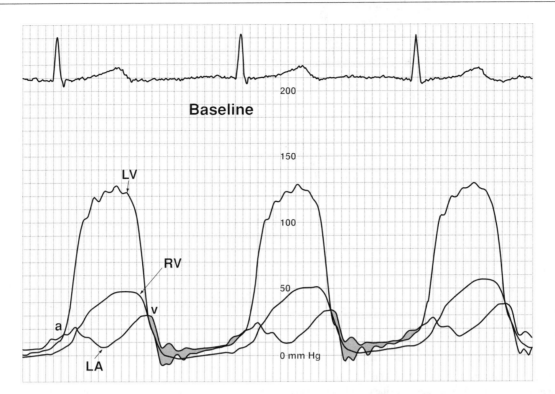

Fig. 28. Mitral stenosis. Pressure tracings in a patient with significant exercise intolerance. The patient was found to have mild mitral stenosis. Rest tracing with a heart rate of approximately 70 beats/min. LV, left ventricular pressure; RV, right ventricular pressure; LA, left atrial pressure. The shaded area represents the pressure gradient across the mitral valve.

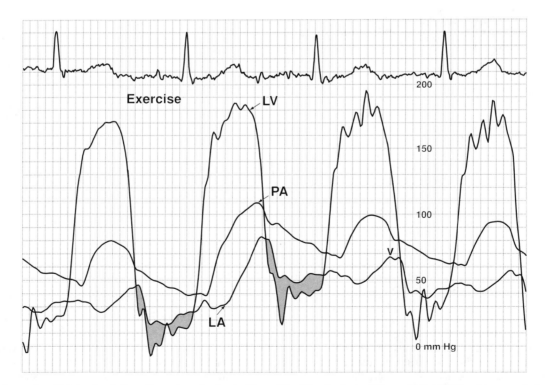

Fig. 28. Effect of exercise. This tracing is from the same patient as in Figure 27. After 4 minutes of exercise, a significant increase in the gradient across the mitral valve was noted. Observe the marked increase in right heart pressures (catheter now in pulmonary artery [PA]) from 50 mm Hg to about 100 mm Hg and the increase in left atrial pressure (LA) (about 30 mm Hg to about 80 mm Hg at the maximal height of the LA "v" wave). The exercise heart rate was approximately 110 beats/min. The shaded area represents the pressure gradient across the mitral valve.

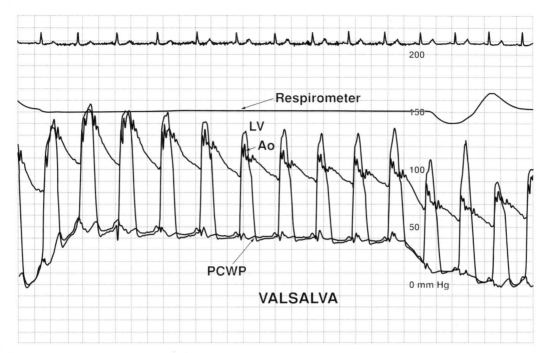

Fig. 30. Hypertrophic obstructive cardiomyopathy. Dynamic left ventricular outflow tract obstruction during phase 2 of the Valsalva maneuver. Note the significant increase in left ventricular (LV) end-diastolic pressure and steady decrease in LV systolic pressure during phase 2 of the Valsalva maneuver along with an increase in the outflow tract gradient. Ao, aorta; PCWP, pulmonary capillary wedge pressure.

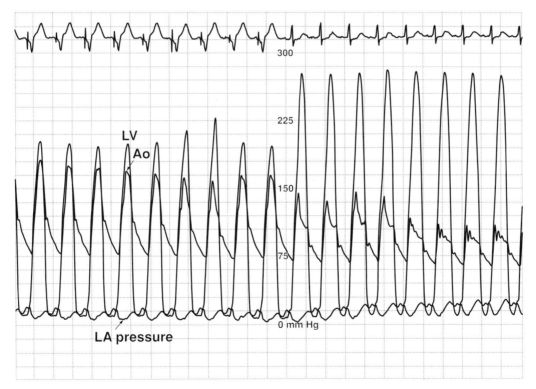

Fig. 31. Effect of pacing on dynamic left ventricular outflow tract gradient. This tracing is from a patient with severe hypertrophic obstructive cardiomy-opathy who was evaluated in the catheterization laboratory to assess whether pacing would be beneficial in decreasing the outflow gradient. Both chambers were paced with varying intervals, and the effect of each pacing regimen was assessed. In the first half of the figure, the patient is being paced in a P-syn-chronized mode with an atrioventricular interval of 100 ms. In the second half of the figure, the pacing is discontinued and the patient is in sinus rhythm. Note the significant worsening of the outflow gradient after the pacing is discontinued. Also note the increase in mean left atrial pressure with discontinua-tion of pacing secondary to worsening of the outflow gradient. LV, left ventricular pressure; LA, left atrial pressure; Ao, aortic pressure.

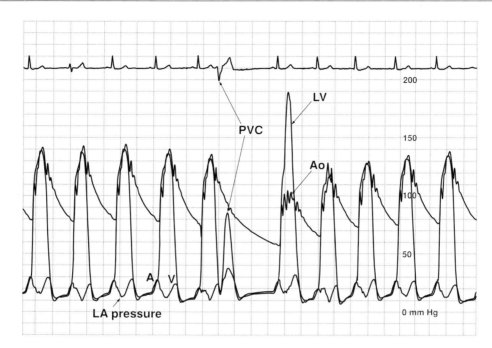

Fig. 32. Brockenbrough sign. The post-extrasystolic behavior of a gradient across the aortic/outflow tract can differentiate between a fixed and a dynamic obstruction. In a patient with hypertrophic obstructive cardiomyopathy, the post-extrasystolic beat demonstrates an increased gradient, resulting in decreased aortic pressure (Ao) even though left ventricular (LV) systolic pressure has increased significantly. This feature is characteristic of dynamic LV outflow tract obstruction and is called the "Brockenbrough sign." In fixed obstruction like aortic stenosis (in the presence of normal LV function), the gradient should not change significantly and the aortic pulse pressure should remain the same or increase slightly. This patient demonstrates an increased gradient for several beats after a premature ventricular contraction (PVC) before it returns to baseline. Also, the dynamic nature of the gradient with beat-to-beat variation should be noted. Note the decrease in the aortic pulse pressure in the post-extrasystolic beat along with the increase in the LV systolic pressure. The increase in left atrial (LA) pressure during the post-extrasystolic beat should also be appreciated. This patient had typical left ventricular outflow type hypertrophic obstructive cardiomyopathy. The Brockenbrough sign can be of immense help in occasional patients who may not have a significant gradient at baseline, especially in the slightly sedated state in the catheterization laboratory.

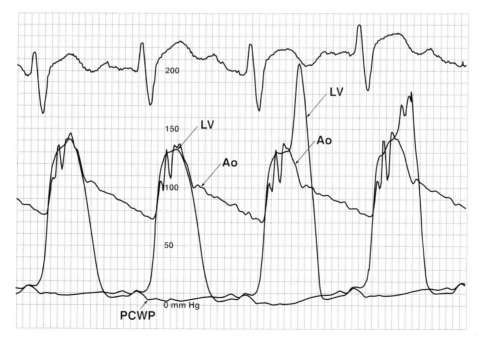

Fig. 33. Artifact. This is a tracing of catheter entrapment. Beat no. 3 is an artifact from left ventricular (LV) catheter entrapment in the small hyperdynamic cavity. The key points that differentiate this from Brockenbrough sign are the absence of premature ventricular contraction and the fact that the aortic pulse pressure (Ao) did not decrease with the apparent increase in the LV systolic pressure.

Constrictive Pericarditis and Restrictive Cardiomyopathy

Cases of constrictive pericarditis and restrictive cardiomyopathy are shown below to highlight the traditional hemodynamic criteria and the more recently recognized dynamic respiratory changes noted in these entities. The traditional hemodynamic criteria are sensitive, but lack adequate specificity to distinguish between constriction and restrictive cardiomyopathy. Dynamic respiratory changes have a high sensitivity and specificity to allow this distinction. In the following cases, significant overlap of the traditional hemodynamic criteria is found in patients with confirmed constrictive pericarditis and restrictive cardiomyopathy. All the tracings are from high-fidelity pressure micromanometers.

Traditional Hemodynamic Criteria for Diagnosing Constrictive Pericarditis in the Catheterization Laboratory

1. Equalization of diastolic pressures (the difference between left ventricular end-diastolic pressure [LVEDP] and right ventricular end-diastolic pressure [RVEDP] ≤ 5 mm Hg).
2. Pulmonary artery systolic pressure < 55 mm Hg.

3. High RVEDP (RVEDP > 1/3 of right ventricular systolic pressure [RVSP]).
4. Dip-and-plateau morphology (left ventricular rapid filling wave > 7 mm Hg).
5. Kussmaul sign (lack of respiratory variations ≤ 3 mm Hg in mean right atrial pressure).

Criteria for Restrictive Cardiomyopathy

1. > 5 mm Hg difference in LVEDP and RVEDP.
2. Pulmonary artery systolic pressure > 55 mm Hg.
3. RVEDP < 1/3 of RVSP.
4. LV rapid filling wave < 7 mm Hg.
5. Normal > 3 mm Hg respiratory variation in mean right atrial pressure.

Dynamic Respiratory Criteria for Constrictive Pericarditis

1. > 5 mm Hg increase in the gradient between early left ventricular diastolic pressure and wedge pressure during inspiration when compared with expiration.
2. Ventricular discordance due to interdependence—at peak inspiration increase in RVSP and decrease in LVSP, and opposite changes during expiration.

Fig. 34. Dissociation of intrathoracic and intracardiac pressures in constrictive pericarditis. The following 3 tracings are from a patient with surgically proven constrictive pericarditis. Simultaneous recordings of left ventricular and pulmonary capillary wedge pressures demonstrating dissociation of intrathoracic and intracardiac pressures. Note the decrease in early diastolic gradient with inspiration (Insp) (beat marked "1") and the increase with expiration (Exp) (beat marked "2"). Also note the dip-and-plateau morphology of left ventricular (LV) diastolic pressures. The nasal respirometer tracing is also shown. PAW, pulmonary artery wedge.

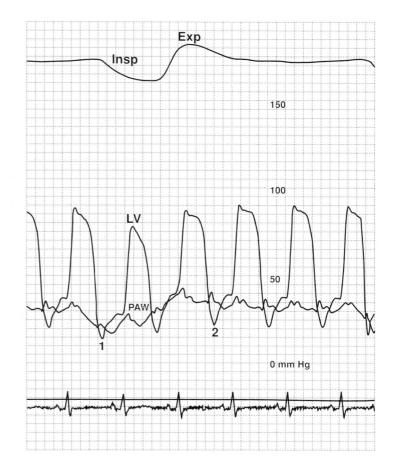

Fig. 35. Ventricular interdependence in constrictive pericarditis. Simultaneous recordings of left ventricular (LV), right ventricular (RV), and right atrial pressures demonstrating ventricular interdependence. Note the discordance in LV and RV systolic pressures with respiration (beats 1 and 2). Other criteria of constrictive pericarditis are also seen, e.g., a marked "W" or "M" pattern in the right atrial pressure tracing, absence of decrease in right atrial pressure with inspiration (Kussmaul sign), right ventricular end-diastolic pressure (RVEDP) > 1/3 of right ventricular systolic pressure (RVSP), and equalization of pressures (< 5 mm difference in left ventricular end-diastolic pressure and RVEDP). However, the RVSP (and, therefore, pulmonary artery systolic pressure, in the absence of RV outflow gradient) is slightly above 55 mm Hg. The nasal respirometer tracing is also shown. Exp, expiration; Insp, inspiration.

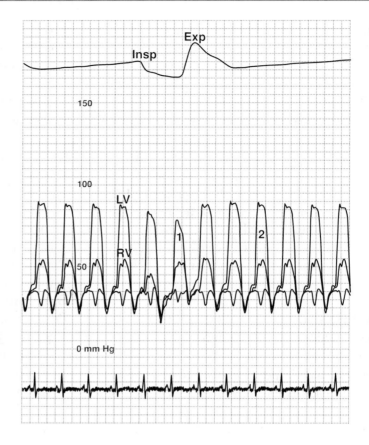

Fig. 36. Hemodynamic tracings in constrictive pericarditis. Higher paper speed (100 mm/s) simultaneous recordings of left ventricular (LV), right ventricular (RV), and right atrial (RA) pressures demonstrating ventricular interdependence. Note the decrease in RV systolic pressure during the first beat and a marked rise in the next ejection at peak inspiration (beat 1) while LV systolic pressure decreases. Note the rapid x and y descents in the RA tracing. The nasal respirometer tracing is shown at the top. Exp, expiration; Insp, inspiration.

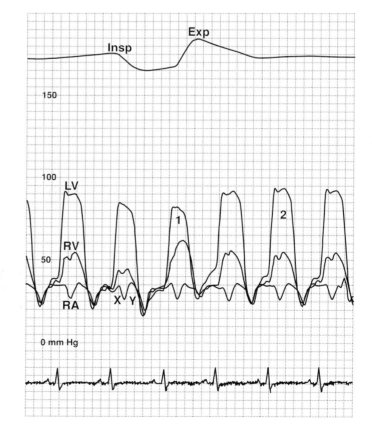

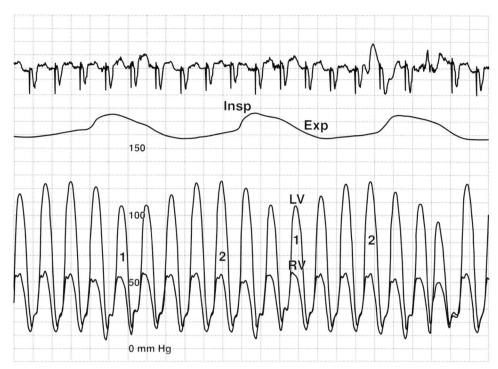

Fig. 37. Simultaneous recordings of left ventricular (LV) and right ventricular (RV) pressure demonstrating subtle ventricular discordance in constrictive pericarditis. This ventricular discordance is more subtle than that seen in Figure 36 and makes the point that ventricular discordance may not be as marked as shown in the Figure 36. There are significant changes in LV systolic pressure, whereas those of RV systolic pressure are more subtle but definitely in the *opposite direction*. At peak inspiration (beat 1), LV systolic pressure is significantly lower, but RV systolic pressure is slightly higher than peak expiration (beat 2), although not markedly so. This is absence of concordance, that is, ventricular discordance. The nasal respirometer tracing is shown at the top. Exp, expiration; Insp, inspiration.

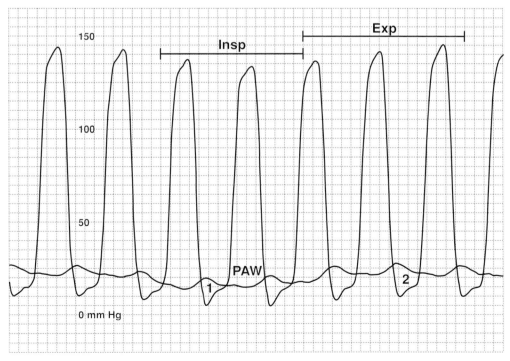

Fig. 38. Restrictive filling in restrictive cardiomyopathy. This tracing is from a patient with idiopathic restrictive cardiomyopathy. Simultaneous recordings of left ventricular and pulmonary capillary wedge pressures demonstrate the lack of dissociation of intrathoracic and intracardiac pressures. Both tracings are from high-fidelity micromanometer catheters. Note the nearly constant early diastolic gradient with respiration (beat 1 vs. 2). Exp, expiration; Insp, inspiration; PAW, pulmonary artery wedge.

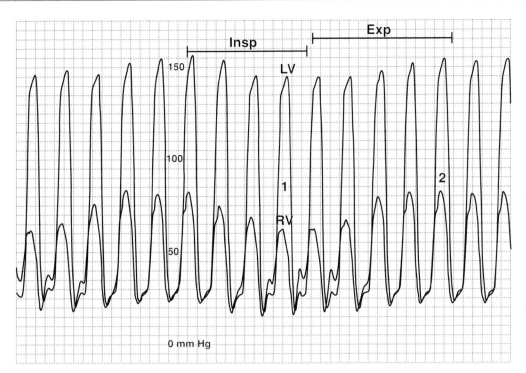

Fig. 39. Simultaneous recordings (from the same patient as in Figure 38) of left ventricular (LV) and right ventricular (RV) pressures demonstrating the absence of ventricular interdependence. Note the concordance in LV and RV systolic pressures with respiration. With inspiration (Insp), the LV and RV systolic pressures decrease and increase in concordance during expiration (Exp) (beat 1 vs. 2). Other features of note are RV systolic pressure (i.e., pulmonary systolic pressure) > 55 mm Hg, RV end-diastolic pressure < 1/3 of RV systolic pressure, dip-and-plateau morphology of diastolic pressures.

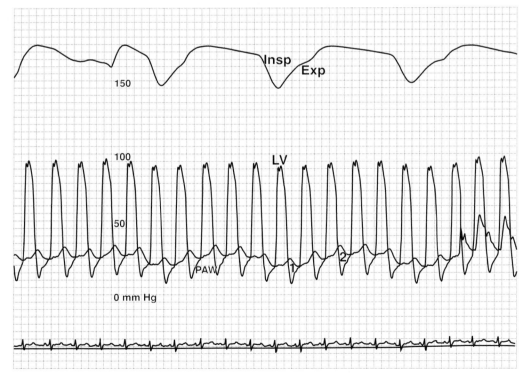

Fig. 40. Tracing from a patient with systemic amyloidosis who had biopsy-proven cardiac involvement resulting in restrictive cardiomyopathy. Simultaneous high-fidelity recordings of left ventricular (LV) and pulmonary capillary wedge pressures demonstrating lack of dissociation of intrathoracic and intracardiac pressures. Note the constant early diastolic gradient (< 5 mm Hg change) with respiration (beat 1 vs. 2) and the wedge balloon deflation showing the pulmonary artery pressure in the last 3 beats. The nasal respirometer tracing is shown at the top. Exp, expiration; Insp, inspiration; PAW, pulmonary artery wedge.

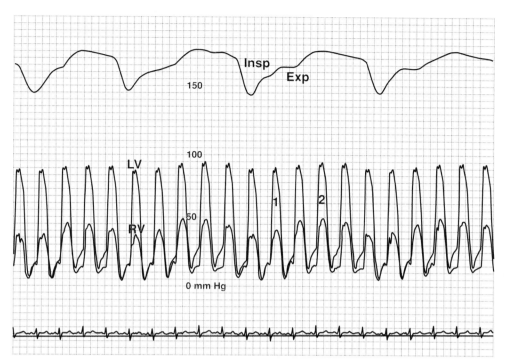

Fig. 41. Simultaneous high-fidelity recordings (from the same patient as in Figure 40) of left ventricular (LV) and right ventricular (RV) pressures demonstrating the absence of ventricular interdependence. Note the concordance in LV and RV pressures and increase with expiration (beat 2). Also note the dip-and-plateau morphology of diastolic pressures, pulmonary artery pressure 55 mm Hg, and RV end-diastolic pressure ≥ 1/3 of the RV systolic pressure—all the traditional criteria thought to be consistent with constriction. The nasal respirometer tracing is shown at the top. Exp, expiration; Insp, inspiration.

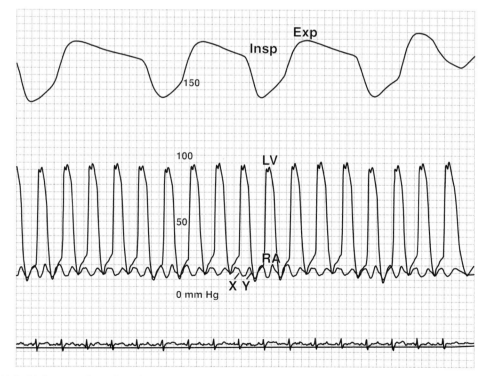

Fig. 42. Simultaneous high-fidelity recordings (from the same patient as in Figures 40 and 41) of left ventricular (LV) and right atrial (RA) pressures. Note the marked "W" or "M" pattern in the RA pressure tracing, with prominent x and y descents and no decrease with inspiration (Insp) (Kussmaul sign). Also note the equalization of RA and LV diastolic pressures. In summary, this patient has most of the traditional criteria of constrictive pericarditis; however, the dynamic respiratory criteria clearly demonstrate that the patient has restriction and not constrictive pericarditis. The nasal respirometer tracing is shown at the top. Exp, expiration.

Notes

Chapter 52

Diagnostic Coronary Angiography and Ventriculography

Peter B. Berger, M.D.

> The principles of angiography and correct image evaluation (rather than the technical details of the procedure) are emphasized in the Cardiology Boards.

Coronary Angiography

Indications for Coronary Angiography

Coronary angiography is used primarily to diagnose obstructive coronary artery disease or plan treatment when the diagnosis is not in doubt. The coronary artery disease most frequently diagnosed is atherosclerosis, but other diseases of the coronary arteries that may be diagnosed with coronary angiography include congenital anomalies of the origin of coronary arteries, coronary fistulas, coronary spasm, coronary emboli, coronary arteritis, and myocardial bridging.

Contraindications to Coronary Angiography

Virtually the only absolute contraindication to coronary angiography is the refusal of a patient to consent to the procedure. Relative contraindications include the presence of correctable electrolyte abnormalities or drug toxicity (e.g., hyperkalemia, digitalis toxicity), febrile illness, acute renal failure, decompensated heart failure, severe allergy to radiographic contrast agents, anticoagulated state or a severe bleeding diathesis, severe uncontrolled hypertension, and pregnancy. Despite the presence of these conditions, it still may be appropriate to proceed with coronary angiography

if the patient risk-benefit ratio is favorable, that is, the information gained from angiography outweighs the risk of performing it.

- Virtually the only absolute contraindication to coronary angiography is the refusal of a patient to consent to the procedure.

Vascular Access for Angiography

The percutaneous femoral artery approach is the most commonly used approach. Direct exposure of the brachial artery and the percutaneous brachial or radial artery approach are used less often. The radial artery is used increasingly in Europe, especially for coronary artery interventions, but this still accounts for a small proportion of cases in the United States.

Catheterization laboratories in which the brachial approach is used most often have a frequency of vascular complications similar to or only slightly higher than that of laboratories using the more common femoral artery approach.

Complications of Coronary Angiography

Major Complications

The major complications of coronary angiography include death, myocardial infarction, and stroke, each of which occurs in about 1 patient per 1,000. The two main risk factors for major adverse events with coronary angiography are left main coronary artery disease and aortic stenosis. Patients with critical left main coronary stenosis have a 20-fold higher risk of death with coronary angiography than those with single-vessel disease. Other important risk factors include increased age, severe angina at rest, left ventricular dysfunction, previous stroke, and severe noncardiac disease (including renal insufficiency, cerebrovascular and peripheral vascular disease, and pulmonary insufficiency). Approximately one-half of the complications that occur within 24 hours after coronary angiography are believed to be "pseudocomplications," in that the "complications" may have occurred during the same period had angiography not been performed.

- The two main risk factors for major adverse coronary artery events with coronary angiography are left main coronary artery disease and aortic stenosis.
- One-half of the complications that occur within 24 hours after coronary angiography are believed to be "pseudocomplications," in that the "complications" may have occurred during the same period had angiography not been performed.

Minor Complications
Other complications include local complications at the vascular access site; the type of complication seen depends on the vascular approach. Complications of percutaneous femoral artery access include hemorrhage, distal embolization, false aneurysm, and local injury to the femoral nerve. Femoral vein thrombosis resulting from compression of the femoral vein during sheath removal has been reported. Complications associated with direct exposure of the brachial artery include thrombosis of the brachial artery. Injury to the brachial nerve, local hemorrhage, and infection may also occur. Percutaneous access of the brachial artery is associated more commonly with hemorrhage than with thrombosis. Significant vascular complications occur in approximately 1% of patients undergoing diagnostic angiography.

- Significant vascular complications occur in approximately 1% of patients undergoing diagnostic angiography.

Arrhythmias During Angiography
Arrhythmias and vasovagal complications occur in approximately 1% of patients and have been reported to occur more frequently with high osmolar than with low osmolar contrast agents. These complications are usually self-limited, but if need be, they generally can be treated readily with electrical cardioversion or defibrillation or the administration of atropine. Pulmonary edema may develop during angiography, most commonly as a result of increased intravascular volume due to the contrast agent, a cardiac complication (i.e., an acute myocardial infarction), or the recumbent position.

Rare Complications
Coronary artery dissection is rare. It generally is preventable by meticulous attention to pressure waveforms and avoidance of overly vigorous injection of the contrast agent.

Coronary artery spasm from a reaction to the catheter tip generally is not clinically significant and usually responds to removal of the catheter. Nitroglycerin (sublingual or intracoronary) may be required.

Contrast Reactions
Serious reactions to contrast agents can mimic an anaphylactic reaction but are immunologically distinct. These reactions, called " anaphylactoid reactions," are rare. They can be treated with immediate administration intravenously of antihistamines and corticosteroids. Anaphylactoid reactions are more likely to occur in patients with a history of allergy to contrast agents and can be minimized by prophylactically administering the above drugs and using low ionic agents.

Renal Failure After Angiography
Renal failure from nephrotoxic contrast agents can be reduced by delaying angiography in patients with acute renal failure, avoiding the concomitant administration of other nephrotoxins, and, most importantly, reducing the volume of contrast agent administered. This can be accomplished by minimizing the number of angiographic views taken and using biplane angiography in patients with preexisting renal disease, who are at increased risk for acute renal failure. Lactic acidosis that is frequently fatal may occur after angiography in diabetic patients taking metformin.

Protamine Reactions
Severe protamine reactions that simulate anaphylaxis occur infrequently but may result in shortness of breath, hypotension, flushing, and flank pain. Protamine is given to reverse the effect of intravenous heparin, which is

administered in many catheterization laboratories (in doses ranging from 2,500 to 5,000 units) to reduce the risk of thromboembolic complications of the procedure. Such reactions are more likely to occur in patients who have received NPH insulin, because of previous exposure to protamine contained in NPH insulin. Thus, the use of protamine should be avoided in such patients. Patients with an allergy to fish are also at increased risk.

The risks of coronary angiography have been so low in recent years that most coronary angiographic studies are performed on an outpatient basis unless the patient's cardiac condition or other illness requires hospitalization the night before or after the procedure (or both).

Precatheterization Evaluation

Each patient is evaluated before angiography is performed. This should include review of the medical history, physical examination, review of recent blood tests (potassium and creatinine levels and activated partial thromboplastin time or international normalized ratio, when appropriate), electrocardiography, and review of previous coronary angiograms, when available. The risks and benefits of the procedure must be explained to the patient so that the patient may give informed consent for the procedure.

Cannulation of the Coronary Arteries

After arterial access is obtained, the coronary catheter is advanced around the aortic arch to the ascending aorta where the coronary arteries arise. Catheters are advanced under fluoroscopic visualization either over a guidewire or with continuous pressure monitoring. Preformed catheters designed to engage the coronary arteries with minimal manipulation are used in most catheterization laboratories; they successfully engage the native vessels in 80% to 90% of cases. Unusual sizes or special shapes are successful in the rest of the cases. In patients with bypass grafts, various specially shaped catheters have been designed to engage left and right saphenous vein bypass grafts and the internal mammary arteries. Different-shaped catheters must be used from the brachial approach and, in particular, from the right brachial approach, because the catheters will not curve along the aortic arch and be naturally guided to the coronary ostia, as are catheters advanced from the femoral arteries and, often, from the left brachial artery.

Contrast Agents

Contrast agents are generally classified as low osmolar agents and high osmolar agents. Low osmolar agents cause less nausea and vomiting, fewer anaphylactoid reactions, less myocardial depression, fewer tachyarrhythmias and bradyarrhythmias, and less congestive heart failure. They have not been shown to be less nephrotoxic than high osmolar agents. High osmolar agents are considerably less expensive and have anticoagulant properties, in comparison with low osmolar agents.

Coronary Artery Anatomy

Dominance

Coronary artery dominance is defined by the artery that gives rise to the posterior descending artery. In approximately 86% of patients, it is the right coronary artery (Fig. 1). In 7% of patients, the circumflex artery is dominant, and 7% of patients have codominant arteries, with both the right coronary artery and the circumflex artery supplying the posterior descending artery. There is no particular clinical significance to whether a patient is right dominant, left dominant, or codominant.

Coronary Arteries

The left main artery is 5 to 10 mm in diameter and generally less than 4 cm long. It bifurcates into the left anterior descending artery and circumflex artery. It may also trifurcate into those branches plus a ramus intermedius artery.

The left anterior descending artery lies in the anterior interventricular groove. It usually wraps around the apex of the left ventricle; its terminal branches reach those of the right posterior descending artery. Diagonal branches supply the lateral wall, and septal branches supply the interventricular septum.

The circumflex artery lies in the left atrioventricular groove. Its terminal branches reach those of the right posterolateral artery. Obtuse marginal branches supply the lateral wall of the left ventricle.

The right coronary artery lies in the right atrioventricular groove. Proximally, it generally gives off the conus artery (50% of patients), the sinoatrial nodal artery (55% of cases), and acute marginal branches to the right ventricle. Frequently, these branches arise from their own coronary ostium in the right coronary sinus. Distally, it most commonly bifurcates into the posterior descending artery and posterolateral artery.

Coronary Artery Anomalies

Coronary artery anomalies are found on 1.0% to 1.5% of coronary angiograms (Table 1). Of these, 90% are abnormalities

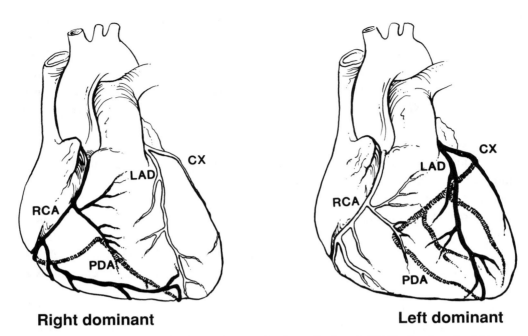

Right dominant   **Left dominant**

Fig. 1. Coronary artery dominance. In right coronary dominance, the posterior descending branch (PDA) arises from the right coronary artery (RCA). In left dominance, the right coronary artery is a diminutive vessel, and the posterior descending artery arises as a continuation of the left atrioventricular groove artery, a branch of the circumflex (CX) system. LAD, left anterior descending artery. (From Giuliani ER, Gersh BJ, McGoon MD, Hayes DL, Schaff HV [editors]: *Mayo Clinic Practice of Cardiology*. Third edition. Mosby, 1996, p 341. By permission of Mayo Foundation.)

in the origin or distribution of a coronary artery and 10% are abnormal fistulas. Coronary anomalies are often classified as benign or clinically significant; most of them are benign.

Benign Coronary Artery Anomalies
The most common are separate ostia of the left anterior descending and circumflex arteries. These occur in 0.4% to 1% of patients and may be associated with a bicuspid aortic valve.

The circumflex artery may arise from the right coronary sinus or as an early branch of the right coronary artery. When present, the circumflex artery virtually always travels behind the aorta to lie in the left atrioventricular groove (Fig. 2).

Rarely, there may be no circumflex artery; in this case, a superdominant right coronary artery supplies the entire left atrioventricular groove and left posterolateral wall.

Although these anomalies are benign, they must be recognized by the angiographer.

Clinically Significant Anomalies
The most common is a coronary artery that originates from the contralateral aortic sinus (that is, the left main or left anterior descending coronary artery from the right sinus of

Valsalva or the right coronary artery from the left sinus of Valsalva). It is important to identify the course as it relates to the great vessels, because if it courses between the aorta and the pulmonary artery, symptoms may occur. In tetralogy of Fallot, the left anterior descending artery arises from the right coronary artery in 4% of patients.

A coronary artery may arise from the pulmonary artery. Most commonly, this is the left main coronary artery, less commonly the left anterior descending artery, and least commonly the right coronary artery. Nearly 90% of patients with these anomalies die during infancy. If the patient survives, the anomalous artery fills retrogradely through collaterals and drains into the pulmonary artery (left-to-right shunt). This condition may cause angina, infarction, and heart failure; it warrants surgical repair (ligation and grafting or reanastomosis to the aorta or subclavian artery).

Coronary Fistula
A coronary artery fistula is an abnormal connection between one of the coronary arteries and another structure, most commonly a venous structure or chamber on the right side of the heart. The right coronary artery is the site of the fistula in 55% of patients. The majority of coronary artery fistulas

Table 1.—Coronary Artery Anomalies Among 126,595 Angiograms

Type of anomaly	Incidence, %	Anomalies, %
Benign (80%)		
Separate, adjacent LAD and LCx ostia	0.40	30.0
LCx		
LCx origin from RSV or RCA	0.40	30.0
Anomalous origin from PSV	< 0.01	0.3
Anomalous origin from aorta		
LMCA	0.01	1.0
RCA	0.15	10.0
Absent LCx	0.003	0.2
Small fistulae	0.10	10.0
Clinically significant (20%)		
Origin of coronary artery from opposite aortic sinus		
LMCA from RSV	0.02	1.0
LAD from RSV	0.03	2.0
RCA from LSV	0.10	10.0
Anomalous origin from pulmonary artery		
LMCA	< 0.01	< 1.0
LAD or RCA	< 0.01	< 1.0
Single coronary artery	0.05	3.0
Multiple or large coronary fistulae	0.05	3.0

LAD, left anterior descending; LCx, left circumflex; LMCA, left main coronary artery; LSV, left sinus of Valsalva; PSV, posterior sinus of Valsalva; RCA, right coronary artery; RSV, right sinus of Valsalva.
Modified from Giuliani ER, Gersh BJ, McGoon MD, Hayes DL, Schaff HV (editors): *Mayo Clinic Practice of Cardiology*. Third edition. Mosby, 1996, p 342. By permission of Mayo Foundation.

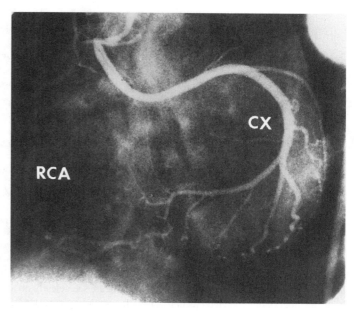

Fig. 2. Anomalous origin of the circumflex coronary artery (CX) from the right coronary artery (RCA). This anomaly occurs in 0.4% of cases. The circumflex branch arises from or near the ostium of the right coronary artery and courses posteriorly to supply the obtuse margin of the heart. (From Giuliani ER, Gersh BJ, McGoon MD, Hayes DL, Schaff HV [editors]: *Mayo Clinic Practice of Cardiology*. Third edition. Mosby, 1996, p 342. By permission of Mayo Foundation.)

- Coronary artery dominance is defined by the artery that gives rise to the posterior descending artery.
- In tetralogy of Fallot, the left anterior descending artery arises from the right coronary artery in 4% of patients.

Angiographic Views

The primary aim of angiography is to visualize all segments of the coronary arteries and their branches (and bypass grafts, if present) in at least two orthogonal views. Stenoses of the coronary arteries must be seen without foreshortening and without being obscured by overlapping branches. To do this, multiple projections must be used combining cranial and caudal angulation with right and left angulation. Standard views are generally selected that, in most patients, lay out the coronary arteries adequately. However, the standard views must be altered in many patients depending on their individual coronary artery anatomy and body habitus and may need to be supplemented by individualized views as well.

The four views of the left coronary arteries and two views of the right coronary artery in Figures 3 to 8 are the most commonly encountered views and the views from which one is expected to identify the major coronary arteries and their major branches. Figure 9 shows coronary artery bridging.

empty into the right ventricle, right atrium, or coronary sinus. Less common are fistulas that empty into the pulmonary artery, left atrium, or left ventricle. Generally, the shunt is small, the myocardial blood flow to the terminal branches of the involved coronary artery is not compromised, and the patients are asymptomatic. However, if the shunt is large, pulmonary hypertension, congestive heart failure, bacterial endocarditis, rupture, and myocardial ischemia in the terminal portion of the involved coronary artery can occur.

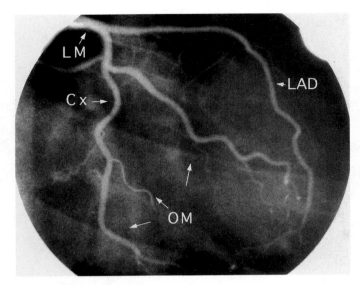

Fig. 3. The circumflex artery (Cx) and its branches are seen clearly on a right anterior oblique caudal projection of the left coronary system. LAD, left anterior descending artery; LM, left main coronary artery; OM, obtuse marginal branches.

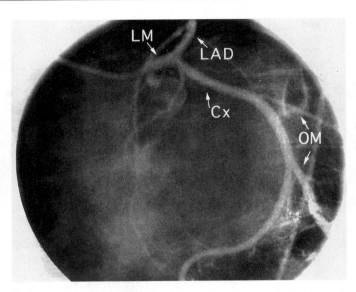

Fig. 4. The distal left main coronary artery (LM), the proximal left anterior descending artery (LAD), and the circumflex artery (Cx) and its branches (especially the proximal portion of its branches) are seen clearly on a left anterior oblique caudal view (termed the "spider view" because it looks somewhat like a spider). OM, obtuse marginal branches.

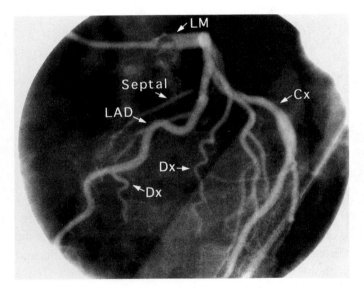

Fig. 5. The left anterior oblique cranial view shows the left anterior descending coronary artery (LAD) and diagonal branches (Dx). (Other abbreviations as in Figure 3.)

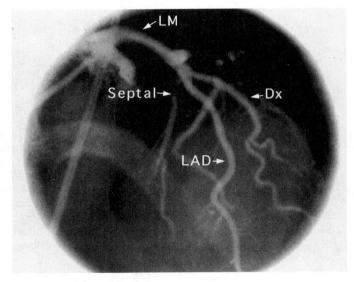

Fig. 6. A right anterior oblique cranial view nicely lays out the LAD and its branches. (Abbreviations as in Figure 5.)

Coronary Artery Lesions

The grading of coronary artery stenoses is usually expressed as a percentage of the nearest normal segment of the same artery. For example, the lumen of an artery reduced to 20% of normal is expressed as an 80% stenosis. Because stenoses are often eccentric, orthogonal views must be obtained. When the degree of stenosis appears to differ significantly in orthogonal views, the most severe stenosis is commonly reported. However, some cardiologists report the average stenosis in the two views. Quantitative computer-assisted methods of quantifying coronary artery stenoses have been advocated because of their greater accuracy and reproducibility but have not yet become part of routine practice because of the time and expense associated with these methods.

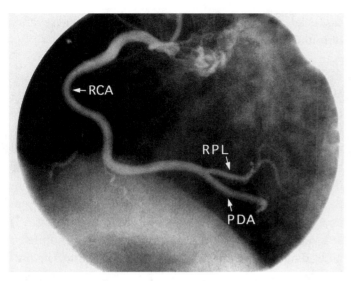

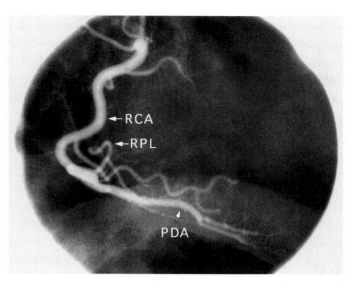

Fig. 7. A left anterior oblique projection of the right coronary artery (RCA) (a dominant right coronary artery) clearly shows the artery and its two main branches, the right posterolateral (RPL) and the posterior descending (PDA) arteries.

Fig. 8. A right anterior oblique projection shows the main portion of the right coronary artery (RCA) and the posterior descending artery (PDA), but individualized views with cranial or caudal angulation are often required to show the right posterolateral (RPL) branch well.

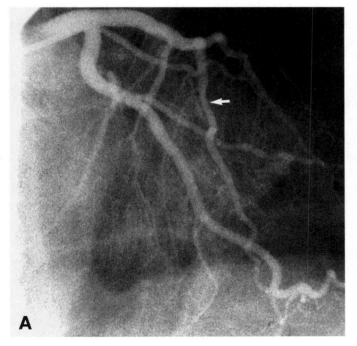

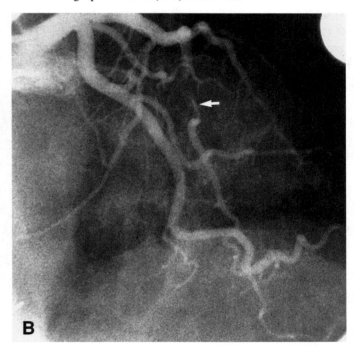

Fig. 9. Coronary artery bridging. *A*, Right anterior oblique view of the left coronary artery in diastole. The left anterior descending coronary artery is only minimally narrowed (*arrow*). *B*, Systolic frame showing obliteration of the middle left anterior descending coronary artery (*arrow*) due to muscular bridging. (From Giuliani ER, Gersh BJ, McGoon MD, Hayes DL, Schaff HV [editors]: *Mayo Clinic Practice of Cardiology*. Third edition. Mosby, 1996, p 345. By permission of Mayo Foundation.)

Limitations of Coronary Angiography

It must always be remembered that a coronary angiogram is a "luminogram" and cannot be used to assess changes in wall thickness, a cardinal feature of atherosclerosis. It relies on the presence of a normal segment of coronary artery, which may not exist, with which to compare a diseased segment. The absence of a normal segment will serve to underestimate the severity and extent of atherosclerosis. Furthermore, measurements of luminal diameter do not take into account any intraluminal obstruction that may be present because of thrombus or protruding tissue due to a ruptured plaque; these can be suggested only indirectly by the presence of certain characteristic angiographic features such as haziness, a mobile object in the vessel lumen, and the appearance of contrast agent on three sides of an unopacified filling defect. Intravascular ultrasonography and angioscopy are able to provide important information about coronary arteries when the limitations of coronary angiography become relevant in the management of a patient.

Special Interventions

In patients with minimal coronary artery disease in whom coronary artery spasm is suspected, it may be appropriate to administer medications that may be useful in making this diagnosis. Until recently, ergonovine, a stimulator of the α-adrenergic and serotonin receptors in coronary vascular smooth muscle, was the drug used for this purpose, but it has been withdrawn from the U.S. market. Methylergonovine (Methergine) is proving to be a suitable substitute. Acetycholine is an endothelium-dependent vasodilator that may cause vasoconstriction in patients with abnormal endothelial function. It reportedly is safer and more sensitive than intravenous ergonovine. Intracoronary nitroglycerin and, in some patients, intracoronary verapamil may be required to reverse vasoconstriction should it occur with any of these drugs.

Left Ventriculography

Technique

At most medical centers, the assessment of left ventricular myocardial abnormalities is part of the evaluation of patients who are undergoing coronary angiography. A catheter is advanced to the aortic root, and the aortic valve is crossed retrogradely in a 30° right anterior oblique (RAO) projection. The catheter is placed in a stable position in the left ventricle, and left ventricular pressure is measured. The catheter then is connected to a power injector, and the contrast agent is injected through the catheter into the left ventricle. Biplane (as opposed to monoplane) images of the ventriculogram are preferred (generally, 30° RAO and 60° LAO), which are more comprehensive and provide a much more accurate assessment of the posterior left ventricle than the RAO view alone.

Indications for Ventriculography

Indications for left ventriculography include the need to assess left ventricular function or the presence and severity of mitral regurgitation.

Contraindications to Ventriculography

With so many alternative ways of determining left ventricular function, including echocardiography and radionuclide ventriculography, patients at particularly high risk for ventriculography might best have ventricular function assessed by one of these other techniques. High-risk patients include those with 1) severe symptomatic aortic stenosis and, in particular, congestive heart failure or angina at rest; 2) severe congestive heart failure or angina at rest from any cause; 3) left ventricular thrombus, particularly if it is mobile or protruding into the left ventricle; and 4) endocarditis involving the aortic and possibly even the mitral valve. Patients with mechanical aortic valve prostheses should not undergo passage of a catheter retrogradely through the prostheses, but ventriculography can still be performed via a transseptal approach or, if both mechanical mitral and aortic valve prostheses are present, via direct left ventricular puncture through the left chest wall.

Assessment of Ejection Fraction and Wall Motion

Determination of left ventricular ejection fraction depends on defining the endocardial contours of the ventricle at end-systole and end-diastole, accurate calibration, and assumptions about the shape of the left ventricle. The left ventricle is assumed to be a prolate sphere-ellipsoid with minor axes that are equal. The accuracy and reproducibility of ventriculography have been well demonstrated. Analysis of the different myocardial segments is more subjective and generally involves assigning a wall motion score to each of the ventricular segments (Fig. 10). Wall motion (the motion of each myocardial region) is classified as normal, mildly hypokinetic, moderately hypokinetic, severely hypokinetic, akinetic, or dyskinetic. If an inexperienced observer is uncertain about the motion of a myocardial segment, it may be helpful to manually trace the end-diastolic and end-systolic contours of the ventricle and superimpose them to aid in the assessment.

Figures 11 through 16 are examples of uncommon abnormalities demonstrated by ventriculography.

Left Ventricular Wall Segment Analysis

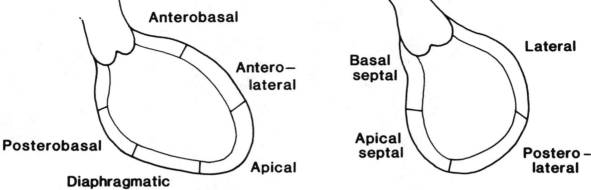

Fig. 10. Analysis of left ventricular wall motion. The outline of the left ventricular cavity in the right anterior oblique (RAO) (*left*) and left anterior oblique (LAO) (*right*) views is demonstrated. The RAO view shows anterobasal, anterolateral, apical, diaphragmatic, and posterobasal segments. The LAO view shows lateral, posterolateral, apical septal, and basal septal segments. (From Giuliani ER, Gersh BJ, McGoon MD, Hayes DL, Schaff HV [editors]: *Mayo Clinic Practice of Cardiology.* Third edition. Mosby, 1996, p 357. By permission of Mayo Foundation.)

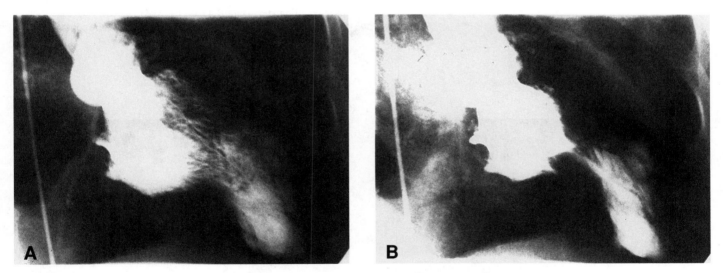

Fig. 11. Right anterior oblique ventriculograms of hypertrophic cardiomyopathy. Diastole (*A*) and systole (*B*) with midcavity obliteration.

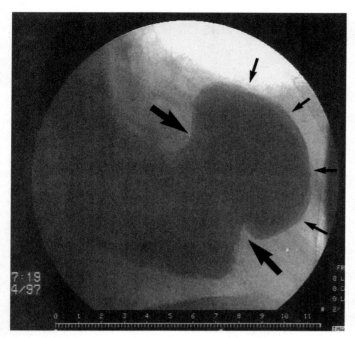

Fig. 12. Pseudoaneurysm of left ventricle (*thin arrows*) with well-defined neck (*thick arrows*). (Courtesy of Dr. Andre Lapeyre.)

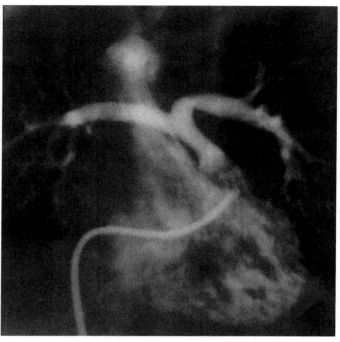

Fig. 13. Right ventriculogram demonstrating anatomy of tetralogy of Fallot. The pulmonary arteries are hypoplastic. The right ventricle is enlarged. The aorta fills with contrast material through the interventricular communication. (From Giuliani ER, Gersh BJ, McGoon MD, Hayes DL, Schaff HV [editors]: *Mayo Clinic Practice of Cardiology*. Third edition. Mosby, 1996, p 1606. By permission of Mayo Foundation.)

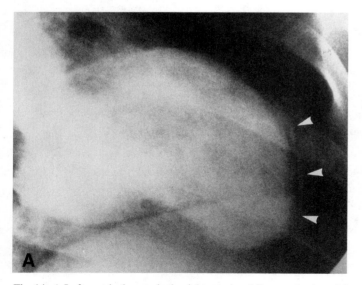

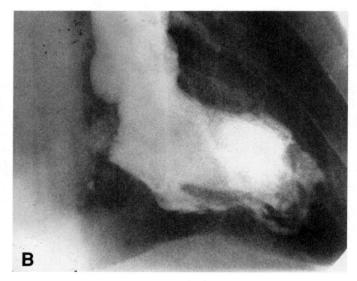

Fig. 14. *A*, Left ventriculogram in the right anterior oblique projection. A large anteroapical left ventricular aneurysm is present. A thin rim of calcification (*arrowheads*) is present along the anterolateral wall. The posterobasal and anterobasal segments showed systolic inward motion, but the remaining segments were dyskinetic. *B*, Anteroapical aneurysm with extensive apical mural thrombus. (From Giuliani ER, Gersh BJ, McGoon MD, Hayes DL, Schaff HV [editors]: *Mayo Clinic Practice of Cardiology*. Third edition. Mosby, 1996, p 359. By permission of Mayo Foundation.)

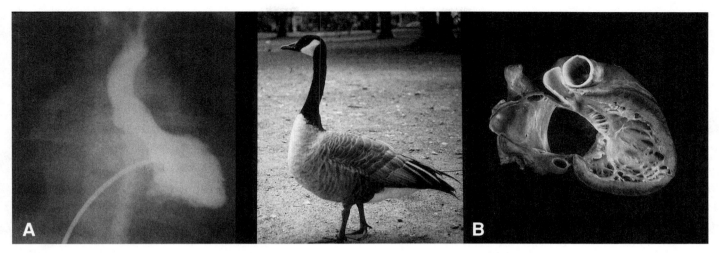

Fig. 15. *A*, Left ventriculogram demonstrating typical appearance in complete atrioventricular canal. *B*, Pathologic specimen. "Gooseneck" appearance of pathologic specimen and angiogram is apparent. (From Giuliani ER, Gersh BJ, McGoon MD, Hayes DL, Schaff HV [editors]: *Mayo Clinic Practice of Cardiology*. Third edition. Mosby, 1996, p 1570. By permission of Mayo Foundation.)

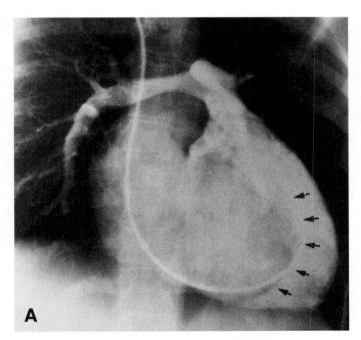

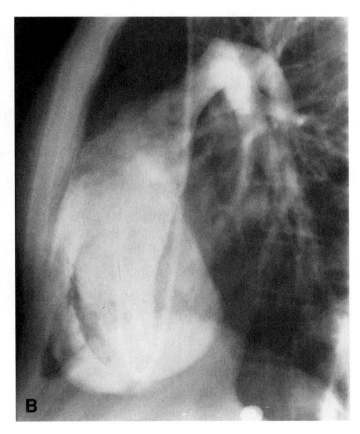

Fig. 16. Anteroposterior (*A*) and lateral (*B*) right ventriculograms from 21-year-old woman with Ebstein anomaly. Anteroposterior view shows large sail-like anterior leaflet (*arrows*) displaced well to left of spine. Severe tricuspid regurgitation is evident. Lateral projection displays pronounced anterior displacement of abnormal anterior tricuspid leaflet. (From *Mayo Clin Proc* 54:163-173, 1979. By permission of Mayo Foundation.)

Questions

Multiple Choice (choose the one best answer)

1. Which of the following is *incorrect* regarding a patient who has had an anaphylactoid reaction to a contrast agent in the past?
   a. Is at increased risk for a second anaphylactoid reaction if exposed again to a contrast agent
   b. The likelihood of a second anaphylactoid reaction can be reduced by the use of a low osmolar contrast agent
   c. The likelihood of a second anaphylactoid reaction can be reduced by the administration of corticosteroids before the second procedure
   d. May have been exposed to NPH insulin in the past, because NPH insulin increases the likelihood of an anaphylactoid contrast reaction

2. Most coronary artery anomalies
   a. Are clinically significant
   b. Are abnormal fistula connections between the coronary arteries and other cardiac structures
   c. Are identified in children
   d. Should be directly visualized by the angiographer

3. Ventriculography
   a. Must be performed in both left anterior oblique and right anterior oblique views to visualize the left ventricle
   b. Can be used to quantify aortic regurgitation
   c. Is associated with a significantly higher risk of complications than coronary angiography
   d. Permits the accurate and reproducible assessment of both mitral regurgitation and left ventricular wall motion abnormalities

4. Coronary angiography is indicated in all the following *except*:
   a. Stable class 3 angina refractory to medical therapy
   b. Uncertainty about the cause of chest pain that is suggestive of coronary spasm
   c. A recent myocardial infarction treated with thrombolytic therapy
   d. Mild angina in a patient with a positive exercise test who is scheduled for an aortic aneurysm repair

Answers

1. Answer d

The risk of an anaphylactoid reaction to contrast media is increased if a previous reaction has occurred but is not related to use of NPH insulin.

2. Answer d

Coronary artery anomalies are frequently incidental findings but should always be visualized.

3. Answer a

Biplane ventriculography is needed for complete visualization of the left ventricle.

4. Answer c

There is no definitive evidence that routine coronary angiography after thrombolytic therapy for myocardial infarction improves prognosis.

Chapter 53

Atlas of Coronary Angiograms, Ventriculograms, and Aortograms

Daniel J. Tiede, M.D.
Stuart T. Higano, M.D.
Joseph G. Murphy, M.D.

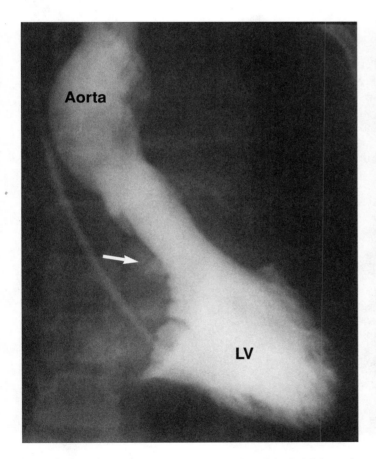

Fig. 1. RAO view. The catheter passed through the atrial septal defect and mitral valve from the right side of the heart into the left ventricle (*LV*). Left ventriculogram of primum atrial septal defect with typical gooseneck deformity of LV outflow tract (*arrow*).

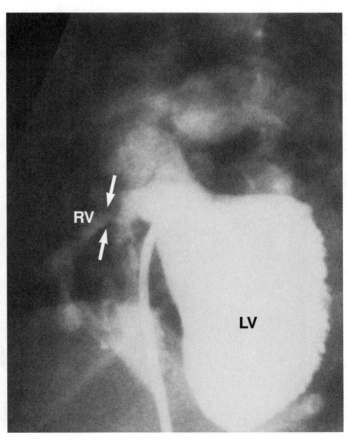

Fig. 2. LAO view. Left ventriculogram in membranous ventricular septal defect (between *arrows*). *LV*, left ventricle; *RV*, right ventricle.

The images in this atlas are typical of ones that may be shown on Cardiology Examinations. The atlas is not exhaustive for all examination images.

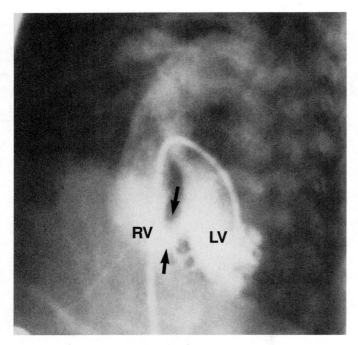

Fig. 3. LAO view. Left ventriculogram showing large muscular ventricular septal defect (*arrows*). RV, right ventricle.

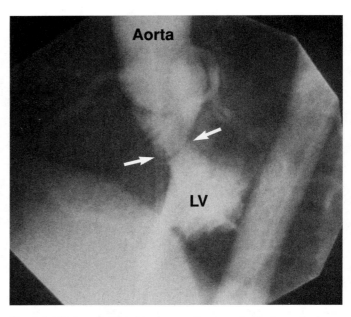

Fig. 4. LAO view. Left ventriculogram showing subvalvular aortic stenosis (between *arrows*). LV, left ventricle.

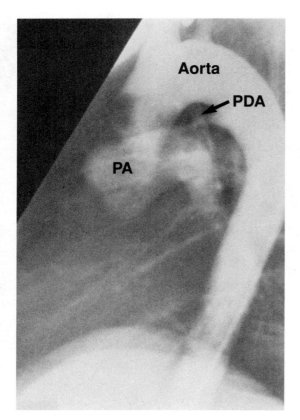

Fig. 5. Aortogram showing a patent ductus arteriosus (PDA) with a significant left-to-right shunt. PA, pulmonary artery.

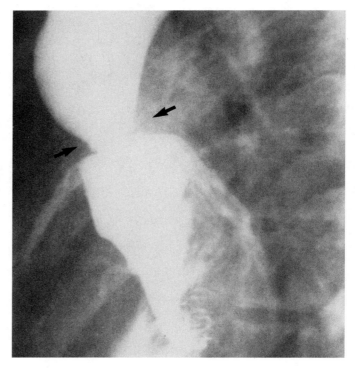

Fig. 6. LAO view. Left ventriculogram showing supravalvular aortic stenosis (*arrows*) (Williams syndrome). Other features (not shown) are pulmonary valve stenosis and infundibular stenosis.

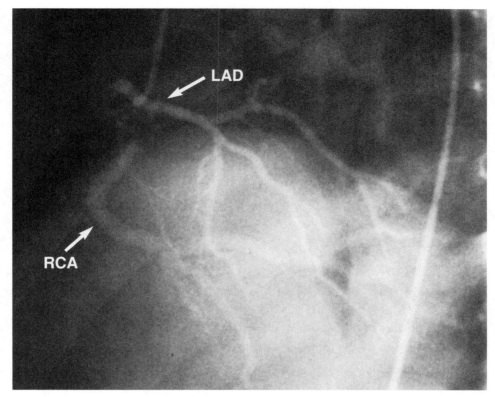

Fig. 7. Abnormal takeoff of the left anterior descending coronary artery (*LAD*) from the right coronary sinus in a patient with tetralogy of Fallot. *RCA*, right coronary artery.

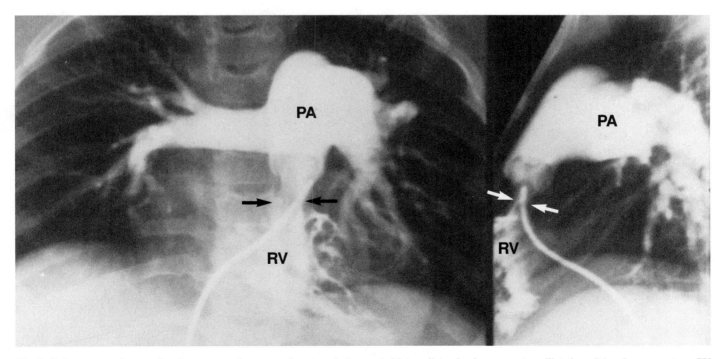

Fig. 8. Pulmonary angiogram showing severe pulmonary valve stenosis (*arrows*). Note unilateral pulmonary artery dilatation. *PA*, pulmonary artery; *RV*, right ventricle.

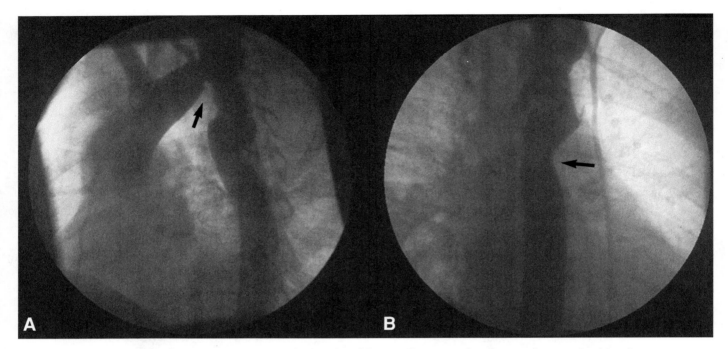

Fig. 9. *A*, LAO and, *B*, AP views of aortic injection. Note mild dilatation of the ascending aorta and moderate aortic coarctation (*arrow*).

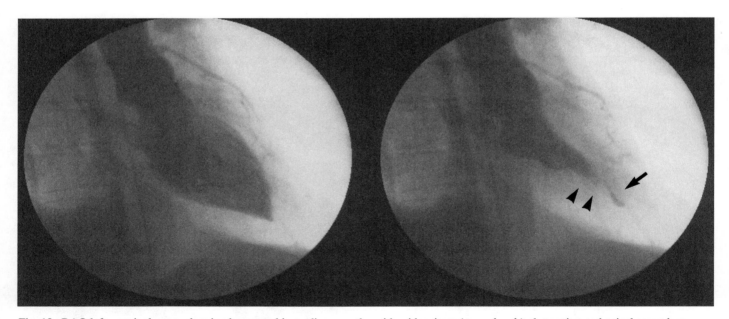

Fig. 10. RAO left ventriculogram showing hypertrophic cardiomyopathy with midcavitary (*arrowheads*) obstruction and apical secondary cavity (*arrow*).

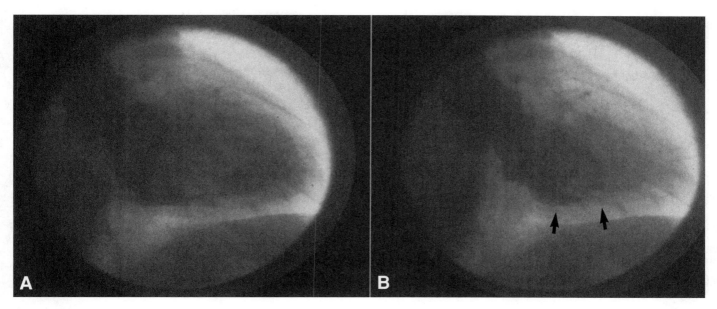

Fig. 11. RAO view of left ventriculogram in, *A*, diastole and, *B*, systole. Moderate left ventricular dilatation and dysfunction. Severe hypokinesis of diaphragmatic, posterobasal, and posterolateral segments (*arrows*).

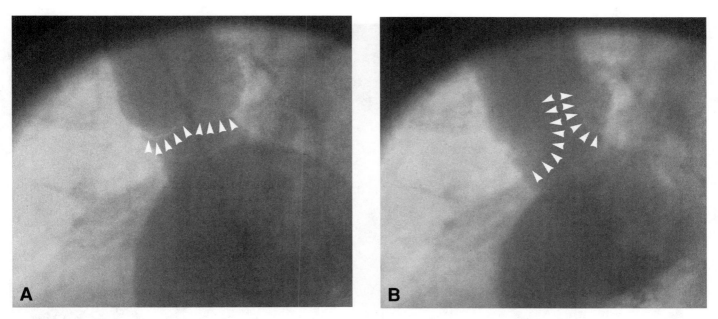

Fig. 12. LAO view of left ventriculogram (magnified) showing normal aortic valve leaflets (*arrowheads*) in, *A*, diastole and, *B*, systole.

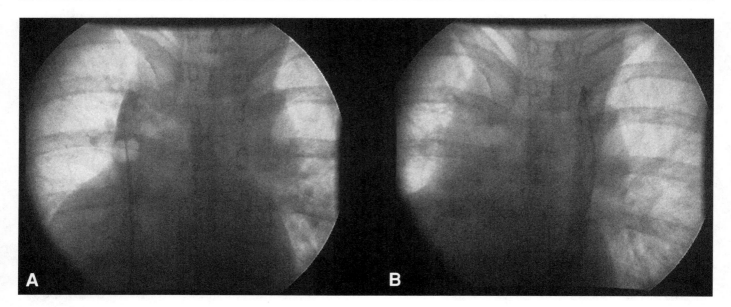

Fig. 13. Dextrocardia (situs solitus). *A*, Catheter in inferior vena cava to right atrium to coronary sinus to left superior vena cava. *B*, Catheter from inferior vena cava to right atrium to right superior vena cava.

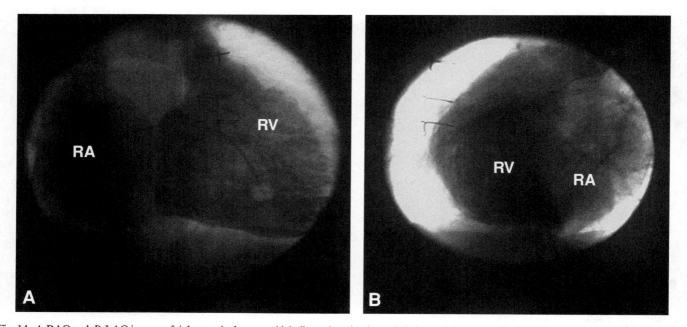

Fig. 14. *A*, RAO and, *B*, LAO images of right ventriculogram with balloon-tipped catheter. Moderate right ventricular (*RV*) dilatation and hypokinesis. Severe tricuspid regurgitation and moderate right atrial (*RA*) enlargement. Note sternal wires. LAO view superimposes RA and RV.

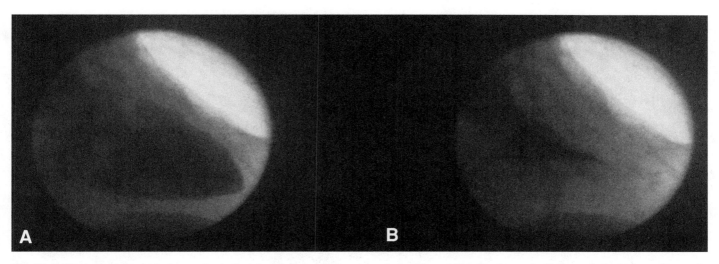

Fig. 15. RAO view of left ventriculogram in, *A*, diastole and, *B*, systole showing apical cavitary obliteration from apical left ventricular hypertrophy or apical variant hypertrophic cardiomyopathy.

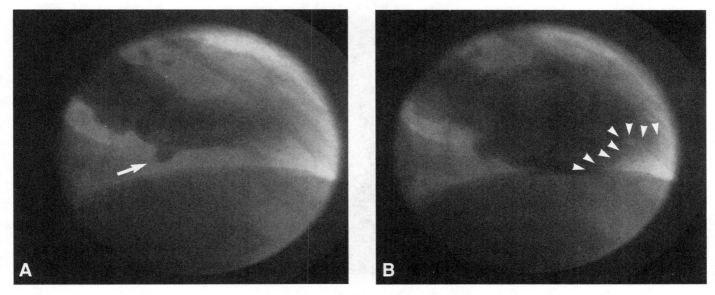

Fig. 16. RAO left ventriculogram. A, Mitral valve prolapse (*arrow*) without regurgitation. B, Apical filling defect suspicious for mural thrombus (*arrowheads*).

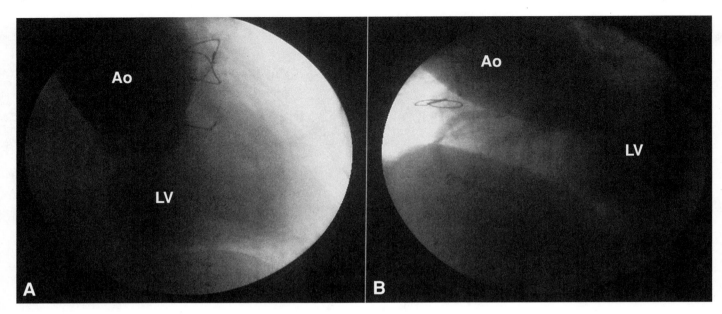

Fig. 17. *A*, RAO and, *B*, LAO views of aortic injection showing moderately severe dilatation of the aortic root (*Ao*) and probable bicuspid aortic valve with severe aortic regurgitation. Note indirect filling of saphenous vein graft to the right coronary artery. Sternal wires are present. *LV*, left ventricle.

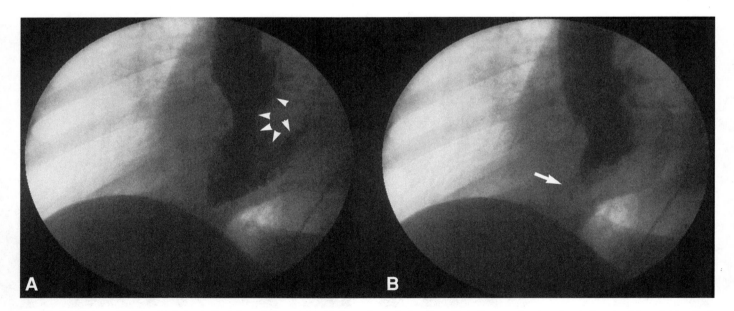

Fig. 18. LAO view of left ventricle in, *A*, diastole and, *B*, systole with hyperdynamic function. Note the prominent washout of contrast from brisk mitral inflow (*arrowheads* in *A*); this likely represents high left atrial pressure (i.e., restrictive filling pattern). Also note hypertrophic cardiomyopathy with mid-cavitary obstruction and apical cavity obliteration (*arrow* in *B*).

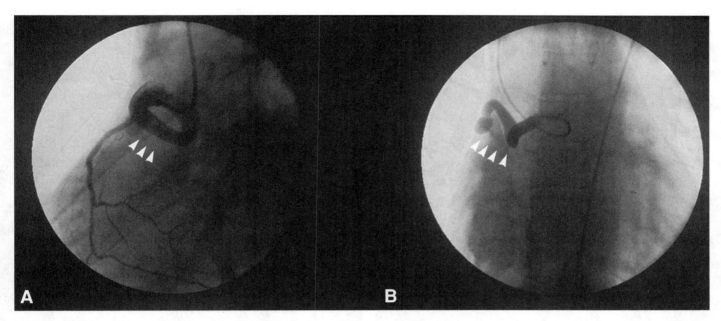

Fig. 19. *A*, LAO and, *B*, AP view of right coronary artery injection showing large fistula from right coronary artery to right atrium. *Arrowheads*, jet of flow.

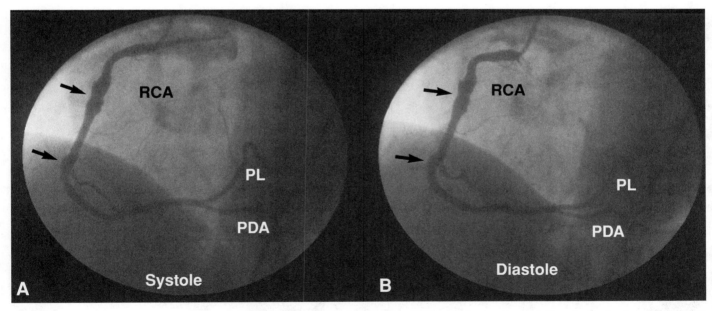

Fig. 20. LAO view in, *A*, systole and, *B*, diastole showing fixation of mid-right coronary (*RCA*), distal posterolateral (*PL*), and posterior descending (*PDA*) arteries from constrictive pericarditis. Note moderate ectasia/aneurysm (*arrows*) of mid-RCA.

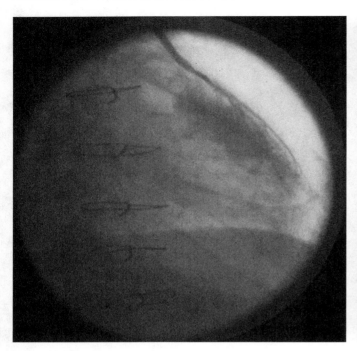

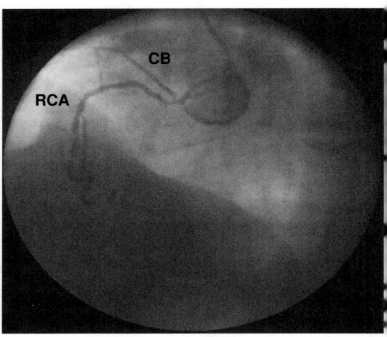

Fig. 21. AP view of saphenous vein graft to first diagonal artery. A large myocardial "blush" is present after percutaneous transluminal coronary angioplasty of the graft. This likely occurred because of microembolization of the microcirculation.

Fig. 22. LAO view of codominant right coronary artery (*RCA*) and severe stenoses of the ostial and mid RCA and conus branch (*CB*). Note contrast agent filling the right sinus of Valsalva.

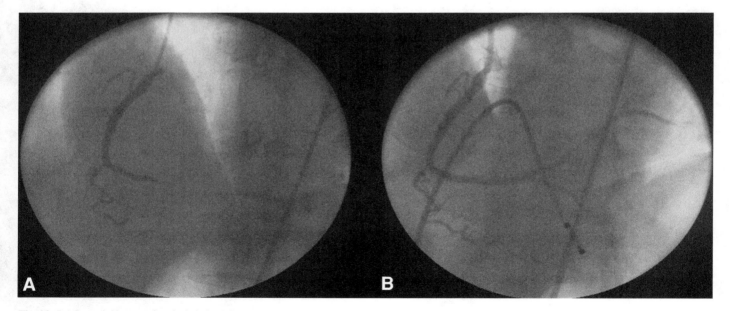

Fig. 23. LAO cranial image of occluded distal right coronary artery. Hazy tapered occlusion suggests thrombus. *B*, During percutaneous transluminal coronary angioplasty (PTCA) there was moderate distal embolization and slow reflow phenomenon. Note placement of temporary pacemaker in right ventricular apex for post-PTCA bradycardia and hypotension (Bezold-Jarisch reflex).

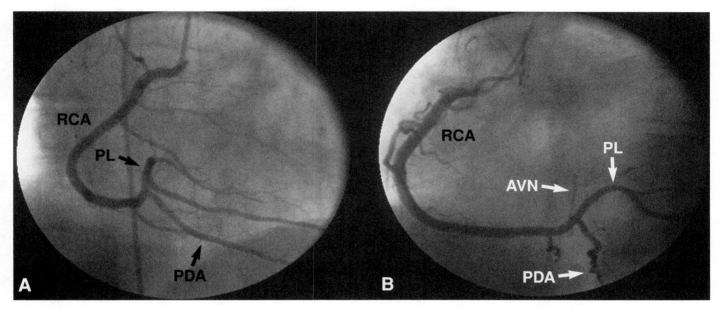

Fig. 24. *A*, RAO and, *B*, LAO views showing normal right coronary artery (*RCA*) (right dominant), right posterolateral artery (*PL*), posterior descending artery branch (*PDA*), and atrioventricular artery (*AVN*) (determining dominance).

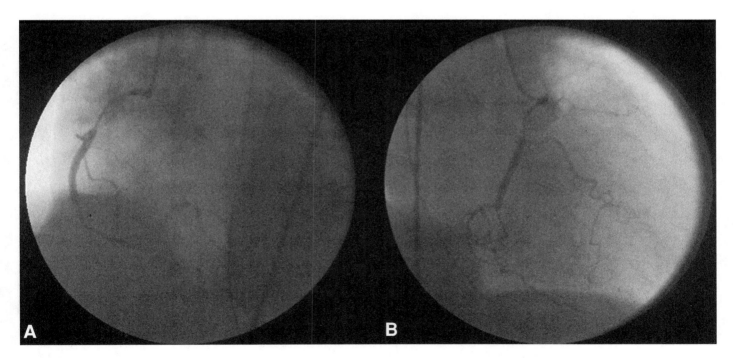

Fig. 25. *A*, LAO and, *B*, RAO views of right coronary artery with diffuse severe spasm except in stented segment (midsection of the artery).

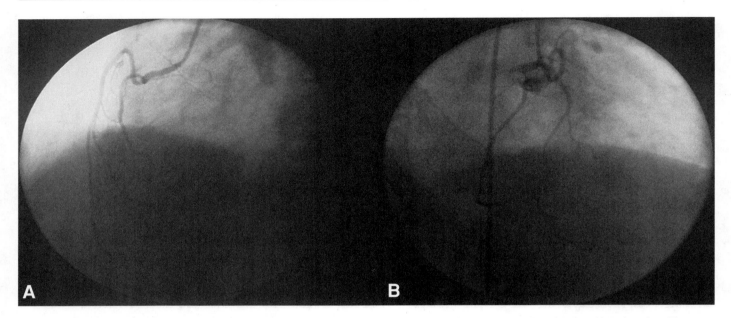

Fig. 26. *A*, LAO and, *B*, RAO views of normal nondominant right coronary artery. Note the diminutive size, predisposing to catheter damping. The artery does not supply the diaphragmatic myocardium. Also note the "shepherd's crook" bend in the proximal right coronary artery.

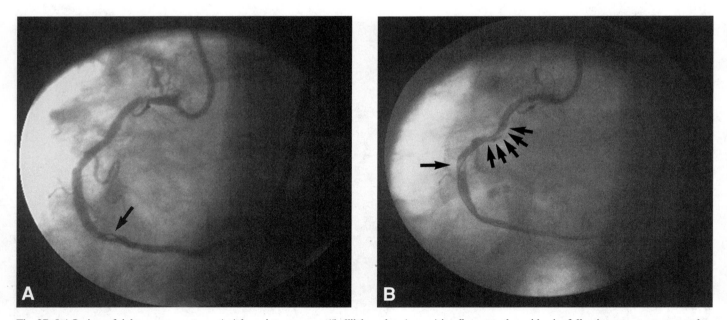

Fig. 27. LAO view of right coronary artery. *A*, A large intracoronary "ball" thrombus (*arrow*) is adherent to the guidewire following percutaneous transluminal coronary angioplasty (PTCA) for acute myocardial infarction. The thrombus was entwined in a second wire and removed successfully without complication. *B*, Note large post-PTCA dissection (*arrows*).

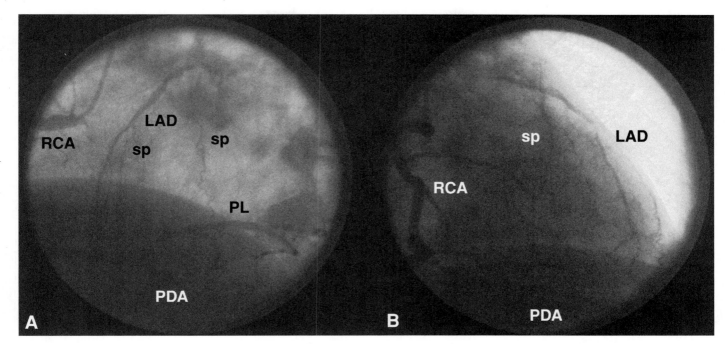

Fig. 28. *A*, LAO and, *B*, RAO views of right coronary artery (*RCA*) injection. Note mild stenoses of RCA. The left anterior descending artery (*LAD*) fills retrogradely via collateral vessels to the distal LAD and septal perforators (sp). The LAD is occluded proximally and moderate disease is scattered throughout it. *PL*, posterolateral artery; *PDA*, posterior descending artery.

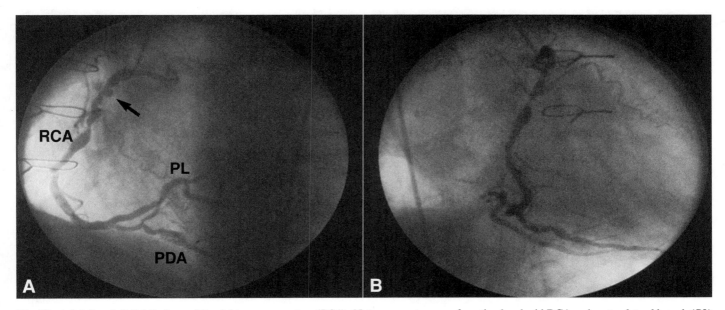

Fig. 29. *A*, LAO and, *B*, RAO views of the right coronary artery (*RCA*). Note severe stenoses of proximal and mid-RCA and posterolateral branch (*PL*) and atherosclerotic ulcer of the proximal RCA (*arrow*). Mild vessel ectasia vs. post-stenotic dilatation. *PDA*, posterior descending artery.

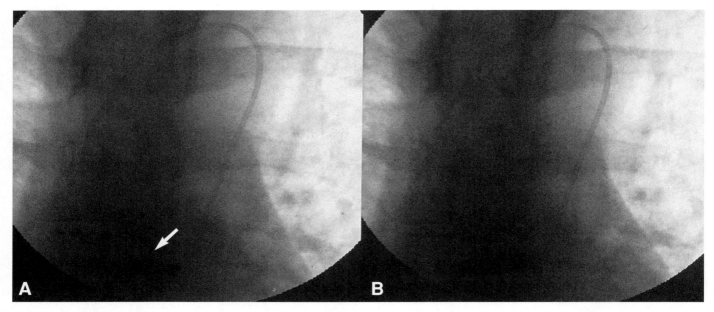

Fig. 30. Tilting disk mechanical prosthetic valve, *A*, open and, *B*, closed. Pigtail catheter is in the ascending aorta. *Arrow*, leaflet.

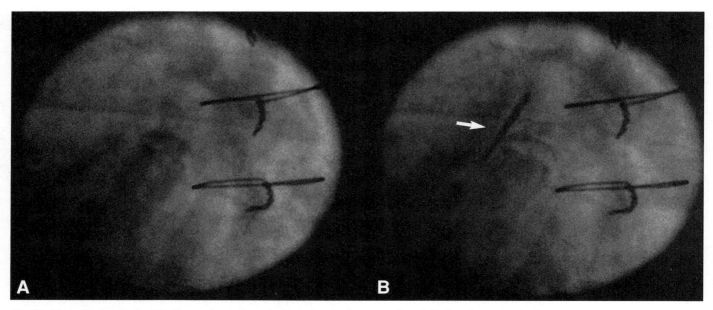

Fig. 31. Normally functioning bileaflet mechanical prosthetic aortic valve in, *A*, systole and, *B*, diastole. *Arrow*, leaflet.

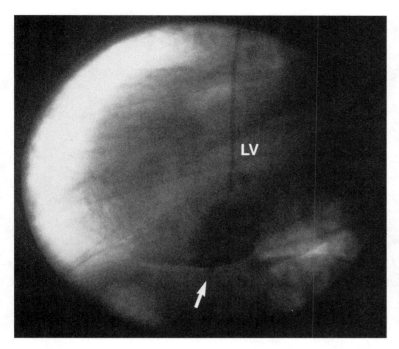

Fig. 32. LAO view of left ventriculogram. Myocardial infarction-induced ventriculoseptal defect. Intraventricular septum is seen as filling defect. Small inferior wall rupture (small jet immediately below catheter) (*arrow*). *LV*, left ventricle.

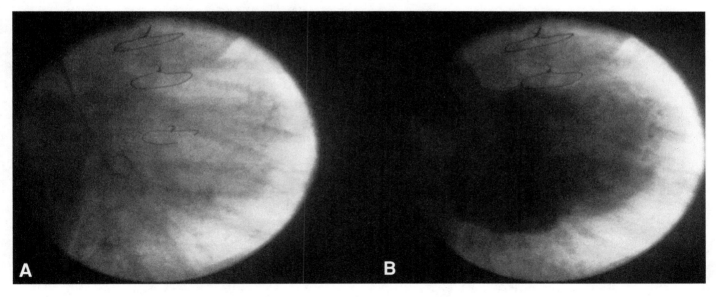

Fig. 33. RAO view of left ventriculogram showing apical mural calcification compatable with old mural thrombus or calcified myocardial infarction scar or calcified ventricular aneurysm. *A*, Before injection of contrast agent and, *B*, during ventriculogram.

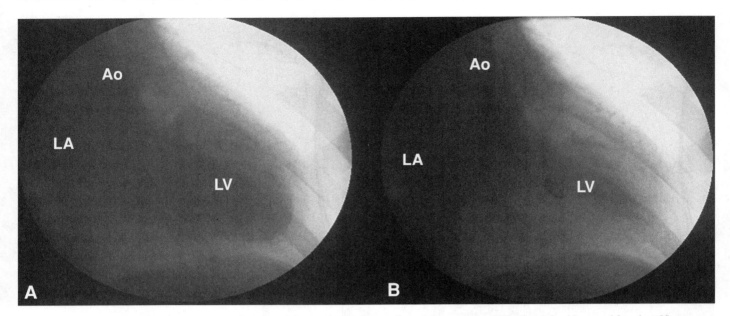

Fig. 34. RAO view of left ventriculogram in, *A*, diastole and, *B*, systole showing moderate left ventricular (*LV*) dilatation with normal function. Note severe mitral regurgitation. *Ao*, aorta; *LA*, left atrium.

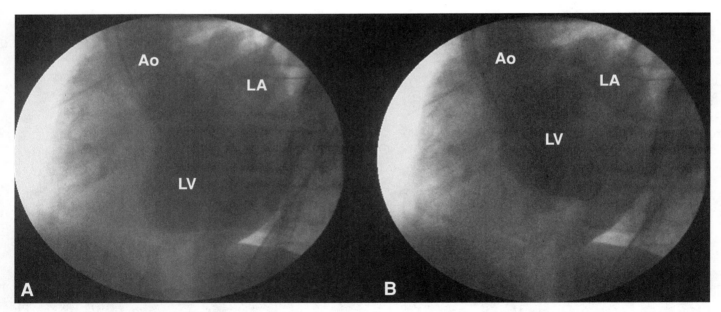

Fig. 35. LAO view of left ventriculogram in, *A*, diastole and, *B*, systole showing moderate left ventricular (*LV*) dilatation with normal function. Note severe mitral regurgitation. *Ao*, aorta; *LA*, left atrium.

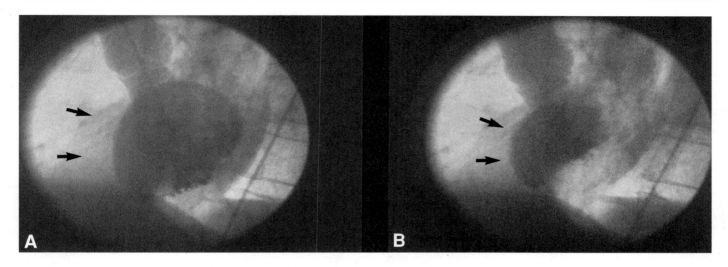

Fig. 36. LAO view of left ventriculogram in, *A*, diastole and, *B*, systole showing akinesis of the anteroapical wall segment (*arrows*).

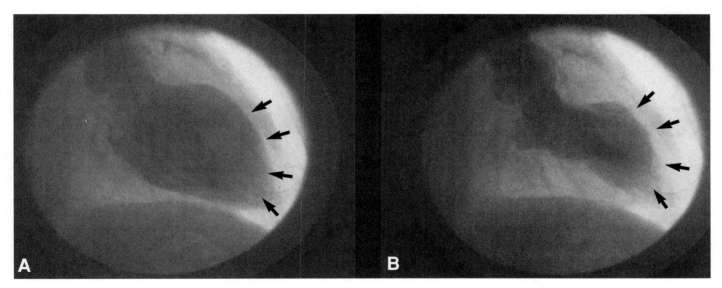

Fig. 37. RAO view of left ventriculogram in, *A*, diastole and, *B*, systole. The left ventricle has normal size but moderately reduced function. Note akinesis of the anterolateral and apical wall segments (*arrows*).

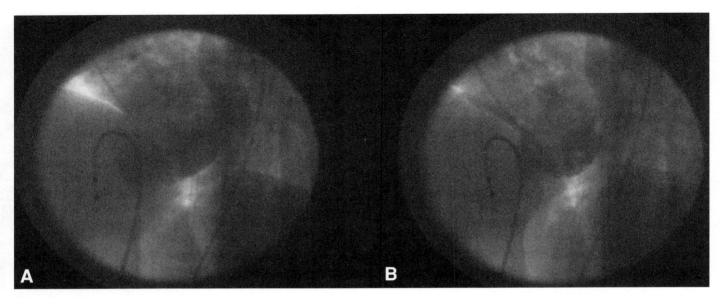

Fig. 38. LAO view of left ventriculogram in, *A*, diastole and, *B*, systole. Note normal size of the left ventricle and akinesis of the posterobasal and posterolateral wall segments. A temporary pacemaker has been placed in the right ventricular apex via the inferior vena cava.

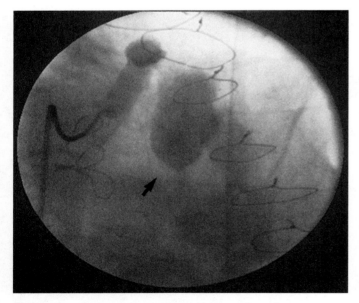

Fig. 39. Large aneurysm (*arrow*) of a saphenous vein graft.

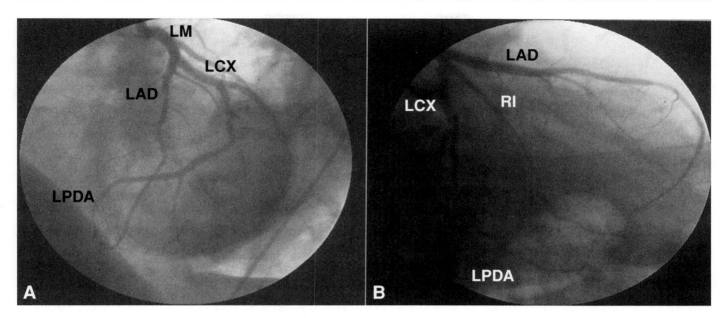

Fig. 40. *A,* LAO cranial and, *B,* RAO caudal views showing (left dominant) normal left main (*LM*), left anterior descending (*LAD*), left circumflex (*LCX*), and ramus intermedius (*RI*) arteries. Note left posterior descending arery (*LPDA*) wrapping around from LCX to the inferoseptal wall, meeting the wrap-around LAD.

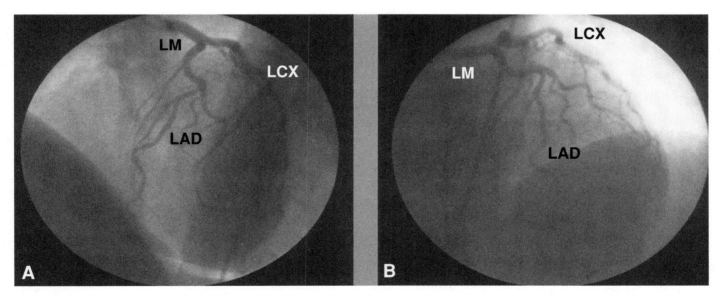

Fig. 41. *A,* LAO and, *B,* RAO cranial views of left main (*LM*) injection showing normal left anterior descending (*LAD*) and nondominant left circumflex (*LCX*) arteries and age-related tortuosity.

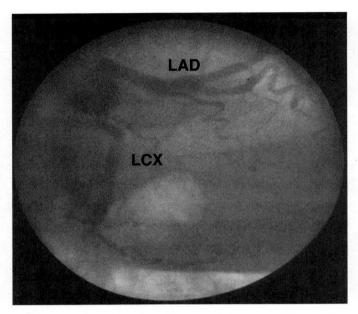

Fig. 42. RAO caudal view of moderate ectasia/aneurysmal disease of the left circumflex (*LCX*) and left anterior descending (*LAD*) arteries.

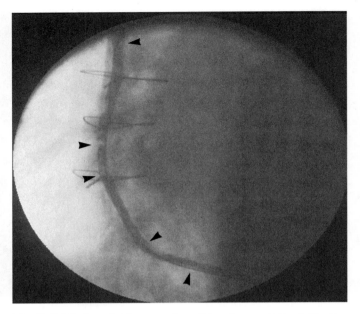

Fig. 43. LAO view of saphenous vein graft to unknown site (probably distal right coronary artery). Extensive intraluminal thrombus appears as multiple hazy filling defects (*arrowheads*).

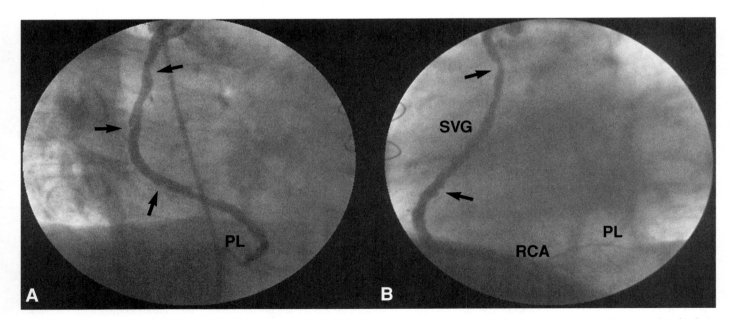

Fig. 44. Saphenous vein graft (*SVG*) to distal right coronary artery (*RCA*). Note moderate stenoses in graft body (*single arrow*) with atherosclerotic ulcer (*double arrow*). *PL*, posterolateral artery.

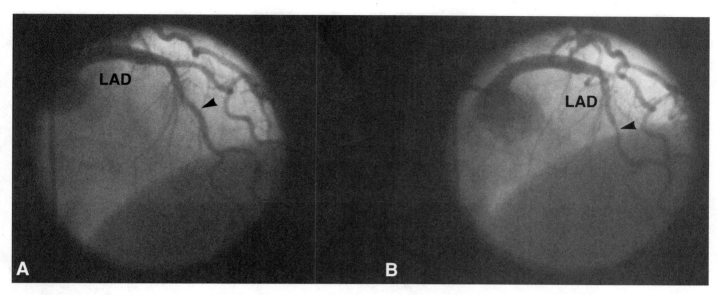

Fig. 45. Moderate bridging (*arrowheads*) of the mid-left anterior descending artery (*LAD*). *RAO*, right anterior oblique artery.

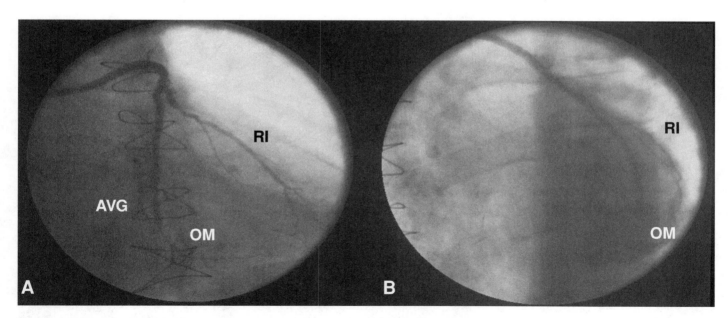

Fig. 46. Normal sequential saphenous vein graft to ramus intermedius artery (*RI*) and obtuse marginal (*OM*). Note total occlusion of the distal left circumflex (no retrograde flow beyond the origin of OM and atrioventricular groove branch artery [*AVG*]).

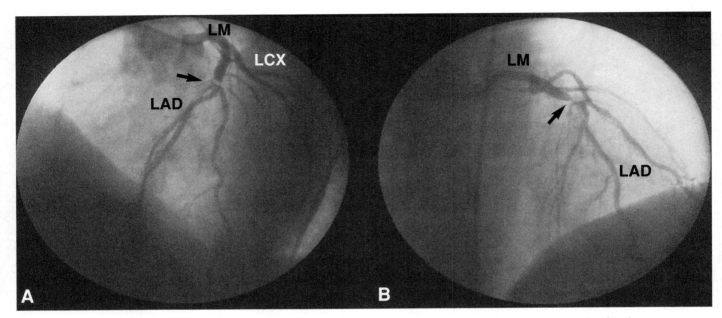

Fig. 47. *A*, LAO and, *B*, RAO cranial views of severe stenosis (*arrow*) of the proximal left anterior descending artery (*LAD*). *LM*, left main coronary artery; *LCX*, left circumflex artery.

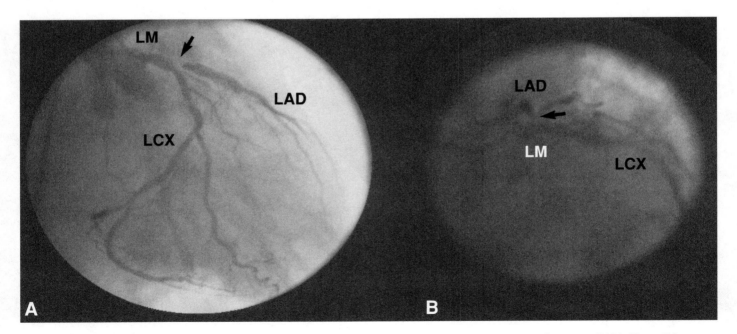

Fig. 48. *A*, RAO and, *B*, LAO caudal views showing severe stenosis (*arrow*) of the origin of the left anterior descending artery (*LAD*). Note mild stenoses of the left circumflex artery (*LCX*). *LM*, left main coronary artery.

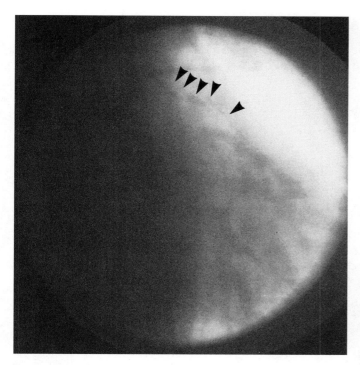

Fig. 49. RAO cranial view showing heavy calcification (*arrowheads*) of the proximal left anterior descending artery.

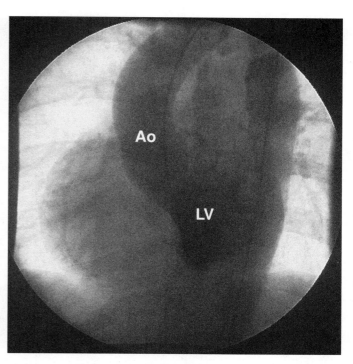

Fig. 50. RAO view of aortic injection showing severe aortic regurgitation. Note the equal density of the aorta (*Ao*) and left ventricle (*LV*). Note relatively normal left ventricular size.

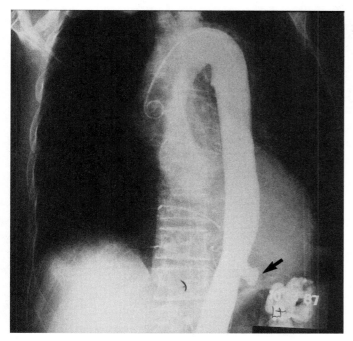

Fig. 51. AP view of aortic injection showing large perforating atherosclerotic ulcer (*arrow*).

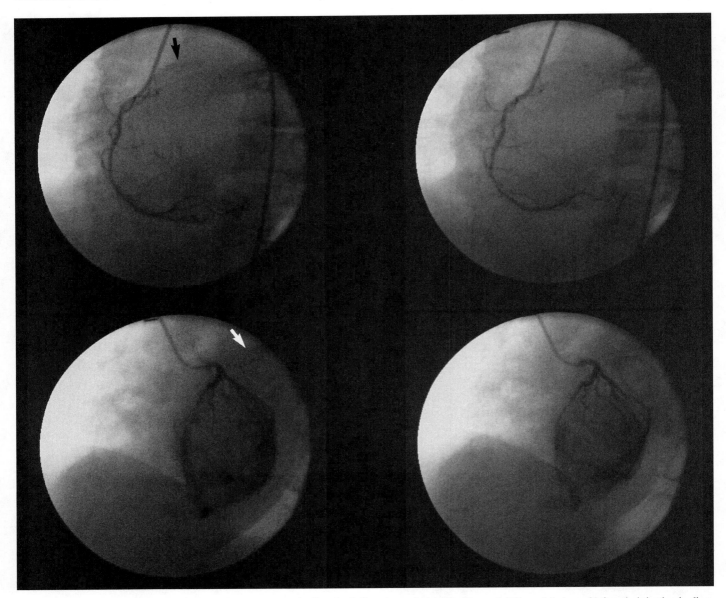

Fig. 52. *Upper*, LAO view of dominant right coronary artery in diastole (*left*) and systole (*right*). *Lower*, LAO cranial view of left main injection in diastole (*left*) and systole (*right*). Fixation of the right coronary artery and branches and the distal left circumflex artery is due to constrictive pericarditis. *Arrows*, Neovascularization of the pericarditis.

Chapter 54

Coronary Artery Physiology

Intracoronary Ultrasonography, Doppler and Pressure Techniques

Stuart T. Higano, M.D.

Normal Physiology

Myocardial Oxygen Consumption

The principal function of the coronary arteries is to provide oxygen and nutrients to the myocardium. Myocardial oxygen consumption ($M\dot{V}o_2$) is equal to the product of coronary blood flow and the arteriovenous oxygen gradient across the coronary vascular bed, that is, arterial oxygen content minus coronary sinus oxygen content. In the resting state, myocardial oxygen extraction is near maximum and coronary sinus oxygen saturations are typically 30% or less (or $Po_2 < 20$ mm Hg). Because myocardial oxygen extraction is already near maximum, $M\dot{V}o_2$ can increase only by increasing coronary blood flow. $M\dot{V}o_2$ is dependent on coronary blood flow, and changes in $M\dot{V}o_2$ closely parallel changes in coronary blood flow. Important determinants of $M\dot{V}o_2$ are heart rate, inotropic state (contractility), and intramyocardial wall stress. $M\dot{V}o_2$ can be approximated clinically by the product of systolic blood pressure and heart rate (called the "rate-pressure product"). The rate-pressure product is an estimate of $M\dot{V}o_2$ (and, thus, coronary blood flow) and is frequently used during exercise testing.

- $M\dot{V}o_2$ can be approximated clinically by the product of systolic blood pressure and heart rate.
- In the resting state, myocardial oxygen extraction is near maximal.
- Important determinants of $M\dot{V}o_2$ are heart rate, inotropic state (contractility), and intramyocardial wall stress.

Coronary Blood Flow Regulation

During rest, normal coronary blood flow is approximately 60 to 90 mL/min per 100 g of myocardium. It can be affected by metabolic, autonomic, and mechanical factors. The most important metabolic factors include adenosine, prostaglandins, and endothelial-derived factors (the vasodilator endothelial-derived relaxing factor, which is thought to be nitric oxide, and the vasoconstrictor endothelin). Oxygen and potassium also have a role in regulating coronary blood flow. Of the agents released from myocardial cells, adenosine is probably the most important. Adenosine results from the breakdown of high-energy phosphates (adenosine triphosphate [ATP]) and, thus, accumulates during ischemia. During times of low oxygen tension, the reduced form of nicotinamide adenine dinucleotide (NADH) is low and ATP cannot be regenerated.

The contribution of the autonomic nervous system to the control of coronary blood flow is likely small. Changes in coronary blood flow with either sympathetic or parasympathetic stimulation are due predominantly to the accompanying changes in loading conditions and contractility.

Mechanical factors have a major effect on coronary blood flow. During myocardial contraction, intramyocardial pressure increases, causing compression of small vessels and a reduction, or "throttling," of coronary blood flow. The result is a predominant diastolic blood flow pattern (Fig. 1). Approximately 60% of coronary blood flow occurs during diastole in the left coronary artery. The situation is opposite in the proximal right coronary artery, where there is much less vessel compression during low-pressure right ventricular contraction, with the result that there is much less reduction in blood flow during systole. Blood flow in the proximal right coronary artery during systole is nearly equal to that during diastole. However, in the distal right coronary artery (beyond the right ventricular marginal branches), coronary blood flow predominantly perfuses the inferior left ventricle, and diastolic flow again predominates.

The myocardial compressive effects are greater in the subendocardial layer than in the subepicardial layer, thus making the subendocardium at increased risk for ischemia. During maximal vasodilatation, myocardial perfusion is regulated primarily by coronary perfusion pressure and myocardial compressive effects. When coronary blood flow is reduced, as from an epicardial coronary artery stenosis, the subendocardial layer is the first region of the myocardium to become ischemic. Subendocardial ischemia can be detected clinically with ST-segment depression on an electrocardiogram. Although flow may be adequate at rest, subendocardial ischemia may occur with exercise or stress. This effect can be particularly pronounced in hypertrophied left ventricles, even with normal coronary arteries (see below).

Diastolic Pressure-Time Index

Coronary blood flow is closely correlated with the diastolic pressure-time index, which is the average difference between aortic and left ventricular cavity pressure times the duration of diastole (i.e., it is the area between diastolic aortic pressure and left ventricular pressure). The diastolic pressure-time index can be altered by changes in aortic diastolic pressure, left ventricular diastolic pressure, and length of diastole. Coronary blood flow is decreased by systemic hypotension (by decreasing aortic diastolic pressure), increased left ventricular end-diastolic pressure (by increasing left ventricular diastolic pressure), and tachycardia (by shortening diastole). Coronary blood flow can be augmented by increased systemic pressure, decreased left ventricular end-diastolic pressure, and slowing of the heart rate. Intra-aortic balloon pumping can augment coronary blood flow by increasing aortic diastolic pressure.

Myocardial Sinusoids

The coronary circulation drains primarily through the coronary sinus and cardiac veins (Fig. 2). A small portion of the venous return drains into the thebesian veins and myocardial sinusoids, which empty directly into the chambers of the

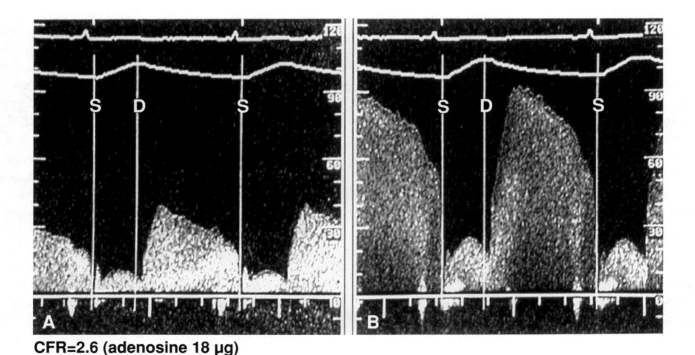

CFR=2.6 (adenosine 18 µg)

Fig. 1. Intracoronary Doppler velocities from the left anterior descending coronary artery showing predominant diastolic flow. *S*, onset of systole; *D*, onset of diastole. Heart rate and aortic pressure are shown. *A*, Flow during basal conditions and, *B*, flow after microvessel vasodilatation with adenosine. Coronary flow reserve (CFR) is the ratio of maximal diastolic flow to basal diastolic flow in the coronary vessel. (From Giuliani ER, Gersh BJ, McGoon MD, Hayes DL, Schaff HV [editors]: *Mayo Clinic Practice of Cardiology*. Third edition. Mosby, 1996, p 1054. By permission of Mayo Foundation.)

left side of the heart. A small right-to-left shunt occurs at this level, even in normal subjects. The sinusoids provide the basis for transmyocardial laser revascularization, an experimental technique for myocardial revascularization. The laser opens up channels between the left ventricular chamber and the sinusoids, allowing oxygenated blood to flow into the capillaries retrogradely.

- Approximately 60% of coronary blood flow occurs during diastole in the left coronary artery.
- Blood flow in the proximal right coronary artery during systole is nearly equal to that during diastole.
- Coronary blood flow is decreased by systemic hypotension, increased left ventricular end-diastolic pressure, and tachycardia.

Autoregulation of Coronary Blood Flow

During resting conditions, coronary blood flow is maintained at a fairly constant level over a range of aortic pressures by the process of autoregulation (Fig. 3). As aortic pressure decreases, coronary blood flow is maintained by dilatation of the resistance vessels. The resistance vessels, or arterioles, are small vessels proximal to the capillaries and are below the resolution of coronary angiography. The converse occurs with an increase in aortic pressure. Therefore, during normal resting conditions, coronary blood flow is pressure-independent. At either extreme, however, autoregulation is

overcome and coronary blood flow becomes pressure-dependent. At low perfusion pressures, the resistance vessels are dilated maximally and any additional decrease in pressure results in a linear decrease in blood flow. At pressures less than 70 mm Hg, the pressure-flow relationship becomes linear, with blood flow decreasing in direct proportion to the decrease in perfusion pressure. At very high perfusion pressures, vasoconstriction is maximal and an additional increase in pressure results in a linear increase in blood flow. At extremely low perfusion pressures (approximately 20 mm Hg), blood flow ceases altogether. This effect is called the "vascular waterfall phenomenon," which is caused by the compressive effects of extravascular intramyocardial pressure. The pressure at which flow ceases is called the "critical closure pressure," or "the critical flow pressure."

- During normal resting conditions, coronary blood flow is pressure-independent.
- At pressures less than 70 mm Hg, blood flow decreases in direct proportion to the decrease in perfusion pressure.

Coronary Flow Reserve

With physical or mental stress, the metabolic demands of the myocardium increase and coronary blood flow must increase to increase $M\dot{V}o_2$. Coronary blood flow increases through dilatation of resistance vessels. When the resistance vessels are dilated maximally, coronary blood flow

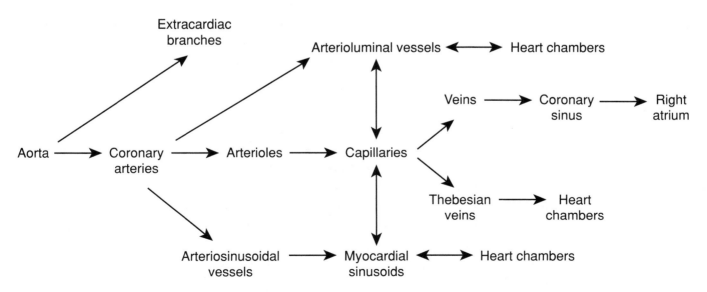

Fig. 2. Diagram of the coronary circulation. (From Mountcastle VB [editor]: *Medical Physiology.* Fourteenth edition. CV Mosby Company, 1980, p 1098. By permission of the publisher.)

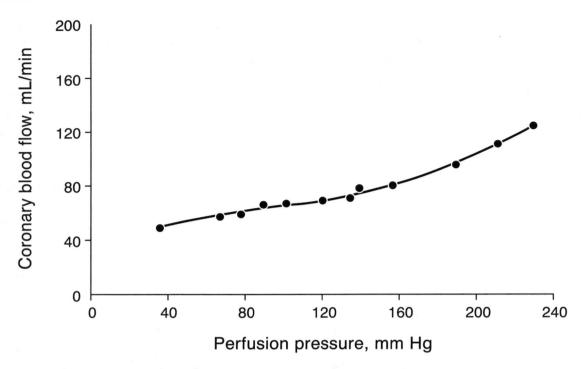

Fig. 3. Autoregulation demonstrated by changes in perfusion pressure. (Modified from *Ann N Y Acad Sci* 80:365-383, 1959. By permission of the New York Academy of Sciences.)

cannot be increased further without an increase in aortic pressure. The vessels proximal to the resistance vessels (i.e., the epicardial and prearteriolar vessels) offer only minimal resistance to coronary blood flow. The ratio of maximal blood flow to resting (or basal) blood flow is termed the "coronary flow reserve" (CFR) (Fig. 4 and Table 1):

$$CFR = \frac{\text{Maximal Coronary Blood Flow}}{\text{Resting Coronary Blood Flow}}$$

Coronary flow reserve, also called the "absolute flow reserve," is a measure of the ability to augment blood flow with stress. It can be measured easily with intra-coronary Doppler techniques. Maximal vasodilatation is produced with vasodilators such as adenosine, papaverine, or dipyridamole. Adenosine has been the easiest to use because of its short half-life, ability to promote maximal vasodilatation, and safety profile. Bradycardia and complete heart block can occur, particularly with injections into the right coronary artery, but are rare at the recommended doses. Papaverine has a longer half-life and can prolong the QT interval, rarely resulting in life-threatening arrhythmias.

- Coronary blood flow increases through dilatation of resistance vessels.
- Maximal vasodilatation is produced with vasodilators such as adenosine, papaverine, and dipyridamole.

Endothelial Function

The endothelium comprises the single layer of cells between the vascular smooth muscle and the blood and circulating components. It is the largest "organ" in the body, with approximately one trillion cells, a total surface area equivalent to six tennis courts, and a total weight greater than that of the liver. Although the endothelium functions as a semiper-meable membrane, its role in coronary artery physiology is more complex (Table 2). A normally functioning endothelium is essential for maintaining normal coronary blood flow. The increase in coronary blood flow with both physical and mental stress is caused largely by endothelial-dependent changes in vasomotor tone. A healthy endothelium is also important for preventing coronary artery disease.

The endothelium continuously produces substances to modulate vascular tone, including nitric oxide, prostacyclin, and endothelial-derived contracting factors such as endothelin. The relaxing factor produced by the endothelium and originally called "endothelium-derived relaxing factor," or

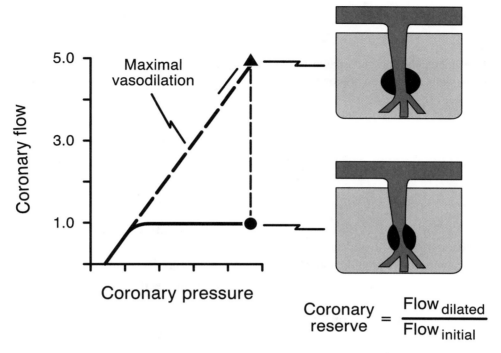

$$\text{Coronary reserve} = \frac{\text{Flow}_{dilated}}{\text{Flow}_{initial}}$$

Fig. 4. Coronary flow reserve. (From *J Am Coll Cardiol* 16:763-769, 1990. By permission of the American College of Cardiology.)

"EDRF," was identified subsequently as nitric oxide. The endothelium produces nitric oxide when the enzyme nitric oxide synthase metabolizes L-arginine; both nitric oxide and citrulline are produced during the metabolism of L-arginine by nitric oxide synthase. Endothelial cells are stimulated to produce nitric oxide by several factors, including acetylcholine, histamine, bradykinin, and platelet-derived substances. Fluid shear stress also stimulates the release of nitric oxide and undoubtedly contributes to the arterial remodeling that occurs with changes in coronary blood flow states. Nitric oxide also increases cyclic guanosine monophosphate (GMP) levels, which mediate vasorelaxation and platelet inhibition. L-Arginine has been used as a "nitrate-donor" to drive nitric oxide synthase and, thus,

Table 1.—Comparison of Three Types of Coronary Flow Reserve

	Absolute flow reserve	Relative flow reserve	Fractional flow reserve
Definition	Ratio of hyperemic to resting flow	Ratio of hyperemic flow in the stenotic region to hyperemic flow in a normal region	Ratio of hyperemic flow in the stenotic region to hyperemic flow in that same region if no lesion is present
Independent of driving pressure	-	+	+
Easily applicable in humans	+	±	+
Applicable to 3-vessel disease	+	-	+
Assessment of collateral flow	±	-	+
Unequivocal reference value	-	+	+

From *Cathet Cardiovasc Diagn* 33:250-261, 1994. By permission of Wiley-Liss.

Table 2.—Functions of the Endothelium

Regulate vasomotor tone
Nonthrombogenic surface and regulate thrombosis/fibrinolysis
Regulate vascular cell growth by production of growth factors
 and inhibitors
Regulate leukocyte and platelet adhesion
Modulate lipid oxidation
Selectively permeable barrier
Modulate thrombogenic response

promote nitric oxide production. The endothelial cells also produce endothelin, a vasoactive peptide that directly stimulates receptors on smooth muscle cells. Endothelin, one of the most potent vasoconstrictors known, is produced in response to endothelial cell stimulation by thrombin, transforming growth factor-β, interleukin-1, epinephrine, antidiuretic hormone, and angiotensin II. The endothelium also can convert angiotensin to angiotensin II through tissue-bound angiotensin-converting enzyme, which also causes vasoconstriction.

● A normally functioning endothelium is essential for maintaining normal coronary blood flow.
● Endothelin is one of the most potent vasoconstrictors known.

Altered Coronary Physiology

Obstructive Coronary Disease

Essentially all the clinical manifestations of obstructive coronary artery disease (coronary atherosclerosis and, rarely, vasculitis or emboli) are caused by altered coronary artery physiology and the myocardial ischemia that results. Coronary artery stenoses deform the column of blood flowing within the coronary artery. Although minor luminal irregularities have little effect on blood flow, more severe stenoses may cause significant transstenotic pressure gradients. The result is a reduction in the perfusion pressures distal to the stenoses. Resting blood flow is maintained by vasodilatation of the resistance vessels (Fig. 5), also called "autoregulation." Although this mechanism maintains resting coronary blood flow, the maximal coronary blood flow will be compromised. Furthermore, any attempt to increase flow across the stenosis increases the pressure gradient.

Autoregulation fails when the severity of the stenosis severely decreases the distal pressure beyond the lower limits of autoregulation. At this point, resting coronary blood flow will be decreased, resulting in resting myocardial ischemia and rest angina. Myocardial viability can be maintained with coronary blood flow as low as 10 to 20 mL/min per 100 g if the mechanical activity and metabolic needs of the heart are reduced (as during hypothermic cardioplegia).

● Myocardial viability can be maintained with coronary blood flow as low as 10 to 20 mL/min per 100 g.

Nonobstructive Coronary Artery Disease

Endothelial Dysfunction

Endothelial dysfunction precedes clinical atherosclerosis and has been detected in patients with normal findings on angiography and intravascular ultrasonography, although microscopic abnormalities likely are present in the endothelial cells. The relationship of endothelial dysfunction to cardiovascular disease is complex. Endothelial dysfunction can be considered the initial pathophysiologic step in the development of atherosclerosis. Several factors cause endothelial dysfunction: hyperlipidemia, cigarette smoking, uncontrolled hypertension, and loss of estrogen in postmenopausal women. Oxidized low-density lipoprotein is internalized by endothelial cells and transported into the intima. It inhibits nitric oxide-dependent relaxation, stimulates the formation of endothelin, and may impair the L-arginine/nitric oxide pathway.

Endothelial dysfunction can be detected in the coronary arteries of humans by selective infusion of acetylcholine into the coronary arteries (see below). With normally functioning endothelium, acetylcholine stimulates the production and release of nitric oxide, which results in vasodilatation and increased coronary blood flow. With endothelial dysfunction, acetylcholine acts directly on smooth muscle cells and causes vasoconstriction; this is called "paradoxical vasoconstriction." If endothelial cell dysfunction is detected, it can be treated with angiotensin-converting enzyme inhibitors, hypolipidemic agents (to decrease low-density lipoprotein to less than 100 mg/dL), estrogen replacement therapy (in postmenopausal women without contraindications), new experimental nitric oxide donors, smoking cessation, and agents to control hypertension. Fish oils and antioxidants have also been used.

● Endothelial dysfunction can be considered the initial pathophysiologic step in the development of atherosclerosis.

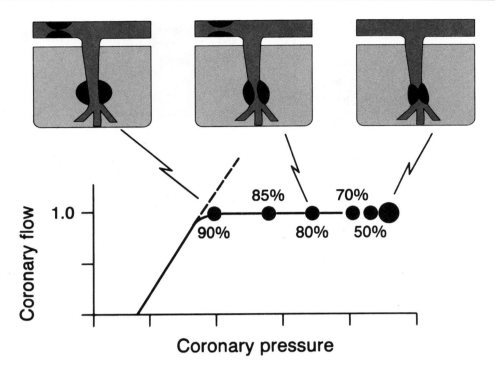

Fig. 5. Effect of stenosis severity on resting flow. (From *J Am Coll Cardiol* 16:763-769, 1990. By permission of the American College of Cardiology.)

- With normally functioning endothelium, acetylcholine stimulates the production and release of nitric oxide, which results in vasodilatation and increased coronary blood flow.

Overload States

Any increase in the workload of the heart increases $M\dot{V}o_2$, whereas coronary blood flow increases in parallel with $M\dot{V}o_2$. Acute pressure overload increases $M\dot{V}o_2$ more than acute volume overload, although most volume overloads include some element of pressure overload.

Chronic overload results in myocardial hypertrophy, with pressure overload causing concentric hypertrophy and volume overload causing eccentric or dilated hypertrophy. The degree of hypertrophy is related to the workload of the heart or $M\dot{V}o_2$ (and, thus, coronary blood flow). Therefore, coronary blood flow per unit of myocardium (milliliters/minute per 100 g) is frequently normal in hypertrophic states. The increased resting flow often results in a decreased coronary flow reserve. In the pressure-overloaded heart, maldistributions in coronary blood flow occur because of increased compressive forces in the subendocardial layer. Even in patients with normal coronary angiographic findings, decreased subendocardial flow can result in angina pectoris and exercise-induced ST-segment depression, a finding often seen in aortic stenosis, hypertrophic cardiomyopathy, and hypertensive left ventricular hypertrophy.

Intravascular Ultrasonography

Although coronary angiography is considered the reference standard for coronary artery imaging, it has several inherent limitations. Angiography is a silhouette technique that detects only arterial disease that indents the luminal column of contrast; it reveals little else about the atherosclerotic plaque. When a normal proximal reference segment does not exist, as in diffuse atherosclerotic disease, it is difficult to detect and to quantitate atherosclerosis with angiography. Angiography also underestimates the amount of atherosclerosis when compensatory arterial enlargement occurs, that is, expansion of the artery at the site of an atherosclerotic plaque. Intimal lesions frequently escape detection by angiography, including angioplasty-induced microfractures, intimal dissections, and mural thrombus. Intravascular ultrasonography improves on the angiographic assessment of coronary arteries by allowing better visualization and quantitation of plaque.

Catheter Technology

Small intracoronary ultrasound catheters provide high-resolution cross-sectional images of the coronary arteries. Catheters as small as 2.6 French, or 0.86 mm (0.33 mm/French size) in diameter, can easily reach the distal segments of the coronary arteries in most patients. The two types of intravascular ultrasound catheters are the mechanical and the solid-state. The mechanical catheters have a rotating ultrasound crystal in the catheter tip. Most systems have a rotating core driven by a motor outside the body. The solid-state catheters have a phased-array or a dynamic-aperture array, with 64 ultrasound crystals arranged around the circumference of the catheter tip, each activated sequentially to produce a rotating ultrasound beam. By using either a mechanical rotating system or a solid-state phased-array system, the ultrasound beam is rotated around the circumference of the catheter at approximately 1,800 rpm. Excellent arterial images can be obtained with both systems; however, only the mechanical systems are subject to nonuniform rotational defects (NURD).

Image Recognition on Intravascular Ultrasonography

The rotating ultrasound beam produces two-dimensional cross-sectional images of the coronary arteries that are analogous to histologic sections (Fig. 6). High-frequency ultrasound transducers (20 to 40 MHz) are used, and they yield high-resolution images. Often, the three layers of the artery (intima, media, and adventitia) can be imaged. Normal intima may not be visible with intracoronary ultrasonography if it is less than 175 µm thick. Luminal area, wall thickness, and plaque size can be measured accurately. Also, the location of the plaque, concentric or eccentric, can be determined. The atherosclerotic plaque can also be characterized according to its fibrous, lipid, and calcium content. Calcium appears bright and echogenic and results in shadowing of the far field (Fig. 7). Lipid plaques typically are sonolucent or dark-appearing. Fibrous plaques have a heterogeneous appearance. Patients with unstable angina more often have soft, lipid-laden plaques. Coronary artery calcification detected with intravascular ultrasonography is predictive of a worse outcome with percutaneous transluminal coronary angioplasty (PTCA) (larger and more frequent dissections) and directional coronary atherectomy (less tissue removed with superficial calcium). An intraluminal thrombus and dissection also can be imaged with intracoronary ultrasonography (Fig. 8).

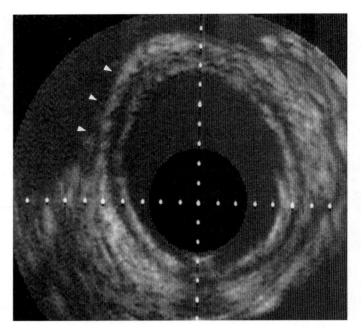

Fig. 6. Intravascular ultrasonographic image of a normal coronary artery. The three mural layers (intima, media, adventitia) are readily apparent. (From *J Am Coll Cardiol* 16:145-154, 1990. By permission of the American College of Cardiology.)

- Coronary artery calcification detected with intravascular ultrasonography is predictive of a worse outcome with PTCA.

Clinical Utility of Intravascular Ultrasonography

Coronary angiography generates an overview of the coronary arterial tree, whereas intravascular ultrasonography provides an in-depth view of a specific portion of the coronary vasculature. Intravascular ultrasonography is useful for detecting mild coronary atherosclerotic disease, assessing an angiographically indeterminate lesion, and assessing coronary stenoses before and after catheter-based coronary artery interventions. Coronary artery disease in transplanted hearts is studied best with intravascular ultrasonography because of the diffuse nature of the disease, which makes it difficult to detect with angiography. Left main coronary artery lesions, which often are difficult to quantitate with angiography because of overlapping branches, diffuse disease, or the ostial location of the disease, are ideally suited for study with intravascular ultrasonography (Fig. 9).

Studies have shown that balloon angioplasty is more likely to result in significant dissection if intravascular ultrasonography reveals heavy arterial calcification. If the calcification is superficial, directional atherectomy will have

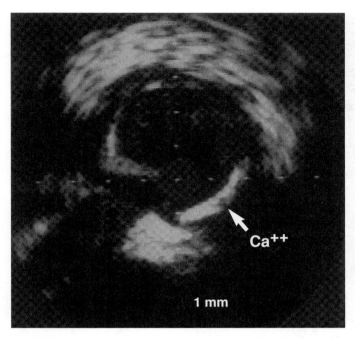

Fig. 7. Intravascular ultrasonographic image of a calcified atherosclerotic plaque adjacent to a septal perforator branch. Calcium (Ca^{++}) is echogenic (bright) and shadows the far field. (From Giuliani ER, Gersh BJ, McGoon MD, Hayes DL, Schaff HV [editors]: *Mayo Clinic Practice of Cardiology*. Third edition. Mosby, 1996, p 1051. By permission of Mayo Foundation.)

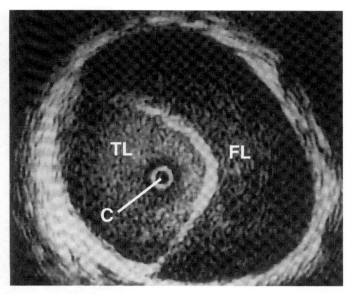

Fig. 8. Intravascular ultrasound image of an aortic dissection. The catheter (C) is in the true lumen (TL). FL, false lumen. (From Giuliani ER, Gersh BJ, McGoon MD, Hayes DL, Schaff HV [editors]: *Mayo Clinic Practice of Cardiology*. Third edition. Mosby, 1996, p 1053. By permission of Mayo Foundation.)

difficulty cutting the tissue, and minimal amounts of plaque will be removed. However, these lesions are ideally suited for treatment with rotational atherectomy (Rotablator). After balloon angioplasty, lesions with certain intravascular ultrasonographic features appear to be at high risk for subsequent restenosis.

The Guidance by Ultrasound Imaging for Decision Endpoints (GUIDE) trial demonstrated that increased plaque burden and smaller lumen areas after PTCA resulted in higher restenosis rates. The Clinical Outcomes with Ultrasound Trial (CLOUT) demonstrated that intravascular ultrasonography could be used to appropriately oversize PTCA balloons, resulting in improved lumen dimensions without an increase in dissection rate. The investigators concluded that the intravascular ultrasonographic demonstration of atheromatous remodeling permits the safe use of balloons traditionally considered oversized, resulting in significantly improved luminal dimensions without increased rates of dissection or ischemic complications. Whether the larger luminal dimensions will translate into improved restenosis rates is not known.

Intravascular ultrasonography also has been used to assist with stent placement. Intravascular ultrasonography can detect stent deployment abnormalities that often are not detected with angiography, including incomplete stent expansion, incomplete stent apposition, articulation site prolapse, and inlet or outlet stenoses. It initially was thought that routine intravascular ultrasonography was needed to detect these abnormalities, thus allowing for safe stenting with aspirin and ticlopidine alone, without warfarin. However, subsequent studies have shown that the routine use of high-pressure balloon inflations within the stent also results in a low subacute stent thrombosis rate when used with aspirin and ticlopidine without the need for routine intravascular ultrasonography. Intravascular ultrasonography has been critical to our understanding of optimal stent deployment techniques. Intravascular ultrasonography has shown that the original deployment techniques (i.e., normal balloon sizes and low deployment pressures) frequently resulted in suboptimal stent deployment, leading to stent thrombosis. The role of intravascular ultrasonography for optimizing stent deployment and reducing restenosis is controversial and is the topic of intense research. Several studies have shown that acute stent dimensions can be improved with intravascular ultrasonographic guidance. Whether these improved dimensions translate into reduced restenosis rates is not known.

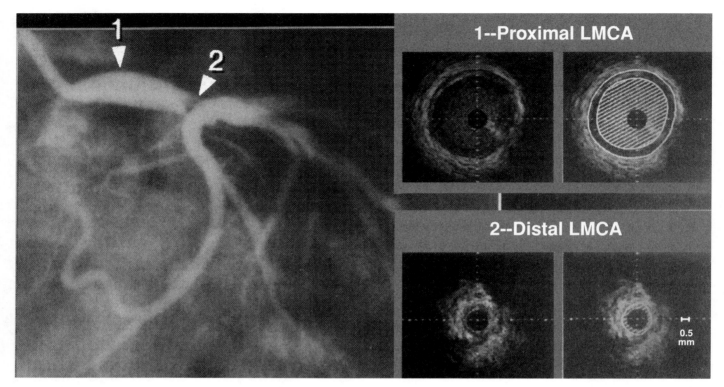

Fig. 9. Coronary angiogram and left main coronary artery (LMCA) intravascular sonograms. *Left*, right anterior oblique view of an indeterminate lesion in the distal LMCA. *Right*, intravascular ultrasound images from the proximal (1) and distal (2) LMCA. The distal LMCA has an 80% area stenosis. Hatched area represents the luminal area. The internal and external elastic membranes are outlined. A, adventitia; M, media. (From *Mayo Clin Proc* 68:134-140, 1993. By permission of Mayo Foundation for Medical Education and Research.)

- Cardiac transplant coronary artery disease is studied best with intravascular ultrasonography because of the diffuse nature of the disease.

- Intravascular ultrasonography can detect stent abnormalities that often are not detected with angiography.

Intracoronary Doppler Measurements

Doppler Technology

Recent developments in Doppler catheter and guidewire technology have made measurement of coronary blood flow velocity in cardiac catheterization laboratories practical, safe, and reproducible. Doppler catheters, 3F (0.99 mm), are placed in the proximal coronary circulation with angioplasty guidewires. The size of the catheters currently available prevents their being placed distal to coronary artery stenoses. Also, because of their large size, they may impair coronary blood flow by occupying a large portion of the coronary lumen.

Doppler guidewires are 0.014 to 0.018 inch (0.36 to 0.46 mm) in diameter and can measure coronary blood flow

velocities distal to coronary artery stenoses without impairing blood flow. Thus, to characterize accurately the effect of the stenosis on blood flow, velocities distal to the stenosis must be measured with a Doppler guidewire. Measurement of proximal flow velocities also includes flow that is shunted away by any branch vessels proximal to the stenosis. Therefore, in response to maximal vasodilatation, the proximal flow velocity response represents an integrated response combining both ischemic and nonischemic myocardium.

The Doppler guidewire is an angioplasty guidewire with a Doppler crystal incorporated in its tip. Ultrasound is emitted from the tip of the guidewire in a pulsed-wave fashion. Between pulses, the frequency of the returning, or reflected, ultrasound is recorded at a specific time after the initial pulse. The specific timing of the received ultrasound determines the depth of the sample volume. In the system currently available, the sample volume depth is 5 mm from the guidewire tip. The returning frequency is analyzed relative to the emitted frequency. The frequency will be shifted upward or downward depending on the velocity of its reflector in the sample volume. In the coronary arteries, erythrocytes act as the primary ultrasound reflectors in the moving stream of blood. The ultrasound emitted from the guidewire tip also diverges from the axis of the guidewire by 12.5 degrees, in effect emitting a spray or cone of ultrasound. The effect allows the ultrasound beam to intersect the center of the stream of flow even if it is placed slightly eccentrically in the artery. Although this may add some error in the Doppler equation, the maximal error should be approximately 10%.

Coronary flow velocity is not equivalent to coronary blood flow. Coronary blood flow can be calculated from measurements of coronary flow velocity and coronary cross-sectional area with the hydraulic equation (flow = velocity x area). Several theoretical issues remain a problem. For example, liquids flowing in a tube have characteristic velocity profiles, with zero velocities at the edges and peak velocities near the center of the stream of flow. The Doppler guidewire measures across the entire velocity profile and records the highest velocity flowing in the velocity profile. If this velocity is used in the hydraulic equation, coronary blood flow will be overestimated because the peak velocity is an over-representation of all the velocities flowing in the parabolic velocity profile. A spatial average velocity is required to measure accurately absolute coronary blood flow. If we assume a true parabolic velocity profile, the average velocity is half the peak velocity and flow can be measured with a modified hydraulic equation (flow = 1/2 velocity x area). With this assumption, coronary blood flow can be measured with a high degree of accuracy. Measurement of absolute flow is not required for coronary flow reserve measurements. If we assume that the flow area remains constant and the shape of the velocity profile does not change, coronary flow reserve simplifies to a ratio of the flow velocities.

- Coronary blood flow can be calculated from measurements of coronary flow velocity and coronary cross-sectional area with the hydraulic equation (flow = velocity x area).

Indications for Intracoronary Doppler Measurements

Indeterminate Coronary Stenoses
Despite a comprehensive angiographic evaluation, coronary stenoses may remain indeterminate. Indeterminate lesions may be angiographically or physiologically indeterminate.

Angiographically indeterminate lesions occur when there are overlapping branches, bifurcations, contrast streaming, or ostial lesions. Physiologically indeterminate lesions are ones that are well seen on angiography but are of intermediate severity, in the 50% to 70% range; they also are called "intermediate lesions." Angiographically indeterminate lesions usually require additional anatomical definition, as with intravascular ultrasonography. Physiologically indeterminate lesions are evaluated best with additional physiologic testing, as with intracoronary Doppler technique. Intermediate lesions can be assessed by the following Doppler measurements:

Diastolic-to-Systolic Velocity Ratio
Normally, coronary blood flow occurs predominantly during diastole, when the effect of myocardial contraction on the small vessels is minimal. During systole, myocardial contraction and vessel compression increase coronary resistance and blood flow is decreased. The diastolic-to-systolic velocity ratio is usually greater than 2. However, when coronary stenosis is present, the effect of systolic contraction on overall coronary resistance is less and the diastolic-to-systolic velocity ratio is reduced. Investigators have used a ratio less than 1.7 to indicate significant stenosis in the left anterior descending coronary artery. Contraction of the normal right ventricle occurs at a lower pressure and has less of an effect on systolic flow. Flow in the normal proximal right coronary artery occurs equally in diastole and systole, and the above criteria are not valid.

Proximal-to-Distal Velocity Ratio
A decrease in velocity distal to a stenosis implies the presence of significant stenosis. For this to be true, there must be a branch vessel proximal to the stenosis to divert flow. In a nonbranching segment such as a bypass graft, the volumetric flow is equivalent above and below the stenosis and, thus, the velocities are equivalent regardless of the severity of the stenosis. If the flow area is reduced, the velocities may be higher distal to the stenosis. Most coronary arterial trees have many branches, and coronary blood flow can be diverted to branches proximal to the stenosis, resulting in a decrease in resting flow distal to the stenosis. A proximal-to-distal velocity ratio greater than 1.7 has been correlated with a pressure gradient greater than 30 mm Hg. However, when compared with adenosine stress sestamibi imaging, the agreement between the Doppler-derived proximal-to-distal velocity ratio and stress imaging was only 48%.

Coronary Flow Reserve

The hallmark of coronary stenosis is its effect on coronary flow augmentation with stress. Coronary flow reserve is defined as the ratio of the maximally augmented coronary flow velocity to resting flow velocity. Previous studies have shown that the normal coronary flow reserve in animals is 3.5 to 5.0. However, with the Doppler guidewire, it has been suggested that normal coronary flow reserve should be 2.0 or greater. The reason for this discrepancy is unclear. However, if a value greater than 2.0 is used for normal coronary flow reserve, there is an 89% agreement between the results of Doppler-derived coronary flow reserve and adenosine stress sestamibi imaging. Doppler-derived coronary flow reserve is influenced by changes in resting myocardial flow, as might occur with post-PTCA reactive hyperemia and changes in heart rate, preload, and contractility.

Chest Pain and Normal Coronary Arteries

The incidence of angiographically normal coronary arteries in patients with angina is approximately 10% to 30%. Although angiography provides an excellent *anatomical* road map of the coronary arteries, it gives little information about the physiology of the coronary circulation. Many of these patients have noncardiac causes of their pain (Table 3), but many others have objective evidence of cardiac ischemia, including exercise- or pacing-induced ST-segment depression, scintigraphic perfusion defects (30% to 40%), stress-induced left ventricular dysfunction (systolic, 70% to 75%; diastolic, 50%), myocardial lactate production (50%), and decreased coronary sinus O_2 saturation (20%). A reduced coronary flow reserve has also been demonstrated in a high percentage of these patients. The mechanism of cardiac ischemia in this syndrome is unclear but centers on two hypotheses: endothelial dysfunction and prearteriolar defect. Prearterioles function as conduit vessels that carry blood from the epicardial vessels to the arterioles. Unlike arterioles, prearterioles are not under metabolic regulation and, thus, do not respond to myocardial ischemia. Endothelial dysfunction may also limit flow during hyperemia, with excessive vasoconstrictor tone. Both exercise and mental stress require normal endothelial cell function for coronary vasodilatation. Both hypotheses may explain chest pain in some patients.

Patients with typical angina and normal coronary arteriograms may benefit from additional assessment of their endothelial function and microcirculation. Such a "functional angiogram" is performed with an intracoronay Doppler guidewire and an infusion catheter. Graded concentrations

Table 3.—Noncardiac Causes of Chest Pain

Psychiatric
    Panic disorders
    Depression
    Anxiety
    Hypochondriasis
Gastrointestinal
    Esophageal spasm
    Peptic ulcer disease
    Gallbladder disease
Musculoskeletal
    Costochondritis
    Herpes zoster
    Arthritis
    Fibromyalgia
Respiratory
    Reactive airways
    Pulmonary embolism
    Pulmonary hypertension
    Pleurisy

of acetylcholine (10^{-6}, 10^{-5}, and 10^{-4} M) are infused selectively into the left anterior descending coronary artery for 3 minutes. Doppler velocities, hemodynamics, and angiographic images are obtained at baseline and with each concentration of acetylcholine as well as with nitroglycerin. A normal response to acetylcholine is vasodilatation. Paradoxical vasoconstriction indicates endothelial dysfunction. Coronary flow reserve is also measured (as described above). Use of vasoactive medications (calcium channel blockers, nitrates, and angiotensin-converting enzyme inhibitors) must be discontinued before the test is performed.

Patients can be stratified into four groups: normal physiology, endothelial cell dysfunction, impaired vasodilatory reserve, and combined defects. Patients with normal results can be reassured. Those with endothelial cell dysfunction can be treated as outlined above, and those with impaired vasodilatory reserve can be treated empirically with conventional antianginal agents, angiotensin-converting enzyme inhibitors, α-blockers, and xanthine derivatives. Imipramine has also been used to treat heightened visceral pain sensitivity.

Although the long-term prognosis for patients with normal coronary angiograms is good, there are subsets (e.g., those with left bundle branch block) with a worse prognosis. Patients with endothelial dysfunction may also be a group that has a poor long-term prognosis, because it is an early stage in the development of atherosclerosis.

Coronary Interventions

The main purpose of coronary interventions is to improve the coronary flow physiology and, thereby, improve symptoms. Physiologic improvement after PTCA has been documented in the Doppler Endpoints Balloon Angioplasty Trial Europe (DEBATE) study. In this study, patients with good angiographic results (quantitative coronary angiography stenosis < 35%) and normal Doppler coronary flow reserve (< 2.5) had a very low incidence of major adverse cardiac events, equivalent to that seen with the optimal stent results achieved in the BENESTENT trial. However, only about 20% of the study population had both angiographic and Doppler coronary flow reserve success. Whether additional treatment for the other patients would improve their outcome is not known. This is an area of active investigation.

Intracoronary Pressure Measurements

In assessing coronary stenosis, the important physiologic component, in addition to flow velocity, is the pressure gradient produced by the stenosis. Translesional pressure gradients were used routinely in the early days of coronary intervention. However, a simple resting translesional pressure gradient alone is inadequate for assessing the physiologic significance of a coronary stenosis. The gradient is highly dependent on aortic pressure, and similar resting gradients can have widely differing implications, given different aortic pressures. Furthermore, a pressure gradient alone gives no information about the ability of the artery to augment flow. The distal coronary pressure during hyperemia can be used to derive the fractional flow reserve, a highly useful measurement of the physiologic effect of a stenosis.

Pressure Guidewires

Pressure guidewires are available, in sizes comparable to those of angioplasty guidewires (0.014 to 0.018 inch), for accurate measurement of distal coronary pressure. Their small size will not cause significant obstruction unless the luminal area is quite small (0.10 to 0.16 mm^2). Pressure gradients can be measured by comparing the aortic pressure (guiding catheter) with the distal coronary pressure (pressure guidewire). The gradient during hyperemia can also be assessed with adenosine (140 µg/kg per minute intravenously or 18 to 30 µg injected into the left coronary artery or 6 to 12

µg injected into the right coronary artery). The gradient equals the difference between the mean pressures in the aorta and the distal coronary segment. Phasic pressures are not used to calculate the gradient, although most of the gradients noted to have a mildly stenotic plaque will be seen during diastole.

Myocardial Fractional Flow Reserve

Myocardial fractional flow reserve (FFR$_{myo}$) is defined as the ratio of the hyperemic flow in a diseased target artery and the hyperemic flow in the same target artery if no lesion is present (Table 1). The FFR$_{myo}$ expresses a given hyperemic flow as a fraction of the normal hyperemic flow and can easily be obtained with distal coronary pressure measurements during hyperemia. It is assumed that during hyperemia small resistance vessels are maximally dilated and constant. In normal coronary arteries, the distal pressure equals the aortic pressure during hyperemia and the FFR$_{myo}$ is equal to 1. Values less than 0.75 indicate physiologically significant lesions and are predictive of abnormal findings on noninvasive function tests.

In contrast to absolute coronary flow reserve measured with Doppler methods, FFR$_{myo}$ is nearly independent of loading factors, and it does not vary appreciably with changing heart rate (atrial pacing), blood pressure (nitroprusside), or contraction (dobutamine) (Table 1).

Indications for Intracoronary Pressure Measurements

Indeterminate Coronary Stenoses

Intermediate severity stenoses in the 40% to 70% diameter stenosis range are often difficult to assess in a cardiac catheterization laboratory. Frequently, these patients are referred for noninvasive functional testing before considering percutaneous coronary revascularization. The lesions can be assessed physiologically with pressure measurements and the FFR$_{myo}$ in a manner similar to Doppler guidewire and the coronary flow reserve. Several studies have examined the correlation between the FFR$_{myo}$ and noninvasive tests of myocardial ischemia. An FFR$_{myo}$ of 0.75 appears to define lesions that produce ischemia on noninvasive tests. That is, if a vessel cannot produce at least 75% of the expected normal hyperemic flow, ischemia will usually result.

Coronary Interventions

Information about the use of pressure measurements after coronary interventions is limited. Preliminary data suggest that after PTCA, patients with a low FFR_{myo} value (from 0.75 to 0.90) and adequate angiographic results (< 30% residual stenosis by quantitative coronary angiography) have an increased restenosis rate compared with patients with higher FFR_{myo} values (> 0.90). A higher FFR_{myo} value reduces the restenosis rate from approximately 30% to 12%, thereby making stenting unnecessary (Table 4). Stents typically have higher FFR_{myo} values after high-pressure inflation.

- Resting pressure gradients are less useful than hyperemic pressure gradients.
- The myocardial fractional flow reserve (FFR_{myo}) is the ratio of the hyperemic flow through an artery with a lesion in question divided by the normal expected hyperemic flow through the same artery if the lesion were not present.
- FFR_{myo} < 0.75 is predictive of ischemia on noninvasive testing.

Table 4.—Use of Myocardial Fractional Flow Reserve (FFR_{myo}) for Assessing Results of Percutaneous Transluminal Coronary Angioplasty (PTCA)

FFR_{myo}	Result and anticipated outcome
< 0.75	Unsuccessful
0.75-0.90	Moderately successful
	Restenosis rate approximately 30%
	Consider additional PTCA or stent
> 0.90	Excellent
	Restenosis rate approximately 12%
	No benefit from stent

Questions

Multiple Choice (choose the one best answer)

1-6. The pressure-flow diagram demonstrates coronary flow both at rest and during maximal hyperemia. Select the one letter on the diagram (a, b, c, d, e, and x) that best describes the coronary pressure-flow relationship in the following conditions (position x represents normal resting flow).

1. Gastrointestinal hemorrhage with mild hypotension
2. A 59-year-old patient at rest with obstructive coronary artery disease and stable exertional angina
3. Maximal exertion in a patient with entirely normal coronary arteries
4. Maximal exertion in a patient with obstructive coronary artery disease
5. Acute myocardial infarction with ST-segment elevation
6. Unstable angina with new ST-segment depression

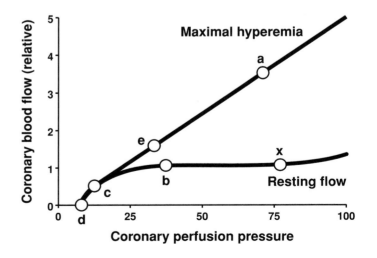

Questions 1-6

7. A 58-year-old man presents with chest pain. Coronary angiography reveals a 60% diameter stenosis in the mid left anterior descending coronary artery. Which of the following intracoronary ultrasonographic or Doppler measurements is the most sensitive for determining if this intermediate stenosis is hemodynamically significant?
   a. Luminal area
   b. Proximal-to-distal velocity ratio
   c. Coronary flow reserve
   d. Percent plaque area in the stenosis
   e. Absolute coronary flow

8. All the following are obligate coronary vasodilators *except*:
   a. Nitroglycerin
   b. Nitric oxide
   c. Acetylcholine
   d. Hypoxia
   e. Hypercapnia

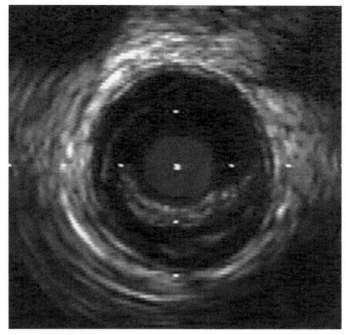

Question 9

9. A 65-year-old man with unstable angina has a high-grade stenosis in the left circumflex artery. The lesion is dilated successfully, with a residual 20% diameter stenosis on angiography and without any appreciable dissection. Intracoronary ultrasonography was performed and images were obtained within the angioplasty site (see figure at right). The intracoronary ultrasonographic image shows:
   a. Calcification
   b. Dissection
   c. Bridging
   d. Thrombus
   e. Hematoma

10. A 62-year-old man with unstable angina has a high-grade stenosis in the proximal left anterior descending artery. Primary stenting was performed, and the stent was post-dilated to 18 atmospheres. Intracoronary ultrasonography was performed to assess adequacy of stent deployment. Images were obtained within the stent and at the proximal and distal stent margins (see figure at right). On the basis of the intracoronary ultrasonographic image, the most appropriate next step would be:
   a. Additional percutaneous transluminal coronary angioplasty (PTCA)
   b. Intracoronary thrombolysis
   c. Directional atherectomy
   d. Stent
   e. Medical therapy

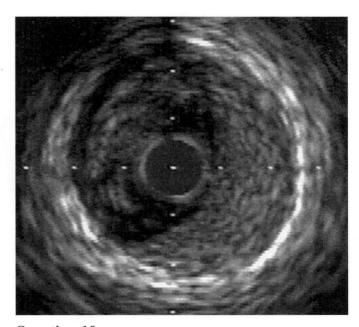

Question 10

11. A 62-year-old man had a stent placed in a complex lesion in the right coronary artery. There was also a 50% to 70% indeterminate lesion in a large obtuse marginal branch. Hyperemic coronary pressures are shown below distal to the stenosis and proximal to the stenosis. On the basis of these tracings, the most appropriate management would be:
    a. PTCA of the obtuse marginal branch
    b. Stent the obtuse marginal branch
    c. GP IIb/IIIa inhibitor
    d. Medical treatment
    e. Intracoronary ultrasonographic evaluation of the lesion

12. All the following have a role in controlling coronary blood flow *except*:
    a. Adenosine
    b. Minimal lumen diameter
    c. Prostaglandins
    d. Nitric oxide
    e. Arterial oxygen saturation

13. The following features may be seen in coronary stenoses that are physiologically significant (i.e., typically result in myocardial ischemia with stress) *except*:
    a. Minimal lumen diameter (angiography) = 0.5 mm
    b. Percent area stenosis (intravascular ultrasonography) = 70%
    c. Coronary flow reserve (Doppler) = 1.6
    d. Myocardial fractional flow reserve (FFR_{myo}) (pressure) = 0.70
    e. Translesional pressure gradient = 50 mm Hg

Match each of the following questions (14 to 18) with the appropriate image (a to e on the facing page)
    14. Normal coronary artery
    15. Coronary dissection
    16. Stent
    17. Soft plaque
    18. Calcified plaque

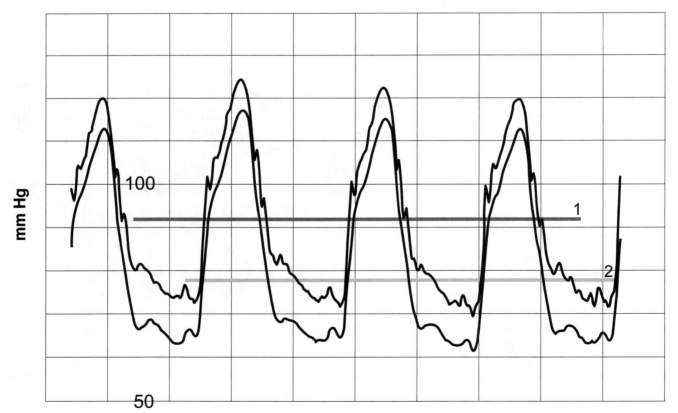

1, Mean arterial pressure; 2, mean distal (transstenotic) pressure.

Question 11

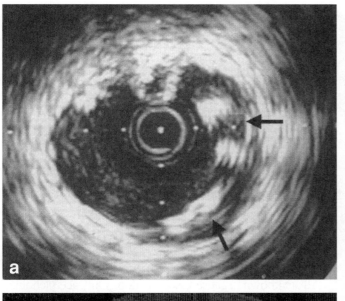

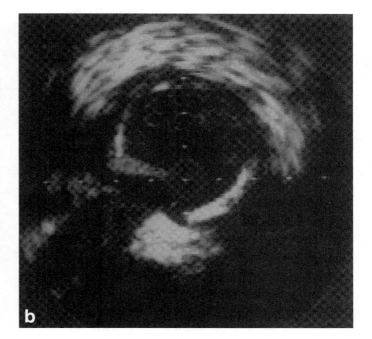

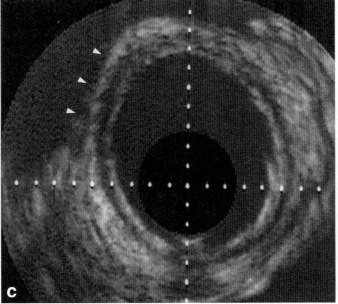

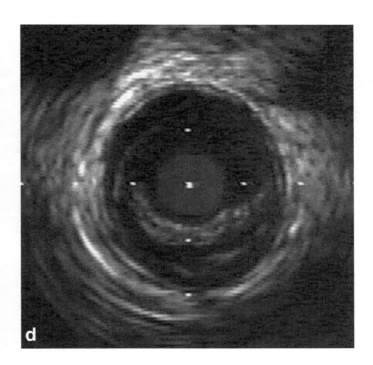

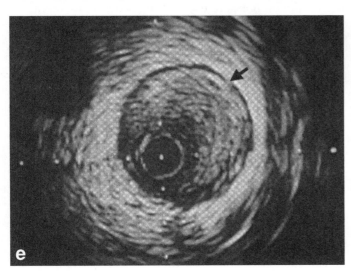

Questions 14-18. *a* and *e* from Pepine CJ, Hill JA, Lambert CR (editors): *Diagnostic and Therapeutic Cardiac Catheterization.* Third edition. Williams & Wilkins, 1998, p 311. By permission of the publisher.

Answers

1. Answer b

The volume loss from the gastrointestinal hemorrhage has decreased aortic pressure and, therefore, coronary perfusion pressure, which is defined as aortic pressure minus right atrial pressure. However, resting flow is maintained because of autoregulation. Severe hypotension could result in a reduction in resting flow and myocardial ischemia.

2. Answer b

The 59-year-old patient with stable angina has normal flow at rest but at a reduced perfusion pressure. The obstructing coronary artery disease results in a reduction in the distal coronary perfusion pressure, similar to that in the patient with the gastrointestinal hemorrhage. Autoregulation maintains resting coronary blood flow. With exertion, coronary blood flow is inadequate, resulting in ischemia and angina because a portion of the microcirculatory reserve was used up to maintain resting flow.

3. Answer a

The increased myocardial demand that occurs during maximal exercise can result in a three- to fivefold increase in coronary blood flow within normal coronary arteries, with minimal changes in perfusion pressure.

4. Answer e

See Answer 2. Resting coronary flow begins at position b with obstructive coronary artery disease. Exercise increases coronary blood flow, further increasing the transstenotic pressure gradient. The result is that maximal hyperemic flow is significantly reduced and is inadequate to prevent ischemia.

5. Answer d

Acute myocardial infarction with ST-segment elevation (injury pattern) implies an acute occlusive thrombus with TIMI 0 flow. In this situation, the distal coronary perfusion pressure would be severely reduced. The presence of collateral flow might limit the reduction in distal perfusion pressure and help maintain coronary blood flow. However, in these situations, an acute injury pattern does not usually develop but rather the patient has a non-Q-wave infarction or may, in fact, be asymptomatic.

6. Answer c

Unstable angina with ST-segment depression (ischemia pattern) implies a reduction in coronary blood flow but not an absence of flow. Again, the distal perfusion pressure is reduced.

7. Answer c

Coronary flow reserve is the most sensitive measurement for determining the hemodynamic significance of an intermediate stenosis. The anatomical measurements made with intracoronary ultrasonography are useful for assessing the quantitative and qualitative aspects of atherosclerosis but are less accurate for determining physiology. Proximal-to-distal velocity ratio is one measurement of lesion severity, but it has been shown to be less accurate than coronary flow reserve.

8. Answer c

All are known to cause vasodilatation. Only acetylcholine can also be a vasoconstrictor if the endothelium is dysfunctional or absent and nitric oxide cannot be produced. In this case, it is not an obligate vasodilator.

9. Answer b

The intracoronary ultrasonographic image shows a dissection in the PTCA site at the 3 to 9 o'clock position. Dissections are seen more commonly with intracoronary ultrasonography than with angiography. There are no bright echoes with shadowing and/or reverberations, so calcium is not likely to be present. The appearance would be atypical for thrombus or hematoma formation. Myocardial bridging should show some elliptical deformation of the vessel during systole.

10. Answer d

The intracoronary ultrasonographic image shows dissection distal to the stent which likely was caused by the high inflation pressure used during stent deployment. A crescentic rim of intramural hematoma at the 1 to 7 o'clock position, which has slightly increased echogenicity, is seen around the circumference of the vessel, with compromise of the vessel lumen. Stenting is needed to manage this complication. Although there is thrombus within the false lumen, thrombolysis has a limited role in treating this entity.

11. Answer d

Mean aortic pressure is 92 mm Hg and mean distal transstenotic pressure is 78 mm Hg during hyperemia, so the myocardial fractional flow reserve is 0.85 and greater than the value (0.75) used to predict an abnormal noninvasive functional test result. A value of 0.85 means that this artery can supply 85% of the normal hyperemic flow.

Intracoronary ultrasonography may show a large amount of atherosclerosis, especially if there has also been compensatory enlargement of the vessel; however, this method is not useful in determining the physiologic significance of the lesion. A GP IIb/IIIa inhibitor may have been indicated for the right coronary artery lesion, but not for the obtuse marginal lesion, "on the basis of these tracings."

12. Answer b

Adenosine, arterial oxygen saturation, prostaglandins, and nitric oxide are all metabolic components that assist in controlling coronary artery blood flow. Minimal lumen diameter of a tight coronary stenosis may affect coronary blood flow but does not have a role in controlling it.

13. Answer b

An $FFR_{myo} < 0.75$ and a Doppler coronary flow reserve < 2.0 would be predictive of abnormal results on noninvasive functional testing. A minimal lumen diameter of 0.5 indicates quite a small lumen, even in a small vessel, and would be expected to be physiologically significant. A resting translesional gradient is much less useful than the hyperemic gradient. Nonetheless, a gradient of 50 mm Hg is very large and would be expected to result in ischemia with stress. However, the percent area stenosis with intravascular ultrasonography is not likely to be predictive of the physiologic behavior of the stenosis. Compensatory enlargement or remodeling at the lesion site may result in an increase in the percent area stenosis even when the lumen area is well preserved and the physiology is normal.

14. Answer c

15. Answer d

16. Answer a

17. Answer e

18. Answer b

Notes

Chapter 55

Applied Anatomy of the Heart and Great Vessels

Joseph G. Murphy, M.D.

This chapter reviews important topics in cardiovascular anatomy that pertain to the practice of clinical cardiology. The format of the chapter is to describe briefly the anatomy followed by the clinical significance in italic type.

Mediastinum

The mediastinum contains, in addition to the heart and great vessels, the distal portion of the trachea, right and left bronchi, esophagus, thymus, autonomic nerves (cardiac and splanchnic, left recurrent laryngeal, and bilateral vagal and phrenic), various small arteries (such as bronchial and esophageal) and veins (such as bronchial, azygos, and hemiazygos), lymph nodes, cardiopulmonary lymphatics, and thoracic duct.

Enlargement of a cardiac chamber or great vessel may displace or compress an adjacent noncardiac structure. An enlarged left atrium may displace the left bronchus superiorly and the esophagus rightward. An aberrant retroesophageal right subclavian artery indents the esophagus posteriorly and may cause dysphagia. Mediastinal neoplasms can compress the atria, superior vena cava, or pulmonary veins.

Pericardium

The pericardium surrounds the heart and consists of fibrous and serous portions. The fibrous pericardium forms a tough outer sac, which envelops the heart and attaches to the great vessels. The ascending aorta, pulmonary artery, terminal 2 to 4 cm of superior vena cava, and short lengths of the pulmonary veins and inferior vena cava are intrapericardial (Fig. 1).

*The fibrous pericardium is inelastic and limits the diastolic distention of the heart during exercise. Cardiac enlargement or **chronic** pericardial effusions, both of which develop slowly, will stretch the fibrous pericardium. However, the fibrous pericardium cannot stretch **acutely**, and the rapid accumulation of as little as 200 mL of fluid may produce fatal cardiac tamponade. Hemopericardium results from perforation of either the heart or the intrapericardial great vessels.*

The serous pericardium is a delicate mesothelial layer that lines the inner aspect of the fibrous pericardium (parietal pericardium) and the outer surface of the heart and intrapericardial great vessels (visceral pericardium). The visceral pericardium, or epicardium, contains the coronary arteries and veins, autonomic nerves, lymphatic channels, and variable amounts of adipose tissue.

Sections of the text in italic type are topics related to pathology.

An atlas illustrating the anatomy of the heart is at the end of the chapter (Plates 1-24).

Modified from Edwards WD: Applied anatomy of the heart. In Giuliani ER, Gersh BJ, McGoon MD, Hayes DL, Schaff HV (editors): *Mayo Clinic Practice of Cardiology.* Third edition. Mosby, 1996, pp 422-489. By permission of Mayo Foundation.

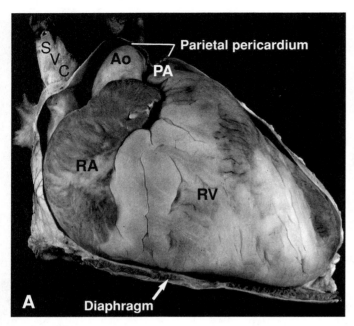

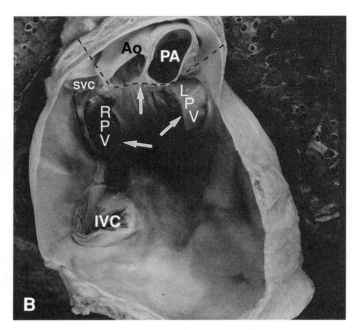

Fig. 1. Parietal pericardium. *A*, Anterior portion of the parietal pericardium has been removed to show the intrapericardial segments of the great arteries and superior vena cava. (Anterior view from 16-year-old boy.) *B*, Heart has been removed from posterior portion of parietal pericardium to show the great vessels, the transverse sinus (*dashed line*), and the oblique sinus (*arrows*). (Anterior view from 13-year-old boy.) (See Appendix at end of chapter for abbreviations.) (*A* from *Mayo Clin Proc* 56:479-497, 1981. By permission of Mayo Foundation.)

In obese subjects, excessive epicardial depot fat may encase the heart, but because pericardial fat is liquid at body temperature, cardiac motion is generally unhindered.

Focal epicardial fibrosis along the anterior right ventricle or posterobasal left ventricle (so-called soldiers' patches) may result from old pericarditis or perhaps from the trauma of an enlarged heart's impact against the sternum or calcified descending thoracic aorta.

Between the great arteries (aorta and pulmonary artery) and the atria is a tunnel-like transverse sinus (Fig. 1). Posteriorly, the pericardial reflection forms an inverted U-shaped cul-de-sac known as the oblique sinus. The ligament of Marshall is a pericardial fold that contains the embryonic remnants of the left superior vena cava.

A sequential saphenous vein bypass graft to the left coronary system may be positioned posteriorly through the transverse sinus. A persistent left superior vena cava will occupy the expected site of the ligament of Marshall, along the junction between the appendage and body of the left atrium.

Between the parietal and visceral layers of the serous pericardium is the pericardial cavity, which normally contains 10 to 20 mL of serous fluid that allows the tissue surfaces to glide over each other with minimal friction.

Thick and roughened surfaces associated with fibrinous pericarditis lead to an auscultatory friction rub, and

organization of such an exudate may result in fibrous adhesions between the epicardium and the parietal pericardium. Focal adhesions are usually unimportant, but occasionally they may allow the accumulation of loculated fluid or, rarely, tamponade of an individual cardiac chamber, usually the right ventricle. After cardiac surgery, the opened pericardial cavity may become sealed again if the parietal pericardium adheres to the sternum; in this setting, the raw pericardial surfaces, which are lined by fibrovascular granulation tissue, may ooze enough blood to cause cardiac tamponade.

Densely fibrotic adhesions, with or without calcification, can hinder cardiac motion and may restrict cardiac filling. The pericardium is thickened in subjects with chronic constriction but not necessarily so in persons with constriction that develops relatively rapidly. In the setting of constrictive pericarditis, surgical excision of only the anterior pericardium (between the phrenic nerves) is often inadequate, because the remaining pericardium surrounds enough of the heart to maintain constriction.

Most postoperative pericardial adhesions are usually functionally unimportant, but they may obscure the location of the coronary arteries at subsequent cardiac operation.

Other pericardial conditions include congenital cysts or diverticula of the pericardium, or the parietal pericardium may be focally deficient or absent.

- The fibrous pericardium cannot adequately stretch acutely, and the rapid accumulation of as little as 200 mL of fluid may produce fatal cardiac tamponade.
- A sequential saphenous vein bypass graft to the left coronary system may be positioned posteriorly through the transverse sinus.

Great Veins

Bilaterally, the subclavian and internal jugular veins merge to form bilateral innominate (or brachiocephalic) veins. The latter then join to form the superior vena cava (or superior caval vein) (Fig. 2).

Superior Vena Cava

The right internal jugular vein, right innominate vein, and superior vena cava afford a relatively straight intravascular route to the right atrium and tricuspid orifice. Accordingly, this route may be used for passage of a stiff endomyocardial bioptome across the tricuspid valve and into the right ventricular apex to obtain a cardiac biopsy specimen. Similarly, both temporary and permanent transvenous pacemaker leads are inserted via either the subclavian or the internal jugular vein and are threaded into the right ventricular apex.

Catheters and pacemakers within the innominate veins and superior vena cava become partially coated with thrombus and may be associated with thrombotic venous obstruction, pulmonary thromboembolism, or secondary infection. Mediastinal neoplasms, fibrosis, and aortic aneurysms may compress the thin-walled veins and result in the superior vena caval syndrome.

Inferior Vena Cava

The inferior vena cava receives systemic venous drainage from the legs and retroperitoneal viscera and, at the level of the liver, from the intra-abdominal systemic venous drainage (portal circulation) via the hepatic veins.

The inferior vena cava, which is retroperitoneal, may become trapped and compressed between the vertebral column posteriorly and either an adjacent retroperitoneal structure (for example, an abdominal aortic aneurysm) or an intraperitoneal structure (for example, a neoplasm) and thereby produce the inferior vena caval syndrome.

Venous thrombi in the lower extremities may extend into the inferior vena cava or may become dislodged and embolize to the right heart and pulmonary circulation.

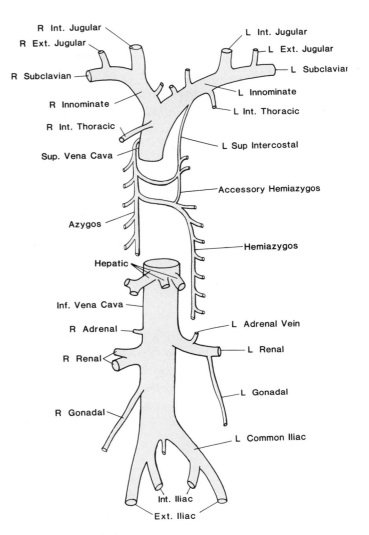

Fig. 2. Systemic veins, excluding the portal circulation. (See Appendix at end of chapter for abbreviations.)

Renal cell carcinomas may extend intravascularly within the renal veins and inferior vena cava and may even form tethered intracavitary right-sided cardiac masses. Hepatocellular carcinomas often involve the hepatic veins and occasionally may enter the suprahepatic inferior vena cava or right atrium.

The superior and inferior pulmonary veins from each lung enter the left atrium. The proximal 1 to 3 cm of the pulmonary veins contain cardiac muscle within the media and may thereby function like sphincters during atrial systole as well as when significant mitral valve disease exists.

The thin-walled and low-pressure pulmonary veins may be compressed extrinsically by mediastinal neoplasms or fibrosis. Rarely, a primary neoplasm may cause luminal obstruction in the major pulmonary veins.

Congenital Abnormalities of the Venous System

Congenital anomalies of the systemic veins include a persistent left superior vena cava (with or without a left innominate vein) joining the coronary sinus or, rarely, the left atrium; an unroofed or absent coronary sinus; a large right sinus venosus valve (so-called cor triatriatum dexter); azygos continuity of the inferior vena cava; and bilateral subrenal inferior venae cavae.

Anomalous Venous Connection

In total anomalous pulmonary venous connection, the confluence of pulmonary veins does not join the left atrium but rather maintains connection to derivatives of the cardinal or umbilicovitelline veins, such as the left innominate vein, coronary sinus, or ductus venosus. An interatrial communication must also be present.

In partial anomalous pulmonary venous connection, only some veins (usually from the right lung) lack left atrial connections. Connection of the right pulmonary veins to the right atrium commonly accompanies sinus venosus atrial septal defects, whereas connection of these veins to the suprahepatic inferior vena cava is usually part of the scimitar syndrome.

Cor Triatriatum

Cor triatriatum (sinistrum) results when the junction between common pulmonary vein and left atrium is stenotic. A fenestrated membranous or muscular shelf subdivides the left atrium into a posterosuperior chamber, which receives the pulmonary veins, and an anteroinferior chamber, which contains the atrial appendage and mitral orifice.

- Mediastinal neoplasms, fibrosis, and aortic aneurysms may compress the thin-walled veins and result in the superior vena caval syndrome.
- The inferior vena cava may become trapped and compressed between the vertebral column posteriorly and either an adjacent retroperitoneal structure or an intraperitoneal structure and thereby produce the inferior vena caval syndrome.
- The thin-walled low-pressure pulmonary veins may be compressed extrinsically by mediastinal neoplasms or fibrosis.
- Connection of one (usually the upper) or both right pulmonary veins to the right atrium commonly accompanies sinus venosus atrial septal defects.

Cardiac Chambers

Right Atrium

The right atrium, along with the superior vena cava, forms the right lateral border of the frontal chest radiographic cardiac silhouette. It receives the systemic venous return from the superior and inferior venae cavae and receives most of the coronary venous return via the coronary sinus and numerous small thebesian veins. The ostium of the inferior vena cava is bordered anteriorly by a crescentic eustachian valve, which may be large and fenestrated and form a so-called Chiari net. The coronary sinus ostium is partly shielded by a fenestrated thebesian valve. The right atrium consists of a free wall and septum.

Its free wall has a smooth-walled posterior portion, which receives the caval and coronary sinus blood flow, and a muscular anterolateral portion, which contains ridge-like pectinate muscles and a large pyramid-shaped appendage. Separating the two regions is a prominent C-shaped muscle bundle, the crista terminalis (or terminal crest). The right atrial appendage abuts the right aortic sinus and overlies the proximal right coronary artery.

The thickness of the right atrial free wall varies considerably. The atrial wall between the pectinate muscles is paper-thin and can be perforated by a stiff catheter.

When atrial enlargement and stasis to blood flow occur, mural thrombi may form within the recesses between the pectinate muscles, particularly in the atrial appendage. Indwelling cardiac catheters or pacemaker wires tend to injure the endocardium at the cavoatrial junction and are often associated with shallow linear mural thrombi. An atrial pacing lead can be inserted into the muscle bundles within the appendage.

Atrial Septum

The atrial septum has interatrial and atrioventricular components (Fig. 3). The interatrial portion contains the fossa ovalis (or oval fossa), which includes an arch-shaped outer muscular rim (the limbus or limb) and a central fibrous membrane (the valve). In contrast to the fossa ovalis, the foramen ovale (or oval foramen, which is patent throughout fetal life) represents a potential interatrial passageway, which courses between the anterosuperior limbic rim and the valve of the fossa ovalis and then through the natural valvular perforation (ostium secundum, or second ostium) into the left atrium. In approximately two-thirds of subjects, the foramen ovale closes anatomically during the first year of life as the valve of the fossa ovalis becomes permanently sealed

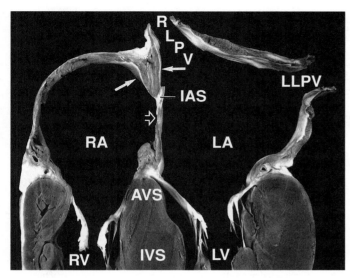

Fig. 3. Atrial anatomy. The atrioventricular septum lies anterior to the inter-atrial septum and posterior to the interventricular septum; note also the infolded nature of the limbus (*arrows*) and the relative thinness of the valve of the fossa ovalis (*open arrow*). (Four-chamber view from 15-year-old boy.) (See Appendix at end of chapter for abbreviations.)

to the limbus. In the remaining third, this flap-valve closes functionally only when left atrial pressure exceeds right atrial pressure; this constitutes a so-called valvular-competent patent foramen ovale.

Through a patent foramen ovale, systemic venous emboli may enter the systemic arterial circulation. Such paradoxic emboli may be thrombotic (e.g., from the legs) or non-thrombotic (e.g., air emboli).

Pronounced atrial dilatation may so stretch the atrial septum that the limbus no longer covers the ostium secundum in the valve of the fossa ovalis. As a result, interatrial shunting may occur across the valvular-incompetent patent foramen ovale (acquired atrial septal defect). In some subjects, aneurysms of the valve of the fossa ovalis may develop and may undulate during the cardiac cycle. Atrial dilatation also stimulates the release of natriuretic peptide.

The atrioventricular component of the atrial septum, which separates the right atrium from the left ventricle, is primarily muscular but also has a small fibrous component (the atrioventricular portion of the membranous septum).

Triangle of Koch

The atrioventricular septum corresponds to the triangle of Koch, an important anatomical landmark that contains the atrioventricular node and bundle; it is bound by the septal tricuspid annulus, the coronary sinus ostium, and the tendon of Todaro.

Tendon of Todaro

The tendon of Todaro is a subendocardial fibrous cord that extends from the eustachian-thebesian valvular commissure to the anteroseptal tricuspid commissure (at the membranous septum); it very roughly corresponds to the level of the mitral annulus.

The thickness of the atrial septum varies considerably. The valve of the fossa ovalis is a paper-thin translucent membrane at birth but becomes more fibrotic with time and may achieve a thickness of 1 to 2 mm. The limbus of the fossa ovalis ranges from 4 to 8 mm in thickness; however, lipomatous hypertrophy may produce a bulging mass more than three times this thickness. The muscular atrioventricular septum forms the summit of the ventricular septum and may range from 5 to 10 mm in thickness; this may be greatly increased in the setting of hypertrophic cardiomyopathy or concentric left ventricular hypertrophy. The membranous septum generally is less than 1 mm thick.

Left Atrium

The left atrium, a posterior midline chamber, receives pulmonary venous blood and expels it across the mitral orifice and into the left ventricle. The esophagus and descending thoracic aorta abut the left atrial wall. Thus, the left atrium, atrial septum, and mitral valve are particularly well visualized with transesophageal echocardiography. The body of the left atrium does not contribute to the frontal cardiac silhouette; however, the left atrial appendage, when enlarged, may form the portion of the left cardiac border between the left ventricle and the pulmonary trunk. Normally the appendage, shaped like a windsock, abuts the pulmonary artery and overlies the bifurcation of the left main coronary artery.

With chronic obstruction to left atrial emptying (for example, rheumatic mitral stenosis), the dilated left atrium may shift the atrial septum rightward and in severe cases may actually form the right cardiac border roentgeno-graphically. Moreover, the esophagus can be shifted rightward, and the left bronchus may be elevated. Mural thrombi often develop within the atrial appendage or, less commonly, the atrial body, and in severe cases can virtually fill the chamber except for small channels leading from the pulmonary veins to the mitral orifice. In contrast to left atrial mural thrombi, which tend to involve the free wall, most myxomas arise from the left side of the atrial septum.

Comparison of Atria

The right atrial free wall contains a crista terminalis and pectinate muscles, whereas the left atrial free wall has neither.

The right atrial appendage is large and pyramidal, in contrast to the windsock-like left atrial appendage. Finally, the atrial septum is characterized by the fossa ovalis on the right side and by the ostium secundum on the left.

Owing to hemodynamic streaming within the right atrium during intrauterine life, superior vena caval blood is directed toward the tricuspid orifice, and inferior vena caval blood, carrying well-oxygenated placental blood, is directed by the eustachian valve toward the foramen ovale. As a result, the most-well-oxygenated blood in the fetal circulation is directed, via the left heart, to the coronary arteries, the upper extremities, and the brain. Even postnatally, the superior vena cava maintains its orientation toward the tricuspid annulus, and the inferior vena cava maintains its orientation toward the atrial septum (Fig. 4).

Consequently, an endomyocardial biopsy specimen of the right ventricular apex is much more easily obtained via a superior vena caval approach than an inferior vena caval approach. In contrast, the passage of a catheter from the right atrium into the left atrium via the foramen ovale is much more easily performed via an inferior vena caval approach. In subjects in whom the foramen ovale is anatomically sealed, the valve of the fossa ovalis may be intentionally perforated (transseptal approach); however, this membrane becomes thicker and more fibrotic with age.

Atrial Septal Defect

A secundum atrial septal defect involves the fossa ovalis region of the interatrial septum. It is the most common form of atrial septal defect and often is an isolated anomaly.

A primum atrial septal defect involves the atrioventricular septum and represents a malformation of the endocardial cushions; it is almost invariably associated with mitral and tricuspid abnormalities, particularly a cleft in the anterior mitral leaflet.

A sinus venosus atrial septal defect involves the posterior aspect of the atrial septum and is usually associated with anomalous right atrial connection of the right pulmonary veins. A coronary sinus atrial septal defect is usually associated with an absent (unroofed) coronary sinus and connection of the left superior vena cava to the left atrium.

- Most myxomas arise from the left side of the atrial septum.
- A secundum atrial septal defect involves the fossa ovalis region of the interatrial septum.
- A coronary sinus atrial septal defect is usually associated

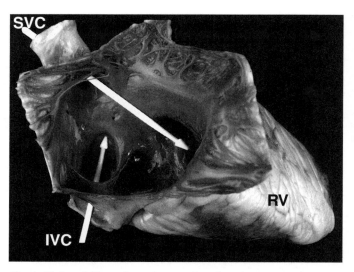

Fig. 4. Right atrial hemodynamic streaming. Superior vena caval blood is directed toward the tricuspid orifice, and inferior vena caval blood is directed toward the fossa ovalis. (Opened right atrium from 31-year-old man.) (See Appendix at end of chapter for abbreviations.) (From Edwards WD: Anatomy of the cardiovascular system. In *Clinical Medicine*. Vol. 6, Chap 1. Spittell JA Jr [editor]. Harper & Row Publishers, 1984, p 8. By permission of Lippincott-Raven Publishers.)

with an absent coronary sinus and connection of the left superior vena cava to the left atrium.

Right Ventricle

The right ventricle does not contribute to the borders of the frontal cardiac silhouette roentgenographically. It is crescent-shaped in short-axis and triangular-shaped when viewed in long-axis.

Conditions, such as pulmonary hypertension, that impose a pressure overload on the right ventricle cause straightening of the ventricular septum such that both ventricles attain a D shape on cross-section. In extreme cases, such as Ebstein's anomaly or total anomalous pulmonary venous connection, leftward bowing of the ventricular septum may result not only in a circular right ventricle and crescentic left ventricle but also in possible obstruction of the left ventricular outflow tract.

The right ventricular chamber consists of three regions— inlet, trabecular, and outlet. The inlet region receives the tricuspid valve and its cordal and papillary muscle attachments. A complex meshwork of muscle bundles characterizes the anteroapical trabecular region. In contrast, the outlet region is smoother-walled and is also known as the infundibulum, conus, or right ventricular outflow tract. Along the outflow tract, an arch of muscle separates the tricuspid and pulmonary valves. The arch consists of a parietal band, outlet septum, and septal band (Fig. 5), known collectively as the crista supraventricularis (supraventricular crest).

During right ventricular endomyocardial biopsy, the bioptome is directed septally, not only to avoid injury to the cardiac conduction system and tricuspid apparatus but also to prevent possible perforation of the relatively thin free wall. Tissue is more often procured from the meshwork of apical trabeculations than from the septal surface per se. When permanent transvenous pacemaker electrodes are inserted into the right ventricle, the apical trabeculations trap the tined tip and thereby prevent dislodgment.

During vigorous cardiopulmonary resuscitation in which ribs are fractured, the jagged-edged bones may be forced through the parietal pericardium, anteriorly, and may lacerate an epicardial coronary artery or may perforate the right atrial or ventricular free wall. Furthermore, if cardiopulmonary resuscitation is exerted along the midsternum rather than the xiphoid area, the right ventricular outflow tract may be compressed and this can result in high right ventricular pressure, which may produce apical rupture.

Left Ventricle

The left ventricle forms the left border of the frontal cardiac silhouette roentgenographically. It is circular in short-axis views and is approximated in three dimensions by a truncated ellipsoid.

Pressure Overload

Conditions such as aortic stenosis and chronic hypertension, which impose a pressure overload on the left ventricle, induce concentric left ventricular hypertrophy without appreciable dilatation. Although the short-axis chamber diameter does not increase significantly, the wall thickness generally increases 25% to 75%, and the heart weight may double or triple.

Volume Overload

Disorders that impose a volume overload on the left ventricle, such as chronic aortic or mitral regurgitation or dilated cardiomyopathy, are attended not only by hypertrophy but also by chamber dilatation. They thereby produce a globoid heart with increased base-apex and short-axis dimensions. Although the heart weight may double or triple, the left ventricular wall thickness generally remains within the normal range because of the thinning effect of dilatation. Accordingly, when the left ventricle is dilated, wall thickness cannot be used as a reliable indicator of hypertrophy (Fig. 6). The term "volume hypertrophy" is favored in this situation. Hypertrophy, with or without chamber dilatation, decreases myocardial compliance and impairs diastolic filling.

Like the right ventricle, the left ventricle can be divided into inlet, apical, and outlet regions. The inlet receives the mitral valve apparatus, the apex contains fine trabeculations, and the outlet is angled away from the remainder of

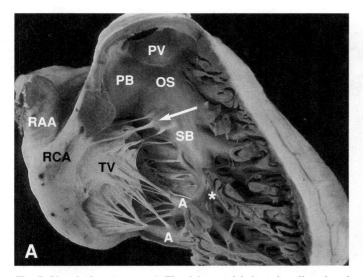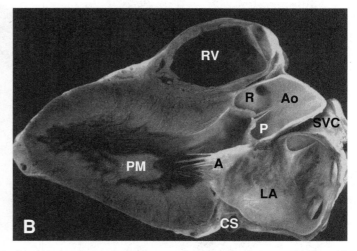

Fig. 5. Ventricular anatomy. *A*, The right ventricle has a heavily trabeculated anteroapical region and exhibits muscular separation between the tricuspid and pulmonary valves. *Moderator band; *arrow*, papillary muscle of the conus. *B*, In contrast, the left ventricle (shown in long-axis) has fine apical trabeculations and is characterized by direct continuity between the mitral and aortic valves. (See Appendix at end of chapter for abbreviations.) (*A*, from Schapira JN, Charuzi Y, Davidson RM [editors]: *Two-Dimensional Echocardiography*. Williams & Wilkins Company, 1982, p 131. By permission of Mayo Foundation.)

the chamber. Inflow and outflow tracts are separated by the anterior mitral leaflet, which forms an intracavitary curtain between the two (Fig. 5).

The anterior mitral leaflet is also in direct contact, at its annulus, with the left and posterior aortic valve cusps. For comparison, the membranous septum abuts the right and posterior aortic cusps, and the outlet septum lies beneath the right and left aortic cusps.

For practical purposes, the base-apex length of the left ventricle is divided into thirds—basal (corresponding to the mitral leaflets and tendinous cords), midventricular (corresponding to the mitral papillary muscles), and apical levels. Each level is then further divided into segments, thus forming the basis for regional analysis of the left ventricle (for example, the evaluation of regional wall motion abnormalities) (Fig. 7 and Table 1).

Hypertrophic cardiomyopathy is characterized by asymmetric (nonconcentric) left ventricular hypertrophy that disproportionately involves the septum. Cardiac amyloid may mimic hypertrophic cardiomyopathy.

In the normal elderly heart, left ventricular geometry is altered (septum is more sigmoid in shape) and in concert with mild fibrosis and calcification of the aortic and mitral valves may contribute to the low-grade systolic ejection murmurs that are so common in the elderly. With advancing age, the aortic annulus dilates appreciably and tilts rightward and less posteriorly, thereby altering the shape and direction of the left ventricular outflow tract, which may simulate hypertrophic cardiomyopathy.

Left ventricular trabeculae carneae are small, and permanent apical entrapment of a tined transvenous pacemaker electrode is difficult to achieve and may necessitate the placement of epicardial electrodes (for example, in patients with corrected transposition of the great arteries or with complete transposition of the great arteries and a previous Mustard or Senning operation).

When left ventricular endomyocardial biopsy is performed, care must be taken not to injure the mitral apparatus or left bundle branch and not to perforate the apex.

In some persons, apical or anteroseptal trabeculae carneae may form a prominent spongy meshwork that may be misinterpreted as apical mural thrombus on imaging studies.

Comparison of Ventricles

Normally, left ventricular wall thickness is three to four times that of the right ventricle. In short-axis, the left ventricle is circular and the right is crescentic. Whereas the tricuspid and pulmonary valves are separated from one another, the mitral and aortic valves are in direct continuity. The right ventricular apex is much more heavily trabeculated than the left.

By two-dimensional echocardiography, ventricular morphology is best inferred by the morphology of the atrioventricular valves, particularly by differences in their annular levels at the cardiac crux (Fig. 3).

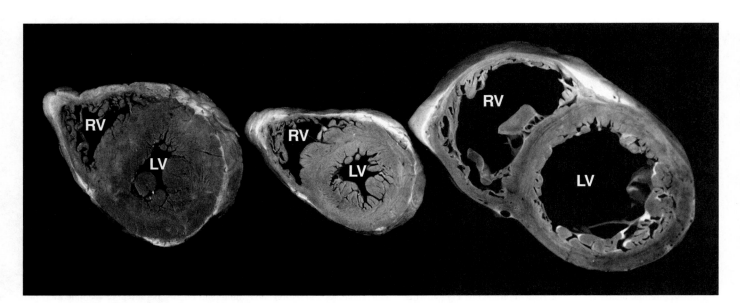

Fig. 6. Compared with a normal heart (center), the heart with pressure hypertrophy (left) has a thick left ventricular wall, but the heart with volume hypertrophy (right) has a normal wall thickness. Both hypertrophied hearts weighed more than twice normal. (Left, from 64-year-old man with aortic stenosis. Right, from 50-year-old man with idiopathic dilated cardiomyopathy.) (See Appendix at end of chapter for abbreviations.)

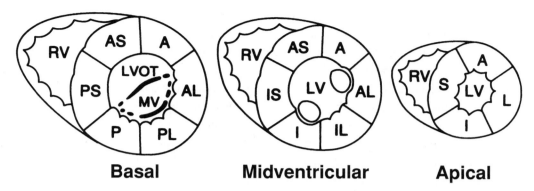

Fig. 7. Regional analysis of the left ventricle. Short-axis views show the recommended 16-segment system. (See Appendix at end of chapter for abbreviations.)

Ventricular Septal Defect

The most common ventricular septal defect, either isolated or associated with other cardiac anomalies, is the membranous (perimembranous) type, which involves the membranous septum. An infundibular (outlet; supracristal; subarterial) ventricular septal defect is commonly encountered in tetralogy of Fallot and truncus arteriosus. A malalignment ventricular septal defect occurs when one of the great arteries overrides the septum and attains biventricular origin, or both great arteries arise from one ventricle. Muscular defects involve the muscular septum and can be solitary or multiple (so-called Swiss cheese septum). A defect of the atrioventricular septum is considered to be an atrioventricular canal defect, and straddling of an atrioventricular valve most commonly occurs across a defect of this type.

Tetralogy of Fallot

Within the spectrum of cyanotic congenital heart disease is a group of anomalies that share in common a maldevelopment of the conotruncal septum. Tetralogy of Fallot, the most common anomaly in this group, results from displacement of the infundibular septum and is characterized by a large malalignment ventricular septal defect, an overriding aorta, and variable degrees of infundibular and valvular pulmonary stenosis. When the pulmonary valve is atretic, pulmonary blood flow may come from the ductus arteriosus or systemic collateral arteries.

Transposition of the Great Arteries

Complete transposition of the great arteries is associated with abnormal conotruncal septation and parallel rather than intertwined great arteries, such that the aorta arises from the right ventricle and the pulmonary artery emanates from the left ventricle; a ventricular septal defect is present in about one-third of cases.

Truncus Arteriosus

Truncus arteriosus implies absent conotruncal septation and is characterized by a single arterial trunk from which the aorta, pulmonary arteries, and coronary arteries arise; the ventricular septal defect is of membranous or infundibular type.

Double-Outlet Right Ventricle

Double-outlet right ventricle is characterized by the origin of both great arteries from the right ventricle, a malalignment ventricular septal defect, and infundibular septal displacement that differs from the type observed in tetralogy.

Myocyte Response to Injury

Myocardial cells are by volume one-half contractile elements and one-third mitochondria. They are exquisitely sensitive to oxygen deprivation, and ischemia represents the most common form of myocardial injury. Other injurious agents include viruses, chemicals, and excessive cardiac workload (volume or pressure).

Table 1.—Percentage of Regional Left Ventricular (LV) Mass

Level	% LV volume per segment	No. of segments	Total, %
Basal	7.2	6	43
Middle	6.0	6	36
Apical	5.3	4	21

The heart has only a limited response to stress or injury. Adaptive responses include hypertrophy and dilatation, whereas sublethal cellular injury is characterized by various degenerative changes. Necrosis is the histologic hallmark of lethal cellular injury, and it elicits an inflammatory response with subsequent healing by scar formation.

Hypertrophy of cardiac muscle cells is accompanied by degenerative changes, an increase in interstitial collagen, and a decrease in ventricular compliance. In dilated hearts, hypertrophied myocytes are also stretched, but with relatively normal diameters. In dilated hearts, the best histologic indicators of hypertrophy are nuclear alterations.

Acute myocardial ischemia is characterized by intense sarcoplasmic staining with eosin dyes, prominent sarcoplasmic contraction bands, and, occasionally, stretched and wavy myocardial cells. When ischemic cells are irreversibly injured, the changes of coagulative necrosis appear. Nuclei fade away (karyolysis) or fragment (karyorrhexis), and the sarcoplasm develops a glassy homogeneous appearance, although in many cases the cross-striations remain intact for several days. Necrotic myocardium elicits an inflammatory infiltrate of neutrophils and macrophages, which serves histologically to differentiate acute infarction from acute ischemia. Because myocardial cells cannot replicate, healing is by organization, with scar formation.

Cardiac Valves

Atrioventricular Valves

The right (tricuspid) and left (mitral) atrioventricular valves have five components, three of which form the valvular apparatus (annulus, leaflets, commissures) and two of which form the tensor apparatus (chordae tendineae and papillary muscles).

Valve Annulus

The annulus of each atrioventricular valve is saddle-shaped. As part of the fibrous cardiac skeleton at the base of the heart, each annulus electrically insulates atrium from ventricle. Since the tricuspid annulus is an incomplete fibrous ring, loose connective tissue maintains insulation at the points of fibrous discontinuity. The mitral annulus, in contrast, constitutes a continuous ring of fibrous tissue.

Valve Leaflet

The valve leaflets are delicate fibrous tissue flaps that close the anatomical valvular orifice during ventricular systole (Fig. 8). The leading edge of each leaflet is its free edge, and its serrated appearance results from direct cordal insertions into this border. The closing edge, in contrast, represents a slightly thickened nodular ridge several millimeters above the free edge. When the valve closes, apposing leaflets contact one another along their closing edges, and interdigitation of these nodular ridges ensures a competent seal. Each leaflet comprises two major layers—namely, the fibrosa, which forms the strong structural backbone of the valve, and the spongiosa, which acts as a shock absorber along the atrial surface, particularly at the closing edge (rough zone), where one leaflet coapts with an adjacent leaflet.

Chordae Tendineae

The chordae tendineae are strong, fibrous tendinous cords that act as guidewires to anchor and support the leaflets. They restrict excessive valvular excursion during ventricular systole and thereby prevent valvular prolapse into the atria. Most tendinous cords branch one or more times, so that generally more than 100 cords insert into the free edge of each atrioventricular valve. By virtue of these numerous cordal insertions, the force of systolic ventricular blood is evenly distributed throughout the undersurface of each leaflet.

Papillary Muscles

The papillary muscles, which may have multiple heads, are conical mounds of ventricular muscle that receive the majority of the tendinous cords. Because of their position directly beneath a commissure, each papillary muscle receives cords from two adjacent leaflets. As a result, papillary muscle contraction tends to pull the two leaflets toward each other and thereby facilitates valve closure.

In the elderly, mild mitral annular dilatation may occur, with or without atrial dilatation. Leaflets become thicker, with increasing nodularity of the rough zone and with mild hooding deformity of the entire leaflet. Contributing to the latter is a decrease in ventricular base-apex length which makes the thickened cords appear relatively longer than necessary, thus simulating mitral valve prolapse.

Tricuspid Valve

The plane of the tricuspid annulus faces toward the right ventricular apex. Along the free wall, the annulus inserts into the atrioventricular junction, whereas along the septum, it separates the atrioventricular and interventricular portions of the septum.

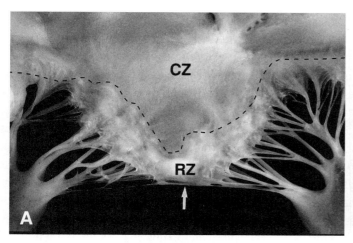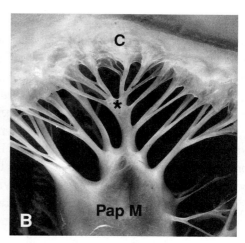

Fig. 8. Components of an atrioventricular valve (from the mitral valve of an 8-year-old girl). *A*, Each leaflet has a large clear zone (*CZ*) and a smaller rough zone (*RZ*) between its free edge (*arrow*) and closing edge (*dotted line*). *B*, Each commissure (*C*) separates two leaflets and overlies a papillary muscle (*Pap M*); a fan-like commissural tendinous cord (***) connects the tip of the papillary muscle to the commissure.

In living subjects, the tricuspid annular circumference varies with the cardiac cycle: it is maximum during ventricular diastole (about 11 cm^2) and decreases by about 30% during ventricular systole. The reduction in area is due to contraction of the underlying basal right ventricular myocardium, since the incomplete tricuspid annulus cannot adequately constrict by itself.

The three tricuspid leaflets are not always well separated from one another. The septal (medial) leaflet lies parallel to the ventricular septum, and the posterior (inferior) leaflet lies parallel to the diaphragmatic aspect of the right ventricular free wall. In contrast, the anterior (anterosuperior) tricuspid leaflet forms a large sail-like intracavitary curtain that partially separates the inflow tract from the outflow tract.

Because of differences in leaflet size and cordal length, the excursion of the posterior and septal leaflets is less than that of the anterior leaflet. In the setting of annular dilatation, leaflet excursion is inadequate to effect central coaptation, and valvular incompetence results. Because the tricuspid annulus is incomplete, and because the basal right ventricular myocardium forms a subjacent muscular ring, dilatation of the right ventricle commonly produces annular dilatation and tricuspid regurgitation. Right atrial dilatation alone, as in constrictive pericarditis, usually does not cause significant tricuspid insufficiency.

Valvular incompetence also may be observed in conditions that limit leaflet and cordal excursion, such as rheumatic disease (fibrosis and scar retraction), carcinoid endocardial plaques (thickening and retraction), and eosinophilic endomyocardial diseases (thrombotic adherence to the underlying myocardium). In normal hearts, mild degrees of tricuspid regurgitation commonly exist.

Tricuspid stenosis involves commissural and cordal fusion and may occur in rheumatic or carcinoid heart disease.

Mitral Valve

Mitral Annulus

The plane of the mitral annulus faces toward the left ventricular apex. The orifice changes shape during the cardiac cycle, from elliptical during ventricular systole to more circular during diastole. In living subjects, the normal mitral annular circumference is maximum during ventricular diastole (about 7 cm^2) and decreases 10% to 15% during systole.

Mitral annular calcification almost invariably involves only the posterior mitral leaflet and forms a C-shaped ring of annular and subannular calcium which may impede basal ventricular contraction and thereby produce mitral regurgitation. Similarly, inadequate basal ventricular contraction may contribute to valvular incompetence in the setting of pronounced left ventricular dilatation; however, because only part of the mitral annulus is in direct contact with the basal ventricular myocardium, dilatation of the ventricle rarely increases annular circumference more than 25%.

Secondary left atrial dilatation may contribute to the progression of preexisting mitral incompetence by displacing the posterior leaflet and its annulus and thereby hindering the excursion of this taut leaflet.

Mitral Leaflets

The mitral leaflets form a continuous funnel-shaped veil with two prominent indentations, the anterolateral and posteromedial commissures. Although the two commissures do not extend entirely to the annulus, they effectively separate the two leaflets. In contrast to the three other cardiac valves, which each comprise three leaflets or cusps, the mitral valve has only two leaflets. At midleaflet level, the mitral orifice is elliptic or football-shaped, and its long axis aligns with the two commissures and their papillary muscles.

Although the anterior leaflet occupies only about 35% of the annular circumference, its leaflet area is almost identical to the area of the posterior leaflet, about 5 cm^2. The total mitral leaflet surface area is 10 cm^2, nearly twice that necessary to close the systolic annular orifice, 5.2 cm^2. However, some folding of leaflet tissue is needed to ensure a competent seal, and the normal leaflets are not as redundant as they might appear.

The myxomatous (or floppy) mitral valve is characterized by annular dilatation, stretched tendinous cords, and redundant hooded folds of leaflet tissue, which are prone to prolapse, incomplete coaptation, cordal rupture, and mitral regurgitation. In contrast, rheumatic mitral insufficiency results from scar retraction of leaflets and cords. In the setting of infective endocarditis, virulent organisms may perforate the leaflet tissue and produce acute mitral regurgitation. In hypertrophic cardiomyopathy, the anterior mitral leaflet contacts the ventricular septum during systole and contributes both to left ventricular outflow tract obstruction and to mitral incompetence.

In chronic aortic insufficiency, the regurgitant stream may impact on the anterior mitral leaflet and produce not only a fibrotic jet lesion but also the leaflet flutter and premature valve closure that are so characteristic echocardiographically.

Papillary Muscles

A fan-shaped cord emanates from the tip of each of the two papillary muscles and inserts into its overlying commissure and into both adjacent leaflets (Fig. 8B). Similarly, a smaller commissural cord inserts into each minor commissure between their posterior scallops. Two particularly prominent cords insert along each half of the ventricular surface of the anterior mitral leaflet, and these so-called strut cords offer additional support for this mid-cavitary leaflet that also forms part of the wall of the left ventricular outflow tract. Cordal length is generally 1 to 2 cm.

Rheumatic mitral stenosis is characterized by cordal and commissural fusion, which obliterate the secondary intercordal orifices and narrow the primary valve orifice. Cordal rupture may occur in a myxomatous (floppy) valve, an infected valve, or, rarely, an apparently normal valve and lead to acute mitral regurgitation.

The mitral papillary muscles occupy the middle third of the left ventricular base-apex length. Two prominent muscles originate from the anterolateral and posteromedial (inferomedial) free wall, beneath their respective mitral commissures. Trabeculations not only anchor the papillary muscles but also may form a muscle bridge between the two papillary groups and thereby contribute to valve closure.

The anterolateral muscle is a single structure with a midline groove in 70% to 85% of cases, whereas the posteromedial muscle is multiple or is bifid or trifid in 60% to 70%. The anterolateral muscle is generally larger and extends closer to the annulus than the posteromedial muscle. Occasionally, an accessory papillary muscle is interposed between the two major muscles along the free wall. No papillary muscles or tendinous cords originate from the septum and terminate on the mitral leaflets. However, in about 50% of subjects, one or more cord-like structures, known as left ventricular false tendons, or pseudotendons, arise from a papillary muscle and insert either onto the septal surface or onto the opposite papillary muscle.

Chronic postinfarction mitral regurgitation is associated with papillary muscle atrophy and scarring, thinning and scarring of the subjacent left ventricular free wall, and left ventricular dilatation. Acute postinfarction mitral regurgitation may be associated with rupture of a papillary muscle (almost invariably the posteromedial) and can involve the entire muscle or only one of its multiple heads.

Competent function of the mitral valve requires the harmonious interaction of all valvular components, including the left atrium and left ventricle.

- Right atrial dilatation alone usually does not cause significant tricuspid insufficiency.
- In normal hearts, mild degrees of tricuspid regurgitation commonly exist.
- Secondary left atrial dilatation may contribute to the progression of preexisting mitral incompetence.
- In hypertrophic cardiomyopathy, the anterior mitral leaflet may contact the ventricular septum during systole and contribute both to left ventricular outflow tract obstruction and to mitral incompetence.
- Chronic postinfarction mitral incompetence is associated with papillary muscle atrophy and scarring.

Semilunar Valves

The right (pulmonary) and left (aortic) semilunar valves, in contrast to the atrioventricular valves, have no tensor apparatus and, therefore, are structurally simpler valves. They consist of annulus, cusps, and commissures. Behind each cusp is an outpouching of the arterial root, known as a sinus (of Valsalva). There are three aortic sinuses and three pulmonary sinuses, which impart a cloverleaf shape to the arterial roots.

The annuli of the semilunar valves are part of the fibrous cardiac skeleton. They are nonplanar structures, shaped like a triradiate crown.

The cusps are half-moon-shaped (semilunar), pocket-like flaps of delicate fibrous tissue which close the valvular orifice during ventricular diastole. The leading edge of each cusp is its free edge. The closing edge, in contrast, represents a slightly thickened ridge that lies a few millimeters below the free edge, along the ventricular surface of the cusp. At the center of each cusp, the closing edge meets the free edge and forms a small fibrous mound, the nodule of Arantius. When the valve closes, apposing cusps contact one another along the surfaces between their free and closing edges (that is, the lunular areas), forming a competent seal.

Like the atrioventricular valves, the semilunar valves contain two major layers histologically. The fibrosa forms the structural backbone of the valve and is continuous with the annulus, whereas the spongiosa acts more as a shock absorber along the ventricular surface, especially at the closing edge. Cusps contain little elastic tissue and, accordingly, have no appreciable elastic recoil. The opening and closing of the semilunar valves is a passive process that entails cusp excursion and annulocuspid hinge-like motion.

In the elderly, degenerative changes in the aortic valve may result in low-grade systolic ejection murmurs. The closing edges become thickened and, along the nodules of Arantius, may form whisker-like projections called Lambl's excrescences. Lunular fenestrations also tend to develop with increasing age.

Disease processes that tend to increase cusp rigidity, such as fibrosis or calcification, or that lead to commissural fusion, such as rheumatic valvulitis, tend to narrow the effective valvular orifice and, as a consequence, produce stenosis. In contrast, processes that straighten the cuspid line between commissures and thereby hold the commissures open, such as arterial root dilatation or rheumatic cuspid scar retraction, tend to produce regurgitation.

Pulmonary Valve

The plane of the pulmonary annulus faces toward the left midscapula with an area of about 3.5 cm^2. The cusps are usually similar in size, although minor variations are commonly observed.

Pulmonary incompetence occurs in conditions that produce dilatation of the pulmonary artery and annulus, such as pulmonary hypertension or heart failure. Combined pulmonary stenosis and incompetence are features of carcinoid heart disease, in which the annulus becomes constricted and stenotic and in which the cusps are also retracted and insufficient. Pure pulmonary stenosis is almost always congenital in origin.

Aortic Valve

The plane of the aortic valve faces the right shoulder. In the living subject, the normal aortic annular area averages about 3 cm^2.

Unoperated symptomatic aortic stenosis has a worse prognosis than many malignancies. The vast majority of stenotic aortic valves are calcified. Most commonly, the valve represents either degenerative (senile) calcification or a calcified congenitally bicuspid valve. Only rarely are heavily calcified valves the site of active infective endocarditis.

Aortic root dilatation stretches open the commissures and thereby produces aortic insufficiency in either a tricuspid or a bicuspid aortic valve. Acute aortic regurgitation may be produced by infective aortic endocarditis with cuspid perforation or by acute aortic dissection with commissural prolapse. Chronic aortic regurgitation with coexistent aortic stenosis is most commonly associated with postrheumatic cuspid retraction, which yields a fixed triangular orifice.

Among cases of infective endocarditis, perhaps none present so varied a clinical spectrum as those associated with aortic annular abscesses. The possible clinical presentations depend to a great extent on the particular cusp(s) involved. Subvalvular extension may involve the anterior mitral leaflet, left bundle branch, or ventricular septal myocardium; involvement of the ventricular septal myocardium may produce a large abscess cavity or result in rupture into a ventricular chamber with the formation of either an aorto-right ventricular or aorto-left ventricular fistula. An aortic annular abscess may expand laterally and enter the pericardial cavity and thereby produce purulent pericarditis or fatal hemopericardium, or it may burrow into adjacent cardiac chambers or vessels and produce various fistulas (aorto-right atrial, aorto-left atrial, or aortopulmonary).

Fibrous Cardiac Skeleton

At the base of the heart, the fibrous cardiac skeleton encircles the four cardiac valves. It comprises not only the four valvular annuli but also their intervalvular collagenous attachments (the right and left fibrous trigones, the intervalvular fibrosa, and the conus ligament) and the membranous septum and tendon of Todaro. This fibrous scaffold is firmly anchored to the ventricles but is rather loosely attached to the atria. Thus, the cardiac skeleton not only electrically insulates the atria from the ventricles but also supports the cardiac valves and provides a firm foundation against which the ventricles may contract.

Because of the intervalvular attachments of the fibrous cardiac skeleton, disease or surgery on one valve can affect the size, shape, position, or relative angulation of its neighboring valves and also can affect the adjacent coronary arteries or cardiac conduction system. Tricuspid annuloplasty or replacement may be complicated by injury to the right coronary artery or atrioventricular conduction tissues, whereas mitral valve replacement may be attended by trauma to the circumflex coronary artery, coronary sinus, or aortic valve. At aortic valve replacement, the anterior mitral leaflet, left bundle branch, or coronary ostia may be injured inadvertently.

Most congenital anomalies of the pulmonary valve are associated with stenosis. Isolated pulmonary stenosis is almost always due to a dome-shaped acommissural valve, with congenital fusion of all three commissures. However, forms of pulmonary stenosis which are associated with other cardiac malformations, such as tetralogy of Fallot, usually result from a bicuspid or unicommissural valve (often with a hypoplastic annulus) or from a dysplastic valve with three thickened cusps.

Congenitally bicuspid aortic valves affect 1% to 2% of the general population and constitute the most common form of congenital heart disease. Although they usually are neither stenotic nor insufficient at birth, most bicuspid valves will become stenotic during adulthood as the cusps calcify, and some will become insufficient as a result of infective endocarditis or aortic root dilatation. In contrast, the congenitally unicommissural aortic valve is usually stenotic at birth and becomes progressively more obstructive as calcification develops in adulthood. Aortic atresia is associated with the hypoplastic left heart syndrome and is usually fatal during the first week of life. All congenital anomalies of the aortic valve are much more common in males than in females.

In truncus arteriosus, the truncal valve most commonly comprises three cusps and resembles a normal aortic valve. However, it may be quadricuspid, bicuspid, or, rarely, pentacuspid and may contain one or more raphes; such nontricuspid valves are often incompetent, particularly if the truncal root is dilated.

- Disease processes that tend to increase cusp rigidity tend to narrow the effective valvular orifice and produce stenosis.
- Processes that straighten the cuspid line between commissures tend to produce regurgitation.
- Pulmonary incompetence occurs in conditions that produce dilatation of the pulmonary trunk and annulus, such as pulmonary hypertension or heart failure.
- Pure pulmonary stenosis is almost always congenital in origin.
- An aortic annular abscess may expand laterally and enter the pericardial cavity.
- Congenitally bicuspid aortic valves affect 1% to 2% of the general population.

Figure 9 shows the anatomy of the heart as seen on magnetic resonance imaging.

Great Arteries

Pulmonary Arteries

The pulmonary artery arises anteriorly and to the left of the ascending aorta and is directed toward the left shoulder. In adults, it is slightly greater in diameter than the ascending aorta, although its wall thickness is roughly half that of the aorta. At the bifurcation, the right pulmonary artery travels horizontally beneath the aortic arch and behind the superior vena cava, and the left pulmonary artery courses over the left main bronchus (Fig. 10). The main and left pulmonary arteries contribute to the left border of the frontal cardiac silhouette roentgenographically.

In pulmonary hypertension, especially in children with pliable tracheobronchial cartilage, the tense and dilated pulmonary arteries can compress the left bronchus and the left upper and right middle lobar bronchi and thereby contribute to recurrent bronchopneumonia in those lobes. Furthermore, the dilated pulmonary artery may displace the aortic arch rightward and secondarily produce tracheal indentation and, occasionally, hoarseness as a result of compression of the left recurrent laryngeal nerve.

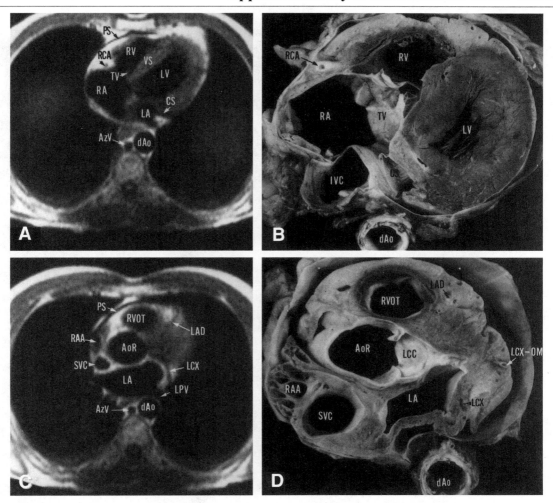

Fig. 9. Transverse (*A* through *D*), sagittal (*E* through *H*), and coronal (*I* through *L*) planes of the heart shown in analogous magnetic resonance images (at left) and anatomic sections (at right). aAo, ascending aorta; Ao, aortic arch; AoR, aortic root; AV, aortic valve; AzV, azygos vein; CS, coronary sinus; dAo, descending thoracic aorta; IA, innominate artery; LA, left atrium; LAA, left atrial appendage; LAD, left anterior descending coronary artery; LB, left bronchus; LCC, left coronary cusp; LCCA, left common carotid artery; LCX, left circumflex coronary artery; LCX-OM, left circumflex coronary artery, obtuse marginal branch; LIV, left innominate vein; LLPV, left lower pulmonary vein; LMA, left main coronary artery; LPA, left pulmonary artery; LPV, left pulmonary vein; LSA, left subclavian artery; LSV, left subclavian vein; LUPV, left upper pulmonary vein; LV, left ventricle; MPA, main pulmonary artery; MV, mitral valve; PS, pericardial sac; PV, pulmonary valve; RA, right atrium; RAA, right atrial appendage; RCA, right coronary artery; RCCA, right common carotid artery; RIV, right innominate vein; RJV, right internal jugular vein; RPA, right pulmonary artery; RSV, right subclavian vein; RV, right ventricle; RVOT, right ventricular outflow tract; SVC, superior vena cava; T, trachea; TV, tricuspid valve; VS, ventricular septum. (From *Mayo Clin Proc* 62:573-583, 1987. By permission of Mayo Foundation.)

Aorta

The aorta arises at the level of the aortic valve annulus and terminates at the aortic bifurcation, approximately at the level of the umbilicus and the fourth lumbar vertebra. The aorta has four major divisions: ascending aorta, aortic arch, descending thoracic aorta, and abdominal aorta (Fig. 11).

The ascending aorta lies almost entirely within the pericardial sac and includes sinus and tubular portions, which are demarcated by the aortic sinotubular junction. The aortic valve leaflets are related to the three sinuses, and the right and left coronary arteries arise from the right and left aortic sinuses, respectively. The ascending aorta lies posterior and to the right of the pulmonary artery.

With age or with the development of atherosclerosis, the aortic sinotubular junction can become heavily calcified, particularly above the right cusp, and may produce coronary ostial stenosis. Among the causes of aortic root dilatation, perhaps aging, mucoid medial degeneration (so-called cystic medial necrosis), and chronic hypertension are the most common and may produce an ascending aortic aneurysm, aortic valvular regurgitation, or acute aortic dissection.

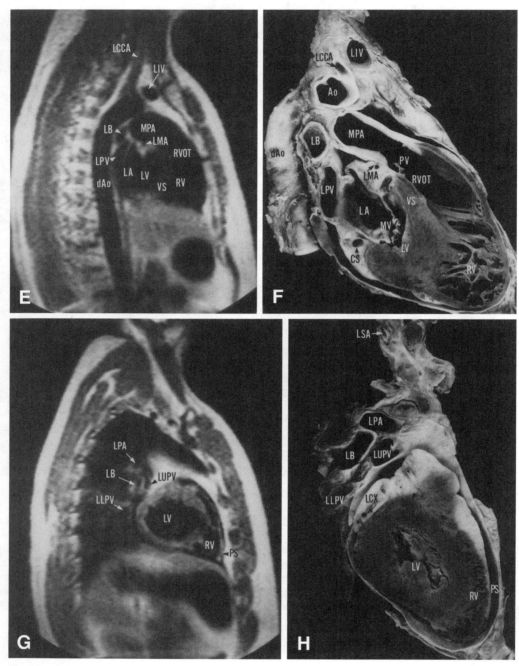

Fig. 9 continued

The aortic arch travels over the right pulmonary artery and the left bronchus. From its superior aspect emanate the innominate (or brachiocephalic), left common carotid, and left subclavian arteries, in that order. In 11% of subjects, the innominate and left common carotid arteries form a common ostium, and in 5%, the left vertebral artery arises directly from the aortic arch, between the left common carotid and left subclavian arteries. The ligamentum arteriosum represents the obstructed fibrotic or fibrocalcific remnant of the fetal ductus arteriosus (ductal artery), which joins the proximal left pulmonary artery to the undersurface of the aortic arch. The aortic arch contributes to the left superior border of the frontal cardiac silhouette and forms the roentgenographic aortic knob.

Aortic Dissection

When aortic dissections do not involve the ascending aorta (type III or type B), the intimal tear is commonly near the

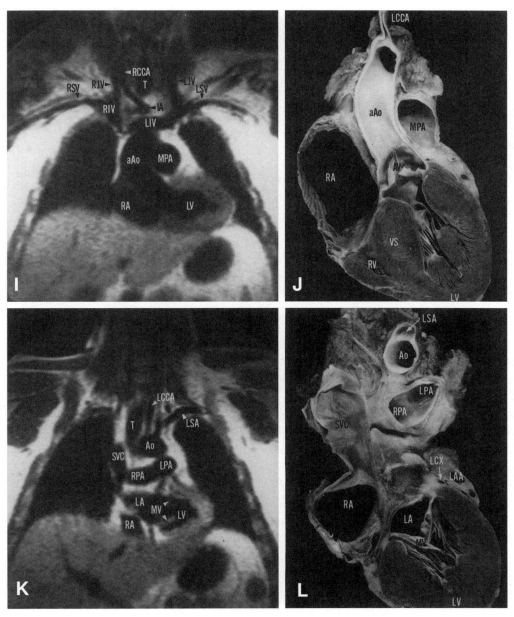

Fig. 9 continued

ligamentum arteriosum or the ostium of the left subclavian artery. By virtue of severe torsional and shear stresses placed on the heart and great vessels during nonpenetrating decelerative chest trauma, as can occur in motor vehicle accidents, the aorta may be transected at the junction between the aortic arch and the descending thoracic aorta. When the tear is incomplete, a posttraumatic pseudoaneurysm can develop with time. Aneurysms of the aortic arch may be associated with hypertension, atherosclerosis, or aortitis, or they may be idiopathic.

Descending Thoracic Aorta

The descending thoracic aorta abuts the left anterior surface of the vertebral column and lies adjacent to the esophagus and the left atrium. Its posterolateral branches are the bilateral intercostal arteries, and its anterior branches include the bronchial, esophageal, mediastinal, pericardial, and superior phrenic arteries. The bronchial arteries, most commonly two left and one right, nourish the bronchial walls and the pulmonary arterial and venous walls. Uncommonly, bronchial arteries may arise from intercostal or subclavian

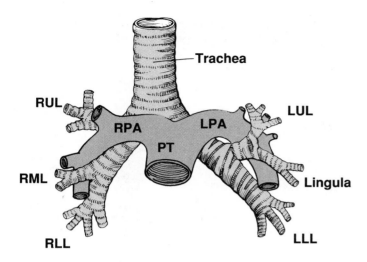

Fig. 10. Pulmonary and bronchial arteries. The right and left pulmonary arteries do not exhibit mirror-image symmetry. (See Appendix at end of chapter for abbreviations.)

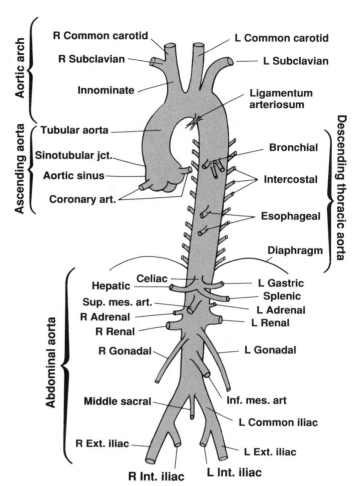

Fig. 11. Systemic arteries. The aorta may be divided into ascending, arch, descending thoracic, and abdominal regions. (See Appendix at end of chapter for abbreviations.)

arteries or, rarely, from a coronary artery. The bronchial veins drain not only into the azygos and hemiazygos veins but also into the pulmonary veins.

If the bronchial circulation is adequate, pulmonary emboli usually do not cause pulmonary infarction. In several forms of pulmonary hypertension, the bronchial arteries become quite enlarged and tortuous.

Aneurysms of the descending thoracic aorta may be associated with aortic dissection, aortitis, atherosclerosis, hypertension, or trauma. They may or may not extend below the diaphragm.

Abdominal Aorta

The abdominal aorta travels along the left anterior surface of the vertebral column and lies adjacent to the inferior vena cava. The major lateral (retroperitoneal) branches include the renal, adrenal, right and left lumbar, and inferior phrenic arteries. The gonadal arteries arise somewhat more anteriorly but remain retroperitoneal. The intraperitoneal branches arise anteriorly and include the celiac artery (with its left gastric, splenic, and hepatic branches) and the superior and inferior mesenteric arteries. The distal aortic branches include the right and left common iliac arteries and a small middle sacral artery.

Atherosclerotic abdominal aortic aneurysms are most commonly infrarenal. They tend to bulge anteriorly and thereby stretch and compress the gonadal and inferior mesenteric arteries. Such aneurysms are generally filled with laminated thrombus and so their residual lumens often

appear normal or even narrowed rather than dilated. Rupture of an atherosclerotic abdominal aortic aneurysm may be associated with extensive retroperitoneal hemorrhage, with or without intraperitoneal hemorrhage.

Aortopulmonary Window

An aortopulmonary septal defect represents a large opening between the ascending aorta and the pulmonary trunk and hemodynamically resembles a patent ductus arteriosus. Rarely, one pulmonary artery may originate from the ascending aorta or ductus arteriosus, while the other arises normally from the pulmonary trunk. Congenital stenosis of the pulmonary arteries is usually associated with maternal rubella during the first trimester. In pulmonary atresia with ventricular septal defect, the pulmonary arteries may be derived from the right or left ductus arteriosus and from bronchial or other systemic collateral arteries (analogous to total anomalous pulmonary venous connection).

Aortic Arch Congenital Abnormalities

Various anomalies result from faulty development of the aortic arches. A right aortic arch results from persistence of the right fourth aortic arch and disappearance of its left counterpart; it most commonly accompanies tetralogy of Fallot, pulmonary atresia with ventricular septal defect, and truncus arteriosus. A double aortic arch results from persistence of both fourth aortic arches. An aberrant retro-esophageal right subclavian artery is a relatively common anomaly, which may cause dysphagia; it probably results from persistence of the right dorsal aorta and resorption of the right fourth aortic arch.

Ductus Arteriosus

The patent ductus arteriosus may be isolated or may accompany other cardiac malformations. A left ductus arteriosus joins the proximal left pulmonary artery to the aortic arch, whereas a right ductus arteriosus joins the proximal right pulmonary artery to the right subclavian artery; in cases of right aortic arch with mirror-image brachiocephalic branching, the opposite pertains.

Coarctation of the Aorta

Coarctation of the aorta represents an obstructive infolded ridge just distal to the left subclavian artery and opposite the ductus arteriosus; it is associated with a congenitally bicuspid aortic valve in at least half of the cases.

- Acute aortic dissection is commonly associated with an intimal tear above the right aortic cusp and with eventual rupture into the pericardial sac.
- When aortic dissections do not involve the ascending aorta (type III or type B), the intimal tear is commonly near the ligamentum arteriosum or the ostium of the left subclavian artery.

Coronary Circulation

Right Coronary Artery

The right coronary artery arises nearly perpendicularly from the right aortic sinus. In 50% of subjects, one or more conus arteries also originate from the right aortic sinus, anterior to the right coronary ostium. Rarely, the descending septal artery or the sinus nodal artery may originate directly from the aorta.

The left coronary artery arises from the left aortic sinus and tends to arise at an acute angle and to travel parallel to the aortic sinus wall. When the left main artery is exceptionally short, its ostium may assume a double-barrel appearance.

Among the various causes of coronary ostial stenosis, perhaps the most common is degenerative calcification of the aortic sinotubular junction, which often affects the right aortic sinus. Stenosis of the right coronary ostium occurs six to eight times more often than that of the left. Aortitis associated with syphilis or ankylosing spondylitis also may be complicated by coronary ostial obstruction. Iatrogenic ostial injury may complicate coronary arteriography, intra-operative coronary perfusion, or aortic valve replacement.

The right coronary artery travels within the right atrioventricular sulcus (or groove) (Fig. 12). In 50% of subjects, the first anterior branch is the conus artery, which nourishes the right ventricular outflow tract; in the remainder, this artery arises independently from the right aortic sinus. The descending septal artery, which arises from the proximal right coronary artery or, rarely, from the conus artery or right aortic sinus, supplies the infundibular septum and, in some individuals, the distal atrioventricular (His) bundle. Along the acute cardiac margin, from base to apex, courses a prominent acute marginal branch, and between this vessel and the conus artery, several smaller marginal branches arise and travel parallel to the acute margin; these vessels nourish the lateral two-thirds of the anterior right entricular free wall.

Beyond the acute margin, along the inferior surface of the heart, the length of the right coronary artery varies inversely with that of the circumflex coronary artery. However, in 90% of human hearts, the right coronary artery gives rise not only to the posterior descending artery, which travels in the inferior interventricular sulcus, but also to branches that supply the inferior left ventricular free wall. Accordingly, these arteries nourish the inferior third of the ventricular septum (the inlet septum), including the right bundle branch and the posterior portion of the left bundle branch, and the inferior left ventricular free wall, including the posteromedial mitral papillary muscle.

Left Main Coronary Artery

The left main coronary artery travels between the pulmonary artery and the left atrium and is covered in part by the left atrial appendage. In two-thirds of subjects, it bifurcates into left anterior descending and circumflex branches, and in the remaining one-third, it trifurcates into the aforementioned

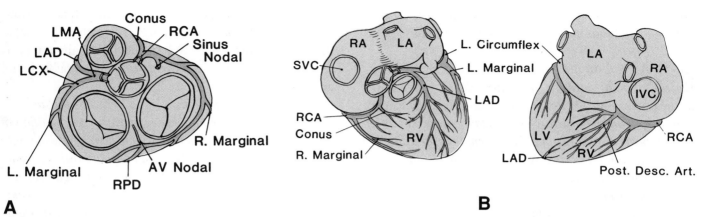

A   **B**

Fig. 12. Coronary arteries. *A*, Base of heart. *B*, Superior and inferior views of the heart. (See Appendix at end of chapter for abbreviations.)

branches and an intermediate artery (ramus intermedius), which follows a course similar to that of either the first diagonal or first marginal branch.

Left Anterior Descending Coronary Artery

The left anterior descending coronary artery travels within the anterior interventricular sulcus (or groove) and, after wrapping around the apex, may ascend a variable distance along the inferior interventricular sulcus. Septal perforating branches nourish not only the anterosuperior two-thirds and entire apical one-third of the ventricular septum but also the atrioventricular (His) bundle and the right and anterior left bundle branches. The proximal septal perforators anastomose with the descending septal artery. Epicardial branches, called diagonals, nourish the anterior left ventricular free wall and the medial third of the anterior right ventricular free wall. Myocardial bridges may be demonstrated angiographically in 12% of subjects and almost invariably involve the anterior descending artery; they produce critical systolic luminal narrowing in only 1% to 2% of hearts and probably have a benign prognosis in most cases.

Left Circumflex Coronary Artery

The (left) circumflex coronary artery travels within the left atrioventricular sulcus (or groove) and often terminates just beyond the obtuse marginal branch. The circumflex artery nourishes the lateral left ventricular free wall; however, in the 10% of subjects in whom the circumflex artery gives rise to the posterior descending branch, it also supplies the inferior left ventricular free wall and the inferior third of the ventricular septum. The circumflex and anterior descending arteries nourish the anterolateral mitral papillary muscles, and the circumflex and right coronary arteries supply the

posteromedial mitral papillary muscles.

The four major epicardial coronary arteries occupy only two planes of the heart. The right and circumflex arteries delineate the plane of the atrioventricular sulcus (cardiac base), and the left main artery and anterior and posterior descending arteries delineate the plane of the ventricular septum.

The origin of the posterior descending artery determines the blood supply to the inferior portion of the left ventricle and thereby defines coronary dominance. In 70% of hearts, the right coronary artery crosses the crux and gives rise to this branch, and right coronary dominance pertains. In 10%, the circumflex coronary artery terminates as the posterior descending branch and thereby establishes left coronary dominance. Both the right and circumflex arteries supply the cardiac crux in the remaining 20% and constitute so-called shared coronary dominance. The dominant coronary artery, however, does *not* supply most of the left ventricular myocardium. In subjects with right coronary dominance, for example, the anterior descending artery supplies about 45% of the left ventricle and the circumflex and right coronary arteries nourish about 20% and 35%, respectively.

Blood Supply of the Cardiac Conduction System

The sinus nodal artery arises from the right coronary artery in 60% of subjects and from the circumflex artery in 40%, but its artery of origin does not depend on patterns of coronary arterial dominance. The atrioventricular nodal artery originates from the dominant artery and, accordingly, arises from the right coronary in 90% and the circumflex in 10%. The atrioventricular nodal artery and the first septal perforator of the anterior descending artery offer dual blood supply to the atrioventricular (His) bundle. Other septal perforating branches of the anterior descending artery supply the anterior aspect of the left bundle branch, and septal perforators of the posterior descending branch, an extension of the dominant artery, supply the posteroinferior portion of the left bundle branch. The right bundle branch receives a dual blood supply from the septal perforators of the anterior and posterior descending arteries.

Coronary Collateral Circulation

In the human heart, the major epicardial coronary arteries communicate with one another by means of anastomotic channels 50 to 200 μm in diameter. Normally, these small collateral arteries afford very little blood flow. However, if arterial obstruction induces a pressure gradient across such a channel, then with time the collateral vessel may dilate and provide an avenue for significant blood flow beyond the stenotic lesion. Such functional collaterals may develop between the terminal branches of two coronary arteries, between the side branches of two arteries, between branches of the same artery, or within the same branch (via the vasa vasorum). They are most numerous in the ventricular septum (between septal perforators of anterior and posterior descending arteries), in the ventricular apex (between anterior descending septal perforators), in the anterior right ventricular free wall (between anterior descending and right or conus arteries), in the anterolateral left ventricular free wall (between anterior descending diagonals and circumflex marginals), at the cardiac crux (between the right and circumflex arteries), and along the atria (Kugel's artery between right and circumflex arteries). Smaller subendocardial anastomoses also exist.

The most common sites for high-grade atherosclerotic lesions are the proximal one-half of the anterior descending and circumflex arteries and the origin and entire length of the right coronary artery. The distribution and severity of atherosclerotic plaques do not differ significantly among patients with angina pectoris, acute myocardial infarction, end-stage ischemic heart disease, or sudden death.

Congenital malformations of the coronary arteries include anomalous ostial origin, anomalous arterial branching patterns, and anomalous arterial anastomoses.

Coronary Veins

The venous circulation of the heart comprises a coronary sinus system, an anterior cardiac venous system, and the thebesian venous system (Fig. 13). Small thebesian veins drain directly into a cardiac chamber, particularly the right atrium or right ventricle; the ostia of these veins are easily recognized along the relatively smooth atrial walls but are difficult to identify in the trabeculated ventricles.

During cardiac electrophysiologic studies among patients with Wolff-Parkinson-White syndrome and left-sided bypass tracts, a catheter electrode may be positioned within the coronary sinus and great cardiac vein, adjacent to the mitral annulus, to localize the aberrant conduction pathways.

Cardiac Lymphatics

Myocardial lymphatics drain toward the epicardial surface, where they are joined by lymphatic channels from the conduction system, atria, and valves. Larger epicardial lymphatics then travel in a retrograde manner with the coronary arteries back to the aortic root, where a confluence of right and left cardiac lymphatics drains into a pretracheal lymph node and eventually empties into the right lymphatic duct.

The coronary veins and cardiac lymphatics work in concert to remove excess fluid from the myocardial interstitium and pericardial sac. Accordingly, obstruction of either system or of both systems may result in myocardial edema and pericardial effusion.

Cardiac Conduction System

Sinus Node

The sinus node is the primary pacemaker of the heart. It is an epicardial structure that measures approximately 15 by 5 by 2 mm and is located in the sulcus terminalis (intercavarum) near the superior cavoatrial junction (Fig. 14). Through its center passes a relatively large sinus nodal artery. Sinus nodal function is greatly influenced by numerous sympathetic and parasympathetic nerves that terminate within its boundaries.

Histologically, the sinus node consists of specialized cardiac muscle cells embedded within a prominent collagenous stroma. Its myocardial cells are smaller than ventricular muscle cells and contain only scant contractile elements. Ultrastructurally, the sinus node comprises transitional cells and variable numbers of P cells centrally and atrial myocardial cells peripherally. The P cells are thought to be the source of normal cardiac impulse formation.

Because the sinus node occupies an epicardial position, its function may be affected by pericarditis or metastatic neoplasms. In the setting of cardiac amyloidosis, the sinus node may be involved by extensive fibrosis or amyloid deposition. Although the sinus node is rarely infarcted, its function can be altered by adjacent atrial infarction.

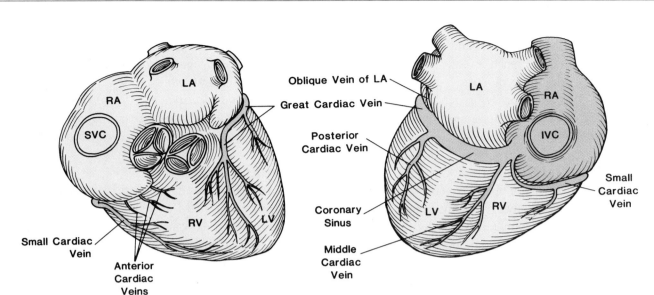

Fig. 13. Coronary veins. Superior and inferior views of the heart. (See Appendix at end of chapter for abbreviations.)

Internodal Tracts

There are no morphologically distinct conduction pathways between the sinus and the atrioventricular nodes by light microscopy, but electrophysiologic studies support the concept of three functional preferential conduction pathways. By ultrastructural studies, some investigators have observed specialized cardiac muscle cells in these internodal tracts.

Lipomatous hypertrophy of the atrial septum may interfere with internodal conduction and induce various atrial arrhythmias. Because the functional preferential pathways travel only in the limbus and not in the valve of the fossa ovalis, internodal conduction disturbances do not occur with intentional septal perforation at cardiac catheterization (transseptal approach), with the Rashkind balloon atrial septostomy, or with the Blalock-Hanlon partial (posterior) atrial septectomy. With the Mustard operation for complete transposition of the great arteries, in which the entire atrial septum is resected and in which the surgical atriotomy may disrupt the crista terminalis, severe disturbances of internodal conduction may result.

Atrioventricular Node

The atrioventricular node is a subendocardial right atrial structure that measures approximately 6 by 4 by 1.5 mm. It is located within the triangle of Koch (bordered by the tendon of Todaro, septal tricuspid annulus, and coronary sinus ostium) and abuts the right fibrous trigone (central fibrous body). The atrioventricular nodal artery courses near the node but not necessarily through it. Sympathetic and parasympathetic nerves enter the atrioventricular node and greatly influence its function.

Like the sinus node, the atrioventricular node histologically consists of a complex interwoven pattern of small specialized cardiac muscle cells within a fibrous stroma. With advanced age, the atrioventricular node acquires progressively more fibrous tissue, although not as extensively as the sinus node.

The so-called mesothelioma of the atrioventricular node is a small and rare primary neoplasm which, by virtue of its position, produces various arrhythmias and may cause sudden death. Metastatic neoplasms may rarely infiltrate the atrioventricular node but do not necessarily alter its function. Sarcoid granulomas tend to involve the basal ventricular myocardium and may destroy the atrioventricular conduction system. Because of its subendocardial position, the atrioventricular node may be ablated nonsurgically at the time of electrophysiologic study.

Atrioventricular Bundle

The atrioventricular (His) bundle arises from the distal portion of the atrioventricular node and courses through the central fibrous body to the summit of the muscular ventricular septum, adjacent to the membranous septum. It affords the only normal physiologic avenue for electrical conduction between ventricles. By virtue of its position within the central fibrous body (right fibrous trigone), the

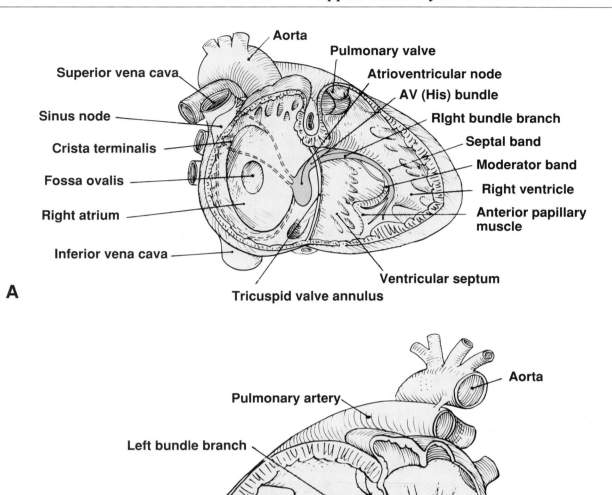

Fig. 14. Cardiac conduction system. *A*, Right heart. The sinus and AV nodes are both right atrial structures. *B*, Left heart. The left bundle branch forms a broad sheet that does not divide into distinct anterior and posterior fascicles. (From Edwards WD: Anatomy of the cardiovascular system. In *Clinical Medicine*. Vol. 6, Chap 1. Spittell JA Jr [editor]. Harper & Row Publishers, 1984, p 8. By permission of Lippincott-Raven Publishers.)

atrioventricular bundle is closely related to the annuli of the aortic, mitral, and tricuspid valves. The atrioventricular bundle has a dual blood supply—from the atrioventricular nodal artery and the first septal perforating branch of the anterior descending artery. In some subjects, a septal branch of the proximal right coronary artery also nourishes the atrioventricular bundle.

The atrioventricular bundle is made up of numerous parallel bundles of specialized cardiac muscle cells, which are separated by delicate fibrous septa. The entire atrioventricular bundle is insulated by a collagenous sheath. With increasing age, the fibrous septa become thicker, and the functional elements may be partially replaced by adipose tissue. Ultrastructurally, the atrioventricular bundle contains Purkinje cells and ventricular myocardial cells in parallel arrangement.

In some subjects, alternate conduction pathways exist between the atria and the ventricles, either within the existing atrioventricular conduction system or elsewhere along the fibrous cardiac skeleton, and may produce various arrhythmias. Atrionodal bypass tracts (of James) connect the atria to the distal atrioventricular node, and atriofascicular tracts (of Breckenmacher) connect the atria to the atrioventricular bundle. Nodoventricular and fasciculoventricular bypass fibers (of Mahaim) connect the atrioventricular node and atrioventricular bundle, respectively, to the underlying ventricular septal summit. These bypass fibers are quite commonly observed histologically and are apparently nonfunctional in most persons, although they may produce ventricular preexcitation in some instances.

Ventricular preexcitation is usually associated with aberrant atrioventricular bypass tracts that bridge the tricuspid or mitral annuli. These tracts often travel within the adipose tissue of the atrioventricular sulcus rather than through a defect in the valvular annuli. Such bypass tracts can be single or multiple and may be identified by electrophysiologic mapping.

Acquired complete heart block may involve the atrioventricular node and bundle or both bundle branches. That occurring with acute myocardial infarction is usually transient and more commonly complicates inferoseptal than anteroseptal infarction. Usually the atrioventricular node and atrioventricular bundle are edematous, or the bundle branches are focally infarcted. Acute heart block also can complicate aortic infective endocarditis. Chronic heart block may be associated with ischemic heart disease or with fibrocalcific disorders of the aortic or mitral valves, but it is most commonly due to idiopathic fibrosis of the atrioventricular bundle and bilateral bundle branches. Heart block may also complicate aortic or mitral valve replacement.

Congenital complete heart block presents as persistent bradycardia in utero and can represent an isolated anomaly or may accompany other cardiac malformations. It results from interruption of atrioventricular conduction pathways, either at the junction between atrial muscle and the atrioventricular node or at the junction between the atrioventricular node and the atrioventricular bundle. The different embryologic origins of these three regions account for the specific sites of disrupted conduction tissue.

Bundle Branches

As an extension of the atrioventricular bundle, the right bundle branch forms a cordlike structure, approximately 50 mm in length and 1 mm in diameter, which courses along the septal and moderator bands to the level of the anterior tricuspid papillary muscle. The left bundle branch forms a broad fenestrated sheet of conduction fibers which spreads along the septal subendocardium of the left ventricle and separates incompletely and variably into two or three indistinct fascicles. The fascicles travel toward the left ventricular apex and both mitral papillary muscle groups. The bundle branches are nourished by septal perforators arising from the anterior and posterior descending coronary arteries. Histologically, the bundle branches consist of parallel tracts of specialized cardiac muscle cells which are insulated by a delicate fibrous sheath. Ultrastructurally, Purkinje cells and ventricular myocardial cells form the bundle branches.

Right bundle branch block may be idiopathic or be associated with ischemic heart disease, chronic systemic hypertension, or pulmonary hypertension. Right ventriculotomy usually produces the electrocardiographic features of right bundle branch block, even though the bundle may not have been transected.

Chronic left bundle branch block may be associated with fibrocalcific degeneration of the ventricular septal summit as a result of chronic ischemia, left ventricular hypertension, calcification of the aortic or mitral valves, or any form of cardiomyopathy.

- The sinus node comprises transitional cells and variable numbers of P cells centrally and atrial myocardial cells peripherally.
- With the Mustard operation for complete transposition of the great arteries, in which the entire atrial septum is resected, severe disturbances of internodal conduction may result.
- The atrioventricular bundle has a dual blood supply—from the atrioventricular nodal artery and the first septal perforating branch of the anterior descending artery.
- Acute heart block may complicate aortic infective endocarditis.

Cardiac Innervation

Because the embryonic heart tube first forms in the future neck region, its autonomic innervation also arises from this level. From the cervical ganglia originate three pairs of cervical sympathetic cardiac nerves, which intermingle as they join the cardiac plexus, between the great arteries and the tracheal bifurcation. Several thoracic sympathetic cardiac nerves arise from the upper thoracic ganglia and also join the cardiac plexus. From the parasympathetic vagus nerves emanate the superior and inferior cervical vagal cardiac nerves and the thoracic vagal cardiac nerves, which likewise interweave within the cardiac plexus. The various sympathetic and parasympathetic nerves then descend from this plexus onto the heart and thereby innervate the coronary arteries, cardiac conduction system, and myocardium. Furthermore, afferent nerves concerned with pain and various reflexes ascend from the heart toward the cardiac plexus.

The transplanted human heart is completely denervated and responds only to circulating (humoral) substances and not to autonomic impulses. Similarly, afferent pathways are also lost, including pain tracts and various reflexes. Consequently, if chronic cardiac transplant rejection produces diffuse coronary arterial obstruction, subsequent myocardial ischemia and infarction will be asymptomatic.

The asplenia syndrome is characterized by bilateral right-sided symmetry and is generally associated with right atrial isomerism, right pulmonary isomerism, abdominal situs ambiguus, and, in some instances, bilateral sinus nodes. In contrast, the sinus node may be congenitally absent or malpositioned in cases of polysplenia with left atrial isomerism.

- The transplanted heart is completely denervated and responds only to circulating (humoral) substances and not to autonomic impulses.
- Congenital complete heart block may present as persistent bradycardia in utero.

Appendix

Abbreviations Used in Figures

A	Anterior	Mes	Mesenteric
Ao	Aorta	MV	Mitral valve
Art.	Artery	OS	Outlet septum
AL	Anterolateral	P	Posterior
AS	Anteroseptal	PA	Pulmonary artery
AV	Atrioventricular	PB	Parietal band
AVS	AV septum	PL	Posterolateral
CS	Coronary sinus	PM	Posteromedial
Desc	Descending	Post.	Posterior
Ext	External	PS	Posteroseptal
I	Inferior	PT	Pulmonary trunk
IAS	Interatrial septum	PV	Pulmonary valve
IL	Inferolateral	R	Right
Inf	Inferior	RA	Right atrium
Int	Internal	RAA	Right atrial appendage
IS	Inferoseptal (Fig. 7 only)	RCA	Right coronary artery
IVC	Inferior vena cava	RLL	Right lower lobe
IVS	Interventricular septum	RLPV	Right lower pulmonary vein
L	Left	RML	Right middle lobe
LA	Left atrium	RPA	Right pulmonary artery
LAD	Left anterior descending coronary artery	RPD	Right posterior descending coronary artery
LCX	Left circumflex coronary artery	RPV	Right pulmonary vein
LLL	Left lower lobe	RUL	Right upper lobe
LLPV	Left lower pulmonary vein	RV	Right ventricle
LMA	Left main coronary artery	S	Septal
LPA	Left pulmonary artery	SB	Septal band
LPV	Left pulmonary vein	Sup	Superior
LUL	Left upper lobe	SVC	Superior vena cava
LV	Left ventricle	TV	Tricuspid valve
LVOT	Left ventricular outflow tract		

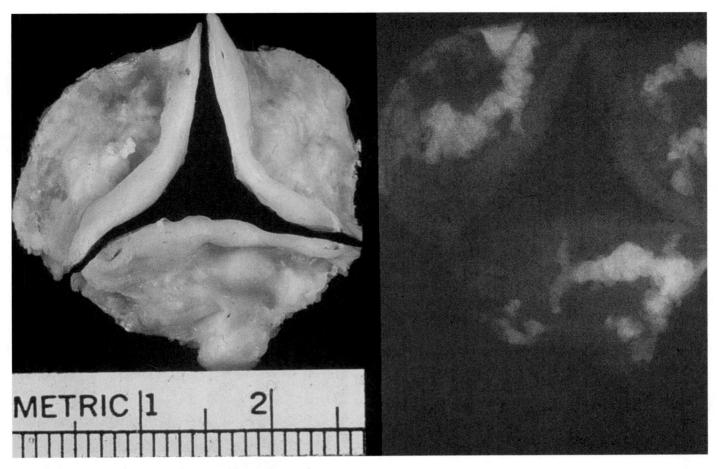

Plate 1. Calcification of aortic valve in degenerative aortic stenosis.

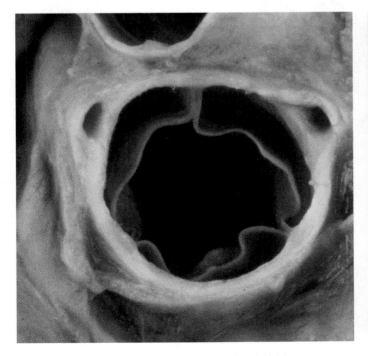
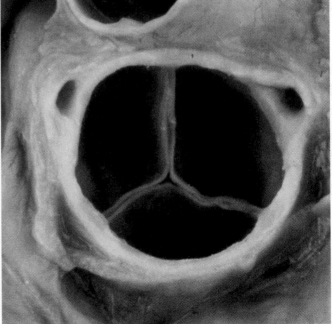

Plate 2. Normal aortic valve, opened (left) and closed (right).

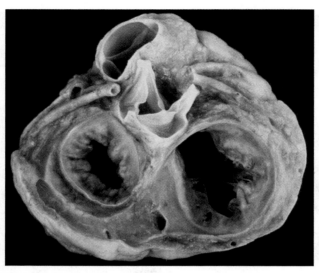

Plate 3. Four valves at base of heart.

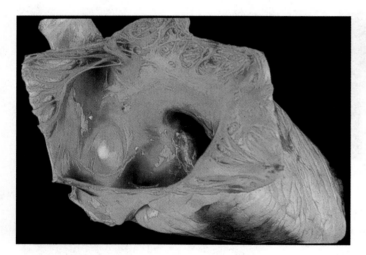

Plate 4. Thin valve of foramen ovale (transilluminated).

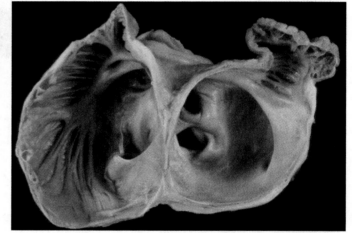

Plate 5. Normal atria.

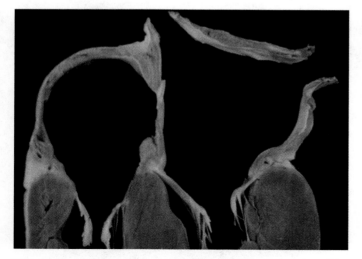

Plate 6. Tricuspid and mitral valves in profile on four-chamber view of the heart. Note that the normal tricuspid valve takes origin below that of the mitral valve, allowing the possibility of a right atrial-to-left ventricular shunt.

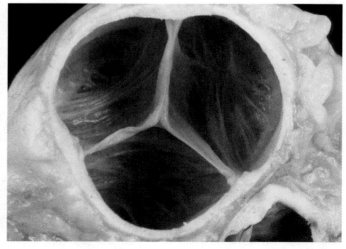

Plate 7. Pulmonary valve.

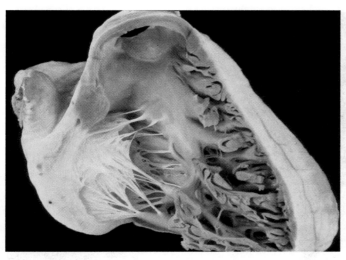

Plate 8. Right ventricle, showing marked trabeculation and tricuspid valve.

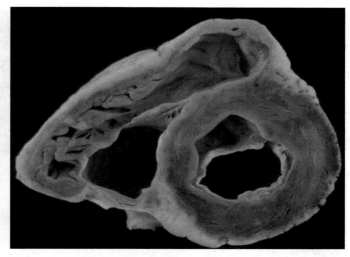

Plate 9. Mitral valve leaflets and annulus (short-axis).

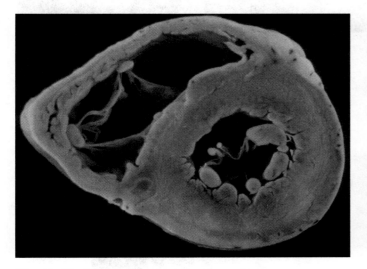

Plate 10. Mitral valve papillary muscles (short-axis).

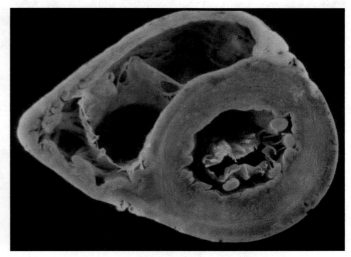

Plate 11. Mitral valve leaflets and chords (short-axis).

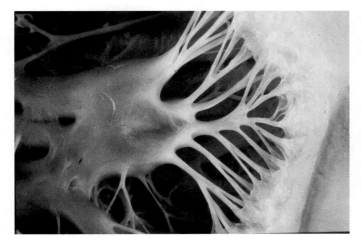

Plate 12. Mitral valve commissural cords.

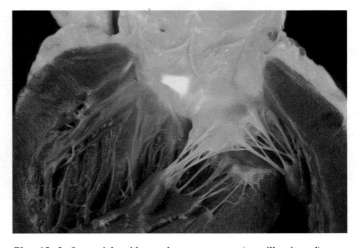

Plate 13. Left ventricle with membranous septum (transilluminated).

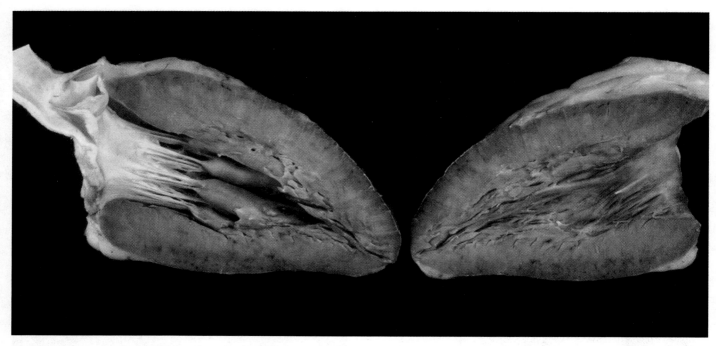

Plate 14. Left ventricle (free wall and septum) with mitral valve on free wall.

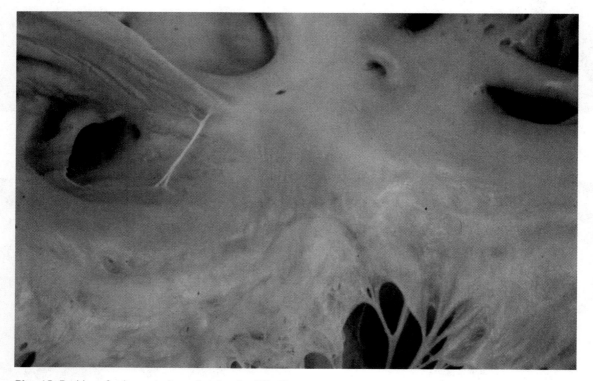

Plate 15. Position of atrioventricular node (triangle of Koch).

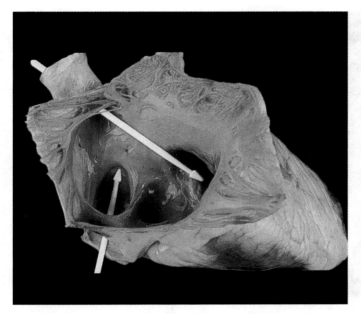

Plate 16. Right atrium, showing hemodynamic streaming (superior vena cava to tricuspid valve to inferior vena cava to foramen ovale).

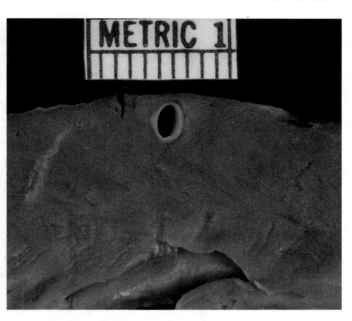

Plate 17. Myocardial bridge, left anterior descending coronary artery.

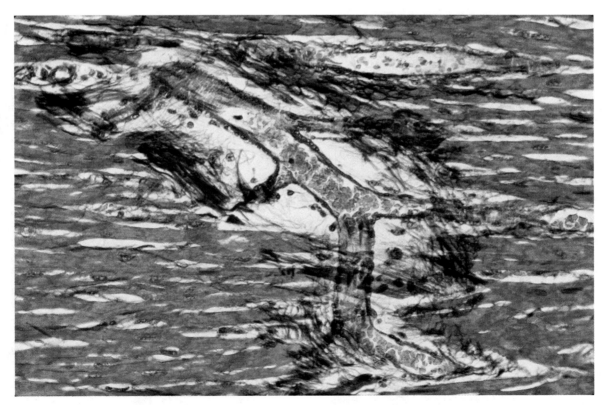

Plate 18. Myocardial arteriole.

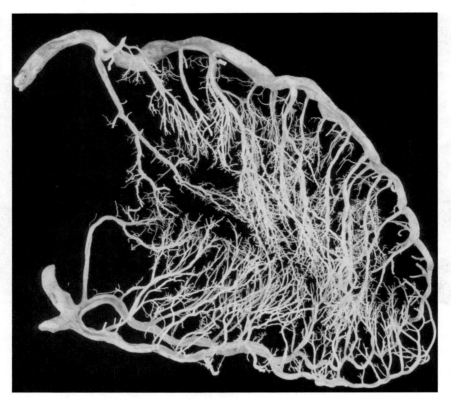

Plate 19. Septal perforators (coronary cast).

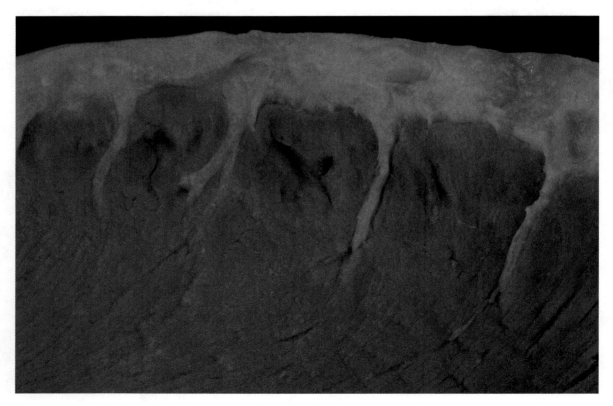

Plate 20. Left anterior descending coronary artery with septal perforators.

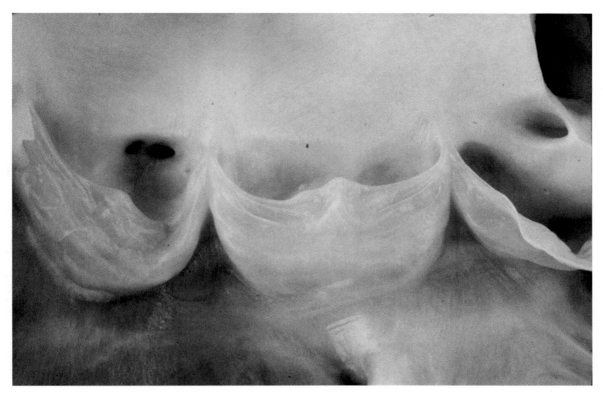

Plate 21. Coronary ostia (conus, right, and left).

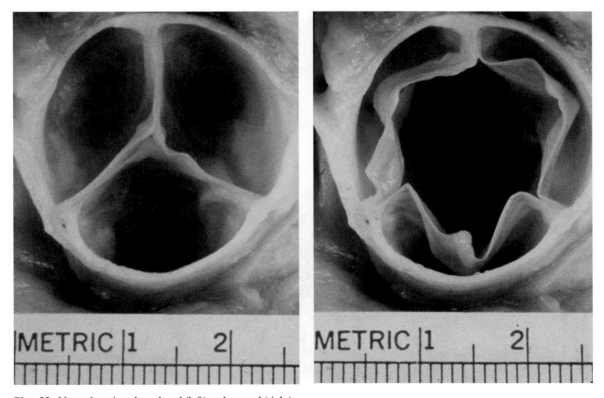

Plate 22. Normal aortic valve, closed (left) and opened (right).

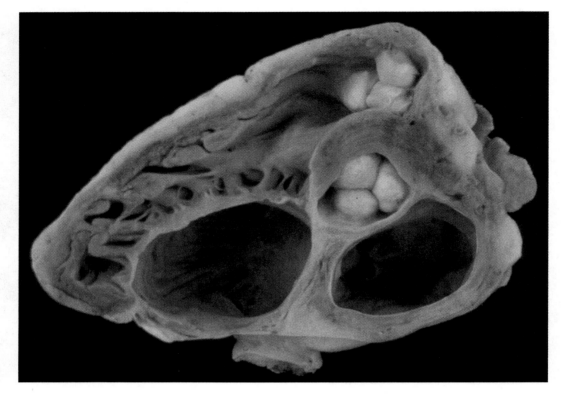

Plate 23. Aortic valve (from below).

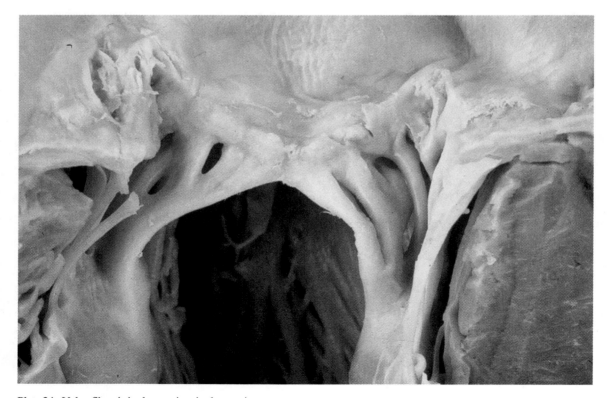

Plate 24. Valve fibrosis in rheumatic mitral stenosis.

Chapter 56

Cardiac Radiography

Jerome F. Breen, M.D.
Mark J. Callahan, M.D.

The conventional upright posteroanterior (PA) and lateral x-ray projections of the chest are obtained with high kilovoltage technique at maximal inspiration to permit short exposure times, which freeze cardiac motion. Interstitial markings are accentuated on a poor inspiratory effort film. A tube-to-film distance of at least 6 feet minimizes distortion and magnification.

Chest radiographs that show cardiac abnormality are a very important part of cardiology examinations.

Always take a systematic approach to reading chest radiographs. Always identify the border-forming structures of the heart on both the frontal and lateral views. Use the pulmonary blood vessels to help explain all abnormal contours.

Always try to compare a chest radiograph with any available previous study.

In a postoperative patient, suspect new abnormalities on chest films to be related to the surgical procedure.

If a CT or MRI scan is shown on the Cardiology Boards, look carefully for pericardial or aortic disease.

Cardiac Silhouette/Chambers

The image of the heart and great vessels on the chest radiograph is a two-dimensional display of dynamic three-dimensional structures (Fig. 1-10). The cardiovascular silhouette varies not only with the abnormality but also with body habitus, age, respiratory depth, cardiac cycle, and position of the patient.

Posteroanterior (PA) Projection

The right mediastinal contour consists of a straight upper vertical border formed by the superior vena cava and a smooth convex lower cardiac contour formed by the right atrium. Occasionally, a short segment of inferior vena cava may be seen where the right atrium meets the diaphragm.

The normal left mediastinal contour is formed by a series of convexities: from superior to inferior, the aortic knob, the pulmonary trunk, and the left ventricle abutting the diaphragm. Rarely, the left atrial appendage can be projected between the pulmonary trunk and the left ventricle in the normal heart, primarily in young females. The shape of the pulmonary trunk segment varies with age and body habitus. Most frequently, this segment is only slightly convex; however, it can be prominent in women 20 to 40 years old and straight or even concave in older patients and still be within normal limits. Occasionally, the cardiophrenic junction of the cardiac silhouette is not formed by the left ventricle but by a fat pad. Less common is a border-forming fat pad in the right cardiophrenic angle which should not be confused with a cardiac mass.

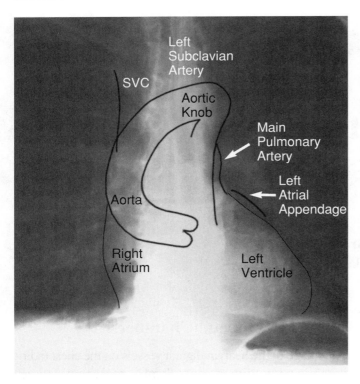

Fig. 1. PA projection of the heart. *SVC*, superior vena cava.

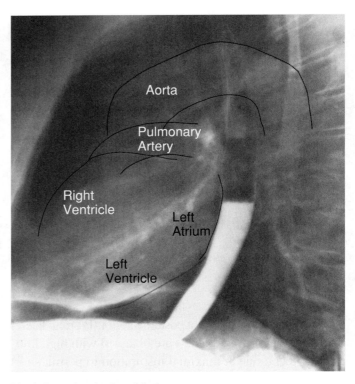

Fig. 2. Lateral projection of the heart.

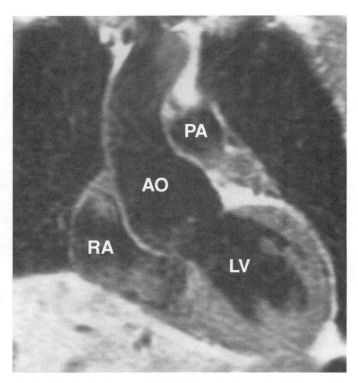

Fig. 3. Magnetic resonance imaging of the heart in the frontal plane. *AO*, aorta; *LV*, left ventricle; *PA*, pulmonary artery; *RA*, right atrium.

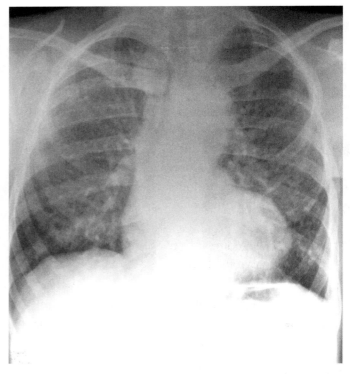

Fig. 4. Tetralogy of Fallot. Indentation in the region of the left pulmonary artery and elevation of the apex due to right ventricular hypertrophy give rise to a "boot-shaped" contour, typical for this condition. (From Schattenberg TT: Chest x-ray films in heart disease. In *Clinical Medicine*. Vol 6. *Cardiovascular Diseases*. Edited by JA Spittell Jr. Harper & Row, Publishers, 1982, chap 33, pp 1-13. By permission of Lippincott-Raven Publishers.)

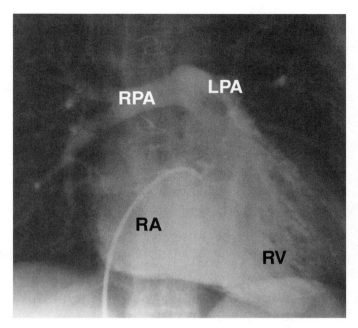

Fig. 5. Angiogram demonstrating the relative positions of the right heart chambers on the PA projection. *LPA*, left pulmonary artery; *RA*, right atrium; *RPA*, right pulmonary artery; *RV*, right ventricle.

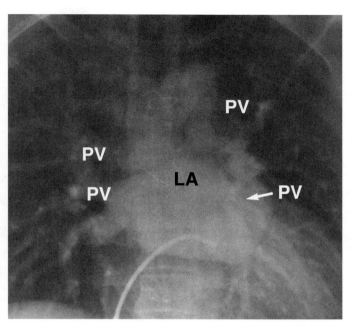

Fig. 6. Angiogram demonstrating the drainage of the pulmonary veins into the left atrium. *LA*, left atrium; *PV*, pulmonary vein.

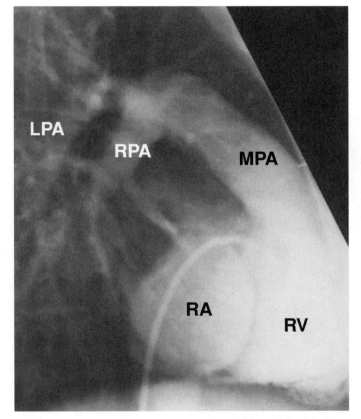

Fig. 7. Angiogram demonstrating the relative positions of the right heart chambers on the lateral projection. *LPA*, left pulmonary artery; *MPA*, main pulmonary artery; *RA*, right atrium; *RPA*, right pulmonary artery; *RV*, right ventricle.

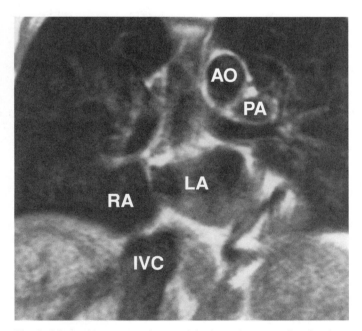

Fig. 8. Magnetic resonance image of the heart demonstrating the close anatomical relationship of right and left atria (*RA* and *LA*), aorta (*AO*), and pulmonary artery (*PA*). *IVC*, inferior vena cava.

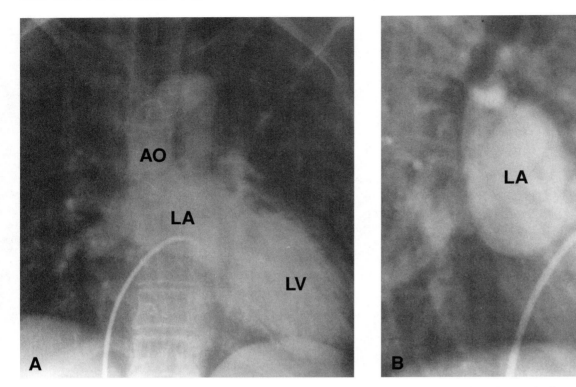

Fig. 9. Angiograms demonstrating the relative position of the left heart chambers on frontal (*A*) and lateral (*B*) projections. *AO*, aorta; *LA*, left atrium; *LV*, left ventricle.

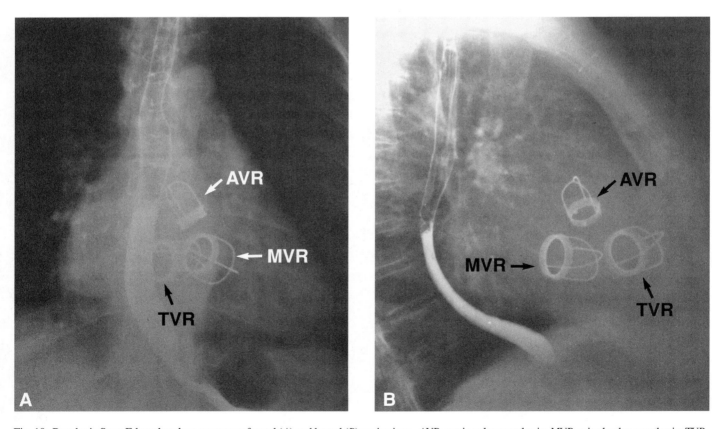

Fig. 10. Prosthetic Starr-Edwards valves as seen on frontal (*A*) and lateral (*B*) projections. *AVR*, aortic valve prosthesis; *MVR*, mitral valve prosthesis; *TVR*, tricuspid valve prosthesis.

- A normal left atrial appendage may be seen projecting between the pulmonary trunk and left ventricle, especially in young females.
- The left cardiophrenic junction may be formed by a fat pad and give a false impression of cardiomegaly.

Lateral Projection

It is routine that the patient's left side is positioned against the film cassette to minimize distortion of the heart due to geometric magnification. Superiorly, the anterior border is formed by the ascending aorta posterior to the retrosternal air space; inferiorly, the right ventricle and right ventricular outflow tract abut the sternum and blend into the main pulmonary artery, which then courses posteriorly to its bifurcation. The posterior cardiac contour is formed by the left atrium superiorly beneath the carina and the left ventricle curving inferiorly to the diaphragm, where the straight vertical edge of the inferior vena cava is often apparent within the thorax as it enters the right atrium.

Heart Size on Chest Radiographs

The cardiothoracic ratio (CTR)—the ratio of the transverse cardiac diameter to the maximal internal diameter of the thorax at the level of the diaphragm on an upright PA chest radiograph—corrects for body size and magnification produced by slight differences in radiographic techniques. In adults, a CTR greater than 0.5 is considered to represent cardiomegaly. In aortic regurgitation, the left ventricle is often enlarged downward rather than horizontally. A high diaphragm position, as seen with obesity or shallow inspiration, will produce an erroneous CTR greater than 0.5. Pectus excavatum and the absence of pericardium displace the heart posteriorly and rotate the apex laterally, resulting in a CTR greater than 0.5 in the presence of a normal-sized heart. Large pericardial fat pads may give a falsely increased CTR. Because of these factors, one can be misled if relying on the CTR alone to diagnose cardiomegaly; however, it does serve as a baseline for future comparisons.

A CTR > 0.5 with a normal heart size occurs with
- Absent pericardium
- Pectus excavatum
- Obesity
- Poor inspiration

Generalized Cardiac Enlargement

Global heart enlargement, with maintenance of an otherwise normal cardiac contour, usually is due to diffuse myocardial disease, abnormal volume or pressure overload as a consequence of valvular heart disease, hyperthyroidism, hypothyroidism, or anemia. Pericardial effusions also produce generalized enlargement of the cardiac silhouette (Fig. 11). Asymmetric enlargement with left ventricular prominence can be seen in the late stages of essential hypertension and other left-sided obstructive lesions with secondary left ventricular failure or in left-sided regurgitant valvular lesions (Fig. 12).

Left Atrial Enlargement

The left atrium sits just below the angle of the carina, in proximity with the left bronchus and esophagus; thus, enlargement is readily reflected by the displacement of these neighboring structures. Enlargement usually produces a double density behind the right atrial margin on a frontal projection as the left atrium bulges out from the mediastinum into the right lung. Occasionally, a double density can be seen in the presence of a normal-sized left atrium in patients with a prominent right pulmonary venous confluence.

Additional signs of left atrial enlargement on the PA projection include upward and posterior displacement of the left main bronchus, resulting in a less acute carinal angle. Enlargement of the left atrial appendage initially causes straightening and, subsequently, a convexity in the upper left cardiac contour. In the presence of a giant left atrium, the left atrium itself may project beyond the right atrium and form a portion of the right cardiac contour. On the

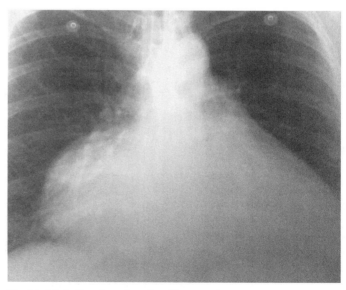

Fig. 11. Markedly enlarged cardiac silhouette primarily due to a large malignant pericardial effusion resulting from a sarcoma invading the heart chambers on the right.

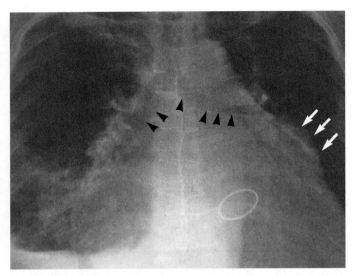

Fig. 12. Multichamber cardiac enlargement resulting from rheumatic heart disease. The left atrium is the most dilated chamber. Note the prominence of the left atrial appendage (*arrows*) and marked splaying of the carina (*arrowheads*). A Hancock valve has been placed in the mitral position.

lateral projection, left atrial enlargement can be recognized by posterior and upward displacement of the left main stem bronchus. The left atrium itself enlarges upward and posteriorly to form an increasing convex density.

- Signs of left atrial enlargement—
    "Double density" of right heart border
    Upward and posterior displacement of left main
        bronchus—widening of carinal angle

Isolated left atrial enlargement most commonly is due to mitral valve stenosis caused by rheumatic heart disease (Fig. 13 and 14). Left atrial myxoma and cor triatriatum can also cause isolated left atrial enlargement. Isolated enlargement of the left atrial appendage or apparent enlargement due to a pericardial defect and focal herniation of the appendage may cause a localized bulge in the upper left cardiac contour without other signs of left atrial dilatation. Left atrial enlargement in combination with additional chamber involvement may be produced by various conditions, such as left ventricular failure, left-sided obstructive lesions, and certain shunts (e.g., ventricular septal defect, patent ductus arteriosus, and aortopulmonary window). However, left atrial enlargement is not seen with simple atrial septal defects. When left atrial enlargement is marked, it most often is due to rheumatic valvular disease.

- Isolated left atrial enlargement—
    Mitral valve disease
    Rarely, cor triatriatum or left atrial myxoma
- Left atrial enlargement does not occur with simple atrial septal defects.

Left Ventricular Enlargement
Left ventricular enlargement can be due to dilatation or hypertrophy or both. Considerable hypertrophy must be present to cause the cardiac shadow to enlarge appreciably. The classic appearance of left ventricular hypertrophy

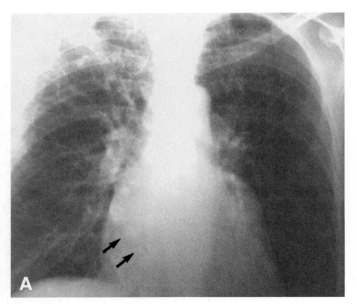
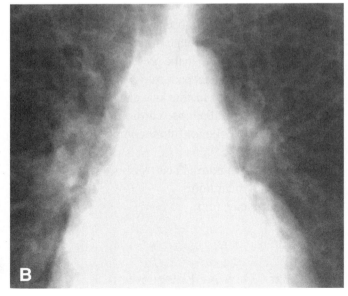

Fig. 13. Mitral stenosis resulting in left atrial enlargement, pulmonary venous hypertension, and right ventricular dilatation. Note the double density projected over the right atrium (*arrows*) because of dilatation of the left atrium.

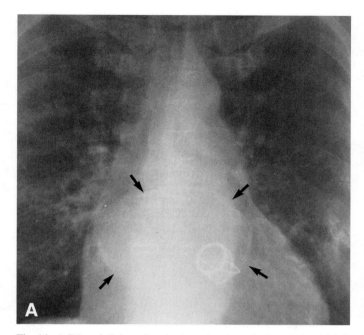 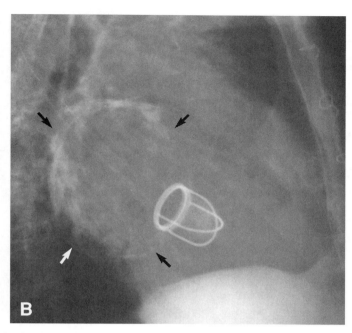

Fig. 14. *A*, PA and, *B*, lateral projections showing mitral stenosis with left atrial enlargement (*arrows*) and calcification of the atrial wall.

on the PA projection is rounding of the cardiac apex, with downward and lateral displacement without cardiac enlargement. Left ventricular dilatation causes an increase in the transverse diameter of the heart and CTR, together with an apparent increase in the length of the left heart border. The cardiac apex may be displaced to the extent that it projects below the diaphragm. On the lateral projection, dilatation increases the posterior convexity of the left ventricular contour, which will project behind the edge of the vertical inferior vena cava. Obstruction to left ventricular emptying or increased afterload, as caused by systemic hypertension, aortic coarctation, or aortic valve stenosis, leads to hypertrophy initially, with rounding of the cardiac apex (Fig. 15). Left ventricular dilatation with cardiac failure may follow. Dilated cardiomyopathy, especially ischemic cardiomyopathy, primarily enlarges the left ventricle. Aortic valve regurgitation and mitral valve regurgitation enlarge the left ventricle and are associated with dilatation of the aorta and left atrium, respectively. Left ventricular aneurysms, usually the result of a previous myocardial infarction, occasionally result in a localized bulge that projects beyond the normal ventricular contour or an angulation of the left ventricular contour (Fig. 16). A large apical aneurysm can appear similar to simple left ventricular chamber dilatation. Sometimes with true aneurysms of the left ventricle, the heart appears

normal in size and contour. False aneurysms often are paracardiac in location, posterior and inferior to the left ventricle. All cardiac chambers have been reported to be involved with aneurysm formation, although atrial aneurysms are extremely rare.

- In the absence of heart failure, left ventricular hypertrophy must be massive before the heart shadow enlarges.

Right Atrial Enlargement

Isolated right atrial enlargement is detected best on a frontal film. Enlargement is to the right and causes increased fullness and convexity of the right cardiac contour and angulation of the junction of the superior vena cava and right atrium. There may be associated dilatation of the superior and inferior venae cavae that causes widening of the right superior mediastinum and an additional border in the right cardiophrenic angle. On the lateral projection, right atrial dilatation is often difficult to appreciate. It causes a "filling-in" of the retrosternal clear space anteriorly and superiorly, with the cardiac silhouette extending behind the sternum more than one-third the way above the cardiophrenic angle, similar to that seen with right ventricular enlargement. There may be a double density that merges with the inferior vena caval shadow, which may be a slightly convex structure. Left atrial enlargement can be simulated by marked right atrial dilatation.

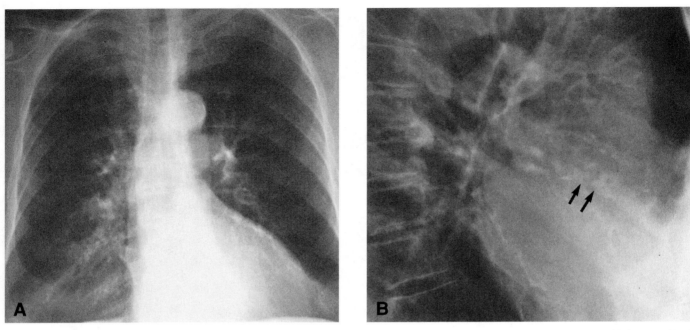

Fig. 15. *A*, PA and, *B*, lateral projections of an enlarged left ventricle with dilatation of the ascending aorta due to combined aortic insufficiency and aortic stenosis. The aortic valve is calcified (*arrows*) and the pulmonary arteries are enlarged in this patient, who also has chronic obstructive pulmonary disease.

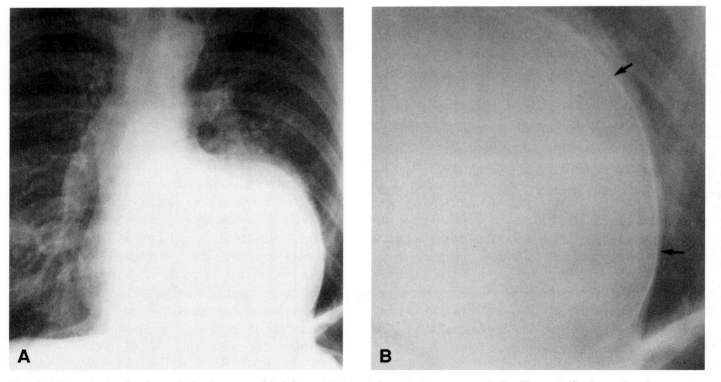

Fig. 16. *A*, PA projection showing marked enlargement of the left ventricle due to left ventricular aneurysm. *B*, Curvilinear calcification outlines the aneurysm (*arrows*).

- Right atrial enlargement "fills in" the retrosternal clear space on the lateral projection.

Isolated right atrial enlargement is uncommon and usually is due to tricuspid stenosis or right atrial tumor. Right atrial dilatation associated with other chamber enlargement, primarily right ventricular enlargement, can be seen in several conditions, such as tricuspid regurgitation, pulmonary arterial hypertension, shunts to the right atrium, and cardiomyopathies (Fig. 17 and 18). Marked isolated right atrial enlargement resulting in a "box-shaped" heart is seen in Ebstein's malformation of the tricuspid valve (Fig. 19). This configuration of the heart is the result of marked angulation at the superior vena caval-right atrial junction as the right atrium enlarges.

- Ebstein's anomaly causes a "box-shaped" heart.

Right Ventricular Enlargement

The right ventricle enlarges by broadening its triangular shape in the superior and leftward direction. With increasing right ventricular enlargement, the entire heart rotates to the left around its long axis and displaces the left ventricle posteriorly. This displacement causes increased convexity of the left upper heart border and elevation of the cardiac apex. The rotation also makes the pulmonary trunk appear relatively small. With marked dilatation, the right ventricle

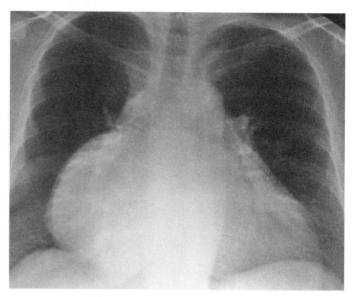

Fig. 17. Marked right atrial dilatation and right ventricular dilatation due to severe tricuspid regurgitation related to traumatic injury of the tricuspid valve.

may form the left heart border on the PA projection.

On the lateral projection, the right ventricle extends cranially behind the sternum, with increased bulk anteriorly. Normally, the heart does not extend more than one-third of the distance from the cardiophrenic angle to the sternal angle or the level of the carina; however, normal extension can vary with body habitus. Isolated right ventricular enlargement

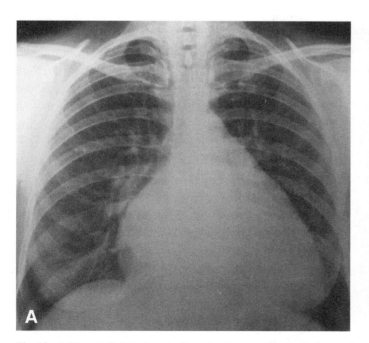

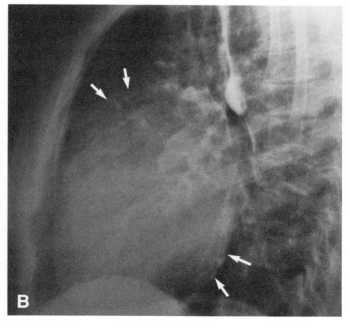

Fig. 18. *A*, PA and, *B*, lateral projections showing combined mitral stenosis and mitral insufficiency resulting in left atrial enlargement, marked right ventricular enlargement, and slight left ventricular enlargement. The dilated ventricles (*arrows*) are appreciated best on the lateral view.

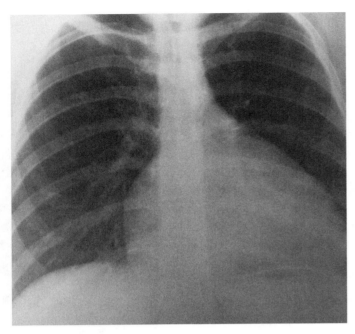

Fig. 19. Enlarged "box-shaped" heart with decreased pulmonary vascularity typical of the Ebstein anomaly.

is very unusual. More typically, there is associated prominence of the right atrium and pulmonary trunk.

Pulmonary Vasculature

Because the pulmonary vasculature reflects the physiologic effects of a cardiac lesion, it provides important clues to the diagnosis. Radiographic abnormalities are primarily the result of an increase in pulmonary blood flow or an obstruction to flow somewhere in the pulmonary circuit.

Normal Pulmonary Blood Flow

The pulmonary arteries and veins extend outward from each hilum in an orderly branching fashion, with gradual tapering peripherally. The hilar density is composed of the proximal pulmonary arteries, with the left hilum normally projecting more cranially than the right one because of the course of the left pulmonary artery over the left main bronchus. In the upper lobes, the veins and arteries are essentially parallel, with the veins lying lateral to their corresponding arteries. The major arteries and veins in the lower lung fields cross each other, with the veins taking a more horizontal course toward the left atrium. In the upright position, there is increased flow to the base of the lungs (largely due to the effects of gravity), which causes

the lower-lobe vessels to increase in size. It may be difficult to identify the apical vessels clearly because pulmonary flow to the apices is negligible in the upright position. Therefore, position has a marked effect on flow distribution.

Increased Pulmonary Blood Flow

As pulmonary flow increases, the pulmonary vessels, both arteries and veins, become enlarged. These enlarged vessels become apparent when pulmonary flow is approximately twice normal. The "over-circulation" pattern may be symmetric or asymmetric. High-output states with increased circulating blood volume, such as anemia, pregnancy, thyrotoxicosis, overhydration, and fever, result in a symmetric increase in vascularity, as do various congenital defects characterized by left-to-right shunts (Fig. 20 and 21). An asymmetric increase in pulmonary flow may be congenital in origin (e.g., pulmonary arteriovenous malformation, anomalous origin of a pulmonary artery) but is more commonly the result of surgical intervention to create a systemic-to-pulmonary shunt to improve pulmonary blood flow in the presence of severe pulmonary stenosis or atresia (e.g., a Blalock-Taussig shunt).

Decreased Pulmonary Blood Flow

Essentially all the linear shadows in the normal lung fields are due to pulmonary vasculature. When flow and, therefore, vessel size are diminished, the lung fields appear abnormally radiolucent. Both symmetric and asymmetric patterns of abnormal vascularity can be observed. Generalized undercirculation can be due to an obstructive lesion in the right heart, as in tetralogy of Fallot, pulmonary atresia, right ventricular tumor, or tricuspid valve atresia. Small-caliber pulmonary vessels with relatively hyperlucent lungs and a small heart are evidence of a marked decrease in the circulating blood volume (e.g., in Addison disease, hemorrhage). Chronic obstructive pulmonary disease (COPD) may result in generalized lung destruction or, more commonly, a patchy distribution of decreased vascularity. Segmental and asymmetric decreases in pulmonary vascularity are seen with pulmonary embolic disease (Westermark sign), segmental COPD, partial pneumonectomy, and branch pulmonary artery stenoses (Fig. 22). Rarely, postinflammatory changes (e.g., granulomatous mediastinitis), extrinsic compression (e.g., aortic aneurysm), and congenital hypoplasia as seen in the scimitar syndrome result in areas of decreased pulmonary flow. Bronchial collateral circulation may become prominent, with a somewhat disordered pattern, when there is a decrease in

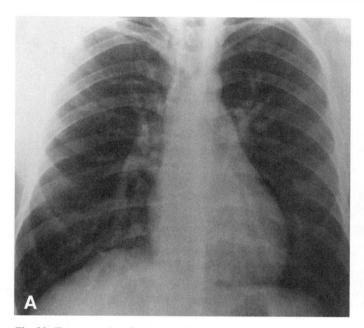
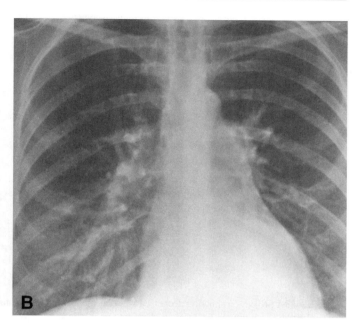

Fig. 20. Two examples of patients with atrial septal defects. *A*, Mild right ventricular dilatation in an asymptomatic patient. *B*, More prominent shunt vascularity and cardiac enlargement in a patient with very mild dyspnea on exertion.

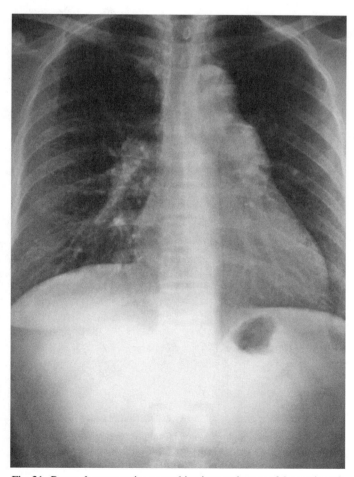

Fig. 21. Patent ductus arteriosus resulting in prominence of the aortic arch and shunt vascularity. There is mild left ventricular enlargement.

pulmonary artery blood flow, and occasionally, it gives the illusion that the overall vascularity is actually normal or even increased. Small hila in tetralogy of Fallot or pulmonary atresia and loss of the normal branching pattern of pulmonary vasculature should be evident on the chest radiograph.

● If the lung hila are small, consider tetralogy of Fallot or pulmonary atresia.

Increased Resistance to Pulmonary Blood Flow

Pulmonary hypertension with redistribution of flow is the result of increased resistance in the pulmonary circuit. Recognition of the various redistribution patterns seen on chest radiographs often allows the level of the increased resistance and the possible underlying abnormality to be identified.

Pulmonary Venous Hypertension

Lesions acting beyond the pulmonary capillary level result in elevation of the pulmonary venous pressure. Left ventricular dysfunction and mitral valve disease are the most common causes of pulmonary venous hypertension; other obstructive lesions at the left atrial level (e.g., atrial myxoma, cor triatriatum, thrombus) or pulmonary vein level (e.g., stenosis, veno-occlusive disease, or thrombosis) are relatively rare.

Initially, because of the increase in venous pressure, venous dilatation occurs throughout the lungs. However,

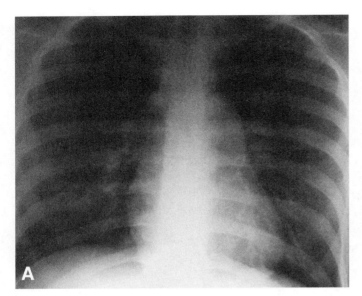
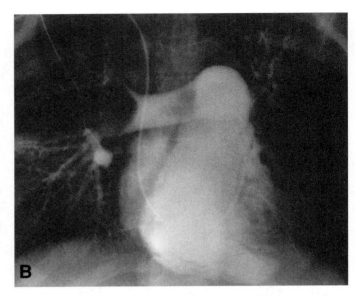

Fig. 22. *A,* PA projection showing decreased vascular markings in both lungs, most marked in the right upper lobe. *B,* The angiogram demonstrates large bilateral emboli, resulting in little flow to the right upper lobe and left lower lobe.

the radiographic pattern typically seen is that of prominent upper lung vessels, both arteries and veins. This phenomenon is thought to be due to a localized segmental reflex initiated by the increase in pulmonary venous pressure above a critical level of about 10 to 15 mm Hg. An additional factor is the accumulation of fluid around compressible small vessels when plasma oncotic pressure is exceeded by pulmonary venous pressure. When a person is in the upright position, the pressure in the lower lung is greater because of hydrostatic forces; therefore, vasoconstriction of both arteries and veins occurs here first and increases resistance to flow, thereby reducing the circulatory volume through these vessels. To overcome the increased resistance and to maintain a gradient in the presence of increased pulmonary venous pressure, the pulmonary artery pressure must increase, resulting in increased flow to the apices. The diverted pulmonary flow increases the size and visibility of the upper-lobe vessels (Fig. 23). As pulmonary venous hypertension increases to the order of 25 mm Hg, there is increased transudation of plasma from the lower lung capillaries that results in interstitial edema. In addition to obscuring further the now smaller and crowded lower-lobe vessels, this transudation results in the radiographic appearance of septal lines (Kerley lines), which are due to fluid within the interlobular septa (Fig. 24). Still further increase in pulmonary venous pressure results in transudation of plasma into the alveoli, producing classic alveolar edema when the pressure exceeds 30 mm Hg.

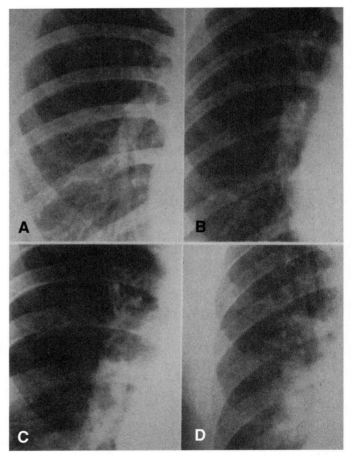

Fig. 23. *A-D,* Serial radiographs demonstrating development of pulmonary venous hypertension continuing on to florid pulmonary edema in a patient with a large myocardial infarction. Note the progressive redistribution of the prominence of the pulmonary vessels to the right upper lobe. The hilar vessels become much less distinct as the edema develops.

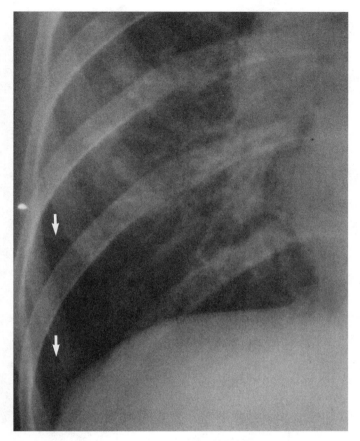

Fig. 24. Interstitial edema with appearance of Kerley lines (*arrows*) due to fluid within the interlobular septa.

Pulmonary Arterial Hypertension

Increased resistance at the pulmonary capillary or arteriolar level increases pulmonary artery pressure. The causes of pulmonary arterial hypertension include 1) obstructive processes (e.g., chronic pulmonary emboli, idiopathic or primary pulmonary arterial hypertension, pulmonary schistosomiasis), 2) obliterative processes (e.g., pulmonary fibrosis, COPD), 3) constrictive processes (e.g., chronic hypoxia), and 4) increased flow as seen in large left-to-right shunts with development of Eisenmenger syndrome (Fig. 25 and 26). Radiographically, pulmonary arteries are dilated centrally, with an abrupt disparity in the caliber of the central and intrapulmonary arteries or "pruning" of the intrapulmonary branches. This uneven response is thought to be due to constriction of the muscular intrapulmonary branches in response to the increased intraluminal pressures, with dilatation of the more elastic central arteries.

- The classic chest radiographic findings in pulmonary arterial hypertension are dilated distal proximal pulmonary arteries and "pruning" of intrapulmonary branches.

Pericardial Disease

Normal pericardium is seldom identified on plain chest radiographs. It may be visible as a sharp line at the cardiac apex, outlined by epicardial and mediastinal fat.

Pericardial Effusion

A pericardial stripe wider than 2 mm that parallels the lower heart border, usually in the lateral projection and best identified in the sternophrenic angle, is diagnostic of a pericardial effusion. The only clue to a relatively small effusion may be a noticeable change in heart size compared with that on previous films. The classic "water flask" configuration of a large effusion may not be present, and the appearance of the cardiac silhouette may be identical to that in dilated cardiomyopathy with no significant distortion other than enlargement. A large heart with a prominent superior vena cava and azygos vein in combination with decreased pulmonary vasculature should raise the question of cardiac tamponade. Acutely, a relatively small effusion can cause tamponade with minimal enlargement of the cardiac shadow.

Pericardial Calcification

Constrictive pericarditis may occur as the end result of pericarditis and pericardial effusion of any cause. Calcification of the pericardium is highly suggestive but not pathognomonic of constrictive pericarditis. More than 50% of patients with constrictive pericarditis do not show calcifications on the plain chest film. Calcifications are found frequently on the anterior and diaphragmatic surfaces, but they may be over any part of the heart. Linear or plaque-like calcifications, often best seen on the lateral view, are typically projected over the right ventricle or the atrioventricular groove (Fig. 27). The entire heart may appear encased in a shell. The calcification may be quite dense and thick.

- More than 50% of patients with constrictive pericarditis do not show pericardial calcification.

Pericardial Defects

Congenital or surgical absence of the pericardium may result in changes in the cardiac contours. Congenital absence is more commonly left-sided and rarely right-sided. Partial defects may allow a portion of the heart (usually the left atrial appendage in congenital defects) to herniate outside the pericardial sac, with the herniated portion producing a bulge in the contour of the heart. "Complete" absence of the

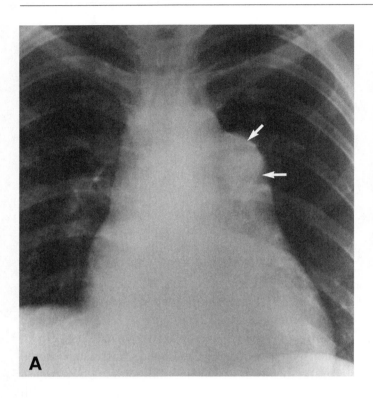

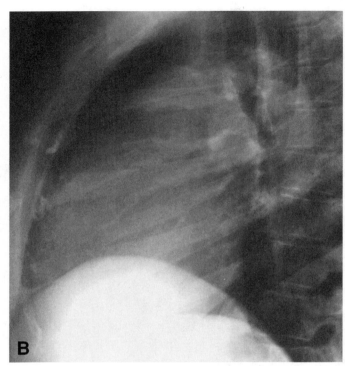

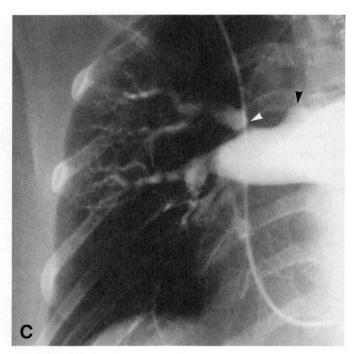

Fig. 25. Pulmonary hypertension due to chronic pulmonary emboli. Note the central pulmonary artery enlargement (*arrows*) (*A*) and right ventricular dilatation seen best in the lateral projection (*B*). The angiogram demonstrates classic arterial occlusions and stenoses (*arrowheads*) (*C*).

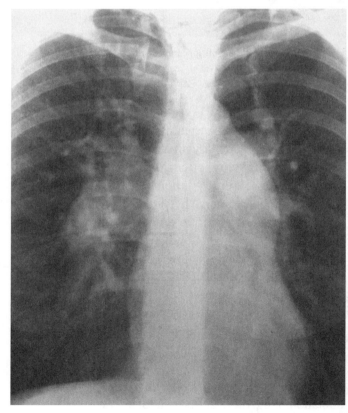

Fig. 26. Marked enlargement of the pulmonary arteries centrally secondary to Eisenmenger syndrome caused by long-standing atrial septal defect.

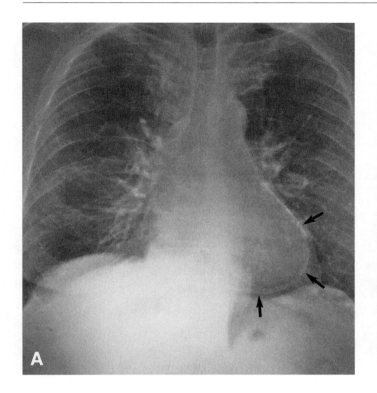

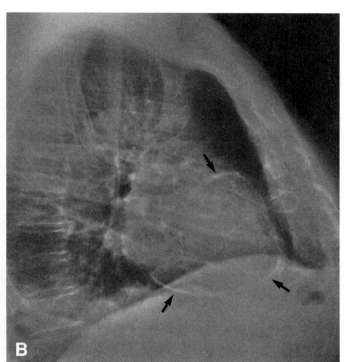

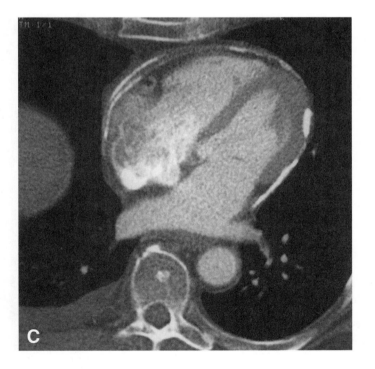

Fig. 27. *A* and *B*, Plain films showing constrictive pericarditis with circumferential pericardial calcifications (*arrows*). Note the pulmonary venous hypertension and right pleural effusion. *C*, Computed tomographic image through the mid ventricles better demonstrates the circumferential nature of the relatively coarse calcifications.

pericardium is actually a unilateral defect and nearly always left-sided. The heart appears shifted to the left without a shift in the trachea (Fig. 28). The left cardiac contour has an elongated appearance. The pulmonary artery often appears prominent and sharply defined. A somewhat similar appearance is seen on the frontal projection when the heart is rotated because of compression of the chest wall in patients with pectus excavatum deformity.

- Partial or "complete" absence of the pericardium is usually left-sided.

Cardiac Masses

The role of plain chest radiographs in the identification of cardiac masses is often limited. Radiologic manifestations are dependent on tumor size and location as well as type. With many intracavitary and intramural tumors of even moderate size, no changes are seen on plain films unless hemodynamic alterations are produced, such as the mimicking of mitral stenosis by a left atrial myxoma. Left ventricular aneurysms, pericardial cysts, extracardiac mediastinal masses, loculated pericardial cysts, and loculated pericardial effusions are all causes of abnormal contours that can be indistinguishable from neoplasms (Fig. 29 and 30). The presence of calcification may help in the detection of a mass, but calcification patterns are not specific, and differentiation from calcification of thrombus or normal structures usually requires additional imaging modalities.

Aortic Disease

The aortic knob, representing the foreshortened transverse aortic arch, is the only border-forming portion of the normal thoracic aorta that is otherwise hidden within the mediastinum. The descending thoracic aorta parallels the thoracic spine on the left. With the development of atherosclerotic aortic disease, unfolding and ectasia (dilatation and elongation) of the aorta occur. As the descending aorta swings into the left chest, more and more of the contour becomes silhouetted by lung; on the lateral projection, a portion of the descending aorta

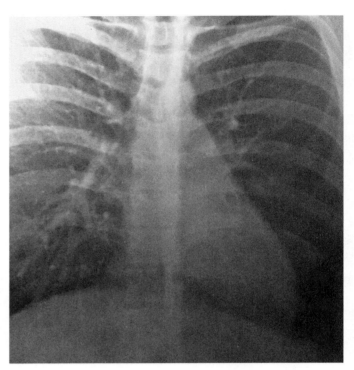

Fig. 28. Absence of pericardium resulting in displacement of the cardiac apex to the left, mimicking an oblique projection.

may be demonstrated, and only then is a clue to the presence of an aneurysm obtained. Unfolding or ectasia of the ascending aorta produces a convexity of the right superior mediastinum. These findings may be indistinguishable from those present with an aortic aneurysm. The most common finding of an aortic aneurysm on a frontal chest radiograph is widening of the superior mediastinum (Fig. 31). Other chest film findings suggestive of a thoracic aortic aneurysm, whether atherosclerotic, luetic, dissecting, or traumatic, include displacement or compression (or both) of the trachea and esophagus either to the left and posteriorly by an aneurysm of the ascending aorta or to the right and anteriorly by an aneurysm of the descending aorta. Calcification in the aorta is a common finding in atherosclerotic aortic disease. Because the aorta is largely hidden by the mediastinal silhouette, the cross-sectional modalities, such as computed tomography and magnetic resonance imaging, provide greater detail in the evaluation and follow-up of aortic disease (Fig. 32-34).

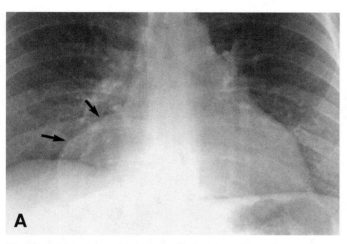
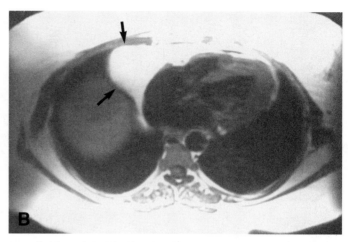

Fig. 29. *A*, Mass (*arrows*) in right cardiophrenic angle consistent with a prominent cardiac fat pad. *B*, The high signal of adipose tissue (*arrows*) is demonstrated with magnetic resonance imaging of this region.

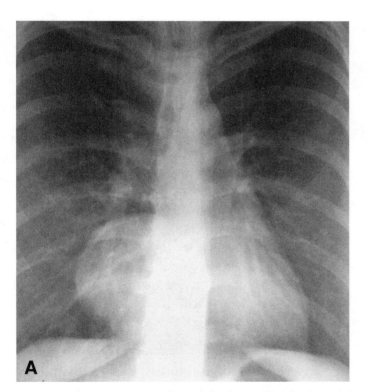
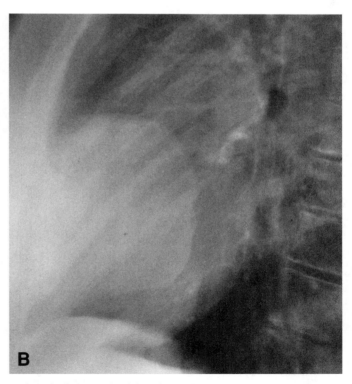

Fig. 30. *A*, PA and, *B*, lateral projections showing a well-defined rounded mass projected adjacent to the right atrium. The heart and pulmonary vasculature are otherwise normal. Appearance is typical of a pericardial cyst.

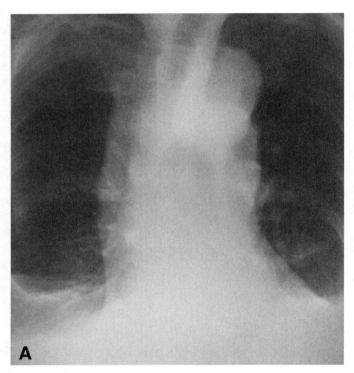 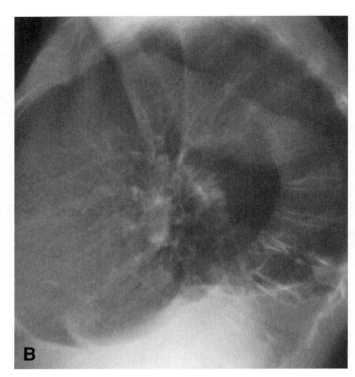

Fig. 31. *A*, PA and, *B*, lateral projections showing marked enlargement of the aortic knob and widening of the mediastinum due to a large ascending aortic aneurysm. The size of the ascending aorta is appreciated better on the lateral view. The patient has significant aortic regurgitation with bilateral pleural effusions.

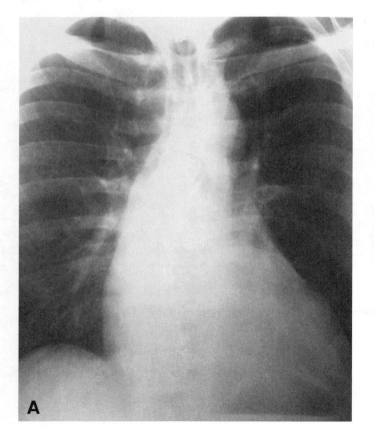 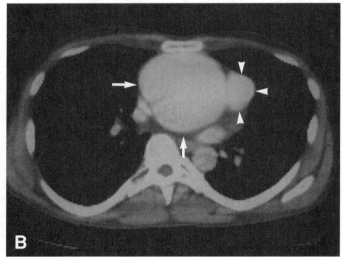

Fig. 32. *A*, PA projection showing marked enlargement of the ascending aorta caused by a dissecting aneurysm. *B*, This is appreciated better on a computed tomographic scan. Note discrepancy in size between the ascending aorta (*arrows*) and the main pulmonary artery (*arrowheads*).

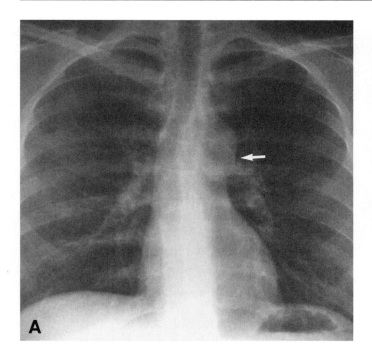

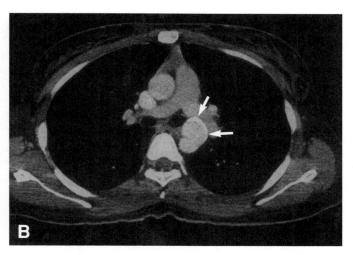

Fig. 33. *A*, Enlargement of the aortic arch containing curvilinear calcification (*arrow*). *B*, Computed tomographic scan demonstrates better the small pseudoaneurysm containing peripheral calcification (*arrows*), the result of remote trauma.

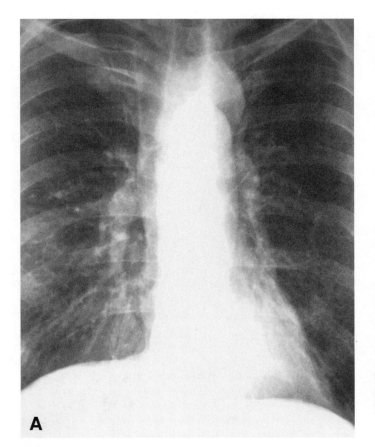

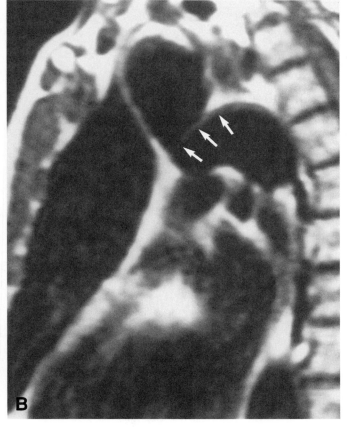

Fig. 34. *A*, Double contour to the aortic arch typical of coarctation. *B*, A magnetic resonance image nicely demonstrates the focal narrowing and resulting kinking (*arrows*) of the proximal descending aorta.

Questions

Multiple Choice (choose the one best answer)

1. These two patients have the same condition. What is it?
   a. Left ventricular aneurysms
   b. Normal chest radiographs, but the patients are poorly positioned for the studies
   c. Absent pericardium
   d. Dilated cardiomyopathy
   e. Pulmonary hypertension

2. What is the diagnosis?
   a. Calcified left ventricular aneurysms
   b. Left atrial calcification due to mitral stenosis
   c. Dense mitral annulus calcification
   d. Pericardial calcification
   e. Calcified pleural plaques

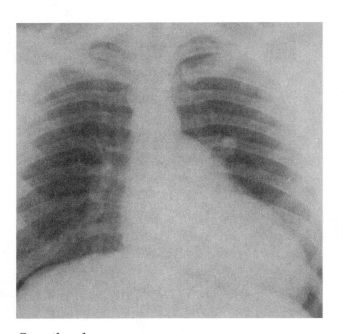
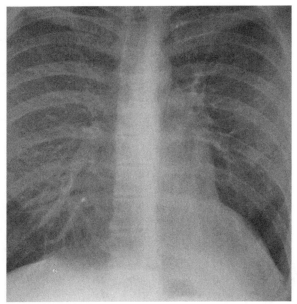

Question 1

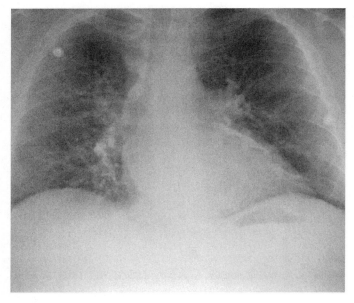
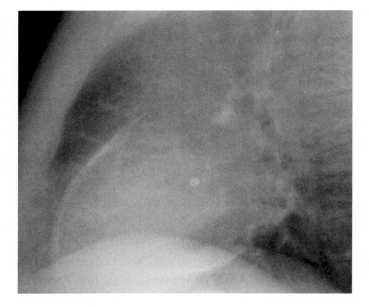

Question 2

3. These four patients all have the same condition. What is it?
   a. Ventricular septal defect
   b. Atrial septal defect
   c. Patent ductus arteriosus
   d. Chronic pulmonary emboli
   e. Left ventricular failure with pulmonary venous hypertension

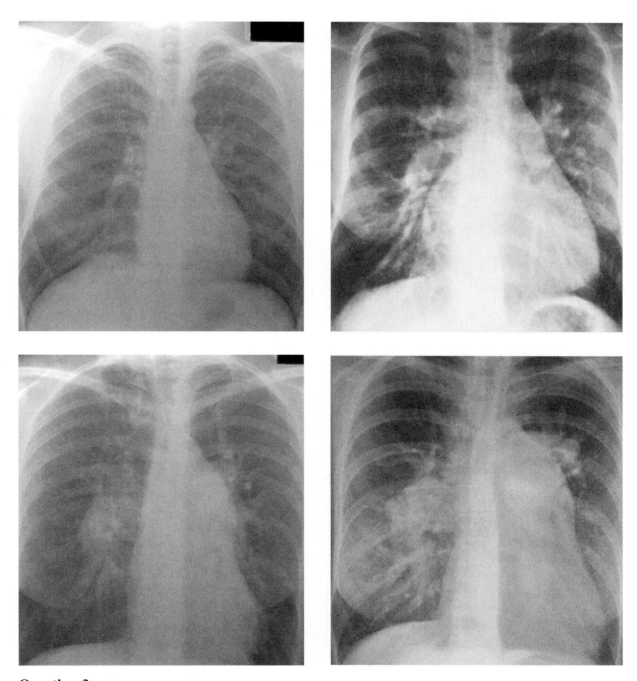

Question 3

4. What is the diagnosis?
   a. Type A dissection
   b. Type B dissection
   c. Traumatic aortic transection
   d. Syphilis
   e. Penetrating aortic ulcer

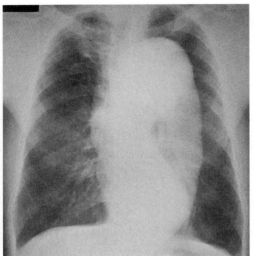

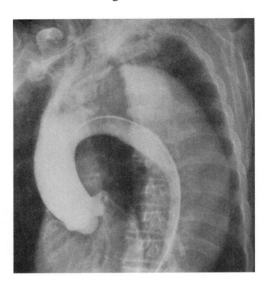

Question 4

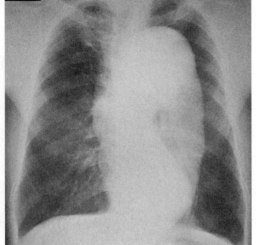

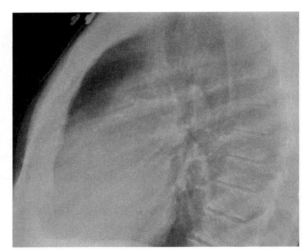

Question 5

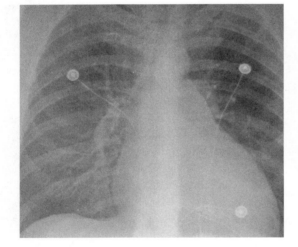

5. Which chamber is massively enlarged?
   a. Left ventricle
   b. Right ventricle
   c. Left atrium
   d. Right atrium

6. This patient has radiographic findings of which of the following conditions?
   a. Mitral stenosis
   b. Aneurysm of the left atrial appendage
   c. Left atrial myxoma
   d. Cor triatriatum

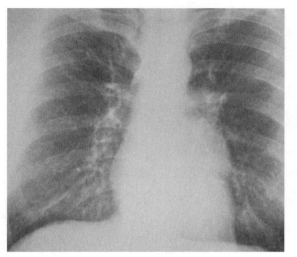

Question 6

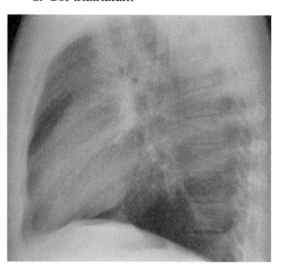

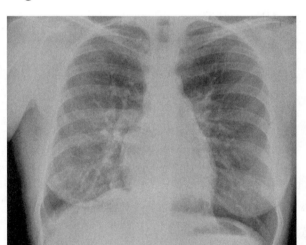

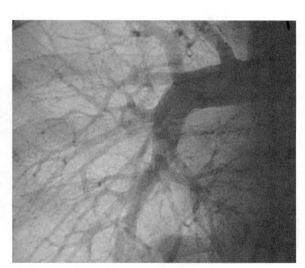

Question 7

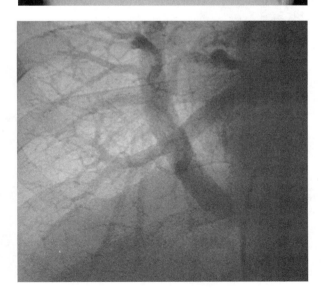

7. What is the diagnosis?
   a. Normal findings
   b. Partial anomalous return of the right upper lobe pulmonary vein
   c. Scimitar syndrome
   d. Arteriovenous fistula
   e. Total anomalous venous return below the diaphragm

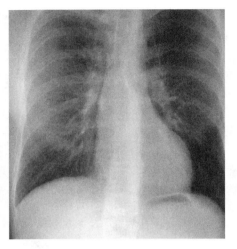

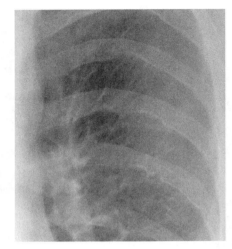

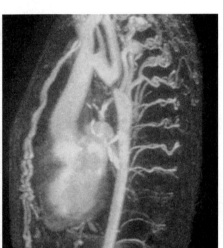

Question 8

8. What is the diagnosis?
   a. Coarctation of the aorta
   b. Pseudocoarctation of the aorta
   c. Type IV truncus arteriosus
   d. Chronic aortic dissection
   e. Arteriovenous malformation of the aorta

9. What is the diagnosis?
   a. Ventricular septal defect
   b. Atrial septal defect

   c. Pulmonary stenosis
   d. Coarctation of the aorta
   e. Patent ductus arteriosus

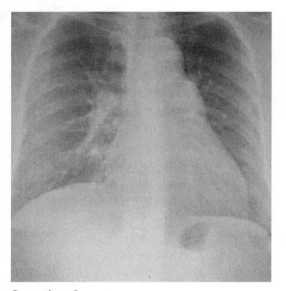

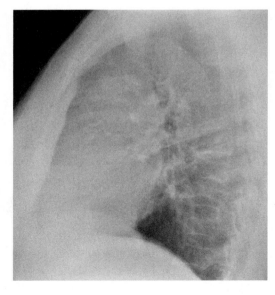

Question 9

10. What is the diagnosis?
    a. Ventricular septal defect
    b. Patent ductus arteriosus
    c. Pulmonary stenosis
    d. Coarctation of the aorta
    e. Truncus arteriosus

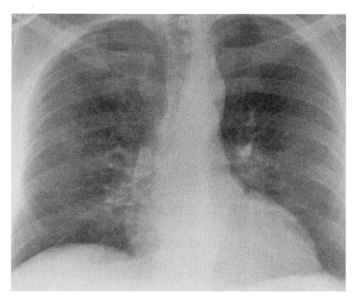 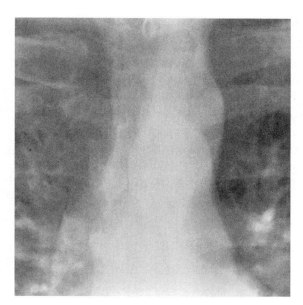

Question 10

Answers

1. Answer c

The heart is shifted to the left but is normal size. The patient is properly positioned. Pectus excavatum also causes this appearance.

2. Answer d

Dense coarse calcification is seen surrounding the heart.

3. Answer b

Four classic examples of patients with atrial septal defect of different severity and duration.

4. Answer b

The dissection flap is not present in the ascending aorta.

5. Answer b

Note how unimpressive the chest radiograph is compared with this patient's computed tomographic scan. The left ventricle is compressed, with flattening of the interventricular septum.

6. Answer b

This patient has an aneurysm of the left atrial appendage. There is no enlargement of the body of the left atrium and no evidence of pulmonary venous or arterial hypertension. The chambers on the right side are not enlarged. Partial absence of the pericardium with a herniated left atrial appendage can also look like this and would be in the differential diagnosis for this patient.

7. Answer c

The chest radiograph and pulmonary angiograms show the classic findings of scimitar syndrome, namely, anomalous connection of the right pulmonary vein(s) to the inferior vena cava, hypoplasia of the right lung, anomalous systemic pulmonary arterial blood supply to the right lung from the aorta, and bronchial abnormalities.

8. Answer a

Coarctation of the aorta. The magnetic resonance image on the right shows the marked narrowing of the descending aorta, with the development of large intercostal collateral vessels. The middle image shows rib notching, a classic radiographic feature of coarctation of the aorta caused by inferior rib erosion due to large collateral intercostal arteries.

9. Answer e

The aorta is prominent along with dilated pulmonary arteries, shunt vascularity, and an enlarged left ventricle.

10. Answer d

The chest radiograph shows an abnormal contour of the aortic arch with a localized indentation at the site of the coarctation to give the "3" sign. Rib notching is absent in this case. The upper curve of the "3" is formed by the left subclavian artery, and the lower half of the curve of the "3" is formed by the post-stenotic dilatation of the aorta.

Chapter 57

Atlas of Radiographs of Congenital Heart Defects

Jerome F. Breen, M.D.
Joseph G. Murphy. M.D.

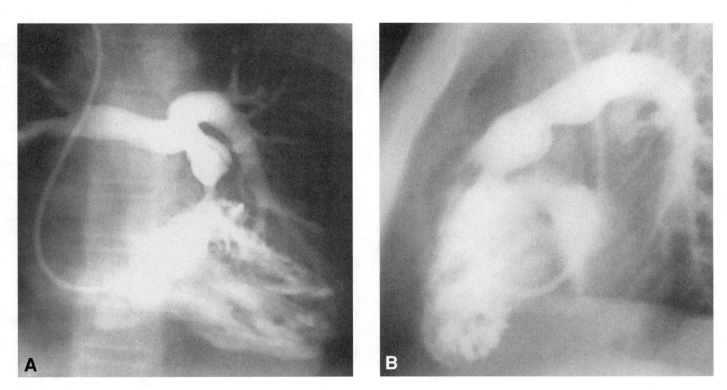

Fig. 1. Tetralogy of Fallot. Right ventriculogram shows marked infundibular stenosis in both frontal (*A*) and lateral (*B*) projections.

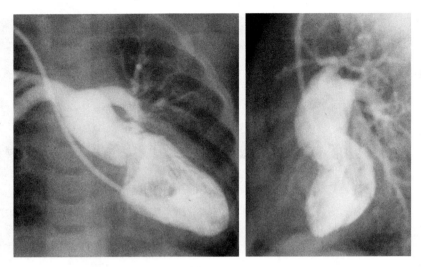

Fig. 2. D-Transposition with intact ventricular septum.

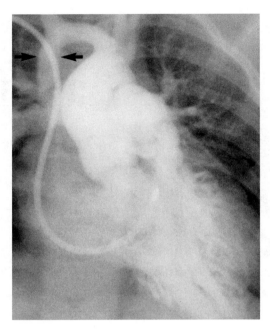

Fig. 3. Tetralogy of Fallot with right subclavian artery-to-right pulmonary artery anastomosis (*arrows*) (right Blalock operation).

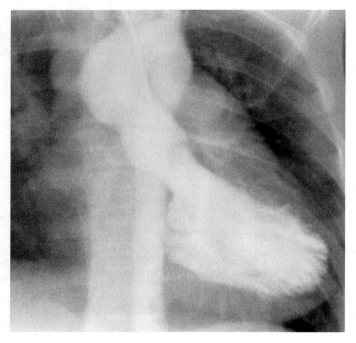

Fig. 4. Partial atrioventricular canal defect. Catheter in left ventricle.

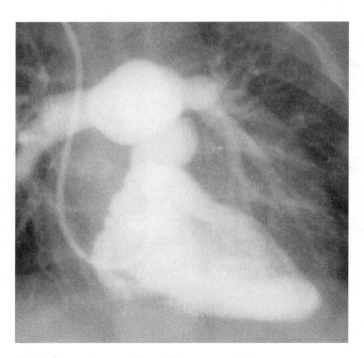

Fig. 5. Corrected transposition with intact ventricular septum.

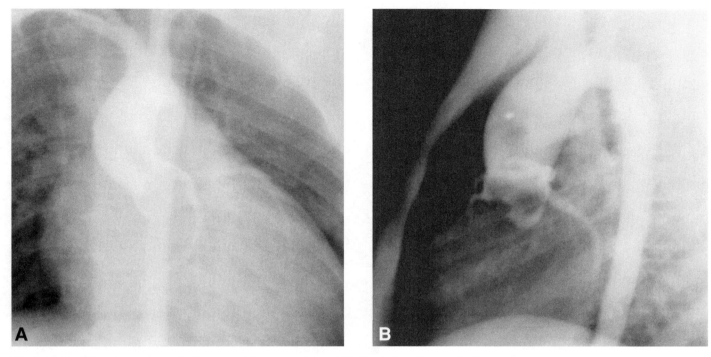

Fig. 6. Congenital aortic stenosis. *A*, Left anterior oblique projection. *B*, Right anterior oblique projection.

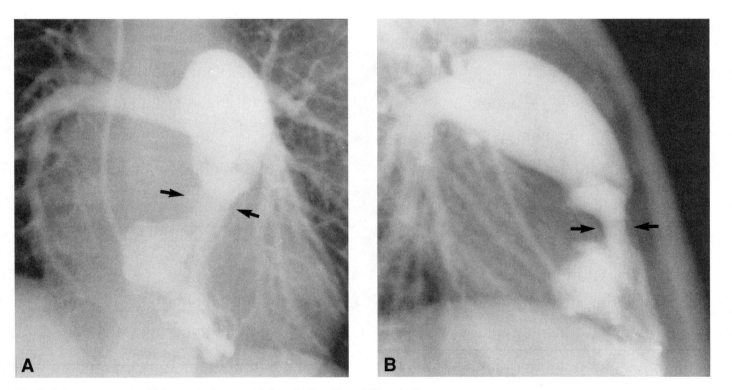

Fig. 7. Pulmonary stenosis. Right ventriculogram with frontal (*A*) and lateral (*B*) projections.

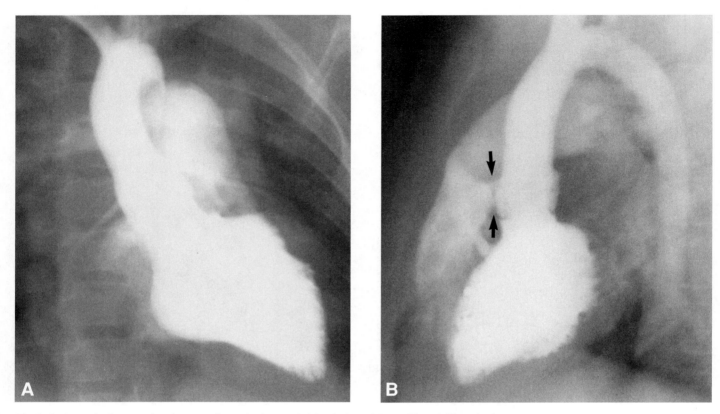

Fig. 8. Left ventriculograms showing a small ventricular septal defect in frontal (*A*) and lateral (*B*) projections.

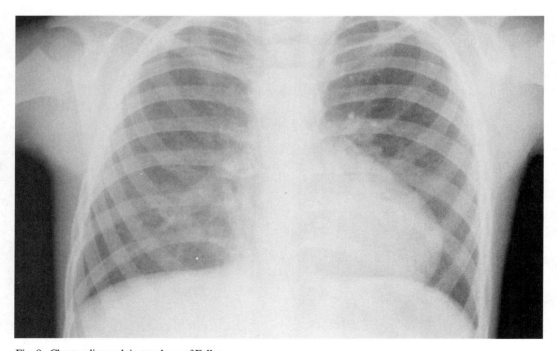

Fig. 9. Chest radiograph in tetralogy of Fallot.

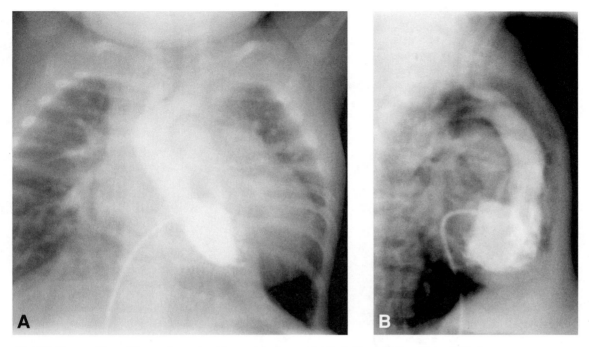

Fig. 10. Transposition of the great vessels with a ventricular septal defect. Frontal (*A*) and lateral (*B*) views.

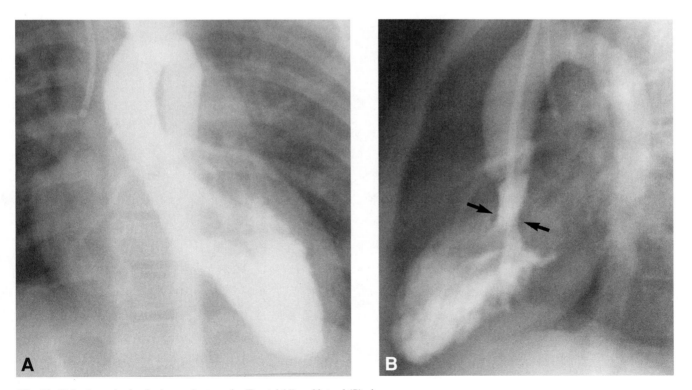

Fig. 11. Valvular and subvalvular aortic stenosis. Frontal (*A*) and lateral (*B*) views.

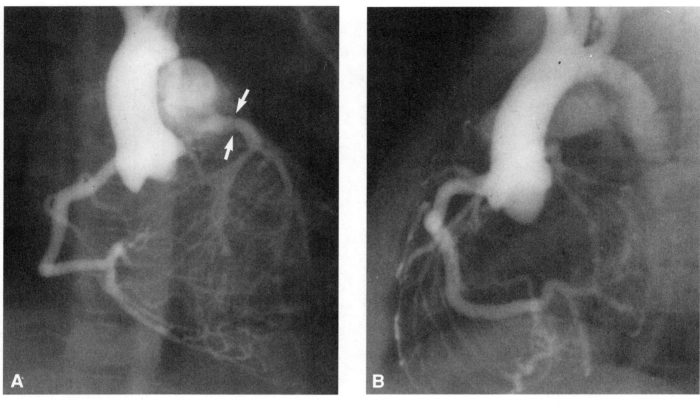

Fig. 12. Origin of the left coronary artery from the pulmonary artery (*arrows*). The right coronary artery arises normally from the right coronary sinus. *A*, Left anterior oblique projection. *B*, Right anterior oblique projection.

Chapter 58

Essential Molecular Biology of Cardiovascular Diseases

Robert D. Simari, M.D.

Basics of Molecular Biology

DNA is the fundamental genetic material of life and specifies the amino acid sequence of the large number of proteins that make up cells. Nucleotides are the building blocks of DNA. DNA consists of nucleotide chains, and each nucleotide consists of a nitrogenous base (purine or pyrimidine), a pentose sugar (2-deoxyribose in DNA and ribose in ribonucleic acid [RNA]), and a phosphate group. The four bases in DNA are adenine (A), guanine (G), cytosine (C), and thymine (T); uridine (U) replaces thymine in RNA (Fig. 1). The nucleotide sequence determines the amino acids encoded. It is the sequence-specific pairing of these nucleotides that is the basis of inheritance of the genetic code. A binds to T and G binds to C: it is from this pairing that the double helical structure of DNA is derived, with its unique ability to reproduce very accurately over many generations (each chain acting as a unique template to which complementary base pairs bind). The genetic information in DNA is transferred to RNA through a process called "transcription" and from RNA to peptides (proteins) through "translation."

- Pyramidines (A and G) bind only to purines (C, T, and U).
- A binds to T.
- G binds to C.
- DNA is double-stranded.
- RNA is single-stranded.

- $DNA \xrightarrow{\text{transcription}} RNA \xrightarrow{\text{translation}} Protein.$

Gene Structure

A gene is a collection of adjacent nucleotides that specify the amino acids of a unique polypeptide. A chromosome is a microscopically visible long thread of DNA that contains many genes. The human genome has 23 pairs of chromosomes (44 autosomal + 2 sex chromosomes) containing about 3 billion base pairs of DNA and approximately 100,000 genes. The primary structure of DNA is determined by its base pair composition (Plate 1). Double-stranded DNA in chromosomes forms a double helical structure that undergoes subsequent supercoiling. Supercoils are additional positive or negative twists that are superimposed on the double helical structure.

A chromosome consists of both nucleic acids and proteins. DNA is complexed with proteins, called "histones," into nucleoprotein fibers, called "chromatin." It is chromatin that gives DNA its beadlike appearance. There are five main classes of histones: H1, H2A, H2B, H3, and H4. Two molecules each of histone H2A, H2B, H3, and H4 form a core, around which 200 base pairs of DNA are wound to form "nucleosomes" (Plate 4). Between nucleosomes, DNA is complexed with histone H1.

A gene contains important structural elements necessary for its function. The "average" gene encodes for 400 amino acids. Genes are divided into "exons" and "introns." Introns

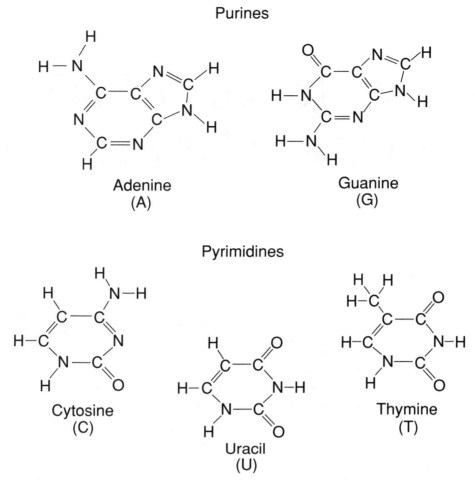

Fig. 1. Chemical structure of purines and pyrimidines.

are DNA sequences whose RNA products are nonfunctional and are removed from messenger RNA (mRNA). Each intron contains specific identifying base pair sequences at its boundaries. In contrast, exons are DNA sequences whose RNA products are fully functional and "exit" from the nucleus and enter the cytoplasm, where they specify specific proteins (Plate 3).

Every nucleic acid chain has an orientation that refers to the orientation of its sugar phosphate backbone. The end that terminates with the 5' carbon is called the "5' end," and the end that terminates with the 3' carbon is called the "3' end." Because double-stranded DNA helices contain identical copies, it is standard to refer to DNA in the 5' to 3' direction. DNA and RNA chains form in the 5' - 3' direction, and proteins are formed in the same direction, which is from the amino to carboxy terminus of the polypeptide chain.

Genes contain DNA sequences that are involved in the control of production of mRNA (transcription) and protein (translation). Promoters are upstream regulatory elements that bind RNA polymerases and the complex of proteins that regulate transcription. Enhancers and suppressors are bidirectional DNA sequences that modulate transcription of DNA and can be found within or at a distance from a gene. At the end of genes are sequences responsible for the termination of transcription and the addition of polyadenylation sequences required for mRNA transport.

From Gene to Protein

The DNA sequence within the exons of a gene and the amino acids that it codes are colinear (Fig. 2). That is, DNA encodes for specific amino acids in a linear fashion, with 3 bases representing 1 amino acid. There is a lack of a 1- to-1 relationship between all possible groups of 3 nucleic acids (codons) and amino acids. Thus, the genetic code is a degenerate code with 64 possible codons specifying only 20 amino acids. Each amino acid has 1 to 6 specifying codons.

Transcription, the formation of RNA from DNA, is a complex process that involves many known and unknown proteins in a highly regulated fashion (Plate 2). Transcription in eukaryotic cells is in three forms, using different RNA polymerases. Transcription that results in mRNA (which makes up only 3% to 5% of total RNA within a cell) is dependent on RNA polymerase II. The RNA polymerases are made up of several subunits and bind DNA sequences (promoters) through separate DNA binding proteins known as "transcription factors." The RNA strand produced by the polymerase is formed upon a single-strand DNA template. This resulting mRNA is complementary to the template DNA.

- A codon is three successive nucleotides of mRNA that code for a single amino acid.
- "STOP" and "START" codons signal the start and termination of protein RNA translation.

The primary mRNA (pre-mRNA) transcript must undergo several processing steps before protein translation can occur in the cytoplasm. The ends of the initial transcript must be modified with methyl capping of the 5' terminal end and polyadenylation of the 3' terminal end. The removal of introns by splicing in the nucleus results in a mature mRNA that is transported to the cytoplasm for translation. Complementary DNA (cDNA) is a product of reverse transcribing mRNA and, as such, does not contain introns.

Translation is the complex interaction between three types of RNA: mRNA acts as a template, ribosomal RNA (rRNA) forms the ribosomes, and transfer RNA (tRNA) acts as a carrier of the amino acids to be incorporated into the polypeptide. mRNA contains the genetic code in the form of codons that identify the sequence of amino acids to be added to the growing polypeptide chain. The resulting protein is then released and can have either an intracellular or extracellular role.

Regulation of Gene Expression

Genes are expressed in a regulated manner throughout an organism. It is this gene regulation that ultimately underlies the variability among cells, tissues, and organisms. Gene expression may be regulated at several levels. Transcriptional regulation modulates the production of mRNA. Translational and post-translational regulation modulate the production and activity of proteins that are expressed.

Regulation of transcription can be direct or indirect. An example of indirect regulation is the effect of modifying

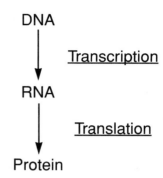

Genetic Paradigm

Fig. 2. The genetic paradigm.

histones by enzymes capable of acetylation or deacetylation of histones that affect the formation of nucleosomes and, thus, the accessibility of RNA polymerases to DNA. A more direct form of regulation is through transcription factors. Transcription factors are specific proteins capable of binding specific DNA sequences and modulating the rate of transcription (Plate 5). Several groups of transcription factors have been identified and are classified by similarities in their protein structure. Zinc finger, helix-loop-helix, and leucine zippers are separate groups of transcription factors known to regulate gene expression.

Translational and post-translational regulation vary in importance with the proteins studied. Some proteins (clotting factors) are made in a precursor form and activated by other proteins (post-translational regulation). Other gene products are regulated either solely or partially at the transcriptional level.

Tools of the Cardiovascular Molecular Biologist

When heated, DNA can be denatured, that is, separated into two complementary strands. With cooling, these strands can be reannealed. Complementary sequences of DNA from other sources, such as short oligonucleotides, can bind in a species-specific manner to single-stranded DNA templates. This binding is referred to as "hybridization."

DNA Techniques

To facilitate handling of short segments of DNA, fragments are often inserted into plasmids, which are circular double-stranded DNA structures (Plate 6). Plasmids have their origin in bacteria and are often associated with the transfer of antibiotic resistance. Plasmids can be used to carry DNA fragments for manipulation and to express genes in vitro or in vivo.

Manipulating DNA Fragments

Portions of DNA, whether genomic or cellular DNA, can be cut, ligated, and extended using a set of powerful enzymes. Restriction endonucleases are bacterial proteins that are capable of cutting DNA at specific DNA sequences (Plate 7). Restriction endonucleases cut within DNA sequences and leave either a 3' or a 5' overlap or blunt ends. Exonucleases are capable of cutting DNA ends that are free in order to tailor recombination events.

Enzymes called "DNA polymerases" can be used to extend DNA fragments. Ligases are capable of joining either blunt or complementary (sticky) ends of DNA, creating a recombinant DNA molecule. This process is often referred to as "cloning."

Analyzing DNA Fragments

The base pair sequence of a fragment of DNA can be determined at a gross or exact level. The use of restriction digests can be very helpful in determining the relative composition of a DNA sequence. Because restriction endonucleases identify specific DNA sequences and the distance between adjacent cuts can be determined with agarose gel electrophoresis, nondetailed maps of DNA fragments can be made.

Sequencing

Sequencing is a powerful tool that enables molecular biologists to create a detailed map containing each base within a portion of DNA. The two classic techniques for sequencing DNA are the Sanger method and the Maxam and Gilbert method. The Sanger method sequences a template DNA using four labeled dideoxynucleotides and a primer (short oligonucleotide complementary to one end). With the use of DNA polymerase, the dideoxynucleotides, when incorporated, terminate the chain. By altering the composition of the dideoxynucleotides, the resulting chains can be identified and, thus, the sequence determined. The Maxam and Gilbert method depends on a series of chemicals that destroy certain bases or combinations of bases. When a portion of radiolabeled DNA is subjected to these reactions and the products are isolated and electrophoresed, the sequences can be inferred.

Southern Blotting

Hybridization of a radiolabeled probe (oligonucleotide) to a template DNA can be used to identify specific DNA fragments (Plate 9). Hybridization to immobilized DNA was first performed by E. M. Southern and is referred to as "Southern blotting." First, a radiolabeled probe is created that is complementary to the target to be identified. Second, the DNA to be analyzed is cut with restriction endonucleases and the resulting fragments are electrophoresed. Third, the DNA is transferred from the agarose to a nylon membrane and fixed to it. Fourth, the probe is hybridized to the membrane. Finally, after washes to remove nonspecific binding, the membrane is exposed to x-ray film. The label exposes the film, identifying specific hybridization to a DNA fragment.

- Southern blotting is used to analyze DNA.
- Northern blotting is used to analyze RNA.
- Western blotting is used to analyze proteins.

Polymerase Chain Reaction

The polymerase chain reaction (PCR) takes advantage of the heat stability of the DNA polymerase from *Thermus aquaticus* (Taq) (Plate 8). The goal of PCR is to amplify a target DNA fragment. The procedure mixes the DNA sample being used as a template, free nucleotides, and the Taq polymerase at 94°C. After DNA denaturation (separation into complementary strands) the temperature is decreased to 55°C, allowing the target sequence to polymerize. This results in an exact copy of the target sequence. Repeating this process 30 to 40 times can generate up to 2^{40} copies of the target DNA. PCR is a powerful tool for amplifying minute portions of DNA for analysis.

- PCR is used to amplify small amounts of DNA.

RNA Techniques

Unlike DNA, which is stable for relatively long periods even at room temperature, RNA is an unstable molecule that is susceptible to degradation from ubiquitous RNAses. Thus, great care is required to obtain and to analyze RNA from cells or tissue. In addition, mRNA representing the genes that are expressed in any cell makes up only a minority of the total RNA within a cell.

Northern Blotting

As with DNA, RNA can be electrophoresed and transferred to membranes and hybridized with labeled probes (Plate 8). These probes can either be DNA or RNA. This process is called "Northern blotting." It provides a means for identifying and quantifying the amount of an RNA species in a sample.

Reverse Transcriptase-Polymerase Chain Reaction
Amplification of mRNA can be performed using reverse transcriptase-PCR (RT-PCR). RT-PCR requires that mRNA undergo reverse transcription to cDNA before the initial amplification steps. This can be performed with a retroviral reverse transcriptase enzyme.

DNA-Protein
As mentioned above, much of the important gene regulation is based on the interactions between proteins and DNA. Techniques have been developed to analyze proteins that bind in a sequence-specific manner to DNA. A popular technique to assess this protein-DNA interaction is the electrophoretic mobility shift assay (EMSA). EMSA is based on the fact that the electrophoretic mobility of DNA fragments bound to protein is delayed compared with that of unbound DNA. Thus, nuclear protein extracts are isolated and exposed to short fragments of radiolabeled double-stranded DNA in a binding buffer. The resulting mixture is electrophoresed and exposed to X-ray film. Unbound DNA runs faster, whereas DNA bound to protein is delayed ("shifted"). Further identification of the bound protein can be pursued by adding to the mixture antibodies specific for the proteins, resulting in further electrophoretic delay ("supershift").

Western Blotting
Western blotting is used to sequence proteins by gel electrophoresis, using antibody probes analogous to Southern blotting for DNA analysis.

Molecular Genetics

The identification of genes associated with disease has been the focus of an enormous effort in biomedical science. Classically, the identification of a disease-related protein led to the development of probes, either nucleic acids or antibodies, with which to screen DNA libraries. The screening of a genomic library can identify the gene associated with the disease (Plate 10). However, the number of diseases for which detailed biochemical defects are known is few.

LOD Score
Without detailed knowledge of the disease protein, positional cloning techniques (gene mapping) can be used to identify disease-related genes. Gene mapping is based on Mendel's laws of genetics, which state that genes sort independently. Thus, truly independent genes should have a 50% chance of association after meiotic sorting. Genes that are tightly linked on a chromosome will have less chance to cross over during meiosis, creating an increased chance of cosegregation (linkage) (Fig. 3 and 4). Linkage analysis is based on the statistical chances that the genes will sort independently. For instance, genes in disparate locations will sort independently, whereas two genes in proximity are less likely to sort independently.

An increasing number of chromosomal markers are available for linkage analysis. Pedigree analysis of families is needed to determine the patterns of coinheritance and the potential linkage with known markers. A likelihood ratio is determined for the coinheritance. For instance, if the likelihood for cosegregation is 1,000:1, the log of the odds ratio (LOD) is 3 (log 1,000 is 3). A LOD score of 3 is the lower limit for statistically significant linkage (95% probability of linkage). After a linkage has been determined, further analysis of the chromosomal region can be performed to isolate the gene of interest.

- LOD score is the statistical chance that the disease gene is colocated near the marker gene.
- A LOD score of 3 corresponds to a probability of linkage of 95% and is the lower limit for significance.

In certain situations, reasonable guesses can be made from the knowledge of a disease which would allow for a list of potential genes that might be responsible for the disease (candidate genes). This candidate approach is improved if linkage data are available to narrow the search to a limited list of reasonable candidates. Some of the genes associated with hypertrophic cardiomyopathy have been identified with the candidate gene approach.

Genetic diseases can be associated with single-gene or multigene abnormalities. Single-gene defects provide a model for understanding the mendelian inheritance of disease (Fig. 5). Autosomally related disorders are associated with abnormalities of the autosomes (non-sex chromosomes). These disorders can be dominant or recessive. Dominant disorders require only one copy (of the two) of the mutant gene to cause the disease. In dominant disorders, a child has a 50% chance of inheriting the gene and, thus, the disease. Penetrance and late or variable expression of the disorder may affect the course of the disease. Autosomal recessive disorders require two mutant copies

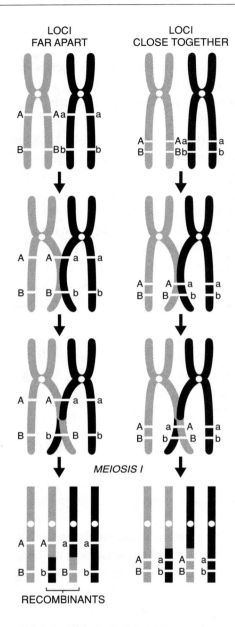

Fig. 3. Segregation of chromosomes depicting differences between close and distant loci.

females to daughters or from males who give their diseased X chromosome exclusively to their daughters. Mutations in the mitochondrial genome are passed from mother to son. Multigenic disorders result from the interaction of multiple genes, and their inheritance pattern is difficult—if not impossible—to discern.

Molecular Basis of Cardiovascular Diseases

Of the many types of diseases that affect the cardiovascular system, an increasing number have been identified to be the result of single-gene or polygenic mutations. Currently, there is a spectrum of cardiac diseases about which the genetic basis is known, including hypertrophic cardiomyopathy (HCM) and the long QT syndrome.

Myocardial Diseases

Hypertrophic Cardiomyopathy
HCM has been recognized as a familial disorder for more than 30 years. It is characterized by great clinical heterogeneity, with architectural disorganization at every level from molecule to ventricle. It also has great genetic heterogeneity. The pattern of inheritance for HCM is autosomal dominant. More than 100 mutations in eight known genetic loci and seven disease genes are associated with HCM. HCM is a disease of sarcomeric proteins, and the genetic variability (defects both within and among genes) may account for the clinical spectrum of disease.

HCM originally was associated with mutations in the β-myosin heavy chain (β-MHC, chromosome 14q11, 30% of patients), α-tropomyosin (chromosome 15q2, 5% of patients), and cardiac troponin T (chromosome 1q3, 15% of patients); however, additions have been made to this list recently, including cardiac myosin-binding protein C (chromosome 11p11.2), essential myosin light chain (chromosome 3), the regulatory myosin light chain (chromosome 12), and cardiac troponin I (chromosome 19). Another locus on chromosome 7q3 has been linked to familial HCM with the Wolff-Parkinson-White syndrome, but the gene responsible has not been identified.

The spectrum of genetic defects associated with HCM has led to the correlation between genotype and phenotype. Clinical studies of β-MHC and cardiac troponin T demonstrated that troponin T mutations may have a significant risk of sudden death in spite of minimal hypertrophy. The

of the gene. A single copy of the mutant gene results in the person being a carrier. The offspring of two carriers have a 1 in 4 chance of having the disease and a 1 in 2 risk of being a carrier.

X-linked disorders result from mutant genes on the X chromosome. Because males have one X chromosome, these disorders act like dominant mutations. In females, they usually act like recessive mutations. Women act as carriers and transmission of disease is only from females to sons. Transmission of carrier status can come from

Cloning disease-related genes

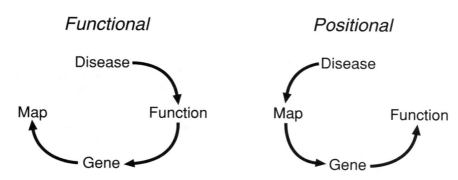

Fig. 4. Functional and positional cloning of disease-related genes.

Arg^{403}Gln mutation in β-MHC has a malignant course similar to that of troponin T defects and more severe than the more benign variant of β-MHC, Val^{606}Met. The development of techniques to screen for these defects clinically in families will allow early detection and better prognosis.

- HCM is associated with mutations in chromosomes 1, 3, 7, 11, 12, 14, 15, and 19.
- Arg^{719}Trp, Arg^{403}Gln, Arg^{453}Cys mutations are associated with a high risk of sudden death.
- Leu^{908}Val mutation is associated with a low risk of sudden death.

Dilated Cardiomyopathy

Dilated cardiomyopathy (DCM) is a primary disorder of the myocardium characterized by increased left ventricular size, decreased ejection fraction, and, in later stages, symptoms of congestive heart failure. In up to 20% to 30% of cases, DCM may have a genetic cause. Some forms of DCM are related to systemic diseases such as muscular dystrophy, whereas others appear as a distinct clinical entity. The understanding of the genetic basis in both types of disease is increasing.

Duchenne muscular dystrophy and its milder form, Becker muscular dystrophy, are associated with defects in the dystrophin gene (*Xp21*); and cardiac involvement is common and is manifested as DCM and heart failure. This is an X-linked disorder. The defective dystrophin gene results in altered expression of dystrophin in cardiac and skeletal muscles. In X-linked DCM, the defect in dystrophin is limited to the myocardium and may be associated with specific mutations within the gene. Other forms of muscular

dystrophy associated with DCM include limb-girdle muscular dystrophy (inherited in an autosomal recessive pattern and associated with defects in the dystrophin-associated glycoprotein complex) and congenital muscular dystrophy (an autosomal dominant disorder associated with defects in laminin).

Genetic defects in DCM not associated with muscular dystrophy have been identified recently. Two unrelated families with DCM have been shown to have mutations in cardiac actin. Unlike HCM, which is associated with deficits in proteins associated with force generation, it has been hypothesized that defects in actin may be associated with deficits in force transmission. Familial DCM is predominantly autosomal dominant in transmission and is frequently asymptomatic and found on screening of family members of an affected person. About 10% of asymptomatic family members will have a normal ejection fraction with an enlarged left ventricular volume.

Mitochondria contain a small amount of DNA that codes for 13 genes involved in mitochondrial metabolism. The Kearns-Sayre syndrome is an example of a mitochondrial cardiomyopathy due to a mitochondrial DNA deletion.

Congenital Heart Disease

Two common examples of the known molecular basis for congenital heart disease are Marfan syndrome and supravalvular aortic stenosis. Marfan syndrome is an autosomal dominant inherited disease with high penetrance characterized by skeletal, cardiovascular, and ocular abnormalities. The incidence of Marfan syndrome is about 1/10,000 births. Premature deaths are due to progressive aortic dilatation with associated aortic insufficiency and aortic dissection. Genetic

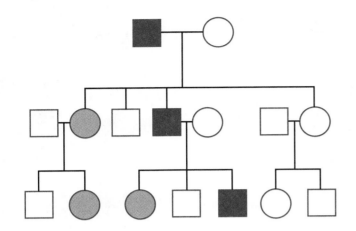

A—Autosomal dominant inheritance

    Multiple generations affected

    Sexes affected equally frequently

    In familial cases, only one parent need be
      affected

    Male-to-male transmission occurs

    Offspring of affected parent have a 50%
      chance of being affected

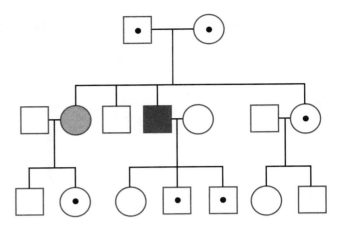

B—Autosomal recessive inheritance

    Single generation affected

    Sexes affected equally frequently

    Each offspring of 2 carriers: 25% affected,
      50% carrier, 25% normal

    2/3 clinically normal offspring are carriers

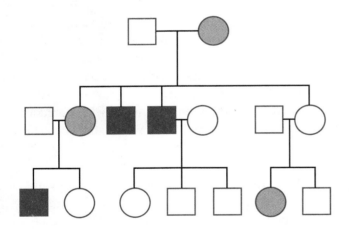

C—Mitochondrial inheritance

    Sexes equally frequently and severely
      affected

    Transmission only through women; offspring
      of affected men are unaffected

    All offspring of affected women may be
      affected

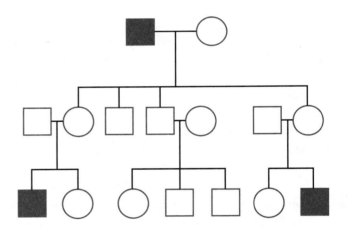

D—X-linked inheritance

    No male-to-male transmission

    All daughters of affected males are carriers

    Sons of carrier mother have 50% chance of
      being affected; daughters have 50% chance
      of being carriers

Fig. 5. *A-D*, Mendelian inheritance patterns. (From Braunwald E [editor]: *Heart Disease: A Textbook of Cardiovascular Medicine*. WB Saunders Company, 1997, p 1654. By permission of the publisher.)

linkage analysis led to the identification of fibrillin as the abnormal protein responsible for this disease. Thirty mutations have been found in the fibrillin gene on chromosome 15 associated with Marfan syndrome.

Linkage analysis has determined that alterations in the elastin gene on chromosome 7 are responsible for supravalvular aortic stenosis. Like Marfan syndrome, this disorder is inherited in an autosomal dominant fashion with high penetrance. Supravalvular aortic stenosis in combination with mental retardation, connective tissue abnormalities, and hypercalcemia is called "Williams syndrome."

Several other single-gene defects are associated with congenital heart disease, including familial atrial septal defects, Holt-Oram syndrome on chromosome 12, and the atrioventricular canal defects associated with Down syndrome. In general, the genetic abnormalities associated with congenital heart disease may result in several clinical presentations.

Arrhythmias

An increasing understanding of the molecular biology of myocardial ion channels has led to a genetic basis of life-threatening arrhythmias in certain patients. The best described model for this is the long QT syndrome. This syndrome, known previously as the "Romano-Ward" and "Jervell Lange-Nielson" syndromes, is a group of related disorders of arrhythmias ("torsades de pointes") associated with prolongation of the QT interval. The long QT syndrome is now recognized to have a distinct genetic basis. More than 35 mutations in four cardiac ion channels are associated with this syndrome.

Arrhythmogenic right ventricular dysplasia (ARVD) is a form of right ventricular cardiomyopathy inherited in an autosomal dominant manner. It is associated with fatty infiltration and fibrosis of the right ventricle, and it may cause sudden death. It is associated with mutations in chromosomes 1 and 14.

The Romano-Ward syndrome is a cluster of disorders inherited in an autosomal dominant pattern associated with at least six genotypes, including mutations in the I_{KS} channel, *HERG* (human ether-a-go-go related gene) I_{KR} channel, and *SCNA5* I_{Na} channel, and unidentified genes for three additional variants. The Jervell and Lange-Nielsen syndrome is an autosomal recessive disorder associated with sensorineural hearing loss and mutations in voltage-gated K channel (*KVLQT1*) and its subunit minK. These genotypes have some associated phenotypic changes on electrocardiography. For example, isolated

prolongation of the ST segment is associated with mutations in the *SCNA5* I_{Na} channel, whereas a double-humped T wave is associated with the *HERG* genotype. In the future as genotype-phenotype relationships are developed, therapy aimed to prevent sudden death in high-risk patients will be a goal.

- Patients with *SCN5A* genotype may benefit from Na$^+$ channel blocking agents.
- Patients with *HERG* may benefit from β-blockers.

Risk Factors for Atherosclerosis

Atherosclerosis is a complex disease associated with acquired and genetic factors. The genetic background is clearly polygeneic and associated with a complex interplay with environmental factors. Of the known risk factors for atherosclerosis, two provide models for a genetic understanding: hyperlipidemia and hyperhomocystinemia.

Hyperlipidemia

One of the most widely understood cardiovascular genetic disorders is associated with familial hypercholesterolemia. Familial hypercholesterolemia is a relatively common cause of increased levels of low-density lipoprotein (LDL) and is associated with a defective LDL receptor gene on chromosome 19. Familial hypercholesterolemia is an autosomal dominant disorder in which the heterozygotes are affected to an intermediate degree. Homozygotes have LDL cholesterol levels of 650 to 1,000 mg/dL and are often affected by coronary atherosclerosis before the age of 10 years. The homozygote phenotype is notable for the presence of planar cutaneous xanthomas. The heterozygotes have LDL levels that are twice normal, and they are at high risk for premature coronary artery disease. At least 150 different mutations of the LDL receptor gene are associated with familial hypercholesterolemia.

The genetic determinants for other abnormalities of lipoprotein metabolism are being studied. The clinical clues to a potential genetic cause for lipoprotein disorders include the presence of premature atherosclerosis in the patient or a first-degree relative, the presence of xanthomas, and extremely high levels of cholesterol (> 300 mg/dL) or triglycerides (> 500 mg/dL).

Hyperhomocystinemia

Hyperhomocystinemia is associated with an increased risk of developing premature vascular disease. Both genetic and nutritional deficiencies can lead to hyperhomocystinemia.

Classic hyperhomocystinemia-homocystinuria is caused by defects in the cystathione β-synthetase gene (chromosome 21q22) and is inherited in an autosomal recessive pattern. Homozygotes have a marfanoid appearance and develop premature vascular disease. Heterozygotes, who appear normal, may have an increased risk of vascular disease. Defects in the gene for 5,10-methylenetetrahydrofolate reductase are also associated with hyperhomocystinemia and premature vascular disease. Treatment with folate and vitamins B_6 and B_{12} can decrease homocystine levels in these patients.

Potential Molecular-Based Therapies for Cardiovascular Disease

Genetically based treatments can be divided into two categories: those dependent on genetic technology for development and those that use genetic material as drugs.

Recombinant Approaches to Drug Development

An example of the importance of recombinant technology in the development of new therapeutics is the development of such revolutionary drugs as recombinant tissue plasminogen activator (r-tPA) and abciximab (ReoPro). The use of r-tPA as a fibrinolytic agent to treat myocardial infarction helped usher in a new age of rapid reperfusion therapy and has been shown in large international trials to decrease mortality. Abciximab, the Fab fragment of a chimeric antibody to the glycoprotein IIb/IIIa receptor on platelets, has proved useful in treating high-risk patients undergoing percutaneous transluminal coronary angioplasty (PTCA).

Gene Therapies for Cardiovascular Disease

Gene transfer is the modulation of foreign or native gene expression by the introduction of new genetic material into a cell or organism. Gene therapy strategies for cardiovascular disease have been limited to somatic cells (non-germline cells). The system with which genes are introduced into cells is known as "vectors." Vectors can contain elements that are both viral and nonviral.

The initial demonstration of vascular gene transfer used plasmid DNA and retroviral vectors to deliver reporter genes to the vasculature. These studies were limited by the low efficiency of gene transfer because retroviral vectors are capable of infecting only dividing cells, which are rarely seen in normal arteries.

The development of adenoviral vectors led to the ability to demonstrate potential therapeutic benefits from vascular gene transfer. Adenoviruses are DNA viruses capable of infecting dividing and nondividing cells. The ability to clone transgenes into replication-deficient adenoviral vectors has resulted in more efficient (yet transient) transgene expression in vascular tissue.

A prime target for gene transfer has been restenosis following PTCA. Restenosis occurs as a result of cellular proliferation, matrix production, thrombosis, and chronic renarrowing. Gene transfer approaches have targeted cellular proliferation as a means to limit restenosis. Gene transfer strategies aimed at killing proliferating cells include the use of the herpesvirus thymidine kinase gene (*tk*) and the prodrug ganciclovir. The *tk* gene product sensitizes infected cells to the killing effects of ganciclovir. Clinical trials using these strategies have been delayed by the lack of effective and safe intracoronary delivery catheters.

Another major target for cardiovascular gene transfer has been the development of strategies to create angiogenesis within ischemic tissue by delivering genes encoding for growth factors. Genes for vascular endothelial growth factor and members of the fibroblast growth factor family have been used for this purpose. Vascular endothelial growth factor is a highly secreted peptide, and as such, the gene can be delivered to relatively few cells within the vessel, resulting in locally increased concentrations of protein.

Suggested Review Reading

1. Papavassiliou AG: Molecular medicine. Transcription factors. *N Engl J Med* 332:45-47, 1995.

2. Rosenthal N: DNA and the genetic code. *N Engl J Med* 331:39-41, 1994.

3. Rosenthal N: Regulation of gene expression. *N Engl J Med* 331:931-933, 1994.

4. Rosenthal N: Tools of the trade—recombinant DNA. *N Engl J Med* 331:315-317, 1994.
Excellent reviews of the basics of molecular biology.

1. Malik MS, Watkins H: The molecular genetics of hypertrophic cardiomyopathy. *Curr Opin Cardiol* 12:295-302, 1997.

2. Marian AJ, Roberts R: Recent advances in the molecular genetics of hypertrophic cardiomyopathy. *Circulation* 92:1336-1347, 1995.

3. Marian AJ, Roberts R: Molecular genetic basis of hypertrophic cardiomyopathy: genetic markers for sudden cardiac death. *J Cardiovasc Electrophysiol* 9:88-99, 1998.

4. Menon AG, Klanke CA, Su YR: Identification of disease genes by positional cloning. *Trends Cardiovasc Med* 4:97-102, 1994.
Reviews of the genetic mutations of hypertrophic cardiomyopathy.

1. Ackerman MJ: The long QT syndrome: ion channel diseases of the heart. *Mayo Clin Proc* 73:250-269, 1998.

2. Olson TM, Michels VV, Thibodeau SN, et al: Actin mutations in dilated cardiomyopathy, a heritable form of heart failure. *Science* 280:750-752, 1998.

3. Towbin JA: The role of cytoskeletal proteins in cardiomyopathies. *Curr Opin Cell Biol* 10:131-139, 1998.
Recent reviews of ion channel mutations in the long QT syndrome.

1. Topol EJ, Califf RM, Weisman HF, et al: Randomised trial of coronary intervention with antibody against platelet IIb/IIIa integrin for reduction of clinical restenosis: results at six months. The EPIC Investigators. *Lancet* 343:881-886, 1994.

Questions

Multiple Choice (choose the one best answer)

1. What carries genetic information from DNA to the ribosomes?
   a. Transfer RNA
   b. Messenger RNA
   c. Ribosomal RNA
   d. Histones

2. What is specific base pair binding of nucleotides from different sources called?
   a. Meiosis
   b. Transcription
   c. Translation
   d. Hybridization

3. What are the proteins that bind DNA sequences to regulate the production of messenger RNA from template DNA called?
   a. Histones
   b. Enhancers
   c. Transcription factors
   d. Ligases

4. What is denaturation?
   a. Formation of germ cells
   b. Cutting of DNA into fragments
   c. Amplification of DNA, as in the polymerase chain reaction (PCR)
   d. Separation of paired strands of DNA as a result of heating

5. If one parent has an autosomal dominant genetic disorder, what are the chances of a male child being affected?
   a. 0%
   b. 25%
   c. 50%
   d. 100%

6. What is Eco RI?
   a. A transcription factor
   b. A gene responsible for hypertrophic cardiomyopathy
   c. Bacteria
   d. A restriction endonuclease

7. Which of the following is used to amplify minute amounts of DNA?
   a. Northern analysis
   b. Ligation
   c. Polymerase chain reaction
   d. Southern analysis

8. Mutations in which genes are associated with dilated cardiomyopathy?
   a. Myosin
   b. Fibrillin
   c. Actin
   d. Troponin T

9. In which gene are mutations found in the greatest percentage of patients with hypertrophic cardiomyopathy?
   a. β-Myosin heavy chain
   b. Elastin
   c. α-Tropomyosin
   d. Troponin T

10. Which gene is associated with classic hyperhomocystinemia?
    a. Cystathione β-synthetase
    b. Fibrillin
    c. Elastin
    d. Troponin T

11. In which cardiovascular disease is genotype prognostic?
    a. Hypertrophic cardiomyopathy
    b. Marfan syndrome
    c. Coronary artery disease
    d. Dilated cardiomyopathy

True/False

12. Genetic therapies for cardiovascular diseases will likely be limited to single-gene disorders.
    a. True
    b. False

Answers

1. Answer b

Transfer RNA (tRNA) carries amino acids to be incorporated into protein and makes up approximately 15% of total cellular RNA. Messenger RNA (mRNA) carries the genetic material from the nucleus to the ribosome for translation into protein and makes up only 3% to 5% of total cellular RNA. Ribosomal RNA (rRNA) consists of two components (50S and 30S) and makes up 80% of cellular RNA. Histones are nuclear proteins that regulate the structure of chromatin.

2. Answer d

Meiosis is the process of cell division to ultimately produce germ cells. Transcription is the synthesis of RNA from a DNA template. Translation is the synthesis of protein on the mRNA template. Hybridization is the pairing of complementary bases from different sources used in many sensitive and specific molecular diagnostic techniques.

3. Answer c

Histones are nuclear proteins that regulate the structure of chromatin. Enhancers are DNA sequences that act to increase transcription which may bind transcription factors. Transcription factors are DNA-binding proteins that regulate the formation of mRNA from template DNA. Ligases are enzymes that ligate pieces of DNA.

4. Answer d

Meiosis results in germ cell production. Digestion of DNA with restriction endonuclease results in cutting of DNA into fragments. PCR requires denaturation to amplify DNA. Denaturation is the separation of complementary strands of DNA by heating. Reannealing of complementary strands occurs with cooling.

5. Answer c

Sex does not affect the inheritance of a dominant trait.

6. Answer d

Eco RI is a restriction endonuclease from *E. coli* and, thus, is capable of sequence-specific cutting of DNA.

7. Answer c

Northern analysis is the process of separating and identifying target messenger RNA. Ligation is the process of joining fragments of DNA using specific enzymes (ligases). Polymerase chain reaction is a process to amplify minute amounts of DNA. Southern analysis is the process of separating and identifying target DNA.

8. Answer c

Mutations in the gene encoding for actin are associated with dilated cardiomyopathy.

9. Answer a

Mutations in the gene for β-myosin heavy chain are associated with 20% to 30% of the families with hypertrophic cardiomyopathy.

10. Answer a

Mutations in the gene for cystathionine β-synthetase are associated with classic hyperhomocystinemia, which is transmitted in an autosomal recessive pattern and associated with premature vascular disease.

11. Answer a

Certain mutations in the gene for β-myosin heavy chain for hypertrophic cardiomyopathy are associated with a greater incidence of sudden death.

12. Answer b

Genetic therapies for cardiovascular diseases currently undergoing clinical trials are not limited to single-gene disorders but are aimed at polygenic and acquired disorders such as ischemic vascular disease.

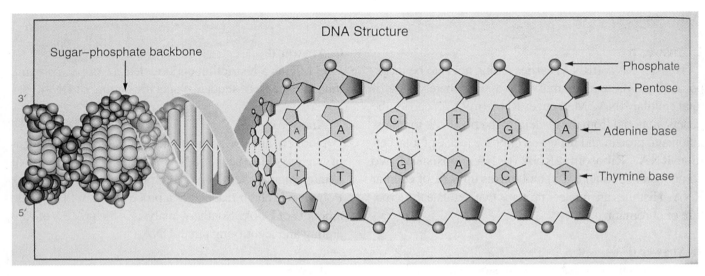

Plate 1. The structure of DNA. (From *N Engl J Med* 331:39-41, 1994. By permission of the Massachusetts Medical Society.)

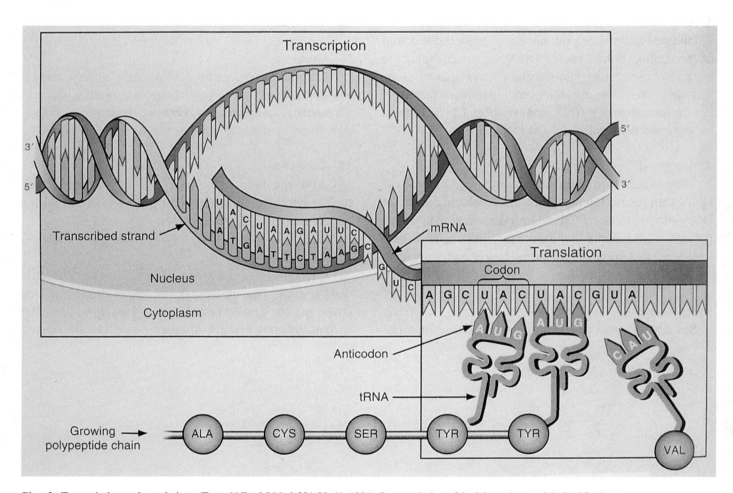

Plate 2. Transcription and translation. (From *N Engl J Med* 331:39-41, 1994. By permission of the Massachusetts Medical Society.)

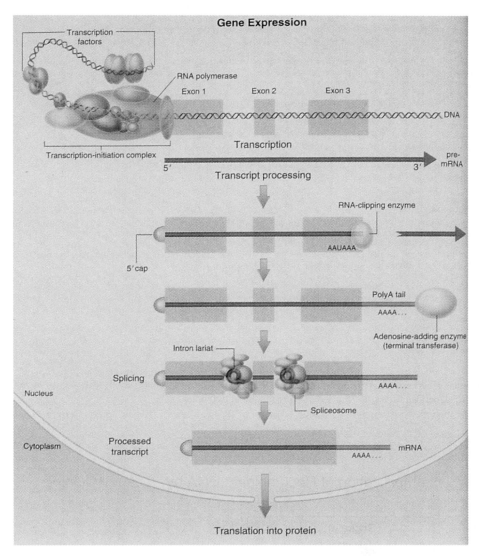

Plate 3. Gene expression. (From *N Engl J Med* 331:931-933, 1994. By permission of the Massachusetts Medical Society.)

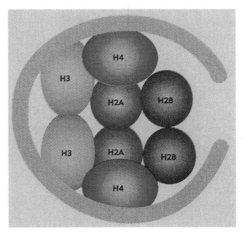

Plate 4. Diagram of nucleosome demonstrating the relationship between histones 2A, 2B, 3, and 4 and associated DNA.

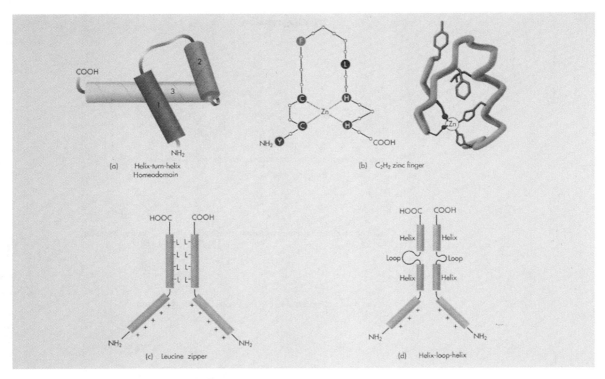

Plate 5. Representative types of transcription factors. (From Watson JD, Gilman M, Witkowski J, et al: *Recombinant DNA*. Second edition. Scientific American Books, 1992, p 164. By permission of the authors.)

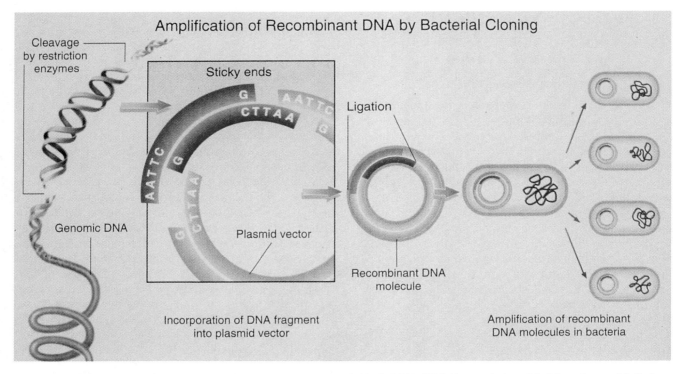

Plate 6. Amplification of DNA by bacterial cloning. (From *N Engl J Med* 331:315-317, 1994. By permission of the Massachusetts Medical Society.)

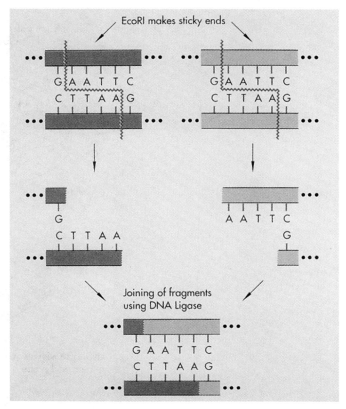

Plate 7. Restriction endonucleases.

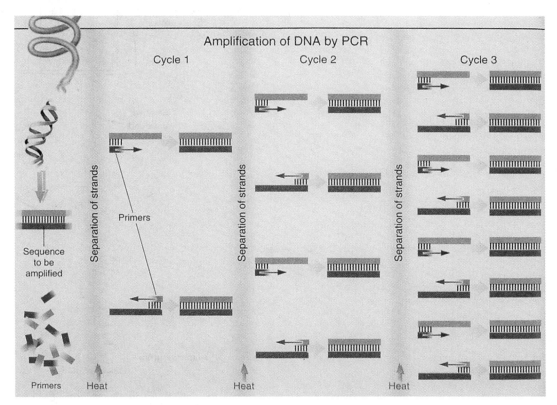

Plate 8. Amplification of DNA by the polymerase chain reaction. (From *N Engl J Med* 331:315-317, 1994. By permission of the Massachusetts Medical Society.)

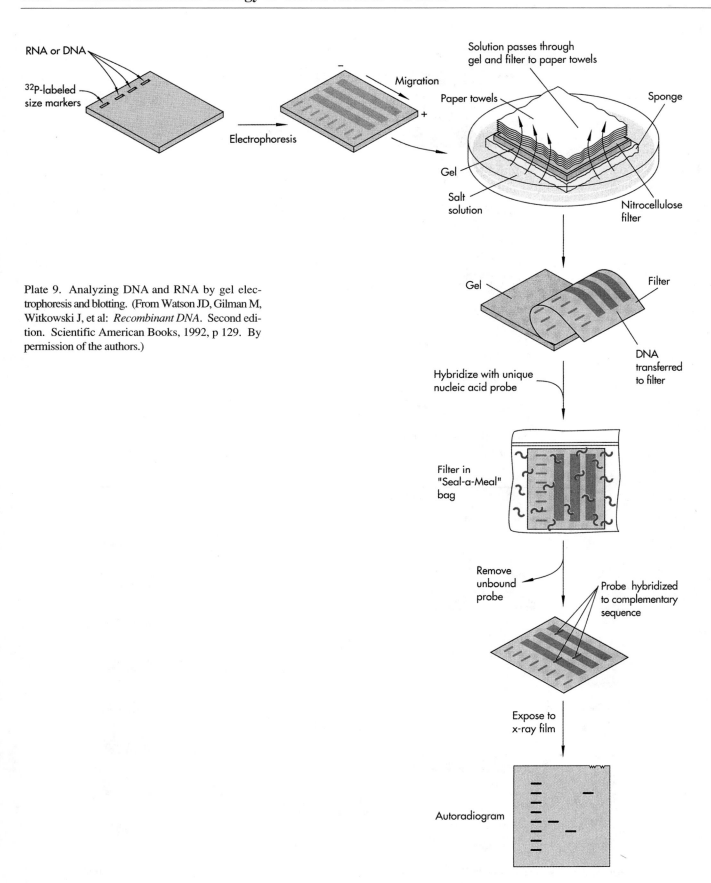

Plate 9. Analyzing DNA and RNA by gel electrophoresis and blotting. (From Watson JD, Gilman M, Witkowski J, et al: *Recombinant DNA*. Second edition. Scientific American Books, 1992, p 129. By permission of the authors.)

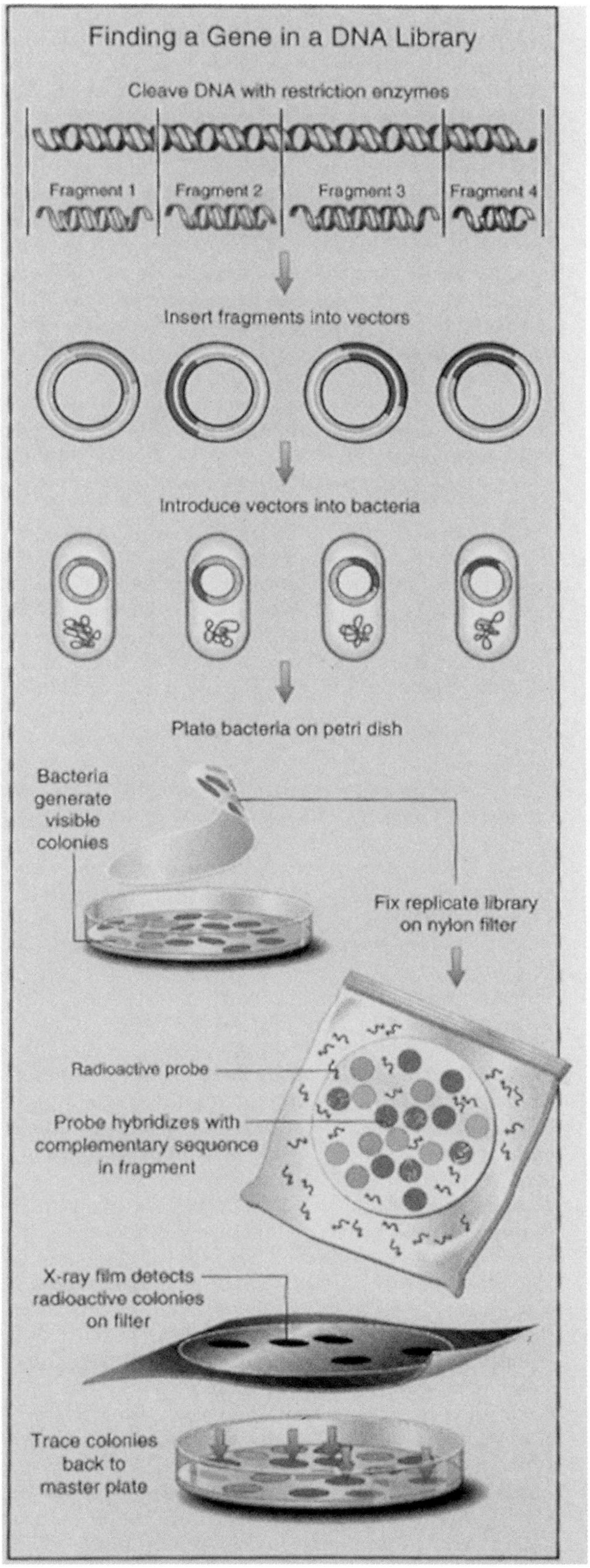

Plate 10. Identifying a gene in a DNA library. (From *N Engl J Med* 331: 599-600, 1994. By permission of the Massachusetts Medical Society.)

Notes

Chapter 59

Peripheral Vascular Disease

Peter C. Spittell, M.D.

Claudication

Patients with occlusive arterial disease of the lower extremity usually have intermittent claudication. The discomfort of intermittent claudication (aching, cramping, or tightness) is always exercise-induced and may involve one or both legs and occurs at a fairly constant walking distance. Relief is obtained by *standing still*. Supine ankle:brachial systolic pressure indices (ABI) before and after treadmill exercise testing can confirm the diagnosis (Table 1). Furthermore, a low ABI is associated with an increased risk of stroke, cardiovascular death, and all-cause mortality.

Pseudoclaudication

Pseudoclaudication is caused by lumbar spinal stenosis and is the condition most commonly confused with intermittent claudication. Pseudoclaudication is usually described as a "paresthetic" discomfort that occurs with standing *and* walking (variable distances). Symptoms almost always are bilateral and relieved by sitting and/or leaning forward. The patient often has a history of chronic back pain or previous lumbosacral spinal surgery. The diagnosis of lumbar spinal stenosis can be confirmed by characteristic findings on electromyography and computed tomography (CT) or magnetic resonance imaging (MRI) of the lumbar spine (Table 2) together with normal or minimally abnormal ABIs before and after exercise.

Table 1.—Grading System for Lower Extremity Occlusive Arterial Disease*

	Supine resting ABI	Post-exercise ABI
Normal	> 1.0	No change or increase
Mild disease	0.8-0.9	> 0.5
Moderate disease	0.5-0.8	> 0.2
Severe disease	< 0.5	< 0.2

ABI, ankle:brachial systolic pressure index.
*After treadmill exercise, 1-2 mph, 10% grade, 5 minutes or symptom-limited.

- The discomfort of intermittent claudication is always exercise-induced.
- Pseudoclaudication is usually described as a "paresthetic" discomfort that occurs with standing *and* walking.

Natural History of Peripheral Vascular Disease

Peripheral vascular disease is associated with significant mortality because of its association with coronary and carotid atherosclerosis. The 5-year mortality rate in patients with intermittent claudication is about 30%, and the major lower extremity amputation rate over 5 years is about 5%. Continued use of tobacco results in a tenfold increase in the risk for major amputation and more than a twofold increase in mortality.

Table 2.—Differential Diagnosis of True Claudication Versus Pseudoclaudication

Feature	Claudication	Pseudoclaudication
Onset	Walking	Standing and walking
Character	Cramp, ache	"Paresthetic"
Bilateral	+/-	+
Walking distance	Fairly constant	More variable
Cause	Atherosclerosis	Spinal stenosis
Relief	Standing still	Sitting down, leaning forward

The location of occlusive arterial disease also affects overall prognosis. Patients with aortoiliac disease have a lower 5-year survival rate (73%) than those with predominantly femoral artery disease (80%). The increased mortality is attributable primarily to cardiac disease. Diabetes mellitus in combination with femoral artery disease results in a further decrease in overall survival and an increased incidence of major amputation.

Diabetic Peripheral Vascular Disease
Diabetic peripheral vascular disease accounts for 60% of leg amputations in the U.S. Over a 25-year period, diabetes mellitus results in a 12-fold increased risk in below-knee amputation. Other clinical features that predict increased risk of limb loss include ischemic rest pain, ischemic ulceration, and gangrene.

Occlusive arterial disease in other locations (e.g., the subclavian artery) is also important, especially in patients being considered for a coronary artery bypass graft and in those who have recurrent angina after having a left internal mammary artery-left anterior descending coronary artery bypass. Stenting of subclavian stenoses may improve myocardial perfusion in patients with internal mammary artery grafts and flow-limiting proximal subclavian stenoses.

- The 5-year mortality rate in patients with intermittent claudication is about 30%.
- Patients with aortoiliac disease have a lower 5-year survival rate than those with predominantly femoral artery disease.

Diagnosis of Peripheral Vascular Disease
Peripheral angiography is not needed to diagnose intermittent claudication. The diagnosis is made clinically. Further quantification can readily be obtained by noninvasive testing (ABI before and after exercise and/or duplex ultrasonography). Angiography is indicated for 1) defining vessel anatomy preoperatively, 2) evaluating therapy, and 3) documenting disease (medicolegal issue). It is also indicated when an "uncommon type" of arterial disease is suspected. More recently, magnetic resonance angiography has been shown to be an accurate alternative to standard angiography; it also is useful in preoperative planning in patients with contraindications to invasive angiography (i.e., renal insufficiency and/or allergy to contrast media) (Fig. 1).

- Peripheral angiography is not needed to diagnose intermittent claudication.

Treatment of Peripheral Vascular Disease
Medical management of intermittent claudication includes discontinuation of tobacco use (all forms), lipid reduction, glucose management in those with diabetes, weight reduc-

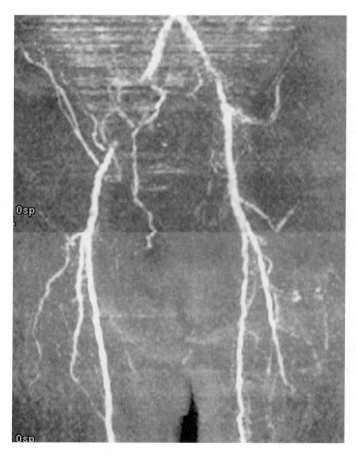

Fig. 1. Magnetic resonance angiography demonstrating high-grade stenosis of left common iliac artery and occlusion of right external iliac artery, with collateral formation.

tion (if obese), foot care and protection, a walking program, pharmacologic therapy, and avoidance of vasoconstrictive drugs.

A regular walking program can result in up to a 400% increase in claudication distance at 3 months. Antiplatelet agents (aspirin, clopidogrel) reduce both the risk of limb loss and the need for surgical revascularization in patients with intermittent claudication. All patients with intermittent claudication should take one of these agents, unless an absolute contraindication exists.

Pentoxifylline (Trental), a methylxanthine, has vasoactive properties, including vasodilation, inhibition of cyclic AMP phosphodiesterase, stimulation of prostacyclin formation, and increased erythrocyte and leukocyte deformability. These properties result in relaxation of vascular smooth muscle, inhibition of platelet aggregation, and decreased blood viscosity. A "target population" of patients with intermittent claudication most likely to benefit from pentoxifylline are those with symptoms present for more than 1 year and an ABI less than 0.8. Only one dosing regimen (400 mg three times daily) is used clinically.

Indications for endovascular or surgical revascularization in a patient with peripheral occlusive arterial disease are "disabling" (lifestyle-limiting) symptoms, diabetes mellitus, rest pain, ischemic ulceration, or gangrene.

Revascularization is elective in nondiabetic patients with intermittent claudication because 1) it does not improve coronary artery or cerebrovascular disease, the major causes of mortality, and consequently does not affect overall long-term survival and 2) the incidence of severe limb-threatening ischemia is relatively low because distal runoff is usually adequate.

Revascularization in patients with rest pain or ischemic ulceration or in those with diabetes mellitus with symptoms

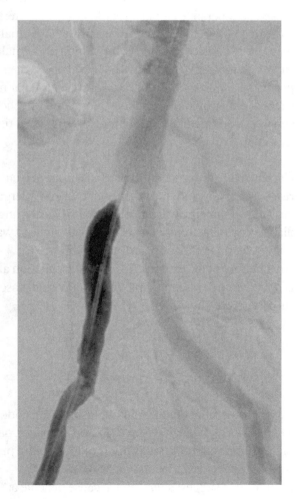

A

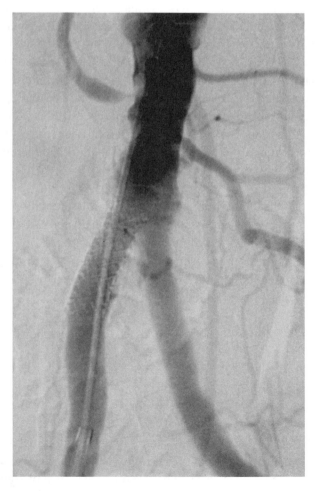

B

Fig. 2. Angiogram demonstrating > 95% stenosis of right common iliac artery before (*A*) and after (*B*) percutaneous transluminal angioplasty and stent placement.

is indicated because 1) the incidence of limb loss is increased without revascularization, 2) surgery may permit a lower anatomical level of amputation, and 3) the risks of the procedure are generally less than the risk of amputation.

Percutaneous transluminal angioplasty (PTA) is an effective alternative to surgical therapy in patients with short, partial occlusions and good distal runoff. The "ideal" lesion for PTA is an iliac stenosis less than 5 cm or a femoropopliteal occlusion or stenosis less than 10 cm in total length (excluding lesions involving the origin of the superficial femoral artery and those affecting the distal-most 2 cm of the popliteal artery). Advantages of PTA over surgery include less morbidity, shorter convalescence, lower cost, and preservation of the saphenous vein for future use. PTA in aortic or iliac disease may also allow for an infrainguinal surgical procedure to be performed at reduced perioperative risk (as compared with intra-abdominal aortic surgery).

Placement of an iliac stent when the hemodynamic results of PTA are inadequate or primary stent placement at the time of initial PTA is being used as treatment in an increasing number of patients (Fig. 2). A recent randomized trial of 279 patients with intermittent claudication with an iliac artery stenosis greater than 50% (proven by angiography) compared direct stent placement with primary angioplasty, with subsequent stent placement only in cases of residual gradient. The difference in the clinical outcomes between the two treatment strategies was not significant at either short-term or long-term follow-up.

- Diabetes mellitus, rest pain, ischemic ulceration, and gangrene are all associated with an increased risk of limb loss in patients with lower extremity arterial occlusive disease. The presence of these features warrants an aggressive approach (angiography followed by endovascular or surgical revascularization).

Renal artery stenosis is discussed in the chapter on hypertension.

Cardiac Risk and Vascular Surgery

Patients with peripheral arterial disease (abdominal aortic aneurysm, lower extremity occlusive arterial disease, and cerebrovascular disease) have a 60% incidence of significant coronary artery disease (> 70% stenosis of one or more epicardial coronary arteries). Up to 30% of patients have

severe correctable three-vessel coronary artery disease with reduced left ventricular function and, thus, are candidates for coronary artery bypass surgery. Clinical markers that identify patients who are at increased risk for a perioperative cardiac event when undergoing vascular surgery include age older than 70 years, angina, diabetes mellitus, ventricular ectopy, pathologic Q waves on the electrocardiogram, and carotid bruit. The perioperative cardiac risk with no clinical markers is 5%; with one to two clinical markers, 15%; and with three clinical markers, 50%.

Noninvasive assessment of cardiac risk before vascular surgery is usually obtained by exercise or pharmacologic stress testing in combination with echocardiography or radionuclide imaging. Pharmacologic stress is used in patients with lower extremity occlusive arterial disease, because these patients cannot achieve an adequate double product on standard exercise testing. The presence of redistribution of thallium-201 or sestamibi or new regional wall motion abnormalities on stress echocardiography predicts an increased perioperative cardiac risk (30% and 50%, respectively). In contrast, the absence of perfusion abnormalities or new stress-induced regional wall motion abnormalities predicts a perioperative cardiac risk of 3% and less than 1%, respectively. An assessment of resting left ventricular function alone, either by radionuclide angiography or echocardiography, is not predictive of perioperative cardiac risk in vascular surgery.

- Clinical markers that identify patients who are at increased risk for a perioperative cardiac event when undergoing vascular surgery include age older than 70 years, angina, diabetes mellitus, ventricular ectopy, pathologic Q waves on the electrocardiogram, and carotid bruit.
- An assessment of resting left ventricular function alone is not predictive of perioperative cardiac risk in vascular surgery.

Acute Arterial Occlusion

The symptoms of acute arterial occlusion are sudden in onset (< 5 hours) and include the "5 Ps": pain, pallor, paresthesia (numbness), poikilothermy (coldness), and pulselessness (absence of peripheral pulses).

Features that suggest a *thrombotic* cause of acute arterial occlusion include previous occlusive disease in the involved limb, occlusive disease involving other extremities, acute aortic dissection, hematologic disease, arteritis, inflammatory bowel disease, neoplasm, and ergotism.

An *embolic* cause of acute arterial occlusion is suggested by the presence of cardiac disease, atrial fibrillation, proximal aneurysm, or atherosclerotic disease.

After confirmation by angiography, the initial therapeutic options for acute arterial occlusion include intra-arterial thrombolysis and surgical therapy (thromboembolectomy). If thrombolytic therapy is used, PTA or surgical therapy is often required subsequently to treat the underlying stenosis (if present) to improve long-term patency rates.

- The "5 Ps" suggestive of acute arterial occlusion include pain, pallor, paresthesia, poikilothermy, and pulselessness.

Aneurysms

Because aneurysms are caused most commonly by atherosclerosis, they are more common in men 60 years or older. Coronary artery and carotid artery occlusive disease are frequent comorbid conditions. Other predisposing factors for aneurysmal disease include hypertension, familial tendency, connective tissue disease, trauma, infection, and inflammatory disease.

Most aneurysms are asymptomatic. Complications of aneurysms include embolization, pressure on surrounding structures, infection, and rupture. Aneurysms of certain arteries develop specific complications more often than other complications. For example, the most common complication of aortic aneurysms is rupture, and a common complication of femoral and popliteal artery aneurysms is embolism. Aortic aneurysms are discussed in the chapter on the aorta.

An iliac artery aneurysm usually occurs in association with an abdominal aortic aneurysm, but it may occur as an isolated finding. Iliac artery aneurysms may cause atheroembolism, obstructive urologic symptoms, unexplained groin or perineal pain, or iliac vein obstruction. CT with intravenous contrast agent or MRI is the preferred diagnostic procedure. Surgical resection is indicated when the aneurysm is symptomatic or larger than 3 cm in diameter.

Popliteal artery aneurysms can be complicated by thrombosis, venous obstruction, embolization, popliteal neuropathy, popliteal thrombophlebitis, rupture, and infection. They are bilateral in 50% of patients, and 40% of patients have one or more aneurysms at other sites, usually of the abdominal aorta. The diagnosis is readily made with

Table 3.—Diagnostic Criteria for Thromboangiitis Obliterans

Age	< 40 years (often < 30 years)
Sex	Males most often
Habits	Tobacco
History	Superficial phlebitis
	Claudication, arch or calf
	Raynaud phenomenon
Examination	Small arteries involved
	Upper extremity involved (positive Allen test)
Laboratory results	Normal glucose, blood cell count, erythrocyte sedimentation rate, lipids, and screening tests for connective tissue disease
Radiography	No arterial calcification

ultrasonography, but angiography is necessary before surgical treatment to evaluate the proximal and distal arterial circulation. When a popliteal aneurysm is diagnosed, surgical therapy is the treatment of choice to prevent serious thromboembolic complications.

Uncommon Types of Occlusive Arterial Disease

The clinical features that suggest an uncommon type of peripheral occlusive arterial disease include young age, acute ischemia without a history of occlusive arterial disease, and involvement of only the upper extremity or digits. Uncommon types of occlusive arterial disease include thromboangiitis obliterans, arteritis associated with connective tissue disease, giant cell arteritis (cranial and Takayasu disease), and occlusive arterial disease due to blunt trauma or arterial entrapment.

Thromboangiitis Obliterans (Buerger Disease)

The diagnostic clinical criteria for thromboangiitis obliterans (Buerger disease) are listed in Table 3. More definitive diagnosis of thromboangiitis obliterans requires angiography, which usually reveals multiple bilateral focal segments of stenosis or occlusion, with normal proximal vessels (Fig. 3). Treatment of thromboangiitis obliterans is the same as for other types of occlusive peripheral arterial disease, with particular emphasis on the need for permanent abstinence

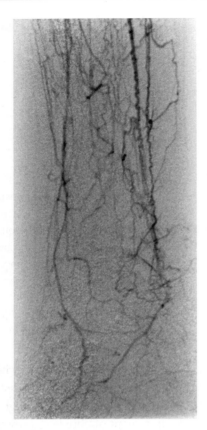

Fig. 3. Angiogram of patient with thromboangiitis obliterans showing characteristic abrupt occlusions, segmental stenoses, and "corkscrew" collaterals of infrapopliteal arteries.

from all forms of tobacco. The activity of the disease will stop permanently with cessation of tobacco use and will resume with further tobacco exposure. Because the arteries involved are small, restoration of pulsatile flow in these patients is usually not a consideration, except in rare patients who are candidates for pedal bypass surgery. Sympathectomy may be useful in severe digital ischemia with ulceration to control pain and to improve cutaneous blood flow.

Popliteal Artery Entrapment

Popliteal artery entrapment occurs most often in young men who have intermittent claudication in the arch of the foot or calf. If the popliteal artery is not already occluded, the finding of diminished pedal pulses with sustained active pedal plantarflexion may be noted. Diagnosis is made by demonstrating on contrast or magnetic resonance angiography medial displacement of the popliteal artery from its normal position in the popliteal space. If untreated, popliteal artery entrapment can lead to post-stenotic dilatation or

thrombosis of the popliteal artery (or both). Treatment is surgical release of the artery from the entrapping muscle and appropriate reconstruction of an occluded or aneurysmal popliteal artery.

Thoracic Outlet Compression Syndrome

Compression of the subclavian artery in the thoracic outlet (thoracic outlet compression syndrome) can occur at several points, but the most common site of compression is in the costoclavicular space between the uppermost rib (cervical rib or first rib) and the clavicle. If the person is symptomatic, the presentation may be any of the following: Raynaud phenomenon in one or more fingers of the ipsilateral hand, digital cyanosis or ulceration, and "claudication" of the arm or forearm. Occlusive arterial disease in the affected arm or hand is readily detected on examination of the arterial pulses and by the Allen test. Compression of the subclavian artery in the thoracic outlet can be demonstrated by noting a decreased or absent pulse in the ipsilateral radial artery during performance of thoracic outlet maneuvers. The diagnosis is confirmed by duplex ultrasonography, magnetic resonance angiography, or angiography, with the involved arm in the neutral and hyperabducted position. Treatment of symptomatic or complicated thoracic outlet compression of the subclavian artery includes surgical resection of the uppermost rib.

- Compression of the subclavian artery in the thoracic outlet can be demonstrated by noting a decreased or absent pulse in the ipsilateral radial artery during performance of the thoracic outlet maneuvers.

It is important to remember that all the connective tissue disorders and giant cell arteritides can involve peripheral arteries, and symptoms of peripheral arterial involvement may dominate the clinical picture. Other than the conservative measures already discussed for ischemic limbs, therapy is directed mainly at the underlying disease. Only after the inflammatory process is controlled should surgical revascularization of chronically ischemic extremities be performed.

Heparin-Induced Thrombocytopenia

Heparin-induced thrombocytopenia affects between 5% and 10% of patients who receive heparin therapy, but the incidence of arterial and/or venous thrombosis is less than 1% or 2%. Heparin-induced thrombocytopenia (type II) typically occurs 5 to 14 days after heparin exposure and is associated with arterial thrombosis (arterial occlusion, ischemic strokes, myocardial infarction) and venous thrombosis (pulmonary embolism, phlegmasia cerulea dolens [venous gangrene], and sagittal sinus thrombosis). The diagnosis of heparin-induced thrombocytopenia is primarily clinical—occurrence of thrombocytopenia during heparin therapy, resolution of thrombocytopenia when heparin therapy is discontinued, and exclusion of other causes of thrombocytopenia—and can be confirmed by demonstration in vitro of a heparin-dependent platelet antibody. Treatment of type II heparin-induced thrombocytopenia includes discontinuation of all forms of heparin exposure (subcutaneous, intravenous, or heparin flushes and heparin-coated catheters) and institution of alternative anticoagulation (thrombin inhibitors or heparinoids).

Vasospastic Disorders

Vasospastic disorders are characterized by episodic color changes of the skin resulting from intermittent spasm of the small arteries and arterioles of the skin and digits. Vasospastic disorders are important because they frequently are a clue to another underlying disorder such as occlusive arterial disease, connective tissue disorders, neurologic disorders, or endocrine disease. Vasospastic disorders also can appear as side effects of drug therapy, specifically of ergot preparations, estrogen replacement therapy, and certain β-blockers.

Raynaud Phenomenon

When Raynaud phenomenon is present, several clinical features can help differentiate primary Raynaud disease from secondary Raynaud phenomenon, as indicated in Table 4.

Primary Raynaud disease is more common in women than men, and its onset usually is before age 40 years. Episodes are characterized by triphasic color changes (white, blue, red). Symptoms are usually bilateral and often symmetric and precipitated by emotion or exposure to cold. Ischemic or gangrenous changes are not present. The absence of any causal condition and the presence of symptoms for at least 2 years are also required for the diagnosis. Raynaud disease is a benign condition, with treatment emphasizing protection from cold exposure and other vasoconstrictive influences. Occasionally, a patient with severe symptoms not controlled by local measures may benefit from a low dose of nifedipine or an α-blocker. Biofeedback can also be an effective measure to control vasospasm and

Table 4.—Comparison of Primary and Secondary Raynaud Phenomenon

	Raynaud phenomenon	
	Primary	Secondary
Age at onset	< 40 yr	> 40 yr
Sex	Women	Men
Bilateral	+	+/-
Symmetric	+	+/-
Toes involved	+	-
Ischemic changes	-	+
Systemic manifestations	-	+

to obviate drug therapy.

Secondary Raynaud phenomenon affects men more often than women, and in most patients the onset is after age 40 years. It is usually unilateral or asymmetric at onset. Associated pulse deficits, ischemic changes, and systemic signs and symptoms are often present. Identification of the underlying cause is basic to appropriate treatment for secondary Raynaud phenomenon.

The initial laboratory evaluation in a patient with Raynaud phenomenon includes complete blood count, erythrocyte sedimentation rate, urinalysis, serum protein electrophoresis, and antinuclear antibody test and tests for cryoglobulin, cryofibrinogen, and cold agglutinins and chest radiography to detect disorders not identified by the medical history and physical examination.

- Primary Raynaud disease is more common in women than men, and its onset usually is before age 40 years.
- Secondary Raynaud phenomenon affects men more often than women, and in most patients, the onset is after age 40 years.

Livedo Reticularis

Livedo reticularis, the bluish mottling of the skin in a lacy reticular pattern, is caused by spasm or occlusion of dermal arterioles. Primary livedo reticularis is idiopathic and not associated with an identifiable underlying disorder. Secondary livedo reticularis is suggested by an abrupt severe onset of symptoms, ischemic changes, and systemic symptoms. Most commonly, it is the result of embolism of atheromatous debris from thrombus in a proximal aneurysm or from proximal atheromatous plaques. The appearance of livedo reticularis in a patient older than

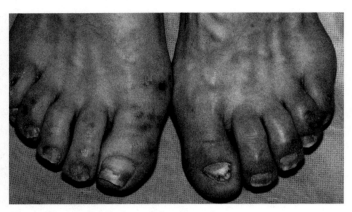

Fig. 4. Characteristic lesions of chronic pernio.

50 years should suggest the possibility of atheroembolism. Other causes of secondary livedo reticularis include connective tissue disease, vasculitis, myeloproliferative disorders, dysproteinemias, reflex sympathetic dystrophy, cold injury, and as a side effect of amantadine hydrochloride (Symmetrel) therapy.

- The appearance of livedo reticularis in a patient older than 50 years should suggest the possibility of atheroembolism.

Chronic Pernio

Chronic pernio is a vasospastic disorder characterized by sensitivity to cold in patients (usually women) with a past history of cold injury. Chronic pernio presents with symmetric blueness of the toes in the autumn and clearing in the spring (Fig. 4). Without treatment, the cyanosis may be accompanied by blistering of the skin of the affected toes. The cyanosis is relieved within a few days after initiating treatment with an α-blocker, which can then be used to prevent recurrences.

Erythromelalgia

Erythromelalgia is the occurrence of red, hot, painful burning fingers or toes (or both) on exposure to warm temperatures or following exercise. It is not a vasospastic disorder but is associated with color change of the skin. It may be primary (idiopathic) or be secondary to an underlying disorder, most commonly myeloproliferative disease, diabetes mellitus, or small fiber neuropathy. Treatment of the primary form includes avoidance of exposure to warm temperatures, aspirin, and a β-blocker (nonselective), which is helpful in some patients. In persons with secondary erythromelalgia, treatment of the underlying disorder usually relieves the symptoms.

Suggested Review Reading

1. Brieger DB, Mak KH, Kottke-Marchant K, et al: Heparin-induced thrombocytopenia. *J Am Coll Cardiol* 31:1449-1459, 1998.
A review of both type I and type II heparin-induced thrombocytopenia, describing incidence, pathogenesis, diagnosis, and treatment.

2. McDaniel MD, Cronenwett JL: Basic data related to the natural history of intermittent claudication. Ann Vasc Surg 3:273-277, 1989.
A concise tabulation of natural history data pertaining to patients with intermittent claudication.

3. Spittell JA Jr: Diagnosis and management of occlusive peripheral arterial disease. Curr Probl Cardiol 15:1-35, 1990.

4. Tetteroo E, van der Graaf Y, Bosch JL, et al: Randomised comparison of primary stent placement versus primary angioplasty followed by selective stent placement in patients with iliac-artery occlusive disease. *Lancet* 351:1153-1159, 1998.
The study demonstrated that selective iliac stent placement, when the post-angioplasty mean pressure gradient across the iliac lesion was greater than 10 mm Hg, had clinical and angiographic outcomes similar to those of primary iliac stent placement.

Questions

Multiple Choice (choose the one best answer)

1. A 64-year-old man comes to the emergency department complaining of sudden onset of severe anterior chest pain radiating to the neck, followed by a syncopal spell. He has a history of systemic hypertension. Two years earlier, a bicuspid aortic valve with mild aortic regurgitation was diagnosed by echocardiography. His only medication is furosemide. Examination reveals a blood pressure of 90/50 mm Hg in both arms and a pulse of 110 beats/min, with a 20-mm Hg paradox. Jugular venous pressure is 18 cm H_2O. There are bibasilar moist rales. The left ventricular impulse is not palpable, and heart sounds are distant. Peripheral pulses are all palpable. Chest radiography reveals cardiomegaly and widening of the superior mediastinum. Electrocardiography reveals sinus tachycardia and low-voltage QRS complexes. The most likely clinical diagnosis in this patient is which of the following?
   a. Pulmonary embolism
   b. Acute myocardial infarction
   c. Pericarditis
   d. Acute aortic dissection
   e. Severe aortic regurgitation and congestive heart failure

2. In a patient with suspected acute aortic dissection, emergency transthoracic echocardiography demonstrates a moderate-sized pericardial effusion and diastolic collapse of the right atrium and right ventricle suggestive of cardiac tamponade. Also present is a 5.2-cm ascending aortic aneurysm. Transesophageal echocardiography identifies an intimal flap in the ascending aorta, transverse aortic arch, and descending thoracic aorta. What is your next step in this patient's management?
   a. Echocardiographically guided pericardiocentesis
   b. Coronary angiography
   c. Medical therapy with fluids and sodium nitroprusside given intravenously
   d. Emergent cardiac surgery
   e. Medical therapy with fluids and β-blockade administered intravenously

3. The most common symptom in acute lower extremity arterial occlusion is which of the following?
   a. Pallor
   b. Paresthesia
   c. Coldness
   d. Pain
   e. Numbness

4. Clinical features of penetrating aortic ulcer include all the following *except*:
   a. Severe chest pain
   b. Systemic hypertension
   c. Pulse deficits
   d. Aortic regurgitation
   e. Neurologic deficits

5. Characteristics of an inflammatory abdominal aortic aneurysm include all the following *except*:
   a. Back pain
   b. Familial tendency
   c. Diarrhea
   d. Increased erythrocyte sedimentation rate
   e. Weight loss

6. Features suggestive of secondary Raynaud syndrome include all the following *except*:
   a. Male sex
   b. Digital gangrene
   c. Positive Allen test
   d. Onset before age 40 years
   e. Systemic symptoms

7. Clinical features of primary antiphospholipid antibody syndrome include all the following *except*:
   a. Recurrent arterial thrombosis
   b. Recurrent spontaneous abortions
   c. Livedo reticularis
   d. Thrombocytosis
   e. Recurrent venous thrombosis

8. Activated protein C resistance is characterized by all the following *except*:
   a. Increased incidence in patients with familial venous thromboembolism
   b. An 80-fold increased incidence of venous thrombosis in heterozygotes
   c. Factor V (Leiden) mutation
   d. Autosomal dominant inheritance
   e. Increased incidence of venous thrombosis in patients taking oral contraceptives

9. Clinical features of lymphedema praecox include all

the following *except*:
a. Bilateral involvement in 50% of patients
b. Onset before age 40 years
c. Female sex
d. Increased incidence of arteriovenous malformations
e. Painless swelling of the involved limb

10. Clinical features of a vertebrobasilar transient ischemic attack include all the following *except*:
a. "Drop" attacks
b. Diplopia
c. Vertigo
d. Aphasia
e. Ataxia

11. Clinical features of incomplete aortic rupture include all the following *except*:
a. Left hemothorax, "apical cap"
b. Sudden deceleration injury
c. Hypertension
d. Rib and clavicle fractures
e. Low risk of rupture in chronic lesions

Answers

1. Answer d

Acute aortic dissection is the most likely clinical diagnosis. Clues to the diagnosis include the patient's history of systemic hypertension and a bicuspid aortic valve, both conditions known to be major risk factors for aortic dissection. The sudden onset of severe chest pain is characteristic of acute aortic dissection. Syncope in association with acute aortic dissection usually signifies cardiac tamponade from rupture of the dissecting hematoma into the pericardial space. Furthermore, the clinical findings of cardiac tamponade in combination with widening of the superior mediastinum on chest radiography support a diagnosis of acute aortic dissection. Pulmonary embolism, pericarditis, and acute myocardial infarction are not associated with widening of the superior mediastinum on chest radiography. Congestive heart failure from isolated severe aortic regurgitation would not account for the sudden onset of severe chest pain.

2. Answer d

Cardiac tamponade resulting from acute aortic dissection is a true surgical emergency. Without surgical treatment, it is the most common cause of death in acute proximal (types I and II, type A) aortic dissection. Echocardiographically guided pericardiocentesis should be avoided in this situation because the withdrawal of pericardial fluid can result in a rapid improvement in left ventricular systolic function and left ventricular dp/dt, resulting in aortic rupture. Instead, a patient with aortic dissection complicated by cardiac tamponade should be taken directly to surgery for institution of cardiopulmonary bypass before evacuation of blood from the pericardial space (*Circulation* 90:2375-2378, 1994).

3. Answer d

The most common presenting symptom in acute arterial occlusion is severe pain in the involved extremity. The other noteworthy but less frequent symptoms and signs of acute arterial occlusion include paresthesia, pallor, absent pulse, and coldness of the involved extremity.

4. Answer c

Penetrating aortic ulcer is characterized clinically by the sudden onset of severe pain in the anterior or posterior chest. Systemic hypertension is the most common associated clinical risk factor. Penetrating aortic ulcers are most common in the descending thoracic aorta but have been reported in the ascending aorta and transverse aortic arch. Neurologic deficits are rare but have been reported, presumably due to involvement of the anterior spinal artery by the intramural hematoma. Dilatation of the ascending aorta resulting in aortic regurgitation can occur from the effects of chronic systemic hypertension. Pulse deficits have not been reported in association with penetrating aortic ulcer.

5. Answer c

Inflammatory abdominal aortic aneurysms comprise approximately 2% to 14% of all abdominal aortic aneurysms. Patients with an inflammatory abdominal aortic aneurysm classically present with abdominal or back pain, malaise, weight loss, and an increased erythrocyte sedimentation rate. Obstructive uropathy is an additional presentation. Diarrhea is not a clinical feature of inflammatory abdominal aortic aneurysm. Preliminary evidence suggests that inflammatory abdominal aortic aneurysm may have a familial component and that current smoking may have a role in the inflammatory process. The diagnosis can be established by computed tomography or magnetic resonance imaging. Treatment is surgical grafting (*J Vasc Surg* 9:643-649, 1989; *J Vasc Surg* 23:860-868, 1996).

6. Answer d

Secondary Raynaud phenomenon is suggested by several clinical features, including male sex, onset of disease after age 40 years, unilateral or asymmetric vascular findings, pulse deficits, ischemic digital changes, and systemic symptoms of an underlying disease.

7. Answer d

Criteria for the diagnosis of antiphospholipid antibody syndrome include both clinical and laboratory findings. Clinical criteria include recurrent venous or arterial thrombosis, recurrent fetal loss, livedo reticularis, and persistent thrombocytopenia. Diagnostic laboratory criteria include the presence of IgG or IgM anticardiolipin antibody and/or lupus anticoagulant. Patients must have at least one clinical and one laboratory finding and the laboratory finding must be positive on at least two occasions more than 3 months apart. The primary antiphospholipid antibody syndrome would not be associated with an underlying autoimmune or infectious disease (*JAMA* 277:1549-1551, 1997).

8. Answer b

Activated protein C resistance (APCR) is an autosomal dominant disorder associated with a mutation in factor V (Leiden). APCR is prevalent in persons with familial or recurrent venous thromoboembolism (20%-50%) and initial idiopathic venous thromboembolism (10%-20%). The risk of venous thromboembolism is increased 80-fold in homozygotes, 8- to 10-fold in heterozygotes. Management of homozygotes with APCR is long-term warfarin anticoagulation. Therapy in heterozygotes must be individualized. Oral contraceptive use is associated with a markedly increased risk of venous thromboembolism in patients with APCR.

9. Answer d

Clinical features of lymphedema praecox include a female predominance (9:1 or 10:1), onset of disease before age 40 years (often before age 20), and involvement of both legs in 50% of patients. The classic clinical presentation is of painless swelling of an extremity in a young woman who is otherwise healthy. Exclusion of lesions in the abdomen and pelvis on the initial clinical encounter is warranted with a clinical examination, Pap smear, and often an ultrasonographic or computed tomographic scan of the pelvis. Lymphedema praecox is not associated with arteriovenous malformations.

10. Answer d

A vertebrobasilar transient ischemic attack is characterized by the sudden onset of one or more of the following symptoms and signs: paresis (1, 2, or 4 limbs), "drop" attacks, numbness of the involved limbs and face, impaired vision (diplopia or bilateral visual field defects), vertigo, nausea, dysarthria, and ataxia. Aphasia is a feature of a carotid territory transient ischemic attack.

11. Answer e

Incomplete rupture of the thoracic aorta usually occurs in association with a sudden, severe deceleration injury. Many patients have associated thoracic, abdominal, and cranial trauma due to the severity of the accident, and many have been thrown from a vehicle. Most patients are hypertensive on initial presentation, and chest radiography frequently demonstrates fractures of the left ribs or clavicle. A left pleural effusion may be present if a significant amount of blood has leaked into the left pleural space. Blood superior to the left upper lobe ("apical cap") can also be seen with incomplete rupture of the isthmus of the thoracic aorta. Once diagnosed, incomplete rupture of the thoracic aorta should be treated with urgent surgical resection, because future risk of rupture is not predictable.

Notes

Chapter 60

Veins and Lymphatics

Peter C. Spittell, M.D.

Edema*

Lower extremity edema is commonly encountered in cardiology practice. Aside from edema due to cardiac disease, other causes of regional edema usually can be identified from characteristic clinical features (Table 1).

Lymphedema

Lymphedema can be primary (idiopathic) or secondary to an underlying disorder. Primary lymphedema (lymphedema praecox) usually affects young women (nine times more frequently than men) and begins before the age of 40 years (often before age 20 years). In women, the symptoms often first appear at the time of menarche or with the first pregnancy. Edema is bilateral in about half the cases (Fig. 1). The initial evaluation of a young woman with lymphedema should include a complete history and physical examination (including pelvic examination and Pap smear) and computed tomography of the pelvis to exclude a neoplastic cause of lymphatic obstruction.

> In a healthy young woman with painless progressive swelling of one or both lower extremities in a pattern consistent with lymphedema, lymphedema praecox is the most likely diagnosis.

Secondary lymphedema is broadly classified into obstructive (postsurgical, postradiation, neoplastic) and inflammatory (infectious) types. Obstructive lymphedema due to neoplasm typically begins after the age of 40 years and is due to pelvic neoplasm or lymphoma. The most frequent cause in men is prostate cancer.

> In a man older than 60 years with painless progressive swelling of one leg, the diagnosis is prostate cancer until proved otherwise.

Inflammatory (infectious) lymphedema occurs as a result of chronic or recurring lymphangitis (or both) or cellulitis. The portal of entry for infection is usually dermatophytosis (tinea pedis) (Fig. 2). The diagnosis of lymphedema can be confirmed noninvasively by lymphoscintigraphy.

Table 1.—Characteristic Clinical Features of Regional Edema

Feature	Venous	Lymphedema	Lipedema
Bilateral	Occasional	Maybe	Always
Foot involved	Yes	Yes	No
Toes involved	No	Yes	No
Thickened skin	No	Yes	No
Stasis changes	Yes	No	No

*The "Questions and Answers" section for this chapter is at the end of the chapter "Peripheral Vascular Disease."

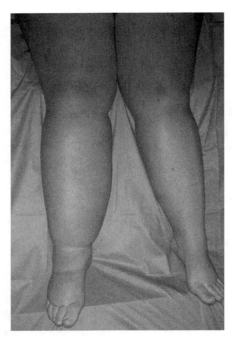

Fig. 1. Young woman with lymphedema praecox of right lower extremity. Note that the edema involves the toes.

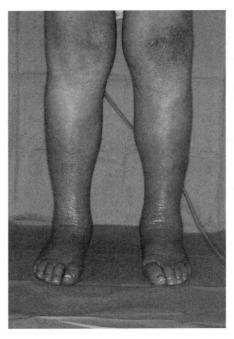

Fig. 2. Inflammatory lymphedema and cellulitis in a man with chronic tinea pedis as portal of entry for bacterial infection.

Medical management of lymphedema includes edema reduction therapy, followed by daily use of custom-fitted, graduated compression (usually 40 to 50 mm Hg compression) elastic support. Antifungal treatment is essential if dermatophytosis is present. Weight reduction in obese patients is also beneficial. Surgical treatment of lymphedema (lymphaticovenous anastomosis, lymphedema reduction surgery) is indicated in highly selected patients.

Venous Disease

Deep vein thrombosis (DVT) is the third most common cardiovascular disease, after acute coronary syndromes and stroke. The overall annual incidence of DVT, which appears to have been relatively constant during the last 15 years, is 48/100,000. Virchow's triad of stasis, hypercoagulability, and vascular endothelial damage contribute in varying degrees to the development of DVT. Risk factors for DVT include immobility, paralysis, recent surgery or trauma (or both), malignancy, cancer chemotherapy, advancing age, family history of DVT, pregnancy, and estrogen use. A major clinical risk factor (immobility, trauma, or recent surgery) is present in approximately one-half of the patients with confirmed DVT. Patients who have total hip or knee replacement surgery have a 40% to 60% risk of DVT without

prophylaxis. A family history of thrombophilia is important, because there are several identifiable and treatable inherited disorders of coagulation. Causes of recurrent DVT are listed in Table 2.

Protein C Deficiency
Protein C deficiency is characterized by recurrent venous thrombosis and is inherited in an autosomal dominant fashion. Episodes of thrombosis are generally spontaneous and usually begin before the age of 30 years. Protein C levels are about 50% of normal. Treatment is lifelong oral anticoagulation, and there is a potential risk of warfarin necrosis. Acquired protein C deficiency can develop postoperatively and in patients with liver disease or disseminated intravascular coagulation. Purpura fulminans occurs in persons homozygous for this condition.

Protein S Deficiency
Protein S deficiency also causes recurrent venous thrombosis and is inherited as an autosomal dominant trait. Onset of episodes usually begins before the age of 35 years, and the episodes are generally spontaneous. Protein S levels are about 50% of normal. Treatment is lifelong oral anticoagulation, and there is no increased risk of warfarin necrosis. Acquired protein S deficiency can occur in association with the nephrotic syndrome, warfarin therapy, pregnancy,

Table 2.—Causes of Recurrent Deep Vein Thrombosis

Primary
   Idiopathic
Secondary
   Neoplasm
   Connective tissue disease
   Inflammatory bowel disease
   Myeloproliferative disorder
   Thromboangiitis obliterans
   Oral contraceptives
Coagulation disorders
   Antithrombin III deficiency
   Protein C deficiency
   Protein S deficiency
   Activated protein C resistance
   Hyperhomocystinemia

antiphospholipid antibody syndrome, and disseminated intravascular coagulation.

Antithrombin III Deficiency

Antithrombin III deficiency, characterized by recurrent venous and arterial thrombosis, is also inherited in an autosomal dominant fashion. The first thrombotic episode is usually after age 20 years and is usually provoked by infection, trauma, surgery, or pregnancy. Antithombin III levels are usually 40% to 60% of normal. Treatment is lifelong oral anticoagulation. In women of childbearing age and in pregnant women, subcutaneous heparin should be used to avoid the teratogenic effects of oral anticoagulation. An acquired form of antithrombin III deficiency can occur in patients with nephrotic syndrome or severe liver disease and in those receiving estrogen therapy.

Factor V Leiden Mutation

Heterozygous carriers of a mutation in factor V that destroys an activated protein C cleavage site (factor V Leiden) are at increased risk for venous thrombosis (i.e., activated protein C resistance). This mutation may occur in 5% to 10% of the general population and may account for as many as 50% of patients with recurrent venous thromboembolism. Recently, a mutation in the prothrombin gene has been identified in some patients with venous thromboembolism.

Hyperhomocystinemia

Hyperhomocystinemia, a disorder of methionine metabolism, is a risk factor for premature atherosclerosis and recurrent DVT. Inherited forms (disorders of transsulfuration and remethylation) and acquired forms (chronic renal failure, organ transplantation, acute lymphoblastic leukemia, psoriasis, vitamin deficiencies [vitamins B_6 and B_{12} and folate], and medications [carbamazepine, phenytoin, theophylline]) can occur. Hyperhomocystinemia is an independent risk factor for stroke, coronary artery disease, peripheral vascular disease, and DVT. Folic acid 0.4 mg/day reduces homocysteine levels, but higher doses of folate are required in patients with chronic renal failure. Screening for hyperhomocystinemia should be considered in patients with premature atherosclerotic disease, a strong family history of premature atherosclerosis, idiopathic DVT, chronic renal failure, systemic lupus erythematosus, or severe psoriasis and in organ transplant recipients.

Clinical Evaluation of Patients With DVT

Symptoms of DVT include leg pain, redness, and swelling, although many patients may be asymptomatic. Signs of DVT include pitting edema, warmth, erythema, tenderness, and a dilated superficial venous pattern in the involved extremity. Although leg veins are the most common site of DVT, upper extremity DVT may occur, especially in patients with a central venous catheter or transvenous permanent pacemaker. Extensive DVT involving an entire extremity may lead to venous gangrene (phlegmasia cerulea dolens), most commonly in association with an underlying malignancy. The clinical diagnosis of DVT is neither sensitive (60% to 80%) nor specific (30% to 72%), and three-fourths of patients who present with suspected acute DVT have other causes of leg pain, such as cellulitis, leg trauma, muscular tear or rupture, postphlebitic syndrome, or Baker cysts. Objective noninvasive tests generally are required to establish a diagnosis of DVT.

Although venography is the reference standard for the diagnosis of DVT and is highly accurate for both proximal and calf DVT, it is invasive, expensive, technically inadequate in about 10% of patients, and may precipitate DVT in approximately 3% of patients. Noninvasive tests for diagnosing DVT are accurate for diagnosing proximal but not calf vein thrombosis. If the results of noninvasive testing are nondiagnostic or are discordant with the clinical assessment, venography is indicated.

Continuous Wave Doppler

Doppler assessment at the bedside, which evaluates each

limb systematically for spontaneous venous flow, phasic flow with respiration, augmentation with distal compression, and venous competence with Valsalva and proximal compression, is useful in the diagnosis of proximal DVT. Doppler examination is relatively insensitive to calf vein thrombosis.

Impedance Plethysmography and Strain-Gauge Outflow Plethysmography

Impedance plethysmography and strain-gauge outflow plethysmography both reliably detect occlusive thrombi in the proximal veins (popliteal, femoral, and iliac veins) but are less reliable in detecting nonocclusive thrombi and are insensitive to calf DVT.

Compression Ultrasonography

Compression ultrasonography (venous noncompressibility is diagnostic of DVT, venous compressibility excludes DVT) is highly sensitive and specific for detecting proximal DVT (Fig. 3).

An approach to clinically suspected DVT is shown in Figure 4.

Treatment options for acute DVT include anticoagulation therapy (heparin, warfarin), thrombolytic therapy, vena caval filter, and surgical thrombectomy. Reduction of limb edema, initially by leg elevation and woven elastic (ACE) wrapping, is an integral part of the initial therapy of acute DVT. When edema reduction has been accomplished, a graduated compression elastic support stocking is required both to control edema and to prevent development of the postphlebitic (post-thrombotic) limb syndrome with venous ulceration. A 30- to 40-mm Hg graduated elastic support garment is usually sufficient. Customized, knee-high, graded compression stockings significantly reduce the occurrence of the postphlebitic syndrome in patients with a first episode of proximal DVT. Additional details of the diagnosis and treatment of DVT are included in the chapter on pulmonary embolism.

Postphlebitic Limb Syndrome

Chronic venous insufficiency (postphlebitic syndrome) is a common disorder that results in significant morbidity. Approximately 30% of patients with DVT develop postphlebitic syndrome within 8 years after the initial DVT. Chronic venous insufficiency most commonly results in swelling, pain, fatigue, and heaviness in the involved extremity. Secondary varicose vein formation, venous stasis

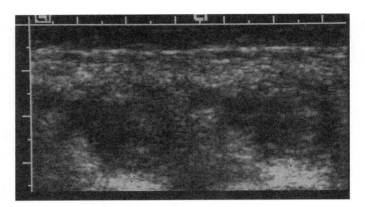

Fig. 3. Compression ultrasonography in a patient with suspected deep vein thrombosis demonstrates noncompressibility of right common femoral vein as evidence of intraluminal thrombus. Echogenic thrombus is visible in common femoral vein (CFV).

changes, and cutaneous ulceration can occur in untreated chronic venous insufficiency. Venous claudication in the setting of previous iliofemoral or vena caval thrombosis causes discomfort, fullness, tiredness, and aching of the extremity during exercise. Unlike intermittent claudication, patients with venous claudication have to sit down and elevate the extremity for relief. Postphlebitic syndrome due to chronic deep venous incompetence is frequently misdiagnosed as recurrent DVT. The correct diagnosis is suggested by the clinical findings of chronic venous insufficiency (edema, venous stasis changes, secondary varicose vein formation) and confirmed by exclusion of new thrombus formation by objective testing (compression ultrasonography). The "side-by-side" comparison of current ultrasonographic studies with previous ultrasonographic or venographic studies is invaluable in documenting new venous thrombosis. Treatment of postphlebitic syndrome initially includes aggressive efforts at edema reduction with woven elastic (ACE) wrapping and pumping devices until edema is reduced, followed by fitting with a graduated compression elastic support stocking (30 to 40 mm Hg). Periodic leg elevation during the day and weight reduction in obese patients are also beneficial.

Leg Ulcer

The etiology of lower extremity ulceration can usually be determined by clinical examination. Clinical features of the four most common types of leg ulcers are summarized in Table 3 and Figure 5.

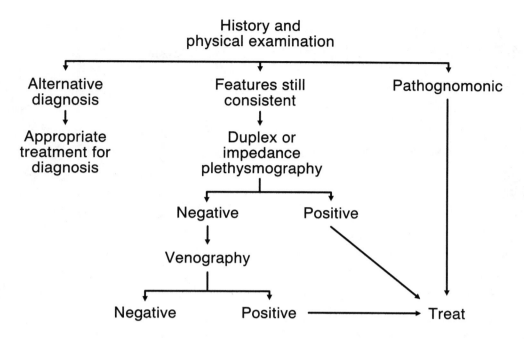

Fig. 4. Algorithm for clinically suspected deep vein thrombosis.

Table 3.—Clinical Features of the Four Most Common Types of Leg Ulcer

Feature	Venous stasis	Arterial	Arteriolar	Neurotrophic
Onset	Trauma +/-	Trauma	Spontaneous	Trauma
Course	Chronic	Progressive	Progressive	Progressive
Pain	No (unless infected)	Yes	Yes	No
Location	Medial leg	Toe, heel, foot	Lateral, posterior leg	Plantar
Surrounding skin	Stasis changes	Atrophic	Normal	Callus
Ulcer				
Edges	Shaggy	Discrete	Serpiginous	Discrete
Base	Healthy	Eschar, pale	Eschar, pale	Healthy or pale

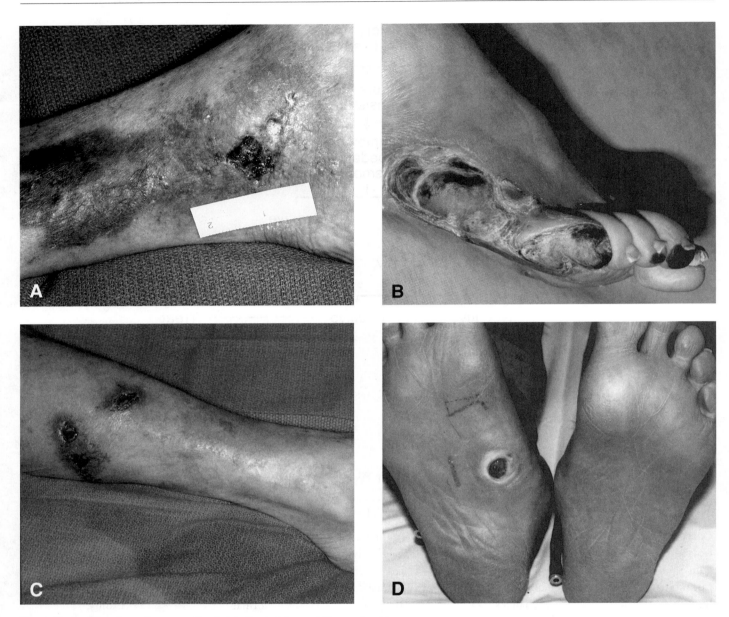

Fig. 5. Types of leg ulcer. *A*, venous; *B*, arterial; *C*, arteriolar; and *D*, neurotrophic.

Suggested Review Reading

1. Anand SS, Wells PS, Hunt D, et al: Does this patient have deep vein thrombosis? *JAMA* 279:1094-1099, 1998.
Recent literature review of the clinical assessment and diagnostic tests and their clinical utility in patients with suspected deep vein thrombosis.

2. Birdwell BG, Raskob GE, Whitsett TL, et al: The clinical validity of normal compression ultrasonography in outpatients suspected of having deep venous thrombosis. *Ann Intern Med* 128:1-7, 1998.
Prospective cohort study of 405 consecutive outpatients with suspected first episode of deep vein thrombosis. A simplified and abbreviated compression ultrasonographic examination of the common femoral and popliteal veins was performed. Ultrasonography had normal results in 335 patients, 2 of whom had deep vein thrombosis during 3 months of follow-up. The authors conclude that it is safe to withhold anticoagulation in outpatients suspected of having first-episode deep vein thrombosis if results of simplified compression ultrasonography are normal at presentation and on a single repeated test performed 5 to 7 days later.

3. Brandjes DP, Buller HR, Heijboer H, et al: Randomised trial of effect of compression stockings in patients with symptomatic proximal-vein thrombosis. *Lancet* 349:759-762, 1997.
Randomized controlled trial of 194 patients with 1st episode of venographically proven proximal deep vein thrombosis. Ninety-six patients were allocated to treatment with graded elastic compression stockings and 98 were allocated to no stockings. Graduated elastic support stockings reduced the incidence of postphlebitic syndrome by up to 50%.

4. Ginsberg JS, Kearon C, Douketis J, et al: The use of D-dimer testing and impedance plethysmographic examination in patients with clinical indications of deep vein thrombosis. *Arch Intern Med* 157:1077-1081, 1997.

5. Kearon C, Julian JA, Newman TE, et al: Noninvasive diagnosis of deep venous thrombosis. McMaster Diagnostic Imaging Practice Guidelines Initiative. *Ann Intern Med* 128:663-677, 1998.
Review of prospective cohort studies and randomized comparison studies of noninvasive diagnostic tests for deep vein thrombosis. The authors conclude that venous ultrasonography is the most accurate noninvasive test for the diagnosis of first symptomatic proximal deep vein thrombosis.

6. Koopman MM, Prandoni P, Piovella F, et al: Treatment of venous thrombosis with intravenous unfractionated heparin administered in the hospital as compared with subcutaneous low-molecular-weight heparin administered at home. *N Engl J Med* 334:682-687, 1996.

7. Levine M, Gent M, Hirsh J, et al: A comparison of low-molecular-weight heparin administered primarily at home with unfractionated heparin administered in the hospital for proximal deep-vein thrombosis. *N Engl J Med* 334:677-681, 1996.

8. Prandoni P, Lensing AW, Cogo A, et al: The long-term clinical course of acute deep venous thrombosis. *Ann Intern Med* 125:1-7, 1996.

9. Schulman S, Granqvist S, Holmstrom M, et al: The duration of oral anticoagulant therapy after a second episode of venous thromboembolism. *N Engl J Med* 336:393-398, 1997.
Randomized controlled trial with 4-year follow-up involving 227 patients with a second episode of acute deep vein thrombosis or pulmonary embolus. Patients were allocated to anticoagulation therapy for 6 months or anticoagulation indefinitely. The incidence of recurrent venous thromboembolism was decreased by 18% in patients receiving indefinite warfarin therapy.

Notes

Chapter 61

Cerebrovascular Disease

Peter C. Spittell, M.D.

Carotid Artery Disease*

Carotid artery disease is common in patients with coronary artery disease and has a wide spectrum of clinical presentations (asymptomatic carotid bruit, transient ischemic attack, reversible ischemic neurologic deficit, or stroke).

An asymptomatic carotid bruit is present in approximately 13% of the population and increases with age. Patients with asymptomatic carotid bruits are at greater risk for cerebral ischemic events than the general population and have a higher overall mortality, primarily because of cardiac death due to associated coronary artery disease and its sequelae. Stroke risk is dependent on the severity of carotid stenosis, with about a 1% per year risk of transient ischemic attack (TIA) and stroke if carotid artery stenosis is 75% or less compared with about 10% for those with stenosis greater than 75%.

TIA is defined as a focal loss of brain function attributed to cerebral ischemia lasting less than 24 hours and localized to a limited region of the brain (Tables 1-3). Stroke is a permanent neurologic deficit. Generally, only 40% of thrombotic strokes are preceded by a TIA. Among patients with a TIA who do not die of another cause within 5 years, one-third will have a stroke, 20% of which occur within the first month after the TIA and 50% within the first year.

- An asymptomatic carotid bruit is present in approximately 13% of the population and increases with age.

- Carotid stenosis severity   1-year risk of TIA/stroke
  - ≤75%   1%
  - >75%   10%

Causes of Stroke

The pathogenesis of stroke includes cardioembolic causes (intracardiac thrombus, intracardiac mass lesions, valvular heart disease, and paradoxic emboli). Other common causes of stroke are large vessel occlusive disease (ascending aorta, aortic arch, major branches of the cerebrovascular circulation) and small vessel disease (diabetes mellitus, hypertension, arteritis). Less common causes include hematologic disease (polycythemia vera, thrombocytosis, leukemia, coagulation factor deficiencies, phospholipid antibody syndromes, cryoglobulinemia, paraproteinemia), and rare causes are air and fat emboli, cortical vein thrombosis, and global hypoperfusion. Risk factors for stroke include hypertension, diabetes mellitus, hyperlipidemia, cigarette smoking, and excessive use of alcohol.

Noninvasive Imaging

Noninvasive evaluation of a carotid bruit includes oculoplethysmography or duplex ultrasonography. Oculoplethysmography measures ocular arterial pressure and is an

*The "Questions and Answers" section for this chapter is at the end of the chapter "Peripheral Vascular Disease."

Table 1.—Clinical Features of Transient Cerebral Ischemia (Transient Ischemic Attack)

Brief--minutes to < 24 hours
Rapid onset
Spontaneous
Focal neurologic signs
Conscious
Normal between attacks

Table 2.—Features of a Transient Ischemic Attack in the Territory of the Carotid Artery

Mono- or hemiparesis
Numbness (unilateral)
Impaired vision (unilateral)
Aphasia, dominant hemisphere
Carotid bruit
Retinal findings (cholesterol emboli)

Table 3.—Features of a Transient Ischemic Attack in the Territory of the Vertebrobasilar System

Limb paresis
Drop attacks
Numbness (limbs and face)
Impaired vision (diplopia or bilateral visual field defects)
Vertigo, nausea
Dysarthria
Ataxia

indirect method of determining whether a hemodynamically significant stenosis is present in the ipsilateral carotid artery. In a study in which oculoplethysmography was used to identify pressure-significant internal carotid artery lesions, persons with an asymptomatic carotid bruit and abnormal oculoplethysmographic results had a twofold greater risk of stroke over 3 years than an age-matched normal population. Limitations of oculoplethysmography include its inability to further localize disease and contraindications in patients with glaucoma or previous ophthalmologic surgery.

Duplex ultrasonography (two-dimensional, pulsed-wave Doppler and color flow Doppler imaging) is able to provide both anatomical and hemodynamic information about the extracranial carotid artery and, currently, is the noninvasive test of choice in the initial evaluation of a patient with carotid occlusive disease. With spectral waveform analysis, duplex ultrasonography can be used to quantify the severity of a carotid artery stenosis into categories of diameter reduction.

Duplex ultrasonography also permits qualitative estimates of the degree of plaque and its location. Evaluation of the subclavian arteries for evidence of occlusive disease or aneurysmal disease and of the vertebral arteries for vessel patency and direction of flow is also possible with ultrasonography.

Angiography

Magnetic resonance angiography (MRA) can accurately diagnose extracranial carotid artery disease and provide details about intracerebral arterial anatomy. MRA is primarily indicated for patients with symptomatic carotid artery disease to exclude intracerebral arterial occlusive disease before carotid endarterectomy. Standard angiography is generally indicated before carotid endarterectomy to define precisely the extent of the extracranial carotid artery disease as well as to determine whether there is associated intracerebral arterial occlusive disease (Fig. 1). Angiography is associated with a stroke risk of about 1%.

Carotid Endarterectomy

Carotid endarterectomy is superior to medical therapy for patients with symptomatic carotid cerebrovascular disease and a high-grade stenosis. This includes carotid territory or retinal TIAs or nondisabling stroke with an ipsilateral high-grade carotid artery stenosis (70% to 99%). Medical therapy is better for persons with mild carotid artery stenosis (0% to 29%), even when symptomatic. The treatment of patients with moderate carotid artery stenosis (30% to 59%) is controversial and must be individualized.

Veterans' Administration Trial
The Veterans' Administration study of 444 males with asymptomatic carotid stenosis greater than 50% on angiography demonstrated that carotid endarterectomy in combination with medical therapy reduced the incidence of ipsilateral neurologic events to 8% (over a mean follow-up of 4 years) in comparison with a 21% event rate with medical therapy alone. However, the combined end point risk

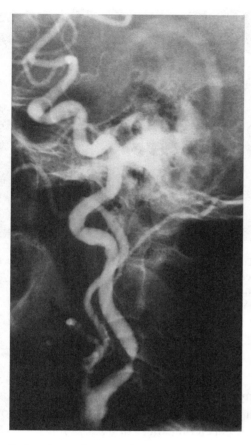

Fig. 1. Cerebral angiogram demonstrating severe stenosis of proximal right internal carotid artery.

of stroke and death was not statistically reduced in this study, emphasizing the need for individualized patient management, because most persons die of their associated coronary artery disease. It should be noted that lowering low-density lipoprotein cholesterol levels with statin medication reduces the stroke risk in patients with coronary artery disease.

Asymptomatic Carotid Atherosclerosis Study Trial

A more recent study (Asymptomatic Carotid Atherosclerosis Study [ACAS]) demonstrated that carotid endarterectomy is superior to medical therapy (aspirin and reduction of risk factors) in persons with *asymptomatic* carotid stenosis greater than 60% if their general health is good and the medical center has a documented combined perioperative morbidity and mortality of less than 3%. When the above criteria were met, the aggregate risk for stroke or death over 5 years was 5% in the surgical group and 11% in the medical group. There was a marked gender effect in this study: the resultant 66% relative

risk reduction in men was statistically significant, but the comparable risk reduction of 17% in women was not statistically significant.

Currently, the approach to a patient with a symptomatic carotid artery stenosis less than 60% is oral anticoagulation for 3 months, followed by antiplatelet therapy (aspirin, clopidogrel) indefinitely. If warfarin is contraindicated, aspirin should be used throughout.

In a patient requiring coronary artery bypass grafting who has significant carotid artery disease, management needs to be individualized. Available data on this group of patients suggest that carotid endarterectomy (when indicated according to the aforementioned conditions) performed simultaneously with coronary artery bypass grafting results in a lower stroke rate than delayed carotid endarterectomy performed within 2 weeks after the coronary artery surgery.

Carotid artery stenting is a promising technique, but to date no randomized trials comparing stenting with endarterectomy have been reported.

- Carotid endarterectomy is superior to medical therapy for persons with *symptomatic* carotid territory or retinal TIAs or nondisabling stroke and ipsilateral high-grade carotid artery stenosis (70% to 99%).
- Carotid endarterectomy is superior to medical therapy in persons with *asymptomatic* carotid stenosis greater than 60% if their general health is good and the medical center has a documented combined perioperative morbidity and mortality of less than 3%.

Although the average risk for stroke or death with carotid endarterectomy is 2% to 5%, in high-risk patients it may be as high as 18%. Percutaneous transfemoral extracranial carotid artery angioplasty (PTA) and carotid artery stenting are possible alternative therapies to carotid endarterectomy in high-risk patients. Reported initial success rates for carotid artery PTA and carotid stenting exceed 95%. Several relatively large nonrandomized series of carotid PTA and carotid stenting have reported clinical embolic complications in up to 10% of patients. Predictors of stroke following carotid artery PTA include advanced age, increased lesion severity, and the length and complexity of the stenosis. Complications include restenosis, stent detachment, and stent distortion. Until a multicenter randomized clinical trial that compares the efficacy of carotid endarterectomy and carotid angioplasty has been completed, insufficient information is available to establish the role of carotid PTA or intravascular stents for internal carotid artery stenosis.

In summary, carotid endarterectomy is beneficial for symptomatic patients with recent nondisabling carotid artery ischemic events and ipsilateral 70% to 99% carotid artery stenosis. Carotid endarterectomy is not beneficial for symptomatic patients with 0% to 29% stenosis. The potential benefit of carotid endarterectomy for symptomatic patients with 30% to 69% stenosis is uncertain. For asymptomatic patients, guidelines for carotid endarterectomy include surgical risk less than 3% and a life expectancy of at least 5 years in the presence of a carotid artery stenosis greater than 60% or a carotid artery stenosis greater than 60% in patients undergoing coronary artery bypass grafting. There are no proven indications for carotid endarterectomy for patients with a surgical risk of 3% or more. However, for patients with a surgical risk of 3% to 5%, an acceptable indication for ipsilateral carotid endarterectomy is stenosis of 75% or greater in the presence of contralateral internal carotid artery stenosis of 75% or greater.

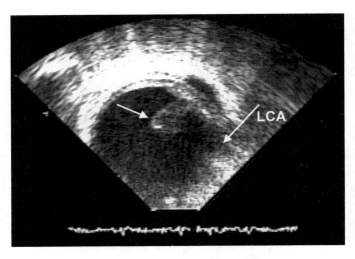

Fig. 2. Transesophageal echocardiography in a patient with recurrent left hemispheric transient ischemic attacks. Transverse view of the distal transverse aortic arch demonstrates large mobile thrombus (*short arrow*) adjacent to origin of the left common carotid artery (*LCA*).

Cerebral Embolism

The identification of atherosclerotic plaque in the thoracic aorta by transesophageal echocardiography is an important finding in patients with cerebral (or systemic) embolic events (Fig. 2). Atherosclerotic plaque thickness greater than 5 mm or mobile thrombus or both predict a high incidence of recurrent embolic events. Many patients with cerebral ischemic events and protruding and mobile atheromas of the thoracic aorta have coexistent carotid artery disease (> 70% stenosis), making precise identification of the source of embolism difficult. Treatment in symptomatic patients with no other identifiable source of embolism is surgical resection of the involved aorta, if the patient's general medical condition permits. Oral anticoagulation treatment for 3 months on the presumption that the friable components will have organized, followed by antiplatelet therapy, is an alternative.

- Many patients with cerebral ischemic events and protruding and mobile atheromas of the thoracic aorta have coexistent carotid artery disease.

Spontaneous Dissection of Cephalic Arteries

Spontaneous dissection of the cervical cephalic arteries is uncommon but important for two reasons: 1) the clinical presentation is characteristic—either hemicrania with oculosympathetic paresis (Horner's syndrome) or hemicrania with delayed focal cerebral ischemic symptoms and 2) the prognosis is good for recovery, and recurrences are rare.

Suggested Review Reading

1. Biller J, Feinberg WM, Castaldo JE, et al: Guidelines for carotid endarterectomy: a statement for healthcare professionals from a Special Writing Group of the Stroke Council, American Heart Association. *Circulation* 97:501-509, 1998.

2. Executive Committee for the Asymptomatic Carotid Atherosclerosis Study: endarterectomy for asymptomatic carotid artery stenosis. JAMA 273:1421-1428, 1995.
Randomized prospective trial of carotid endarterectomy versus medical therapy in asymptomatic patients with greater than 60% stenosis of an internal carotid artery.

Chapter 62

The Aorta

Peter C. Spittell, M.D.

Aortic Atheroembolism

Atheroembolism is characterized by livedo reticularis, blue toes, palpable pulses, hypertension, renal insufficiency, increased erythrocyte sedimentation rate, and eosinophilia (transient). Atheroembolism can occur spontaneously or be due to medication (warfarin or thrombolytic therapy), or to angiographic or surgical procedures. Lower extremity atheroembolism is caused most commonly by abdominal aortic aneurysm or diffuse atherosclerotic disease. In these patients, livedo reticularis and blue toes are bilateral (Fig. 1). Unilateral blue toes suggest that the embolic source is distal to the aortic bifurcation. The treatment of choice is to identify the source of embolism and, if possible, to surgically resect it.

- Atheroembolism is characterized by livedo reticularis, blue toes, palpable pulses, hypertension, renal insufficiency, increased erythrocyte sedimentation rate, and eosinophilia (transient).

Thoracic Aortic Aneurysms

Thoracic aortic aneurysms are caused most commonly by atherosclerosis, but they also occur in patients with systemic hypertension, Marfan syndrome, giant cell arteritis (cranial and Takayasu disease), and infections (syphilis) and as a result of trauma. Most thoracic aortic aneurysms are asymptomatic and are discovered incidentally on chest radiography. Computed tomography (CT), magnetic resonance imaging (MRI), and transesophageal echocardiography (TEE) are all accurate noninvasive techniques for imaging thoracic aortic aneurysms (Fig. 2). Indications for surgical resection include the presence of symptoms, an aneurysm enlarging under observation (particularly if the patient has hypertension), traumatic aneurysm, pseudoaneurysm, and an aneurysm 6 cm or greater in diameter (5.5-6 cm in low-risk patients). In patients with Marfan syndrome, surgery is usually indicated when the ascending aortic diameter exceeds 5 cm.

Abdominal Aortic Aneurysm

Abdominal aortic aneurysm can be diagnosed reliably with ultrasonography, CT, or MRI (Fig. 3). Angiography is not required unless the renal or peripheral arterial circulation needs to be visualized to plan treatment. In a good-risk patient, elective surgical treatment of an abdominal aortic aneurysm should be considered for aneurysms greater than 4 cm in diameter. Elective surgical repair is definitely indicated when the aneurysm diameter is between 4.5 cm and 5.0 cm in good-risk patients. In patients with significant comorbid conditions (pulmonary, cardiac, renal, or liver disease), surgical therapy is individualized. In persons with

The "Questions and Answers" section for this chapter is at the end of the chapter "Peripheral Vascular Disease."
An atlas illustrating pathologic conditions of the aorta is at the end of the chapter (Plates 1-7).

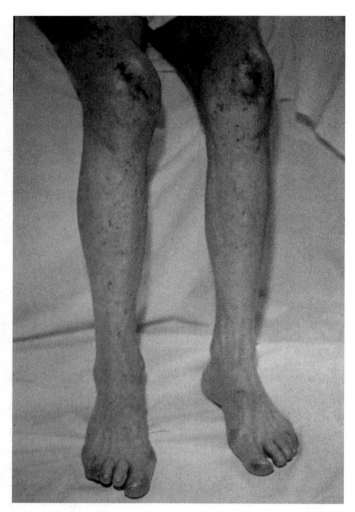

Fig. 1. Livedo reticularis over both patellae and multiple blue toes in a patient with atheroembolism from an abdominal aortic aneurysm.

a large and/or symptomatic abdominal aortic aneurysm whose comorbid condition makes them poor surgical candidates, exclusion of the aneurysm by placement of an intra-luminal stent-anchored polyethylene terephthalate fiber (Dacron) prosthetic graft via retrograde transfemoral cannulation under local anesthesia has given encouraging results in preliminary studies. The role of stent-graft placement in patients who are otherwise good surgical candidates is undefined, and no randomized trial comparing aneurysm surgery to stent-graft placement has been reported.

- Elective surgical repair is definitely indicated when aneurysm diameter is between 4.5 cm and 5.0 cm in good-risk patients.

An inflammatory abdominal aortic aneurysm is suggested

by the triad of back pain, weight loss, and increased erythrocyte sedimentation rate. Obstructive uropathy may occur with ureteral involvement. The findings on CT are diagnostic (Fig. 4). The treatment is surgical resection.

Surgery is also indicated for abdominal aortic aneurysms that are symptomatic, traumatic, or infectious in origin or are rapidly expanding (> 0.5 cm/year).

- An inflammatory abdominal aortic aneurysm is suggested by the triad of back pain, weight loss, and increased erythrocyte sedimentation rate.
- Surgery is indicated for abdominal aortic aneurysms that are greater than 5 cm in diameter, symptomatic, traumatic, or infectious in origin or are rapidly expanding (> 0.5 cm/year).

Aortic Dissection

Etiology
The most common predisposing factors for aortic dissection are advanced age, male gender, hypertension, Marfan syndrome, and congenital abnormalities of the aortic valve (bicuspid or unicuspid valve). When aortic dissection complicates pregnancy, it usually occurs in the third trimester. Iatrogenic aortic dissection, as a result of cardiac surgery or invasive angiographic procedures, can also occur.

Classification
Aortic dissection involving the ascending aorta is designated as "type I" or "type II" (proximal, type A), and dissection confined to the descending thoracic aorta is designated as "type III" (distal, type B) (Fig. 5).

Clinical Features
The acute onset of severe pain (often migratory) in the anterior chest, back, or abdomen occurs in 70% to 80% of patients, and hypertension is present in 60% to 80%. Additional findings include aortic diastolic murmur (15% to 20% of patients), pulse deficits (10% to 40%), and neurologic changes (10% to 30%). Syncope in association with aortic dissection occurs when there is rupture into the pericardial space, producing cardiac tamponade. Congestive heart failure is due most commonly to severe aortic regurgitation. Acute myocardial infarction (most commonly inferior infarction due to right coronary artery ostial dissection) and pericarditis are additional cardiac presentations.

Clues to type I aortic dissection include substernal pain,

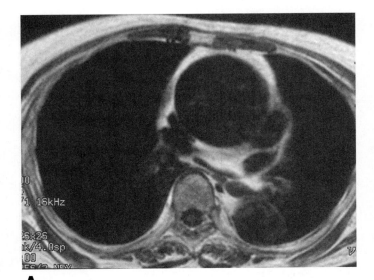

A

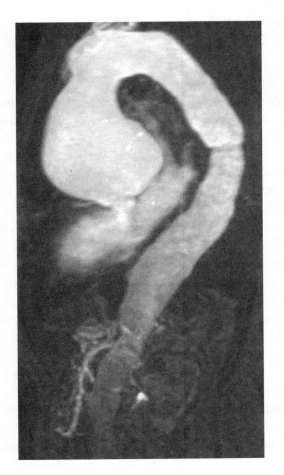

C

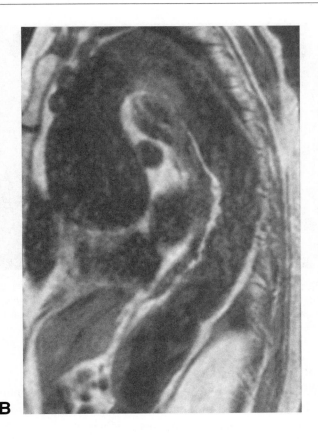

B

Fig. 2. Magnetic resonance imaging/angiography in a patient with asymptomatic thoracic aortic aneurysm. Images in the transverse, *A*, and longitudinal, *B*, planes demonstrate a large aneurysm of the ascending aorta (7.8 cm) and moderate dilatation (4.5 cm) of the descending thoracic aorta. Moderate aortic regurgitation is also demonstrated, *C*.

aortic valve incompetence, decreased pulse or blood pressure in the right arm, decreased right carotid pulse, pericardial friction rub, syncope, ischemic electrocardiographic changes, and Marfan syndrome.

Clues to type III aortic dissection include interscapular pain, hypertension, and left pleural effusion.

● In a patient with a catastrophic presentation, systemic hypertension, and unexplained physical findings of vascular origin—especially in the presence of chest or back pain and an aortic murmur—aortic dissection should always be included in the differential diagnosis, and an appropriate screening test should be performed emergently.

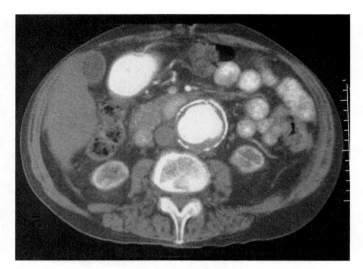

Fig. 3. Computed tomography with intravenous contrast demonstrating a large aneurysm of the infrarenal abdominal aorta. There is a small amount of laminated thrombus within the aneurysm and dense peripheral calcification.

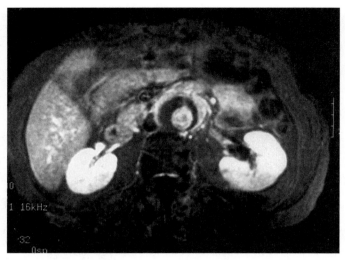

Fig. 4. Computed tomographic scan of abdomen of patient with inflammatory abdominal aortic aneurysm. Note the high attenuation change surrounding the aorta, representing inflammatory change in periaortic retroperitoneal tissue.

Laboratory Tests

Chest radiography may reveal widening of the mediastinum and supracardiac aortic shadow, deviation of the trachea to the right, a discrepancy in diameter between the ascending and descending aorta, and pleural effusion (Fig. 6). Normal findings on chest radiography do not exclude aortic dissection.

Diagnosis

Definitive diagnosis of aortic dissection can be made using any of the following imaging modalities: echocardiography, CT, MRI, and aortography.

Echocardiography

The combination of transthoracic echocardiography (TTE) and TEE can be used to identify an intimal flap, communication between the true and false lumina, a dilated aortic root (> 4.2 cm), thrombus formation, widening of the aortic walls, aortic regurgitation, and pericardial effusion/tamponade. Multiplane techniques have markedly improved the accuracy of TEE (Fig. 7). Advantages of TEE include portability, safety, accuracy, rapid diagnosis, use in patients with hemodynamic instability, and use intraoperatively.

CT

CT can accurately detect the intimal flap, identify two lumina, and demonstrate displaced calcification, size difference between ascending and descending aortic lumina, hemopericardium, pleural effusion, and abdominal aorta involvement (Fig. 8). The disadvantages include nonportability (limiting its use in patients with hemodynamic instability) and the need for intravenous contrast agents.

MRI

MRI is as accurate as CT in the diagnosis of aortic dissection. Demonstration of the intimal flap, entry/exit sites, thrombus formation, aortic regurgitation, pericardial effusion, pleural

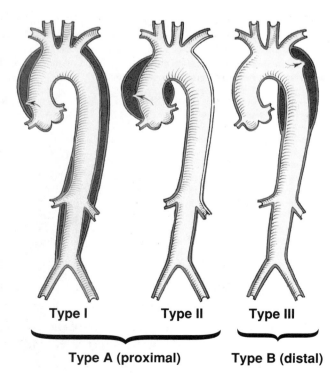

Type I   Type II   Type III

Type A (proximal)   Type B (distal)

Fig. 5. Classification of aortic dissection.

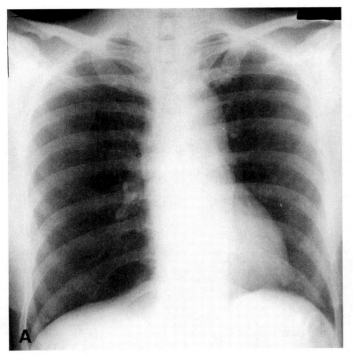 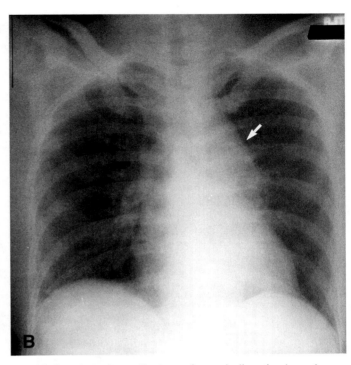

Fig. 6. Chest radiographs of patient before (*A*) and after (*B*) aortic dissection. Note widening of superior mediastinum after aortic dissection (*arrow*).

effusion, and abdominal aorta involvement is possible (Fig. 9). MRI is also able to delineate involvement of aortic arch vessels. Disadvantages of MRI include cost and nonportability.

Aortography

Aortography can accurately diagnose aortic dissection by showing the intimal flap, opacification of the false lumen, and deformity of the true lumen. Also, associated aortic regurgitation and coronary artery anatomy can be visualized. The disadvantages include invasive risks, exposure to intravenous contrast agents, and nonportability.

The choice of test (TTE, TEE, CT, MRI, or aortography) in a patient with suspected acute aortic dissection depends

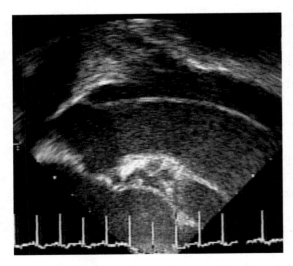

Fig. 7. Transesophageal echocardiographic view of ascending aorta in the longitudinal plane demonstrating an intimal flap originating in right coronary sinus.

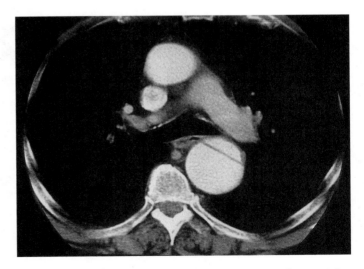

Fig. 8. Computed tomography with intravenous contrast demonstrating dilatation of descending thoracic aorta and an intimal flap. Note the relatively equal opacification of true and false lumina.

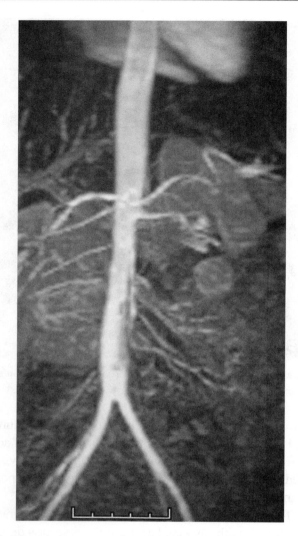

Fig. 9. Magnetic resonance angiography demonstrating dissection of mid and distal abdominal aorta in patient with a remote history of sudden deceleration injury.

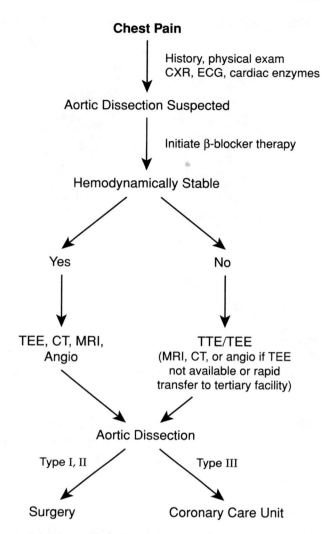

Fig. 10. Initial management of suspected acute aortic dissection. Angio, angiography; CT, computed tomography; CXR, chest radiography; ECG, electrocardiography; TEE, transesophageal echocardiography; TTE, transthoracic echocardiography.

on which is most readily available and the hemodynamic stability of the patient. Currently, our test of choice in suspected acute aortic dissection is the combination of TTE and TEE. The initial management of suspected acute aortic dissection is shown in Figure 10.

The most common cause of death in aortic dissection is rupture into the pericardial space, with cardiac tamponade. Echocardiographically guided pericardiocentesis is associated with an increased risk of aortic rupture and death. Cardiac tamponade due to aortic dissection is a surgical emergency, and generally pericardial fluid should be removed only in the operating room after cardiopulmonary bypass has been instituted. Other causes of death include acute congestive heart failure due to severe aortic regurgitation, rupture

through the aortic adventitia, rupture into the left pleural space, and occlusion of vital arteries. Factors that propagate dissection include "impulse" pulsatile flow and increased mean arterial pressure.

- Cardiac tamponade due to aortic dissection is a surgical emergency, but percutaneous pericardiocentesis should be performed only in cases of imminent death.

Treatment

Pharmacologic therapy should be instituted as soon as the diagnosis of aortic dissection is suspected (see below). Emergent surgery is indicated for types I and II (proximal, type A) aortic dissection. Pharmacologic therapy in the

Table 1.—Initial Pharmacologic Therapy for Aortic Dissection

Hypertensive patients

Sodium nitroprusside intravenously, 2.5 to 5 µg/kg per minute

with

Propranolol intravenously, 1 mg every 4 to 6 hours

(The goal is to have systolic blood pressure < 110 mm Hg—a lower pressure is acceptable if urine output is maintained at least at 25 to 30 mL/hr—until oral medication is started)

or

Intravenous esmolol, metoprolol, or atenolol (in place of propranolol)

or

Intravenous labetalol (in place of sodium nitroprusside and a β-blocker)

Normotensive patients

Propranolol, 1 mg intravenously every 4 to 6 hours

or

20 to 40 mg orally every 6 hours

(Metoprolol, atenolol, or labetalol may be used in place of propranolol)

coronary care unit is the preferred initial treatment for type III (distal, type B) aortic dissection, with delayed surgical therapy (2 to 3 weeks) for selected patients whose general medical condition permits operation.

The initial pharmacologic therapy is outlined in Table 1. When long-term pharmacologic therapy is used for type III aortic dissection, indications for surgery include development of saccular aneurysm, increasing aortic diameter, or symptoms related to chronic dissection.

Penetrating Aortic Ulcer

Penetrating aortic ulcer occurs when an atherosclerotic plaque undergoes ulceration and penetrates the internal elastic lamina. It results in one of four possible consequences: 1) formation of an intramural hematoma, 2) formation of a saccular aneurysm, 3) formation of a pseudoaneurysm, or 4) a transmural rupture (Fig. 11). Penetrating aortic ulcer almost always involves the mid or distal descending thoracic aorta and rarely the ascending or abdominal aorta. The clinical features of penetrating aortic ulcer are similar to those

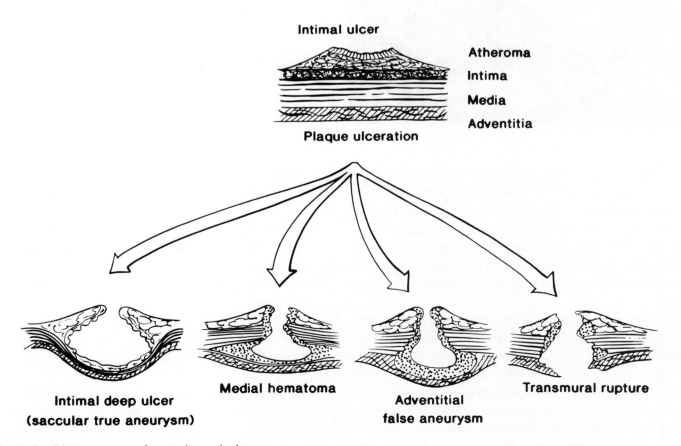

Fig. 11. Possible consequences of penetrating aortic ulcer.

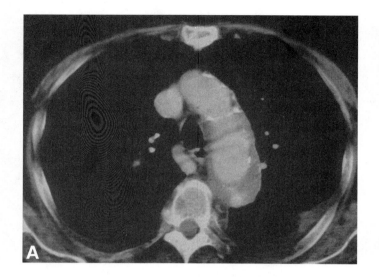

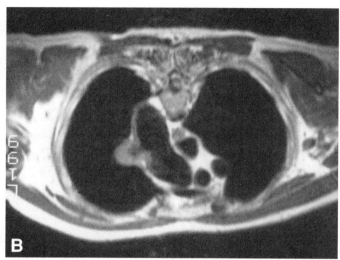

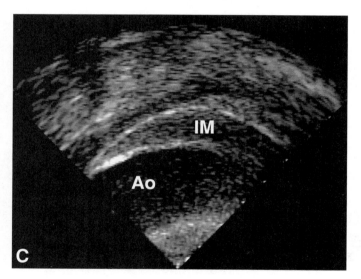

Fig. 12. *A*, Computed tomography with intravenous contrast demonstrating intramural hematoma of transverse aortic arch caused by a penetrating aortic ulcer. *B*, Magnetic resonance image scan demonstrating a penetrating aortic ulcer of transverse aortic arch. *C*, Transesophageal echocardiographic view of transverse aortic arch (transverse plane) demonstrating intramural hematoma (*IM*).

of aortic dissection and include acute onset of pain in the anterior or posterior chest (or both) and hypertension. Pulse deficits, neurologic signs, and acute cardiac disease (aortic regurgitation, myocardial infarction, pericardial effusion) are not seen in penetrating aortic ulcer as they are in classic aortic dissection. The diagnosis of penetrating aortic ulcer can be established with CT, MRI, TEE, or aortography (Fig. 12).

The treatment for penetrating aortic ulcer is usually non-operative if only an intramural hematoma is present. With control of hypertension, the intramural hematoma tends to resolve spontaneously over time. Surgical therapy is indicated for patients who have ascending aortic involvement or develop a saccular aneurysm or a pseudoaneurysm or for patients with intramural hematoma who have persistent symptoms, increasing aortic diameter, or poorly controlled

hypertension. The most common serious complication of surgical therapy for penetrating aortic ulcer is paraplegia.

- Penetrating aortic ulcer occurs when an atherosclerotic plaque undergoes ulceration and penetrates the internal elastic lamina.
- The treatment for penetrating aortic ulcer is usually non-operative.

Incomplete Aortic Rupture

Incomplete rupture of the thoracic aorta (in the region of the aortic isthmus) results from a sudden deceleration injury. It is seen most often in motor vehicle accident victims and should be suspected when there is evidence of trauma to the chest wall, decreased or absent leg pulses, left-sided hemothorax, or widening of the superior mediastinum on chest radiography. These patients usually are hypertensive at initial presentation. The diagnosis can be confirmed with TEE, CT, MRI, or angiography. Treatment is emergent surgical repair in patients who are suitable surgical candidates. At initial presentation, the condition of 40% to 50% of the patients is unstable. No clinical or imaging criteria accurately predict future complete rupture, so even if a patient presents with a chronic incomplete rupture, surgery is still indicated. Most of the patients are young, and the risk of elective surgical repair is low, with an otherwise good prognosis for long-term survival if aortic repair is successful.

- Incomplete rupture of the thoracic aorta (in the region of the aortic isthmus) results from a sudden deceleration injury, frequently a motor vehicle accident.

Suggested Review Reading

1. Dressler FA, Craig WR, Castello R, et al: Mobile aortic atheroma and systemic emboli: efficacy of anticoagulation and influence of plaque morphology on recurrent stroke. *J Am Coll Cardiol* 31:134-138, 1998. *Transesophageal echocardiographic study of 31 patients with a history of systemic emboli demonstrated a high incidence of recurrent vascular events when mobile thrombus was present (regardless of thrombus size) and improved outcome with oral anticoagulation with coumadin.*

2. Ernst CB: Abdominal aortic aneurysm. *N Engl J Med* 328:1167-1172, 1993.

3. Harris JA, Bis KG, Glover JL, et al: Penetrating atherosclerotic ulcers of the aorta. *J Vasc Surg* 19:90-98, 1994. *Review of the natural history and optimal imaging modality of penetrating atherosclerotic ulcers of the aorta. Most patients can be managed medically and many demonstrate progressive aortic enlargement on serial imaging. Aortic dissection, aortic rupture, and embolization were less common outcomes.*

4. Kouchoukos NT, Dougenis D: Surgery of the thoracic aorta. N Engl J Med 336:1876-1888, 1997.

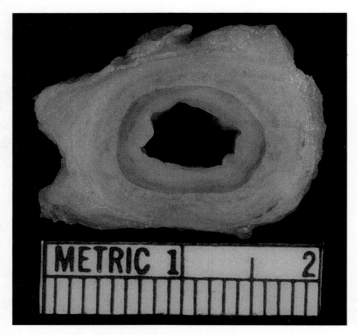

Plate 1. Takayasu arteritis in descending thoracic aorta.

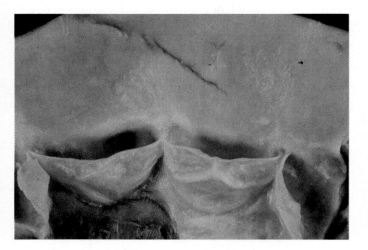

Plate 2. Isolated intimal tear of ascending aorta in giant cell aortitis.

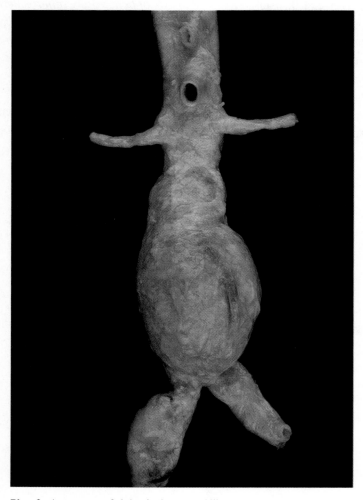

Plate 3. Aneurysms of abdominal aorta and iliac artery.

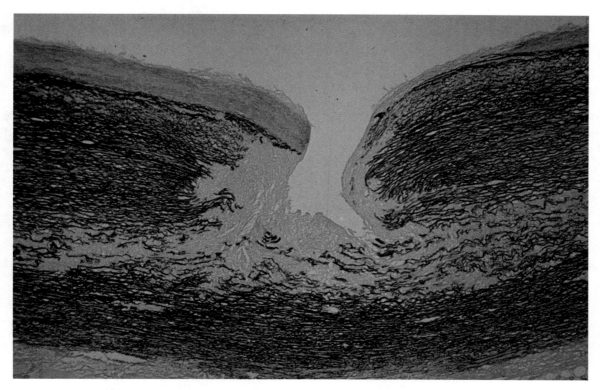

Plate 4. Isolated intimal tear of ascending aorta in giant cell aortitis.

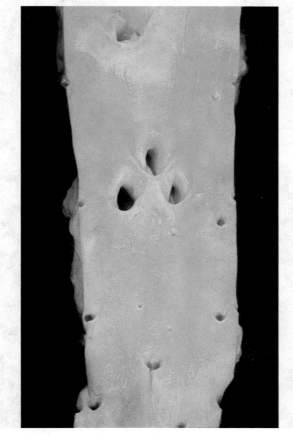

Plate 5. Atherosclerosis of the abdominal aorta.

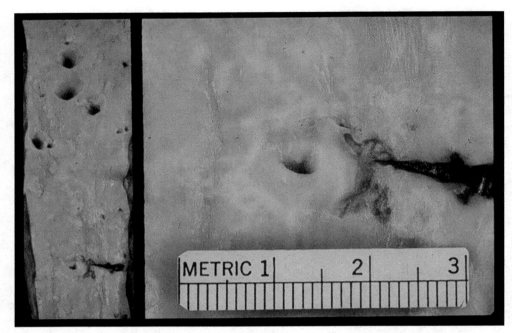

Plate 6. Type III aortic dissection involving the abdominal aorta.

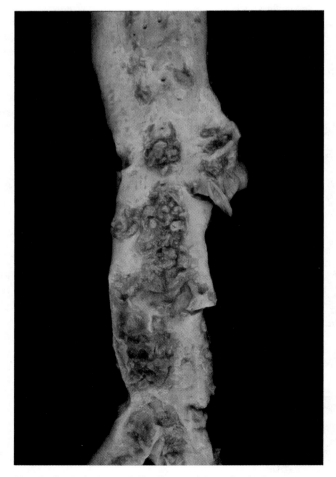

Plate 7. Grade 4 ulcerocalcific disease of the abdominal aorta.

Chapter 63

Adult Congenital Heart Disease

Carole A. Warnes, M.D.

Atrial Septal Defect (ASD)

Secundum ASD

The secundum type of ASD is the most common adult congenital heart defect after bicuspid aortic valve. The defect is in the central portion of the atrial septum and is associated with left-to-right shunting and right ventricular volume overload. Adults are often asymptomatic, and the murmur may be found incidentally on physical examination. The natural history of unrepaired ASD is that atrial fibrillation develops in patients in their 40s or 50s in association with tricuspid regurgitation and often right ventricular failure. Death is usually from heart failure or thromboembolic stroke, although survival into old age occurs in some patients.

Physical Examination

The jugular venous pressure is often normal and the "a" and "v" waves may be equal in amplitude. Other findings are a right ventricular lift, an ejection systolic murmur from the pulmonary area (always less than grade 3/6), fixed splitting of the second heart sound, and a tricuspid diastolic flow rumble if the shunt is large (Qp/Qs more than 2.5 to 1).

Electrocardiography

Typical electrocardiographic findings include an RSR pattern and partial right bundle branch block, often with right-axis deviation.

Chest Radiography (Fig. 1 and 2)

A prominent pulmonary artery, right ventricular enlargement, and pulmonary plethora are found on chest radiographs. Left atrial enlargement does not typically occur unless the patient is older than 40 years or has atrial fibrillation. If left atrial enlargement is present in a young person with an ASD in sinus rhythm, consider a primum ASD in the differential diagnosis or coincidental mitral valve disease.

Diagnosis and Management

The diagnosis of ASD can usually be made with echocardiography, but if the image is suboptimal, transesophageal echocardiography should be performed. Cardiac catheterization is usually unnecessary to confirm an ASD unless coexistent coronary artery disease is suspected. If there is evidence of right ventricular volume overload, the ASD should be closed to prevent right heart failure, paradoxical embolus, and atrial arrhythmia. (Closing an ASD later in life, although still beneficial, is associated with an increased risk of atrial arrhythmias during late follow-up.) Percutaneous device closure of an ASD is now possible, but, to date, no randomized trial of surgical versus device closure of an ASD has been reported.

- The secundum type of ASD is the most common adult congenital heart defect after bicuspid aortic valve.
- Cardiac catheterization is usually unnecessary to confirm an ASD unless coexistent coronary artery disease is suspected.

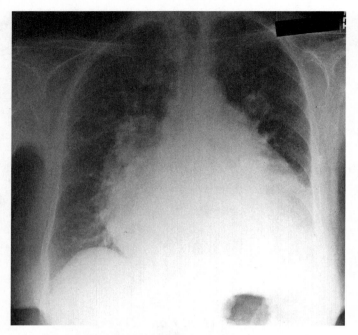

Fig. 1. Chest radiograph showing cardiomegaly and congestive heart fail-ure in an elderly woman with atrial septal defect. (From *Cardiovasc Clin* 10 No 3:161-197, 1980. By permission of FA Davis Company.)

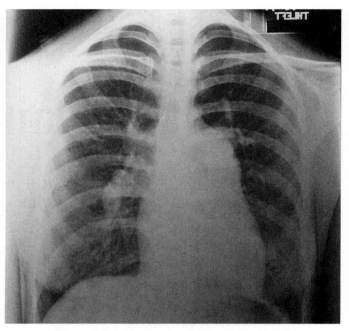

Fig. 2. Chest radiograph of 35-year-old woman with atrial septal defect. There is severe pulmonary vascular obstructive disease with prominence of the main pulmonary artery and decreased peripheral pulmonary vasculari-ty. (From *Cardiovasc Clin* 10 No 3:161-197, 1980. By permission of FA Davis Company.)

Primum ASD

The primum type of ASD is in the lower portion of the atrial septum and is a defect in the atrioventricular septum. Both atrioventricular valves are on the same anatomical level and are congenitally abnormal. Classically, the mitral valve is cleft, but 4% of defects may be associated with double-ori-fice mitral valve. The mitral valve, therefore, has various degrees of regurgitation and may occasionally be stenotic. The septal leaflet of the tricuspid valve often is deficient, with varying degrees of tricuspid regurgitation. The find-ings on physical examination in primum ASD are the same as those for secundum ASD, with the addition of variable signs of mitral regurgitation.

Electrocardiography

Electrocardiography shows left-axis deviation with right bundle branch block. First-degree atrioventricular block occurs in approximately 75% of cases.

Diagnosis

The condition is diagnosed with echocardiography, and car-diac catheterization is usually unnecessary. Because of the elongated ventricular outflow tract, the so-called goose-neck

deformity is produced on angiography. Subaortic stenosis is a recognized association.

Management

Patch closure is used for the ASD, and the mitral cleft is repaired if the valve is regurgitant.

- The findings on physical examination in primum ASD are the same as those for secundum ASD, with the addi-tion of variable signs of mitral regurgitation.

Sinus Venosus ASD

Sinus venosus is a defect in the superior portion of the sep-tum usually associated with anomalous pulmonary vein (classically, the right upper pulmonary vein).

Diagnosis

The diagnosis usually can be made with echocardiography (this may require transesophageal echocardiography), and the pulmonary vein also should be diverted at the time of surgical repair.

- Eisenmenger syndrome develops in approximately 5% of patients with ASD.

Ventricular Septal Defect

Small defects (so-called maladie de Roger) often produce a loud murmur but are of little or no clinical significance apart from the need for endocarditis prophylaxis. Defects can occur at many different areas in the septum, the most common being in the membranous and muscular parts of the septum. These defects have the possibility of closing spontaneously up to about age 20 years. Defects in other positions never close spontaneously (such as subaortic defects, subpulmonary defects, and canal-type defects) (Fig. 3).

Small defects may be associated with a thrill at the left sternal edge, usually in the fourth interspace. The murmur is usually holosystolic, but it may be shorter if it is in the muscular septum because the defect may be occluded during late systole. Large defects also may produce a mitral diastolic flow rumble at the apex, particularly when the shunt has a Qp/Qs more than 2.5 to 1.

- Ventricular septal defect is the most common congenital heart defect to produce the Eisenmenger syndrome.

Patent Ductus Arteriosus

This classically is associated with maternal rubella. A small ductus may be of little or no hemodynamic consequence and is consistent with a normal life span. A patent ductus arteriosus commonly calcifies in adult life.

Physical Examination

Because it produces an "arteriovenous fistula," the pulse pressure is usually wide with a prominent left ventricular impulse and a continuous "machinery murmur" enveloping the second heart sound. This usually is audible beneath the left clavicle in the second intercostal space.

Therapy

In most cases, the patent ductus is ligated because surgical therapy is curative. Thoracoscopic surgical closure is now possible. After ligation, patients do not need endocarditis prophylaxis. Percutaneous device closure of the ductus is an alternative therapy.

Differential Diagnosis

The differential diagnosis of a patent ductus arteriosus includes pulmonary atresia with systemic collateral vessels in a patient with cyanosis, aortopulmonary window, ventricular septal

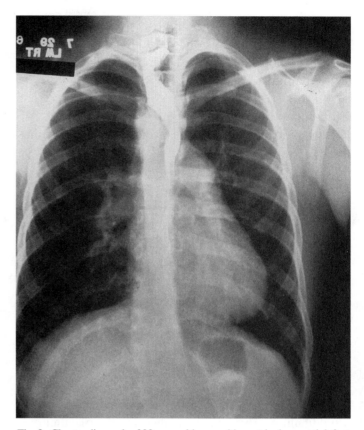

Fig. 3. Chest radiograph of 22-year-old man with ventricular septal defect complicated by pulmonary vascular obstructive disease. Note nearly normal cardiac size with apex tilted upward, marked dilatation of central pulmonary arteries, and decreased peripheral pulmonary vascularity. (From Bonchek LI, Brooks HL [editors]: *Office Management of Medical and Surgical Heart Disease: A Concise Guide for Physicians.* Little, Brown & Company, 1981, pp 183-217. By permission of Lippincott-Raven Publishers.)

defect, and aortic regurgitation. Rarely, coarctation may produce a continuous murmur.

Pulmonary Stenosis

Pulmonary stenosis may be associated with Noonan syndrome, in which case the valve is frequently dysplastic. The condition usually produces few or no symptoms unless the pulmonary stenosis is very severe. Usually the valve remains pliable until well into middle age; thus, an ejection click is common until later life.

Physical Examination

The following features suggest pulmonary stenosis: a prominent "a" wave in the jugular venous pressure, right ventricular lift, ejection click (the earlier the click, the more severe the stenosis), systolic murmur, and delayed pulmonary component of second heart sound (P_2) (absent in severe pulmonary stenosis).

Electrocardiography

Right ventricular hypertrophy is seen on the electrocardiogram.

Chest Radiography

When stenosis is at valve level, there is poststenotic dilatation of the main and left pulmonary arteries, which is a typical radiographic appearance (Fig. 4). Lung fields are oligemic *only* in severe pulmonary stenosis.

Diagnosis and Management

The diagnosis is made from the findings on clinical examination and echocardiography. Severe stenosis is usually a gradient of more than 50 mm Hg (right ventricular pressure more than two-thirds of systemic pressure). Most patients have good results from balloon valvotomy. Often, coexistent subpulmonary stenosis is due to hypertrophy of the infundibulum. This usually regresses with time after pulmonary valvotomy. Midterm results appear to be comparable to those with surgical commissurotomy; hence, balloon valvotomy is now the procedure of choice for treatment of pulmonary stenosis.

- Pulmonary stenosis may be associated with Noonan syndrome, in which case the valve is frequently dysplastic.
- Severe stenosis is usually a gradient of more than 50 mm Hg.
- Balloon valvotomy is now the procedure of choice for treatment of pulmonary stenosis.

Coarctation of the Aorta

Coarctation of the aorta most often is diagnosed in childhood and is usually a discrete narrowing of the aorta just distal to the left subclavian artery. Occasionally there may be an elongated, narrowed thoracic aorta. Coarctation is much more common in males than females and often is associated with a bicuspid aortic valve. It is the most common anomaly associated with Turner syndrome. It also is associated with ventricular septal defect, Shone syndrome, and cerebral aneurysms in the circle of Willis.

It may be noted as an incidental murmur, but if it is not

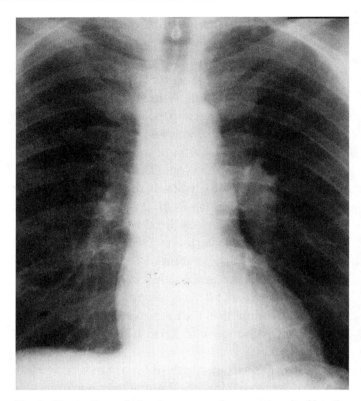

Fig. 4. Chest radiograph showing severe pulmonary stenosis. Note the poststenotic dilatation of the main and left pulmonary arteries, indicating that this is valvular pulmonary stenosis.

detected in childhood it may present with systemic hypertension in adulthood. The narrowing in the aorta produces systemic hypertension above the coarctation and reduced blood pressure below the coarctation in the legs. Sometimes patients present because of signs of hypertension on retinal examination.

As a result of the coarctation, systemic collateral vessels frequently develop from the subclavian, axillary, internal mammary, scapular, and intercostal arteries. It is the intercostal artery collateral vessels that produce the classic rib notching.

Physical Examination

Findings on physical examination include radiofemoral delay and a decrease in blood pressure between the upper and lower extremities. An ejection systolic murmur is present in the second space at the left sternal edge. This occasionally extends into diastole, producing a continuous murmur when the coarctation is severe. Collateral murmurs may be audible and palpable over the thorax and particularly the back over the scapulae. An ejection click may be heard when there is an associated bicuspid aortic valve. The aortic component of the second heart sound (A_2) may be loud, and a fourth heart sound may be present if there is systemic hypertension.

Electrocardiography

Electrocardiography shows varying degrees of left ventricular hypertrophy.

Chest Radiography

Chest radiographs may show the classic "figure-3" sign beneath the aortic knob, which represents dilatation of the aorta above the coarctation and then dilatation below. Rib notching is a variable feature (Fig. 5 and 6).

Complications

The major complications of coarctation include aortic rupture or dissection, coexistent aortic valve disease, left ventricular failure, stroke (due to either systemic hypertension or rupture of a cerebral aneurysm), endocarditis, and endarteritis.

Pregnancy in patients with coarctation is associated with an increased risk of aortic dissection and rupture. The risk of aortic dissection and rupture also is increased in Turner syndrome, even in the absence of coarctation.

Diagnosis

Coarctation of the aorta is diagnosed from findings on physical examination and Doppler echocardiography. Doppler echocardiography at rest may show a limited gradient, and exercise Doppler echocardiography may improve the diagnostic accuracy. If the coarctation is not well visualized, be cautious with the gradient interpretation because collateral vessels may reduce the gradient even when significant coarctation is present. If Doppler echocardiographic imaging is not satisfactory, consider magnetic resonance imaging or aortography.

Treatment

Surgical repair by left lateral thoracotomy is the accepted

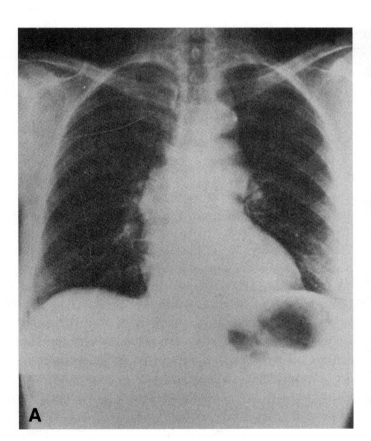
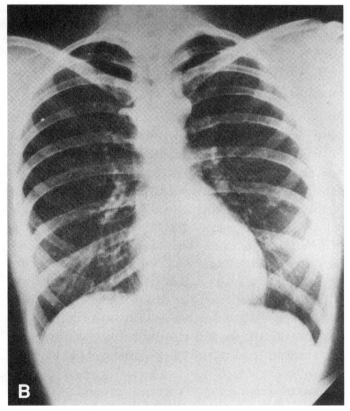

Fig. 5. *A*, Coarctation of aorta with "figure-3" sign seen along upper aspect of left cardiac silhouette; indentation just below aortic arch represents coarcted segment with poststenotic dilatation below this. *B*, No other characteristics of aortic coarctation are present except notching beneath the undersurface of the ribs, evident on the left side. (From Giuliani ER, Gersh BJ, McGoon MD, Hayes DL, Schaff HV [editors]: *Mayo Clinic Practice of Cardiology*. Third edition. Mosby, 1996, p 1575. By permission of Mayo Foundation.)

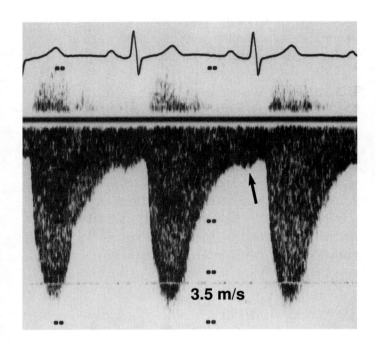
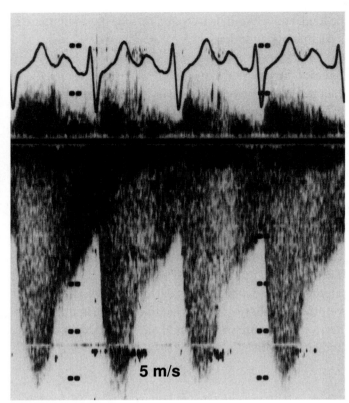

3.5 m/s

5 m/s

Fig. 6. Continuous-wave Doppler recordings down the descending aorta in a patient with coarctation of the aorta. *Left*, Resting recording with a peak systolic velocity of 3.5 m/s indicates a maximal instantaneous gradient of approximately 49 mm Hg. Note the persistence of high velocity (approximately 1 m/s) in diastole (*arrow*). *Right*, With exercise, the peak velocity increases to 5 m/s (100 mm Hg maximal instantaneous gradient) and the diastolic flow also is increased, to 2 m/s. These measurements are consistent with severe coarctation. (From Giuliani ER, Gersh BJ, McGoon MD, Hayes DL, Schaff HV [editors]: *Mayo Clinic Practice of Cardiology*. Third edition. Mosby, 1996, p 1576. By permission of Mayo Foundation.)

treatment. Re-coarctation, however, is possible, and there is still a significant incidence of systemic hypertension (75% at 30 years) after coarctation repair. Balloon angioplasty also has been performed, but it is less successful in patients with higher gradients and also is associated with aneurysm formation.

Even after successful repair of coarctation, the aorta is still abnormal and patients are still at increased risk of dying of dissection and rupture. They also die of premature coronary artery disease, heart failure, and stroke. The earlier the age of repair, the less chance of systemic hypertension and its complications. In one Mayo Clinic series, patients who had operation at younger than 14 years had a 20-year survival rate of 91%, and patients who had operation at age 14 years or older had a reduced 20-year survival rate of 79%.

- Coarctation is much more common in males than females and commonly is associated with a bicuspid aortic valve.
- The major complications of coarctation include aortic rupture or dissection, coexistent aortic valve disease, left ventricular failure, stroke (due to either systemic hyper-

tension or rupture of a cerebral aneurysm), endocarditis, and endarteritis.

Ebstein Anomaly

The major abnormality in Ebstein anomaly is inferior displacement of the tricuspid valve into the right ventricle, producing an "atrialized" right ventricle above and a small right ventricle below, which often has impaired contraction. The degree of displacement is variable, as is the degree of abnormality of the tricuspid valve. The septal leaflet is variably deficient or even absent. The posterior leaflet also often is deficient, and there is a large "sail-like" anterior leaflet that is the hallmark of the condition. Among patients with Ebstein anomaly, 50% have either a patent foramen ovale or a secundum ASD, and 25% have one or more accessory atrioventricular conduction (Wolff-Parkinson-White syndrome) pathways. The anomaly is thought to be associated with maternal lithium ingestion.

Physical Examination

Findings include a low-volume pulse with cool extremities and sometimes peripheral cyanosis reflecting low cardiac output. Central cyanosis may be present if there is an atrial communication. A "v" wave may be present in the jugular venous pressure, although this is uncommon even in the presence of significant tricuspid regurgitation because the large right atrium absorbs the tricuspid regurgitant volume. There is a subtle right ventricular lift. The loud tricuspid component of the first heart sound (T_1) is produced by the sail-like anterior leaflet of the tricuspid valve. The holosystolic murmur of tricuspid regurgitation is often associated with one or more systolic clicks in Ebstein anomaly.

Chest Radiography

Varying degrees of cardiomegaly with marked right atrial enlargement are seen on chest radiographs (Fig. 7 and 8). In contrast to cardiomyopathy, the pedicle is very narrow (small pulmonary artery). Usually, the lung fields are normal or oligemic.

Electrocardiography

Right atrial enlargement produces tall P waves, which may be the largest of any anomaly (Himalayan P waves). Right bundle branch block often is present, or there may be evidence of preexcitation.

Diagnosis and Management

The diagnosis is made with echocardiography. Cardiac catheterization is unnecessary unless coexistent coronary artery disease is suspected. Surgical repair is indicated when 1) patients have functional limitation, 2) the cardiothoracic ratio is more than 60%, 3) an atrial communication is present and the patient is cyanotic (risk of stroke), 4) a bypass tract is present, and 5) there is severe tricuspid regurgitation (especially if the valve is reparable).

Surgical Repair

Surgery consists of closure of the atrial communication, repair of the tricuspid valve if there is sufficient mobility to the anterior leaflet, and plication of the atrialized right ventricle. If the valve is tethered and immobile, tricuspid valve replacement may be necessary.

- Among patients with Ebstein anomaly, 50% have either a patent foramen ovale or a secundum atrial septal defect, and 25% have one or more accessory atrioventricular conduction (Wolff-Parkinson-White syndrome) pathways.

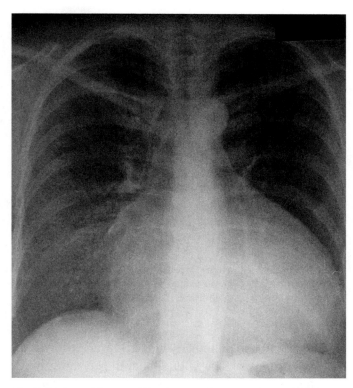

Fig. 7. Patient with severe Ebstein anomaly, severe right atrial enlargement, and huge cardiomegaly with a very narrow pedicle.

Cyanotic Heart Disease

There are many "natural survivors" with cyanotic heart disease who reach adulthood without having had surgery. These include patients with tetralogy of Fallot, anatomical variants with a very large interventricular shunt (single ventricle), pulmonary stenosis with atrial septal defect, Ebstein anomaly with ASD, and Eisenmenger syndrome.

Tetralogy of Fallot

One of the so-called conotruncal abnormalities, tetralogy of Fallot consists of a large subaortic ventricular septal defect and obstruction to the pulmonary outflow, usually at the infundibular level and often at the pulmonary valve level also. This produces right ventricular hypertrophy. In addition, the aorta overrides the ventricular septal defect.

The pressure in the right ventricle is the same as that in the left because of the large ventricular septal defect. The obstruction to pulmonary blood flow causes desaturated blood to be diverted into the aorta, which is often large; thus, the degree of right ventricular obstruction determines the degree of cyanosis. Hence, in childhood, the so-called acyanotic Fallot or the pink tetralogy occurs when there is

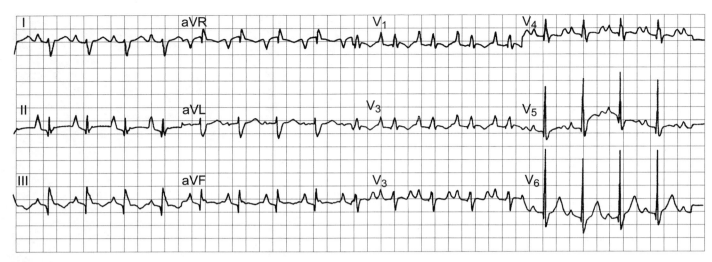

Fig. 8. Electrocardiogram from 15-year-old boy with Ebstein anomaly. Note prominent P wave, prolonged atrioventricular conduction, and delay in right ventricular conduction. (From Giuliani ER, Gersh BJ, McGoon MD, Hayes DL, Schaff HV [editors]: *Mayo Clinic Practice of Cardiology*. Third edition. Mosby, 1996, p 1601. By permission of Mayo Foundation.)

little obstruction to pulmonary blood flow and patients do not have cyanosis. The infundibular hypertrophy, however, tends to be progressive; thus, the cyanosis increases with advancing age.

Most patients have repair in childhood, but occasionally they reach adulthood without surgical intervention. These adult patients do *not* have right ventricular failure until they are at least 40 years of age, unless they have a superimposed arrhythmia.

Physical Examination

Findings on physical examination include varying degrees of cyanosis and clubbing, right ventricular lift, a thrill at the left sternal edge if the pulmonary obstruction is severe, long systolic murmur in the pulmonary area, and absent P_2.

Adult patients who have not had operation may have aortic regurgitation, because the aorta is large and the cusps prolapse into the defect. Aortic regurgitation may be of varying degree. The aortic regurgitant jet may enter the right ventricle, and this may ultimately produce right ventricular failure.

Chest Radiography

Tetralogy of Fallot is associated with right aortic arch (approximately 25% of cases), right ventricular enlargement, concave pulmonary bay, and possibly pulmonary oligemia.

Electrocardiography

Tetralogy of Fallot is associated with right ventricular hypertrophy, usually right-axis deviation, and tall, peaked P waves.

Diagnosis and Management

The diagnosis can usually be made with echocardiography. The coronary anatomy should also be determined because of the increased incidence of anomalous coronary anatomy if surgical correction is being contemplated. If the pulmonary arteries are of adequate size, surgical repair involves closure of the ventricular septal defect and relief of the outflow obstruction. In simple cases, this involves resection of the infundibular muscle, but if the pulmonary annulus is small, it may involve pulmonary valvotomy, right ventricular outflow patch, transannular patch, excision of the pulmonary valve, or placement of a conduit from the right ventricle to the pulmonary artery.

Long-term problems after surgical repair of tetralogy include sudden death due to ventricular arrhythmias (more common after late repair associated with residual hemodynamic abnormalities such as poor right ventricular function, residual ventricular septal defect, residual pulmonary stenosis), thought to result from right ventricular fibrosis; aortic regurgitation and aortic dilatation; right ventricular aneurysm formation at the site of patching of the right ventricular outflow; reoperation (for pulmonary regurgitation or pulmonary stenosis); and infective endocarditis (on aortic valve).

Other patients with tetralogy of Fallot may survive because of earlier palliative shunts that improve pulmonary blood flow and help pulmonary arteries to grow. Types of shunt include Blalock-Taussig (a subclavian artery-to-pulmonary artery anastomosis—can be used on either the right or the left side); Waterston shunt between the ascending aorta and the right pulmonary artery; Potts shunt (descending aorta-to-left pulmonary artery shunt); and a central shunt constructed with a polytetrafluoroethylene (PTFE, Gore-Tex) graft.

Problems with palliative shunts include distortion of the pulmonary arteries, which may kink, thrombose, or occlude, and pulmonary vascular disease when the shunt is too large. Patients with large shunts are at risk of volume overload on the ventricle and ultimately ventricular failure with pulmonary vascular disease. These patients are not accepted for heart-lung transplantation because of the lateral thoracotomy and the profound risk of bleeding.

- Tetralogy of Fallot consists of a large subaortic ventricular septal defect and obstruction to the pulmonary outflow.
- Problems with palliative shunts include distortion of the pulmonary arteries, which may kink, thrombose, or occlude, and pulmonary vascular disease when the shunt is too large.

Other Causes of Cyanosis

Pulmonary Atresia With Ventricular Septal Defect
This is also a conotruncal abnormality and has the same intracardiac anatomy as tetralogy of Fallot, except that the right ventricular outflow tract is blind or atretic. Pulmonary blood flow arises from collateral vessels from the descending aorta which are congenital, patent ductus arteriosus, bronchial collateral vessels, and coronary collateral vessels.

Collateral vessels may be end arteries feeding into the lung tissue directly, or one or more collateral vessels may enter into central pulmonary arteries.

Forty percent of patients with pulmonary atresia have a right aortic arch.

Transposition of the Great Arteries
Patients with transposition of the great arteries have virtually all had surgery by the time they reach adulthood, either in the form of an atrial baffle procedure (Mustard or Senning) or an arterial switch procedure. Long-term complications of atrial baffle procedure are significant because the right ventricle still supports the systemic circulation; hence, right ventricular failure and tricuspid regurgitation are common. Atrial arrhythmias, particularly junctional rhythm and atrial flutter, are also common late in follow-up.

Tricuspid Atresia
Patients with tricuspid atresia have also usually had operation by the time they reach adulthood. The tricuspid valve

is absent, so systemic blood flows from the right atrium to the left atrium. It then enters the left ventricle and reaches the pulmonary artery through a ventricular septal defect into a hypoplastic right ventricle. This pattern occurs when the great arteries are normally related. Most patients have reduced pulmonary blood flow because of a small ventricular septal defect with or without pulmonary stenosis. If the ventricular septal defect is large, there may be pulmonary hypertension.

Single Ventricle
There are many forms and combinations of abnormalities; the most common type in adulthood is a double-inlet left ventricle with pulmonary stenosis. Patients therefore will have cyanosis with *left* ventricular hypertrophy and signs of pulmonary stenosis.

Truncus Arteriosus
In this condition, the pulmonary arteries arise from the aorta, and the intracardiac anatomy is the same as that for pulmonary atresia. The pulmonary arteries are usually not stenosed, and so the clinical features are those of Eisenmenger syndrome. Truncal regurgitation is common.

Total Anomalous Pulmonary Venous Drainage
In this condition, all the pulmonary veins drain to the right atrium or a major systemic vein, producing right-sided volume overload. An atrial communication is obligatory. When the venous confluence connects to the left innominate vein, it produces the "snowman" sign on chest radiography. Total anomalous pulmonary venous drainage is very rare in adulthood.

Corrected Transposition With Ventricular Septal Defect and Pulmonary Stenosis
Corrected transposition (levo [L]-transposition) is an anomaly in which there is atrioventricular discordance and ventriculoarterial discordance. Thus, the right atrium enters into the left ventricle, which ejects into the pulmonary artery. The left atrium enters into the morphologic right ventricle, which ejects into the aorta. Thus, the circulation flows correctly (hence the term "corrected" transposition) but flows through the wrong chambers. Atrioventricular valves travel with the appropriate ventricle; thus, the flimsy tricuspid valve sits at the mouth of the right ventricle in the systemic circulation. The coronary artery pattern is also reversed. The common associated anomalies are ventricular septal defect; abnormalities of the left atrioventricular valve

(tricuspid valve), which is usually regurgitant; and pulmonary stenosis.

Complete heart block is also a common association. Patients may survive to their 50s or 60s if they have corrected transposition and no associated anomalies, but problems often occur because of the morphologic right ventricle supporting the systemic circulation. The presence of an associated defect, particularly left atrioventricular valve regurgitation, usually causes presentation earlier in life. The presence of pulmonary stenosis and ventricular septal defect will produce varying degrees of cyanosis (depending on the severity of the pulmonary stenosis), and the clinical features may resemble those of tetralogy of Fallot.

Electrocardiography
Findings on electrocardiography include absent Q waves in the left precordial leads and Q waves present in the right precordial leads (QR pattern in leads II, III, and V_1).

Chest Radiography
A straight left aortic border (because the aorta does not ascend on the right and the pulmonary trunk is not border-forming on the left) is seen on chest radiographs. The ventricle may show a hump-shaped contour in the region of the left atrial appendage.

Surgical Treatment
The ventricular septal defect, if present, is closed. Relief of pulmonary stenosis may be difficult because of access problems and the danger of producing heart block or damage to the right coronary artery. A conduit is often, therefore, necessary. The left atrioventricular valve cannot be repaired and always needs replacement if regurgitant.

Eisenmenger Syndrome
Babies born with either a large ventricular septal defect or a large patent ductus arteriosus have a large left-to-right shunt in early childhood with increased blood volume and pressure transmitted to the right side of the heart. The result is pulmonary hypertension and subsequent pulmonary vascular disease, which may become established within the first 2 years of life. Rarely, other intracardiac shunts may also result in Eisenmenger physiology. This reversal of the left-to-right shunt causes cyanosis, and the original congenital heart defect then becomes inoperable. Some infants with large shunts never have any decrease in their pulmonary vascular resistance and have pulmonary vascular disease from an early age. The right-to-left shunting associated

with pulmonary hypertension is called Eisenmenger syndrome. It may rarely occur with secundum ASD (< 5% of cases), usually later in life.

Physical Examination
Physical examination reveals the following findings: cyanosis and clubbing, jugular venous pressure that may be normal or with a slightly prominent "a" wave, right ventricular lift, ejection click from the dilated pulmonary artery, *little or no* murmur (pressure in both ventricles is equal), loud P_2 (may be palpable), and variable murmur of pulmonary regurgitation. There may be differential cyanosis between the limbs if the patient has a patent ductus arteriosus.

Electrocardiography
Right ventricular hypertrophy is found on electrocardiography.

Chest Radiography
On chest radiography, the following are findings: prominent central pulmonary arteries (may be calcified; these are sometimes mistaken for lymphadenopathy), right ventricular contour, and peripheral pulmonary artery pruning.

Diagnosis
The diagnosis can be made from the findings on physical examination and echocardiography. Rarely, the shunt is missed because the pressure is equal in both chambers and the ventricular septal defect is overlooked. A patent ductus arteriosus may be difficult to see because there is little blood flow through the ductus. The differential diagnosis of Eisenmenger syndrome is primary pulmonary hypertension, but patients with Eisenmenger syndrome have a much better long-term survival than patients with primary pulmonary hypertension. Death may occur from acute hypoxia or sudden ventricular arrhythmia. Patients frequently experience symptomatic deterioration in their 40s but may survive to their 60s. Vasodilatation should be avoided (such as hot tubs and vasodilator therapy). Patients should be followed for progressive right ventricular dilatation and tricuspid regurgitation, which may herald right ventricular failure. They may become extremely symptomatic with the onset of atrial arrhythmias, and sinus rhythm should be maintained whenever possible. The only effective treatment options for Eisenmenger syndrome are heart-lung transplantation or single-lung transplantation with closure of the defect.

- Patients with Eisenmenger syndrome have a much better long-term survival than patients with primary pulmonary hypertension.
- The only effective treatment options for Eisenmenger syndrome are heart-lung transplantation or single-lung transplantation with closure of the defect.

Hematologic Abnormalities

Patients with cyanosis have increased erythrocytes (it is *not* polycythemia), and management of erythrocytosis may be difficult. Patients with high degrees of erythrocytosis (hemoglobin > 20 g/dL, hematocrit > 65%) may experience symptoms of hyperviscosity (poor concentration, headache, and fatigue). This condition is uncommon with lower hemoglobin levels (unless the patient is dehydrated). Patients therefore should *not* have therapeutic phlebotomy unless the hemoglobin value is more than 20 g/dL. Frequent phlebotomies, in particular, should be avoided, because they destabilize the erythropoiesis and produce a rebound response on behalf of the bone marrow and, ultimately, iron deficiency anemia. When iron-deficient microcytes are produced, this condition not only causes a deterioration in exercise capacity but also, because iron-deficient red cells are less deformable than normal red cells, paradoxically increases the risk of stroke.

Phlebotomy should *never* be performed in patients without concomitant fluid replacement, particularly in patients with Eisenmenger syndrome, who may experience hypotension and even sudden death.

In contrast, although patients with cyanotic heart disease have a slightly increased risk of stroke, they also have hemostatic problems and are at increased risk of bleeding. These hemostatic problems include prolonged prothrombin time, prolonged activated partial thromboplastin time, decreased coagulation factors, decreased platelet count, and abnormal platelet function.

Thus, patients with cyanotic heart disease should never receive anticoagulation therapy unless there is a very strong indication to do so, and, ideally, the international normalized ratio (INR) should be kept on the low side of the therapeutic range.

If a patient with cyanosis is to undergo surgery and the hemoglobin value is more than 20 g/dL, therapeutic phlebotomy with fluid exchange will tend to normalize the hemostatic problems.

Renal Abnormalities

Adults with cyanotic congenital heart disease frequently have abnormal renal function with a reduced glomerular filtration rate, proteinuria, and hyperuricemia. The high uric acid levels are due to a low fractional uric acid excretion and the overproduction of urate from red cell turnover. Hyperuricemia is particularly important when cyanotic patients have cardiac catheterization, and they should *not* be dehydrated around the time of the procedure, particularly because they may require a large amount of imaging contrast, which may induce acute renal failure. Intravenous fluid hydration is indicated in very cyanotic patients, with meticulous attention to fluid balance and good urine output.

Orthopedic Abnormalities

Scoliosis is also much more common in patients with cyanotic heart disease (even in the absence of a lateral thoracotomy). In addition, patients may have a painful arthropathy due to hypertrophic changes in the long bones.

Pulmonary Abnormalities

Patients with Eisenmenger syndrome are at particular risk of hemoptysis (which can be life-threatening and may be due to pulmonary hemorrhage, pulmonary embolus, or in situ pulmonary infarction). In addition, they are prone to vasodilatation, which may prove fatal. Any decrease in blood pressure (such as that produced by vasodilators) may cause increased right-to-left shunting, cerebral hypoxia, and sudden death; thus, patients should not be given vasodilator therapy. Extreme caution must be used when patients with Eisenmenger syndrome are undergoing noncardiac surgery.

- Adults with cyanotic congenital heart disease frequently have abnormal renal function with a reduced glomerular filtration rate, proteinuria, and hyperuricemia.
- Patients with Eisenmenger syndrome are at particular risk of hemoptysis.

Syndromes Associated With Congenital Heart Disease

Syndromes associated with congenital heart disease include the following:

- Down syndrome: atrioventricular septal defects (atrioventricular canal, primum ASD), ventricular septal defect

- Turner syndrome: coarctation of the aorta, bicuspid aortic valve
- Holt-Oram syndrome: secundum ASD
- Marfan syndrome: aortic dilatation, dissection, and rupture; mitral valve prolapse
- Noonan syndrome: pulmonary stenosis

Right aortic arch is associated with the following:
- Pulmonary atresia
- Truncus arteriosus
- Tetralogy of Fallot

With cardiac apex on one side and gastric bubble on the other, consider the following:
- Corrected transposition
- Single ventricle

If both the cardiac apex *and* the gastric bubble are on the right, the heart may be normal (situs inversus totalis)

The Electrocardiogram in ASD

- Right bundle branch block and right-axis deviation: secundum ASD
- Right bundle branch block and left-axis deviation (with or without first-degree atrioventricular block): primum ASD

American Heart Association Recommendations for Endocarditis Prophylaxis

Endocarditis prophylaxis is recommended for all patients with congenital heart disease, with the following exceptions:
- For isolated secundum ASD
- More than 6 months after surgical repair of secundum ASD, ventricular septal defect, patent ductus arteriosus (with no residual defect)

Suggested Review Reading

1. Ammash N, Warnes CA: Cerebrovascular events in adult patients with cyanotic congenital heart disease. *J Am Coll Cardiol* 28:768-772, 1996.
Review of 162 patients with cyanotic congenital heart disease, showing that microcytosis due to iron deficiency anemia is a major predisposing cause of cerebrovascular events. This finding supports a conservative approach toward phlebotomy in patients with cyanosis and an aggressive approach in treating iron deficiency anemia in adults with cyanosis.

2. Cohen M, Fuster V, Steele PM, et al: Coarctation of the aorta. Long-term follow-up and prediction of outcome after surgical correction. *Circulation* 80:840-845, 1989.
The largest study of patients with coarctation of the aorta, describing 646 patients who had repair of isolated coarctation. The study shows that 11% required subsequent cardiovascular operation. There were 87 late deaths, and the mean age at death was 38 years. Late problems included coronary artery disease, heart failure, cerebrovascular accidents, and ruptured aortic aneurysm. Age at the time of initial repair is an important predictor of long-term survival and a predictor of later systemic hypertension. Associated cardiovascular abnormalities requiring subsequent operation are common.

3. Connelly MS, Liu PP, Williams WG, et al: Congenitally corrected transposition of the great arteries in the adult: functional status and complications. *J Am Coll Cardiol* 27:1238-1243, 1996.
Study reviewing the problems of systemic ventricular function in congenitally corrected transposition of the great arteries. The frequency of atrial arrhythmias, which occurred in 36% of survivors, and the problems with atrioventricular block, common in this patient population, are discussed.

4. Driscoll DJ, Offord KP, Feldt RH, et al: Five- to fifteen-year follow-up after Fontan operation. *Circulation* 85:469-496, 1992.

Long-term study of Fontan operation showing 5- and 10-year survival rates of 70% and 60%, respectively. Factors associated with reduced survival are reviewed. At least 20% of survivors have cardiac arrhythmias.

5. Feldt RH, Driscoll DJ, Offord KP, et al: Protein-losing enteropathy after the Fontan operation. *J Thorac Cardiovasc Surg* 112:672-680, 1996.
Review of the incidence and management of protein-losing enteropathy. The poor prognosis of this condition is noted; the 5-year survival rate is approximately 50%.

6. Gewillig M, Wyse RK, de Leval MR, et al: Early and late arrhythmias after the Fontan operation: predisposing factors and clinical consequences. *Br Heart J* 67:72-79, 1992.

7. Konstantinides S, Geibel A, Olschewski M, et al: A comparison of surgical and medical therapy for atrial septal defect in adults. *N Engl J Med* 333:469-473, 1995.
Study suggesting that surgical repair of atrial septal defect in comparison with medical therapy, in patients older than 40 years, increases long-term survival and limits the deterioration of function due to heart failure. The study confirmed, however, that surgically treated patients still need to be followed closely for the onset of atrial arrhythmias to reduce the risk of thromboembolic complications.

8. Perloff JK, Marelli AJ, Miner PD: Risk of stroke in adults with cyanotic congenital heart disease. *Circulation* 87:1954-1959, 1993.

9. Shah D, Azhar M, Oakley CM, et al: Natural history of secundum atrial septal defect in adults after medical or surgical treatment: a historical prospective study. *Br Heart J* 71:224-227, 1994.
Study comparing medically and surgically treated patients who had secundum atrial septal defect and a mean follow-up of 25 years. The study suggested no difference in survival or symptoms between the two groups and no difference in the incidence of new arrhythmias, stroke, or embolic phenomena. This is a controversial study suggesting that the outcome in adults with atrial septal defect was not improved by surgical closure.

10. Van Son JA, Danielson GK, Huhta JC, et al: Late results of systemic atrioventricular valve replacement in corrected transposition. *J Thorac Cardiovasc Surg* 109:642-652, 1995.
Article describes 40 patients with congenitally corrected transposition of the great arteries who had valve replacement. Valve replacement must be considered at the earliest sign of progressive ventricular dysfunction, preferably before the ejection fraction is 40% or less.

Questions

Multiple Choice (choose the one best answer)
1. Which of the following physical findings would *not* be associated with the congenital anomaly shown on this chest radiograph?
   a. Right ventricular lift
   b. Systolic thrill
   c. Diastolic flow rumble
   d. Normal jugular venous pressure
   e. Fixed splitting of the second sound

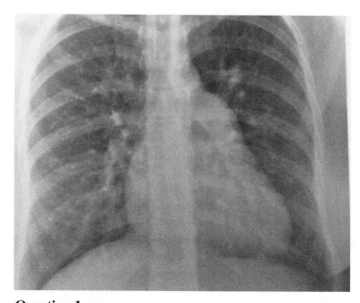

Question 1

2. All the following physical findings would be expected to be associated with the chest radiograph shown below *except*:
   a. A soft P_2
   b. Prominent "v" wave in the jugular venous pressure
   c. Right ventricular lift
   d. Ejection click
   e. Diastolic flow rumble

3. Which one of the following patients needs endocarditis prophylaxis?
   a. Patient with isolated secundum atrial septal defect having dental extraction
   b. Patient with ligated patent ductus arteriosus having cystoscopy
   c. Patient with bicuspid aortic valve, functionally normal, having dental cleaning and scaling
   d. Patient with coarctation having cardiac catheterization
   e. Patient with primum atrial septal defect having transesophageal echocardiography

4. Which one of the following physical findings would *not* be expected in the anomaly shown on the chest radiograph below?
   a. Systolic murmur
   b. Absent pulmonary component (P_2) of the second heart sound

   c. Sustained left ventricular impulse
   d. Systolic click
   e. Right ventricular lift

5. Which one of the following is true of atrial septal defect (ASD)?
   a. Primum ASD is associated with left-axis deviation and left bundle branch block
   b. Secundum ASD is associated with partial right bundle branch block and right-axis deviation
   c. Sinus venosus ASD is associated with the presence of an anomalous left upper pulmonary vein
   d. When closed in a patient younger than 30 years, long-term survival is the same as that for the normal population
   e. Primum ASD is associated with cleft aortic valve

6. Which one of the following does *not* cause a continuous murmur?
   a. Coronary fistula
   b. Patent ductus arteriosus
   c. Sinus of Valsalva-to-right atrial fistula
   d. Ventricular septal defect with pulmonary hypertension
   e. Pulmonary arteriovenous fistula

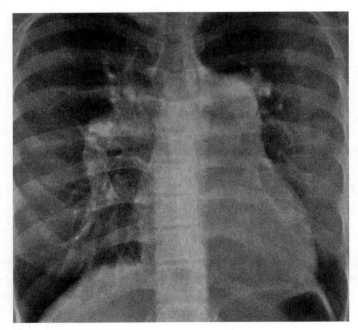

Question 2

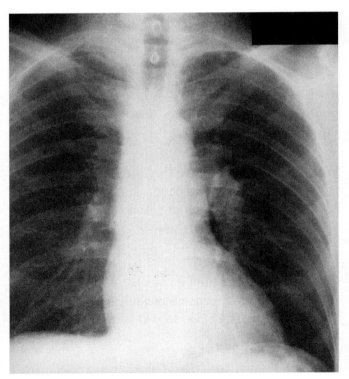

Question 4

7. What is the most likely diagnosis associated with this electrocardiogram?
   a. Coarctation of the aorta
   b. Secundum atrial septal defect
   c. Primum atrial septal defect
   d. Ebstein anomaly
   e. Pulmonary stenosis

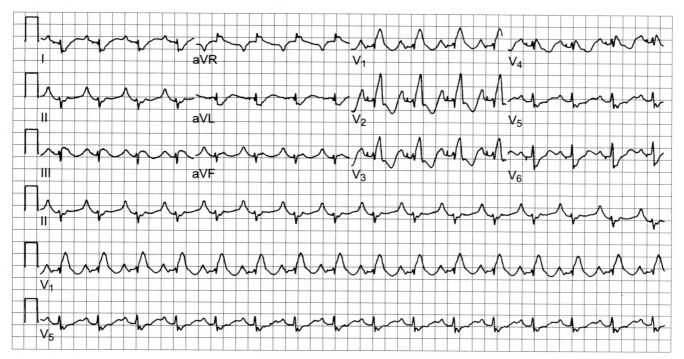

Question 7

8. What is the most likely congenital anomaly shown on this chest radiograph?
   a. Congenitally corrected transposition
   b. Tricuspid atresia
   c. Primum atrial septal defect
   d. Eisenmenger syndrome
   e. Tetralogy of Fallot

9. Long-term complications after repaired tetralogy of Fallot often include all the following *except*:
   a. Aortic regurgitation
   b. Ventricular arrhythmias
   c. Pulmonary regurgitation
   d. Pulmonary hypertension
   e. Right ventricular dysfunction

10. Which one of the following is *not* a feature of the adult patient with severe tetralogy of Fallot?
    a. Systolic thrill
    b. Loud murmur through the ventricular septal defect
    c. Absent P_2
    d. Aortic regurgitation
    e. Right ventricular hypertrophy

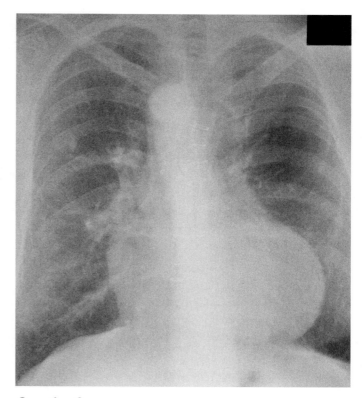

Question 8

11. What congenital anomaly is most likely associated with the electrocardiogram shown below?
    a. Primum atrial septal defect
    b. Ebstein anomaly
    c. Tetralogy of Fallot
    d. Congenitally corrected transposition
    e. Tricuspid atresia

12A. A 19-year-old patient with Eisenmenger physiology due to a ventricular septal defect has a transient ischemic attack. Her hemoglobin value is 19 g/dL, hematocrit value 60%, and creatinine concentration 1.3 mg/dL. Which of the following is true?
    a. Her platelet count is likely to be high

    b. She should receive warfarin for anticoagulation
    c. Her prothrombin time is likely to be prolonged
    d. She should have a therapeutic phlebotomy of 2 units
    e. She should receive heparin for anticoagulation

12B. Results of her physical examination are unchanged from her last clinic evaluation 6 months ago. All of the following tests should be performed *except*:
    a. Echocardiography
    b. Blood cultures
    c. Measurement of the mean corpuscular volume
    d. Cardiac catheterization
    e. Magnetic resonance imaging of the head

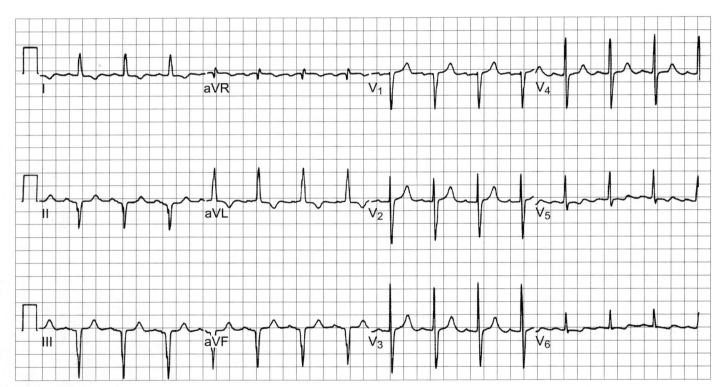

Question 11

Answers

1. Answer b

This is a typical radiograph of a patient with a large secundum atrial septal defect. There is a large heart with a right ventricular contour, a prominent pulmonary artery, and plethora in the lung fields. A diastolic rumble would be expected because of the increased flow across the tricuspid valve. Secundum atrial septal defect is never associated with a systolic thrill.

2. Answer a

This is a typical radiograph from a patient with Eisenmenger syndrome. There is a prominent pulmonary artery and a large right ventricle. The central pulmonary arteries are very large and almost aneurysmal. There is no pulmonary plethora, and indeed peripheral pruning is clearly demonstrated in both lung fields, more marked on the right. Right ventricular lift would be expected because of the right ventricular hypertension, and an ejection click is very common because of the dilated pulmonary artery. An early diastolic murmur from pulmonary regurgitation is also common, as is a palpable P_2 that is very loud on auscultation. Patients do not have loud ejection systolic murmurs because the right ventricular pressure is equal to that of the left.

3. Answer c

Even a patient with a functionally normal bicuspid aortic valve is susceptible to endocarditis and so must be given antibiotic prophylaxis when having dental work. Endocarditis does not develop in patients with an isolated secundum atrial septal defect. Patients who have had a ligated patent ductus arteriosus are considered cured and do not require antibiotic prophylaxis. Coarctation of the aorta is a low-risk lesion for endocarditis, and because cardiac catheterization is a sterile procedure, endocarditis prophylaxis is not required. Transesophageal echocardiography is an atraumatic procedure and does not require routine antibiotic prophylaxis.

4. Answer c

The chest radiograph shows poststenotic dilatation of the main and left pulmonary arteries consistent with severe valvular pulmonary stenosis. Expected physical findings include absent P_2, right ventricular lift, pulmonary ejection click, prominent "a" wave in the jugular venous pulse, and a systolic murmur.

5. Answer b

Primum ASD is associated with left-axis deviation and right bundle branch block. An anomalous right upper pulmonary vein is the usual finding in sinus venosus ASD. ASD needs to be closed before 20 years for a normal survival. Primum ASD is associated with a cleft mitral valve.

6. Answer d

Ventricular septal defect with significant pulmonary hypertension usually has little or no associated murmur because the pressure in the right ventricle is the same as that in the left. All other lesions in this group do cause a continuous murmur.

7. Answer d

This electrocardiogram shows marked right atrial enlargement (Himalayan P waves) and right bundle branch block most consistent with Ebstein anomaly.

8. Answer e

This chest radiograph shows a boot-shaped heart, pulmonary oligemia, and concave pulmonary bay, strongly suggestive of tetralogy of Fallot.

9. Answer d

Pulmonary hypertension is not associated with tetralogy of Fallot because the pulmonary stenosis "protects" the lungs.

10. Answer b

In severe tetralogy of Fallot, the right and left ventricular pressures approximate because of the large ventricular septal defect. Thus, there is little or no murmur through the defect.

11. Answer d

This electrocardiogram shows absent Q waves in the left precordial leads and a QR pattern in leads II, III, and V_1, strongly suggestive of congenitally corrected transposition.

12A. Answer c

Patients with cyanotic heart disease have problems with clotting and are also at increased risk of bleeding. The platelet count is usually low, and platelet function is abnormal. Clotting factors are frequently reduced, and the prothrombin time and accelerated partial thromboplastin time are often prolonged. In patients with Eisenmenger syndrome caused by ventricular septal defect who present with a transient ischemic attack, the possibility of endocarditis and cerebral abscess should always be ruled out. Routine anticoagulation with warfarin is not indicated unless the transient ischemic attacks are recurrent, antiplatelet agents fail, and there is no indication of cerebral abscess. This patient has stable hemoglobin and hematocrit values and should not have a therapeutic phlebotomy. This should be performed only if the hemoglobin value is more than 20 g/dL and the hematocrit value is more than 65%. Therapeutic phlebotomy should be performed only 1 unit at a time and always with concomitant fluid replacement. Anticoagulation with heparin is indicated only if all other causes of transient ischemic attack have been ruled out.

12B. Answer d

It is important to investigate this patient for infective endocarditis (blood culture, echocardiography), cerebral abscess (magnetic resonance imaging), and iron deficiency anemia, which predisposes to transient ischemic attack and stroke.

Chapter 64

Hypertension

Michael J. Hogan, M.D.

Definition

A sustained blood pressure greater than 140 mm Hg systolic and 90 mm Hg diastolic or the requirement for antihypertensive medication defines hypertension. The average of two or more blood pressure readings on at least two occasions after a screening visit is needed to apply this definition.

The patient should be seated with the back straight and the arm supported at heart level. After the subject has rested for 5 minutes, the examiner should measure the pressure with a cuff that encircles, at a minimum, 80% of the upper arm. If a mercury sphygmomanometer is not available, a calibrated aneroid manometer or validated electronic device is adequate.

Classification and Staging

In its sixth report (JNC-VI), the Joint National Committee on Prevention, Detection, Evaluation, and Treatment of High Blood Pressure classified blood pressure in degrees of both normality and stages of hypertension. Although assignment to these blood pressure classes is somewhat arbitrary, increased blood pressure readings reflect the cardiovascular, cerebrovascular, and renal risks across the blood pressure continuum (Table 1). The classifications apply to persons who are not taking antihypertensive medications and who are not acutely ill. When the systolic and diastolic pressures fall in different categories, the physician should select the higher category to stage the patient's hypertension. Staging should be based on the average of two or more blood pressure measurements on two or more occasions after the initial screening.

Epidemiology

Diastolic and, to a greater extent, systolic blood pressure increase with age. After age 65, the increase in systolic pressure becomes more prevalent, with 65% to 75% of the cases of hypertension in the elderly being isolated systolic hypertension (systolic pressure > 160 and diastolic pressure < 95).

The incidence of hypertension and the complication rates vary between sexes and among different ethnic groups. Men are at greater risk for developing hypertension until age 55, when a reversal begins; by age 75, the incidence is greater in women. At all ages, however, the complication

An atlas illustrating pathologic conditions associated with hypertension is at the end of the chapter (Plates 1-7).

Table 1.—Classification of Blood Pressure for Adults Age 18 and Older

Category	Systolic, mm Hg		Diastolic, mm Hg
Optimal	< 120	and	< 80
Normal	< 130	and	< 85
High-normal	130-139	or	85-89
Hypertension			
Stage 1	140-159	or	90-99
Stage 2	160-179	or	100-109
Stage 3	≥ 180	or	≥ 110

Table 2.—Trends in the Awareness, Treatment, and Control of High Blood Pressure in Adults: United States, 1976-94*

	NHANES II (1976-80), % of respondents	NHANES III (Phase 1) 1988-91, % of respondents	NHANES III (Phase 2) 1991-94, % of respondents
Awareness	51	73	68.4
Treatment	31	55	53.6
Control†	10	29	27.4

NHANES, National Health and Nutrition Examination Survey.
*Data are for adults age 18 to 74 years with systolic blood pressure ≥ 140 mm Hg, diastolic blood pressure ≥ 90 mm Hg, or taking antihypertensive medication.
†Systolic blood pressure < 140 mm Hg and diastolic blood pressure < 90 mm Hg.
Modified from Burt V et al. and unpublished NHANES III, phase 2, data provided by the Centers for Disease Control and Prevention, National Center for Health Statistics.

rate is higher in men. For African-Americans, the prevalence of hypertension is among the highest in the world. The prevalence of hypertension in Native Americans equals or exceeds that of the general population. Despite these differences among ethnic groups, the same contributors to hypertension exist.

The National Health and Nutrition Examination Surveys demonstrated increases in awareness, treatment rates, and control rates of hypertension between 1976 and 1991 (Table 2). Of concern is a decrease in each of these items in recent years. These findings mirror a flattening of the curves for the decline in age-adjusted mortality rates for strokes and coronary artery disease in white and African-American men and women.

Detection and Classification of Hypertension

The diagnosis of hypertension requires the demonstration of increased blood pressure on repeated measurements over time. If the patient is taking medications that have a postural effect on blood pressure or the patient reports symptoms compatible with a postural decrease in blood pressure, the examiner should measure the pressure with the patient in the sitting and standing positions.

The recognition that blood pressure measurements made in a doctor's office (or hospital) may be different from those made away from the office has prompted self-measurement of blood pressure by an increasing number of patients or family members and ambulatory monitoring of blood pressure. JNC-VI pointed out that self-measurement can 1) distinguish sustained hypertension from elevations detected by health care providers ("white coat hypertension"), 2)

assess response to treatment programs both in level of control and association between blood pressure and side effects, 3) improve compliance by enhancing patient participation in the health care process, and 4) possibly decrease costs.

Risk Stratification and Treatment Recommendations

A new feature of JNC-VI is the addition of risk stratification as an element in the treatment decision. The Committee selected six major risk factors and five sites of target organ damage on which physicians should base treatment decisions (Table 3). Combining risk stratification with hypertension staging provides a rationale for decisions about when to incorporate pharmacologic therapy with lifestyle modification (Table 4). The committee was careful to recommend lifestyle modification as an adjunct to pharmacologic treatment at all blood pressure levels.

Clinical Evaluation

The examiner should question the subject to determine if one or more of the four major contributors to essential (primary) hypertension is present. These contributors are 1)

Table 3.—Components of Cardiovascular Risk Stratification in Patients With Hypertension*

Major risk factors
    Smoking
    Dyslipidemia
    Diabetes mellitus
    Age older than 60 years
    Sex (men and postmenopausal women)
    Family history of cardiovascular disease: women
      younger than 65 or men younger than 55
Target organ damage/clinical cardiovascular disease
    Heart disease
        Left ventricular hypertrophy
        Angina/previous myocardial infarction
        Previous coronary revascularization
        Heart failure
    Stroke or transient ischemic attack
    Nephropathy
    Peripheral arterial disease
    Retinopathy

obesity, 2) excessive salt intake, 3) excessive alcohol intake, and 4) lack of exercise. Additional information needed to make a diagnosis of essential hypertension includes a family history of hypertension and the duration of the hypertension. Care must be taken to determine whether the patient's knowledge of the duration is accurate (i.e., knowledge of approximately when the increase in pressure occurred).

Although smoking is a recognized risk factor for vascular disease and inhalation of tobacco smoke can acutely increase blood pressure, smoking is not a contributor to chronic hypertension. Caffeine can also increase blood pressure acutely, but it is not a contributor. The acute effects are important to remember and patients should be advised to abstain from caffeine-containing beverages or foods for 1 hour before blood pressure is measured.

The initial examination of a patient with hypertension should focus on measurement of the blood pressure (as described above), assessment of the cardiovascular system, and determination of the extent of target-organ damage. Because the arteriole is the vessel that sustains the major damage from chronic hypertension, funduscopic examination is critical in the initial evaluation of the hypertensive patient and during follow-up to assess the efficacy of treatment. Examination of peripheral pulses can detect obliterative disease that might predispose the patient to renovascular hypertension. Abdominal auscultation is important in this part of the examination. Auscultation of the heart and lungs provides an assessment of the degree of end-organ damage sustained by the heart. Neurologic examination provides insight into the other major area of end-organ damage.

The initial laboratory evaluation should include chest radiography, electrocardiography, and measurement of serum concentrations of sodium, potassium, and creatinine. Historical and clinical features may dictate more specific tests.

Secondary Hypertension

The small percentage of patients with hypertension whose increased blood pressure is due to a definable pathologic process justifies an evaluation only in selected instances. In general, a search for the cause of hypertension should be limited to patients 1) with hypertension of recent or sudden onset, 2) with hypertension resistant to treatment

Table 4.—Risk Factor Stratification and Treatment

Blood pressure stage, mm Hg	Risk group A (no risk factors; no TOD/CCD)	Risk group B (at least one risk factor, not including diabetes; no TOD/CCD)	Risk group C (TOD/CCD and/or diabetes, with or without other risk factors)
High-normal (130-139/85-95)	Lifestyle modification	Lifestyle modification	Drug therapy
Stage 1 (140-159/90-99)	Lifestyle modification (up to 12 mo)	Lifestyle modification (up to 6 mo)	Drug therapy
Stages 2 and 3 (≥160/≥100)	Drug therapy	Drug therapy	Therapy

CCD, clinical cardiovascular disease; TOD, target-organ damage.

(uncontrolled on adequate doses of three medications, one of which is a diuretic), 3) who demonstrate physical findings (e.g., abdominal bruits) or biochemical abnormalities (unprovoked hypokalemia) suggesting a secondary form of hypertension, and 4) who have none of the contributors to essential hypertension.

The list of disease conditions associated with increased blood pressure is long (Table 5) and contains rare diseases seldom encountered in clinical practice. Three causes of secondary hypertension that merit special attention are 1) renovascular hypertension, 2) catecholamine excess states, and 3) mineralocorticoid excess states.

Renovascular Hypertension

Obstruction to blood flow in one or both renal arteries can occur from fibromuscular thickening of the arterial wall or atherosclerotic plaque deposition in the endothelial lining of the vessel. The former usually occurs in women younger than 40 years. Atherosclerotic renovascular disease often occurs coincidently with cerebrovascular, coronary, or peripheral vascular disease.

The sudden onset of hypertension in a young woman who has few contributors to essential hypertension should raise the suspicion that fibromuscular renovascular disease is the cause. Sudden worsening in previously adequate blood pressure control, resistant hypertension, or difficult-to-control hypertension in a patient with evidence of atherosclerotic vascular disease indicates the likelihood of atherosclerotic renovascular hypertension. A caveat for attempting to diagnose renovascular hypertension in the elderly is that the prevalence of renovascular disease increases with age and not all renovascular disease is etiologically related to hypertension. Only after the affected vessel(s) is treated can the diagnosis be made.

Excretory urography, radionuclide renal scanning, and ultrasonography are the procedures most often used to screen for renovascular disease. Each has limited sensitivity (percent of false negatives). In an instance of low probability, a less sensitive diagnostic test may be satisfactory. For patients in whom the probability of a renovascular cause of hypertension is great, angiography is the definitive diagnostic procedure. However, advances in magnetic resonance imaging of blood vessels have brought this technology to the forefront for patients with conditions that make conventional contrast angiography a significant risk (e.g., diabetic nephropathy). The main forms of treatment are angioplasty with or without stent placement and surgical bypass of the affected area.

Table 5.—Secondary Hypertension: Diseases in Which High Blood Pressure May Occur

I. Systolic and diastolic hypertension

Renovascular diseases
  Atherosclerosis
  Fibromuscular disease
  Thrombosis
  Embolism
  Dissecting renal artery aneurysms
  Atherosclerotic renal artery aneurysms
  Extrinsic renal artery compression (from tumors or cysts)
  Congenital hypoplasia of the renal artery
  Neurofibromatosis
  Transplant rejection fibrosis
  Arteriovenous fistulas
  Vasculitis (associated with periarteritis nodosa, systemic lupus erythematosus, scleroderma)
  Intercapillary glomerular sclerosis (Kimmelstiel-Wilson disease)
Renal parenchymal diseases
  Polycystic kidneys
  Glomerulonephritis
    Membranoproliferative
    Acute poststreptococcal
    Chronic membranous
    Focal sclerosing
    Septic embolic
  Chronic pyelonephritis
  Renal cortical atrophy due to vesicoureteral reflux
  Ureteral obstruction
  Prostatic obstruction
  Perirenal hematoma
  Renal vein thrombosis
  Tumors (renin-producing juxtaglomerular cell tumor, Wilms tumor)
  Unclassified end-stage renal disease
  Urate nephropathy
  Analgesic nephropathy
  Postirradiation nephropathy
  Congenital hypoplastic kidney
  Renal trauma
  Liddle syndrome

Table 5 (continued)

Gordon syndrome	Tricyclic antidepressants
Endocrine diseases	Monoamine oxidase inhibitors in conjunction with high
Cushing syndrome	tyramine ingestion
Congenital adrenal hyperplasia (11-hydroxlyase	Ergot alkaloids
deficiency)	Heavy-metal poisons (e.g., lead, arsenic)

Gordon syndrome
Endocrine diseases
  Cushing syndrome
  Congenital adrenal hyperplasia (11-hydroxlyase
    deficiency)
  Hypogonadism and mineralocorticoid excess (17-
    hydroxylase deficiency)
  Primary aldosteronism
  Acromegaly
  Myxedema
  Pheochromocytoma
  Extra-adrenal chromaffin tumors
Central nervous system diseases (neurogenic hypertension)
  Psychogenic
  Increased intracranial pressure
    Encephalitis
    Brain tumors
    Respiratory acidosis
  Acute poliomyelitis
  Polyneuritis
  Spinal cord section
  Familial dysautonomia
  Acute porphyria
Exogenous agents
  Estrogen-containing oral contraceptives
  Sodium
    Sodium chloride
    Sodium bicarbonate
    Sodium-containing medications
  Lithium
  Mineralocorticoids
  Anabolic or adrenogenic steroids
  Nonsteroidal anti-inflammatory drugs
  Direct or indirect sympathomimetics (e.g., ephedrine,
    phenylephrine)

Tricyclic antidepressants
Monoamine oxidase inhibitors in conjunction with high
  tyramine ingestion
Ergot alkaloids
Heavy-metal poisons (e.g., lead, arsenic)
Cyclosporine
Erythropoietin
Street drugs
Miscellaneous
  Coarctation of the aorta
  Toxemia of pregnancy
  Hypercalcemia
  Increased intravascular volume (e.g., polycythemia,
    postoperative state)
  Burns
  Carcinoid syndrome
  Insect stings (e.g., spider, scorpion)
  Rebound hypertension
    Sudden withdrawal of clonidine
    Withdrawal of methyldopa, β-adrenergic receptor
      blockers, postganglionic sympathetic-blocking
      drugs
II. Systolic hypertension with wide pulse pressure
Increased cardiac output or increased stroke volume
  Arteriovenous fistula
  Thyrotoxicosis
  Hyperkinetic heart disease
  Aortic valve insufficiency
  Patent ductus arteriosus
  Paget's disease of bone
  Severe anemia
  Beriberi
Decreased compliance of aorta
  Arteriosclerosis

From Giuliani ER, Gersh BJ, McGoon MD, Hayes DL, Schaff HV (editors): *Mayo Clinic Practice of Cardiology*. Third edition. Mosby, 1996, p 1783. By permission of Mayo Foundation.

Mineralocorticoid Excess

Hypokalemia or an inappropriate low-normal serum potassium concentration in the absence of diuretic therapy should signal the possibility of a mineralocorticoid-excess state. Cushing syndrome, with its attendant clinical picture, may be the cause. Primary aldosteronism, a more common condition, has few clinical features, except for polyuria and musculoskeletal symptoms. The diagnosis of Cushing syndrome rests on the demonstration of persistent nonsup-pressible cortisol secretion. Hypokalemia, increased excretion of aldosterone, and suppression of plasma renin activity in a patient with hypertension support the diagnosis of primary aldosteronism.

Pheochromocytoma

Catecholamine-secreting neoplasms of the adrenal glands (pheochromocytomas) or extra-adrenal chromaffin tissue (paragangliomas) can create some of the more dramatic presentations in patients with hypertension. These tumors most commonly are in the adrenal medulla. They can cause a wide variety of symptoms. The classic symptom triad of headache, diaphoresis, and tachycardia all too frequently is absent in patients with hypertension. Severe hypertension associated with the induction of anesthesia is an often overlooked syndrome in patients with pheochromocytoma. Postural hypotension may also occur. The diagnosis depends on the demonstration of increased excretion of catecholamines or their major metabolites (or both).

Special Circumstances

Hypertension in Pregnancy

When pregnancy supervenes in women with chronic hypertension, treatment with most medications except for angiotensin-converting enzyme inhibitors and angiotensin II blockers may be continued. The appearance of hypertension after the 20th week of gestation represents a different clinical problem. Because the complications of hypertension are related primarily to the duration of uncontrolled hypertension, initiating pharmacologic therapy to treat pregnancy-associated hypertension requires caution. The JNC-VI recommendations for the treatment of pregnancy-associated hypertension are summarized in Table 6.

Hypertensive Crises (Emergencies/Urgencies)

The need for an immediate decrease in blood pressure is rare. Blood pressure itself, unaccompanied by symptoms or signs of progressive end-organ damage, should not dictate the need for immediate reduction. Hypertensive emergencies are instances that require immediate reduction in blood pressure. "Reduction" should not be confused with "normalization."

Hypertensive emergencies requiring an immediate decrease in blood pressure include hypertensive encephalopathy, intracranial hemorrhage, unstable angina pectoris, acute myocardial infarction, acute left ventricular failure with pulmonary edema, aortic dissection, and eclampsia. The treatments of choice for these emergencies are parenteral therapies that have rapid onset and cessation of action. Agents commonly used for immediate reduction of blood pressure are listed in Table 7. The recommendation of JNC-VI for immediate blood pressure reduction in emergency hypertension is to decrease the mean arterial pressure by no more than 25% in the first 2 hours and to no less than 160/100 mm Hg during the next 6 hours. Extreme care must be taken to avoid precipitous decreases in blood pressure that risk renal, cerebral, or coronary ischemia.

Hypertensive urgencies include upper level of stage 3 hypertension, papilledema, progressive target-organ damage, and severe perioperative hypertension. The rapid onset of action of many newer antihypertensive agents may obviate parenteral therapy when the patient can take oral medication.

Pharmacologic Treatment

When lifestyle modifications fail to decrease blood pressure satisfactorily or when the risk stratification criteria outlined above indicate initiation of pharmacologic treatment, various classes of antihypertensive agents are available. The major classes of antihypertensive medications and general considerations for their use are listed in Table 7.

Cost, duration of action, and side effects all affect compliance and, thus, success in controlling hypertension. At each visit the patient should be queried about these issues.

Acknowledgment

This chapter is adapted from the one by Dr. D. J. Wilson for the previous edition of this book.

Table 6.—Antihypertensive Drugs Used in Pregnancy*

The report of the NHBPEP Working Group on High Blood Pressure in Pregnancy permits continuation of drug therapy in women with chronic hypertension (except for ACE inhibitors). In addition, angiotensin II receptor blockers should not be used during pregnancy. In women with chronic hypertension with diastolic levels of 100 mm Hg or greater (lower when end-organ damage or underlying renal disease is present) and in women with acute hypertension when levels are 105 mm Hg or greater, the following agents are suggested:

Suggested drug	Comment (C or D, pregnancy risk[†])
Central α-agonists	Methyldopa (C) is the drug of choice recommended by the NHBPEP Working Group
β-Blockers	Atenolol (C) and metoprolol (C) appear to be safe and effective in late pregnancy. Labetalol (C) also appears to be effective (α- and β-blockers)
Calcium antagonists	Potential synergism with magnesium sulfate may lead to precipitous hypotension (C)
ACE inhibitors, angiotensin II receptor blockers	Can cause fetal abnormalities (including death) and these drugs should not be used in pregnancy (D)
Diuretics	Diuretics (C) are recommended for chronic hypertension if prescribed before gestation or if patients appear to be salt-sensitive. They are not recommended in preeclampsia
Direct vasodilators	Hydralazine (C) is the parenteral drug of choice based on its long history of safety and efficacy (C)

ACE, angiotensin-converting enzyme; NHBPEP, National High Blood Pressure Education Program.
*There are several other antihypertensive drugs for which there are very limited data.
[†]The U.S. Food and Drug Administration classifies pregnancy risk as follows: C, adverse effects in animals; no controlled trials in humans; use if risk appears justified; D, positive evidence of fetal risk.

Table 7.—Drugs Used in the Treatment of Hypertension

Drug class	Mechanism of action	Side effects/adverse reactions	Comments
Thiazides and related diuretics Hydrochlorothiazide Chlorthalidone Metolazone Indapamide	Reduce plasma and extra-cellular fluid and CO initially; long-term peripheral resistance is lowered and CO is normalized	Hypokalemia, hyperuricemia, hypercalcemia, hyperglycemia, hyponatremia, elevated LDL, triglycerides, photosensitivity	Ineffective when serum creatinine > 2.0 Potentiate lithium toxicity Enhance digitalis toxicity Increase warfarin dose
Loop diuretics Bumetanide Ethacrynic acid Furosemide Torsemide	See Thiazides	Hypokalemia, hyperuricemia, hyperglycemia, reversible deafness	Effective when serum creatinine > 2.0 Ethacrynic acid may be used in sulfa or thiazide allergy Do not cause hypercalcemia

Potassium-sparing diuretics
Aldosterone antagonist
  Spironolactone
Aldosterone independent
  Triamterene
  Amiloride
	Weak diuretics which interfere with Na-K, Na-H exchange in distal renal tubule, increased potassium reabsorption	Hyperkalemia, gynecomastia (spironolactone), skin rash	Spironolactone is agent of choice in primary aldosteronism
			Avoid in renal failure
			Caution when used with ACE inhibitors

Table 7 (continued)

Drug class	Mechanism of action	Side effects/adverse reactions	Comments
Adrenergic central α_1-agonists Clonidine Guanabenz Guanfacine Methyldopa	Stimulate central α-receptors which inhibit efferent sympathetic activity	Drowsiness, sedation, dry mouth, fatigue, postural dizziness	Rebound hypertension may occur with abrupt withdrawal, especially when used with high-dose β-blocker therapy Avoid use in unreliable patients
Adrenergic inhibitors-peripheral antagonists Reserpine	Block transport of norepinephrine into storage granules in peripheral neurons, reduce sympathetic tone, deplete tissue catecholamines	Depression, nasal congestion, may aggravate peptic ulcer disease by increasing gastric acid secretion	Contraindicated in patients with a previous history of depression or peptic ulcer disease Inexpensive
Guanadrel Guanethidine	Promote degranulation of catecholamine storage granules in peripheral nerve endings, inhibit norepinephrine release from storage sites	Postural hypotension, fluid retention, diarrhea, retrograde ejaculation, exercise-induced hypotension	Do not penetrate central nervous system Interactions with ephedrine, tricyclic antidepressants, and antihistamines
Adrenergic inhibitors-α-receptor blockers Doxazosin Prazosin Terazosin	Cause vasodilatation by blockade of postsynaptic α_1-receptors	Postural hypotension, syncope (first dose), weakness, palpitation, headache	Reduce voiding symptoms in benign prostatic hypertrophy Favorable effect on HDL and total cholesterol Used in treating pheochromocytoma
Adrenergic inhibitors-β-blockers No ISA Atenolol Betaxolol Bisoprolol Metoprolol Nadolol Propranolol Timolol ISA Acebutolol Pindolol	Non-ISA drugs lower cardiac output, reduce renin release, and decrease central sympathetic outflow ISA drugs do not reduce cardiac output, and cause mild vasodilatation with reduced total peripheral resistance	Bradycardia, bronchospasm, worsening of heart block or CHF, may mask hypoglycemic symptoms, fatigue, insomnia, vivid dreams, may cause or complicate depression, reduced exercise tolerance	Should not be used in patients with asthma, COPD, uncompensated CHF, or sick sinus syndrome Should not be abruptly withdrawn in patients with CAD Drug without ISA lowers HDL and raises triglycerides
Adrenergic inhibitors α/β-Blockers Carvedilol Labetalol	Combined effects of α and β blockade lead to a reduction of TPR, with little effect on CO or heart rate α-Blocking properties generally greater than β-blocker effects	Postural hypotension, head "tingling" or scalp paresthesia with labetalol, nausea with high-dose labetalol, β-blocker side effects	Available as intravenous preparation for treating hypertensive crisis May interfere with urinary tests for pheochromocytoma Appear to be lipid neutral Carvedilol may be of benefit in advanced CHF

Table 7 (continued)

Drug class	Mechanism of action	Side effects/adverse reactions	Comments
ACE inhibitors Benazepril Captopril Enalapril Fosinapril Lisinopril Moexipril Perindopril Quinapril Ramipril Trandolapril	Block angiotensin II formation, promote vasodilatation, lower aldosterone secretion, increase bradykinin and vasodilatory prostaglandins	Cough, rash, angioneurotic edema, dysgeusia, or taste disturbance Hyperkalemia, especially with renal impairment Hypotension with high doses and diuretics Nephrotic-range proteinuria and leukopenia reported with captopril	Contraindicated in 2nd and 3rd trimesters of pregnancy Dose reduction and special monitoring may be required in renal insufficiency Preferred agent for treatment of HBP complicating CHF or diabetes
Angiotensin II receptor blockers Losartan Valsartan	Block the AT_1 receptor in blood vessels, with resultant fall in TPR and blood pressure, lowers aldosterone secretion	Hyperkalemia and deterioration of renal function infrequent but may occur in patients with renal impairment Angioedema may occur	No cough Gradual onset of antihypertensive action Losartan increases uric acid excretion Contraindicated in the 2nd and 3rd trimester of pregnancy
Calcium anatagonists Diltiazem Verapamil Dihydropyridines Amlodipine Felodipine Isradipine Nicardipine Nifedipine Nisoldipine	Block inward movement of Ca ions across cell membranes Smooth muscle relaxation, and vasodilation with reduction in TPR, and preserved or increased CO	Headache, dizziness, edema, constipation Tachycardia and gingival hyperplasia more common with dihydropyridines	Diltiazem and verapamil reduce sinus rate and may cause heart block Digoxin and carbamazepine levels may be increased with verapamil and diltiazem Cyclosporine levels increased with diltiazem, nicardipine, and verapamil
Direct vasodilators Hydralizine Minoxidil	Direct, primarily arteriolar vasodilatation	Tachycardia, flushing, headache, fluid retention Lupus-like reaction with hydralazine Hair growth with minoxidil May cause angina pectoris in patients with CAD	Should be used with a diuretic to minimize pseudotolerance and with a β-blocker to prevent tachycardia Hydralazine subject to phenotypically determined metabolism

ACE, angiotensin-converting enzyme; CAD, coronary artery disease; CHF, congestive heart failure; CO, cardiac output; COPD, chronic obstructive pulmonary disease; HBP, high blood pressure; HDL, high-density lipoprotein; ISA, intrinsic sympathomimetic activity; LDL, low-density lipoprotein; TPR, total peripheral resistance.

Questions

Multiple Choice (choose the one best answer)

1. A 50-year-old man has a 3-decade history of hypertension and repeated episodes of rapid increases in blood pressure necessitating urgent treatment. He is a nonsmoker, does not drink alcohol, and avoids salt, but is sedentary and obese (body mass index is 35). Previous evaluations included a normal isotope renogram, and he recalls collecting urine for 24-hour analysis, but no results from this study are available. Current medications include benazepril (Lotensin), 20 mg twice daily; acebutolol (Sectral), 200 mg/day; terazosin (Hytrin), 5 mg/day; amlodipine (Norvasc), 5 mg/day; potassium chloride (K-Dur), 20 mEq twice daily; and furosemide, 20 mg every other day.

    Physical examination results: blood pressure in right arm 156/90 mm Hg and left arm 148/92 mm Hg (seated) and 134/90 mm Hg (standing); pulse, 72 beats/min; normal fundi on retinoscopy; lungs are clear to auscultation; S_1 and S_2, normal; no murmurs; no S_3 or S_4; no carotid or abdominal bruits; no abdominal masses; all peripheral pulses are normal; and no radiofemoral pulse delay. Laboratory test results: creatinine, 12 mg/dL; Na^+, 143 mEq/L; K^+, 3.6 mEq/L; chest radiography, normal.

    You elect to evaluate this patient with resistant hypertension for the presence of a secondary form of hypertension. What test is most likely to give you the diagnosis?

    a. Blood sampling for plasma renin activity and serum aldosterone
    b. Doppler ultrasonographic examination of the renal arteries
    c. Determination of 24-hour urine excretion of catecholamines
    d. Dobutamine echocardiography
    e. Transesophageal echocardiography

2. A reproductive endocrinologist refers a 34-year-old woman who is 16 weeks pregnant and has an average blood pressure of 160/100 mm Hg. She has no contributing factors to her hypertension (e.g., obesity or excessive salt intake). You would consider all the following medications for this woman to control her hypertension *except*:

    a. Methyldopa
    b. Atenolol
    c. Labetalol
    d. Lisinopril

3. A gynecologist seeks your consultation for a 62-year-old woman with difficult-to-control high blood pressure the morning after she has had a hysterectomy. She had been taking labetalol (100 mg twice daily for 3 years). Two days preoperatively, she stopped taking this medication. With induction of anesthesia, her blood pressure increased to 220/126 mm Hg. Intravenous nitroprusside reduced her blood pressure at operation, but in the recovery room her systolic blood pressure fluctuated between 160 and 230 mm Hg. Your recommendation would be which of the following?

    a. Reinitiate treatment with intravenous labetalol until she is able to take oral medications, and refer her to her primary care provider
    b. Recommend sublingual nifedipine for all systolic pressures greater than 180 mm Hg and obtain an echocardiogram to assess left ventricular function and thickness
    c. Initiate treatment with an α_2-blocker and have the patient collect a 24-hour urine sample for determining the excretion rates of catecholamines
    d. Obtain a renal arteriogram

4. A 62-year-old man returns for a third blood pressure measurement in 2 months. His blood pressure has been increased for the past 3 years, but no treatment was instituted. His father and older brother died of myocardial infarctions at ages 66 and 52 years, respectively. His blood pressure today is 168/100 mm Hg. His cardiovascular examination, including funduscopy, is normal. There are no renal bruits. He is not overweight. Which of the following would be the best recommendation?

    a. Collect urine for measurement of catecholamine excretion
    b. Initiate therapy with either a small-dose potassium-sparing diuretic or β-adrenergic blocker
    c. Continue to observe and measure the blood pressure in 4 weeks
    d. Screen for renovascular disease with Doppler ultrasonography of the renal arteries or isotope renography before starting treatment

5. Each of the following statements about hypertension associated with heart transplant recipients is true *except*:

a. Cyclosporine causes vasoconstriction, possibly by increasing endothelin-1 production and decreasing nitric oxide production

b. The normal circadian rhythm in blood pressure is lost in heart transplant recipients receiving treatment with cyclosporine

c. The hypertension that follows heart transplantation is volume-dependent, and efforts at salt restriction have a positive effect on lowering blood pressure

d. Nicardipine, amlodipine, diltiazem, and verapamil decrease cyclosporine levels, requiring increased cyclosporine doses to maintain adequate immunosuppression

6. Each of the following is a contributing factor to the development of essential hypertension *except*:
   a. Obesity
   b. Alcohol consumption
   c. Salt intake
   d. Cigarette smoking
   e. Lack of exercise

7. You are asked to consult on a 68-year-old man with mild, stable, intermittent claudication and hypertension. In the past year, his blood pressure control has deteriorated despite increasing antihypertensive medication. One month ago, his local physician initiated therapy with an angiotensin-converting enzyme inhibitor. When you see the patient, his blood pressure is 150/90 mm Hg but his creatinine value has increased from 1.5 to 4.6 mg/dL in the month since blood pressure therapy was started. The most likely cause of the patient's clinical deterioration is:
   a. Atheroembolism to the renal arteries
   b. Rapidly progressive arteriolar nephrosclerosis
   c. Obstructive uropathy
   d. Bilateral renal artery stenosis
   e. Improvement in blood pressure control

8. For the treatment of hypertensive emergencies, each of the following is an appropriate regimen *except*:
   a. Sodium nitroprusside (0.25–10 μg/min) as an intravenous infusion
   b. Nitroglycerin (5-100 μg/min) as an intravenous infusion
   c. Enalaprilat (1.25-5 mg) by intravenous injection every 6 hours
   d. Have patient bite on a nifedipine capsule (10 mg) for sublingual absorption or infuse the liquid via a nasogastric tube
   e. Labetalol (0.5-2 mg/min) as an intravenous infusion

9. You are asked to see an 80-year-old woman who resides in a nursing home and has become lethargic and confused but still follows oral instructions. She has a history of hypertension and "heart disease." Her medications include digoxin (Lanoxin), triamterene and hydrochlorothiazide (Maxzide), and nifedipine (Procardia). Despite "forcing fluids," the nursing home staff was unsuccessful in decreasing a recent fever. The medical director prescribed an infusion of dextrose 5% in water. At admission, the patient's blood pressure was 146/90 mm Hg recumbent and 108/60 mm Hg sitting, with an accompanying pulse increase from 70 to 98 beats/min. Cardiac examination is otherwise normal. Pertinent laboratory data are as follows: serum Na$^+$, 118 mEq/L; K$^+$, 2.9 mEq/L; serum creatinine, 1.8 mg/dL; and urine osmolality, 780 mosm/kg. The most prudent course of treatment would be:
   a. Restrict fluids to less than 600 mL/24 hr to treat the syndrome of inappropriate antidiuretic hormone (SIADH) secretion
   b. Perform transesophageal echocardiography to exclude an intracardiac source of cerebral embolism
   c. Feed salted chicken soup and allow water as desired by the patient, rechecking Na$^+$ and K$^+$ concentrations daily
   d. Administer 1 L of hypertonic saline over a 60-minute period

10. You are asked to see a 57-year-old man in whom palpitations developed 18 months ago. His primary physician found the patient hypertensive and documented paroxysmal atrial tachycardia. He prescribed sotalol (Betapace). The episodes of palpitations decreased in frequency, but flushing and headache developed and the hypertension persisted. The local physician measured the patient's metanephrine excretion rate at 12.6 mg/24 hr (normal, < 1.3 mg/24 hr). Your best recommendation for the care of this patient would be:
    a. Obtain a computed tomographic scan of the abdomen, focusing on the adrenal glands
    b. Initiate therapy with dibenzyline to augment the β-adrenergic blockade of sotalol in treating the patient's possible pheochromocytoma
    c. Obtain a total body ^{131}meta-iodobenzylguanidine

(MIBG) scan

d. Measure fractionated catecholamine excretion with high-performance liquid chromatography on the 24-hour urine sample that demonstrated the initial increased metanephrine excretion

e. Obtain an echocardiogram to assess left ventricular function and obtain a surgical consultation

11. An 82-year-old woman with a history of dementia and "borderline" hypertension, previously treated with triamterene and hydrochlorothiazide (Dyazide), was admitted to the coronary care unit from her daughter's home with chest pain and a blood pressure of 224/128 mm Hg. Her blood pressure was controlled with intravenous nitroprusside therapy. Myocardial infarction and aortic dissection were excluded. On dismissal from the coronary care unit, the best course of action would be:

a. Obtain duplex ultrasonographic examination of the renal arteries

b. Substitute captopril (25 mg three times daily) for her previous medications

c. Obtain renal angiography and perform percutaneous angioplasty or stenting for any stenotic lesions found

d. Add atenolol, 25 mg daily, to her diuretic and arrange follow-up blood pressure measurements

12. A 68-year-old woman is referred to you because of hypertension. She last saw a physician 35 years previously at the birth of her last child. Increased blood pressure was discovered during a physical examination performed at the insistence of the patient's children. She has no associated symptoms. Her blood pressure was 178/80 mm Hg and 186/72 mm Hg on two separate occasions. Cardiovascular examination is otherwise normal. All the following statements regarding this patient's case are true *except*:

a. Systolic blood pressure increases with age, and as long as her diastolic pressure is less than 90 mm Hg she is not at increased risk for the complications of hypertension

b. Counsel the patient on the importance of maintaining an ideal body weight, limiting salt intake, and moderating alcohol intake, and begin a graded walking program

c. Treatment with either a β-adrenergic blocker or diuretic is likely to reduce the risk that the patient will have a stroke or heart attack

d. Anemia and thyrotoxicosis should be excluded because either can result in isolated systolic hypertension, and in the elderly the classic symptoms of either disease may be lacking

Answers

1. Answer a

The potassium concentration of 3.6 mEq/L is within the normal range but is inappropriate in the face of significant angiotensin-converting enzyme (ACE) inhibition at the stated dosage of benazepril in combination with potassium supplementation. The diuretic is unlikely to be the cause of this inappropriate potassium concentration in light of the normal sodium concentration of 143 mEq/L, which suggests volume *expansion* and secondary vasopressin (antidiuretic hormone) suppression. The normal creatinine value while receiving an ACE inhibitor and the absence of an abdominal bruit argue against renal artery stenosis.

Coarctation of the aorta is unlikely to present at this age, and the normal chest radiograph and the absence of radiofemoral pulse delay also argue against coarctation of the aorta.

2. Answer d

Fetal abnormalities have been associated with angiotensin-converting enzyme inhibitors and angiotensin II receptor blockers.

3. Answer c

Among the stimuli for catecholamine release from pheochromocytomas (paragangliomas), anesthesia induction is one of the more common. The α_2-blocker is the first line of medical therapy and will not interfere with catecholamine measurement, as will labetalol.

4. Answer b

The patient has stage 2 hypertension and is in risk group B (JNC-VI). β-Adrenergic blockers and diuretics have been shown in outcome studies to lower blood pressure and reduce morbidity and mortality. Therapy should be started now. The patient is unlikely to have secondary hypertension.

5. Answer d

These agents *increase* cyclosporine levels, making it necessary to monitor cyclosporine levels while adjusting the dosage of any of these agents. This can be used to decrease the cyclosporine requirement, thereby reducing treatment costs.

6. Answer d

Although a definite risk factor for the development of coronary and peripheral vascular disease, cigarette smoking is not a contributor to the development of essential hypertension.

7. Answer d

Afferent arteriolar tone is mediated through angiotensin II. Blockade of angiotensin II generation results in afferent arteriolar dilation, which in combination with decreased efferent flow due to the renal artery stenosis results in decreased glomerular filtration and an increase in the serum creatinine value. Because no permanent pathologic changes take place within the kidney in this setting, discontinuance of the angiotensin-converting enzyme inhibitor should result in a return to a pretreatment creatinine concentration.

8. Answer d

Oral absorption of the nifedipine liquid often results in a precipitous decrease in blood pressure. Such a rapid decline in pressure has been associated with myocardial infarction, cerebral ischemic events, and death. All the other suggested pharmacologic treatments are acceptable.

9. Answer c

This scenario suggests an elderly patient with good left ventricular function that is stressed by the decrease in effective intravascular volume brought about by her fever. The use of a thiazide diuretic further decreases her intravascular volume, stimulating both the renin-angiotensin-aldosterone axis and the vasopressin (antidiuretic hormone) secretion. In this setting, both potassium and sodium ion loss occur, and the free water administered exacerbates the hyponatremia further. Treatment should slowly return the effective intravascular volume to its compensated state and resolve the electrolyte abnormalities. Hypertonic saline can cause pontine cerebral injury that is frequently fatal.

10. Answer d

Sotalol is primarily excreted by the kidneys and is measured in the metanephrine assay. The high-pressure liquid chromatography method of measuring catecholamines would not measure this medication and would document or exclude a pheochromocytoma (paraganglioma).

11. Answer d

Patients of this age are likely to have renovascular lesions that may be responsible for increased blood pressure. The patient should be intellectually competent to consent to have an elective invasive procedure such as renal angiography and must be a surgical candidate should there be a major complication with renal artery angioplasty. Angiotensin-converting enzyme inhibition in the elderly can be accompanied by a precipitous decrease in blood pressure and decline in renal function, and the taking of medication three times per day presents a significant compliance burden.

12. Answer a

Isolated systolic hypertension in the elderly is associated with increased cardiovascular, cerebrovascular, and renal morbidity and mortality, and treating it appropriately reduces the risk to that of an age- and sex-adjusted control population.

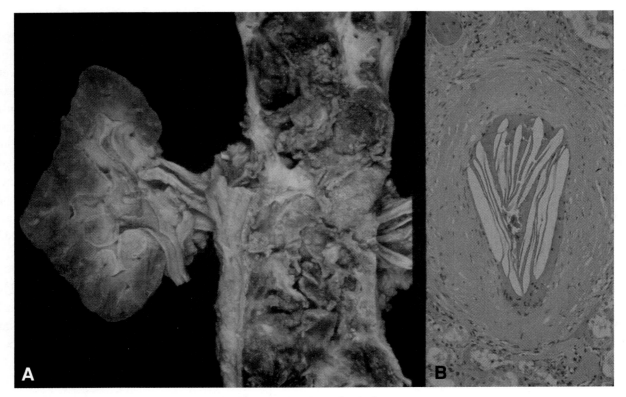

Plate 1. *A*, Atherosclerosis of the descending aorta. *B*, Renal cholesterol emboli.

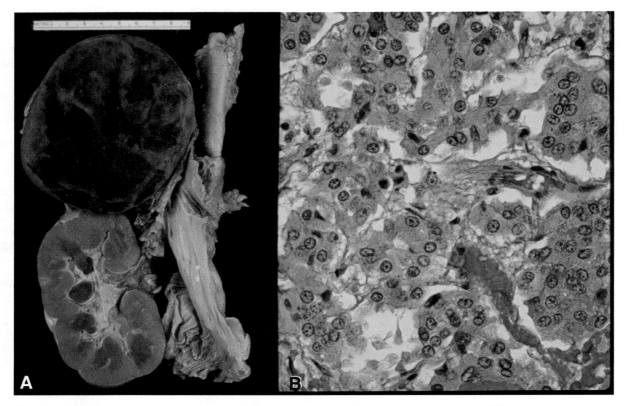

Plate 2. *A*, Gross and, *B*, microscopic specimens of pheochromocytoma of the right adrenal gland. (*B*, x100.)

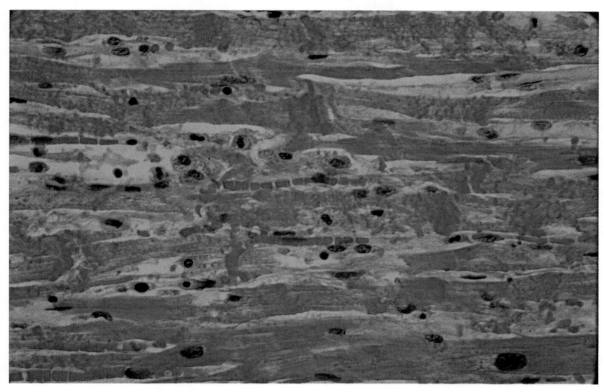

Plate 3. Myocardial cardiotoxicity in pheochromocytoma. (x100.)

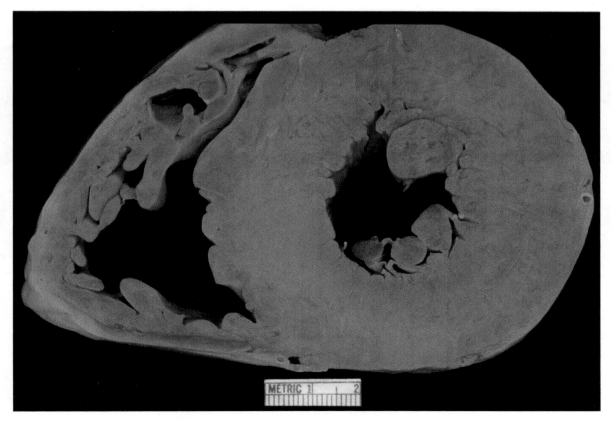

Plate 4. Concentric left ventricular hypertrophy in chronic hypertension.

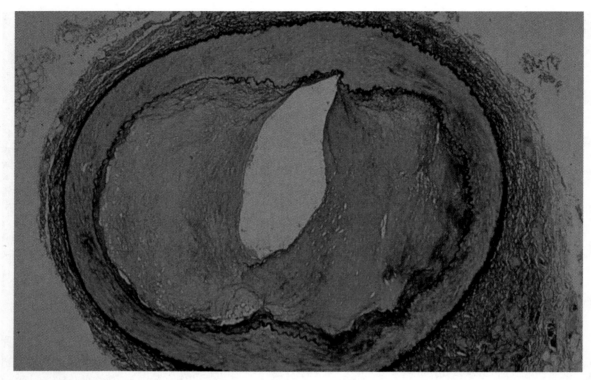

Plate 5. Renal artery atherosclerosis (grade 4).

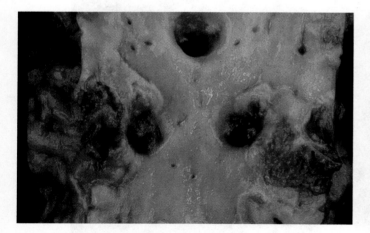

Plate 6. Atherosclerotic narrowing of renal ostia.

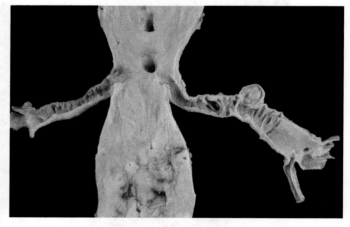

Plate 7. Fibromuscular dysplasia of the renal arteries.

Chapter 65

Medical Ethics for Cardiology Boards

Udaya B. S. Prakash, M.D.
William F. Dunn, M.D.
John G. Park, M.D.

> Medical ethics are the moral principles and practices that govern physician conduct in the treatment of patients. Ethical obligations typically exceed the minimal legal duties of the physician to patients.

Medical ethics cannot be adequately learned from a textbook. The following outline of principles should be considered a guide only. Increasing emphasis is being placed on medical ethics in the certifying and licensing examinations for physicians.

Principles of Medical Ethics

The three major principles are 1) autonomy, 2) beneficence and nonmaleficence, and 3) justice.

Autonomy

Autonomy involves respect for the patient's right to self-determination and implies "decisional capability," that is, the ability to think about the available information and to draw conclusions. Clinical evidence of confusion, disorientation, and psychosis resulting from organic diseases, metabolic disturbances, and iatrogenic causes can adversely affect decision-making ability. In clinical practice, the lack of decisional capability should be proved, and not presumed. Decisionally capable patients have the right to refuse medical therapy, even at the risk of death. If a previously decisionally capable patient had indicated, clearly and convincingly, whether life-sustaining therapy should be administered or withheld in the event of permanent unconsciousness, that wish should be respected, unless it was subsequently clearly rescinded.

- Autonomy: respecting the patient's right to self-determination.
- Autonomy implies "decisional capability" (the right to refuse medical therapy, even at the risk of death).
- Lack of decisional capability should be proved, and not presumed.

Substituted Judgment
This is the ability of family members or other duly appointed person(s) to make therapeutic decisions on behalf of the patient, on the basis of what they believe the patient, if decisionally capable, would have chosen.

Surrogate Decision Maker
The surrogate represents the patient's interests and previously expressed wishes in the context of the medical issues. The surrogate is ideally designated by the patient before the critical illness. One type of surrogate is the durable power

of attorney, in which a legally binding proxy directive authorizes a designated individual to speak on behalf of the patient. The second type of surrogate is the patient's family, physician, or the court. The third type is a moral surrogate (usually a family member) who best knows the patient and has the patient's interest at heart.

- Ideally, a surrogate is designated by a patient before the critical illness.

Living Will
This is a type of "advance directive" or "health-care declaration." This document commonly includes a declaration of "durable power of attorney for health-care matters (proxy)." The living will reflects the patient's autonomy and can aid greatly in medical decision making. Any decisionally capable person 18 years or older can have a living will.

- Living will: a type of "advance directive" or "health-care declaration."
- The living will reflects a patient's autonomy.
- Legal reliability may vary from state to state.

Disclosure
To make the principle of autonomy function, the physician must provide decisionally capable patients with adequate and truthful information on which to base medical decisions. Honesty on the part of the physician is an integral part of patient autonomy. Severity of illness scoring systems hold promise in assisting the physician in quantifying the risk of mortality, thereby providing the patient more precise input to aid in decision making than has been available in the past. Scoring system data should be interpreted, however, only within the clinical context and cautiously until they are widely validated; these systems remain in evolution.

A serious issue is the availability of more than one acceptable form of therapy for a disease. In a patient with a cancer amenable to surgical resection, chemotherapy or radiation may provide a similar long-term outlook, albeit with different complications and side effects. However, the physician may be biased toward one of the three treatments. In this situation, it is the duty of the physician to set aside personal bias and provide detailed information on each treatment and its potential complications and to allow the well-informed patient to express personal preferences.

- Physician must provide decisionally capable patients with adequate and truthful information on which to base

medical decisions.
- Physician must consider ethical issues as well as the patient's values and preferences.
- Honesty is an integral part of autonomy.
- Severity of illness scoring systems may assist in assessment of mortality risk.

Informed Consent
This is voluntary acceptance of physician recommendations by decisionally competent patients or surrogates who have been furnished with ample truthful information regarding risks, benefits, and alternatives and who clearly indicate their comprehension of the information. Informed consent is especially important when performing new, innovative, nonstandard surgical procedures and research procedures. Informed consent from surrogates is necessary to perform an autopsy (except in specific instances such as coroners' cases, in which the decision is made by outside authorities) or to practice intubation, placement of intravascular lines, or other procedures on the newly dead. The amount of information needed by the patient to give informed consent is not that which the physician feels is adequate (Professional Practice Standard) but that which the average prudent person would need to make a decision (Reasonable Person Standard). In rare exceptions, the physician can treat a patient without truly informed consent (e.g., in an emotionally unstable patient who requires urgent treatment, informing the patient of the details may produce further problems). Many "informed consent" forms in clinical use do not meet the Reasonable Person Standard and are therefore of little value morally or legally.

- Amount of information needed by patient is that which the average prudent person would need to make a decision (Reasonable Person Standard).
- Many "informed consent" forms do not meet Reasonable Person Standard and are therefore of little value morally or legally.

Confidentiality
Patient confidentiality provides the patient the right to keep medical information solely within the realm of the physician-patient relationship. The physician is obliged to maintain the medical information in strict confidence. Exceptions to this include instances when data, if not released to appropriate agencies, have the potential to cause greater societal harm. Typical examples include positive results of the human

immunodeficiency virus (HIV) test or a sputum culture that is positive for *Mycobacterium tuberculosis*. Patients who voluntarily request the HIV test should be informed by the physician that the result, if positive, will be automatically reported to the appropriate health agency. Confidentiality may also be breached when patients ask about hereditary diseases in their parents or siblings.

- Physician is obliged to maintain medical information in strict confidence.
- Exceptions include instances when data, if not released to appropriate agencies, may cause greater societal harm (e.g., positive HIV test, positive sputum culture for *Mycobacterium tuberculosis*).

Group-Specific Beliefs
Certain religious practices preclude or compromise accepted medical practices. The principle of autonomy provides that adult patients who refuse life-saving measures (e.g., blood transfusion) should be allowed to maintain their religious practices. However, in cases involving children, the courts have overruled the religious objections.

- Adult patients who refuse life-saving measures (e.g., blood transfusion) should be allowed to maintain their religious practices.

Beneficence and Nonmaleficence
Beneficence is acting to benefit patients by preserving life, restoring health, relieving suffering, and restoring or maintaining function. The physician (acting in good faith) is obligated to help patients attain their own interests and goals as determined by the patient, *not* the physician.

- Beneficence: preservation of life, restoration of health, relief of suffering, and restoration or maintenance of function.

The principle of nonmaleficence is based on "do no harm, prevent harm, and remove harm." This principle addresses unprofessional behavior; verbal, physical, and sexual abuse of patients; and uninformed and undisclosed experimentation on patients with drugs and procedures with the potential to cause harmful side effects. Breach of physician-patient confidentiality which results in harm to the patient is another example of maleficence.

- Nonmaleficence: "do no harm, prevent harm, and remove harm."

Implied Consent
The principle of implied consent is invoked when true informed consent is not possible because the patient (or surrogate) is unable to express a decision regarding treatment, specifically in emergency situations in which physicians are compelled to provide medically necessary therapy, without which harm would result. This clarifies that there is a duty to assist a person in urgent need of care. This principle has been legally accepted, and it provides the physician a legal defense against battery (although not negligence).

- Implied consent is invoked when true informed consent is not possible.

Treatment of Minors
Minors, that is, persons aged 17 years or younger, in all states require parental permission for nonemergency cardiac treatment, with several exceptions. Emancipated minors can be treated without parental permission. This group includes married minors, those in the armed services, students living away from home in college, and those clearly living independent of their parents.

Incurable Disease and Death
The following guidelines are suggested in dealing with incurable disease and death. The patient and family (if the patient so desires) must be provided ample opportunity to talk with the physician and ask questions. An unhurried openness and "willing-to-listen" attitude on the part of the physician are critical for a positive outcome. Patients often find it easier to share their feelings about death with their physician, who is likely to be more objective and less emotional, than with family and friends. Nevertheless, the physician should not remain or appear completely detached from the patient's feelings and emotions. Even an attempt on the part of the physician to enter the "inner" feelings of the patient will have a soothing, if not therapeutic, effect.

- The patient and family must be provided every opportunity to talk with the physician and ask questions.
- An unhurried openness and "willing-to-listen" attitude on the part of the physician are critical for a positive outcome.

The physician should assume the responsibility to furnish or arrange for physical, emotional, and spiritual support. Adequate control of pain, maintenance of human dignity, and close contact with the family are crucial. The emotional and spiritual support available through local clergy (as appropriate, given the patient's personal beliefs) should not be underestimated. At no other time in life is the reality of human mortality so real as in the terminal phases of disease. It is always preferable to allay the anxiety of the dying patient through adequate emotional and spiritual support rather than by sedation. The physician should constantly remind herself or himself that despite all the medical technology that surrounds the patient, the patient must not be dehumanized.

- Adequate pain control, maintenance of human dignity, and close contact with family are crucial.
- Despite all the technology that surrounds the patient, human-to-human contact should be the most important aspect of treatment.
- It is always preferable to allay anxiety by adequate emotional and spiritual support rather than by sedation.

Control of Pain
The principle of beneficence calls for relief of suffering. Adequate analgesia, particularly in patients with incurable disease, is the responsibility of the physician. If death ensues in a terminally ill patient because of respiratory depression from analgesia, the physician has not acted immorally. Patients allowed to die after removal from ventilators are commonly treated in this fashion. Nevertheless, it is necessary to stress that the primary objective of analgesia is relief of pain and not the hastening of death, even in terminally ill patients.

- Beneficence calls for relief of suffering.
- Adequate analgesia, particularly in patients with incurable disease, is the responsibility of the physician.
- Physician has not performed immorally if death in a terminally ill patient is the result of respiratory depression from analgesic therapy; euthanasia is not the goal.

Nonabandonment
Abandonment connotes leaving the patient (for whom the physician has provided—or agreed to provide—health care in the past) without care. This conduct is unacceptable and has been "universally condemned as a serious and punishable infraction of both the legal and ethical obligations that physicians owe patients." In contrast, nonabandonment denotes a requisite ethical obligation of physicians to provide optimal care once the patient and physician mutually agree to enter into a relationship. Noncompliance by the patient, in terms of taking medications or following

a physician's instructions, is not grounds for abandonment. Physicians should strive to respond to the needs of their patients over time, but they should not trespass their own values in the process.

Conflict of Interest
The principle of beneficence requires that the physician not engage in activities that are not in the patient's best interest. Some studies have suggested that physicians' prescribing practices are influenced by financial and other significant rewards from drug companies. If the physician does not ardently avoid areas of potential conflict of interest (because of the principle of beneficence), the result may be maleficence.

Conscientious Objection by the Physician
Physicians may refuse to perform a treatment or procedure that they judge immoral by their moral standards. Treatment should not be refused to patients whom a physician dislikes on moral grounds.

Justice
Every patient deserves and must be provided optimal care as warranted by the underlying medical condition. Allocation of medical resources fairly and according to medical need is the basis for this principle. The decision to provide optimal medical care should be based on the medical need of each patient and the perceived medical benefit to the patient. The patient's social status, ability to pay, or perceived social worth should not dictate the quality or quantity of medical care. The physician's clear-cut responsibility is to the patient's well-being (beneficence). Physicians should not make decisions about individual care of their patients based on larger societal needs. The bedside is not the place to make general policy decisions.

- Justice: allocation of medical resources fairly and according to medical need.
- Physician should not make decisions about individual care of patients based on larger societal needs.

Triage

Triage is a term applied to the decisions made in emergency situations about whom to select for treatment. The moral principle is to do the greatest good for the greatest number of patients. In this situation, preference for treatment is given to moderately and severely injured patients in whom emergency treatment can affect clinical outcome. In patients with minor injuries and those with a high probability of death even with advanced treatment, care is delayed.

Managed Care

Health maintenance organizations are the most common model of managed care. They seek to provide their members with appropriate medical care at generally lower costs than fee-for-service practice models. Incentives for physicians to be cost-conscious and cost-effective are usually part of the practice plan.

Physicians owe a professional responsibility to the patient to investigate symptoms appropriately and to recommend the best therapeutic option even if this is the more expensive option. Never should financial issues be allowed to interfere with the provision of conscientious, high-quality care.

"Do Not Resuscitate" (DNR)

DNR orders affect administration of cardiopulmonary resuscitation (CPR) only; other therapeutic options should not be influenced by the DNR order. Every person whose medical history is unclear or unavailable should receive CPR in the event of cardiopulmonary arrest. CPR is not recommended when it merely prolongs life in a patient with terminal illness or when the fatal outcome is clinically evident.

Of paramount importance are the patient's knowledge of the extent of disease and the prognosis, the physician's estimate of the potential efficacy of CPR, and the wishes of the patient (or surrogate) regarding CPR as a therapeutic tool. The DNR order should be reviewed frequently because clinical circumstances may dictate other measures (e.g., a patient with dilated cardiomyopathy who had initially turned down heart transplantation and wanted to be considered a "DNR candidate" may change her or his mind and now opt for the transplantation). Physicians should discuss the appropriateness of CPR or DNR with patients at high risk for cardiopulmonary arrest and with the terminally ill. The discussion should optimally take place in the outpatient setting, during the initial period of hospitalization, and periodically during hospitalization, if appropriate. DNR orders (and rationale) should be entered in the patient's medical records.

- DNR orders affect CPR only.

- Other therapeutic options should not be influenced by the DNR order.
- Every patient should be considered a candidate for CPR unless clear indications exist otherwise.
- CPR is not recommended when it merely prolongs life in a patient with a terminal illness.
- DNR orders should be reviewed frequently.
- DNR orders (and rationale) should be entered in the patient's medical records.

Withholding and Withdrawing Life Support

This decision may be compatible with beneficence, nonmaleficence, and autonomy. The right of a decisionally capable person to refuse lifesaving hydration and nutrition was upheld by the U.S. Supreme Court, but a surrogate decision maker's right to refuse treatment for decisionally incapable persons can be restricted by states. Brain death is not a necessary requirement for withdrawing or withholding life support. The value of each medical therapy (risk:benefit ratio) should be assessed for each patient. The American Medical Association has issued certain guidelines, and one of them states that a life-sustaining medical intervention can be limited without the consent of the patient or surrogate when the intervention is judged to be futile. The extent to which these guidelines will be upheld by legal authorities is as yet unclear. When appropriate, the withholding or withdrawal of life support is best accomplished with input from more than one experienced clinician and institutional ethics authorities.

- Withholding or withdrawing life support does not conflict with the principles of beneficence, nonmaleficence, and autonomy.
- Brain death is not a necessary requirement for withdrawing or withholding life support.

Persistent Vegetative State

This is a chronic state of unconsciousness (loss of self-awareness) lasting for more than a few weeks, characterized by the presence of wake/sleep cycles, but without behavioral or cerebral metabolic evidence of cognitive function or of being able to respond in a perceptive manner to external events or stimuli. The body retains functions necessary to sustain vegetative survival, if provided nutritional and other supportive measures—note that the U.S. Supreme Court has ruled that there is no distinction between artificial feeding and hydration versus mechanical ventilation.

- Persistent vegetative state: unconsciousness (loss of self-awareness) lasting for more than a few weeks.
- U.S. Supreme Court ruling states that there is no distinction between artificial feeding and hydration versus mechanical ventilation.

Definition of Death

Death is irreversible cessation of circulatory and respiratory function *or* irreversible cessation of all functions of the entire brain, including the brain stem. Clinical criteria (at times substantiated by electroencephalographic testing or assessment of cerebral perfusion) permit the reliable diagnosis of "cerebral death."

The family should be informed of the brain death but should not be asked to decide whether further medical therapy should be continued. One exception is when the patient had earlier directed the family to make certain decisions, such as organ donation, in case of brain death.

Once it is ascertained that the patient is "brain dead" and that no further therapy can be offered, the primary physician, preferably after consultation with another physician involved in the care of the patient, may withdraw supportive measures.

The imminent possibility of harvesting organs for transplantation should in no way affect any of the above-outlined decisions. When organ donation is possible after the determination of brain death, the family should be approached, preferably before cessation of cardiac function, regarding organ donation.

- Death: irreversible cessation of circulatory and respiratory function *or* irreversible cessation of all functions of entire brain, including brain stem.
- Electroencephalography is not necessary to establish death.

Suggested Review Reading

Withholding and Withdrawal of Life-Sustaining Therapies

1. American College of Chest Physicians/Society of Critical Care Medicine Consensus Panel: Ethical and moral guidelines for the initiation, continuation, and withdrawal of intensive care. *Chest* 97:949-958, 1990.
An important ethical consensus statement from these two societies.

2. American Thoracic Society: Withholding and withdrawing life-sustaining therapy. *Am Rev Respir Dis*

144:726-731, 1991.
This official statement of the American Thoracic Society was adopted by its Board of Directors in March 1991.

3. Council on Ethical and Judicial Affairs, American Medical Association: Decisions near the end of life. *JAMA* 267:2229-2233, 1992.
Council report from the American Medical Association concerning end-of-life issues, including pertinent definitions, ethical principles, and Council recommendations.

4. Hakim RB, Teno JM, Harrell FE Jr, Knaus WA, Wenger N, Phillips RS, Layde P, Califf R, Connors AF Jr, Lynn J: Factors associated with do-not-resuscitate orders:

patients' preferences, prognoses, and physicians' judgments. SUPPORT Investigators. Study to Understand Prognoses and Preferences for Outcomes and Risks of Treatment. *Ann Intern Med* 125:284-293, 1996.
Medical treatment decisions should be based on the preferences of informed patients or their proxies and on the expected outcomes of treatment. In this study, do-not-resuscitate orders were written earlier for patients older than 75 years, regardless of prognosis. This suggests that physicians may be placing undue emphasis on age as a predictor of survival in the intensive care unit setting.

5. Hooper SC, Vaughan KJ, Tennant CC, Perz JM: Major depression and refusal of life-sustaining medical treatment in the elderly. *Med J Aust* 165:416-419, 1996.
Moderate or severe major depression in the elderly is associated with a high degree of refusal of life-sustaining treatments. Treatment of the depression leads to increased acceptance of these treatments, particularly if the prognosis is good.

6. Meisel A: Legal myths about terminating life support. *Arch Intern Med* 151:1497-1502, 1991.
Commonly held erroneous beliefs among physicians regarding what the law permits concerning the termination of life support include 1) anything that is not specifically permitted by law is prohibited; 2) termination of life support is murder or suicide; 3) a patient must be terminally ill for life support to be stopped; 4) it is permissible to terminate extraordinary treatments, but not ordinary ones; 5) it is permissible to withhold treatment, but once started, it must be continued; 6) stopping tube feeding is legally different from stopping other treatments; 7) termination of life support requires going to court; and 8) living wills are not legal.

7. Prendergast TJ, Luce JM: Increasing incidence of withholding and withdrawal of life support from the critically ill. *Am J Respir Crit Care Med* 155:15-20, 1997.
In this intensive care unit study, recommendations to withhold or withdraw life support preceded 179 of 200 deaths (90%) in 1992 and 1993, compared with 114 of 224 deaths (51%) in 1987 and 1988. Cardiopulmonary resuscitation was initiated in 10% of deaths in 1992 and 1993 but in only 49% in 1987 and 1988. In 1992 and 1993, 90% of patients who died in the intensive care units did so after a decision to limit therapy, a major change in practice.

8. Snyder JW, Swartz MS: Deciding to terminate treatment: a practical guide for physicians. *J Crit Care* 8:177-185, 1993.
This report provides systematic identification and deliberate assessment criteria for 1) brain death; 2) the nature, extent, cause, prognosis, and reversibility of impairment; 3) the type of treatment to be withheld or withdrawn; 4) the futility of any proposed intervention; 5) the capacity of the patient for health care decision making; 6) the evidence of a patient's wishes; 7) the proper roles of family members, surrogate decision makers, and other health professionals (such as ethics committees). The report emphasizes that applicable policies, ethics, laws, and potential conflicts of interest will enhance efficiency and add value to the decision-making process at the end of life.

9. Sprung CL: Changing attitudes and practices in foregoing life-sustaining treatments. *JAMA* 263:2211-2215, 1990.
This article provides a stark look at the risks of the slippery slope phenomenon in medical ethics, in a historical context. This study also provides a useful review of American legal rulings shaping current ethical norms.

10. The SUPPORT Principal Investigators: A controlled trial to improve care for seriously ill hospitalized patients: the study to understand prognoses and preferences for outcomes and risks of treatments (SUPPORT). *JAMA* 274:1591-1598, 1995.
A 2-year prospective multi-institutional observational study (phase I) with 4,301 patients followed by a 2-year controlled clinical trial (phase II) with 4,804 patients and their physicians randomized by specialty group to the intervention group (n = 2,652) or control group (n = 2,152). In phase I, substantial shortcomings in communication, frequency of aggressive treatment, and the characteristics of hospital death (relative to patient wishes) were found. The phase II intervention (enhanced communication) failed to improve care or patient outcomes.

11. Task Force on Ethics of the Society of Critical Care Medicine: Consensus report on the ethics of foregoing life-sustaining treatments in the critically ill. *Crit Care Med* 18:1435-1439, 1990.
Consensus statement adopted by the Society of Critical Care Medicine regarding the withholding and withdrawing of life support.

Futility

1. Halevy A, Brody BA: A multi-institution collaborative policy on medical futility. *JAMA* 276:571-574, 1996.
A discussion of the flawed definitions of futility, coupled with a report on the creation of a local multi-institution futility policy created by representatives of local ethics committees in the Houston area.

2. Schneiderman LJ, Jecker NS, Jonsen AR: Medical futility: response to critiques. *Ann Intern Med* 125:669-674, 1996.
A relevant discussion regarding the futility debate.

Quality of Life: Quality of life may be significantly improved after open heart surgery, aortic valve replacement, and angioplasty in octogenarians.

1. Kumar P, Zehr KJ, Chang A, Cameron DE, Baumgartner WA: Quality of life in octogenarians after open heart surgery. *Chest* 108:919-926, 1995.

2. Little T, Milner MR, Lee K, Constantine J, Pichard AD, Lindsay J Jr: Late outcome and quality of life following percutaneous transluminal coronary angioplasty in octogenarians. *Cathet Cardiovasc Diagn* 29:261-266, 1993.

3. Olsson M, Janfjall H, Orth-Gomer K, Unden A, Rosenqvist M: Quality of life in octogenarians after valve replacement due to aortic stenosis. A prospective comparison with younger patients. *Eur Heart J* 17:583-589, 1996.

Physician-Assisted Suicide/Euthanasia

1. Quill TE, Meier DE, Block SD, Billings JA: The debate over physician-assisted suicide: empirical data and convergent views. *Ann Intern Med* 128:552-558, 1998.
A discussion of the physician-assisted suicide controversy.

Questions

Multiple Choice (choose the one best answer)

1. A 79-year-old widower with end-stage ischemic cardiomyopathy remains in the cardiac care unit, intubated and ventilated, 10 days after admission for decompensated congestive heart failure with acute respiratory insufficiency. He is receiving 80% oxygen to maintain a saturation of 90%. He remains diaphoretic. Blood pressure is 78/44 mm Hg and pulse is 56 beats/min. A summation gallop is present. The lung examination reveals persisting bilateral pleural effusions and crackles in the lower half of the chest. The left ventricle is dilated, and the ejection fraction is 10%. He is receiving maximal therapy, including intravenous dobutamine. His living will states that he would not want prolonged life support in the face of progressive decline, but his three children, after several discussions, want continued care. What should occur next?
   a. Continued full supportive measures
   b. Search for additional family members with whom to discuss withdrawal of therapy
   c. Withdrawal of support
   d. Legal counsel
   e. Ethics consultation

2. For a patient experiencing cardiac arrest, a brief trial of cardiopulmonary resuscitation is appropriate in which of the following situations?
   a. An 89-year-old woman with restrictive cardiomyopathy due to amyloid heart disease
   b. A 35-year-old man with anoxic encephalopathy-

induced persistent vegetative state after a witnessed out-of-hospital cardiac arrest that occurred while running a marathon

c. A 41-year-old cocaine addict with a large anterior wall myocardial infarction who has stated he does not want to be resuscitated

d. A 55-year-old smoker with a previous inferior wall myocardial infarction who is admitted with a new large anterior wall myocardial infarction in cardiogenic shock and is now experiencing ventricular fibrillation-type cardiac arrest

e. None of the above

3. A 35-year-old man with newly diagnosed renal cell carcinoma metastatic to the myocardium commands his physician not to tell his wife and three children of his poor prognosis, and he indicates that he does not plan to divulge the information either. His wife asks about her husband's condition. Which of the following is an appropriate response?

a. Indicate that her husband is in good health

b. Divulge the patient's true condition and prognosis to his wife

c. Refuse to divulge the patient's condition

d. Send a letter to the patient's home, where the wife will likely read the contents

4. Testing of a patient for human immunodeficiency virus (HIV) is appropriate in which of the following circumstances in the absence of patient consent?

a. A catheterization laboratory nurse receives a needle-stick injury while performing emergency cardiac catheterization on a 65-year-old veteran

b. As a matter of policy in a high-risk endemic urban area, before all coronary arteriography procedures

c. If a third party, such as a patient's spouse, will be in danger if the result is seropositive

d. If the patient is suspected of having HIV-associated heart disease

e. If requested by the patient's insurer

5. As part of a new prosthetic valve application, a company plans to use pericardium harvested from patients undergoing pericardiectomy. Which of the following statements is false regarding the commercial use of human tissue?

a. Profits from the commercial use of human pericardium may be shared with patients

b. The potential for commercial applications must be disclosed to the patient before commercialization of human tissue

c. Human tissue may be used for commercial purposes without patient consent, provided the donor patient cannot be identified from the final product

d. Informed consent must be obtained for commercial use of human tissue

6. Which of the following statements is incorrect regarding "do not resuscitate" (DNR) orders?

a. Subsequent to preparing a living will, a decisionally capable patient may verbally change the DNR directive

b. The DNR order implies that all life-sustaining therapy not be instituted

c. Once written, the order can be changed at any time.

d. The frequency of DNR orders has increased during the past decade in hospitalized patients

7. A 55-year-old man, previously healthy, has an out-of-hospital ventricular fibrillation-type cardiac arrest. A bystander initiated cardiopulmonary resuscitation (CPR), but the patient was unconscious for approximately 45 minutes before defibrillation was performed by the paramedics. The patient was then transferred to the cardiac intensive care unit unresponsive and intubated. Soon after arrival, the patient's hemodynamic status began to deteriorate despite multiple pressors. The physician approached the patient's family members and friends, and the grave prognosis was discussed. The patient's parents insisted that maximal therapy be continued indefinitely. The fiancée (who has lived with the patient for 10 years), however, states that they have had several conversations about this topic and the patient did not wish to be maintained on life support and he valued active life too much to continue such aggressive measures. On further discussion, it becomes clear that the patient has not interacted with the parents for more than 20 years and that his siblings, who remain uncertain in the decision process, have also not interacted with the patient for more than 15 years. Who would be considered the appropriate surrogate decision maker?

a. Parents

b. Siblings

c. Fiancée

d. Take the case to the courts to have a conservator appointed

8. Forgoing therapy should *not* be discussed in which of the following cases?
   a. When the patient has a diagnosis with a grave prognosis
   b. When the burdens of therapy outweigh the benefits
   c. When the quality of the patient's life is expected to be unacceptable to the patient
   d. When a course of therapy that was initially beneficial is no longer efficacious in achieving the goals of the patient
   e. None of the above

9. Which of the following minors *cannot* receive non-emergency cardiac treatments without parental consent?
   a. 17-year-old who lives at home but has a part-time job
   b. 16-year-old who lives in a different state while attending college
   c. 17-year-old who is in the armed forces
   d. 15-year-old who is married
   e. None of the above

10. One week after an out-of-hospital cardiac arrest, an 87-year-old patient in the coronary care unit is maintained in an unconscious state. There is no response to verbal or nonverbal stimuli. The patient is able to trigger the mechanical ventilator. Oculocephalic ("doll's eye") responses are present. All of the following statements are correct *except*:
   a. The patient is in a persistent vegetative state
   b. An electroencephalogram (EEG) is not necessary for accurate prognostication and decision making
   c. The patient is not brain-dead, given the presence of brain stem reflexes

11. You are working for a managed care institution, and a patient is admitted to your intensive care unit because of a hemodynamically unstable myocardial infarction. The patient receives thrombolytics, and after initial stabilization her condition suddenly deteriorates. You would like to take her to the cardiac catheterization laboratory, but the staff is about to start an elective case. Because the patient's insurance has expired, the administrators insist that the patient be given another thrombolytic or be transferred to the next hospital whose catheterization laboratory is open, which is only 1 mile away. What should you do?
   a. Give another thrombolytic and reassess the clinical condition
   b. Call the paramedics and prepare the patient to be transferred while you ride along
   c. Have the catheterization laboratory start the elective case, stabilize the most critical lesion, and then complete the case after your patient undergoes emergency catheterization
   d. Insist on the gravity of the situation and that the elective case be postponed
   e. Discuss the options with the insurance department about reinstatement of the insurance policy

12. An 89-year-old patient with lung cancer metastatic to the brain presents to the hospital after a large, hemodynamically compromising myocardial infarction. The patient had clearly indicated that he did not want to be resuscitated and that he should be kept comfortable. All the members of the staff and the family members are in agreement. You explain that he will be kept comfortable by the use of morphine, but the family members are concerned about the narcotic hastening death. What should you do?
   a. Tell them that narcotics will still be used despite the possibility of respiratory suppression
   b. Tell them that you understand their concern and that you will not use any narcotics
   c. Tell them that despite his clinical condition, the order will be for a low dose of morphine to be given infrequently so as to minimize the chance of respiratory depression
   d. Tell them that despite his clinical condition, the order will be for 1 mg of morphine to be given every 12 hours as a means of minimizing the chance of respiratory depression
   e. Tell them that morphine will be used, but if there are any signs of respiratory depression, naloxone will be used to reverse the effect of morphine

Answers

1. Answer c

The right of a decisionally capable person to refuse life-sustaining therapy has been upheld by the U.S. Supreme Court. A living will is a legal document that serves as testament to the wishes of a decisionally capable individual.

2. Answer e

In general, brief trials at resuscitation, "slow" codes, or half-hearted resuscitation efforts are inappropriate. For patients in whom resuscitation would be physiologically futile, resuscitation should not be started.

3. Answer c

Duty of confidentiality is owed to the patient. Because there is no risk to the patient's wife by not divulging the true diagnosis, his request should not be overruled, however uncomfortable the physician feels.

4. Answer a

HIV testing is permissible without patient consent in the case of a needle-stick injury or mucosal contact by a health-care worker. Screening HIV testing is not appropriate without patient consent. If a third party is in danger, public health authorities should be contacted.

5. Answer d

Consent must be obtained from patients under all circumstances for the commercial use of human tissue.

6. Answer b

A DNR order refers only to cardiopulmonary resuscitation and does not affect other aspects of care, which should be addressed on their own relative merits.

7. Answer c

Although the parents and the siblings are the next of kin, the patient has not interacted with them for more than 15 years. The fiancée, however, has interacted and lived with the patient during the past 10 years, in effect establishing a spousal relationship. Thus, a reasonable assumption is that she would best know the patient's current wishes.

8. Answer e

All of the situations are appropriate for discussing withholding or withdrawal of therapy, according to the Ethics Committee of the Society of Critical Care Medicine.

9. Answer a

For the treatment of minors (17 years old or younger), parental consent is required unless the minor is considered emancipated (married, in the armed services, living away from home in college, and clearly living independent of the parents).

10. Answer a

The persistent vegetative state requires several weeks of observation to establish the diagnosis.

11. Answer d

The concept of justice states that medical resources need to be allocated according to medical need. Because the physician's primary responsibility is the well-being of the patient, the physician must do what is necessary to improve the condition of the patient without considering the patient's social status, ability to pay, perceived social worth, or perceived repercussion from the hospital administrator.

12. Answer a

The American Medical Association, the American Thoracic Society, and the Society of Critical Care Medicine have clearly accepted the practice of using narcotics in terminally ill patients for the purpose of relieving suffering. When used in this clinical situation, the physician is not considered unethical if the use of narcotics hastens death by the narcotic contributing to respiratory depression, if the primary goal is patient comfort from perceived dyspnea or suffering (principle of "double effect").

Notes

Chapter 66

Evidence-Based Medicine and Statistics for the Cardiology Boards

Victor M. Montori, M.D.
Joseph G. Murphy, M.D.

Evidence-Based Medicine

Evidence-based medicine is the careful use of the best available evidence to guide medical decision making. Medical decision making, in turn, consists of three elements: scientific evidence, clinical setting, and patient-physician factors.

Scientific Evidence

The scientific evidence includes information obtained from the patient (history, physical examination, and results of imaging and body fluid studies) interpreted in conjunction with the results of applicable scientific investigations. The levels of evidence are described in Table 1. Large randomized controlled trials and individual patient data meta-analysis occupy the highest levels of evidence, and most important trials in cardiology belong to this level.

The Clinical Setting

The clinical setting is where the clinical decision occurs. This scenario includes constraints due to time as well as to limitations arising from the availability of technology (i.e., primary angioplasty may be better than thrombolysis *if* you have access within a reasonable time to a center that performs the procedure; otherwise, thrombolysis is the preferred treatment).

When the evidence is transferred into clinical practice, the setting in which that practice functions has to be recognized. Practice guidelines should present the evidence and the recommended action but should be interpreted with the individual patient's best interest in mind. Knowledge of the scientific evidence by the physician and its accurate communication and understanding by the patient will shape the clinical decision, but the decision is also influenced by the patient's and physician's previous experiences, fears, and cultural and ethical values (Fig. 1).

Statistics in Cardiology

Statistics can evaluate treatment strategies among groups of similar patients and measure the probability that the observed clinical response is a chance finding. Statistical questions on various medical examinations generally test the candidate's understanding of the basic principles of statistical analysis and the role of these principles in clinical decision making.

Null Hypothesis

The null hypothesis is frequently used in the context of comparing treatment groups (e.g., comparing drugs A and B). The null hypothesis states that no true difference exists between groups and that any observed difference is due to chance alone. The null hypothesis is rejected when the difference between groups is large enough to reach statistical significance (i.e., the probability that the result is due to chance is less than a specific set value).

Table 1.—Levels of Evidence

Grade of recommendation	Level of evidence	Therapy
A	1a	Evidence based on meta-analysis of multiple homogeneous randomized clinical trials
	1b	Evidence based on meta-analysis of individual nonhomogeneous randomized clinical trials but with narrow confidence interval
	1c	Evidence based on historic "all or none" data (all patients died before treatment became available) and on treatment, few or none die
B	2a	Evidence based on meta-analysis of homogeneous cohort studies
	2b	Individual cohort study or lesser quality randomized clinical trials
	2c	"Outcomes" research
	3a	Evidence based on meta-analysis of homogeneous case-control studies
	3b	Individual case-control study
C	4	Case series or lesser quality cohort study or case-control studies
	5	Expert opinion

Data from the Centre for Evidence-Based Medicine, Oxford, UK 1998 (http://cebm.jr2.ox.ac.uk/eboc/eboc.html).

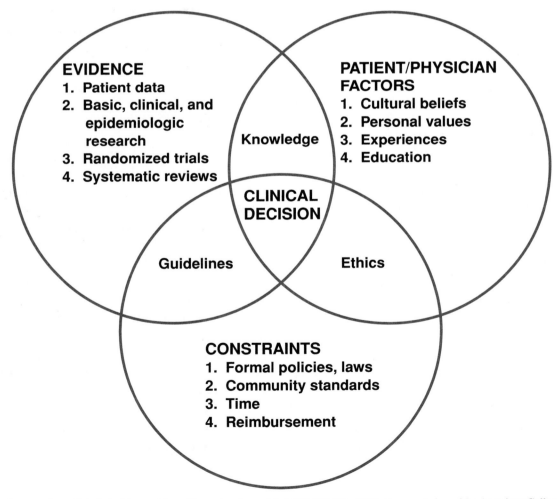

Fig. 1. Factors that enter into clinical decision making. (From *Ann Intern Med* 126:389-391, 1997. By permission of the American College of Physicians.)

Alpha Level

The alpha level of a statistical test is the probability that the test made a type I error and concluded that the observed difference is real (statistically significant) when, in fact, chance explains the observation. The alpha level, or threshold value, for statistical significance is set by the researcher, typically at 0.05 or 0.01 (i.e., there is a 5% or 1% chance that the test will falsely report a significant difference when none exists).

Beta Level

The beta level of a statistical test is the probability that the test made a type II error and concluded that the observed difference is due to chance (not statistically significant) when, in fact, the observed difference is real. The beta level, or threshold value, for statistical significance is set by the researcher, typically at 0.2 or 0.1. The statistical power of a test is the ability to detect a given difference if one exists and is calculated as 1 minus beta. A beta of 0.2 gives a statistical power of 0.8 (i.e., an 80% chance of detecting any difference that exists).

Therapeutic Decisions

The Digitalis Investigation Group (DIG) study of digoxin in patients with heart failure is used below to illustrate how to apply the evidence to therapeutic decisions (*N Engl J Med* 336:525-533, 1997).

Type of Study

The DIG study was a multicenter randomized, double-blinded, placebo-controlled trial of 6,800 patients with heart failure. The mean age at enrollment was 63 years, with a mean follow-up of 37 months. Most patients were men (78%), and all had a left ventricular ejection fraction of 45% or less and were in sinus rhythm. Most patients were taking diuretics and angiotensin-converting enzyme (ACE) inhibitors. The main study outcome evaluated was total mortality; secondary outcomes included, among others, hospitalization for heart failure and digoxin toxicity. The results are summarized in Table 2.

Risk of Death in the DIG Study

The risk of death for all causes in the patients receiving digoxin (experimental event rate) was 1,181/3,397, or 34.7%. The risk in the placebo group (control event rate) is 1,194/3,403, or 35%. The risk difference is 34.7 - 35.0 = -0.3%. In absolute numbers, this is the absolute risk reduction (ARR), 0.3% (Table 3).

The relative risk, or risk ratio (RR), is 34.7/35, or 0.99, with a 95% confidence interval (CI) of 0.91 to 1.07. This confidence interval includes "1," or the possibility that the two true risks can be identical. Therefore, this difference is reported as not statistically significant.

The relative risk reduction (RRR) is 1 minus RR, or 1 minus 0.99, or 0.01. The confidence interval includes a reduction of 0 or no risk reduction.

Risk of Hospitalization in the DIG Study

The risk of hospitalization for worsening heart failure in the patients receiving digoxin is 910/3,391, or 0.27, and the same risk in the subjects receiving placebo is 1,180/3,403, or 0.35. Therefore, the ARR = |0.27 - 0.35| = 0.08.

The RR is 910/1,180, or 0.77 (95% CI, 0.66 to 0.79). The confidence interval does not include 1, so this risk difference is statistically significant.

The RRR = 1 minus RR, or 1 - 0.77 = 0.23. This is often the statistic used in pharmaceutical promotional material because it usually shows the largest effect: "Digoxin causes a 23% reduction in the risk of hospitalization for worsening heart failure." Even though this number is large, if the baseline risk of hospitalization for worsening heart failure is small, a difference of 23% may not have clinical importance.

Table 2.—Results of Digitalis Investigation Group Study

	All deaths	Hospitalization for worsening heart failure	Hospitalization for digoxin toxicity	Total no. of patients randomized
Digoxin	1,181	910	67	3,397
Placebo	1,194	1,180	31	3,403

Table 3.—Summary of Equations

$$ARR = |EER-CER| \qquad RRR = \frac{1-EER}{CER}$$

$$NNT = \frac{1}{ARR} \qquad RR = \frac{EER}{CER}$$

ARR, absolute risk reduction; CER, control event rate; EER, experimental event rate; NNT, number needed to treat; RR, relative risk (or risk ratio); RRR, relative risk reduction.

Number Needed to Treat

A number that better reflects the absolute baseline risks and the difference between them is the "number needed to treat" (NNT). NNT is the number of patients that need to receive the intervention to prevent one bad outcome. This is calculated as the reciprocal of the ARR. For the outcome "hospitalizations for worsening heart failure," the NNT is $1/(8/100) = 13$ (95% CI, 10 to 18). This number is expressed as "13 patients with heart failure who are taking ACE inhibitors and diuretics need to take digoxin for 37 months to prevent one hospitalization because of worsening heart failure." The CI is narrow, and the ends of the CI are clinically equivalent.

The true value for the total population lies within the CI, with 95% certainty. If the CI is wide, careful interpretation of the ends is suggested. This becomes evident when an unfavorable risk-to-benefit ratio arises, while accepting one extreme of the CI as the true value.

In negative studies (those in which the confidence interval crosses the line of no difference or those that show no statistically significant difference), comparing the clinical significance of the low end and the high end might help identify a beneficial trend in those receiving the intervention. This trend may or may not be confirmed by larger trials with narrower confidence intervals. A table (Table 4) with NNT in cardiology can help to compare effect sizes from different interventions.

Number Needed to Harm

A similar concept is the "number needed to harm" (NNH). This is the number of patients who need to receive the intervention for one patient to suffer a bad outcome. We can use the numbers in the fourth column of Table 2 ("Hospitalization for digoxin toxicity"): In this case, the

ARI (absolute risk increase) = $|(67/3,397) - (31/3,403)|$ = $|0.019 - 0.009| = 0.01$, or $1/100$. The NNH is $1/ARI$, or $1/(1/100)$, or 100. This number is expressed as "100 patients with heart failure who are receiving ACE inhibitors and diuretics need to receive digoxin for 37 months for one of them to need hospitalization due to digoxin toxicity."

In summary, for each 100 patients who receive digoxin, approximately 8 will benefit and 1 will be harmed.

Are the Results Applicable to the Care of *This* Patient?

A first approach to answer this question is to look at the inclusion and the exclusion criteria of the published study and compare these with the patient's characteristics. Would my patient be eligible for this study? Because most trials have narrow inclusion criteria, most patients would not be eligible but could still benefit from the intervention.

It is more important to establish what is so different about *this* patient that would render an otherwise efficacious intervention ineffective. The difference between the average study subject and *this* patient can be in any of the categories in Table 5.

For instance, a patient with class I heart failure and a physician-estimated 5% risk of being admitted to the hospital for worsening heart failure in 37 months receives digoxin in addition to an ACE inhibitor and a diuretic. In the DIG study population, this risk of hospitalization was 35%. Therefore, the risk of hospitalization of this patient is about 1/7 that of the average study participant. The NNT for a beneficial outcome in the study (13) needs to be divided by 1/7 to obtain an estimate of the NNT for this patient, or 91.

Thus, the benefit of digoxin for this low-risk patient is less than that for the study patients. Therefore, NNT changes with the patient baseline risk—thus, the frequently observed finding in cardiology that sicker patients generally derive greater benefit from therapeutic interventions and low-risk patients have less to gain.

If the patient has differences that would cause the treatment to be less efficacious (in decreasing the risk of a bad outcome), the NNT would also be higher, reflecting changes in the risk difference. The NNT also changes depending on the length of follow-up, but estimates are less precise because the risk does not necessarily increase linearly with time (sometimes the risk is higher early after the exposure and decreases with time, i.e., the risk of fatal arrhythmias after myocardial infarction).

Table 4.—Numbers Needed to Treat (NNT)

Intervention	Outcome	NNT
Myocardial infarction (MI)		
Streptokinase alone (vs. nothing) ISIS-2	Prevent 1 death at 5 wk	40
Aspirin alone (vs. nothing) ISIS-2	Prevent 1 death at 5 wk	40
Streptokinase + aspirin (vs. nothing) ISIS-2	Prevent 1 death at 5 wk	20
tPA	Hemorrhage stroke	500
Streptokinase	Hemorrhagic stroke	1,000
tPA vs. streptokinase (GUSTO)	Save 1 life with tPA vs. streptokinase	100
Thrombolytic therapy 5 hr earlier	Save 1 life	100
Heart failure		
Enalapril in class IV CHF (NYHA)	Prevent 1 death at 1 yr	6
Enalapril in class I or II CHF (NYHA)	Prevent 1 death at 1 yr	100
Others		
CABG in left main stenosis	Prevent 1 death at 2 yr	6
Carotid endarterectomy in high-grade symptomatic stenosis	Prevent 1 stroke or death in 2 yr	9
Simple antihypertensives for severe hypertension	Prevent 1 stroke, MI, or death in 1 yr	15
Simple antihypertensives for mild hypertension	Prevent 1 stroke, MI, or death in 1 yr	700
Aspirin in unstable angina	Prevent MI or death in 1 yr	25
Aspirin in healthy US physician	Prevent MI or death in 1 yr	500
Treating hypertension in the over-60s	Prevent 1 coronary event	18
Simvastatin vs. placebo in CHD	Prevent 1 coronary death over 5 yr	29
Simvastatin vs. placebo in CHD	Prevent 1 major coronary event over 5 yr	15

CABG, coronary artery bypass grafting; CHD, coronary heart disease; CHF, congestive heart failure; NYHA, New York Heart Association; tPA, tissue plasminogen activator.
From Bandolier at www.jr2.ox.ac.uk/bandolier (Jan. 10, 1999).

In summary, the "number needed to treat" and the "number needed to harm" can describe the results of therapeutic interventions. These numbers are easy to extract from the published reports and are useful in comparing interventions and explaining the efficacy of these interventions to patients. The estimate of the true effect of an intervention should be analyzed in the context of the confidence interval for that estimate. The applicability of a study result should be judged by identifying the differences between the particular patient and the average study subject.

Diagnostic Decisions

In the study of Khan MA, et al. (A normal electrocardiogram precludes the need for left ventriculography in the assessment of coronary artery disease. *Heart* 79: 262-267, 1998), the aim was to "assess whether a normal electrocardiogram (ECG) can identify good left ventricular function and obviate the need for routine left ventriculography in patients undergoing cardiac catheterization for suspected coronary artery disease." The study was a prospective assessment of 391 patients in whom ECG (test) and ventriculography (reference standard) were performed. A cardiologist described the ECG as normal or abnormal and left ventricular function was assessed by ventriculography. The results are summarized in Table 6.

The diagnostic features of the test (ECG) can be described as follows:

Sensitivity

Sensitivity—the proportion of patients with the condition of interest who have a positive test. If the test has a high sensitivity and it is negative, it rules out the disease (SnNout). This is defined by the true positives (a) over the total number of subjects with the condition or true positives (a) + false negatives (b).

Table 5.—Possible Differences Between Average Study Patient and a Particular Patient

Issues	Differences that may diminish treatment response
Biologic	1. Pathophysiologic differences in the illness
	2. Patient differences
Socioeconomic	3. Differences in patient compliance
	4. Differences in provider compliance
Epidemiologic	5. Comorbid conditions that would change the risk:benefit ratio
	6. Differences in untreated patient's risks of adverse outcomes

Modified from JAMA 279:545-549, 1998. By permission of the American Medical Association.

$$Sensitivity = \frac{a}{a+b}$$

$$Sensitivity = 52/54 = 96.3\%$$

Specificity

Specificity—the proportion of patients without the condition of interest who have a negative test. If the test has a high specificity and it is positive, it rules in the disease (SpPin). This is measured by the true negatives (d) over the total number of subjects without the condition, or true negatives (d) + false positives (c).

$$Specificity = \frac{d}{c+d}$$

$$Specificity = 136/337 = 40.4\%$$

Positive Predictive Value

Positive predictive value is the proportion of patients with a positive test result who have the condition of interest. This is defined by true positives (a) over all positives, or true positives (a) and false positives (c).

$$PPV = \frac{a}{a+c}$$

$$PPV = 52/253 = 20.5\%$$

Table 6.—2 x 2 Table Comparing Test and Reference Standard

		Reference standard		
		EF < 50%	EF ≥ 50%	Total
Test	Abnormal ECG	52 / a	201 / c	253 / a+c
	Normal ECG	b / 2	d / 136	b+c / 138
	Total	a+b / 54	c+d / 337	a+b+c+d / 391

ECG, electrocardiogram; EF, ejection fraction.

Negative Predictive Value

Negative predictive value is the proportion of patients with a negative test result who do not have the condition of interest. This is defined by the proportion of true negatives (d) over all negatives, or true negatives (d) + false negatives (b).

$$NPV = \frac{d}{b+d}$$

$$NPV = 136/138 = 98.5\%$$

Likelihood Ratio of a Positive Test (+LR)

This is the ratio of the likelihood of having a positive test in disease and the likelihood of having a positive test in the absence of disease.

$$+LR = (a/a+b)/(c/c+d)$$

$$+LR = \frac{Sensitivity}{1\text{-}Specificity}$$

$$+LR = 1.61$$

Likelihood Ratio of a Negative Test (-LR)

This is the ratio of the likelihood of having a negative test in disease and the likelihood of having a negative test in the absence of disease.

$$-LR = (b/a+b)/(d/c+d)$$

$$-LR = \frac{1\text{-}Sensitivity}{Specificity}$$

$$-LR = 0.09$$

The pretest probability for a low ventricular ejection fraction in a certain patient can be estimated from the history and physical examination data. The post-test probability can be calculated (via odds) by means of knowing the pretest probability and the likelihood ratio.

$$\text{Probability} = \frac{\text{Odds}}{\text{Odds} + 1}$$

Pretest Odds x LR = Post-test Odds

An alternative to this calculation is to use a nomogram (Fig. 2) that relates the LR with the pretest and post-test probabilities. If a test is positive, use the +LR. Note that a +LR is usually greater than 1 and gives a higher post-test probability than the pretest probability. A -LR is usually less than 1 and gives a lower post-test probability than the pretest probability. When the pretest probability is between 30% and 70%, test results with a high LR rule in disease. A very low LR virtually rules out the disease. A test with an LR of 1 does not change the pretest probability of disease after the application of the test.

If a patient has a normal ECG (negative test), the high sensitivity (96.3%) allows us to rule out left ventricular ejection fraction less than 50% (SnNout). The negative predictive value is 98.5%, and the negative likelihood ratio is 0.09.

If the pretest probability of having a low ejection fraction in this patient is 40%, then

Odds = Prob/1-Prob
Pretest Odds = 0.4/(1-0.4) or 0.66
Post-test Odds = Pretest Odds x LR *or*
0.66 x 0.09 = 0.059

$$\text{Post-test Probability} = \frac{0.059}{1 + 0.059} = 5.6\%$$

The nomogram (Fig. 2) also shows a similar result (dashed line). This demonstrates how having a normal ECG moderately decreases the probability of having a low ventricular ejection fraction.

In the study population, the prevalence {a+b/(a+b+c+d)} of an ejection fraction less than 50% is 13.8%. Given the pretest probability of 13.8%, the application of the -LR would give a post-test probability of 1% (solid line on nomogram). The likelihood ratio is independent of the prevalence (as opposed to the predictive value that depends on the prevalence of disease in the study population). If the prevalence that was used to calculate the predicted value is similar to the pretest probability of the condition in the population of interest, then the post-test

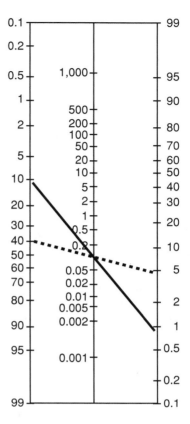

Fig. 2. Nomogram relating likelihood ratio with pre- and post-test probabilities. (From *N Engl J Med* 293:257, 1975. By permission of the Massachusetts Medical Society.)

probability and the predicted value will be similar.

Is a probability of ventricular dysfunction of 5.6% low enough to change the decision to obtain a ventriculogram? Is a probability of 1% low enough?

The "action threshold" is the likelihood of disease above which additional action would cause more good than harm and below which it will cause more harm than benefit. The action threshold justifies performing a test that would move the likelihood of disease above the threshold and change management.

If our test misses patients with a left ventricular ejection fraction less than 50%, this means missing an opportunity to add an ACE inhibitor and to decrease mortality. If 100 patients present with a normal ECG, the negative predictive value indicates that 99 patients will have a normal left ventricular ejection fraction. According to the study, the patient who was missed would have an ejection fraction between 40% and 50% and would not benefit from ACE inhibition. Therefore, the negative test is useful in patients with a low (around 13.8%) pretest probability for an ejection fraction less than 50% because it keeps the likelihood of disease below the action threshold and allows the physician to forego ventriculography (performing ventriculography will expose patients to more harm than benefit).

In patients with a higher pretest probability (i.e., those with a history of anterior myocardial infarction and symptoms and signs of heart failure), the test will not perform as well and more patients with left ventricular dysfunction will be missed (5.6% if the pretest probability is 40%). In this setting, a negative test will keep the likelihood of disease above the action threshold and ventriculography will be performed regardless of the ECG interpretation. This behavior will provide the benefits of ACE inhibition to most patients with a low ejection fraction.

> In summary, diagnostic tests are defined by comparison with a reference standard. A negative high-sensitivity test rules out the disease (SnNout). A positive high-specificity test rules in the disease (SpPin). The predictive values depend on the prevalence of the condition in the study sample. The +LR is Sensitivity/(1-Specificity). The -LR is (1-Sensitivity)/Specificity. LR x Pretest Odds = Post-test Odds. Odds = Probability/(1-Probability). The post-test probability of disease should be above the action threshold for a diagnostic intervention to be more likely to cause benefit than harm.

Trial Evidence for the Practice of Cardiology

The following are examples of well-documented evidence-based treatments in cardiology based primarily on well-conducted randomized clinical trials. The list is not exhaustive.

Preventive Cardiology

Tobacco
Smoking cessation reduces the risk of cardiovascular events.

Lipids
Statins reduce the risk of cardiovascular events in patients with documented ischemic heart disease and hyperlipidemia (4S, CARE trials) and in asymptomatic middle-aged men with hyperlipidemia (WOSCOP)

Physical Exercise
Physical exercise decreases cardiovascular mortality and increases exercise tolerance in patients who have had a myocardial infarction.

Physical exercise decreases symptoms of heart failure in patients with left ventricular dysfunction

Homocysteine
Increased levels of homocysteine may be causally linked to vascular disease. Folate supplementation of the diet reduces serum levels of homocysteine.

Estrogen Replacement Therapy
Estrogen replacement therapy that is initiated for other reasons may be an effective second-line lipid-lowering agent.

Estrogen replacement on its own should not be used for the prevention or treatment of ischemic heart disease (HERS study)

Stable Coronary Artery Disease

Stable angina
β-Blockers prolong life after myocardial infarction (MIAMI Trial).

Coronary Artery Bypass Grafting (CABG) vs. Medical Therapy (ECSS, VA, CASS, MA trials)
CABG is beneficial for symptom relief in medically refractory angina pectoris. In chronic stable angina pectoris, CABG prolongs life more than conventional medical treatment in the following patient subsets: hemodynamically significant left main coronary disease (> 50% stenosis – VA trial), three-vessel disease (> 70%) irrespective of the presence or degree of left ventricular function, two-vessel coronary artery disease in association with left ventricular dysfunction (ejection fraction < 40%), or proximal left anterior descending coronary artery disease (> 70%).

Percutaneous Transluminal Coronary Angioplasty (PTCA) vs. Medical Therapy
PTCA is indicated for symptom relief in patients with myocardial ischemia not responding adequately to conventional antianginal medication.

PTCA is not indicated for treatment of an angiographic stenosis in the absence of spontaneous or exercise-induced myocardial ischemia.

PTCA may be beneficial for severe myocardial ischemia, regardless of symptoms.

PTCA vs. CABG
PTCA and CABG can both provide excellent symptom relief, but PTCA alone leads to the need for repeat revascularization

procedures (either a second PTCA or CABG) more often than CABG.

Intracoronary stenting is associated with less restenosis than PTCA (STRESS and BENESTENT Trials), but it has not been compared directly with CABG in a randomized controlled trial.

CABG may be more beneficial than PTCA in diabetic patients with two- or three-vessel disease. For nondiabetic patients with multivessel disease, CABG and PTCA have similar benefit, but CABG is preferable for high-risk patients and more repeat revascularization procedures will be needed after PTCA.

Acute Ischemic Syndromes

β-Blockers, aspirin, nitrates, and heparin are beneficial in acute ischemic coronary syndromes.

Calcium channel blockers have no documented benefit in acute coronary syndromes in the absence of coronary vasospasm.

Calcium channel blockers and nitrates are the treatment of choice for vasospastic angina.

Aspirin reduces future cardiovascular events in patients after myocardial infarction or stroke and in patients with stable or unstable angina or peripheral vascular disease.

GPIIb/IIIa inhibitors are beneficial in unstable angina and after coronary interventions: abciximab (EPILOG trial), tirofiban (PRISM and PRISM-PLUS trials), integrilin (PURSUIT trial).

Heparin is superior to aspirin alone in unstable angina (Montreal Trial).

Low-molecular-weight heparin (enoxaparin) is superior to unfractionated heparin in unstable angina/non-Q-wave myocardial infarction (ESSENCE Trial).

Early noninvasive management of non-Q-wave myocardial infarction with a later stratification strategy to select patients for invasive investigation is better than an early invasive strategy (VANQUISH Trial).

● Patients in whom medical therapy for unstable angina fails should have coronary angiography.

Acute Myocardial Infarction

Thrombolysis decreases mortality in patients with ST-segment elevation myocardial infarction and in those with new left bundle branch block and symptoms consistent with myocardial infarction. The mortality benefit is greatest in patients who receive early thrombolysis (< 6 hours after coronary artery occlusion), but benefit may still accrue to patients receiving late thrombolysis ((LATE, EMERAS trials). Patients older than 75 years also benefit from thrombolysis.

Thrombolysis is not beneficial in patients with ST-depression myocardial infarction.

β-Blocker treatment should be started in all myocardial infarction patients within 24 hours after the onset of symptoms and continue for at least 2 years, unless contraindicated. ACE inhibitor treatment should be started the first day after myocardial infarction unless contraindicated. The mortality benefit with ACE inhibitors after myocardial infarction is greater in patients with heart failure, anterior myocardial infarction, or left ventricular dysfunction (SAVE, AIRE, TRACE, SMILE trials).

Routine administration of magnesium or lidocaine to myocardial infarction patients is not indicated. Warfarin for 6 months decreases the incidence of cardiac thromboembolism in patients with documented intracavitary thrombus.

Low-dose warfarin in addition to low-dose aspirin did not improve overall outcome after myocardial infarction (CARS Trial).

Primary PTCA is the preferable treatment for acute myocardial infarction in patients at high risk for stroke (GUSTO-1, GUSTO-2, PAMI), in cardiogenic shock, or those with contraindications to thrombolysis.

Heart Failure

Digoxin reduces hospitalizations for heart failure and improves clinical symptoms and exercise capacity (DIG trial).

Vasodilators are beneficial for short-term relief of acute pulmonary edema.

The combination of hydralazine and isosorbide dinitrate is indicated for patients with chronic heart failure who do not tolerate ACE inhibitors (VHeFT-1).

Diuretics reduce symptoms and improve exercise capacity in heart failure but have never been documented to improve survival.

ACE inhibitors decrease mortality and symptoms in patients with symptomatic heart failure and asymptomatic patients with left ventricular dysfunction. (CONSENSUS, SOLVD, SAVE trials).

ACE inhibitors are beneficial for patients after myocardial infarction, especially those with a left ventricular ejection fraction less than 35% (SOLVD) or less than 40% (SAVE).

Inotropic agents provide short-term improvement in symptoms of patients with severe congestive heart failure but do not prolong survival.

β-Blockers improve survival, cardiac function, and symptoms in patients receiving conventional heart failure therapy.

Acute Myocarditis and Dilated Cardiomyopathy

Corticosteroids are beneficial for giant cell myocarditis, hypersensitivity myocarditis, and cardiac sarcoidosis.

Questions

The studies of angiotensin-converting enzyme (ACE) inhibition in heart failure provided the following findings:

    a. CONSENSUS: in patients with New York Heart Association (NYHA) class IV heart failure, 1 year of treatment with enalapril reduced the risk of dying by 36%. The placebo arm experienced a mortality of 52%.

    b. SOLVD I: 25 patients with NYHA class II-III heart failure need to receive enalapril for 1 year to prevent one death. Enalapril reduced the risk of dying at 1 year by 25%.

    c. SOLVD II: in patients with NYHA class I-II heart failure, the 3-year mortality in the placebo group was 16% and 15% in the enalapril group.

1. Which study provides the smallest relative risk reduction?

2. Which study shows the smallest "number needed to treat" (NNT)?

3. Which patients benefit the most from the use of enalapril?

In the study of Khan MA et al. (A normal electrocardiogram precludes the need for left ventriculography in the assessment of coronary artery disease. *Heart* 79:262-267, 1998), the results of a cardiology fellow's assessment of 391 ECG tracings were used to measure the ability of ECG testing to predict normal or abnormal ventricular ejection fraction. The trainee interpreted 170 ECG tracings as normal. The prevalence of an ejection fraction less than 50% in the study population was 13.8%. The ECG as read by the fellow had a specificity of 49.5%.

4. Calculate the negative predictive value and the likelihood ratio for a negative test.

5. You decide to reproduce the study in a population that has a 25% prevalence of an ejection fraction less than 50%. The same fellow will read the ECG tracings. If you decide that ventriculography will be performed if the probability of a low ejection fraction is more than 3%, is it worth having the fellow read the ECG tracings before catheterization to decide whether ventriculography will be performed?

Answers

1. c; 2. a; 3. a

Trial	Placebo	Enalapril	RRR	ARR	NNT*
Consensus	0.52	0.36	0.31	0.16	7
SOLVD I	0.16	0.12	0.25	0.04	25
SOLVD II	0.16	0.15	0.06	0.01	100

*The number needed to treat for 1 year to prevent 1 death, except for SOLVD II in which the observation period was 3 years.

4. Sensitivity = 51/54 = 94.4%; specificity = 49.5%; NPV = 167/170 = 98.2%; -LR = (1 - 0.944)/0.495 = 0.113

5. Pretest odds = 0.25/(1 - 0.25) = 0.33; -LR = 0.113; post-test odds = 0.33 x 0.113 = 0.037. Post-test probability = 0.037/1 + 0.037 = 0.035, or 3.5%. Because this is greater than 3%, the test will not change my decision to perform ventriculography; therefore, the ECG is not worth doing in this population.

	Ejection fraction		
	< 50%	≥ 50%	Total
ECG abnormal	51	170	221
ECG normal	3	167	170
Total	54	337	391

Chapter 67

Heart Disease in the Elderly Patient

Joseph G. Murphy, M.D.
R. Scott Wright, M.D.

> The differences in the presentation and management of cardiovascular disease between the elderly patient and the nonelderly patient are important clinical and examination issues.

Age-Related Changes in Cardiac Anatomy and Physiology

Ventricle

Heart weight increases about 1 g/year between ages 30 and 90 years, probably due to left ventricular hypertrophy secondary to an age-related increase in systolic blood pressure. This results in an increase in both left ventricular mass and wall thickness. In addition to myocardial cell mass, intercellular collagen also increases with age.

Ventricular hypertrophy leads to significant changes in cardiac function with age, including 1) an increase in left ventricular stiffness; 2) reduced filling during early diastole; and 3) a prolonged diastolic isometric relaxation phase. There is a reduction in the length of the left ventricle from apex to base with the development of an S-, or sigmoid-, shaped septum in some patients.

Conduction System

There are marked changes in the conduction system, including loss of 50% to 75% of the pacemaker cells of the sinoatrial node and fibrosis of the specialized conduction tissue of the bundle of His.

Interestingly, some parameters of cardiac function do not change with age, including resting cardiac output, stroke volume, and ejection fraction. Although systolic function is well preserved in the elderly, diastolic function declines as a result of a slowing down of calcium accumulation by the sarcoplasmic reticulum.

- Systolic function is well preserved in the elderly, but diastolic function is impaired.

Atrial Fibrillation

Atrial fibrillation occurs in 5% of women and 6% of men older than 65 years and is frequently asymptomatic. Independent risk factors for a thromboembolic event in patients with atrial fibrillation include age, diabetes, hypertension, a history of heart failure, a prior transient ischemic attack or stroke, an enlarged left atrium, and poor left ventricular function. Warfarin reduces the risk of stroke by about two-thirds. Age is an independent risk factor for hemorrhagic complications with warfarin therapy, as are poorly controlled hypertension and excessive anticoagulation. Overall, the benefits of warfarin therapy outweigh the bleeding risks in the elderly population, and in general warfarin is indicated for the prophylaxis of thromboembolic events in most elderly patients in atrial fibrillation. Aspirin provides some protection from stroke in elderly patients when warfarin anticoagulation is contraindicated.

The diagnosis of atrial fibrillation may be subtle in the elderly. Atrial fibrillation can worsen or precipitate heart failure and angina in the elderly patient, and the worsening or new onset of these symptoms should merit a search for arrhythmias, including atrial fibrillation. Mental status changes, stroke, or a transient ischemic attack also may be the presenting symptoms for new-onset atrial fibrillation. Occult hyperthyroidism, silent myocardial infarction, hypokalemia due to use of a diuretic, alcoholism, and digoxin toxicity may present with atrial fibrillation. Pulmonary disease, including pneumonia, pulmonary embolism, and chronic obstructive lung disease, may precipitate atrial fibrillation, especially if β-agonists are used.

- Atrial fibrillation occurs in 5% of women and 6% of men older than 65 years.
- Age is an independent risk factor for hemorrhagic complications with warfarin therapy in the elderly.
- Warfarin reduces the stroke risk by about two-thirds.

Bradycardias

Aging is associated with an increased occurrence of conduction system fibrosis within the sinus node, atrioventricular node, and bundle branches. Sympathetic and parasympathetic neural influence on the conduction system decreases. Maximal heart rate decreases with age, and sinus bradycardia is common in the elderly even in the absence of cardiac disease. The elderly are more dependent than younger patients on atrial systole to complete late ventricular diastolic filling. Pacemakers are effective therapy for symptomatic bradycardia in the elderly. Dual-chamber pacemakers that allow atrioventricular synchrony are beneficial if sinus rhythm is present, and they may decrease the future occurrence of atrial fibrillation.

- Maximal heart rate decreases with age.

Coronary Artery Disease

Dyspnea is a more common presenting symptom of coronary artery disease in the elderly patient than in the younger patient. A fourth heart sound and a soft mitral regurgitation murmur are frequently present in many elderly patients and are poor predictors of the presence of coronary artery disease. The treatment of coronary artery disease in the elderly is similar to that in younger patients. Coronary artery bypass and percutaneous transluminal coronary angioplasty are both very effective in the elderly but are associated with a somewhat higher morbidity and mortality rate.

- A fourth heart sound and a soft mitral regurgitation murmur are poor predictors of the presence of coronary artery disease in the elderly.

Myocardial Infarction

Myocardial infarction is associated with a higher mortality rate, a higher incidence of congestive cardiac failure, and a higher reinfarction rate in the elderly patient than in the younger patient. Fewer elderly patients with myocardial infarction are eligible for thrombolysis because of contraindications (such as stroke, transient ischemic attack, severe hypertension, bleeding), and in those without contraindications, thrombolytics are used less often because of the higher occurrence of late and atypical presentations of myocardial infarction. The diagnosis of myocardial infarction is more difficult in the elderly; dyspnea and pulmonary edema are the most common presentation symptoms. Electrocardiography frequently is nondiagnostic because of baseline electrocardiographic abnormalities. In the elderly, small myocardial infarctions may be associated with increased levels of creatine kinase-MB without an increase in the total creatine kinase level. Non–Q-wave myocardial infarction, cardiogenic shock, cardiac rupture, and death due to electromechanical dissociation are more common. The size of a first infarct does not increase with age, and death from ventricular fibrillation is less common than in the younger patient with infarction. Both primary angioplasty and thrombolysis are beneficial in the elderly patient with myocardial infarction who has ST-segment elevation, but angioplasty is not associated with the excess rate of stroke that occurs with use of thrombolysis in the elderly. The indications for adjunctive angioplasty after myocardial infarction in the elderly are similar to those in younger patients and include the occurrence of exercise-induced or spontaneous ischemia.

- Elderly patients with myocardial infarction are less often candidates for thrombolysis.
- Primary angioplasty is not associated with the excess stroke rate that occurs with use of thrombolytics in the elderly.

Stress Testing

Treadmill exercise stress testing is less useful in the elderly population because of the higher occurrence of resting ST-segment changes, higher use of digoxin, and the increased incidence of peripheral vascular, orthopedic, and lung disease that limit exercise capacity. The predictive accuracy of a negative stress test is lower in the elderly patient because of the higher occurrence of coronary artery disease. Pharmacologic stress tests (dobutamine, adenosine, or dipyridamole echocardiography or nuclear imaging) are useful in the elderly patient. Stress testing with cardiac imaging has a sensitivity of 80% to 90% and a specificity of 70% to 80%.

- The predictive accuracy of a negative stress test is lower in the elderly patient.

Lipid Management

There is controversy about the value of aggressive lipid management in the elderly patient, and objective data are few. The Scandinavian 4S study documented the benefit of cholesterol reduction with use of simvastatin on cardiac mortality and morbidity in a secondary prevention study that contained elderly patients. Estrogen replacement therapy reduces cardiovascular mortality in postmenopausal women.

Hypertension

The rate of hypertension in persons older than 65 years is approximately 50%. Treating hypertension in the elderly, including isolated systolic hypertension (Systolic Hypertension in the Elderly Program, SHEP trial, which used a thiazide diuretic or a β-blocker), significantly reduces morbidity and mortality. This benefit extends to the primary end point of stroke and the secondary end point of myocardial infarction.

Valvular Heart Disease

Calcific aortic stenosis, usually due to degenerative changes in a tricuspid valve, is the most common valvular heart disease in the elderly. The physical signs of aortic stenosis may be masked in the elderly. The classic parvus and tardus pulse of severe aortic stenosis may be absent because of increased arterial stiffness, and benign systolic murmurs due to aortic sclerosis without stenosis are frequent. Aortic valve replacement is superior to balloon aortic valvuloplasty in all but moribund patients with severe aortic stenosis. Mitral regurgitation due to papillary muscle dysfunction resulting from ischemia and myxomatous degeneration of the mitral valve apparatus are both frequent in the elderly. Mitral stenosis is usually the late result of rheumatic fever. The opening snap of mitral stenosis may be absent in the elderly patient because of valve calcification. The intensity of the first heart sound also may be reduced for similar reasons. Balloon mitral valvuloplasty is less successful in the elderly patient with mitral stenosis because of the increased occurrence of valvular and subvalvular calcification.

- The physical signs of aortic stenosis may be masked in the elderly.
- The opening snap of mitral stenosis may be absent in the elderly.

Congestive Heart Failure

Heart failure may occur in up to 10% of patients older than 80 years, and in many cases it is due to pure diastolic ventricular dysfunction. The elderly are relatively more dependent on the Frank-Starling stretch response and less dependent on heart rate to increase cardiac output in response to exercise. Systolic ventricular dysfunction is usually caused by ischemic, hypertensive, or valvular heart disease. The impaired ability of the kidneys to excrete a fluid challenge also may contribute to fluid overload. The factors that lead to ventricular diastolic dysfunction and heart failure in the elderly include an impaired ventricular relaxation time and an increase in myocardial stiffness, leading to an increase in left ventricular diastolic filling pressure. Echocardiography is the imaging method of choice to diagnose diastolic ventricular dysfunction. Treatment of diastolic ventricular dysfunction is with angiotensin-converting enzyme inhibitors or calcium channel blockers, especially in the setting of hypertension. Diuretics may exacerbate diastolic ventricular dysfunction.

- The elderly are relatively more dependent on the Frank-Starling stretch response and less dependent on heart rate to increase cardiac output.

Cardiac Drugs

Elderly patients in general have a decreased lean body mass, decreased serum proteins, decreased glomerular filtration rate, and decreased hepatic microsomal oxidation compared with nonelderly patients. The rates of left ventricular dysfunction and conduction system disease are higher. Renal clearance of digoxin, quinidine, and procainamide is decreased, and drug toxicity occurs more easily than in younger patients.

In the Cardiac Arrhythmia Suppression Trial (CAST study), the incidence of proarrhythmia was higher in elderly patients than in younger patients with the antiarrhythmic agents flecainide, encainide, and moricizine. Adverse drug reactions are at least doubled in the elderly, and patient compliance with drug regimens is poorer. The elderly have blunted baroreceptor reflexes and diminished β-receptor responsiveness.

- Adverse drug reactions are at least doubled in the elderly.

Chapter 68

Heart Disease in Women

Sharonne N. Hayes, M.D.

Cardiovascular disease is the number one cause of death in women, outnumbering deaths from all other causes combined. Each year almost 500,000 women have myocardial infarction and more than 250,000 die of coronary artery disease. Combined with stroke, hypertension, and other vascular disease, more than 500,000 women die annually of cardiovascular disease (Fig. 1). Although virtually all women can readily quote the lifetime incidence of breast cancer (1 in 9), few realize that 50% (1 in 2) of all women will *die* of cardiovascular disease, compared with 4% (1 in 25) who die of breast cancer. Because of the higher proportion of women in the aging population, each year more women die of cardiovascular disease than men. Whereas the death rate from cardiovascular disease in men has declined steadily during the last 20 years, the rate has remained relatively the same for women (Fig. 2). Black women have a 71% greater age-adjusted death rate from coronary artery disease than white women.

- 50% of women will die of cardiovascular disease.
- The death rate from cardiovascular disease in women has remained relatively unchanged in the last 20 years.

Despite the magnitude of the problem in women, much less information about optimal primary and secondary prevention strategies, diagnostic modalities, and responses to medical and surgical treatments is available for women than for men. This lack of data reflects several factors, including the exclusion of women from many older clinical trials, a lower prevalence of symptomatic coronary artery disease in women than in men until age 70, hormonal effects and gender differences in presenting symptoms, and relative effects of various risk factors. These uncertainties have contributed to inaction and nontreatment of women because of the lack of gender-specific data or to the assumption that data resulting from male-only studies apply equally to women. The inaction and nontreatment approach has led to missed opportunities for life-saving interventions and preventive measures and the assumption of data equivalency approach has led to possibly harmful overly conservative or aggressive measures in women.

A knowledge gap still exists in many areas of cardiovascular care for women; however, the National Institutes of Health no longer funds studies that do not include women subjects unless there is a compelling explanation for not doing so.

Gender Differences Versus Gender Bias

Clear gender differences have been identified in the epidemiology and presentation of disease, risk factor prevalence, physiology, and response to diagnostic tests and interventions (Table 1). Also, there are several factors that solely or predominately affect women, including menopausal status, hormone replacement therapy, oral contraceptives, and pregnancy-related heart disease. During the last decade, several studies have noted important gender differences in

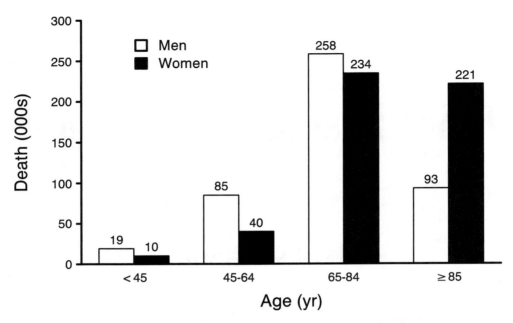

Fig. 1. Death from cardiovascular disease, by age and gender. (Modified from 1998 Heart and Stroke Statistical Update. National Center for Health Statistics and the American Heart Association 1995.)

clinical outcomes and use of diagnostic and therapeutic drugs and interventions, especially in the evaluation and treatment of women with chest pain and myocardial infarction. The concern has been raised that women are evaluated less intensively, underreferred, and not treated as aggressively as men for comparable presentation and disease. In one study, 10 times as many men with abnormal nuclear stress study results were referred to coronary angiography than women with similar results, and women with abnormal test results were more than 4 times as likely to have their symptoms attributed to a psychiatric cause. Other studies have shown little or no difference in the evaluation and management of cardiac disease.

Much of the difference and apparent bias demonstrated in these studies can be attributed to differences in baseline characteristics, but some investigators have been concerned that the almost universally worse outcomes of cardiovascular disease in women cannot be explained completely by

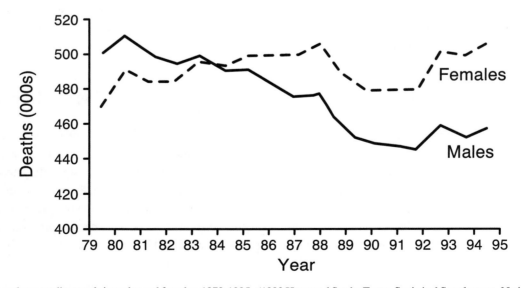

Fig. 2. Cardiovascular mortality trends in males and females, 1979-1995. (1999 Heart and Stroke Facts: Statistical Supplement. National Center for Health Statistics and the American Heart Association 1995.)

Table 1.—Known Gender Differences That May Affect Diagnosis, Treatment, and Outcomes for Heart Disease

Epidemiology and prevalence
Age
Etiology
Presenting symptoms
Risk factor prevalence and strengths
Comorbid conditions
Body and coronary artery size
Menopause and hormonal status
Myocardial responses to aging, blood pressure, and volume loads
Accuracy of diagnostic tests
Physiologic responses to exercise
Response to pharmacologic interventions
Psychosocial/economic factors
Communication style

statistically controlling for older age and comorbid conditions. Other authors contend that the results of these studies demonstrate that women may be receiving more "appropriate" care and that men are being "overtreated," but this view does not adequately explain the vast differences in the rates of diagnostic testing, revascularization procedures, and prescription of therapeutic drugs of proven benefit.

Ischemic Heart Disease

Evaluation of Chest Pain

Despite the important epidemiologic and clinical information on cardiac disease and risk factors that have resulted from the Framingham Study, this long-term longitudinal study is responsible for some of our early misconceptions about coronary artery disease in women. In the early 1970s, the Framingham group reported that more women than men (56% vs. 46%) have angina as their presenting symptom of cardiac disease, but more men who have angina go on to have myocardial infarction (25% vs. 14%). This led to the erroneous conclusion that angina is a benign condition in women. This misconception was clarified with publication of the results of the Coronary Artery Surgery Study (CASS), which showed that even in women with classic anginal symptoms, the rate of normal coronary arteries on angiography is approximately 50%, compared with less than 20% in men. In the Framingham Study, angina was defined clinically without angiographic confirmation of obstructive coronary artery lesions. Women are more likely to have a nonischemic cause of chest pain (mitral valve prolapse-associated chest pain and chest wall pain) that has a benign prognosis. Thus, it is likely that the early Framingham Study included a significant number of women with chest pain of a noncardiac nature who would be expected to have a benign clinical course. Reexamination of the data showed that the prognosis for older women who probably had true ischemia was actually worse than that for men in the Framingham Study.

Presenting Symptoms

On average, women with coronary artery disease present with symptoms, cardiac events, or sudden death 10 years later than men. Although the mechanism for this delay has not been explained completely, it likely is due largely to the protective effects of endogenous estrogen in premenopausal women. Most men and women present with "typical" symptoms of coronary artery disease; however, disproportionately more women present "atypically," with dyspnea, fatigue, or referred pain, perhaps because the characteristic symptoms were derived from studies of populations composed predominately of middle-aged men who are much younger than the majority of women with coronary artery disease. For women, advanced age, lower activity level, and comorbid conditions often contribute to the more frequent occurrence of silent ischemia, dyspnea, and other nonclassic symptoms. Many older women have the impression that coronary artery disease is a "widow maker" or a "man's disease" and attribute their chest pain or dyspnea to a benign cause and delay seeking treatment. Numerous studies have demonstrated that because of late presentation, women are less likely to be eligible for emergency percutaneous transluminal coronary angioplasty (PTCA) or thrombolysis for acute myocardial infarction and often have more advanced anatomical disease on coronary angiography.

- On average, women with coronary artery disease present with symptoms, cardiac events, or sudden death 10 years later than men.
- Women frequently present with atypical cardiac symptoms.

Stress Testing

The noninvasive diagnosis of coronary artery disease in women is challenging. Standard stress electrocardiographic testing is less accurate in women than in men and has led some practitioners to adopt a rather negative approach and to treat women empirically without further investigation or to use invasive testing exclusively. This attitude is not warranted and likely results in poor outcome. Numerous studies have examined the results of exercise electrocardiography in women and have found high false-positive rates in women compared with men, perhaps because of the lower prevalence of coronary artery disease in women until age 70. Also, there is evidence that the lower specificity is related to gender-specific autonomic and sex hormone effects on the electrocardiogram. In older women, failure to achieve an adequate stress level due to deconditioning or orthopedic limitation may adversely affect the sensitivity of an exercise test. Despite these limitations, normal findings on stress electrocardiography at an adequate workload in a woman are a good indicator that flow-limiting coronary artery disease is unlikely.

● Standard stress electrocardiographic testing is less accurate in women than in men.

Because of these limitations, imaging stress tests have gained popularity for women. However, gender-specific artifacts and physiologic responses have been described in both nuclear and echocardiographic stress studies. Historically, women have been underrepresented in studies of imaging stress tests, and the reported sensitivities and specificities have varied widely. Therefore, drawing conclusions about the absolute incremental value of stress imaging over standard stress testing is not possible.

● Gender-specific artifacts and physiologic responses have been described in both nuclear and echocardiographic stress studies.

The standard diagnostic criteria used for interpreting exercise radionuclide angiographic findings have not proved accurate in women. An abnormal result is defined as a lack of increase in ejection fraction with exercise. In men, the increase in stroke volume in response to exercise is caused by an increase in ejection fraction, whereas in women, it is caused by an increase in end-diastolic volume. As a result, up to one-third of women with normal coronary arteries do not have an increase in ejection fraction with exercise. Stress thallium (Tl-201) scintigraphy improves diagnostic accuracy in women, but many of the available studies relied on planar thallium rather than the more commonly used single-photon emission computed tomography. Breast tissue attenuates radioactivity and may produce a false-positive study as a result of artifactual defects in the anterior wall and septum. The use of technetium 99m (Tc 99m) sestamibi imaging, a higher energy radiotracer, reduces the breast tissue attenuation artifact, and limited comparison studies have suggested that thallium and sestamibi have similar test sensitivities, but test specificity may be enhanced by sestamibi imaging. The information available about pharmacologic stress using dipyridamole, adenosine, or dobutamine is limited but suggests that the diagnostic accuracy is similar for men and women.

● Breast tissue may simulate anterior or septal ischemia on thallium imaging.

Exercise echocardiography, although not extensively studied, may improve the accuracy of exercise testing for the diagnosis of heart disease in women. It has been proposed as a cost-effective initial approach to the evaluation of chest pain. Also, it has the advantage of providing information about other causes of chest pain and valvular and myocardial function. Dobutamine echocardiography is safe in women. Preliminary data about its diagnostic accuracy in women compared with men are conflicting, probably reflecting the small number of subjects and the patient population.

Until more studies are reported, no firm guidelines can be offered about specific stress testing modalities in women, because no approach or technique has been shown to be clearly superior. As in men, the pretest probability of disease is likely more important in determining diagnostic accuracy than the specific type of test. If the likelihood of coronary artery disease is low, no stress test is very accurate. If the goal is localization of ischemia or if the resting electrocardiogram is abnormal, imaging techniques should be used. If a woman cannot exercise adequately because of noncardiac factors, the initial stress test should be pharmacologic.

In women with an intermediate probability of coronary artery disease and a normal resting electrocardiogram, standard stress electrocardiography has acceptable sensitivity and specificity. If the results are normal, there is a high negative predictive value regarding the absence of coronary artery disease and the prognosis is good. There are not enough data to demonstrate a clearly superior imaging technique in women, so when this approach is chosen, the type of study should depend on local expertise, patient characteristics, and costs. In women with worrisome symptoms and high pretest probability of coronary artery disease, an argument can be made to proceed directly (without noninvasive testing) to coronary angiography to define anatomy. Coronary angiography is safe in women, and most studies have demonstrated that despite gender differences and rates of referral to angiography, after the anatomy is defined women are revascularized at a rate similar to men.

- In women with an intermediate probability of coronary artery disease and a normal resting electrocardiogram, standard stress electrocardiography has acceptable sensitivity and specificity.

Myocardial Infarction

Numerous studies have demonstrated greater early and late mortality and more complications in women than in men after acute myocardial infarction. However, analysis of several of the larger studies of acute myocardial infarction (GUSTO-I, ISIS-III, TIMI-IIIB) and of several population-based investigations has determined that after baseline differences have been accounted for—especially age and cardiac risk factors—gender is no longer an independent risk factor for death. Women with acute myocardial infarction are older and have more comorbid conditions than men and have increased frequency of all cardiac risk factors except smoking. Diabetes mellitus is more common in women and may account for the increased frequency of silent myocardial infarction. Women may be slightly less likely to present with sudden death but more likely than men to have non-Q-wave myocardial infarction. Also, women are more likely to delay receiving treatment by seeking care at their doctor's office instead of going directly to an emergency department. Other delays in initiating therapy for women, compared with men, once in the hospital have also been observed.

The risk of in-hospital complications (reinfarction, stroke, and myocardial rupture) has been reported to be higher in women, but some of these differences may be related to older age. Women have more heart failure despite better residual left ventricular systolic function, presumably because of diastolic abnormalities. After dismissal, women are less likely to be referred for cardiac rehabilitation and, if referred, are more likely to drop out. When they do participate in cardiac rehabilitation programs, however, they tend to have similar or greater improvement of objective measures of risk factors and fitness than men. Women fare more poorly on quality-of-life scores and have increased anxiety and depression. They tend to have poor psychosocial support and are more likely than men to be in a lower socioeconomic group and to live alone.

All therapies and interventions for the treatment of myocardial infarction that have been found beneficial for men are also beneficial for women, including revascularization by thrombolysis, direct angioplasty or surgery, aspirin, β-blockers, and angiotensin-converting enzyme (ACE) inhibitors. However, numerous studies have demonstrated that women are less likely to have invasive diagnostic and therapeutic procedures when hospitalized for acute coronary syndromes. These differences have not been explained entirely by adjustment for baseline factors, and it appears that this relative "undertreatment" is not benign—women in these studies who had a revascularization procedure had a better prognosis than those who did not.

- Numerous studies have demonstrated greater early and late mortality and more complications in women than in men after acute myocardial infarction.
- Diabetes mellitus is more common in women and may account for the increased frequency of silent myocardial infarction.
- The risk of in-hospital complications (reinfarction, stroke, and myocardial rupture) has been reported to be higher in women, but some of these differences may be related to older age and comorbid conditions.

Coronary Angiography

Several studies have demonstrated that female gender is an independent predictor of a lower likelihood of receiving coronary angiography, even when baseline factors and severity of disease are considered. Because coronary angiography is a prerequisite for catheter- or surgical-based revascularization, women in these studies, de facto, had a lower rate of revascularization. Among men and women who undergo coronary angiography, there appears to be little difference in the subsequent use of angioplasty and bypass surgery, suggesting that once the anatomy is defined, subsequent decisions are based primarily on severity of disease and not gender. Although the appropriate use of coronary angiography is still debated, these studies showed that appropriate cardiac catheterization was associated with low mortality in both men and women and the relative underuse of coronary angiography in women is associated with adverse long-term outcomes.

- Female gender is an independent predictor of a lower likelihood of receiving coronary angiography.

Thrombolysis

Thrombolytic therapy is a well-established approach for revascularization in eligible patients who present early with acute myocardial infarction, with nearly a 30% overall reduction in mortality. There is no evidence for an important gender difference in the fundamental mechanism of action of thrombolytic agents. After adjustment for age and comorbid conditions, women have the same rate of vessel patency, left ventricular ejection fraction, and short- and long-term mortality as men. Women receive thrombolytic therapy much less frequently than men, at least partly because they are more likely to be ineligible at the time of evaluation, because of age, comorbid conditions, and late presentation. However, some studies have demonstrated less use of thrombolysis in eligible women than in men that is not explained by known factors.

Intracerebral hemorrhage is more common in women than in men, perhaps because of smaller body size and lack of thrombolytic dose adjustments. Data suggest that treatment of acute myocardial infarction in women by "direct angioplasty" may result in lower rates of mortality and hemorrhagic stroke than treatment with thrombolysis, whereas both treatments result in similar outcomes in men. Whether female gender is an independent risk for intracerebral hemorrhage or is a result of comorbid conditions and lack of dose adjustment is not known. Although active bleeding at the time of thrombolysis is usually an absolute contraindication to thrombolysis, anecdotal reports from the GUSTO-I trial and others suggest that the risk of severe vaginal bleeding in actively menstruating women is not prohibitively high and is not a sufficient reason to deny women the benefits of thrombolytic therapy.

- Women receive thrombolytic therapy much less frequently than men.
- Intracerebral hemorrhage is more common in women than in men, perhaps because of smaller body size and lack of thrombolytic dose adjustments.

Catheter-Based Revascularization

Early in the interventional era, the procedural success rate for PTCA in women was lower than in men because of the large nonsteerable catheters and balloons and the generally smaller coronary arteries in women. With current technology and equipment, no gender differences in procedural success or restenosis rates have been documented. Nearly all reported series show that women have more severe angina and more concomitant illnesses, including diabetes mellitus,

hypertension, and heart failure, at the time of intervention. When age and these baseline characteristics are considered, there are minimal or no gender differences in short- or long-term survival or rates of myocardial infarction or coronary artery bypass grafting (CABG) whether the interventional procedure is performed for unstable angina, acute myocardial infarction, or electively for stable angina.

Women are more likely than men to have residual angina and to take antianginal medication after PTCA. This difference, also observed after CABG, has not been explained completely. Microvascular disease and abnormalities in coronary flow reserve associated with left ventricular hypertrophy or diabetes mellitus may contribute to this observation.

Few studies have examined newer interventional techniques in women, but directional and excisional coronary atherectomy, excimer laser, and stent implantation appear to have similar rates of long-term survival and restenosis. The results of most reported series have indicated a slightly lower procedural success rate and a higher rate of myocardial infarction and vascular complications in women. This likely reflects difficulties related to the smaller size of the body and the coronary arteries. The differences may be less with improved technology.

PTCA should be offered to women who have the appropriate indications for revascularization and suitable anatomy, without specific concerns for gender.

- Women are more likely than men to have residual angina and to take antianginal medication after PTCA.

Coronary Artery Surgery

According to early results of women who had CABG, women have greater operative and short-term mortality than men. Various explanations for this include technical factors related to smaller body size, more advanced disease at the time of operation, and referral bias. However, population studies and long-term results from the CASS registry and BARI trial have reported similar graft patency and long-term survival benefits in men and women who have surgical revascularization. The rates of perioperative death and complications (myocardial infarction, stroke, and heart failure) are greater for women, but this disparity disappears when baseline factors such as age and heart failure are considered. Women are more likely to have residual angina that requires therapy. Also, women have been more likely than men to require emergent bypass surgery, which is independently associated with higher morbidity and mortality. CABG provides excellent relief of symptoms and comparable survival benefits in women; therefore, concern about increased mortality should not influence referral for surgery in appropriate women.

Pharmacologic Therapy

Aspirin, β-blockers, and ACE inhibitors are underutilized in eligible patients with acute myocardial infarction or left ventricular dysfunction, and women and elderly patients are less likely to receive these beneficial medications, even when coronary artery disease is documented or after myocardial infarction. They more likely are treated with calcium channel blockers, which have no documented survival benefit. Fewer therapeutic interventional studies have been performed in women, but the ones available suggest that women benefit as much or more than men. The ISIS-I and ISIS-II trials demonstrated that improved survival in women receiving β-blockers and aspirin was comparable to that in men, with the greatest benefit accrued by those at highest risk. Trials involving ACE inhibitors generally have shown beneficial effects in women but often less than those in men. Unless contraindications exist, these drugs should be used to treat virtually all women with myocardial infarction.

Established therapies for acute and chronic ischemia have been shown to benefit women, but they have tended to be used later in the course of the disease and to be used less frequently than in men. Outcome likely will improve if ischemia is recognized and treated earlier.

- The ISIS-I and ISIS-II trials demonstrated that improved survival in women receiving β-blockers and aspirin was comparable to that in men.

Noncoronary Cardiovascular Disease

Valvular Heart Disease

Mitral Valve Prolapse

Mitral valve prolapse is commonly associated with female gender. The Framingham Study and others have reported a markedly higher prevalence rate of mitral valve prolapse diagnosed clinically or by M-mode echocardiography in women than in men. However, most studies have suggested that men with mitral valve prolapse are proportionately more likely to develop progressive mitral regurgitation and other complications. The discrepancies between the clinical and echocardiographic diagnoses of mitral valve prolapse

are considerable. More recent studies with two-dimensional echocardiography, which may be less likely to "overcall" the diagnosis of mitral valve prolapse, have questioned the marked female preponderance and have not found any gender difference in the prevalence of mitral valve prolapse.

- Men with mitral valve prolapse are proportionately more likely to develop progressive mitral regurgitation.

Aortic Valve Disease

Gender differences have been observed in aortic valve disease and call into question the generalizability to women of surgical criteria developed in men. Calcific aortic stenosis is predominately a disease of the elderly. Women with aortic stenosis have a different pattern of left ventricular adaptation to the pressure load of aortic stenosis than men, with better preservation of left ventricular systolic function and a concentric pattern of left ventricular hypertrophy. Men more frequently have eccentric hypertrophy and lower systolic function. There are conflicting reports on gender-related differences in mortality after aortic valve replacement for aortic stenosis.

The classic criteria (left ventricular end-diastolic diameter ≥ 70 mm; left ventricular end-systolic diameter ≥ 50 mm) for timing aortic valve replacement for severe chronic aortic regurgitation in men and women have been questioned recently. Women with even advanced severe aortic regurgitation rarely meet established left ventricular diameter surgical criteria, which traditionally have not been adjusted for body size. Even after significant symptoms develop in women, ventricular dimensions tend to be smaller than those of the criteria. Thus, using these criteria for women results in operating late in the clinical course, with resulting poor outcomes. Female gender appears to be an independent risk factor for poor outcome, and the optimal criteria for surgical timing for asymptomatic chronic aortic regurgitation in women are not clear. Surgery should be considered in men and women with more than mild symptoms or with an ejection fraction less than 55%.

- Women with even advanced severe aortic regurgitation rarely meet established left ventricular diameter surgical criteria.

Congestive Heart Failure

The rate of hospitalization for congestive heart failure has increased steadily in the last 20 years. Congestive heart failure affects approximately 20% of the population over age 45. Information about gender differences in prevalence, cause, and optimal therapy of heart failure is sparse and conflicting. The Framingham Study found that the incidence rates of congestive heart failure are higher in men but that the prevalence of congestive heart failure is nearly equal except in the very elderly. Five-year survival was better in women than in men. Hypertension, diabetes mellitus, and valvular heart disease tend to be more common in women with congestive heart failure, whereas coronary artery disease and smoking are more common in men. In the Framingham Study, congestive heart failure was a clinical diagnosis and did not depend on left ventricular ejection fraction being depressed.

Women are more likely to have better left ventricular systolic function than men with similar heart failure symptoms. Symptoms in women have been ascribed to a higher rate of diastolic dysfunction; that is, women tend to be more symptomatic than men with a similar left ventricular ejection fraction. Numerous studies have found ejection fraction to be a powerful predictor of outcome, and the preponderance of diastolic dysfunction in women with symptoms out of proportion to systolic dysfunction may explain their improved outcome compared with that of men with similar symptoms. Many of the major heart failure intervention trials did not include women or had a small proportion of them. Conclusions drawn from these trials must be interpreted carefully, but in the CONSENSUS, SOLVD, and SAVE heart failure trials women received considerably less benefit from ACE inhibitor therapy than men.

Fewer than 20% of cardiac transplantation operations are performed on women, and there appears to be a gender effect on outcome after cardiac transplantation. Women may be at increased risk for death and rejection episodes, but the data are based on small numbers. One possible cause for poor outcomes is the increased frequency of autoimmune disease in women and multiparity, which exposes women to additional antibodies to foreign material. The question of selection bias is open, but one study found that the underrepresentation of women receiving cardiac transplantation is partly a result of more women declining the procedure.

- Heart failure due to diastolic dysfunction is more common in women than in men.
- In the CONSENSUS, SOLVD, and SAVE heart failure trials, women received considerably less benefit from ACE inhibitor therapy than men.

Arrhythmias, Syncope, and Sudden Death

Little gender-specific information is available about the prevalence, presentation, or therapy of cardiac arrhythmias; however, some differences have been observed. Women presenting with syncope tend to be older, have fewer premonitory symptoms, have better left ventricular function, and are less likely to have a cardiac cause of syncope identified. They subsequently tend to have fewer cardiac events. Female survivors of cardiac arrest tend to have better left ventricular function and are less likely to have coronary artery disease as an underlying cause. Also, they are more likely to have dilated cardiomyopathy, valvular heart disease, long QT syndrome, right ventricular dysplasia, coronary vasospasm, or a structurally normal heart. Despite these differences, long-term survival appears to be similar. The rate of defibrillator implantation in women is similar to or lower than that in men. Benefits of defibrillator therapy are less well defined for women, mainly because of the small number of study subjects and events.

- Female survivors of cardiac arrest tend to have better left ventricular function and are less likely to have coronary artery disease as an underlying cause.

Although the prevalence of atrial fibrillation is higher at all ages in men than in women, the much larger population of women over age 75 results in there being a greater number of women than men with atrial fibrillation. It has been estimated that 50% to 55% of all persons and 60% of those older than 75 years who have atrial fibrillation are women. Optimal management of elderly patients with atrial fibrillation has not been firmly established, because they potentially have the most to gain from anticoagulation for stroke prevention but are often at higher risk from the complications of anticoagulation.

- More women than men have atrial fibrillation, probably because of the greater number of elderly women.

Paroxysmal supraventricular tachycardia is believed to be more common in women than in men. Several investigators have described cyclical variation in the frequency and duration of paroxysmal supraventricular tachycardia in premenopausal women, with the highest frequency occurring in the luteal phase of the menstrual cycle when estrogen levels are lowest. The mechanism is not known but may be a function of cyclic body temperature changes, direct or indirect actions of estrogen, or progesterone effects.

Risk Factors

Men and women have the same risk factors for coronary artery disease, but the relative weight of a given risk may be more or less significant in women. Age and a family history of coronary artery disease increase the risk of this disease in women.

Diabetes Mellitus

Diabetes mellitus is a more powerful risk factor for coronary artery disease and heart failure in women than in men and completely negates the protective effect of female gender, even in premenopausal women. The metabolic derangements accompanying diabetes adversely contribute to obesity, lower levels of high-density lipoprotein (HDL) cholesterol, increased levels of triglycerides, abnormal endothelial and coagulation function, and increased risk of hypertension. Diabetes acts synergistically with other risk factors, especially smoking, to markedly increase cardiac risk, and it is an independent risk for subsequent cardiac events and poor outcome after PTCA in women.

- Men and women have the same risk factors for coronary artery disease, but the relative weight of a given risk may be more or less significant in women.
- Diabetes mellitus is a more powerful risk factor for coronary artery disease and heart failure in women than in men.

Tobacco

Cigarette smoking is a significantly stronger risk factor in women than in men. Even passive exposure to smoking has been shown to increase the risk of cardiac disease in women. The number of cigarettes smoked correlates with the risk, and even women who smoke fewer than 5 cigarettes per day have double the risk of coronary artery disease than nonsmokers. Smoking cessation is associated with a significant reduction of risk, and women with coronary artery disease who continue to smoke have significant progression of atherosclerosis and are at increased risk for recurrent events and repeat revascularization. As a public health issue, this is critical because more teenage girls and young women report greater cigarette use than boys, at least partly as a weight-control measure. Hispanic women and women with fewer than 12 years of education also have increased rates of smoking. In general, men have been more successful at smoking cessation efforts. Addressing these issues will be important to reduce smoking and the accompanying risk in women.

- Cigarette smoking is a significantly stronger risk factor in women than in men.

Hypertension

Women make up 60% of all those in the U.S. who have hypertension. The prevalence of hypertension is greater in men than in women until age 60. In black and Hispanic persons older than 60 years and in white people older than 70, the age-specific hypertension rate is higher in women than in men, with women older than 80 having rates 14% higher than men. Blood pressure tends to increase throughout life in men and women, but before age 60, women have lower systolic and diastolic blood pressure than men. Subsequently, systolic blood pressure increases more steeply in women and surpasses that of men. As a result, older women are more likely to have isolated systolic hypertension.

Although the exact cause of hypertension in most men and women is not known, several types of hypertension exclusively or disproportionately affect women. Renal artery stenosis caused by fibromuscular dysplasia has a strong female preponderance (8:1) and should be considered when hypertension occurs in a woman younger than 40, is difficult to control, or occurs in a woman who had a pregnancy complicated by severe hypertension. Ingestion of currently available oral contraceptive agents is associated with an increase in blood pressure, although not as commonly as with first-generation agents. This increase is usually mild and rarely requires discontinuation of the oral contraceptive agent. However, blood pressure should be monitored after a woman starts taking an oral contraceptive, and the association between increased blood pressure and oral contraceptives should be recognized in women who present with hypertension while taking these agents.

Hypertension and left ventricular hypertrophy both are stronger relative risk factors for stroke and congestive heart failure in women than in men, and the Framingham data have shown that the presence of left ventricular hypertrophy removes the survival advantage of female gender. Although women were underrepresented in early hypertension treatment trials, subsequent trials and analyses have concluded that no real gender differences exist in relative risk reduction for stroke and cardiovascular events from the treatment of hypertension. Absolute risk reductions are lower in women because the baseline risk of events is lower. Current guidelines from the Joint National Committee on the Treatment of Hypertension-VI (JNC-VI) are not gender-specific, and it appears that women with hypertension benefit from therapy and should be treated as aggressively as men.

- Older women are more likely to have isolated systolic hypertension.
- Hypertension and left ventricular hypertrophy both are stronger relative risk factors for stroke and congestive heart failure in women than in men.

Hyperlipidemia

Serum levels of total cholesterol in women increase steadily from the mid-30s to age 55 to 60. Low-density lipoprotein (LDL) cholesterol levels remain lower than those in men until approximately age 50, at which age the levels in men stabilize and are surpassed by those in women (Fig. 3). This increase in cholesterol coincides with the average age of menopause and likely contributes to the observed increase in cardiac events in older women. Hyperlipidemia in women is associated with increased risk of coronary artery disease. Women younger than 65 years with a total cholesterol level greater than 240 mg/dL, LDL cholesterol greater than 160 mg/dL, or HDL cholesterol less than 50 mg/dL have a relative risk of a cardiac event that is 2 to 3 times that of women without hyperlipidemia. Although a low HDL cholesterol level remains a strong risk factor in women older than 65, the relationship of total cholesterol and LDL cholesterol and coronary artery disease in older women is not as strong. There are conflicting data for women about the independent risk associated with increased triglyceride levels. These risks appear similar to those reported for men.

Often, primary prevention hyperlipidemia trials have excluded women and the elderly; therefore, there is little information on which to base therapeutic decisions. The 1993 National Cholesterol Education Program–Adult Treatment Panel-II (NCEP–ATP-II) acknowledged gender differences and estrogen status in calculating the risk for coronary artery disease. For premenopausal women without coronary artery disease, there are insufficient data to recommend early or aggressive pharmacologic therapy unless multiple risks are present. Dietary and exercise counseling and appropriate follow-up should be advised. Postmenopausal women without known coronary artery disease and hypercholesterolemia or a low HDL cholesterol level may be considered for estrogen replacement therapy, which may obviate additional pharmacologic therapy. The Air Force/Texas Coronary Atherosclerosis Prevention Study (AFCAPS/TexCAPS) randomly assigned almost 1,000 postmenopausal women with no known vascular disease, average total cholesterol levels, and low-average HDL cholesterol levels to placebo or treatment with lovastatin and found a 46% reduction in cardiovascular events in treated women. Although the study was not powered to detect treatment differences in mortality end points, the study is important because it showed similar or greater reduction of events in women than in men and demonstrated risk reduction from lipid modification in a relatively low-risk group that otherwise would not be treated according to current

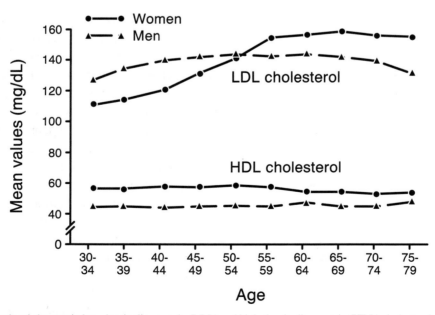

Fig. 3. Age- and gender-related changes in low-density lipoprotein (LDL) and high-density lipoprotein (HDL) cholesterol. After age 50, women have higher LDL cholesterol than men, and the HDL cholesterol advantage diminishes. (Modified from *Nutr Rev* 46:68-78, 1988. By permission of International Life Sciences Institute.)

NCEP–ATP-II guidelines.

Compared with the paucity of primary prevention data, there is strong evidence from well-designed randomized trials to support aggressive treatment of increased cholesterol levels in women with known cardiovascular disease. The Cholesterol and Recurrent Events (CARE) Trial randomized men and women with recent myocardial infarction and "normal" LDL cholesterol levels (115 to 174 mg/dL) to treatment with pravastatin or placebo. Treated men and women both had a significant reduction in all end points (Fig. 4), including cardiac death, myocardial infarction, and revascularization. Subgroup analysis demonstrated an even greater reduction in risk for coronary events in women than in men (46% vs. 20%), and the benefit was observed much earlier in the follow-up period. Higher baseline LDL levels were associated with greater risk reductions. The Scandinavian Simvastatin Survival Study (4S) randomly assigned hyperlipidemic patients with coronary artery disease to treatment or placebo. The risk reductions for major coronary events were similar in men and women (34% vs. 35%, respectively). Other studies have demonstrated similar reductions in LDL cholesterol levels and progression of coronary atherosclerosis with treatment in women and men.

- There is strong evidence from well-designed randomized trials to support aggressive treatment of increased cholesterol levels in women with known cardiovascular disease.

These studies provide evidence to support the use of the current NCEP–ATP-II guidelines for secondary prevention of coronary artery disease in women, with a goal LDL cholesterol level of less than 100 mg/dL. Although not specifically designed to do so, no study has suggested significant gender differences in the efficacy of dietary intervention or lipid-lowering drugs. The NCEP–ATP-II guidelines do not consider estrogen a first-line lipid-lowering drug, but many clinicians believe that it should be strongly considered as such in postmenopausal women with hypercholesterolemia and low HDL cholesterol levels. Combination therapy with estrogen and 3-hydroxy-3-methylglutaryl-coenzyme A (HMG-CoA) reductase inhibitors has been shown to have beneficial and complementary effects on various lipoprotein subfractions and is reasonable depending on baseline lipid status.

Risk Factors Unique to Women

Oral contraceptives are one of the most effective methods for pregnancy prevention, but women who took first-generation high-dose agents had an increased rate of myocardial infarction and thrombotic events. There was a clear synergy between first-generation oral contraceptives and cigarette smoking that led to a marked increase in the risk for myocardial infarction in smokers—believed to be via a thrombotic rather than an atherosclerotic mechanism. Studies of the cardiovascular effects of oral contraceptives have been hampered by the rare occurrence of clinical events in this young, generally

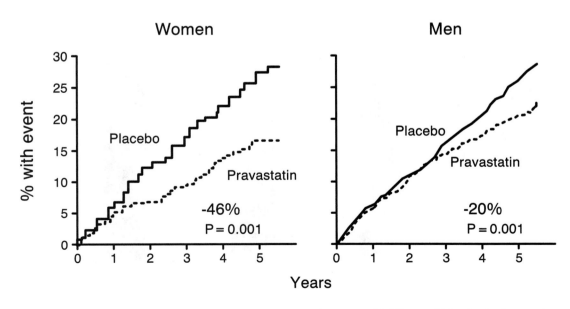

Fig. 4. The effect of pravastatin on recurrent coronary events in 576 postmenopausal women and 3,583 men. Risk reduction in treated women was greater than that of treated men and occurred earlier in the treatment period. (From *J Am Coll Cardiol* 32:140-146, 1998. By permission of the American College of Cardiology.)

healthy population of women and by changes in oral contraceptive formulations. Current oral contraceptive formulations, with a markedly lower estrogen content, have been associated with much lower rates of myocardial infarction, and it appears that there is little or no increased risk in nonsmoking women taking oral contraceptives and no increased risk in those who previously took them. There is insufficient information about the risk of stroke, and although a small excess risk of ischemic stroke cannot be excluded, a large risk appears unlikely. Smokers, especially those older than 35 years, should quit smoking and, if unable to do so, should use an alternative birth control method.

Oral contraceptives are associated with increased blood pressure, and some women may become overtly hypertensive. If hypertension occurs while a woman is taking an oral contraceptive, the drug should be discontinued and blood pressure should be monitored to assure return to normal. In most cases, the increase in blood pressure promptly resolves after discontinuation of oral contraceptives. Previous use of oral contraceptives is not associated with increased risk of myocardial infarction or hypertension. An increased incidence of deep vein thrombosis and pulmonary embolus has been observed in women taking oral contraceptives. The incidence is less with current oral contraceptive formulations than it was for older high-dose drugs, with a relative risk of approximately 2. This increased risk should be put into perspective, because the absolute risk for thromboembolic events is very low in premenopausal women and must be balanced with the risks associated with pregnancy. The risk of pregnancy-related thromboembolic events and stroke is as much as 3 times higher than that associated with oral contraceptives. Overall, oral contraceptives appear to be safe and effective and to have a low risk of adverse effects in young, nonsmoking women.

Menopause and Hormone Replacement Therapy

Decreasing levels of estrogen at menopause are associated with several adverse effects on cardiac risk factors, including increased total cholesterol level, LDL cholesterol level, Lp(a), circulating procoagulants, and homocysteine and decreased HDL cholesterol levels. These changes are responsible at least partly for the observed acceleration of cardiovascular events after menopause (Fig. 5). Premenopausal women who have had bilateral oophorectomy and do not receive estrogen replacement have more than twice the risk of myocardial infarction than those who receive estrogen. Most women experience "perimenopause" for several years before cessation of menses, at an average age of 51 years, and can expect to live approximately one-third of their lives after menopause.

- Premenopausal women who have had bilateral oophorectomy and do not receive estrogen replacement have more than twice the risk of myocardial infarction than those who receive estrogen.

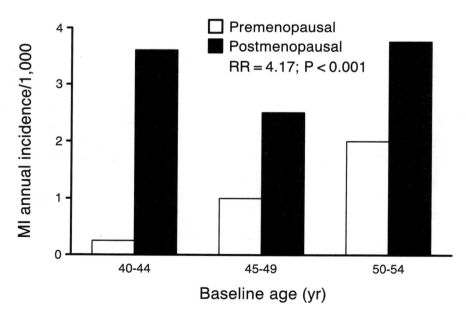

Fig. 5. Menopausal status as a risk for coronary artery disease. Note that the risk for women younger than 55 years, even postmenopausal women, is low. MI, myocardial infarction. (From *Arch Intern Med* 155:57-61, 1995. By permission of the American Medical Association.)

Postmenopausal estrogen replacement has been associated with reduced cardiovascular risk. Considerable primary epidemiologic data and meta-analyses, including the Lipid Research Clinic program and the Nurses' Health Study, indicate risk reductions of 40% to 50% for coronary artery disease in women who choose to take postmenopausal hormone replacement therapy. The data for stroke reduction by estrogen is less robust, but a similar risk reduction has been shown. These data are observational and not from prospective randomized trials, but there has been remarkable uniformity and consistency in the results. There is considerable interest in the possible role of postmenopausal hormonal replacement therapy as a potential intervention to prevent coronary artery disease.

Numerous biologically plausible mechanisms whereby estrogen favorably affects risk factors or physiologic responses have been elucidated. Estrogen reverses many of the unfavorable physiologic changes that occur at menopause. Lipid effects are prominent, but the mechanisms are incompletely understood. Orally administered estrogen decreases LDL cholesterol by 10% to 20%, increases HDL cholesterol by 10% to 30%, and lowers Lp(a) by 25% to 50%. Triglycerides are increased by 20% or more (Fig. 6). The atherogenicity of the triglyceride increase is controversial because of purported differences in the catabolic pathways of the high molecular weight, very low density lipoprotein (VLDL) that is induced by hormone replacement therapy. Transdermal administration of estrogen has little or no effect on lipoprotein levels, suggesting that the liver effects of estrogen absorbed through the gut are responsible for these changes. These favorable effects are also seen when estrogen is combined with progestational agents, but the increase in HDL levels is often blunted. Limited data suggest that the use of micronized progesterone, compared with medroxyprogesterone, blunts the estrogen-induced increase in HDL cholesterol less, while maintaining protection against endometrial hyperplasia.

The balance of the effects of estrogen is likely due to several direct and indirect vascular and hemostatic effects (Fig. 7). Estrogen receptors have been identified in the coronary artery. Although supraphysiologic concentrations of estrogen may directly cause smooth muscle relaxation in conductance coronary arteries, physiologic levels enhance endothelial function by potentiating endothelial-dependent vasodilatation. Estrogen appears to stimulate nitric oxide release, perhaps by up-regulating nitric oxide synthase, and reduces release of endothelial-derived constriction factors such as endothelin-1. The paradoxical acetylcholine-induced coronary vasoconstriction observed in women with vascular disease is decreased and acetylcholine-stimulated increases in coronary flow and vessel diameter are enhanced. Calcium channel blocking properties of estrogen have also

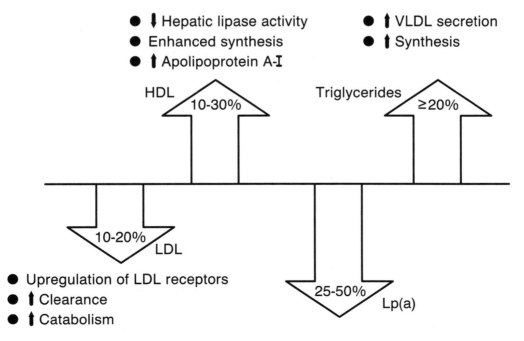

Fig. 6. Effects of estrogen on lipoproteins and proposed mechanisms. HDL, high-density lipoprotein; LDL, low-density lipoprotein; VLDL, very low-density lipoprotein.

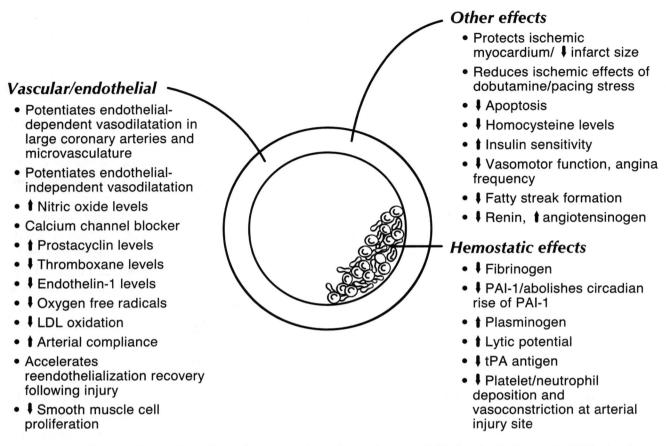

Vascular/endothelial

- Potentiates endothelial-dependent vasodilatation in large coronary arteries and microvasculature
- Potentiates endothelial-independent vasodilatation
- ↑ Nitric oxide levels
- Calcium channel blocker
- ↑ Prostacyclin levels
- ↓ Thromboxane levels
- ↓ Endothelin-1 levels
- ↓ Oxygen free radicals
- ↓ LDL oxidation
- ↑ Arterial compliance
- Accelerates reendothelialization recovery following injury
- ↓ Smooth muscle cell proliferation

Other effects

- Protects ischemic myocardium/ ↓ infarct size
- Reduces ischemic effects of dobutamine/pacing stress
- ↓ Apoptosis
- ↓ Homocysteine levels
- ↑ Insulin sensitivity
- ↓ Vasomotor function, angina frequency
- ↓ Fatty streak formation
- ↓ Renin, ↑ angiotensinogen

Hemostatic effects

- ↓ Fibrinogen
- ↓ PAI-1/abolishes circadian rise of PAI-1
- ↑ Plasminogen
- ↑ Lytic potential
- ↓ tPA antigen
- ↓ Platelet/neutrophil deposition and vasoconstriction at arterial injury site

Fig. 7. Potential beneficial non-lipid-mediated effects of estrogen on the cardiovascular system. LDL, low-density lipoprotein; PAI-1, plasminogen activator inhibitor; tPA, tissue plasminogen activator.

been observed. These favorable effects may be responsible for the improved performance on stress tests of women with coronary artery disease who are taking estrogen.

Estrogen is associated with several favorable changes in hemostatic factors. Fibrinogen, plasminogen activator inhibitor (PAI)-1, and tissue plasminogen activator (t-PA) antigen levels are almost 50% lower in postmenopausal women taking estrogen than in those not receiving treatment. Fibrinolytic potential is enhanced. Some of these effects may be due to the antioxidant properties of estrogen. Estrogen has been observed to decrease the rate of LDL oxidation to more dense atherogenic particles. Estrogen suppresses the proliferation of intimal cells and smooth muscle, reduces platelet and neutrophil deposition at sites of arterial injury, increases prostacyclin levels, and decreases ACE levels. Homocysteine levels are approximately 50% lower in postmenopausal women receiving estrogen replacement than in those not receiving treatment. Estrogen has no significant effect on blood pressure or rate of weight gain after menopause.

Despite the impressive benefits reported for coronary artery disease risk in these observational trials, the data of any nonrandomized, nonprospective study have to be interpreted carefully. This is especially important because the first randomized, blinded, placebo-controlled trial of estrogen for secondary prevention of coronary events did *not* show any significant reduction in cardiac risk.

The Heart and Estrogen/Progesterone Replacement Study (HERS) enrolled 2,763 postmenopausal women younger than 80 years with definite coronary artery disease and an intact uterus to receive continuous-combined estrogen and medroxyprogesterone or placebo. The average follow-up was 4.1 years and was 100% complete. No significant differences were observed for any of the cardiovascular outcomes; that is, combination hormone replacement therapy did *not* reduce cardiovascular events as expected from results of previous observational trials. The unexpected results of HERS has made this already complicated issue more complex. The validity of previous epidemiologic studies has been called into question for several reasons. In most of the previous studies, conjugated equine estrogen (Premarin) was the only estrogen formulation used and the doses were often higher than those currently recommended. The use of a progestational agent in women with a uterus was not routine and, therefore, does not reflect current practice or address the concern that the addition of progestins antagonizes part or all of the beneficial effects of estrogen. The women in HERS received continuous medroxyprogesterone, which blunts the beneficial lipid effects and has other potential adverse physiologic effects. Selection bias, or "the healthy user" effect, is also of concern. In many of the previous studies, the women receiving hormone replacement had achieved a higher educational and socioeconomic level and had fewer cardiac risk factors than those not receiving this therapy and, thus, were already at lower risk for cardiovascular disease. Also, compliance with a medical regimen is associated with other healthy lifestyle patterns and better outcomes. Sicker women and those with less access to medical care may not have been considered candidates for estrogen replacement therapy, further skewing the data and exaggerating the benefits of estrogen.

The data from HERS is especially troubling because these high-risk study participants would have been expected, from the results of previous trials, to receive the greatest risk reduction from hormone replacement therapy. There was a nonsignificant trend toward lower mortality late in the study period, which may reflect the beneficial lipid effects observed in the hormone replacement therapy group. The results of this trial should not be extrapolated to other patient populations, that is, patients without coronary artery disease or without a uterus or receiving other hormone replacement therapy formulations (estrogen alone or cyclic estrogen and progestin). The results of HERS indicate that hormone replacement therapy should not be recommended to women with coronary artery disease solely for cardioprotection. Several large randomized prospective trials to assess the role of estrogen replacement therapy for primary and secondary prevention of coronary heart disease and all-cause mortality, such as the Women's Health Study, are under way and will be reported in several years.

Noncardiac Risks and Benefits of Hormone Replacement Therapy

All women with suspected coronary artery disease should have their hormonal status assessed as a risk factor. The decision to start hormone replacement therapy must be individualized and based on the risk for coronary artery disease, breast cancer, and fracture and on hysterectomy status, life expectancy, and side effects (Table 2). The patient's wishes and concerns need to be strongly considered and discussed. Observed noncardiac benefits of estrogen replacement therapy include a decrease in postmenopausal symptoms, osteoporotic fractures, colon cancer, urinary incontinence, and Alzheimer's disease. However, concern about the risk of breast cancer prevents many women from considering hormone replacement therapy. Results of epidemiologic studies have been contradictory, but it appears that estrogen therapy for more than 5 to 10 years is associated with an increased relative risk of breast cancer of 1.2 to 1.5, which is similar to that imparted by early menarche and nulliparity. Previous estrogen therapy is not associated with increased risk, and the mortality from breast cancer does not appear to be increased by hormone replacement therapy. Breast cancer risk must be put into perspective because cardiovascular disease kills more women than breast cancer at all ages (Fig. 8).

Unopposed estrogen is associated with significantly increased risk of endometrial hyperplasia and cancer. The excess risk of cancer is eliminated with the addition of progestin; therefore, unopposed estrogen is recommended only for women who have had a hysterectomy.

Venous thromboembolism and pulmonary embolus have been associated with estrogen replacement. The increase in relative risk of venous thromboembolism appears to be 2 to 4 (2.9 in HERS). This risk appears higher during the first year of treatment and affects those currently receiving

Table 2.—Contraindications and Relative Contraindications to Hormone Replacement Therapy

Contraindications
    Unexplained vaginal bleeding
    Recent vascular thrombosis
    Carcinoma of the breast
    Most endometrial cancers
Relative contraindications/conditions requiring additional considerations or monitoring
    Hypertriglyceridemia
    Active liver disease/impaired liver function
    Thrombophlebitis
    Seizure disorder
    Uterine leiomyomas
    Endometriosis
    Migraine headaches
    Gallbladder disease
    History of breast cancer
    History of endometrial cancer

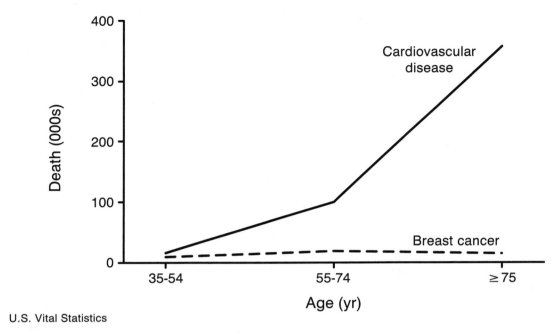

Fig. 8. Comparison of deaths from cardiovascular disease and breast cancer, by age.

treatment but not those who formerly received it. The women affected may have unidentified coagulopathies or other predisposing risk factors, because no consistent adverse effects on the clotting system have been identified. The absolute incidence is low, but women experiencing venous thromboembolism while receiving hormone replacement therapy should be evaluated for the presence of coagulopathy.

Selective estrogen receptor modulators (SERMs) are a class of synthetic tissue-specific estrogens ("designer estrogens") formulated to provide the beneficial action of estrogen without the risks and side effects. Tamoxifen (used for prevention and treatment of breast cancer) and raloxifene (approved for the treatment of osteoporosis) are the most commonly used SERMs, and both of them have favorable effects on lipoprotein and homocysteine levels. These drugs do not have significant beneficial effects on HDL cholesterol, and the observed improvements in the lipid profile are less than those observed with oral estrogen. Currently, the role of SERMs in preventing cardiovascular disease is unclear and further study is warranted.

Hormone Replacement Therapy Recommendations

Currently, no consensus exists about the role of postmenopausal hormone replacement therapy in the prevention of coronary artery disease. Recommendations are evolving as new data are published.

Hypercholesterolemia

The National Cholesterol Education Program (NCEP-II) guidelines now include postmenopausal status as a coronary artery disease risk factor in the assessment of therapy for hyperlipidemia. Estrogen replacement therapy may be considered as the initial/primary therapy of hypercholesterolemia in postmenopausal women because of both its efficacy and relatively low cost. It has complementary effects on the lipid profile when combined with statins. Statins should be given as initial therapy for hyperlipidemia in women with vascular disease.

Secondary Prevention

On the basis of the results of HERS, hormone replacement therapy should not be recommended to women with documented coronary artery disease solely for cardioprotection. If noncardiac indications exist, hormone replacement therapy may be prescribed but the increased risk of venous thromboembolism should be discussed. All other proven therapies (aspirin, β-blockers, statins, ACE inhibitors) should be used maximally. Many of the HERS participants did not receive optimal treatment at baseline with these therapies.

For example, the average LDL cholesterol was 145 mg/dL, fewer than 50% of the women were taking lipid-lowering drugs, and fewer than 35% were taking β-blockers.

Primary Prevention

Adequate data to support widespread use of estrogen replacement therapy in postmenopausal women for primary prevention of coronary artery disease do not exist. Although this approach possibly would decrease significantly the incidence of coronary artery disease, it also would unnecessarily expose many women at low risk for coronary artery disease to hormone side effects and risk of breast cancer. Additional recommendations must await large randomized

trials. Until then, postmenopausal women should have the plasma levels of lipids measured. If hypercholesterolemia is present and no contraindications exist (e.g., breast cancer), hormone replacement therapy may be considered as initial therapy. If the lipid levels are satisfactory but other strong risks for coronary artery disease exist (family or smoking history or diabetes mellitus), estrogen replacement therapy might also be considered.

Many questions remain unanswered and include determining the optimal duration of therapy, route of administration, and choice of progestin and the benefit/risk profile in certain populations, for example, patients with hypertriglyceridemia or treated breast cancer.

Suggested Review Reading

1. Hulley S, Grady D, Bush T, et al: Randomized trial of estrogen plus progestin for secondary prevention of coronary heart disease in postmenopausal women. *JAMA* 280:605-613, 1998.
The first reported randomized, blinded, placebo-controlled secondary prevention trial of postmenopausal hormone replacement therapy found no overall cardiovascular benefit from continuous combined estrogen and medroxyprogesterone therapy. Thromboembolic events were increased. Based on this trial, this treatment is not recommended solely for cardioprotection in women with known coronary artery disease.

2. Klodas E, Enriquez-Sarano M, Tajik AJ, et al: Surgery for aortic regurgitation in women. Contrasting indications and outcomes compared with men. *Circulation* 94:2472-2478, 1996.
Women compared with men have a poorer outcome after aortic valve replacement for aortic regurgitation. Current criteria for timing of surgical intervention may not be applicable to women.

3. Mosca L, Manson JE, Sutherland SE, et al: Cardiovascular disease in women: a statement for healthcare professionals from the American Heart Association. *Circulation* 96:2468-2482, 1997.
A comprehensive review of current issues in the diagnosis and treatment of cardiovascular disease in women.

4. Stone GW, Grines CL, Browne KF, et al: Comparison of in-hospital outcome in men versus women treated by either thrombolytic therapy or primary coronary angioplasty for acute myocardial infarction. *Am J Cardiol* 75:987-992, 1995.
This study suggests that women who undergo thrombolysis for myocardial infarction have a worse outcome than those who undergo primary PTCA.

5. Goldberg RJ, Gorak EJ, Yarzebski J, et al: A communitywide perspective of sex differences and temporal trends in the incidence and survival rates after acute myocardial infarction and out-of-hospital deaths caused by coronary heart disease. *Circulation* 87:1947-1953, 1993.

6. Hochman JS, McCabe CH, Stone PH, et al: Outcome and profile of women and men presenting with acute coronary syndromes: a report from TIMI IIIB. TIMI Investigators. Thrombolysis in Myocardial Infarction. *J Am Coll Cardiol* 30:141-148, 1997.

7. Lee KL, Woodlief LH, Topol EJ, et al: Predictors of 30-day mortality in the era of reperfusion for acute myocardial infarction. Results from an international trial of 41,021 patients. *Circulation* 91:1659-1668, 1995.

8. Malacrida R, Genoni M, Maggioni AP, et al: A comparison of the early outcome of acute myocardial infarction in women and men. *N Engl J Med* 338:8-14, 1998.

References 5-8: Results of these large studies, including GUSTO-I, TIMI, and ISIS-III, regarding mortality after myocardial infarction indicate little or no independent contribution of gender on mortality. In these studies, age and comorbid illness were the strongest predictors of mortality.

9. Bell MR, Grill DE, Garratt KN, et al: Long-term outcome of women compared with men after successful coronary angioplasty. *Circulation* 91:2876-2881, 1995.

10. Jacobs AK, Kelsey SF, Brooks MM, et al: Better outcome for women compared with men undergoing coronary revascularization: a report from the Bypass Angioplasty Revascularization Investigation (BARI). *Circulation* 98:1279-1285, 1998.

11. Keelan ET, Nunez BD, Grill DE, et al: Comparison of immediate and long-term outcome of coronary angioplasty performed for unstable angina and rest pain in men and women. *Mayo Clin Proc* 72:5-12, 1997.

12. Welty FK, Mittleman MA, Healy RW, et al: Similar results of percutaneous transluminal coronary angioplasty for women and men with postmyocardial infarction ischemia. *J Am Coll Cardiol* 23:35-39, 1994.

References 9-12: Studies demonstrating similar short-term results and long-term outcomes of men and women undergoing PTCA and CABG for various indications.

13. Downs JR, Clearfield M, Weis S, et al: Primary prevention of acute coronary events with lovastatin in men and women with average cholesterol levels: results of AFCAPS/TexCAPS. Air Force/Texas Coronary Atherosclerosis Prevention Study. *JAMA* 279:1615-1622, 1998.

14. Lewis SJ, Sacks FM, Mitchell JS, et al: Effect of pravastatin on cardiovascular events in women after myocardial infarction: the Cholesterol and Recurrent Events (CARE) Trial. *J Am Coll Cardiol* 32:140-146, 1998.

15. Miettinen TA, Pyorala K, Olsson AG, et al: Cholesterol-lowering therapy in women and elderly patients with myocardial infarction or angina pectoris: findings from the Scandinavian Simvastatin Survival Study (4S). *Circulation* 96:4211-4218, 1997.

16. O'Brien T, Nguyen TT: Lipids and lipoproteins in women. *Mayo Clin Proc* 72:235-244, 1997.

17. Sacks FM, Pfeffer MA, Moye LA, et al: The effect of pravastatin on coronary events after myocardial infarction in patients with average cholesterol levels. *N Engl J Med* 335:1001-1009, 1996.

References 13-17: Treatment of hyperlipidemia in women reduces subsequent cardiac events and mortality in women with known cardiovascular diseases as well as in primary prevention.

18. Gilligan DM, Quyyumi AA, Cannon RO III: Effects of physiological levels of estrogen on coronary vasomotor function in postmenopausal women. *Circulation* 89:2545-2551, 1994.

19. Grodstein F, Stampfer MJ, Manson JE, et al: Postmenopausal estrogen and progestin use and the risk of cardiovascular disease. *N Engl J Med* 335:453-461, 1996.

20. Stampfer MJ, Colditz GA, Willett WC, et al: Postmenopausal estrogen therapy and cardiovascular disease: ten-year follow-up from the Nurses' Health Study. *N Engl J Med* 325:756-762, 1991.

21. The Writing Group for the PEPI Trial: Effects of estrogen or estrogen/progestin regimens on heart disease risk factors in postmenopausal women. The Postmenopausal Estrogen/Progestin Interventions (PEPI) Trial. *JAMA* 273:199-208, 1995.

References 18-21: Observational trial data regarding cardiac risk and mortality reduction with hormone replacement therapy and possible biologic mechanisms.

Questions

True/False

1. Myocardial infarction in premenopausal women is rare.
   a. True
   b. False

2. Standard stress electrocardiographic testing is no longer considered an appropriate diagnostic test in women because of high false-positive rates.
   a. True
   b. False

3. Women are more likely than men to have silent myocardial infarction.
   a. True
   b. False

4. Thrombolytic therapy for women with acute myocardial infarction is more cost-effective and associated with better outcomes than emergent percutaneous transluminal coronary angioplasty (PTCA).
   a. True
   b. False

5. There are insufficient data to support long-term aspirin use in women with coronary artery disease.
   a. True
   b. False

Multiple Choice (choose the one best answer)

6. Several cardiac risk factors are adversely affected at menopause. Postmenopausal estrogen replacement may reduce cardiac risk by:
   a. Increasing HDL cholesterol levels
   b. Increasing plasminogen activator inhibitor (PAI)-1 levels
   c. Enhancing LDL oxidation
   d. Lowering triglyceride levels
   e. Lowering insulin requirements in women with diabetes mellitus

7. Women with congestive heart failure, compared with men, exhibit all the following *except*:
   a. Tend to have better left ventricular systolic function
   b. Have a generally better prognosis with similar symptoms
   c. Are more likely to have significant valvular disease
   d. Benefit more from angiotensin-converting enzyme (ACE) inhibition therapy

Answers

1. Answer a

The incidence of myocardial infarction in premenopausal women is less than 2/1,000 women per year. Smoking markedly increases the risk.

2. Answer b

Women have higher false-positive rates on stress electrocardiography than men. Although data are lacking about the optimal approach to assessing chest pain in women, initial stress electrocardiographic testing in women who have normal baseline electrocardiographic findings and who are able to exercise is a very reasonable strategy. Negative findings on stress electrocardiography at a good workload have excellent negative predictive value.

3. Answer a

Investigators do not know why women have more silent myocardial infarctions. The higher incidence of diabetes mellitus among women and the possible lack of recognition of symptoms by patients and physicians may be contributory.

4. Answer b

Revascularization by thrombolysis and percutaneous transluminal coronary angioplasty (PTCA) have been shown to improve outcome in women with acute myocardial infarction. Women have a higher rate of stroke after thrombolytic therapy than men, and some small randomized studies have shown better outcomes in women who receive emergent PTCA rather than thrombolysis for acute myocardial infarction. Until more definitive comparison data are available, women with acute myocardial infarction should be considered for urgent revascularization by whatever method is available at the treating institution. Emergent PTCA should be strongly considered where facilities exist for rapid treatment.

5. Answer b

Several secondary prevention trials have shown reduction of recurrent myocardial infarction rates in women taking aspirin. The data are less robust for primary prevention but suggestive of benefit.

6. Answer a

HDL cholesterol is increased by up to 20% in women receiving estrogen replacement therapy. PAI-1 levels and LDL oxidation are decreased and triglyceride levels usually increase. No studies have demonstrated reduced insulin requirements in diabetics who start estrogen replacement therapy.

7. Answer d

Women with congestive heart failure tend to have better preserved left ventricular systolic function than men with similar symptoms and, perhaps because of this, have a better prognosis. Valvular heart disease is more often a cause of congestive heart failure in women than in men. Most trials have found similar or less benefit conferred by angiotensin-converting enzyme (ACE) inhibitor therapy in women than in men with congestive heart failure.

Chapter 69

Cardiac Trauma

Joseph G. Murphy, M.D.
Thomas P. Nobrega, M.D.

> Cardiac trauma is increasing in incidence in clinical practice and is usually a minor topic on the Cardiology Boards.

Penetrating cardiac injury is due primarily to knife or gunshot injuries, whereas blunt cardiac injury is usually due to automobile or motorcycle accidents or industrial incidents. Iatrogenic cardiac trauma also may occur as a result of cardiopulmonary resuscitation, endomyocardial biopsy, or the use of intravascular catheters, including Swan-Ganz catheters (Table 1). Males between the ages of 15 and 35 are the most common victims of cardiac trauma.

- Nonpenetrating cardiac trauma usually results from automobile or industrial injuries, whereas penetrating cardiac injuries usually result from knife or gunshot wounds.
- 50% of patients with traumatic penetrating cardiac injury die rapidly, usually before hospitalization.

Penetrating Cardiac Injury

Penetrating cardiac trauma most commonly affects the right ventricle, followed in order by the left ventricle, right atrium, and left atrium. Cardiac injury may occur from direct injury or indirectly from rib fractures that puncture the cardiac chambers. The principal consequences of perforating cardiac injury are cardiac tamponade and exsanguinating hemorrhage, both of which lead to death rapidly if they are not treated on an emergency basis. Whether cardiac tamponade develops will depend on the chamber penetrated, the size of the penetration, and whether the pericardium is also lacerated. The left ventricle is usually capable of sealing a small hole because of the thickness of the surrounding muscle, whereas a perforation of the right atrium or right ventricle usually leads to rapid hemopericardium. If the pericardium also is opened by the initial injury, tamponade usually will be prevented and the bleeding will present as a hemothorax. Occasionally, the pericardial tear also may act as a flap valve and prevent blood drainage into the pleural space and lead to tamponade. The signs and treatment of pericardial tamponade are discussed in the chapter on pericardial disease.

- Cardiac injury may occur from direct injury or indirectly from rib fractures that puncture the cardiac chambers.

Blunt Cardiac Injury

Nonpenetrating cardiac trauma may result from a direct force on the chest wall or indirectly from pressure on the

---

An atlas illustrating pathologic conditions associated with cardiac trauma is at the end of the chapter (Plates 1-7).

Table 1.—Traumatic Cardiac Lesions

I. Pericardial
    A. Hemorrhagic pericarditis
    B. Pericardial laceration
        1. Asymptomatic
        2. Herniation with cardiac strangulation
    C. Tamponade
        1. Rupture of pericardial vessel
        2. Rupture of coronary artery
        3. Rupture of cardiac chamber
    D. Purulent pericarditis, due to associated rupture of esophagus
    E. Pneumopericardium
    F. Recurrent pericarditis
    G. Constrictive pericarditis
    H. Intrapericardial diaphragmatic hernia
II. Myocardial
    A. Contusion
        1. Subepicardial
        2. Subendocardial
        3. Transmural
    B. Ischemic infarction, secondary to traumatic occlusion of coronary artery
    C. Myocardial hematoma
    D. Myocardial laceration
    E. Myocardial rupture
        1. Ventricular
        2. Ventricular septum
        3. Atrial
        4. Atrial septum
        5. Papillary muscles
    F. Aneurysm
    G. Pseudoaneurysm
    H. Diffuse calcification ("myocarditis ossificans")
III. Endocardial
    A. Thrombus
        1. Asymptomatic
        2. Systemic or pulmonary emboli
IV. Valvular
    A. Atrioventricular valves
        1. Chordal rupture
        2. Papillary muscle rupture
        3. Torn leaflet
    B. Semilunar valves
        1. Avulsion of cusp
        2. Avulsion of commissure
        3. Torn cusp
        4. Intimal tear in adjacent aorta with cusp displacement
        5. Sinus of Valsalva aneurysm with cusp displacement

Table 1 (continued)

V. Coronary artery
    A. Intimal tear/thrombosis
    B. Laceration
    C. Arteriovenous fistula
    D. Arteriocameral fistula
VI. Aorta and pulmonary artery
    A. Rupture
        1. Pseudoaneurysm (with varying amounts of circumference involved)
        2. Exsanguination
    B. Aneurysm

From Giuliani ER, Gersh BJ, McGoon MD, Hayes DL, Schaff HV (editors): *Mayo Clinic Practice of Cardiology.* Third edition. Mosby, 1996, p 1699. By permission of Mayo Foundation.

abdomen displacing a large volume of blood suddenly into the heart. Both forms of injury are frequent in automobile accidents. Nonpenetrating cardiac trauma may result in myocardial contusions; chamber or vessel lacerations; rupture of chordae tendineae, papillary muscles, or cardiac valves; pericarditis; pericardial lacerations; and, rarely, the late development of constrictive pericarditis.

Myocardial Contusion

Myocardial contusion is primarily a histologic diagnosis, and there are no definitive clinical criteria for establishing this diagnosis. A high level of suspicion is important, but currently available diagnostic tests have limited sensitivity or specificity to establish or exclude the diagnosis. Although late complications from blunt cardiac trauma may occur in a small number of patients, in the majority of patients with cardiac trauma who present with stable vital signs, a short period of electrocardiographic monitoring (about 24 hours) is usually sufficient to determine whether arrhythmia or heart failure will develop. Sudden cardiac death due to ventricular fibrillation may occur with low-energy impact to the chest wall (such as from a baseball impact) if the blow coincides with a narrow window of time during cardiac repolarization. Damage to the coronary artery may result in occlusion, laceration, or, more rarely, fistula formation. Rupture of the intraventricular septum, myocardial aneurysm, and pseudoaneurysm formation also have been reported.

- Damage to the coronary artery may result in occlusion, laceration, or, more rarely, fistula formation.

Medical Cardiac Injury

External cardiac massage frequently results in nondisplaced rib fractures and may also lead to rupture of the left ventricle or right ventricle if performed too vigorously, especially in the setting of a recent myocardial infarction when softening of the myocardium has occurred. Other complications include rupture of the papillary muscles that support the tricuspid valve, resulting in severe tricuspid regurgitation, and, more rarely, rupture of the aorta. Penetrating cardiac injuries caused by medical trauma occur during endomyo-cardial biopsy of the right ventricle or after perforation with a temporary pacemaker wire. Dissection of the aorta or coronary ostia may occur during coronary angiography. In rare cases, coronary angioplasty has resulted in coronary artery rupture and tamponade. Intra-aortic balloon coun-terpulsation also may cause aortic dissection, but it is more likely to cause thromboembolic complications as a result of pulsation against the atheromatous plaques in the aorta. Indwelling venous catheters may migrate and perforate the pulmonary arteries, and improper use of balloon-tipped pulmonary artery catheters may lead to branch pulmonary artery rupture and intrapulmonary hemorrhage.

Diagnosis of Cardiac Injury

Cardiac trauma must always be suspected in the setting of blunt or penetrating trauma to the chest or abdomen. A rapid assessment of the patient (airways, breathing, circu-lation [ABC]), neck veins, and extremities, looking for clues to tamponade or hemorrhagic shock, is mandatory. Cardiac contusion is frequently unrecognized. Myocardial contusion may lead to regional wall motion abnormalities and asso-ciated hemorrhagic infiltrate and myocyte necrosis on histologic examination. Acute heart failure and ventricular arrhythmias may occur, but they usually resolve within hours or days. Cardiac injury can occur in the absence of sternal or rib fractures or other significant chest injuries. In cases of blunt cardiac injury, the electrocardiogram may show 1) nonspecific ST-T wave changes, 2) electrocardio-graphic changes of acute pericarditis, or 3) pathologic Q waves. An increase in the creatine kinase-MB enzyme level confirms the presence of cardiac injury, but a false-positive increase also may occur with very severe skeletal muscle injury. Cardiac enzyme levels may be normal even with extensive cardiac injury and may result in acute heart failure.

Echocardiography is the imaging method of choice for identification of cardiac injury (Fig. 1). The findings include pericardial contusion, pericardial tamponade, regional wall motion abnormalities, chamber enlargement, valvular incom-petence, and the presence of intracardiac shunts. An adequate transthoracic echocardiographic examination is not possible in up to 30% of trauma victims, and transesophageal echocar-diography may be needed. Transesophageal echocardiog-raphy may not be possible in patients with cervical, maxillary, or mandibular injuries (Fig. 2).

- Cardiac injury can occur in the absence of sternal or rib fractures or other significant chest injuries.
- Echocardiography is the imaging method of choice for identification of cardiac injury.

Treatment of Cardiac Injury

Emergency pericardiocentesis for cardiac tamponade may be life-saving if the patient is hemodynamically unstable. Echocardiography-guided pericardiocentesis is preferred if immediately available. Emergency thoracotomy is the treat-ment of choice for severe hemorrhage due to cardiac trauma. Lesser degrees of cardiac contusion may be managed con-servatively. For hypotensive patients who have multiple-injury trauma and do not respond to fluids, consider cardiac tamponade or ventricular hypokinesia—both conditions are easily diagnosed with echocardiography. Inotropic agents and intra-aortic balloon counterpulsation (provided there is no aortic injury) may be beneficial in patients with ventricular hypokinesia due to myocardial contusion. Traumatic rupture of the atrial or ventricular septum or major valve injury generally requires surgical repair. Traumatic cardiac rupture due to blunt trauma occurs most commonly in the right or left ventricle. Late cardiac rupture may occur from contu-sion complicated by intramyocardial hemorrhage, necrosis, and softening. Emergency operation is the treatment of choice for patients with cardiac rupture. Patients who present with pseudoaneurysm formation should have surgical repair because future rupture is unpredictable.

Damage to Intracardiac Structures

The aortic valve is the most frequently damaged valve in nonpenetrating chest injuries. Patients with underlying valvular heart disease are considered to be at a higher risk than those without preexisting disease. Aortic or mitral

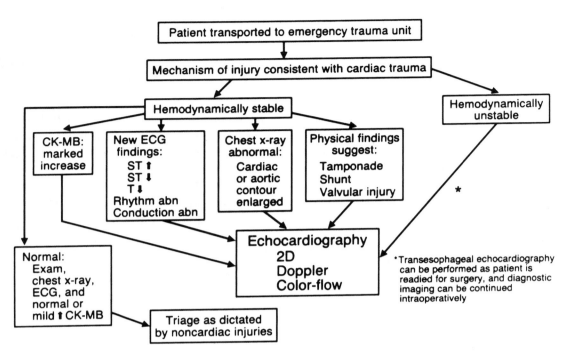

Fig. 1. Use of echocardiography in patients with potential cardiac trauma. abn, abnormality; CK, creatine kinase; 2D, two-dimensional; ECG, electrocardiography; exam, examination. (From Giuliani ER, Gersh BJ, McGoon MD, Hayes DL, Schaff HV [editors]: *Mayo Clinic Practice of Cardiology*. Third edition. Mosby, 1996, p 1713. By permission of Mayo Foundation.)

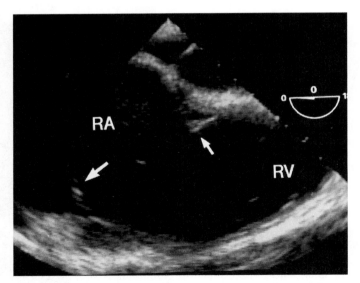

Fig. 2. Traumatic right ventricular contusion and tricuspid valve disruption; modified right ventricular inflow view at 0° multiplane imaging. The right ventricle (*RV*) is markedly enlarged and was nearly akinetic on real-time examination. The anterior tricuspid leaflet (*large arrow*) is unsupported and flail; both the anterior and the septal (*small arrow*) leaflets are dwarfed by profound tricuspid annular dilatation, which is responsible for an expansive gap between the noncoapting leaflets. *RA*, right atrium. (From Freeman WK, Seward JB, Khandheria BK, Tajik AJ [editors]: *Transesophageal Echocardiography*. Little, Brown and Company, 1994, p 566. By permission of Mayo Foundation.)

incompetence due to valve leaflet tears usually presents early and worsens with time. Tricuspid valve injury is unique in that it may be recognized only years after the original injury. Aortic incompetence may result from a combination of damage to the aortic wall and damage to the valve leaflets, and it may improve when perivalvular edema and hemorrhage subside. Sudden traumatic obstruction to left ventricular outflow during systole may result in papillary muscle or mitral valve rupture. The risk of cardiac valve injury is dependent on the time at which the injury occurs during the cardiac cycle. Injury during systole damages the mitral valve, whereas injury during diastole damages the aortic valve. Severe abdominal injury, even in the absence of chest trauma, may result in tricuspid valve or right ventricular papillary muscle rupture. Definitive treatment for significant valve injury is valve replacement or repair. Injury to the coronary arteries from blunt or penetrating trauma may lead to coronary occlusion and myocardial infarction. Left ventricular pseudoaneurysm or aneurysm formation may result from coronary trauma. Atrioventricular fistula formation is a rare complication of penetrating trauma and most commonly affects the right coronary artery. The fistula may extend from the right coronary artery into the coronary sinus, the great cardiac vein, the right ventricle, or the right atrium.

- The risk of cardiac valve injury is dependent on the time at which the injury occurs during the cardiac cycle.
- Atrioventricular fistula formation is a rare complication of penetrating trauma and most commonly affects the right coronary artery.

Injury to the Aorta and Great Vessels

Rupture of the aorta is the most frequent nonpenetrating injury to the great vessels and occurs in about 8,000 cases annually in the United States. Traumatic rupture of the aorta occurs after rapid deceleration injuries such as falls or automobile accidents. Traumatic aortic rupture is present in about 20% of patients who die of injuries from motor vehicle accidents each year. The site of the aortic tear is usually the junction of the aortic arch and the descending aorta at a point where the descending aorta is fixed to the spine by the intercostal arteries. This injury is usually fatal in 80% to 90% of patients, but survival has been reported with emergency cardiac operation. Partial rupture of the aorta is associated with increased arterial pressure in the upper extremities, decreased arterial pressure in the lower extremities, and evidence of widening of the superior mediastinum on chest radiography or computed tomography. Pseudoaneurysm of the aorta tends to expand and rupture, but it also may contain thrombus that embolizes to distant sites. Fistulas may form to adjoining structures. Transesophageal echocardiography,

computed tomography, and aortic angiography are the imaging methods of choice in cases of suspected aortic injuries (Fig. 3). The commonest angiographic findings are an intimal flap and a pseudoaneurysm. With aggressive surgical intervention, about 80% of patients who reach a hospital will survive; without surgery, 2% to 5% of patients will develop a chronic pseudoaneurysm.

- The site of the aortic tear is usually the junction of the aortic arch and the descending aorta.

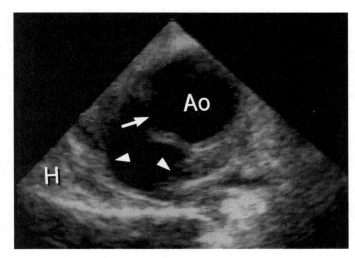

Fig. 3. Traumatic rupture of the descending thoracic aorta after a motor vehicle accident; transverse transesophageal echocardiographic plane. A large rent in the aorta (*Ao*) is clearly visualized (*arrow*) communicating with an adjacent para-aortic space (*arrowheads*); there is also hematoma formation (*H*). (From Freeman WK, Seward JB, Khandheria BK, Tajik AJ [editors]: *Transesophageal Echocardiography.* Little, Brown and Company, 1994, p 458. By permission of Mayo Foundation.)

Suggested Review Reading

1. Karalis DG, Victor MF, Davis GA, et al: The role of echocardiography in blunt chest trauma: a transthoracic and transesophageal echocardiographic study. *J Trauma* 36:53-58, 1994.
This is a prospective review of 105 patients with severe blunt chest trauma assessing the utility of both transthoracic and transesophageal echocardiography.

2. Link MS, Wang PJ, Pandian NG, et al: An experimental model of sudden death due to low-energy chest-wall impact. *N Engl J Med* 338:1805-1811, 1998.
Ventricular fibrillation was induced in a pig model by precise timing of the chest wall impact. The work has implications for sports-related injuries.

3. Rosenthal MA, Ellis JI: Cardiac and mediastinal trauma. *Emerg Med Clin North Am* 13:887-902, 1995.
This is a thorough overview of cardiac trauma and has helpful management algorithms for both blunt and penetrating cardiac trauma.

4. Roxburgh JC: Myocardial contusion. *Injury* 27:603-605, 1996.
This is a brief review of myocardial contusion.

Questions

Multiple Choice (choose the one best answer)

1. The most commonly injured chamber in survivors of blunt cardiac rupture is:
   a. Left atrium
   b. Right atrium
   c. Right ventricle
   d. Left ventricle

2. In penetrating cardiac trauma, the most commonly injured chamber is:
   a. Left atrium
   b. Right atrium
   c. Right ventricle
   d. Left ventricle

3. In experimental models of sudden death due to blunt chest trauma, the frequency of ventricular fibrillation is closely dependent on:
   a. The phase of respiration at the time of impact
   b. The timing with respect to electrical repolarization
   c. The shape of the object striking the chest
   d. The heart rate
   e. Serum magnesium level

4. Myocardial contusion should be considered in which of the following situations?
   a. Blunt chest trauma
   b. Lower abdominal trauma
   c. Crush injury to the lower body
   d. All of the above

5. In a hemodynamically unstable patient with suspected cardiac trauma, which of the following diagnostic tests should be performed as soon as possible?
   a. Electrocardiography
   b. Chest radiography
   c. Echocardiography
   d. Cardiac enzyme determinations

6. All of the following statements regarding the management of patients with suspected myocardial contusion are true *except*:
   a. The use of inotropes may extend the area of injury
   b. If patients are hemodynamically stable and have normal electrocardiograms, telemetry monitoring is nonetheless indicated
   c. Management of pump failure should be directed at unloading the right ventricle

Answers

1. Answer b

2. Answer c

Its anatomical position and relatively thin wall make the right atrium more vulnerable to rupture. The anatomical position of the right ventricle makes it more vulnerable to penetrating trauma.

3. Answer b

Both the hardness of the object and the timing with respect to repolarization influence the frequency of ventricular fibrillation.

4. Answer d

The heart may be injured directly, by compression between bony structures, or by displacement of lower abdominal contents from below.

5. Answer c

Echocardiography is an important part of the evaluation of patients with suspected cardiac trauma. It allows rapid assessment of, for example, pump function, pericardial fluid, and valvular disruption.

6. Answer a

Unlike myocardial infarction, the use of inotropes in myocardial contusion will not extend the area of injury because of the nature of the condition of myocardial contusion.

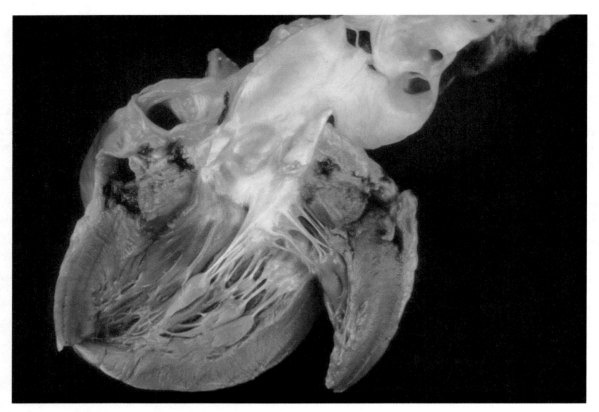

Plate 1. Motor vehicle accident resulting in cardiac trauma and fatal hemopericardium.

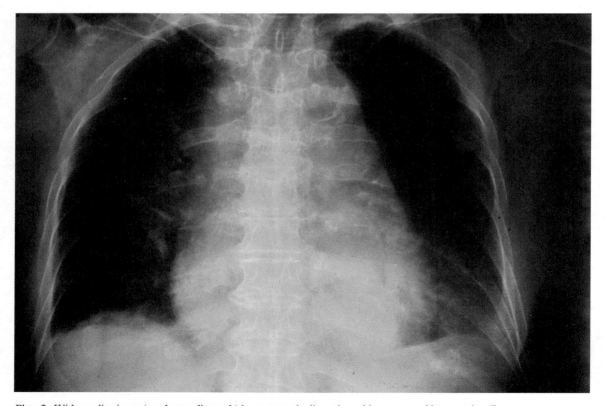

Plate 2. Wide mediastinum (on chest radiograph) in acute aortic dissection with rupture and hemopericardium.

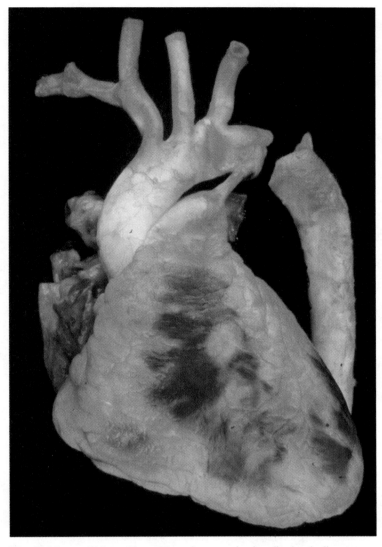

Plate 3. Motor vehicle accident with aortic transection just distal to the ligamentum arteriosum.

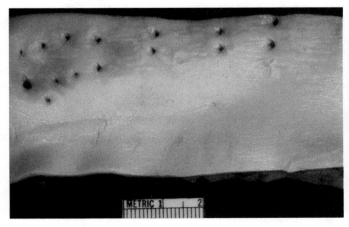

Plate 4. Shallow tears of descending thoracic aorta after a motor vehicle accident.

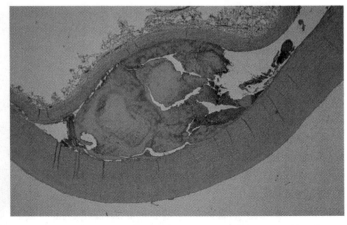

Plate 5. Dissection of proximal descending thoracic aorta resulting from a motor vehicle accident. (x5.)

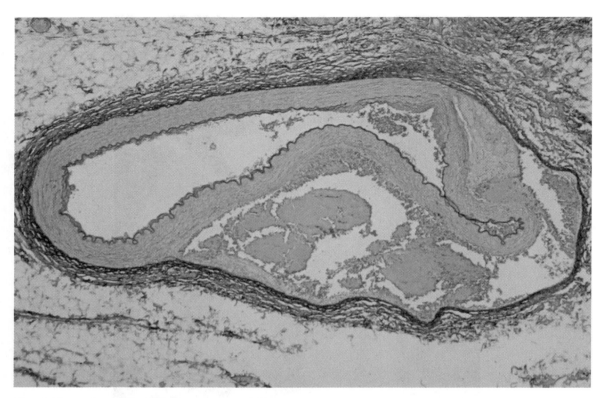

Plate 6. Traumatic rupture of right coronary artery. (x5.)

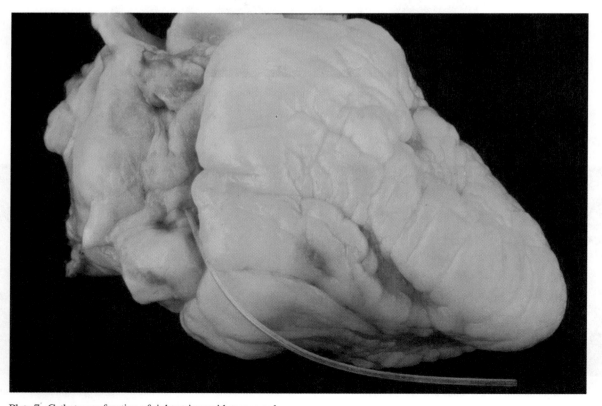

Plate 7. Catheter perforation of right atrium with tamponade.

Chapter 70

Neoplastic Heart Disease

Joseph G. Murphy, M.D.
William K. Freeman, M.D.

Primary tumors of the heart are exceedingly rare, accounting for less than 5% of all cardiac tumors; the remaining 95% of tumors are metastatic tumors to the heart. The most common primary cardiac tumors in adults are myxomas (usually occurring in the left atrium, Fig. 1), followed by lipomas and fibroelastomas (Table 1). The most common cardiac tumor in children is rhabdomyoma.

- Primary cardiac tumors are 5% of all cardiac tumors.
- Metastatic cardiac tumors are 95% of all cardiac tumors.
- The most common primary cardiac tumors in adults are myxomas.

Clinical Features of Cardiac Tumors

Cardiac myxoma may result in systemic symptoms, largely due to embolic phenomenon or its secretion of interleukin-6 (IL-6). Constitutional symptoms include fever and weight loss. Embolic phenomena are due to tumor fragmentation and thromboembolism from the tumor surface. These embolic episodes may mimic systemic vasculitis or infective endocarditis. Right-sided cardiac tumors may result in recurrent pulmonary emboli. The most common presenting symptoms of left-sided cardiac myxomas are dyspnea on exertion, paroxysmal nocturnal dyspnea, and fever, but sudden death and hemoptysis also may occur. The most common physical finding with a left atrial myxoma is a mitral diastolic murmur (similar to mitral stenosis but without the opening snap) (Table 2) or a mitral systolic murmur due to mitral incompetence.

Table 1.—Common Types of Primary Tumors of the Heart

Benign (75%)
    Myxoma
    Rhabdomyoma
    Fibroma
    Lipoma and lipomatous hypertrophy of the atrial septum
    Atrioventricular node tumor
    Papillary fibroelastoma
    Hemangioma
Malignant (25%)
    Angiosarcoma
    Rhabdomyosarcoma
    Fibrosarcoma

From Giuliani ER, Gersh BJ, McGoon MD, Hayes DL, Schaff HV (editors): *Mayo Clinic Practice of Cardiology*. Third edition. Mosby, 1996, p 1675. By permission of Mayo Foundation.

Other features include an added heart sound or tumor plop, atrial fibrillation, clubbing, and Raynaud phenomenon. Left atrial tumors may mimic mitral stenosis or incompetence, endocarditis, or vasculitis. Right atrial tumors may mimic Ebstein anomaly, atrial septal defect, or constrictive pericarditis (Fig. 2). Left ventricular tumors may mimic aortic stenosis or hypertrophic obstructive cardiomyopathy, and right ventricular tumors may mimic pulmonary stenosis, pulmonary hypertension, or pulmonary emboli.

The most common malignant cardiac tumor in adults is angiosarcoma. In children, rhabdomyosarcoma is the most

An atlas illustrating pathologic conditions associated with neoplastic heart disease is at the end of the chapter (Plates 1-8).

common malignant tumor. A malignant lymphoma may occasionally develop in the adult heart.

The locations of cardiac myxomas are listed in Table 3.

- Cardiac myxoma results in systemic symptoms, largely due to its secretion of interleukin-6 (IL-6).
- Right atrial tumors may mimic Ebstein anomaly, atrial septal defect, or constrictive pericarditis.

Familial Cardiac Tumors

The familial cardiac myxoma syndromes constitute approximately 10% of myxomas and have an autosomal dominant transmission.

In Carney syndrome, myxomas arise in noncardiac locations (usually breast or skin), pigmentation of the skin occurs (usually lentigines or pigmented nevi), and there may be endocrine tumors, including pituitary adenomas, adrenocortical disease, or testicular tumors. Other syndromes include the NAME syndrome (*n*evi, *a*trial myxoma, *m*yxoid neurofibroma, and *e*phelides) and the LAMB syndrome (*l*entigines, *a*trial *m*yxoma, and *b*lue nevi). Familial cardiac myxoma syndromes differ from nonfamilial (sporadic) myxomas in that they occur in younger patients, have less of a female preponderance, are frequently multiple, are more frequently recurrent postoperatively, and occur more often in a ventricular site. Familial myxomas are associated with freckling and noncardiac tumors in approximately two-thirds of cases and with endocrine tumors in one-third of cases. Cardiac rhabdomyomas are associated with the tuberous

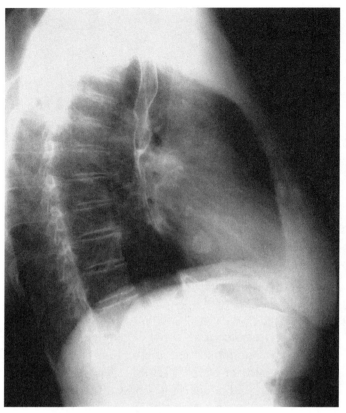

Fig. 1. Lateral chest radiograph demonstrating calcified left atrial myxoma. (From Giuliani ER, Gersh BJ, McGoon MD, Hayes DL, Schaff HV [editors]: *Mayo Clinic Practice of Cardiology*. Third edition. Mosby, 1996, p 1679. By permission of Mayo Foundation.)

sclerosis syndrome, which is characterized by hematomas in multiple organs, epilepsy, mental deficiency, and adenoma sebaceum. Cardiac fibromas are benign connective tissue

Table 2.—Features Differentiating Left Atrial Myxoma From Mitral Valve Disease

Parameter	Myxoma	Mitral valve disease
History	Short duration	Chronic
	Associated constitutional symptoms	No associated constitutional symptoms
	Syncope occasionally noted	Syncope rare
Symptoms	Occasionally episodic	Progressive
Physical examination	Tumor "plop"	Opening snap
	Murmurs varying with position	Murmurs constant
	Associated valve disease unusual	Associated valve disease common
Electrocardiogram	Sinus rhythm	Atrial fibrillation
Chest radiograph	Tumor calcification	Valve calcification
	Left atrium small	Left atrium enlarged
Echocardiogram	Characteristic findings	Characteristic findings

From Giuliani ER, Gersh BJ, McGoon MD, Hayes DL, Schaff HV (editors): *Mayo Clinic Practice of Cardiology*. Third edition. Mosby, 1996, p 1681. By permission of Mayo Foundation.

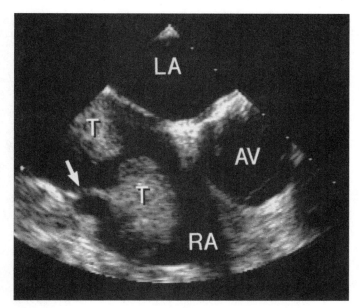

Fig. 2. Multicentric right atrial myxomas; modified basal transverse transesophageal echocardiography plane. Two of three right atrial myxomas (*T*) are visible in this plane. The larger has a well-defined slender stalk (*arrow*) attaching the tumor to the lateral wall of the right atrium (*RA*). The smaller myxoma has a broad-based attachment to the posterior atrial septum. *AV*, aortic valve; *LA*, left atrium. (From Freeman WK, Seward JB, Khandheria BK, Tajik AJ [editors]: *Transesophageal Echocardiography*. Little, Brown and Company, 1994, p 342. By permission of Mayo Foundation.)

tumors that occur predominantly in children. Imaging of cardiac tumors is usually with echocardiography, Imatron computed tomography, or magnetic resonance imaging. Atrial myxomas may recur in approximately 5% of patients. Malignant cardiac tumors have a uniformly poor prognosis.

- NAME syndrome (*n*evi, *a*trial myxoma, *m*yxoid neurofibroma, and *e*phelides).
- LAMB syndrome (*l*entigines, *a*trial *m*yxoma, and *b*lue nevi).

Lipomatous Hypertrophy of the Atrial Septum

Lipomatous hypertrophy of the atrial septum, although not a true tumor, is the accumulation of nonencapsulated adipose tissue (both fetal and adult type) within the atrial septum (Fig. 3). This can lead to massive atrial septal hypertrophy that may protrude into the right atrium. It is more common in elderly, obese women. Lipomatous hypertrophy of the atrial septum has been variably associated with supraventricular arrhythmias. The diagnosis is usually made with echocardiography.

Table 3.—Locations of Cardiac Myxomas

Location	%
Left atrium	75
Right atrium	15
Right ventricle	5
Left ventricle	5

Mesothelioma of the Atrioventricular Node

The mesothelioma of the atrioventricular node is a cystic tumor usually diagnosed at autopsy. It is a rare cause of sudden death due to complete heart block, ventricular fibrillation, or cardiac tamponade.

Papillary Fibroelastoma

Papillary fibroelastomas are benign tumors that arise from the cardiac valves (Fig. 4). They may cause valvular incompetence, coronary obstruction if located on the arterial side of the aortic valve, and thromboembolic complications. Surgical excision is curative.

Metastatic Cardiac Tumors

Metastatic tumors of the heart, predominantly from carcinoma of lung and breast, malignant melanoma, and the leukemias and lymphomas, constitute the majority of cardiac tumors, outnumbering primary cardiac tumors approximately 20 to 1.

Pericardial metastasis presenting with pericarditis is the most common symptom of metastatic heart disease. Less commonly the patient may have an asymptomatic pericardial effusion detected on chest radiography or echocardiography. If the pericardial fluid collects rapidly, the patient may present with pericardial tamponade. Myocardial metastasis is frequent in patients dying of widespread carcinomatosis, but it is rarely diagnosed before death. Endomyocardial and valve metastases may mimic primary cardiac tumors, but they are rare.

Neoplastic Pericarditis

At autopsy, approximately 10% of patients dying of malignancy have pericardial involvement, 5% of which have myocardial metastases. Table 4 lists tumors that can cause neoplastic pericarditis.

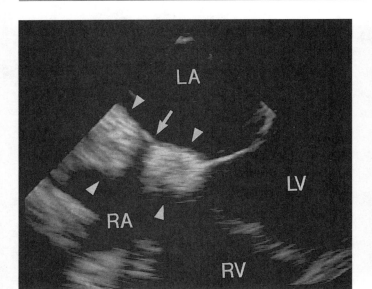

Fig. 3. Lipomatous hypertrophy of the atrial septum; transverse transesophageal echocardiography plane, four-chamber view. Extensive fatty tissue accumulation within the atrial septum (*arrowheads*) spares the fossa ovalis membrane (*arrow*), imparting the typical dumbbell appearance of lipomatous atrial septal hypertrophy. *LA*, left atrium; *LV*, left ventricle; *RA*, right atrium; *RV*, right ventricle. (From Freeman WK, Seward JB, Khandheria BK, Tajik AJ [editors]: *Transesophageal Echocardiography*. Little, Brown and Company, 1994, p 349. By permission of Mayo Foundation.)

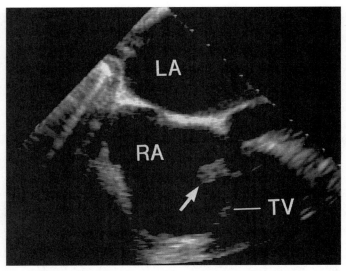

Fig. 4. Papillary fibroelastoma of the tricuspid valve; transverse transesophageal echocardiography plane. A broad-based mass (*arrow*) is attached to the atrial surface of the septal leaflet of the tricuspid valve. The "shimmering" mobility of its fronds on real-time examination was typical of papillary fibroelastoma. *LA*, left atrium; *RA*, right atrium; *TV*, tricuspid valve. (From Freeman WK, Seward JB, Khandheria BK, Tajik AJ [editors]: *Transesophageal Echocardiography*. Little, Brown and Company, 1994, p 350. By permission of Mayo Foundation.)

Nephroblastoma (Wilms tumor) and neuroblastoma are additional causes of neoplastic pericarditis in children.

Primary pericardial tumors are very rare. They include mesothelioma (associated with asbestos exposure), pheochromocytoma, and sarcomas (fibrosarcoma, liposarcoma, angiosarcoma).

A hemorrhagic pericardial effusion may be due to extramedullary intrapericardial hematopoiesis in chronic myeloid leukemia and myelomonocytic leukemic blast crisis.

Small nonprogressive, asymptomatic pericardial effusions may occur in 50% of patients with breast cancer, probably as a result of lymphatic obstruction.

Carcinoma of the bronchus and breast spreads to the heart primarily via lymphatics but also by direct extension and, more rarely, via the pulmonary veins (bronchogenic carcinoma). Carcinoma of the testis and kidney may spread via the venous system and lead to intracardiac metastasis.

Myocardial metastasis may be clinically asymptomatic or may present with nonspecific ST-T wave changes, cardiac arrhythmias, heart block, or myocardial dysfunction. Echocardiography is the most commonly used imaging method in suspected cardiac metastatic disease, but magnetic resonance imaging and computed Imatron tomography imaging are also valuable. Pericardiocentesis under echocardiographic guidance allows diagnosis of pericardial metastases in 70% to 80% of patients.

Treatment of pericardial metastasis is usually palliative, but radiation therapy and chemotherapy are valuable. Malignant pericardial effusion can be treated in the short term by an indwelling drainage catheter and more long term by a pericardial window. Surgical pericardiectomy may be required if the pericardial window obstructs. In patients with acquired immunodeficiency syndrome (AIDS), cardiac tumors may be due to non-Hodgkin lymphoma or metastatic Kaposi sarcoma.

Table 4.—Tumors That Cause Neoplastic Pericarditis

Tumor	%
Lung carcinoma	40
Breast carcinoma	20
Hodgkin disease, leukemia, lymphomas	15
Other carcinoma	10
Melanoma	5
Sarcoma	5
Others	5

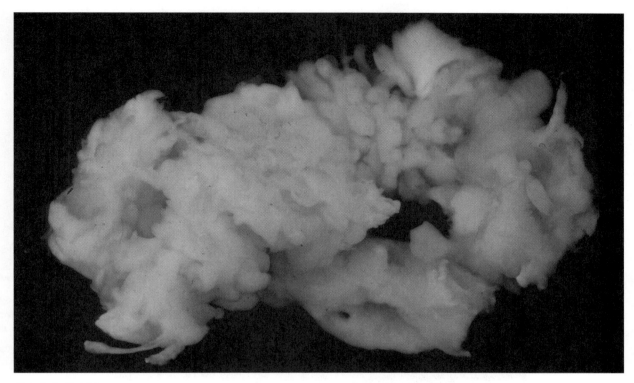

Plate 1. Left atrial myxoma.

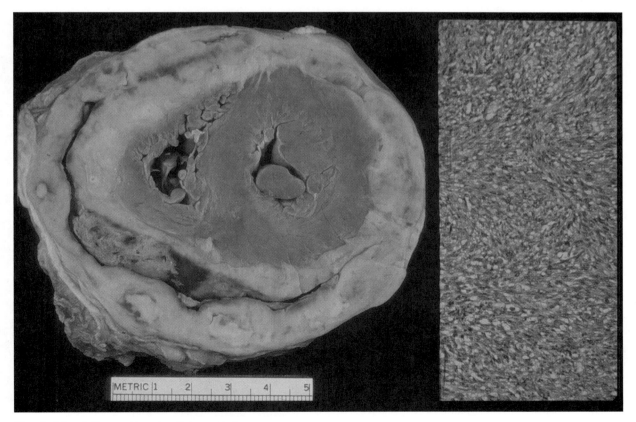

Plate 2. Mesothelioma with pericardial constriction.

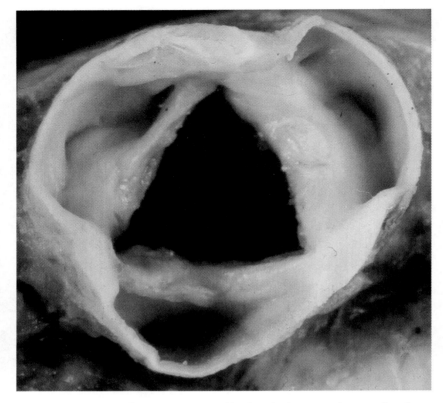

Plate 3. Carcinoid heart disease causing a combination of pulmonary valve stenosis and incompetence.

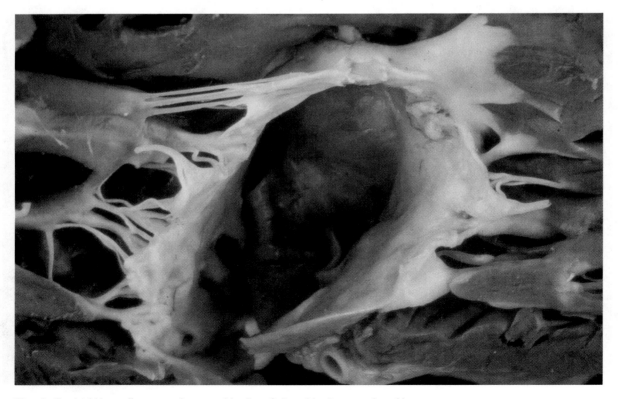

Plate 4. Carcinoid heart disease causing a combination of tricuspid valve stenosis and incompetence.

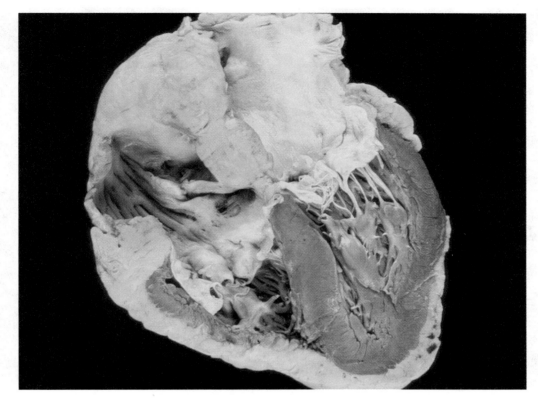

Plate 5. Lipomatous hypertrophy of atrial septum.

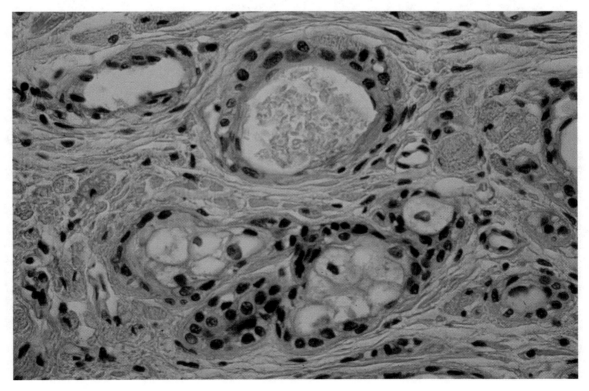

Plate 6. Mesothelioma of atrioventricular node associated with sudden death.

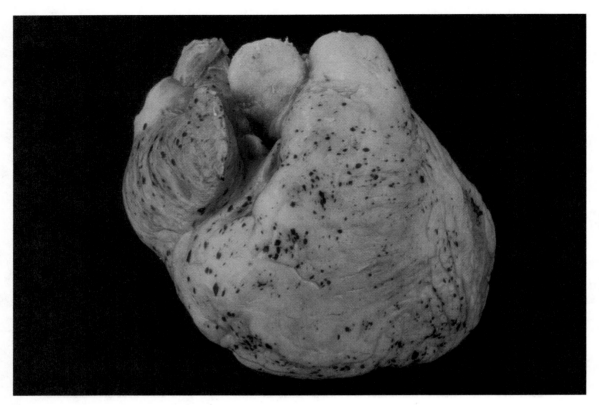

Plate 7. Metastatic melanoma affecting the epicardial surface of the heart.

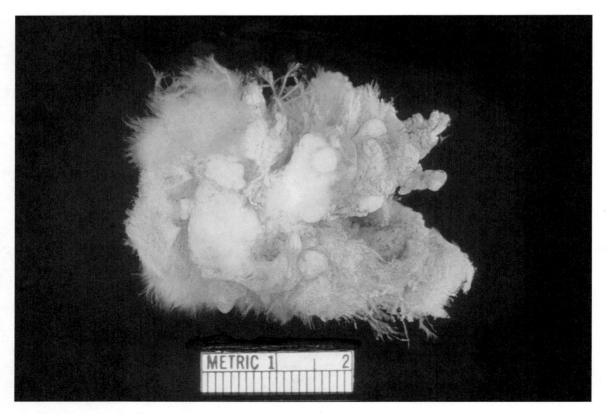

Plate 8. Papillary fibroelastoma of mitral papillary muscle.

Chapter 71

Systemic Disease and the Heart

Marian T. McEvoy, M.D.
Joseph G. Murphy, M.D.

The effects of systemic diseases on the heart are an important area to review for the Cardiology and Internal Medicine Examinations. This chapter is not exhaustive but concentrates on the areas most likely to be tested in these examinations. Most questions in this area ask about clinical management problems that require knowledge of the effect of systemic diseases on the heart. An important question is how the systemic disease modifies either the diagnosis or the management of the cardiac problem and how the cardiac disease, in turn, modifies the approach to the systemic disease.

Neurologic Disease

Cardiac involvement in neurologic disease is unusual; the most important examples are summarized below.

Friedreich Ataxia

Friedreich ataxia is an autosomal recessive neurologic disorder associated with hypertrophic type cardiomyopathy and, less commonly, dilated cardiomyopathy. The hypertrophic cardiomyopathy seen in Friedreich ataxia differs from the usual type in that septal myofibrillary disarray is absent, malignant ventricular arrhythmias are rare,

and left ventricular systolic and diastolic function remain relatively normal. Concentric left ventricular hypertrophy is more common than asymmetric septal hypertrophy. A dilated cardiomyopathy may also be seen in Friedreich ataxia and has a poor prognosis.

• The hypertrophic cardiomyopathy seen with Friedreich ataxia is more benign than the more common form.

Duchenne Muscular Dystrophy

Duchenne muscular dystrophy is an X-linked recessive disorder that affects all muscle types. It is characterized by the absence of the protein dystrophin normally found on the sarcolemma of muscle cells. This disease selectively involves the posterobasal and posterolateral left ventricular wall, including the posterolateral papillary muscle, with relative sparing of the atria, right ventricle, septum, and the anterior wall of the left ventricle. Cardiac involvement also includes atrial and ventricular arrhythmias, especially inappropriate sinus tachycardia or atrial flutter, a malignant arrhythmia when encountered in childhood, because of 1:1 atrioventricular node conduction at this age. Electrocardiography (ECG) shows tall precordial R waves with deep Q waves in leads I, aVL, V_5, and V_6. Muscle levels of creatine kinase are increased. Female carriers of the Duchenne muscular dystrophy gene also have abnormal

An atlas of systemic disease manifestations is found at the end of the chapter (Plates 1-8).

muscle levels of creatine kinase and abnormal ECG findings. Diaphragmatic and intercostal respiratory muscle weakness and kyphoscoliosis lead to impaired respiration, and cardiac failure is common during the late stages of the disease. Procainamide is contraindicated and may make muscle weakness worse. Becker muscular dystrophy is considered a variant of Duchenne muscular dystrophy characterized by the presence of an abnormal dystrophin protein rather than its absence. Cardiac and skeletal muscle involvement are milder, but cardiac failure, cardiomyopathy, and ventricular and atrial arrhythmias may occur.

- Duchenne muscular dystrophy preferentially involves the posterobasal and posterolateral left ventricular wall and is associated with inappropriate sinus tachycardia and atrial flutter.

Myotonic Muscular Dystrophy

Myotonic muscular dystrophy is an autosomal dominant genetic muscle disorder characterized by delayed relaxation of skeletal muscles after contraction. Cardiac involvement is usually limited to conduction system disturbances, but heart failure rarely occurs. All degrees of heart block are seen. Deep abnormal Q waves may be seen in the ECG in the absence of myocardial infarction.

Other Neurologic Diseases

Kearns-Sayre syndrome is a genetic disease transmitted through mitochondrial DNA and characterized by progressive external ophthalmoplegia, pigmentary retinopathy, and heart block that frequently requires permanent pacemaker implantation.

Guillain-Barré syndrome is a nonhereditary demyelinating neuropathy associated with autonomic dysfunction and, rarely, sudden death that is probably due to cardiac arrhythmias.

Head injuries and cerebral hemorrhage may be associated with marked ECG changes, including QT prolongation, prominent U waves, ST-segment elevation or depression, and deep symmetrical T-wave inversion in the precordial leads.

Endocrine and Metabolic Disease

Acromegaly

Acromegaly is associated with cardiomegaly, hypertension, focal myocardial fibrosis, lymphocytic myocarditis, premature atherosclerosis, and a specific acromegalic cardiomyopathy. Cardiomegaly is the result of growth hormone stimulation and hypertension and is associated with myocardial fibrosis and degeneration of myofibrils. Acromegalic cardiomyopathy complicated by heart failure is poorly responsive to conventional heart failure treatment but may respond to octreotide. The hypertension of acromegaly is a low renin-type hypertension due to plasma volume expansion, which responds well to diuretics and sodium restriction.

Hyperthyroidism

Thyroid hormone has effects on the heart similar to those of β-adrenergic receptor stimulation. In hyperthyroidism, the heart is hyperdynamic, with an increase in heart rate, systolic blood pressure, cardiac output, and stroke volume and a decrease in systemic vascular resistance. Atrial fibrillation is the most common serious arrhythmia in hyperthyroidism, occurring in 25% of patients. Atrial fibrillation is problematic because of increased atrioventricular node conduction and relative refractoriness to digoxin. β-Blockers are the drug of choice in this situation pending definitive treatment of the underlying condition. About 40% of patients have spontaneous reversion from atrial fibrillation to sinus rhythm when they become euthyroid. Always check for occult hyperthyroidism in patients with unexplained new-onset atrial fibrillation. Ventricular arrhythmias, heart failure, or, more rarely, conduction disturbances may also occur in association with hyperthyroidism.

Hypothyroidism

Hypothyroidism is associated with a decrease in heart rate, ventricular contractility, and cardiac output but an increase in systemic vascular resistance and systemic blood pressure. It may also be associated with pericardial effusion and an abnormal lipid profile (increase in low-density lipoprotein cholesterol and triglycerides).

Cushing Syndrome

Cushing syndrome results from glucocorticoid excess due to ACTH-producing adenomas of the pituitary. Other causes include ectopic ACTH-producing tumors and primary adrenal tumors. Iatrogenic Cushing disease may be caused by the therapeutic use of steroids. Cushing syndrome is associated with hyperkalemia, systemic hypertension, and left ventricular hypertrophy. The hypertension of Cushing syndrome is relatively resistant to conventional antihypertensive medications but may respond to ketoconazole because of its inhibitory effect on adrenal enzymes.

Addison Disease

Addison disease or other causes of adrenal insufficiency, including abrupt withdrawal of steroid medication, is associated with arterial hypotension, postural hypotension, and syncope. Specific electrocardiographic (ECG) changes, low-voltage ECG, prolonged QT interval, and sinus bradycardia may occur.

Hyperaldosteronism

This is the result of excess secretion of aldosterone. It is associated with hypokalemia and hypertension.

Fabry Disease

This is an X-linked recessive lysosomal storage disorder that results in glycosphingolipid infiltration of the heart, skin, brain, and kidneys. Infiltration of cardiac myocytes results in ventricular hypertrophy and dysfunction, myocardial ishemia and infarction, endothelial dysfunction, valve thickening and incompetence, and arrhythmias.

Refsum Disease

This is an autosomal recessive neurodegenerative disorder due to accumulation of phytanic acid that these patients cannot metabolize. Cardiac involvement includes conduction disorders (atrioventricular node and bundle branch), arrhythmias, and an increased occurrence of sudden death.

Glycogen Storage Diseases

In type II glycogen storage disease (Pompe disease) and type III disease, cardiomyopathy due to myocardial deposition of abnormal glycogen occurs, leading to cardiomyopathy.

Amyloidosis

Amyloid infiltration of the heart may occur in many of the inherited amyloidoses and lead to cardiomyopathy with features of restrictive, dilated, and hypertrophic variants. The prognosis is poor without cardiac transplantation. Cardiac amyloidosis may also occur with minimal or no systemic involvement.

Connective Tissue Disease

Rheumatoid Arthritis

Rheumatoid arthritis may be associated with involvement of all cardiac structures, including the pericardium, valves, myocardium, conduction system, coronary arteries, aorta, and pulmonary circulation. Rheumatoid arthritis can cause both granulomatous and nongranulomatous inflammation of the leaflets of cardiac valves, rarely leading to severe mitral or aortic valve incompetence. The myocardium may be involved by an inflammatory myocarditis or by the deposition of amyloid. The pericarditis of rheumatoid arthritis is characterized by a low glucose value and complement depletion in the pericardial fluid. Constrictive pericarditis rarely occurs. Rheumatoid nodules may be deposited in the conduction system, leading to all degrees of heart block. Aortitis and pulmonary hypertension due to pulmonary vasculitis are rare complications.

- The pericarditis of rheumatoid arthritis is characterized by a low glucose value and complement depletion.

Systemic Lupus Erythematosus

Systemic lupus erythematosus can involve all cardiac structures. Special features of cardiac involvement in systemic lupus erythematosus include nonbacterial endocarditis, antiphospholipid antibody syndrome, and congenital heart block in the offspring of mothers with subacute cutaneous lupus erythematosus.

The offspring of mothers with anti-Ro and anti-La antibodies are at risk for the development of both myocarditis and inflammation and fibrosis of the conduction system, leading to congenital heart block. Treating the mother with corticosteroids may be beneficial if fetal complete heart block is detected utrasonographically.

- The offspring of mothers with anti-Ro and anti-La antibodies are at risk for the development of congenital heart block.

Polymyositis

Polymyositis is associated with myocarditis, pericarditis, and conduction system disease. Myocarditis is rare in the absence of systemic myositis but may respond to systemically administered corticosteroids, hence the importance of endomyocardial biopsy if myocarditis is suspected in polymyositis. All degrees of conduction system disease may be seen with polymyositis. Pericarditis, rarely leading to constrictive pericarditis, may occur.

Ankylosing Spondylitis

Ankylosing spondylitis is associated with aortic incompetence in up to 10% of patients and, more rarely, mitral valve prolapse and mitral regurgitation. Histologically there is an infiltrate of lymphocytes and plasma cells in the aortic wall and around the vasa vasorum, with resultant shortening and thickening of the aortic valve leaflets and aortic root dilatation. Conduction system disease due to both fibrosis and acute inflammation may occur.

Scleroderma

Pericardial disease (pericarditis, pericardial effusions, tamponade, constrictive pericarditis) and pulmonary hypertension are the classic cardiac complications associated with diffuse scleroderma, although conduction system disease and myocardial fibrosis also occur. Patients with CREST syndrome (calcinosis cutis, Raynaud phenomenon, esophageal dysfunction, sclerodactyly, and telangiectasia) are at higher risk for cardiac complications, particularly pericarditis, than patients with uncomplicated scleroderma.

Relapsing Polychondritis

Relapsing polychondritis is associated with aneurysms of the ascending aorta and with aortic incompetence due to inflammation of cartilaginous supporting tissues. Vasculitis of large- and medium-sized arteries, including the coronary vessels, may also occur.

Reiter Syndrome

Reiter syndrome is associated with aortitis, aortic incompetence, heart block, and pericarditis.

Behçet Disease

Behçet disease is associated with aneurysms of the arch vessels and abdominal aorta, aortitis, and aortic incompetence.

Churg-Strauss Syndrome

Classically, Churg-Strauss syndrome is associated with eosinophilic myocarditis and restrictive cardiomyopathy; however, acute pericarditis, constrictive pericarditis, myocardial infarction, arrhythmias, and heart failure may also occur.

Polyarteritis Nodosa

Polyarteritis nodosa is associated with arteritis and aneurysm formation of the epicardial coronary arteries. Myocarditis and pericarditis may also occur.

Hematology/Oncology Diseases

Anemia

Chronic anemia leads to a compensatory increase in cardiac output due to increased venous preload and decreased systemic vascular resistance. Venous return and systemic catecholamines increase, and, rarely, high-output cardiac failure occurs. Left ventricular dilatation and hypertrophy try to maintain an increased stroke volume. Anemia lowers the threshold for angina and may cause nonspecific ST changes even in the absence of cardiac disease. The rapidity of the development of anemia is a major determinant of symptoms. Severe anemia may cause abnormal findings on a cardiac examination, including a hyperdynamic apex, systolic flow murmurs across the aortic and pulmonary valves, diastolic flow murmurs across the mitral and tricuspid valves, and third and fourth heart sounds.

Thalassemia

Thalassemia frequently is associated with systemic iron overload and myocardial iron deposition due to extravascular hemolysis and multiple blood transfusions. This leads to systolic and diastolic ventricular dysfunction, with eventual heart failure. Recurrent pericarditis, pericardial effusions, and, rarely, pericardial tamponade may occur. Heart block may occur because of iron deposition in the atrioventricular node. Chronic anemia is common in thalassemia, and transfusions are frequently required. Chelation agents significantly reduce the occurrence of transfusion-associated cardiac dysfunction.

Sickle Cell Disease

Sickle cell disease is associated with chronic anemia, heart failure, myocardial infarction, and pulmonary infarction. Myocardial infarction in the absence of coronary atherosclerosis occurs because of in situ thrombosis of sickled cells. Sickling is aggravated by high oxygen extraction by the myocardium. Papillary muscle infarction is a well-recognized complication of sickle cell disease. Pulmonary infarction can result from thrombosis in situ as well as from pulmonary emboli and can predispose to recurrent pulmonary infections. Cardiac complications due to iron overload are less common in sickle cell disease than in thalassemia.

Primary Hemochromatosis

Primary hemochromatosis is a genetic disorder of increased iron absorption that results in an increase in the serum level of iron and ferritin and a decrease in total iron binding capacity. Cardiac manifestations include atrial and ventricular arrhythmias, heart block, biventricular enlargement, restrictive cardiomyopathy, and heart failure. Repeated phlebotomy is protective against the cardiac complications of hemochromatosis if started before organ damage has occurred. When phlebotomy is initiated later in the course of the disease, it may reduce organ dysfunction.

Cardiac Radiation Damage

Cardiac radiation damage occurs after irradiation of the mediastinum, usually for Hodgkin or non-Hodgkin lymphoma. All cardiac structures can be damaged, and the initial cardiac symptoms may develop years to decades after irradiation. All forms of pericarditis may occur, including acute pericarditis with or without effusion, chronic pericarditis, effusive-constrictive pericarditis, and constrictive pericarditis. Asymptomatic pericardial thickening without signs of constriction is a common late finding in patients who had mediastinal (mantle) irradiation in the past.

Cardiac irradiation may cause an acute or, more likely, chronic valvulitis that results in valve stenosis or incompetence. Dilated cardiomyopathy due to myocardial microsvasculature damage is a late consequence of cardiac irradiation. Cardiac irradiation can cause significant endothelial damage of the coronary arteries, leading to nonatherosclerotic coronary artery disease. Irradiation in childhood increases fourfold the relative risk of myocardial infarction in adulthood. Irradiation during childhood and the concomitant use of anthracycline chemotherapy agents increase the risk of myocardial damage.

Cancer Chemotherapy

The anthracyclines, including daunorubicin and doxorubicin, are the major causes of chemotherapy-induced cardiomyopathy. The probability of developing cardiomyopathy is dependent on the cumulative dose of medication administered. The risk of cardiomyopathy is less than 1% up to 400 mg/m^2 but increases to 7% at 550 mg/m^2 and to more than 15% at 700 mg/m^2. Preexisting cardiac disease, concomitant use of cyclophosphamide, previous chest irradiation, or age older than 70 years all increase the risk of cardiomyopathy. All patients requiring anthracycline chemotherapy should have a baseline evaluation of ventricular function. If the ejection fraction is 50% or greater, the risk of cardiomyopathy is small, but the ejection fraction should be determined again after dose levels of 300 mg/m^2 and 400 mg/m^2 and after each subsequent dose of doxorubicin. Chemotherapy should be stopped if the ejection fraction decreases by 10% or more or to less than 50%.

In patients with a baseline ventricular dysfunction, chemotherapy should not be initiated if the ejection fraction is 30% or less. If it is between 30% and 50%, chemotherapy can be administered provided the ejection fraction remains greater than 30% and does not decrease by more than 10% from baseline. Children are more sensitive than adults to the adverse effects of chemotherapy, even with a surface area-adjusted dose, and for unknown reasons, females are more sensitive than males.

Cyclophosphamide administered in a high dose is associated with hemorrhagic myocarditis, cardiomyopathy, and pericardial effusion. Paclitaxel (Taxol) may cause atrioventricular block and bundle branch block, and 5-fluorouracil is associated with coronary vasospasm, angina pectoris, and, rarely, myocardial infarction or myocarditis. Interleukin-2 is associated with capillary leak syndrome and, rarely, myocarditis. Cardiomyopathy is a rare reported association of interferon-α therapy.

Cocaine

Cocaine has numerous adverse cardiovascular effects. Many of these effects are related to the sympathomimetic effect of cocaine, which is due to blockage of reuptake of catecholamines in sympathetic nerve terminals. Cocaine has been associated with acute myocardial infarction, sudden cardiac death, noninfarction chest pain, myocarditis, and cardiomyopathy. Hypertension is often a prominent feature because of systemic vasoconstriction. Other effects include accelerated atherosclerosis, subarachnoid hemorrhage, and aortic dissection. Supraventricular and ventricular arrhythmias are common. β-Blockers should be avoided because of the risk of further vasoconstriction due to unopposed vasoconstrictor effects. Labetalol (combined α- and β-blockers) may be used, as may nitrates and calcium channel blockers. Lidocaine used to treat ventricular arrhythmias may precipitate seizures.

Specific Syndromes With Cardiac Involvement

Kartagener Syndrome

This syndrome is caused by an autosomal recessive genetic disorder that affects microtubule function. Clinically, it is characterized by situs inversus, including dextrocardia, bronchiectasis, sinusitis, and sterility due to abnormal sperm and cilia.

Marfan Syndrome

Marfan syndrome is an autosomal dominant disorder characterized by musculoskeletal, cardiovascular, and ocular abnormalities. Cardiac involvement includes mitral valve prolapse leading to mitral regurgitation, aortic root dilatation leading to aortic regurgitation, aortic aneurysm, aortic dissection, and rupture. This syndrome is caused by a genetic mutation in the fibrillin gene. Two important clinical points are that, first, the risk of aortic dissection and rupture increases significantly during pregnancy, especially in women with at least moderate aortic root dilatation before pregnancy. Second, all patients with Marfan syndrome should receive β-blockers, which have been reported to decrease the rate of aortic root expansion and the risk of aortic rupture. Aortic replacement should be considered in asymptomatic patients with an aortic root diameters of 6 cm or greater.

Ehlers-Danlos Syndrome

This is an autosomal dominant disorder associated with hyperextensile joints, spontaneous pneumothoraces, scoliosis, arthritis, and cardiovascular abnormalities that include mitral and tricuspid valve prolapse, aortic root dilatation and rupture, and dissection and rupture of other major arteries. Marked variation in the risk of cardiovascular abnormalities is found among the different forms of this syndrome, of which at least 15 are known.

Pseudoxanthoma Elasticum

This condition is associated with yellow skin papules, angioid streaks in the retina, and cardiovascular disease. Coronary arteries, peripheral arteries, cardiac valves, and the cardiac conduction system may all be affected in this disease, resulting in a high risk of atherosclerosis even in the absence of traditional risk factors, valve incompetence, and heart block.

Osteogenesis Imperfecta

Osteogenesis imperfecta is characterized by findings of blue sclera, increased bony fragility, and hearing loss and is associated with mitral valve prolapse and aortic incompetence.

Noonan Syndrome

This syndrome is characterized by impaired mental abilities, characteristic facies, hypertrophic cardiomyopathy, pulmonary valve stenosis or infundibular stenosis, peripheral pulmonary artery stenosis, patent ductus arteriosus, atrial septal defect, and tetralogy of Fallot.

Williams Syndrome

This syndrome is characterized by mental impairment, characteristic facies, supravalvular aortic stenosis, peripheral pulmonary artery stenosis, ventricular septal defect, atrial septal defect, major artery stenoses, and unexplained hypercalcemia in infancy.

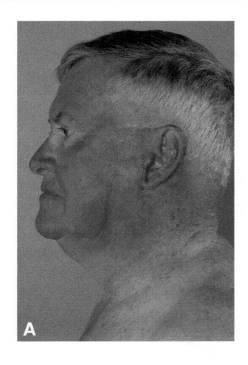

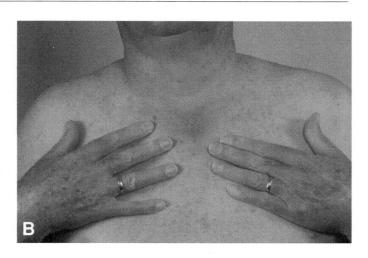

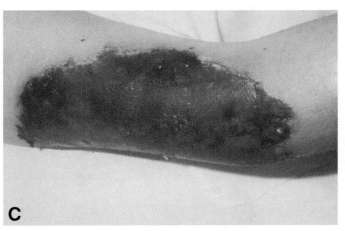

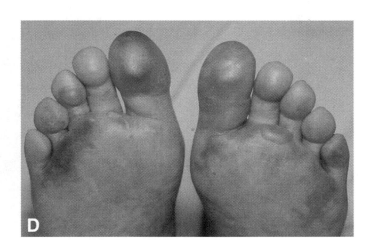

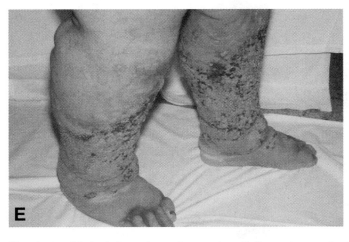

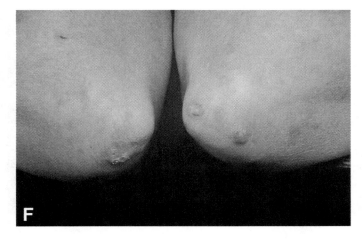

Plate 1. *A* and *B*, Amiodarone hyperpigmentation. *C*, Coumarin necrosis. *D*, Thrombotic coagulopathy. *E*, Chronic lymphedema. *F*, Churg-Strauss granuloma.

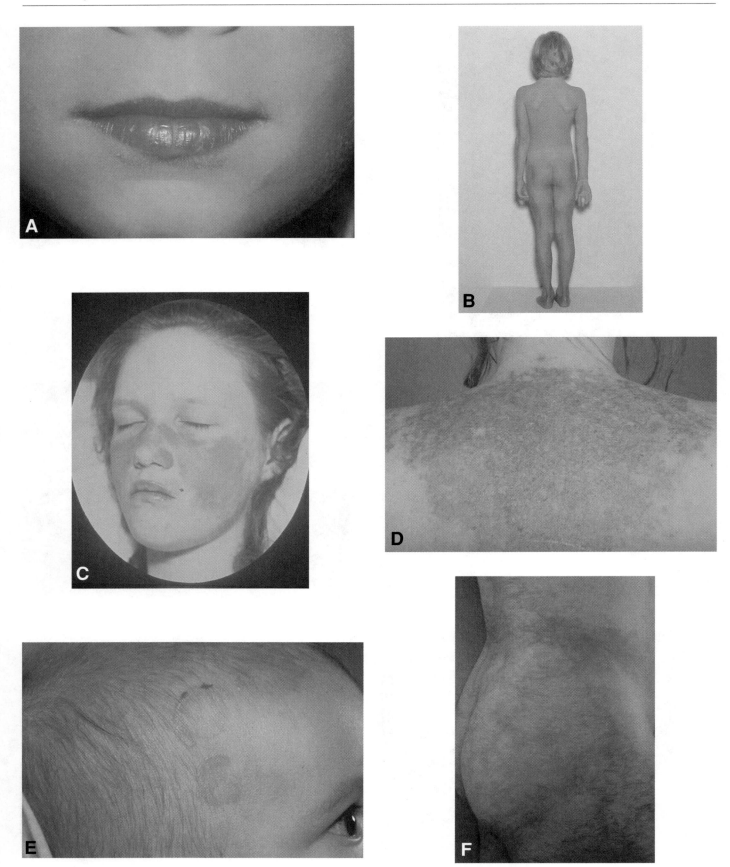

Plate 2.   *A* and *B*, Kawasaki syndrome.   *C* and *D*, Lupus erythematosus, systemic.   *E*, Neonatal lupus.   *F*, Livedo reticularis.

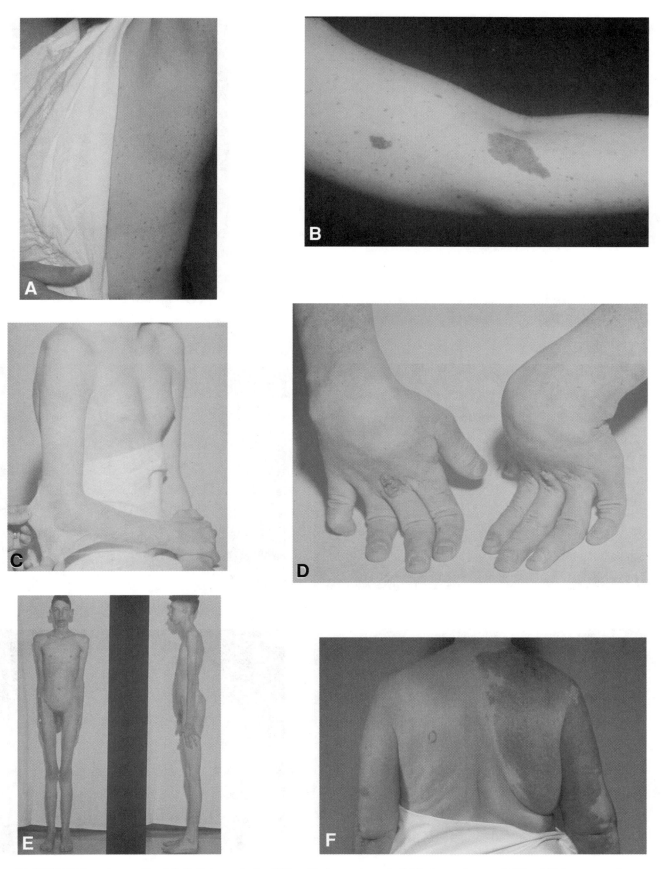

Plate 3. *A* and *B*, LEOPARD syndrome. *C* and *D*, Cutis hyperelastica (Ehlers-Danlos syndrome). *E*, Marfan syndrome. *F*, Klippel-Trénaunay syndrome.

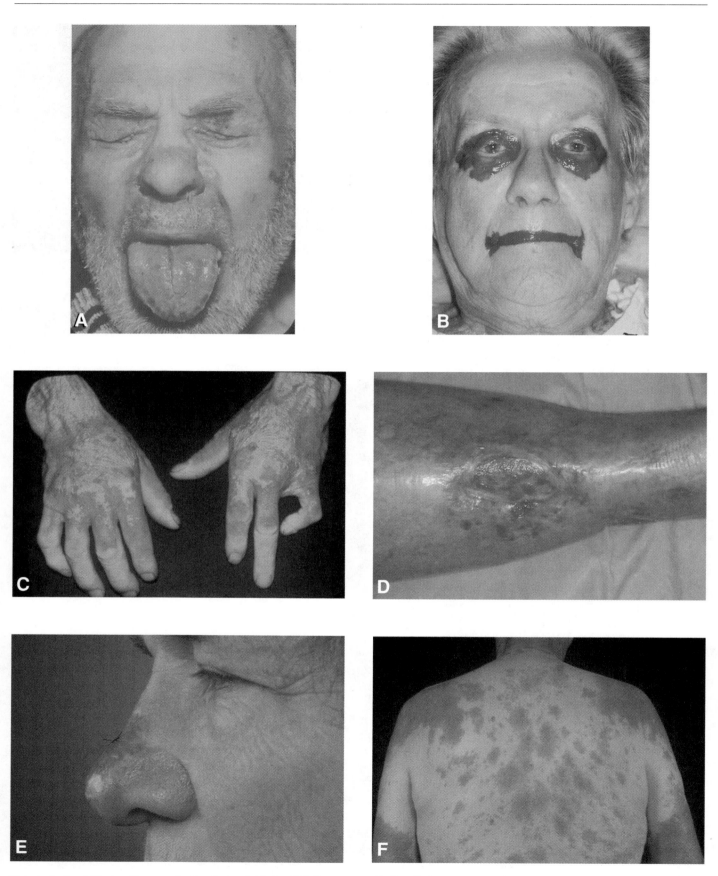

Plate 4. *A*, Amyloidosis with macroglossia. *B*, Amyloidosis. *C*, Pellagra, acute. *D*, Cryofibrinogenemia. *E*, Sarcoidosis/lupus pernio. *F*, Sarcoidosis.

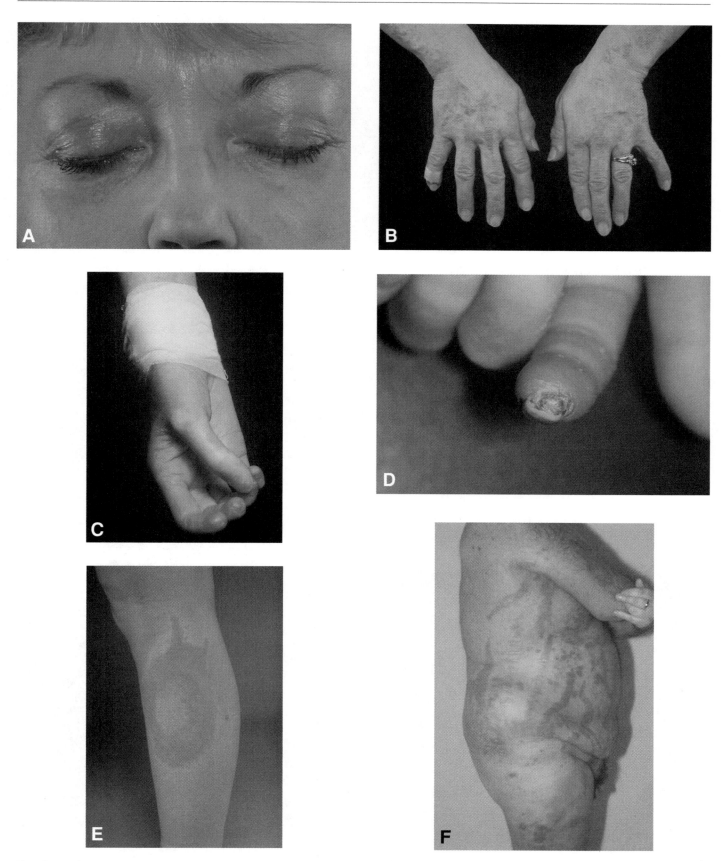

Plate 5. *A* and *B*, Dermatomyositis. *C*, Scleroderma/Raynaud phenomenon. *D*, Scleroderma, systemic. *E*, Erythema chronicum migrans. *F*, Exogenous Cushing disease.

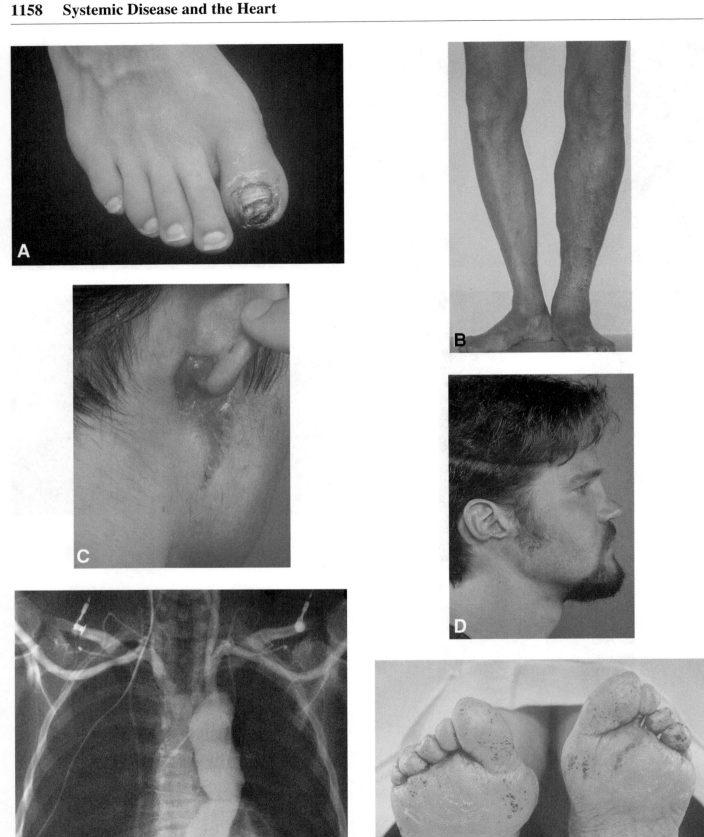

Plate 6. *A*, Buerger disease (thromboangiitis obliterans). *B*, Arteriovenous fistula. *C* and *D*, Wegener granulomatosis. *E*, Takayasu vasculitis. *F*, Vasculitis.

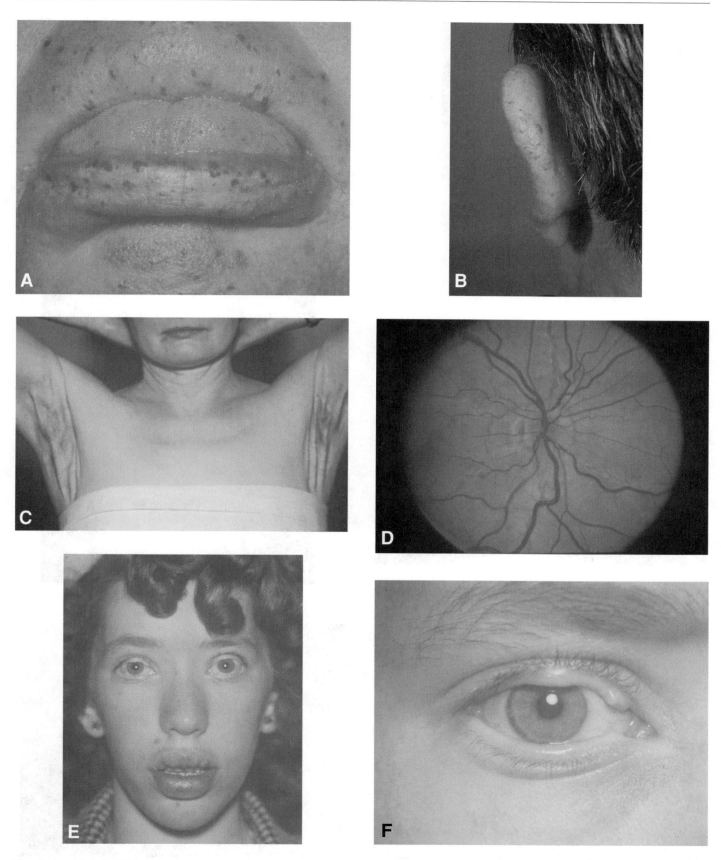

Plate 7. *A* and *B*, Osler-Weber-Rendu disease. *C*, Pseudoxanthoma elasticum. *D*, Angioid streak in pseudoxanthoma elasticum. *E* and *F*, Neuroma in multiple endocrine neoplasia type 3, associated with pheochromocytoma.

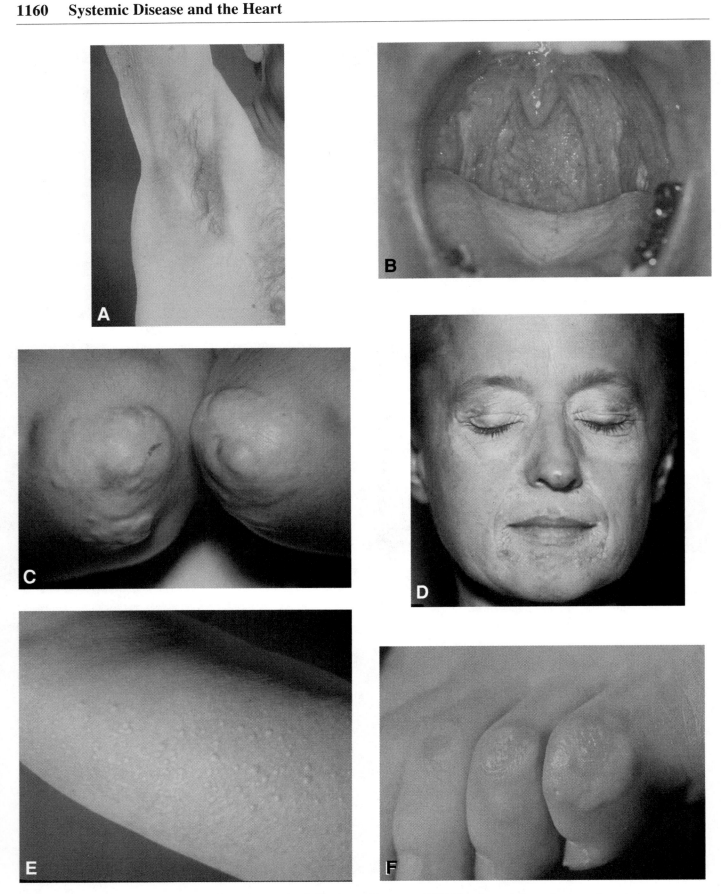

Plate 8. *A* and *B*, Diffuse-plane normolipemic xanthomatosis. *C*, Xanthoma tuberosum. *D-F*, Biliary hypercholesterolemic xanthomatosis.

Chapter 72

Essentials of Pharmacokinetics and Pharmacodynamics

Aleksandar Jovanovic, Ph.D.
Sofija Jovanovic, D.V.M., Ph.D.
Peter A. Brady, M.D.
Arshad Jahangir, M.D.
Andre Terzic, M.D., Ph.D.

A rational approach to pharmacotherapy combines the principles of pharmacokinetics and pharmacodynamics (Fig. 1).

- Pharmacokinetics describes what happens to a drug after it has been administered and includes drug absorption, distribution, and elimination.
- Pharmacodynamics describes the principles of drug action and includes the interaction between a drug and target site (receptor, membrane, etc.).

Pharmacokinetics

The pharmacokinetic processes of absorption, distribution, and elimination determine how rapidly, in what concentration, and for how long the drug will appear at the target site.

Absorption

To reach the site of action, drugs must be absorbed from the site of administration by crossing cell membranes. This commonly occurs by diffusion through the lipid bilayer, although carrier-mediated transport for some drugs may be involved. The ability of a drug to diffuse depends on its size, lipid solubility, and charge. Absorption is more efficient for small, lipid-soluble, and electrically neutral molecules. However, many drugs are either bases or acids, and their ionic charge depends on the pH of the surrounding fluid. In addition to the physicochemical characteristics of the drug, the absorption rate can also be modified by drug formulation.

"Bioavailability" is defined as the fraction of the unchanged drug that is absorbed into the systemic circulation. Bioavailability is equal to 100% following intravenous administration. After other routes of administration, drugs usually are incompletely absorbed, and, thus, only a fraction of the administered dose can reach the systemic circulation. After oral administration and absorption across the gut, drugs can be metabolized in the gut wall or liver before reaching the systemic circulation. This can contribute to a reduction in the bioavailability. Drug metabolism that occurs en route from the gut lumen to the systemic circulation is referred to as "first-pass metabolism." Variations in first-pass metabolism have been reported between persons. Importantly, in patients with severe liver disease, a decrease in first-pass metabolism can lead to an unexpectedly high bioavailability.

Distribution

After absorption, drugs are distributed within the body. Distribution depends on drug liposolubility, drug binding to plasma protein, drug pK, and regional blood flow. Body compartments in which a drug may be distributed are listed in Table 1.

The "volume of distribution" (Vd) is the volume of body fluid in which a drug distributes. It can be calculated using the amount of drug in the body and the plasma concentration of the drug. If plasma concentration is low, the volume of distribution will be high, and vice versa.

Pharmacokinetics

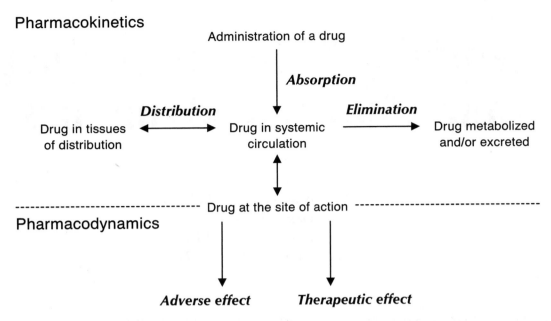

Fig. 1. Primary pharmacokinetic and pharmacodynamic processes. The concentration of a drug achieved at the site of action links pharmacokinetic with pharmacodynamic processes.

Binding to Plasma Proteins

In the blood, a proportion of the drug is bound to plasma proteins, mainly albumin (acidic drugs) and α_1-glycoprotein (basic drugs). Only the unbound (free) fraction distributes, because the protein-bound complex is too large to cross membranes. Thus, only the unbound form is responsible for clinical effects. Changes in protein binding (e.g., due to displacement interactions) will lead to a transient increase in the free drug concentration, as in warfarin displacement by certain antibiotics.

Table 1.—Major Body Compartments in Which Drugs May Be Distributed

Compartment	Drug
Blood (0.08 L/kg) or plasma (0.04 L/kg)	Large molecules bound to plasma proteins (heparin)
Extracellular space (0.2 L/kg)	Large water-soluble molecules (mannitol)
Total body water (0.6 L/kg)	Small water-soluble molecules (ethanol)
Fat (0.3 L/kg)	Lipid-soluble molecules (inhalational anesthetics)
Bone (0.07 L/kg)	Ions (fluoride)

Elimination

Drugs are eliminated from the body by two principal mechanisms: liver metabolism and renal excretion. In principle, drug metabolism inactivates the drug and increases the rate of renal elimination. It should be pointed out that drug-metabolizing enzymes have been exploited to convert inactive prodrugs into pharmacologically active molecules, as with enalaprilat.

Drug Metabolism

Metabolism of drugs in the liver occurs in two phases. Phase 1 involves mainly oxidation (rarely reduction or hydrolysis) generating a more ionic compound. Phase 2 involves conjugation, usually with glucuronic acid and sulphate. Phase 1 oxidation can occur through hydroxylation, oxygenation, dealkylation, or deamination. These reactions are catalyzed by oxidases of the endoplasmic reticulum, which include cytochrome P-450 and cytochrome b_5, with corresponding reductase enzymes. Phase 2 metabolism involves addition of a small molecule to the phase 1 metabolite, which usually leads to a loss of pharmacologic activity. Certain drugs may promote their own metabolism or induce metabolism of other drugs. Conversely, some drugs may inhibit drug metabolism. Drug interactions at the level of metabolism can be of clinical relevance, such as liver enzyme induction by rifampicin.

"Drug clearance" is defined as the volume of blood cleared

of the drug per unit of time and is used to describe drug elimination. Clearance (Cl) of a drug can be calculated as follows:

$$Cl = 0.69 \times \frac{\text{Volume of Drug Distribution}}{t_{1/2}}$$

where $t_{1/2}$ is the half-life of the drug. The half-life of a drug is the time required to halve the amount of the drug in the body. The rate of elimination can be calculated as

$$\text{Clearance} \times \text{Drug Concentration in Plasma}$$

The concentration of a drug in the blood most commonly decreases in an exponential manner, that is, through first-order kinetics (Fig. 2).

Pharmacodynamics

Modern pharmacotherapy is based on understanding the targets of drug action and the quantitative aspects of drug-receptor interaction.

Targets of Drug Action

To produce a pharmacologic response, a drug interacts with one or more constituents on the target cell. Most drugs produce their effects by binding to proteins; notable exceptions of this include general anesthetics, alcohol, and certain antitumor and antimicrobial drugs that may interact with nonprotein cellular targets such as lipids or DNA molecules. The most common drug targets are enzymes, transporters, ion channels, and receptors. In contrast to other targets, receptors are coupled to signal transduction cascades through which they regulate distant cellular functions. Receptors are located either within the plasmalemma or in subcellular compartments, including the cytosol and nucleus. A receptor can be coupled to a target protein directly or through intermediate molecules, including guanosine triphosphate (GTP)-binding proteins. Thus, a drug may modulate enzyme activity, translocation of molecules by carriers, or ion permeance through ion conductance or may activate and block receptors.

Quantitative Aspects of Drug-Target Interaction

The relationship between drug amount and response can be described as follows:

$$E = (E_{max} \cdot C)/(C + EC_{50})$$

Where E is the response elicited by concentration (C) of the drug at the target site, E_{max} is the maximal response that can be achieved by the drug, and EC_{50} is the concentration of the drug that produces 50% of the maximal response. A concentration-response relationship is usually plotted with drug effect on the ordinate and drug concentration (log scale) on the abscissa (Fig. 3).

The "affinity" reflects the ability of a drug to bind to a receptor and can be described by K_A, the dissociation constant of the drug-receptor complex, as follows:

$$\text{Affinity} = \frac{1}{K_A}$$

Thus, a higher K_A reflects a lower affinity of a drug for a receptor, whereas a lower K_A reflects a higher affinity. The ability of a drug to activate a receptor reflects the intrinsic activity of the drug. A "full agonist" is defined as a drug with intrinsic activity (= 1). A "partial agonist" is a drug with partial intrinsic activity (< 1). An "antagonist" is a drug lacking intrinsic activity (= 0) but exhibiting an affinity for the receptor (Fig. 4).

The response of a tissue to a drug depends on

$$\text{Response} = f \cdot \frac{(\varepsilon \cdot N_{tot} \cdot A)}{(A + K_A)}$$

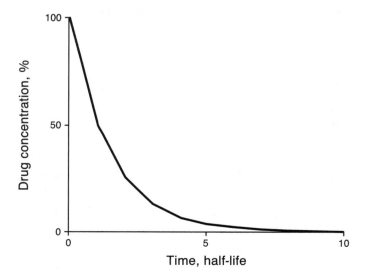

Fig. 2. Plot of plasma concentration against time, expressed as half-life, of a drug with first-order kinetics.

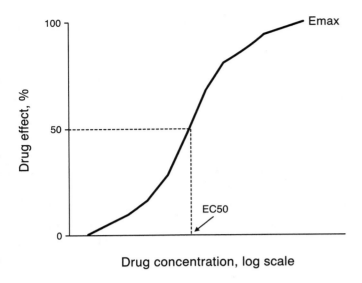

Fig. 3. Concentration-response curve. E_{max} is maximal response that can be achieved by the drug, and EC_{50} is the half-maximal response.

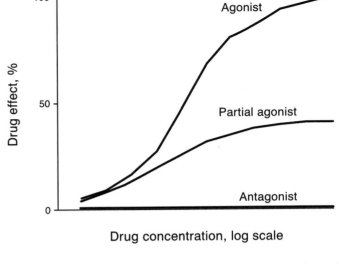

Fig. 4. Concentration-response curves of an agonist, partial agonist, and antagonist.

Where f is the transducer function (which is a tissue property), ε is the intrinsic activity (which is characteristic of the drug-receptor complex), N_{tot} is the number of available receptors, A is the drug concentration, and K_A is the dissociation constant of the drug-receptor complex (the concentration of drug required to occupy 50% of available receptors).

"Potency" and "efficacy" describe a drug in terms of its therapeutic effect (Fig. 5). Potency relates to the EC_{50}, and efficacy to E_{max}.

In Figure 5, drug A is more potent than drug B. Thus, a lesser amount of drug A is required to produce the same response as drug B. However, drugs A and B have the same efficacy, that is, they achieve the same E_{max}. Potency largely determines the dose that needs to be administered to achieve the desired effect. Thus, low potency is important only if the drug has to be administered in inconveniently large amounts. In contrast to drugs A and B, drug C has a lower efficacy (Fig. 5). Efficacy largely determines the magnitude of the achievable therapeutic effect. In addition to the intrinsic activity of the drug, other factors such as pharmacokinetic variables of the drug, the characteristics of the receptor-effector system involved, and the drug's propensity to cause a toxic effect ultimately define the clinical effectiveness of a drug.

Despite their usefulness in characterizing the actions of a drug, concentration-response curves may have limitations in their applications in clinical decision making. For example, such curves may be difficult to use if the expected outcome of treatment is a discrete "either-or" ("quantal" response), such as prevention of arrhythmia or death. In this regard, the dose of a drug required to produce a specified effect can be deduced using a large number of subjects (or experimental animals) and plotting the cumulative frequency of distribution of responder against the log of the dose (Fig. 6).

The quantal dose-response curve is characterized by a median effective dose (ED_{50}), which is the dose that produces the specified therapeutic effect in 50% of persons. Quantal dose-effect curves may also be used to generate information about the margin of safety to be expected for a tested drug. The dose required to produce a toxic effect in 50% of animals is called the "median toxic dose" (TD_{50}) (Fig. 6). If the toxic effect is so extreme as to cause death of the animal population, then this variable is called "median lethal dose" (LD_{50}). A measure that relates the dose of a drug required to produce a desired effect to the dose of the same drug that produces a toxic effect is termed "therapeutic index." In animal studies, the therapeutic index is defined as TD_{50}/ED_{50}. In humans, drug trials and clinical practice reveal the range of effective versus toxic doses. The clinically acceptable risk of toxicity strongly depends on the severity of the disease being treated.

A toxic effect of a drug may be mediated through interaction with the same receptors responsible for the therapeutic effect (e.g., postural hypotension induced by prazosin). Alternatively, an adverse effect could be due to action through

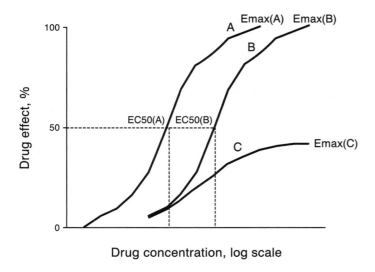

Fig. 5. Relationships between concentration and effect of drugs with different potencies and efficacies.

the same receptors but in different tissues or in different effector pathways (e.g., digitalis glycosides augment cardiac contractility but also produce cardiac arrhythmia, gastrointestinal effects, and changes in vision mediated by inhibition of Na^+/K^+ ATPase in different cell types). In addition, adverse effects may be the consequence of interaction with different types of receptors (antipsychotic drugs exhibit therapeutic effect through action on dopamine receptors, but they may decrease blood pressure through action on adrenergic receptors).

Rational Dosage Regimen

After a drug class has been selected for treating a clinical condition, a rational dosage regimen is required to individualize pharmacotherapy. A rational dosage regimen is based on achieving a target concentration at the site of drug action that will produce the desired therapeutic effect.

Pharmacokinetic Considerations

In most clinical situations, drugs are administered in such a way as to maintain a steady-state concentration of the drug in the body; that is, each dose is given to replace the amount of drug that has been eliminated since the preceding dose. At steady-state, the dosing rate ("rate-in") should equal the rate of elimination ("rate-out"). Therefore,

$$\text{Maintenance Dosing Rate} = Cl \times TC$$

Where Cl is clearance and TC is the target concentration. If the bioavailability of the drug is less than 1, then the dosing rate (DR) needs to be divided by F, the drug bioavailability. The maintenance dose is calculated as follows:

$$MD = DR \times DI$$

Where MD is the maintenance dose, DR is the dosing rate, and DI is the dosing interval that equals the time elapsed between 2 doses. It may be desirable to administer a loading dose that promptly increases the concentration of a drug

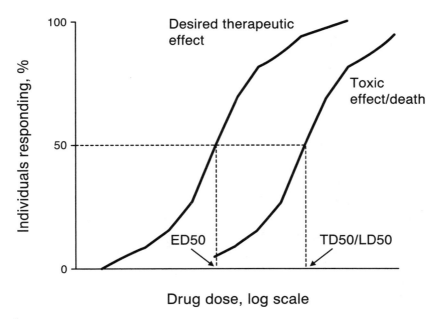

Fig. 6. Quantal dose-response plot.

to the target concentration. Loading dose (LD) can be calculated from the equation

$$LD = Vd \times TC$$

Where Vd is the volume of distribution (see above) and TC is the target concentration.

The pharmacokinetic variables that may affect dosage regimens include absorption, clearance, volume of distribution, and drug half-life. The most frequent cause of underdosage or overdosage is inadequate patient compliance. This can be determined by measuring the concentration of the drug in the blood. If compliance is adequate, other causes of absorption alteration should be considered. Kidney, liver, or heart failure would decrease the clearance of a drug. In the elderly, the relative decrease in skeletal muscle mass tends to produce a smaller volume of distribution of a drug. The volume of distribution can be overestimated in obese patients if dosage is based on body weight but the drug used does not distribute into fatty tissue. Also, abnormal accumulation of fluid (edema, ascites, pleural effusion) can markedly increase the volume of distribution of certain drugs. Changes in drug clearance and volume of distribution alter the half-life of a drug.

Clinical Monitoring of Dosage

In many cases, the action of a drug can be monitored by clinical observation and dosage regimens modified accordingly. Measurement of drug concentration in the blood can be performed to help optimize therapy. In this regard, the physician should address the following questions:

1) Is the patient responding to therapy or showing symptoms of toxicity?

2) Does the concentration measured in the blood reflect the administered dose? Is the concentration within the therapeutic or target range?

3) If the patient is not responding or manifests adverse effects, how should the therapy be modified? Should the drug be discontinued?

Pharmacodynamic Considerations

If increasing the dose of a drug in a particular patient does not lead to further changes in the clinical response, it is possible that a maximal effect of a drug has been reached (see above). Recognition of a maximal drug effect is important in avoiding further increase in dosage that could increase the risk of toxicity. Failure of therapy can be due to changes in the sensitivity of a target organ to a drug. This can be detected by measuring therapeutic drug concentrations in a patient whose response is not adequate to the administered therapy. This may result from an abnormal condition or a disease state, down-regulation of target receptors, or drug-drug interaction.

Questions

Multiple Choice (choose the one best answer)

1. A drug administered by the intravenous route has a bioavailability of:
   a. 0
   b. 1
   c. >1
   d. <1

2. First-pass metabolism of a drug depends on:
   a. Hepatic clearance and hepatic blood flow
   b. Renal clearance and renal blood flow
   c. Hepatic clearance and renal blood flow
   d. Renal clearance and hepatic blood flow

3. Calculation of the rate of elimination requires knowledge of the:
   a. Bioavailability and concentration of drug in the plasma
   b. Clearance and concentration of drug in the plasma
   c. Volume of distribution and concentration of drug in the plasma
   d. Volume of distribution and clearance of the drug

4. The affinity of a drug to its receptor is best described by the:
   a. Maximal effect of the drug
   b. Mean effective concentration of the drug
   c. Dissociation constant of the drug receptor-complex
   d. Intrinsic activity of the drug

5. A partial agonist has the following intrinsic activity:
   a. 0
   b. 1
   c. >1
   d. <1

6. The efficacy of a drug is best described by the:
   a. Maximal effect of the drug
   b. Median effective dose
   c. Dissociation constant of the drug receptor-complex
   d. Clearance of the drug

7. Calculation of the loading dose requires knowledge of the:
   a. Clearance and volume of distribution
   b. Clearance and target concentration
   c. Dosing rate and dosing interval
   d. Volume of distribution and target concentration

8. Calculation of the maintenance dose of a drug requires knowledge of the:
   a. Bioavailability of a drug and clearance
   b. Bioavailability of a drug and target concentration
   c. Clearance and target concentration
   d. Clearance and volume of distribution

9. When the concentration of a drug in plasma is within the therapeutic range, failure of therapy is most likely due to:
   a. Poor patient compliance
   b. Kidney or liver failure
   c. Altered volume of distribution of the drug
   d. Changes of sensitivity of target organ to a drug

Answers

1. Answer b

2. Answer a

3. Answer b

4. Answer c

5. Answer d

6. Answer a

7. Answer d

8. Answer c

9. Answer d

Notes

Chapter 73

Antiarrhythmic Drugs

Robert F. Rea, M.D.

General Principles of Antiarrhythmic Drug Action

"Pharmacokinetics" describes the absorption, distribution, metabolism, and elimination of a drug, and "pharmacodynamics" describes the effect of the drug on the patient. Although the two are related (drug effect commonly parallels drug level), drug effect(s) may be altered by comorbid conditions, concurrent drug use, age, liver and kidney function, and other patient variables.

Levels of antiarrhythmic drugs may fluctuate over the dosing interval, and this may affect arrhythmia suppression. Equally important is the affinity of the drug for the myocardial cell membrane or receptor, where it acts. This affinity is not constant; that is, the drug binds and unbinds even during a constant blood level. The determinants of receptor binding include the association and dissociation constants of the drug and the fraction of time a given cell receptor (typically an ion channel) exists in the rested, inactivated, or active state, and the affinity of the drug for the specific receptor state. This concept, called the "modulated receptor hypothesis," is illustrated in Figure 1.

An associated concept is that of "use dependency," illustrated in Figure 2. Drugs that bind preferentially to active channels (open block) demonstrate direct use dependency; that is, they bind more avidly the more often the channel is active. These drugs are ideal for treatment of paroxysmal tachyarrhythmias, because the episodic rapid heart rates effectively increase drug effect during the episodes, with less drug effect seen during normal, nontachycardic rhythms.

However, many drugs exhibit reverse use dependency; that is, they bind more avidly to rested channels (closed block). Thus, their effect is amplified in the setting of bradycardias and diminished during tachycardias. An example is sotalol, which not only exhibits reverse use dependency but, because of its β-blocking effect, also slows heart rate, further potentiating the drug effect (and proarrhythmic tendency).

Antiarrhythmic Drug Classification

Antiarrhythmic drugs are frequently classified according to the Vaughan Williams system. Class I drugs are predominantly sodium channel blockers, class II drugs are β-adrenergic receptor blockers, class III drugs prolong action potential duration, and class IV drugs are calcium channel blockers.

Class I drugs are subdivided into IA, IB, and IC on the basis of the extent of sodium channel blockade, with class IC agents most potent, IB least potent, and IA intermediate, with respect to this drug action. Remember C > A > B for "most to least" potent sodium channel blockade.

- **C > A > B** for "most to least" potent sodium channel blockade.

1169

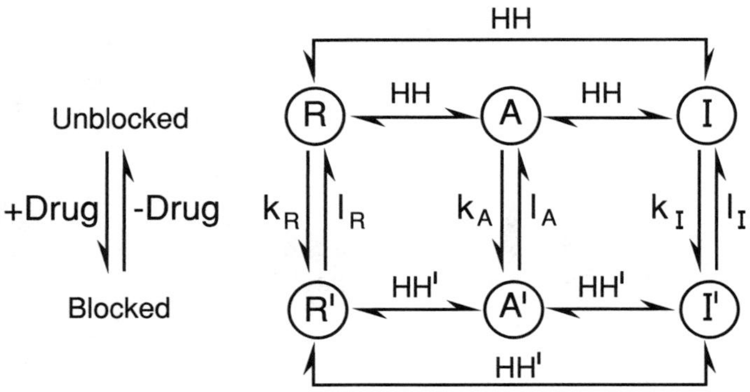

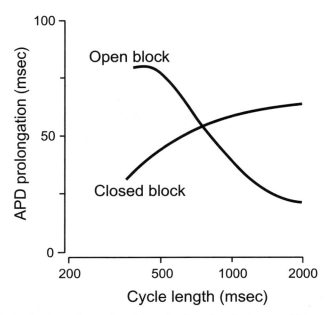

Fig. 1. Diagram of modulated receptor mechanism of action of antiarrhythmic drugs. HH = standard Hodgkin-Huxley rate constants; HH´ = same but voltage-dependence altered by drug binding; k_R, k_A, k_I represent association rate constants; l_R, l_A, l_I represent the dissociation rate constants for the respective fractions. (From *Circulation* 75:514-520, 1987. By permission of the American Heart Association.)

Fig. 2. Plot of opposite rate dependency of prolongation of action potential duration for an agent blocking open or closed channels. Open state blocking drug exhibits use-dependent prolongation of action potential duration, whereas the closed state blocker exhibits reverse use dependence. (From *Circulation* 81:686-690, 1990. By permission of the American Heart Association.)

The pharmacokinetics of antiarrhythmic drugs; their effects on pacing threshold, digoxin level, and warfarin; their removal by dialysis; and their common side effects are summarized in Tables 1 to 5 in the Appendix.

An alternative classification of antiarrhythmic drugs based on membrane channels, receptors, and cardiac ion pumps has been proposed by the Task Force of the Working Group on Arrhythmias of the European Society of Cardiology (Fig. 3).

Proarrhythmia

The tendency of antiarrhythmic drugs to facilitate the emergence of new arrhythmias is heightened in the presence of structural heart disease. The results of a meta-analysis of drug trials following myocardial infarction are shown in Figure 4. The only drug class that definitively showed a mortality benefit was β-blockers. Although amiodarone was of borderline benefit, it was not associated with increased mortality.

In general, the proarrhythmic tendency of antiarrhythmic drugs is potentiated in the presence of structural heart disease of any type, most importantly in the presence of systolic left ventricular dysfunction. This is especially true for class IC drugs, as emphasized in the Cardiac Arrhythmia Suppression Trial (CAST).

Important clinical pointers in proarrhythmia prevention.
1. With class IA drugs, proarrhythmia is dose-independent; most studies suggest that proarrhythmia occurs with normal or subtherapeutic drug levels. Clinically, it is important to follow the corrected QT interval on the electrocardiogram (ECG). Although there are no firm guidelines, QT prolongation beyond 500 ms generally is cause to decrease drug dose or to abandon this drug class. The paradox is that some degree of QT prolongation is indicative of antiarrhythmic drug effect, that is, prolongation of repolarization.
2. With class IC drugs, proarrhythmia may be provoked by increased heart rates; hence, the common clinical practice of performing exercise tests after drug loading. Some studies have suggested the proarrhythmia with class IC may be reversed or attenuated with β-adrenergic blocking agents.
3. With class III drugs, proarrhythmia typically is dose-dependent, especially with sotalol. The development of bradycardia, QT prolongation, and ventricular ectopy with marked QT prolongation following the post-extrasystolic pause is cause for concern.

Quinidine (Class IA)

Quinidine is an isomer of quinine, an antimalarial drug.

Hemodynamics of Quinidine
The α-adrenergic blocking property of quinidine in addition to its direct vasorelaxant effect causes peripheral

Drug	Channels						Receptors				Pumps	Clinical effects			ECG effects		
	Na			Ca	K	I_f	α	β	M₂	P	Na-K ATPase	LV function	Sinus rate	Extra-cardiac	PR interval	QRS width	JT interval
	Fast	Med.	Slow														
Lidocaine	○ (Low)											→	→	△			↓
Mexiletine	○ (Low)											→	→	△			↓
Tocainide	○ (Low)											→	→	●			↓
Moricizine	● (High)											↓	→	○		↑	
Procainamide		●			△							↓	→	●	↑	↑	↑
Disopyramide		●			△				○			↓	→	△	↑↓	↑	↑
Quinidine		●			△		○		○			→	↑	△	↑↓	↑	↑
Propafenone		●						△				↓	↓	○	↑	↑	
Flecainide			●		○							↓	→	○	↑	↑	
Encainide			●									↓	→	○	↑	↑	
Bepridil	○			●	△							?	↓	○			↑
Verapamil	○			●			△					↓	↓	○	↑		
Diltiazem				△								↓	↓	○	↑		
Bretylium					●		◨	◨				→	↓	○			↑
Sotalol					●			●				↓	↓	○	↑		↑
Amiodarone	○			○	●		△	△				→	↓	●	↑		↑
Alinidine				△		●						?	↓	●			
Nadolol								●				↓	↓	○	↑		
Propranolol	○							●				↓	↓	○	↑		
Atropine									●			→	↑	△	↓		
Adenosine										□		?	↓	○	↑		
Digoxin									□		●	↑	↓	●	↑		↓

Relative potency of block:
○ Low   △ Moderate   ● High   □ Agonist   ◨ Agonist/Antagonist

Fig. 3. The Sicilian Gambit approach to antiarrhythmic therapy. (Modified from *Circulation* 84:1831-1851, 1991. By permission of the American Heart Association and Knoll Pharmaceutical Company.)

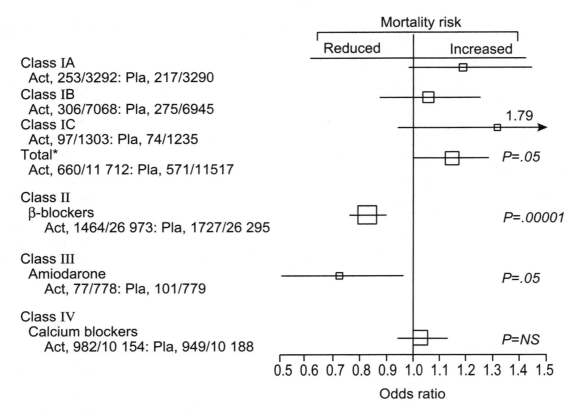

Fig. 4. Effects of antiarrhythmic agents on mortality. Typical odds ratio (OR) by classes (I, II, III, and IV) and subclasses (IA, IB, and IC). Areas of squares are proportional to the variance for each trial or group of trials. Bars indicate 95% confidence intervals. Portions to the left of vertical line (corresponding to OR < 1.0) indicate reduced risk with treatment; portions to the right of vertical line indicate increased risk with treatment. Mortality data (number of deaths/number allocated treatment) are provided for active treatment (Act) and placebo or control (Pla). Note that in the trials of class I agents there was an overall increased risk (with excesses observed in classes IA, IB, and IC). The use of classes II and III significantly reduced risk, and with class IV there was a nonsignificant trend toward excess risk. Asterisk indicates that data from a small trial of three class I agents (quinidine, disopyramide, and mexiletine), excluded from data for the individual subclasses, have been included in overall class I data. (From *JAMA* 270:1589-1595, 1993. By permission of the American Medical Association.)

vasodilatation, leading to orthostatic hypotension and reflex sinus tachycardia. Quinidine does not cause a clinically important negative inotropic effect, even in the setting of severe ventricular dysfunction. The vagolytic effect of this drug can enhance conduction through the atrioventricular (AV) node, and the ventricular response during atrial fibrillation or flutter may increase. This may be fatal during atrial flutter, when slowing of the atrial rate and faster AV nodal conduction can combine to create a 1:1 AV response—thus, the importance of beginning treatment with an AV nodal blocking drug before starting treatment with quinidine.

- The vagolytic effect of quinidine can enhance conduction through the AV node and can be fatal if used alone without an AV node blocking agent (digoxin, β-blocker, calcium channel blocker).

Drug Interactions of Quinidine

Digoxin levels are increased (doubled in many cases) because of decreased tissue binding (lower volume of distribution) and decreased renal and biliary clearance. The increased digoxin level reaches a steady state in 48 hours. The digoxin dose should be halved when treatment with quinidine is started. The anticoagulant effect of warfarin may be increased. An increased neuromuscular blocking effect may be seen when quinidine is given in combination with either depolarizing or nondepolarizing skeletal muscle relaxants. Quinidine inhibits cytochrome $P450_{db1}$ and, thus, decreases the metabolism of propranolol, metoprolol, and propafenone. Theoretically, the proarrhythmic potential of quinidine may be increased when it is given in combination with other drugs that can prolong repolarization (e.g., other class IA or III antiarrhythmic agents).

Heparin displaces quinidine and increases the unbound

fraction in plasma. Verapamil can increase quinidine levels by decreasing its metabolism. Cimetidine increases quinidine levels by decreasing nonrenal clearance by almost 50%, thus prolonging its half-life from 6.5 to 10 hours. Amiodarone increases quinidine levels and also has a compounding effect on prolonging repolarization.

Quinidine concentrations may decrease when phenobarbital, phenytoin, or rifampin are given, because of increased hepatic metabolism. Nifedipine reportedly increases quinidine clearance.

- Quinidine interacts with digoxin, warfarin, heparin, muscle relaxants, propranolol, metoprolol, propafenone, calcium channel blockers, cimetidine, and enzyme-inducing drugs (phenobarbital, phenytoin, rifampin).

Side Effects of Quinidine

About one-third of patients treated with quinidine develop gastrointestinal side effects, most commonly abdominal cramping and diarrhea. Rash is common. "Cinchonism" consists of decreased hearing, tinnitus, and blurred vision, but it can include delirium when severe. Thrombocytopenia

and Coombs'-positive hemolytic anemia can occur; the former usually resolves within 9 days after use of the drug is discontinued but can persist for more than a month. Lupus syndrome with development of antihistone antibodies has been reported. Granulomatous hepatitis may rarely be seen. At toxic levels of quinidine, severe QRS widening and ventricular arrhythmias may occur. These effects may be reversed with the infusion of sodium lactate or sodium bicarbonate.

- About one-third of patients treated with quinidine develop gastrointestinal side effects.
- Other, rarer, noncardiac side effects with quinidine are rash, cinchonism, thrombocytopenia, hemolytic anemia, lupus syndrome, and granulomatous hepatitis.

Proarrhythmia With Quinidine

Quinidine syncope, most frequently due to ventricular tachycardia, has been reported, with an incidence of 0.5% to 4.4%. Quinidine-induced ventricular fibrillation is an early event, with a median occurrence at 3 days after starting treatment for all class IA drugs. A concordance rate of 31% for drug-induced

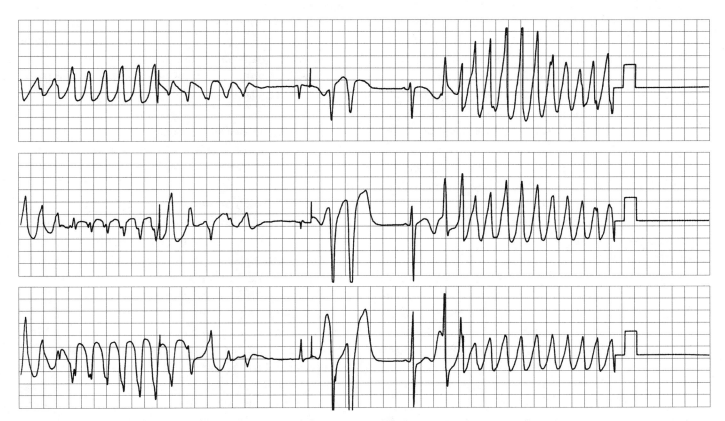

Fig. 5. Torsades de pointes showing the long QT interval, the characteristic QRS peaks that appear to twist around the baseline, the short-long-short R-R cycles that characteristically precede this rhythm, and the paroxysmal bursts of wide complex ventricular tachycardia.

ventricular fibrillation is observed among the class IA drugs. Thus, when torsades de pointes or ventricular fibrillation occurs with any class IA agent, it is prudent to avoid using another drug from the same class. Torsades de pointes (Fig. 5) is well known to occur as a side effect of quinidine, and pause-dependent early afterdepolarizations have been recorded in persons who have this arrhythmia.

- The toxic effects of quinidine may be reversed with the infusion of sodium lactate or sodium bicarbonate.
- A concordance rate of 31% for drug-induced ventricular fibrillation is observed between the class IA drugs.

The results of a meta-analysis of six randomized trials of quinidine in the treatment of atrial fibrillation suggest increased mortality among patients taking the drug. Total mortality was 2.9% for those receiving quinidine, compared with 0.8% in the placebo groups. Sudden death was known to have occurred in only 0.8% of the quinidine group. The empiric use of quinidine in patients who have cardiac arrest has been associated with an increased incidence of subsequent sudden death in comparison with those receiving no treatment.

The serious problem of proarrhythmia argues for in-hospital continuous ECG monitoring during the initiation of antiarrhythmic drug therapy. This is particularly so for class IA drugs in which the proarrhythmic response appears to be idiosyncratic and not necessarily related to the type of arrhythmia being treated or the presence of underlying cardiac disease. When so initiated, the early proarrhythmic response to quinidine is 0.6%. When the QT_c is prolonged more than 500 ms, the antiarrhythmic drug should be stopped to prevent proarrhythmia. Proarrhythmia due to quinidine may occur at normal QT intervals. Plasma levels of quinidine or its metabolites do not predict proarrhythmia and frequently are in or below the therapeutic range. Hypokalemia facilitates induction of early afterdepolarizations by quinidine in vitro and probably predisposes to development of torsades de pointes during clinical use.

Torsades de pointes due to antiarrhythmic drug therapy can be treated with magnesium or isoproterenol and/or temporary pacing at 100 to 110 pulses/min. Early afterdepolarizations are suppressed by these interventions, and because triggered activity may be the mechanism of torsades de pointes, this may explain the antiarrhythmic effect.

- Plasma levels of quinidine or its metabolites do not predict proarrhythmia.
- Hypokalemia probably predisposes to torsades de pointes in patients taking quinidine.

Procainamide (Class IA)

Procainamide is a congener of procaine, a ganglionic blocking agent with membrane-stabilizing properties.

Hemodynamics of Procainamide
Hypotension can occur during intravenous administration of procainamide because of decreased sympathetic efferent activity (likely caused by ganglionic blockade), an effect shared with procainamide's parent compound procaine. In most patients, procainamide has no significant hemodynamic effect when given orally. In a study of patients with severe heart failure, procainamide caused a 17% decrease in cardiac index and no change in left ventricular filling pressure after a single oral dose. Worsening of heart failure symptoms occurred in 10% of patients.

Drug Interactions of Procainamide
Cimetidine can double procainamide levels by decreasing renal clearance; ranitidine has no effect. Neuromuscular side effects may be seen when procainamide is given to patients with myasthenia gravis or when given concomitantly with aminoglycosides. Alcohol decreases procainamide levels by increasing hepatic clearance. Amiodarone increases procainamide levels. Trimethoprim decreases renal clearance and increases plasma levels. The proarrhythmic potential of procainamide may be increased, theoretically, when it is given in combination with other drugs that prolong repolarization (e.g., other class IA or III antiarrhythmic agents).

- Cimetidine can double procainamide levels.
- Procainamide also interacts with aminoglycosides, alcohol, amiodarone, and trimethoprim.

Side Effects of Procainamide
Gastrointestinal side effects limit the use of procainamide in about 25% of patients and are dose-related. Rash, fever, Raynaud phenomenon, agranulocytosis, Coombs'-positive hemolytic anemia (rarely), depression, and psychosis may occur. Cholestatic jaundice has been reported.

Drug-induced lupus erythematosus syndrome associated with procainamide therapy has been recognized since 1962. Antinuclear antibodies form in about 80% of patients, with most patients serologically converting in the first 6 months of therapy. Clinical lupus develops in 30% of patients taking the drug long-term. Signs and symptoms include fever, arthralgias, myalgias, serositis, pulmonary infiltrates, and hepatomegaly. This drug-induced lupus differs from the idiopathic form in that renal, bone marrow, and central nervous system involvement rarely occur. Antibodies to histones have been reported in two-thirds of affected patients, and antibodies to DNA may be detected. Antibodies to double-stranded DNA are detected much less frequently than in the idiopathic form of lupus. Persons who are "slow acetylators" of procainamide develop antibodies and lupus syndrome sooner and at lower cumulative doses than do "rapid acetylators." N-acetylprocainamide, the major metabolite of procainamide, is not thought to produce the lupus syndrome, and patients with procainamide-induced lupus have had resolution of their symptoms when treatment was switched to N-acetylprocainamide.

- Gastrointestinal side effects occur in 25% of patients taking procainamide.
- Persons who are "slow acetylators" of procainamide develop antibodies and lupus syndrome sooner and at lower cumulative doses than do "rapid acetylators."
- Other noncardiac side effects of procainamide are rash, fever, Raynaud phenomenon, agranulocytosis, hemolytic anemia, depression, psychosis, and cholestatic jaundice.

Proarrhythmia With Procainamide

Torsades de pointes can occur as a result of the effects of procainamide on repolarization. Although not extensively studied, the incidence of torsades de pointes with procainamide is probably less than with quinidine. When treatment is initiated during continuous monitoring, early proarrhythmia with procainamide is rare. When used empirically as treatment after cardiac arrest, procainamide has been associated with an increased rate of sudden death, as compared with nontreated patients.

Disopyramide (Class IA)

Hemodynamics of Disopyramide

A strong negative inotropic effect is seen with disopyramide. This effect is related directly to the plasma level of the drug and is seen predominantly in patients with underlying left ventricular dysfunction. The negative inotropic effect precludes the use of disopyramide in patients with ventricular dysfunction and a history of systolic congestive heart failure. A study of 100 patients taking disopyramide orally showed that pulmonary edema occurred in 55% of those with a history of congestive heart failure and in only 3% of those with no such history. Conversely, in the setting of diastolic dysfunction, ventricular performance may be improved. The negative inotropic effect of disopyramide is so significant that it has been used successfully to treat hypertrophic obstructive cardiomyopathy.

- A strong negative inotropic effect is seen with disopyramide, and heart failure may be precipitated in those with decreased left ventricular dysfunction.

Drug Interactions of Disopyramide

Phenobarbital, phenytoin, and rifampin increase hepatic metabolism of disopyramide and can decrease its plasma level. The negative inotropic effect of some drugs (e.g., β-adrenergic blockers) has an additive effect when they are used in combination with disopyramide. The pharmacokinetics of disopyramide are not altered by cimetidine. Erythromycin can increase disopyramide levels by inhibiting hepatic mono-N-dealkylation, and this has led to torsades de pointes. The proarrhythmic potential, theoretically, may be increased when disopyramide is given in combination with other drugs that can prolong repolarization (e.g., other class IA or III antiarrhythmic agents).

- Erythromycin can increase disopyramide levels.
- Enzyme-inducing drugs can decrease plasma disopyramide levels.

Side Effects of Disopyramide

Anticholinergic side effects occur in 29% of patients taking disopyramide and include dry mouth, blurred vision, constipation, and urinary retention. The bladder effects typically are seen in older men and can be counteracted with bethanechol. A sustained-release preparation of pyridostigmine at doses of 90 mg every 12 hours to 180 mg every 8 hours prevents or diminishes the anticholinergic effects of disopyramide and allows higher tolerated doses of the drug.

Disopyramide-induced hypoglycemia has been reported and may be due to enhanced secretion of insulin. Predisposing factors appear to include advanced age, malnutrition, and chronic renal failure. Other reported side effects include nausea, vomiting, rash, cholestatic jaundice, and agranulocytosis.

Disopyramide caused regular uterine contractions in all 10 near-term pregnant women in whom it was studied.

- Anticholinergic side effects occur in 29% of patients taking disopyramide.
- Disopyramide-induced hypoglycemia has been reported and may be due to enhanced secretion of insulin.

Proarrhythmia With Disopyramide

As with other drugs that prolong repolarization, disopyramide can cause ventricular fibrillation and torsades de pointes, although its propensity appears to be less than that of quinidine. In a large series of patients with ventricular arrhythmias who began disopyramide therapy while being continuously monitored, serious proarrhythmia was an unusual event.

Lidocaine (Class IB)

Hemodynamics of Lidocaine

Typically, lidocaine does not alter hemodynamics. In some patients with left ventricular dysfunction, depressed cardiac function can be seen transiently during the administration of a bolus of the drug.

Drug Interactions of Lidocaine

Propranolol, metoprolol, and cimetidine each decrease hepatic blood flow and, consequently, the metabolism of lidocaine, producing up to an 80% increase in the plasma level of the drug. Ranitidine does not affect lidocaine levels. Phenobarbital decreases the plasma concentration of lidocaine.

- Propranolol, metoprolol, and cimetidine each decrease the metabolism of lidocaine.

Side Effects of Lidocaine

The central nervous system side effects of lidocaine predominate and include perioral numbness, paresthesias, diplopia, hyperacusis, slurred speech, altered consciousness, seizures, respiratory arrest, and coma. Infra-His conduction block has been reported in some patients with preexisting conduction system disease. Sinus node depression has occurred in patients with underlying sinus node disease.

Proarrhythmia With Lidocaine

Theoretically, lidocaine may cause arrhythmias by slowing conduction without causing block. Clinically relevant proarrhythmias due to lidocaine are not a concern.

Mexiletine (Class IB)

Mexiletine was developed originally as an anticonvulsant agent and subsequently was found to have antiarrhythmic properties. Knowing this helps one to understand some of the untoward side effects mexiletine has on the central nervous system.

Hemodynamics of Mexiletine

Generally, mexiletine has little effect on heart rate, blood pressure, cardiac output, or intracardiac pressures. In patients with severe left ventricular dysfunction, mexiletine may cause an increase in pulmonary capillary wedge pressure, but this effect is variable. Ejection fraction is generally unaltered by mexiletine in patients with structural heart disease. In patients with a history of congestive heart failure, exacerbation occurred in only 2%.

Drug Interactions of Mexiletine

The metabolism of mexiletine is enhanced by phenytoin, phenobarbital, and rifampin. Levels of mexiletine can be increased by reduced hepatic metabolism caused by cimetidine, chloramphenicol, and isoniazid. Theophylline levels increase a mean of 65% with mexiletine. Digoxin levels and warfarin effects are unchanged by mexiletine. Side effects may be seen at lower doses when mexiletine treatment is begun before lidocaine therapy is discontinued.

- Theophylline levels increase a mean of 65% with mexiletine.
- Digoxin and warfarin are unaffected by mexiletine.

Side Effects of Mexiletine

Gastrointestinal and central nervous system side effects are the most prominent ones associated with mexiletine and are dose- and concentration-related. Tremor is typically the first sign of central nervous system toxicity, but blurred vision, dysarthria, ataxia, and confusion may occur. The tremor caused by mexiletine often responds to treatment with β-adrenergic blocking drugs. Thrombocytopenia rarely has been reported. Increased liver function tests and other blood dyscrasias are rare.

- Mexiletine may cause significant central nervous system side effects.

Proarrhythmia With Mexiletine

The incidence of serious proarrhythmia due to mexiletine reportedly is 1.3% in patients being treated for ventricular tachycardia or fibrillation.

Tocainide (Class IB)

Tocainide, a lidocaine analog, was developed as an oral equivalent of lidocaine that could be used for long-term arrhythmia suppression.

Hemodynamics of Tocainide

Tocainide is well tolerated hemodynamically by most patients. In patients with a history of congestive heart failure, exacerbation occurs in 3.7%. In a study of patients with severe heart failure, tocainide caused an 18% decrease in cardiac index and a 26% increase in left ventricular filling pressure after a single oral dose. Worsening of symptoms occurred in 33%.

Drug Interactions of Tocainide

Cimetidine, but not ranitidine, decreases the bioavailability of tocainide; elimination rate is not affected. Side effects may be seen at lower doses when tocainide treatment is initiated before lidocaine therapy is discontinued. Otherwise, no significant drug interactions have been reported for tocainide.

Side Effects of Tocainide

Adverse reactions have been reported in 30% to 40% of patients and necessitate discontinuation of tocainide treatment in 10% to 20%. As with mexiletine, nausea and vomiting and central nervous system side effects predominate and are related to the dose and plasma concentration. These adverse effects may be reduced by administering tocainide with meals, because this results in lower peak plasma concentrations, as discussed above. Agranulocytosis has been estimated to occur with an incidence of 0.18%; periodic leukocyte counts are recommended for patients receiving tocainide. Pneumonitis and pulmonary fibrosis have been reported, with an estimated incidence of 0.11%. Skin rash and more serious dermatologic reactions may occur.

- Noncardiac side effects of tocainide include agranulocytosis, pneumonitis, and pulmonary fibrosis.

Proarrhythmia With Tocainide

Serious proarrhythmia is rare with tocainide. Torsades de pointes would not be expected to occur with tocainide and has not been reported. Ventricular fibrillation rarely has been reported to be caused by tocainide.

Phenytoin (Class IB)

The initial, and still major, use of phenytoin is for seizures.

Hemodynamics of Phenytoin

Hypotension can occur during intravenous administration of phenytoin, but this may be caused partly by the diluent in the intravenous preparation. A significant ventricular depressant effect is not known to occur with phenytoin. Sinus node dysfunction can worsen with phenytoin treatment in patients with underlying sinus disease.

Drug Interactions of Phenytoin

Through induction of hepatic enzymes, phenytoin increases the metabolism of many drugs, including quinidine, disopyramide, lidocaine, mexiletine, and theophylline. Phenytoin levels are increased by isoniazid, chloramphenicol, disulfiram, and some sulfonamides. Antacids decrease the absorption of phenytoin.

Side Effects of Phenytoin

Central nervous system side effects, particularly nystagmus and ataxia, occur in a concentration-dependent manner with phenytoin. Rash, nausea, blood dyscrasias, lupus syndrome, peripheral neuropathy, hyperglycemia, lymphadenopathy, Stevens-Johnson syndrome, hirsutism, and osteomalacia may be seen. Gingival hyperplasia can occur, with an incidence of about 50%, but eliminating preexisting periodontal disease at the initiation of therapy and practicing thorough oral hygiene can prevent this reaction. Extravasation during intravenous administration can cause serious tissue damage, including limb loss.

A rare but important reaction is phenytoin hypersensitivity syndrome, which is characterized by fever, skin lesions (ranging from acneiform to erythema multiforme), lymphadenopathy, hepatosplenomegaly, and leukocytosis with eosinophilia. It occurs more frequently in black than in white patients and may be fatal. Corticosteroids have been used with success.

- Noncardiac side effects of phenytoin include central nervous system side effects, lupus syndrome, blood dyscrasias, peripheral neuropathy, gingival hypertrophy, rash, lymphadenopathy, hirsutism, and osteomalacia.

Proarrhythmia With Phenytoin

The propensity for phenytoin to produce arrhythmogenesis appears to be low and is not well described.

Moricizine (Class IC)

Moricizine, a phenothiazine derivative, was widely used in Russia and Europe before gaining approval in the U.S. Its initial promise was unrealized because of excess mortality in the moricizine-treated group in CAST II.

Hemodynamics of Moricizine

Symptomatic ventricular dysfunction does not occur with moricizine if the patient does not have a history of congestive heart failure; however, among patients with such a history, worsening of symptoms has been reported in 4.8%.

Drug Interactions of Moricizine

Cimetidine decreases moricizine clearance, which leads to increased levels of the drug. Clearance of theophylline is increased 40% to 70% by moricizine and, thus, higher doses of theophylline may be needed. Moricizine has no interaction with digoxin level or warfarin effect.

- Cimetidine and theophylline interact with moricizine.

Side Effects of Moricizine

Moricizine treatment is discontinued in 7% to 11% of patients because of its side effects. Central nervous system and gastrointestinal side effects are the predominant adverse reactions, and dizziness, nausea, and headache are the most common complaints. Fever, abdominal pain, diarrhea, altered mental state, thrombocytopenia (0.2%), increased liver function tests (0.7%), and conduction abnormalities also have been reported with moricizine. Moricizine does not block dopamine receptors, and so even though it is a phenothiazine derivative, it does not cause Parkinson-like symptoms.

- Central nervous system and gastrointestinal side effects are the prominent side effects with moricizine.

Proarrhythmia With Moricizine

Moricizine was used in the CAST II trial, and this portion of the study was halted early because of an increased incidence of mortality during the initial 14 days of therapy with moricizine in comparison with placebo. Initial reports stated an incidence of early proarrhythmia with moricizine of 3.2% in 908 patients treated for ventricular arrhythmias. Since then, proarrhythmia rates of 15% to 27% have been reported and appear to be related to the severity of the presenting arrhythmia and ventricular dysfunction. In some patients, proarrhythmia can be produced by exercise.

Flecainide (Class IC)

Flecainide was developed as a fluorinated congener of procainamide.

Hemodynamics of Flecainide

Heart rate typically is unaffected by flecainide except in the presence of sinus node disease. Flecainide has a negative inotropic effect similar to that of disopyramide. Flecainide exacerbated congestive heart failure in 16% of patients with a history of this condition and in 6% of those without such a history. No effect on ejection fraction was detected in patients with a left ventricular ejection fraction greater than 50% at baseline. Flecainide is not recommended for patients with severe ventricular systolic dysfunction or a history of congestive heart failure. It may be useful in patients with diastolic dysfunction and arrhythmias.

Drug Interactions of Flecainide

Flecainide increases digoxin levels by a mean of 25% through decreased drug clearance. Flecainide levels are increased by amiodarone and cimetidine. Both propranolol and flecainide levels are mildly (< 30%) increased when these drugs are given concomitantly. Quinidine inhibits hepatic metabolism of flecainide and increases the elimination half-life about 20%.

- Flecainide levels are increased by amiodarone and cimetidine.

Side Effects of Flecainide

Flecainide treatment reportedly had to be discontinued in 13% of patients because of side effects. Central nervous system reactions include blurred vision, headache, and ataxia. Congestive heart failure can be provoked in patients with underlying reduced ventricular function.

Proarrhythmia With Flecainide

Flecainide was used in CAST, which tested the hypothesis that suppression of ventricular ectopy after myocardial infarction decreases the incidence of sudden death. The trial was discontinued early when results showed that mortality was higher among patients treated with flecainide or encainide, as compared with those treated with placebo (Fig. 6 and 7). In that trial, proarrhythmia was not just an early event; the mortality curves for drug and placebo continued to diverge throughout follow-up. When used for treatment of ventricular arrhythmias, flecainide has more

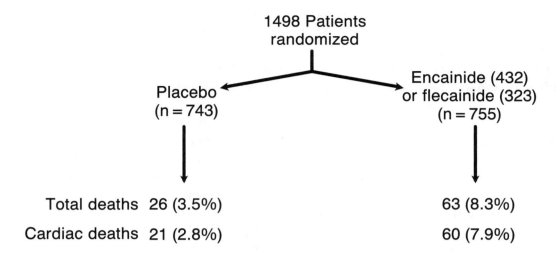

Fig. 6. Cardiac Arrhythmia Suppression Trial. Mortality figures for patients assigned to active drug versus placebo, at 10-month mean follow-up. (From *Patients at Risk for Sudden Cardiac Death: Outcome Studies*. Minneapolis: Medtronics, 1998. By permission of the publisher.)

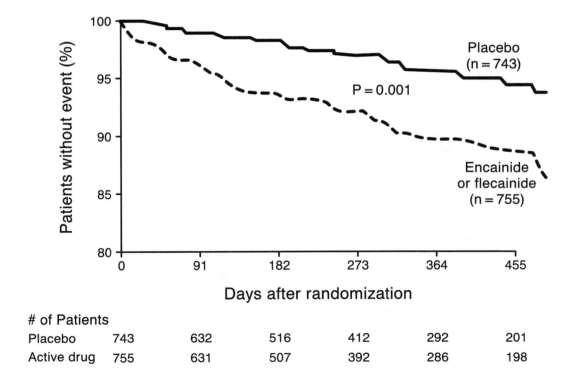

Fig. 7. Cardiac Arrhythmia Suppression Trial. Prognosis of post-myocardial infarction patients treated with placebo vs. encainide/flecainide. Event is defined as death or cardiac arrest due to arrhythmia. (From *Patients at Risk for Sudden Cardiac Death: Outcome Studies*. Minneapolis: Medtronics, 1998. By permission of the publisher.)

proarrhythmic potential when the underlying rhythm disorder is sustained ventricular tachycardia. Reduced left ventricular function probably also predisposes to arrhythmogenesis. Because of the significant use-dependent effects of the drug, proarrhythmia can sometimes occur with exertion; therefore, exercise testing is recommended before hospital dismissal after achieving steady state with flecainide. β-Adrenergic blockade has been used successfully to treat proarrhythmia due to flecainide.

Ventricular proarrhythmia due to flecainide is rare in the treatment of paroxysmal atrial fibrillation or paroxysmal supraventricular tachycardia. Only a few cases of serious proarrhythmia have been reported in patients with normal hearts who received flecainide for supraventricular arrhythmias. In a series of 55 patients treated with flecainide for paroxysmal atrial fibrillation, atrial proarrhythmia was 5%.

- Flecainide has more proarrhythmic potential when the underlying rhythm disorder is sustained ventricular tachycardia.

Propafenone

Propafenone is structurally related to β-adrenergic antagonists and has β-blocker properties.

Hemodynamics of Propafenone
Although resting sinus rate is usually unchanged with propafenone, the response to exercise is blunted. Propafenone has a negative inotropic effect that is due at least partly to its β-adrenergic and calcium channel blocking activity. In patients with a history of congestive heart failure, exacerbation occurred in 9.3%. The ejection fraction did not deteriorate in 10 patients with a left ventricular ejection fraction greater than 45% at baseline. However, a decrease in ejection fraction can be seen in patients with compromised ventricular function. This negative inotropic property is less pronounced than that of disopyramide and flecainide. Systolic blood pressure may decrease in some patients after taking an oral dose of propafenone.

As noted above, propafenone is related to and shares properties with β-blockers. About 7% of the U.S. population lacks P450$_{db1}$ enzyme activity that results in metabolism to 5-hydroxypropafenone, which has less β-blockade than the parent compound. In this group, levels of propafenone

are higher, levels of 5-hydroxypropafenone are lower, and physiologic β-blockade is increased.

Drug Interactions of Propafenone
Propafenone increases digoxin levels an average of 83%, possibly because of a decrease in nonrenal clearance and volume of distribution (but the mechanism is not known). Warfarin clearance is decreased with propafenone, leading to an increased anticoagulant effect (prothrombin time increased up to 44% in one small series). Propranolol and metoprolol are both metabolized by the cytochrome P450$_{db1}$ system, and their levels are increased in the presence of propafenone, which is metabolized by this enzyme. Theophylline, cyclosporine, and desipramine levels are increased by propafenone.

Phenytoin, phenobarbital, and rifampin increase the metabolism of propafenone. Quinidine blocks the cytochrome P450$_{db1}$ system and inhibits the conversion of propafenone to 5-hydroxypropafenone in "extensive metabolizers." Cimetidine causes an increase in propafenone levels that results in a small but significant lengthening of the QRS.

- Propafenone increases digoxin levels an average of 83%.
- Propafenone increases the anticoagulant effect of warfarin.

Side Effects of Propafenone
Nausea, dizziness, and a metallic taste (especially with dairy products) are the most common side effects of propafenone. Blurred vision, paresthesias, constipation, increased liver function tests, exacerbation of asthma (probably due to the β-adrenergic blocking effect), and conduction abnormalities may occur. Central nervous system side effects appear to be related to propafenone plasma concentration and are more frequent in "poor metabolizers." Overall, about 10% to 25% of patients discontinue propafenone treatment because of its side effects.

Proarrhythmia With Propafenone
Polymorphic ventricular tachycardia and ventricular fibrillation have been reported shortly after initiation of propafenone therapy. Incessant ventricular tachycardia may also occur. The incidence of serious proarrhythmia with propafenone treatment of ventricular arrhythmias is about 5%. Molar sodium lactate reportedly reverses the arrhythmogenic effect of propafenone. In the treatment of atrial arrhythmias, propafenone can sometimes cause atrial flutter, with 1:1 AV conduction when AV nodal block is not accomplished. Ventricular proarrhythmia occurring with

propafenone treatment of supraventricular arrhythmias in patients with structurally normal hearts is exceedingly rare. This latter situation may be one in which initiation of antiarrhythmic drug therapy in an outpatient setting can be contemplated. Obtaining an ECG and an exercise test upon attainment of steady state is still recommended.

Amiodarone (Class III)

Amiodarone was developed initially as an antianginal agent and subsequently was found to have powerful and complex antiarrhythmic actions. The initial enthusiasm generated from European medical centers was tempered when pulmonary and hepatic toxic effects were documented. Nonetheless, amiodarone is widely used, and because of multicenter trials of its use to prevent sudden death in diverse patient groups (EMIAT, CAMIAT, AVID, STAT-CHF, and GESICA), it will continue to be widely used.

Hemodynamics of Amiodarone
With amiodarone taken orally, there is no change in left ventricular ejection fraction, even in patients with reduced ventricular function. In fact, STAT-CHF demonstrated an increase in ejection fraction and a decrease in hospitalization rates for patients with congestive heart failure who received amiodarone. Amiodarone given intravenously, recently approved for treatment of life-threatening ventricular arrhythmias, may cause hypotension in higher dose ranges.

Drug Interactions of Amiodarone
Amiodarone increases digoxin concentration (dose should be halved), warfarin effect (dose should be reduced by 1/3 to 1/2), and cyclosporine concentration. Because amiodarone has β-blocking and calcium channel blocking activity, there may be an additive effect when it is given in combination with drugs possessing these characteristics.

Side Effects of Amiodarone
Amiodarone can cause many side effects, and the most important ones to be aware of are pulmonary toxicity, hepatotoxicity, and thyrotoxicity, both hyperthyroidism (rare) and hypothyroidism (more common). Pulmonary toxicity may present as dyspnea, nonproductive cough, fever, or pleuritic chest pain or merely with asymptomatic changes on a chest radiograph. Other side effects to be aware of include photosensitivity, blue discoloration of the skin, and corneal

microdeposits (which rarely cause a problem).

● Noncardiac side effects of amiodarone are common and can be life-threatening.

Proarrhythmia With Amiodarone
Amiodarone may cause life-threatening ventricular arrhythmias, including ventricular fibrillation and torsades de pointes—a 4% incidence among patients being treated for ventricular arrhythmias in one reported series. However, it is probably less proarrhythmic than other antiarrhythmic agents.

Clinical Trials of Amiodarone
Because of its relatively safe proarrhythmic profile and multiplicity of cellular effects (essentially all cardiac class effects have been reported), amiodarone has been the subject of several important clinical trials in which it was used prophylactically rather than for treatment of a specific arrhythmia. These trials can be divided roughly into studies of patients after myocardial infarction (EMIAT, CAMIAT, and others) and studies of patients with heart failure (STAT-CHF and GESICA).

CAMIAT

CAMIAT (Canadian Amiodarone Myocardial Infarction Arrhythmia Trial) randomized 1,202 patients after myocardial infarction who had 10 or more ventricular premature depolarizations per hour or one or more runs of ventricular tachycardia on ambulatory ECG to receive amiodarone or placebo (Fig. 8-10). Over a 1.79-year follow-up, resuscitated ventricular fibrillation or arrhythmic death occurred in 6.0% of patients in the placebo group and 3.3% in the amiodarone group ($P = 0.016$). *It was concluded that amiodarone reduces ventricular fibrillation and arrhythmic death after myocardial infarction with frequent or repetitive ventricular premature complexes. The absolute risk reduction was greatest in patients with a previous myocardial infarction or congestive heart failure.*

EMIAT

EMIAT (European Myocardial Infarct Amiodarone Arrhythmia Trial) randomized 1,486 patients with ischemic ventricular dysfunction after myocardial infarction (ejection fraction $\leq 40\%$) (Fig. 11-13). Over a 21-month follow-up,

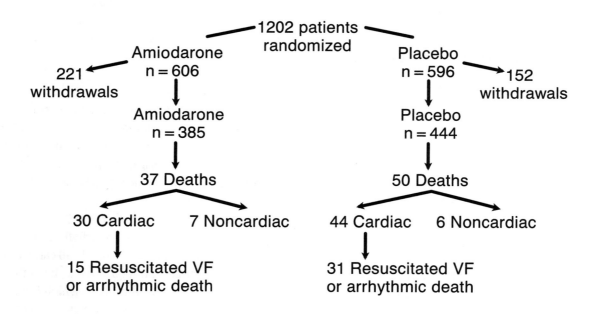

Fig. 8. Canadian Amiodarone Myocardial Infarction Arrhythmia Trial. Outcome events for patients randomized to amiodarone versus placebo. VF, ventricular fibrillation. (From *Patients at Risk for Sudden Cardiac Death: Outcome Studies*. Minneapolis: Medtronics, 1998. By permission of the publisher.)

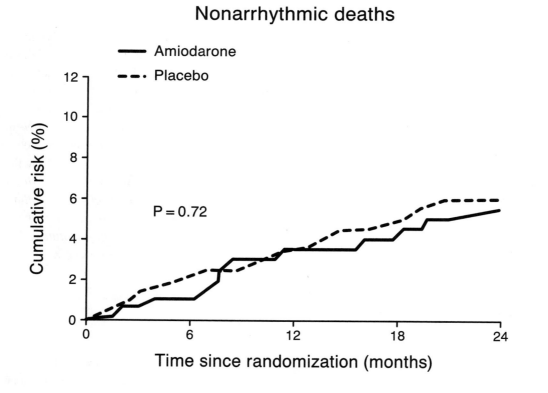

Fig. 9. Canadian Amiodarone Myocardial Infarction Arrhythmia Trial. Nonarrhythmic death rates. (From *Lancet* 349:675-682, 1997. By permission of The Lancet.)

All-cause mortality

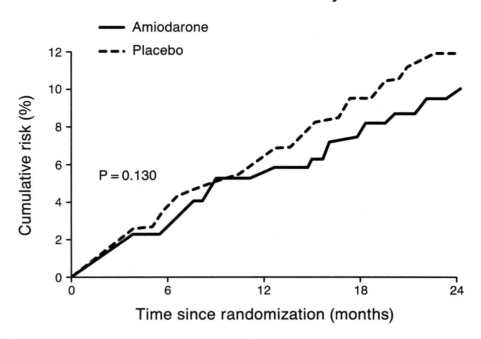

Fig. 10. Canadian Amiodarone Myocardial Infarction Arrhythmia Trial. All-cause mortality rates. (From *Lancet* 349:675-682, 1997. By permission of The Lancet.)

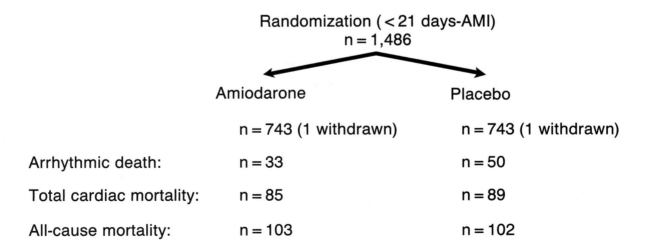

Fig. 11. European Myocardial Infarct Amiodarone Arrhythmia Trial. Outcome events for patients randomized to amiodarone versus placebo. AMI, anterior myocardial infarction. (From *Patients at Risk for Sudden Cardiac Death: Outcome Studies*. Minneapolis: Medtronics, 1998. By permission of the publisher.)

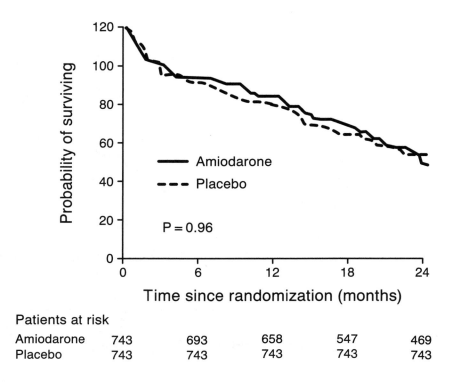

Fig. 12. European Myocardial Infarct Amiodarone Arrhythmia Trial. Kaplan-Meier estimates of all-cause mortality by group. (From *Lancet* 349:667-674, 1997. By permission of The Lancet.)

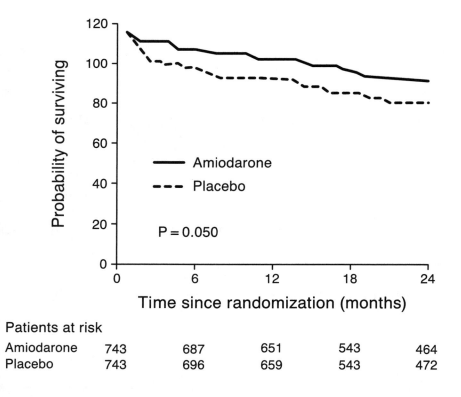

Fig. 13. European Myocardial Infarct Amiodarone Arrhythmia Trial. Kaplan-Meier estimates of arrhythmic deaths and resuscitated cardiac arrest by group. (From *Lancet* 349:667-674, 1997. By permission of The Lancet.)

all-cause and cardiac mortality were similar in both groups (~ 14%), although there was a 35% decrease in arrhythmic deaths in patients receiving amiodarone. *Amiodarone therapy in this group of patients was not supported by the study.*

The conclusions of these trials differ, as did their entry criteria. CAMIAT focused on ventricular ectopy, whereas EMIAT focused on ventricular dysfunction. Clearly, patients in EMIAT were sicker, with substantially greater overall mortality. Interestingly, the details in CAMIAT indicate that, like EMIAT, all-cause mortality was unaffected by amiodarone. The ultimate message from these trials is ambiguous, but amiodarone at the very least was shown to be no worse than placebo, supporting at a minimum its use in patients who require antiarrhythmic therapy for other reasons.

GESICA Trial

GESICA (Grupo de Estudio de la Sobrevida en la Insuficiencia Cardiaca en Argentina) randomized in a nonblinded fashion 516 patients with heart failure to standard heart failure treatment with or without a low dose (300 mg/day) of amiodarone (Fig. 14-16). At 2-year follow-up,

there were significant decreases in overall deaths (28%), arrhythmic deaths (27%), and deaths due to heart failure (23%) in patients receiving amiodarone. *It was concluded that amiodarone is an effective treatment for decreasing mortality among patients with severe heart failure.*

STAT-CHF Trial

STAT-CHF (Survival Trial of Antiarrhythmic Therapy in Congestive Heart Failure) randomized in a blinded fashion 674 patients with heart failure *and* ≥ 10 ventricular premature depolarizations per hour *and* an ejection fraction of 40% or less to amiodarone or placebo (Fig. 17 and 18). At 2-year follow-up, there was a significant effect of amiodarone on overall survival or incidence of sudden death. Of interest, ejection fraction was improved with amiodarone, and there was a trend for improved mortality in the subset (~ 1/3) with nonischemic cardiomyopathy.

Like EMIAT and CAMIAT, the GESICA and STAT-CHF studies had different entry criteria and different conclusions. Of importance, about 2/3 of patients in GESICA and about 1/3 in STAT-CHF had nonischemic cardiomyopathy. This raises the possibility that the benefit of amiodarone may be

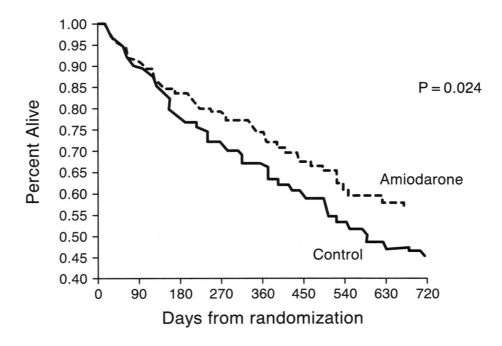

Fig. 14. Grupo de Estudio de la Sobrevida en la Insuficiencia Cardiaca en Argentina. Two-year mortality due to all causes. (From *Lancet* 344:493-498, 1994. By permission of The Lancet.)

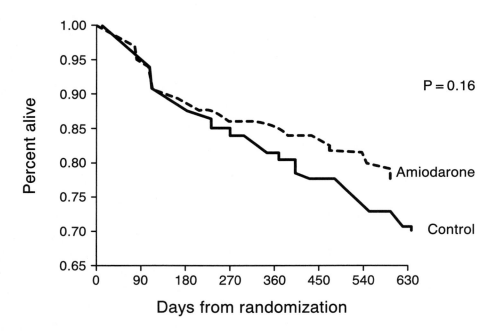

Fig. 15. Grupo de Estudio de la Sobrevida en la Insuficiencia Cardiaca en Argentina. Mortality due to progressive heart failure. (From *Lancet* 344:493-498, 1994. By permission of The Lancet.)

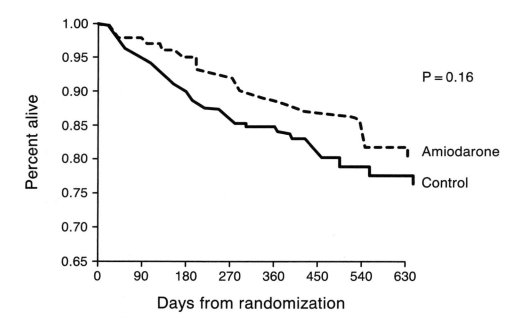

Fig. 16. Grupo de Estudio de la Sobrevida en la Insuficiencia Cardiaca en Argentina. Mortality due to sudden death. (From *Lancet* 344:493-498, 1994. By permission of The Lancet.)

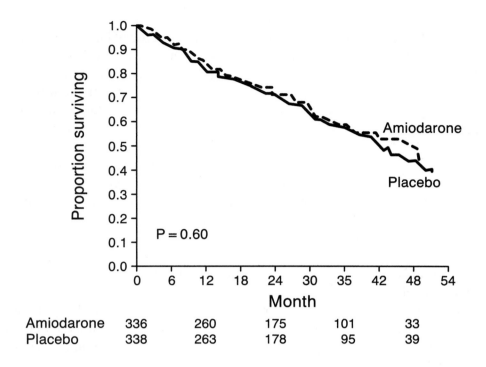

Amiodarone	336	260	175	101	33
Placebo	338	263	178	95	39

Fig. 17. Survival Trial of Antiarrhythmic Therapy in Congestive Heart Failure. Comparison of amiodarone versus placebo for decrease of overall mortality in patients with congestive heart failure. (From *N Engl J Med* 333:77-82, 1995. By permission of Massachusetts Medical Society.)

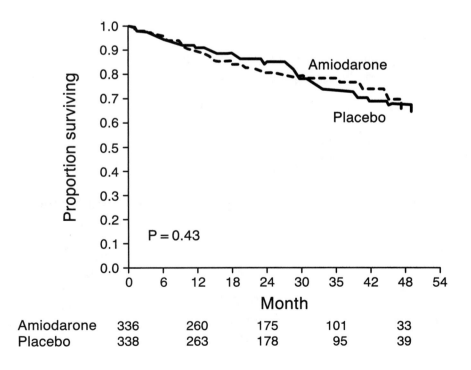

Amiodarone	336	260	175	101	33
Placebo	338	263	178	95	39

Fig. 18. Survival Trial of Antiarrhythmic Therapy in Congestive Heart Failure. Comparison of amiodarone versus placebo for decrease in the incidence of sudden death. (From *N Engl J Med* 333:77-82, 1995. By permission of Massachusetts Medical Society.)

greatest in the nonischemic subgroup, as suggested by the post-hoc analysis in STAT-CHF. Also, it is clear from both studies that amiodarone improved ejection fraction and heart failure, although the mechanism is unclear.

Sotalol (Class III)

Hemodynamics of Sotalol
Sotalol is a potent β-adrenergic blocker that causes significant bradycardia and worsening of left ventricular dysfunction. In patients with hypertension, it has an antihypertensive effect.

Drug Interactions of Sotalol
The β-blocking effect of sotalol may cause interactions with other drugs that have either β-blocking properties or AV nodal inhibitory effects such as digoxin or nonvascular selective calcium channel blockers such as verapamil and diltiazem.

Side Effects of Sotalol
Fatigue is a prominent side effect of sotalol. Most of its side effects are related to its β-blocking effect.

Proarrhythmia With Sotalol
The QT lengthening caused by sotalol can result in ventricular fibrillation or torsades de pointes. Proarrhythmia rates of 3% to 5% have been reported. Its use in patients prone to hypokalemia/hypomagnesemia (i.e., those taking diuretics) and use of higher dose ranges (> 160 mg twice daily) are associated with heightened proarrhythmia. Note that the proarrhythmic effect seen with sotalol is dose-related, unlike that with quinidine, procainamide, and disopyramide. The SWORD (Survival With Oral d-Sotalol) trial evaluated d-sotalol, a purely potassium blocker with no β-blocking effect, in 3,121 patients with left ventricular dysfunction and a recent myocardial infarction or recent heart failure and a remote myocardial infarction. d-Sotalol increased mortality among these high-risk patients after myocardial infarction (Fig. 19 and 20).

Bretylium (Class III)

Bretylium is rarely used and then only in the setting of recurrent ventricular tachycardia or fibrillation, having failed lidocaine, procainamide, and DC cardioversion.

Hemodynamics of Bretylium
Bretylium causes an initial norepinephrine release, with subsequent depletion of norepinephrine from sympathetic nerve terminals. This results in increased blood pressure, followed by orthostatic hypotension. This feature has inhibited attempts to develop long-acting oral congeners.

Side Effects of Bretylium
Orthostatic hypotension can occur with bretylium and may

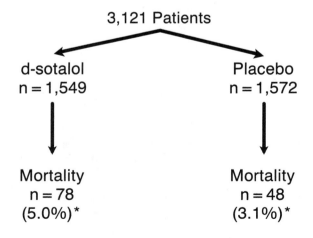

Fig. 19. Survival With Oral d-Sotalol Trial. Mortality figures for patients assigned to d-sotalol versus placebo. F/U, follow-up. (From *Patients at Risk for Sudden Cardiac Death: Outcome Studies*. Minneapolis: Medtronics, 1998. By permission of the publisher.)

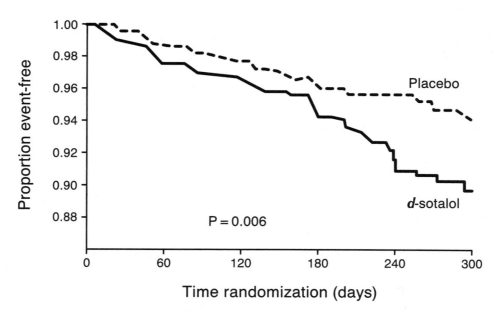

Fig. 20. Survival With Oral *d*-Sotalol Trial. Event-free survival for patients randomized to placebo or *d*-sotalol. (From *Lancet* 348:7-12, 1996. By permission of The Lancet.)

take days to resolve. There may be nausea and vomiting during delivery of the initial bolus.

Proarrhythmia With Bretylium
There may be an initial worsening of arrhythmias because of norepinephrine release.

Ibutilide (Class III)

Ibutilide, a class III intravenous agent, is used for chemical conversion of atrial fibrillation and flutter to sinus rhythm.

Hemodynamics of Ibutilide
Ibutilide is a novel class III drug that prolongs action potential duration in the atrium by blocking the outward repolarizing potassium current (delayed K rectifier). It has scant hemodynamic effect.

Side Effects of Ibutilide
The drug is administered as a 1-mg bolus and repeated at 10 minutes if conversion has not occurred. It has few extracardiac side effects.

Proarrhythmia With Ibutilide
Proarrhythmia is the Achilles' heel of ibutilide. In one

series, 6 of 157 patients developed polymorphic ventricular tachycardia and 4 required cardioversion because of hemodynamic collapse. Underlying impairment of left ventricular function and prolonged baseline QT interval may be risk factors for proarrhythmia.

Adenosine (Unclassified)

Adenosine has long been understood to be an endogenous modulator of smooth muscle tone and cardiac electrophysiologic properties. Its use in pharmacologic doses for arrhythmias has revolutionized acute treatment of supraventricular tachycardia in emergency departments, clinics, and hospitals. It also is effective in rare ventricular tachycardias that result from triggered activity. Adenosine is used to evaluate coronary flow reserve in patients with coronary artery disease and to treat the "no-reflow" and "slow-flow" phenomena seen after coronary artery interventional procedures.

Hemodynamics of Adenosine
Intravenously administered adenosine has a short duration of action (1 to 5 seconds), and the hemodynamic effects (i.e., sinus tachycardia, increased systolic arterial pressure, and decreased diastolic arterial pressure) are similarly short. The direct vasodilator effect of the drug is offset by sympathetic

excitation via its actions on chemoreceptors and other visceral receptors. Hyperventilation occurs because of chemoreceptor stimulation. The adenosine effect will be augmented in patients taking dipyridamole and diminished in those taking theophylline compounds; this reflects inhibition of adenosine uptake by dipyridamole and block of adenosine receptors by theophylline. Denervated hearts are supersensitive to the electrophysiologic effects of adenosine.

Side Effects of Adenosine

Patients almost uniformly complain of chest pain and dyspnea with the injection of adenosine. However, these abate within seconds.

Proarrhythmia With Adenosine

An underappreciated problem with adenosine is its tendency to promote atrial fibrillation, which can be sustained in susceptible patients. This can be a problem in patients with a bypass tract-mediated narrow QRS supraventricular tachycardia that is converted to preexcited atrial fibrillation (atrial fibrillation that is conducted to the ventricle over the bypass tract), a more worrisome rhythm. Sinus bradycardia and arrest can also occur. Ventricular proarrhythmia usually consists of ventricular premature contractions and nonsustained ventricular tachycardia, but ventricular fibrillation can occur. Because of the short duration of action of adenosine, supraventricular tachycardia may recur within minutes after administration of the drug.

- The adenosine effect will be augmented in patients taking dipyridamole and diminished in those taking theophylline compounds.
- Denervated hearts are supersensitive to the electrophysiologic effects of adenosine.

Examination Strategy

The pharmacology and pharmacokinetics of antiarrhythmic drugs are clinically important and are a very "testable" area for the Cardiology Boards, because many objective facts are known about drugs. Although it may be debated about when to use a specific drug, there usually is a definite answer about the pharmacologic properties of a given compound. Particular attention should be paid to drug metabolism, half-life, elimination route, effect on surface electrocardiographic intervals, drug interactions, and side effects. Although any cardiac drug currently approved by the FDA may be included in a test question, the ones most important for the Cardiology Boards are quinidine, procainamide, lidocaine, flecainide, propafenone, amiodarone, and sotalol. However, it is best to learn about each drug—if time permits. Encainide should be considered only as it relates to the conclusions of the Cardiac Arrhythmia Suppression Trial: its pharmacology is not important for the Cardiology Boards. Important examination topics include proarrhythmia, amiodarone trials, and drug side effects.

Suggested Review Reading

General Concepts of Antiarrhythmic Drug Action

1. Hondeghem LM: Antiarrhythmic agents: modulated receptor applications. *Circulation* 75:514-520, 1987.

2. Hondeghem LM, Snyders DJ: Class III antiarrhythmic agents have a lot of potential but a long way to go. Reduced effectiveness and dangers of reverse use dependence. *Circulation* 81:686-690, 1990.
These two well-written articles explain the dynamic nature of antiarrhythmic drug action.

Proarrhythmia

1. The Cardiac Arrhythmia Suppression Trial (CAST) Investigators: Preliminary report: effect of encainide and flecainide on mortality in a randomized trial of arrhythmia suppression after myocardial infarction. *N Engl J Med* 321:406-412, 1989.

2. Coplen SE, Antman EM, Berlin JA, et al: Efficacy and safety of quinidine therapy for maintenance of sinus rhythm after cardioversion. A meta-analysis of randomized control trials. *Circulation* 82:1106-1116, 1990.
Another meta-analysis, but focusing on presumed ventricular proarrhythmia in patients treated for atrial fibrillation.

3. Echt DS, Liebson PR, Mitchell LB, et al: Mortality and morbidity in patients receiving encainide, flecainide, or placebo: The Cardiac Arrhythmia Suppression Trial. *N Engl J Med* 324:781-788, 1991.
References 1 and 3 are milestones in the development of modern arrhythmology. They point up the proarrhythmic tendency of antiarrhythmic drugs in the post-myocardial infarction period.

4. Roden DM: Risks and benefits of antiarrhythmic therapy. *N Engl J Med* 331:785-791, 1994.
Excellent overview of the concepts of pro- and anti-arrhythmic drug actions.

5. Teo KK, Yusuf S, Furberg CD: Effects of prophylactic antiarrhythmic drug therapy in acute myocardial infarction. An overview of results from randomized controlled trials. JAMA 270:1589-1595, 1993.
A sobering review of pharmacologic attempts to limit arrhythmic events after myocardial infarction.

Reviews of Individual Drugs

1. Belardinelli L, Lerman BB: Electrophysiological basis for the use of adenosine in the diagnosis and treatment of cardiac arrhythmias. *Br Heart J* 63:3-4, 1990.

2. Campbell RW: Mexiletine. *N Engl J Med* 316:29-34, 1987.

3. Clyne CA, Estes NA III, Wang PJ: Moricizine. N Engl J Med 327:255-260, 1992.

4. Ellenbogen KA, Stambler BS, Wood MA, et al: Efficacy of intravenous ibutilide for rapid termination of atrial fibrillation and atrial flutter: a dose-response study. *J Am Coll Cardiol* 28:130-136, 1996.
The first randomized trial of ibutilide for atrial fibrillation and flutter.

5. Funck-Brentano C, Kroemer HK, Lee JT, et al: Propafenone. *N Engl J Med* 322:518-525, 1990.

6. Hohnloser SH, Woosley RL: Sotalol. *N Engl J Med* 331:31-38, 1994.

7. Roden DM, Woosley RL: Drug therapy. Tocainide. *N Engl J Med* 315:41-45, 1986.

References 2, 3, 5, and 7 are concise reviews of individual agents and are worth keeping at hand.

8. Waldo AL, Camm AJ, deRuyter H, et al: Effect of *d*-sotalol on mortality in patients with left ventricular dysfunction after recent and remote myocardial infarction. *Lancet* 348:7-12, 1996.
d-Sotalol lacks the β-adrenergic blocking property of racemic sotalol. It was thought that the elimination of the bradycardic effect (potentiating reverse-use dependency) would also eliminate some of the proarrhythmia of this class III drug. However, in this trial, treatment with d-sotalol worsened outcome.

Amiodarone
Amiodarone is a chapter in itself and is fertile territory for board questions. It is now used for atrial fibrillation and by many for prevention of sudden death.

1. The Antiarrhythmics Versus Implantable Defibrillators (AVID) Investigators: A comparison of antiarrhythmic-drug therapy with implantable defibrillators in patients resuscitated from near-fatal ventricular arrhythmias. *N Engl J Med* 337:1576-1583, 1997.
An important study comparing implantable cardiac defibrillators with amiodarone or sotalol in patients with ventricular tachycardia or ventricular fibrillation. Implantable cardiac defibrillators were shown to be superior.

2. Cairns JA, Connolly SJ, Roberts R, et al: Randomised trial of outcome after myocardial infarction in patients with frequent or repetitive ventricular premature depolarisations: CAMIAT. Lancet 349:675-682, 1997.

3. Daoud EG, Strickberger SA, Man KC, et al: Preoperative amiodarone as prophylaxis against atrial fibrillation after heart surgery. *N Engl J Med* 337:1785-1791, 1997.
An interesting study of amiodarone given perioperatively for atrial fibrillation prophylaxis. This highlights the resurgence of interest in and use of amiodarone.

4. Doval HC, Nul DR, Grancelli HO, et al: Randomised trial of low-dose amiodarone in severe congestive heart failure. *Lancet* 344:493-498, 1994.

5. Galve E, Rius T, Ballester R, et al: Intravenous amiodarone in treatment of recent-onset atrial fibrillation: results of a randomized, controlled study. *J Am Coll Cardiol* 27:1079-1082, 1996.

Intravenous amiodarone is shown to be of little use compared with placebo for treatment of recent-onset atrial fibrillation.

6. Julian DG, Camm AJ, Frangin G, et al: Randomised trial of effect of amiodarone on mortality in patients with left-ventricular dysfunction after recent myocardial infarction: EMIAT. *Lancet* 349:667-674, 1997.

References 2 and 6 are two studies of amiodarone after myocardial infarction with slightly different entry criteria and different conclusions.

7. Levine JH, Massumi A, Scheinman MM, et al: Intravenous amiodarone for recurrent sustained hypotensive ventricular tachyarrhythmias. *J Am Coll Cardiol* 27:67-75, 1996.

Key reference on intravenous amiodarone.

8. Mason JW: Amiodarone. *N Engl J Med* 316:455-466, 1987.

Excellent general overview.

9. Singh SN, Fletcher RD, Fisher SG, et al: Amiodarone in patients with congestive heart failure and asymptomatic ventricular arrhythmia. Survival Trial of Antiarrhythmic Therapy in Congestive Heart Failure. *N Engl J Med* 333:77-82, 1995.

References 4 and 9 are two important studies of amiodarone in heart failure. It is suggested from GESICA and a post-hoc analysis of STAT-CHF that amiodarone may have a survival benefit in dilated, nonischemic cardiomyopathy.

Appendix

Table 1.—Pharmacokinetics of Antiarrhythmic Drugs

Drug	Bioavail-ability, %	Protein binding, %	Time to peak concentration, hr	Elimination half-time, hr	Therapeutic range, µg/mL	Elimination route
Quinidine	70-85	70-95	1-4	6-8	2-5	Liver
Procainamide	70-95	15-20	0.5-1.5	3-5	4-12	Liver & kidney
Disopyramide	85	Variable	2	4-8	2-5	Liver & kidney
Lidocaine	---	50-80	---	1-4	1.5-5.0	Liver
Mexiletine	90	70	2-4	8-16	0.75-2.0	Liver
Tocainide	>90	10-50	1.0-1.5	11	5-12	Liver & kidney
Phenytoin	55-90	90	8-12	24	10-20	Liver
Moricizine	38	95	0.8-2.0	2-6	NA	Liver
Flecainide	95	30-40	2-4	12-27	0.2-1.0	Liver & kidney
Propafenone	5-50	95	2-3	2-4	0.2-1.0[*]	Liver
Amiodarone	35-65	96	3-7	30-100 days	1-2.5	Liver
Sotalol	100	0	2-4	7-18	~2.5	Kidney
Bretylium	---		---	5-10	NA	Kidney

NA, not applicable.
*Plasma levels for guiding propafenone therapy may not be useful.

Table 2.—Effect of Antiarrhythmic Drugs on Pacing Threshold and Energy Required for Defibrillation

Drug	Pacing	Defibrillation
Quinidine	Increased at high concentrations	Possible increase at very high dose
Procainamide	Increased at high concentrations	No effect
Disopyramide	Increased at toxic concentrations	Not studied
Lidocaine	Variably, no effect or increased	Increased
Mexiletine	Variably, no effect or increased	Variably, no effect or increased (case report)
Tocainide	No effect	Not studied
Phenytoin	Not studied	Increased
Moricizine	Not studied	No effect
Flecainide	Increased	Variably, no effect or increased
Propafenone	Increased	Variably, increased or decreased
Amiodarone	No effect	Increased
Sotalol	No effect	Decreased
Bretylium	Not studied	Not studied

Table 3.—Impact of Antiarrhythmic Drugs on Digoxin Level and Warfarin Effect

Drug	Digoxin	Warfarin
Quinidine	Increased	Increased
Procainamide	No effect	No effect
Disopyramide	No effect	Possible increase
Lidocaine	No effect	No effect
Mexiletine	No effect	No effect
Tocainide	No effect	No effect
Phenytoin	No effect	No effect
Moricizine	No effect	No effect
Flecainide	Increased	No effect
Propafenone	Increased	Increased
Amiodarone	Increased	Increased
Sotalol	No effect	No effect
Bretylium	No effect	No effect

Table 4.—Removal of Antiarrhythmic Drugs by Hemodialysis and Peritoneal Dialysis

Drug	Hemodialysis	Peritoneal dialysis
Quinidine	No	No
Procainamide	Yes	No
Disopyramide	Yes	No
Lidocaine	No	No
Mexiletine	No	No
Tocainide	Yes	No
Phenytoin	No	No
Moricizine	No	No
Flecainide	No	No
Propafenone	No	No
Amiodarone	No	No
Sotalol	Yes	?
Bretylium	?	?

Table 5.—Common and/or Important Side Effects of Antiarrhythmic Drugs

Drug	Side effect
Quinidine	GI, hemolytic anemia, thrombocytopenia, rash, hypotension (α-adrenergic blockade), lupus syndrome (rare), proarrhythmia
Procainamide	Gastrointestinal, lupus syndrome, rash, leukopenia, proarrhythmia
Disopyramide	Anticholinergic (constipation, dry mouth, blurred vision, urinary retention), CHF exacerbation, proarrhythmia
Lidocaine	CNS (at higher levels)
Mexiletine	CNS, GI, proarrhythmia (rare)
Tocainide	CNS, GI, proarrhythmia (rare), pulmonary fibrosis, leukopenia
Phenytoin	CNS (at higher levels), aplastic anemia, lupus syndrome, peripheral neuropathy, hyperglycemia, lymphadenopathy, Stevens-Johnson syndrome, hirsutism, osteomalacia
Flecainide	CNS (at higher levels), CHF exacerbation, proarrhythmia
Propafenone	CNS (at higher levels), metallic taste, asthma exacerbation (β-adrenergic blockade), proarrhythmia
Moricizine	CNS (at higher levels), proarrhythmia
Amiodarone	Pulmonary fibrosis, hypo- or hyperthyroidism, hepatitis/cirrhosis, blue skin, corneal microdeposits, bradycardia, proarrhythmia
Sotalol	Fatigue, bradycardia, proarrhythmia
Bretylium	Orthostatic hypotension (norepinephrine depletion), nausea/vomiting

CHF, congestive heart failure; CNS, central nervous system; GI, gastrointestinal.

Questions

Multiple Choice (choose the one best answer)

1. Which of the following antiarrhythmic drugs is the most potent sodium channel blocker?
   a. Quinidine
   b. Procainamide
   c. Sotalol
   d. Flecainide

2. The proarrhythmic effect of which of the following antiarrhythmic agents is most directly correlated with drug dose?
   a. Disopyramide
   b. Sotalol
   c. Lidocaine
   d. Procainamide

3. Amiodarone used prophylactically in patients with heart failure is most likely to improve survival in which of the following groups?
   a. Ischemic cardiomyopathy, ejection fraction > 40%
   b. Nonischemic cardiomyopathy, ejection fraction > 40%
   c. Ischemic cardiomyopathy, ejection fraction < 40%
   d. Nonischemic cardiomyopathy, ejection fraction < 40%

4. Use dependence refers to which of the following concepts?
   a. The effect of an antiarrhythmic drug is increased with repeated use over time

b. The effect of an antiarrhythmic drug is related directly to the frequency with which the ion channel affected is in the closed state

c. The effect of an antiarrhythmic drug is related directly to the frequency with which the ion channel affected is in the open state

d. The effect of an antiarrhythmic drug is related directly to the frequency with which the ion channel affected is in the rested state

5. Proarrhythmia with which of the following drugs may emerge with increased heart rates?
   a. Procainamide
   b. Mexiletine
   c. Propafenone
   d. Sotalol

6. The Cardiac Arrhythmia Suppression Trial (CAST) tested which of the following hypotheses?
   a. The presence of ventricular ectopy after myocardial infarction is an adverse prognostic sign
   b. Drug suppression of asymptomatic ventricular ectopy after myocardial infarction improves mortality
   c. Amiodarone improves mortality in patients with ventricular ectopy after myocardial infarction
   d. Amiodarone improves mortality in patients with ventricular ectopy and heart failure

7. Amiodarone enhances the effect of which of the following drugs?
   a. Warfarin
   b. Digoxin
   c. Cyclosporine
   d. All the above

8. Lidocaine levels are increased by drugs that decrease hepatic blood flow. Which of the following drugs do not increase lidocaine levels?
   a. Propranolol
   b. Metoprolol
   c. Ranitidine
   d. Cimetidine

9. Prolongation of the PR interval on the electrocardiogram would be most likely with which of the following drugs?
   a. Lidocaine
   b. Quinidine
   c. Propafenone
   d. Ibutilide

10. All the following drugs may increase the energy requirements for ventricular defibrillation *except*:
    a. Sotalol
    b. Amiodarone
    c. Lidocaine
    d. Mexiletine
    e. Tocainide

11. Antiarrhythmic drug use in renal failure is problematic. Which of the following drugs has no important renal elimination?
    a. Quinidine
    b. Procainamide
    c. Sotalol
    d. Bretylium

12. Prolongation of the QT interval on the electrocardiogram would be expected with all the following drugs *except*:
    a. Lidocaine
    b. Amiodarone
    c. Ibutilide
    d. Propafenone
    e. Procainamide

Answers

1. Answer d

2. Answer b

3. Answer d

4. Answer c

5. Answer c

6. Answer b

7. Answer d

8. Answer c

9. Answer c

10. Answer a

11. Answer a

12. Answer a

Chapter 74

Angiotensin-Converting Enzyme Inhibitors

Peter A. Brady, M.D.

Angiotensin-Converting Enzyme

Angiotensin-converting enzyme (ACE) regulates the balance between two opposing systems that modulate blood pressure: the renin-angiotensin system (RAS) and the kallikrein-kinin system (Fig. 1). ACE exists in the blood and other body fluids as well as in tissues. Increased activity of the RAS leads to salt and water retention and increased vascular tone, which increases blood pressure. Activation of the kallikrein-kinin system leads to the formation of bradykinin, which promotes vasodilatation and natriuresis.

RAS activation occurs under three main conditions: 1) decreased delivery of sodium to the renal macula densa, 2) a decrease in renal perfusion, and 3) sympathetic stimulation leading to release of renin by renal juxtaglomerular cells. Renin acts on angiotensinogen, a prohormone, which leads to the formation of angiotensin I. Angiotensin I is acted upon by ACE to produce angiotensin II. The actions of angiotensin II are mediated mainly by type 1 angiotensin receptors (AT_1). Angiotensin II induces intense vasoconstriction through direct action on vascular smooth muscle cells. It also causes vasoconstriction indirectly through stimulation of the sympathetic nervous system, both centrally and peripherally. Angiotensin II increases circulating plasma volume by stimulating the release of aldosterone from the adrenal cortex, which promotes retention of salt and water, and release of antidiuretic hormone (ADH), or vasopressin, from the posterior pituitary, which promotes fluid retention. In tissues, angiotensin II promotes cellular migration, proliferation, and growth. Such actions may be important in the pathogenesis of certain disease states, for example, myocardial hypertrophy.

ACE increases degradation of bradykinin. In the cardiovascular system, bradykinin promotes vasodilatation through the production of arachidonic acid and its metabolites and nitric oxide by vascular endothelium. In the kidney, bradykinin promotes natriuresis through direct action on the renal tubules. Thus, bradykinin acts to oppose many of the actions of angiotensin II.

The inhibition of ACE alters the balance between RAS and the kallikrein-kinin system in favor of vasodilatation and natriuresis and may have beneficial antiproliferative and antihypertrophic effects.

Pharmacology of Angiotensin-Converting Enzyme Inhibitors

ACE inhibitors differ in potency, bioavailability, plasma half-life, and route of elimination. Most available ACE inhibitors are prodrugs that require esterification in the liver before they become active. This property increases bioavailability. ACE inhibitors can be divided into three groups on the basis of their chemical structure: sulfhydryl-containing (captopril), phosphinyl-containing (fosinopril), and carboxyl-containing (enalapril, lisinopril, trandolapril, benazepril, and ramipril). Captopril, the first clinically available ACE inhibitor, differs from the others by having the shortest plasma half-life.

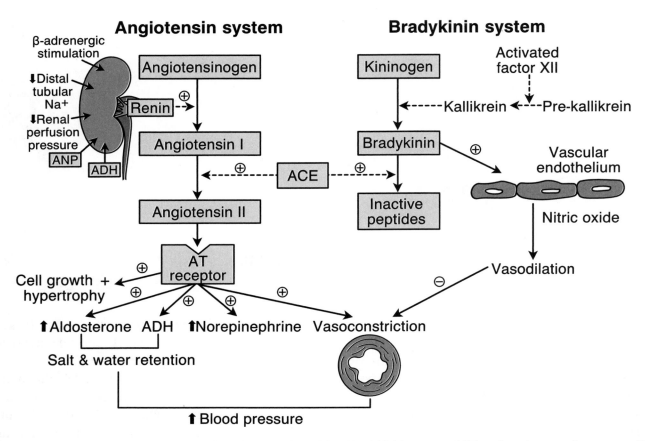

Fig. 1. Regulation of blood pressure by the renin-angiotensin and kallikrein-kinen (bradykinin) systems. ACE, angiotensin-converting enzyme; ADH, antidiuretic hormone; ANP, atrial natriuretic peptide; AT, angiotensin.

Evidence suggests that the sulfhydryl-containing moiety may confer additional properties such as free-radical scavenging and effects on prostaglandins. Because most ACE inhibitors are excreted by the kidneys, dosages need to be reduced in patients with renal dysfunction. Exceptions are fosinopril and trandolapril, which are also excreted by the liver.

Hemodynamic Effects of ACE Inhibitors

ACE inhibitors decrease systemic vascular resistance, with little change in heart rate. In normotensive and hypertensive persons with normal left ventricular function, ACE inhibitors have minimal effect on cardiac output or pulmonary capillary wedge pressure. In systolic dysfunction, ACE inhibitors reduce afterload, preload, and systolic wall stress such that cardiac output increases without an increase in heart rate. The lack of a heart rate response with ACE inhibitors is believed to be due to an effect of these agents on baroreceptor activity as well as inhibition of the normal tonic influence of angiotensin II on the sympathetic nervous system.

It is in contrast to the rate-slowing effects of some calcium channel blockers and direct-acting vasodilators, which may be associated with a compensatory increase in heart rate.

Clinical Indications for ACE Inhibitors

Hypertension
ACE inhibitors lower mean systolic and diastolic pressures in hypertensive patients as well as in salt-depleted normotensive patients. The decrease in pressure correlates with plasma renin activity and angiotensin levels such that the largest pressure decrease is observed in patients with the highest plasma renin activity. With chronic use of these agents, additional blood pressure lowering occurs independently of plasma renin activity and may involve increased production of vasodilatory prostaglandins by the kallikrein-kinin system.

Currently, ACE inhibitors are first-line therapy only for patients with hypertension and concomitant congestive heart failure or documented systolic dysfunction or patients with type 1 (insulin-dependent) diabetes mellitus with proteinuria (Joint National Committee for the Detection, Evaluation, and Treatment of High Blood Pressure [JNC-VI]). However, recent data suggest that patients with hypertension and non-insulin-dependent diabetes mellitus may also benefit from ACE inhibitors. The effect of ACE inhibitors on mortality among patients with uncomplicated essential hypertension is unknown. Clinical trials, including the Captopril Prevention Project and the Antihypertensive and Lipid-Lowering Treatment to Prevent Heart Attack Trial (ALLHAT) are under way.

Congestive Heart Failure

Several large prospective randomized placebo-controlled trials have demonstrated that treatment with ACE inhibitors reduces mortality among patients with ventricular dysfunction, even when asymptomatic (Table 1). Reduced mortality is due primarily to a reduction in the progression toward clinical heart failure. However, a reduction in the incidence of sudden death and fatal myocardial infarction has also been observed. The effect of ACE inhibitors on mortality among patients with predominant diastolic dysfunction is unknown. Because ACE inhibitors reverse left ventricular hypertrophy, they may also be beneficial in this group.

Myocardial Infarction

Treatment with ACE inhibitors should be beneficial following myocardial infarction for several reasons: 1) they prevent activation of the RAS, which occurs after myocardial infarction, especially in patients with congestive heart failure, 2) they have an antiadrenergic action, and 3) they favorably affect the ventricular remodeling that begins soon after myocardial infarction and involves both infarcted and non-infarcted areas of myocardium, leading to progressive ventricular dilatation and increased left ventricular wall stress. Acutely, ventricular remodeling maintains stroke volume despite reduced myocardial fiber shortening. However, chronically, it results in increased wall stress and altered ventricular loading, leading to further ventricular enlargement and, ultimately, to clinical congestive heart failure.

Eight prospective randomized trials have examined the use of ACE inhibitors in myocardial infarction. These trials may be divided into 1) those in which ACE inhibitors were given to all patients in a randomized fashion (GISSI-3, ISIS-4, and CONSENSUS II and the Chinese Captopril Trial) (Table 2) and 2) those that required evidence of symptomatic or asymptomatic left ventricular dysfunction before randomization (SAVE, AIRE, TRACE, SMILE) (Table 3).

In ISIS-4 and GISSI-3, captopril and lisinopril versus placebo resulted in a 6% and 11% reduction in mortality, respectively, beyond that achieved with thrombolysis and current standard therapy. Another 17% reduction occurred when lisinopril was combined with nitrates given intravenously. In contrast, in CONSENSUS II, enalaprilat given intravenously in the first 24 hours after myocardial infarction was associated with a trend toward increased mortality (nonsignificant). This may have been due to the greater frequency of hypotension observed in this study. These data support the use of oral ACE inhibitors in patients in the early phase of myocardial infarction if hypotension can be avoided.

In the AIRE study, ramipril was given to patients with clinically evident congestive heart failure and resulted in a mortality reduction of 27% over 15 months of follow-up. In the SAVE study, captopril was given to patients with reduced

Table 1.—Clinical Trials of Angiotensin-Converting Enzyme (ACE) Inhibitors in Congestive Heart Failure (CHF) and Left Ventricular Dysfunction

Trial*	Population	ACE inhibitor	Outcome
CONSENSUS	NYHA class IV	Enalapril vs. placebo	Decreased mortality and CHF
SOLVD-T[†]	NYHA classes II and III	Enalapril vs. placebo	Decreased mortality and CHF[†]
V-HeFT II	NYHA classes II and III	Enalapril vs. hydralazine, isosorbide dinitrate	Decreased mortality and sudden death
SOLVD-P[†]	Asymptomatic left ventricular dysfunction	Enalapril vs. placebo	Decreased mortality, CHF, and hospitalizations

NYHA, New York Heart Association.

*Full names of trials: CONSENSUS, Cooperative North Scandinavian Enalapril Survival Study; SOLVD, Studies on Left Ventricular Dysfunction (P, prevention, and T, treatment): V-HeFT, Veterans Administration Heart Failure Trial.

[†]Duration of follow-up varied between 5 months and 6 years.

systolic function (ejection fraction < 40%) 3 days after infarction for a mean of 42 months and resulted in a 19% reduction in all-cause mortality, a 22% reduction in progression to overt congestive heart failure, and a 22% reduction in first hospitalization for heart failure. In the TRACE study, trandolapril was given to patients with decreased systolic function (ejection fraction < 35%) starting 3 to 7 days after myocardial infarction and continuing for 2 to 4 years. This study included patients with clinically evident ischemia or congestive heart failure (i.e., patients who were excluded from the SAVE trial). Mortality was reduced by 22%.

Prevention of Reinfarction and Coronary Ischemic Events

An interesting—but unexpected—finding of the SAVE trial was that captopril reduced the frequency of reinfarction. The mechanism of this is not known. One hypothesis is that ACE inhibitors may augment the protective effect of bradykinin on vascular endothelium and promote fibrinolysis. Also, evidence suggests that these inhibitors may slow the progression of atherosclerosis. Ongoing trials are investigating this important question.

Which Patients Should Receive ACE Inhibitors After Myocardial Infarction: Summary of Recent Recommendations

On the basis of data from the trials described in Tables 2 and 3, the American College of Cardiology/American Heart Association Task Force have designated ACE inhibitors a class I indication (a condition for which there is good evidence that a given treatment is beneficial) to be given within the first 24 hours after anterior wall myocardial infarction or in those with clinical heart failure. A class IIa indication (a condition in which the weight of evidence is in favor of efficacy) is other patients within the first 24 hours after acute myocardial infarction. These recommendations assume the absence of significant hypotension or a clear-cut contraindication to the use of ACE inhibitors. For patients given ACE inhibitors in a nonselective manner, indications to continue therapy may be reassessed before dismissal or at first follow-up. Patients most likely to benefit from early and continued use of these agents include those with a history of hypertension, diabetes, or previous myocardial infarction or who have anterior electrocardiographic changes, a high resting heart rate, pulmonary congestion, or left ventricular systolic dysfunction.

ACE Inhibitors in African-Americans

ACE inhibitors are less efficacious in African-American patients than in matched white patients, particularly compared with the efficacy of L-type calcium channel blockers (nifedipine, verapamil, and diltiazem). Thus, higher doses of ACE inhibitors may be required. One explanation for this is that renin levels often are lower in hypertensive blacks than whites. This explanation is supported by the finding that coadministration of diuretics, which increase plasma renin activity, abolishes racial differences in the response to ACE inhibitors. Too few data exist on clinical outcomes in African-Americans to recommend specific guidelines for treatment.

Table 2.—Clinical Trials in Which Angiotensin-Converting Enzyme (ACE) Inhibitors Were Given to All Patients After Myocardial Infarction

Trial*	ACE inhibitor	Time of initial dose	Duration	Outcome
GISSI-3	Lisinopril vs. nitrates	24 hr	6 wk	Decreased mortality
ISIS-4	Captopril vs. placebo	24 hr	28 days	Decreased mortality
CONSENSUS II	Enalaprilat/enalapril vs. placebo	24 hr	40-180 days	No improvement in survival, hypotension with enalaprilat

*Full names of the trials: CONSENSUS, Cooperative North Scandinavian Enalapril Survival Study; GISSI, Gruppo Italino per lo Studio della Streptochinasi nell'Infarcto Miocardico; ISIS, International Study for Infarct Survival.

Table 3.—Clinical Trials in Which Angiotensin-Converting Enzyme (ACE) Inhibitors Were Given to Selected Patients After Myocardial Infarction (MI)

Trial*	Population	ACE inhibitor	Time of initial dose	Duration	Outcome
SAVE	MI, decreased LV function	Captopril vs. placebo	3-16 days	24-60 mo	Decreased mortality
AIRE	MI with CHF	Ramipril vs. placebo	3-10 days	≥ 6 mo	Decreased mortality
TRACE	MI, decreased LV function	Trandolapril vs. placebo	3-7 days	24-50 mo	Decreased mortality
SMILE	MI	Zofenopril vs. placebo	24 hr	6 wk	Decreased mortality

CHF, congestive heart failure; LV, left ventricular; LVEF, LV ejection fraction.
*Full names of trials: AIRE, Acute Infarction Ramipril Efficacy; SAVE, Survival and Ventricular Enlargement; SMILE, Survival of Myocardial Infarction Long-Term Evaluation; TRACE, Trandolapril Cardiac Evaluation.

Contraindications to ACE Inhibitors

Adverse effects of ACE inhibitors are listed in Table 4, and drug interactions of these agents are given in Table 5. The following are contraindications to treatment with ACE inhibitors:

- Severe inoperable bilateral renal artery stenosis
- Preexisting hypotension
- Fixed or dynamic left ventricular outflow tract obstruction
- Pregnancy
- Uncontrolled hyperkalemia

Angiotensin Receptor Blocking Agents

Angiotensin (AT_1) receptor blocking agents block the final common pathway of angiotensin II action. Thus, they block the action of angiotensin II produced by pathways independently of the RAS system (e.g., chymase and cathepsin) or produced locally in different tissues. They have no effect on bradykinin metabolism. Available clinical data suggest that AT_1 blockers are safe, well tolerated, and at least as effective as ACE inhibitors. Like ACE inhibitors, AT_1 blockers are also less efficacious in African-Americans, probably through a similar mechanism.

Clinical Trials of AT_1 Blockers
The ELITE (Evaluation of Losartan in the Elderly) trial suggested that AT_1 blockers may be more effective and better tolerated than ACE inhibitors in patients with congestive heart failure. Fewer patients taking losartan withdrew from treatment because of adverse events than patients taking captopril (12.2% vs. 20.8%). Fourteen patients in the captopril group withdrew from treatment because of cough compared with none in the losartan group.

Losartan was also associated with better survival than captopril. Newer agents such as irbesartan have been tested recently in clinical trials and appear to produce sustained hemodynamic benefit and functional improvement in patients with congestive heart failure. Preliminary data from the RESOLVD (Randomized Evaluation of Strategies for Left Ventricular Dysfunction) pilot study using another AT_1 blocker, candesartan cilexitil, in various doses in conjunction with enalapril (20 mg) suggest that combination therapy with AT_1 blockers and ACE inhibitors may have additional hemodynamic benefit in congestive heart failure compared with either agent alone.

ACE and Neutral Endopeptidase Inhibitors

Neutral endopeptidase catalyzes the degradation of endogenous vasodilator peptides, including atrial natriuretic peptide and brain natriuretic peptide, substance P, and bradykinin. Currently, interest is focused on whether combinations of neutral endopeptidase inhibitors, ACE inhibitors, or endothelin-1 receptor blockade may be beneficial in certain patients.

Table 4.—Adverse Effects of Angiotensin-Converting Enzyme Inhibitors

Class effects	
Hypotension	Increased frequency in renin-dependent states, e.g., low Na^+ intake and concomitant diuretic use
Cough	Incidence, 10%-40%
	Dose-dependent, mechanism unknown but possibly related to bradykinin or substance P; often necessitates cessation of therapy
Hyperkalemia	Frequent and usually minor, stabilizes after 1st week
Renal failure	Most often due to decreased renal perfusion, e.g., renal artery stenosis or low output state
Teratogenic	2nd and 3rd trimesters
	ACE inhibitors must be discontinued *immediately* if pregnancy is confirmed or suspected
Angioedema	Rare, 1-2/1,000; usually occurs 1st month but may appear later
Dysgeusia	Abnormal taste
Sulfhydryl-related effects	
Neutropenia	Rare (< 0.05%), higher incidence in patients with collagen vascular diseases
Rash	1%, usually maculopapular, pruritic; rarely exfoliative dermatitis
Proteinuria	1% of patients receiving captopril, but paradoxically captopril will decrease proteinuria in diabetic nephropathy

Table 5.—Drug Interactions of Angiotensin-Converting Enzyme (ACE) Inhibitors

Drug	Comment
Potassium	Potassium supplements, potassium-sparing diuretics, and salt substitutes should be used with caution or discontinued because of the potassium-sparing effect of aldosterone suppression
Diuretics	Increased sensitivity to hypotensive effects of ACE inhibitors because of higher baseline renin levels
Nonsteroidal anti-inflammatory drugs	May decrease antihypertensive action of ACE inhibitors, more common in the presence of low renin levels

Suggested Review Reading

1. ACE Inhibitor Myocardial Infarction Collaborative Group: Indications for ACE inhibitors in the early treatment of acute myocardial infarction: systematic overview of individual data from 100,000 patients in randomized trials. *Circulation* 97:2202-2212, 1998.

2. Ryan TJ, Anderson JL, Antman EM, et al: ACC/AHA guidelines for the management of patients with acute myocardial infarction. A report of the American College of Cardiology/American Heart Association Task Force on Practice Guidelines (Committee on Management of Acute Myocardial Infarction). *J Am Coll Cardiol* 28:1328-1428, 1996.

Questions

Multiple Choice (choose the one best answer)

1. True statements about angiotensin-converting enzyme (ACE) inhibitors include:
   a. Equally effective in all patient groups
   b. Result in complete blockade of the effects of angiotensin II
   c. Individual ACE inhibitors have a similar efficacy
   d. Are best used in combination with β-blockers to prevent reflex tachycardia
   e. Have minimal effect on cardiac output in patients with normal ventricular function

2. All the following are true about the vascular effects of angiotensin-converting enzyme (ACE) inhibitors *except*:
   a. ACE inhibitors directly increase synthesis and release of plasminogen activator inhibitor-I

   b. Angiotensin II enhances activity of the sympathetic nervous system
   c. ACE inhibitors decrease the progression of atherosclerosis in some animal models
   d. ACE inhibitors have antithrombotic effects

3. True statements about adverse effects of angiotensin-converting enzyme (ACE) inhibitors include:
   a. Most adverse effects of ACE inhibitors can be attributed to decreased production of angiotensin II
   b. Increase in K^+ levels above normal in the first week after starting treatment with ACE inhibitors is often an early sign of renal dysfunction requiring discontinuation of the treatment
   c. Increase in K^+ levels above normal in the first week after starting treatment with ACE inhibitors is normal
   d. Only sulfhydryl-containing ACE inhibitors have embryopathic effects

Answers

1. Answer e

ACE inhibitors are less effective in African-Americans than in other populations, and they do not cause complete blockade of angiotensin II. Individual ACE inhibitors have different bioavailability and efficacy profiles. Use of ACE inhibitors is not associated with tachycardia. The agents have minimal effect on cardiac output in normotensive patients and those with normal ventricular function. They do not cause reflex tachycardia.

2. Answer a

Plasminogen activator inhibitor-1 inhibits endogenous

fibrinolytic peptides such as tissue plasminogen activator and is increased by angiotensin II. Therefore, it would be expected to be decreased by ACE inhibitors. Angiotensin II enhances the activity of the sympathetic nervous system by several mechanisms, including blockade of norepinephrine reuptake and facilitation of norepinephrine release.

3. Answer c

Angiotensin II levels are decreased by ACE inhibitors. All ACE inhibitors are potentially harmful in pregnancy and should be discontinued immediately.

Notes

Chapter 75

Diuretics

Peter A. Brady, M.D.
Joseph G. Murphy, M.D.

Diuretics act on the kidney to promote excretion of sodium and water. They are classified according to their site of action (Fig. 1). The three main groups of diuretics used clinically are loop diuretics, thiazides, and potassium-sparing diuretics. Except for thiazides, all diuretics must be transported to the luminal side of the nephron to act. Transportation may be blocked by organic acids that accumulate in renal failure. This explains the decreased efficacy of diuretics in renal failure and why progressively larger doses of drug are needed to induce diuresis.

Loop Diuretics

The loop diuretics are furosemide (Lasix), bumetanide (Bumex), and ethacrynic acid (Edecrin).

Pharmacology
Loop diuretics inhibit the $Na^+/K^+/2 Cl^-$ cotransporter, which transports chloride ions across luminal cells of the ascending limb of the loop of Henle. Because the site of action is on the intraluminal side of the nephron, loop diuretics must first be excreted by the proximal tubule. Cotransport inhibition results in increased intraluminal concentration of Na^+, K^+, Cl^-, and H^+ which are lost in the urine, leading to, respectively, hyponatremia, hypokalemia, hypochloremia, and alkalosis. The side effects of loop diuretics are listed in Table 1.

Clinical Indications
Acute pulmonary edema and symptomatic heart failure are the most frequent indications for a loop diuretic. It is interesting to note that no randomized controlled study has been performed that documents a survival benefit of diuretics in heart failure. In general, diuretics should be used for class III and IV heart failure in combination with angiotensin-converting enzyme (ACE) inhibitors and institution of dietary salt restriction. Diuretics may also be required in class II heart failure if significant edema is present.

Loop diuretics have excellent clinical efficacy because they 1) induce higher sodium (and, thus, water loss) than other diuretics, 2) promote diuresis, even in the presence of low glomerular filtration rate (GFR), and 3) cause venodilation, which reduces ventricular preload.

ACE inhibitors have replaced diuretics as the first-line agent in patients with mild congestive heart failure. Angiotensin II and antidiuretic hormone (ADH), which are increased in congestive heart failure through activation of the renin angiotensin system, oppose the action of loop diuretics. Therefore, in general, ACE inhibitors or angiotensin I receptor blocker (AT_1) should be initiated before starting treatment with a diuretic. "Dilutional" hyponatremia may occur because of sodium loss and relative water retention due to increased activation of angiotensin II and ADH and is best treated by a combination of water restriction, low-dose diuretics, and ACE inhibitors.

In patients presenting with acute pulmonary edema, either furosemide (Lasix), 40 mg intravenously, or bumetanide (Bumex), 1 mg intravenously, is the diuretic of first choice. Larger doses of loop diuretics may be administered subsequently if needed.

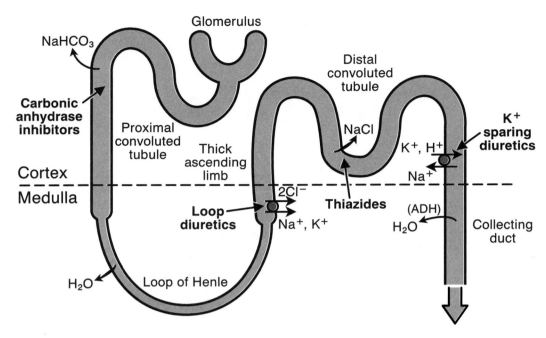

Fig. 1. Sites of action of diuretics used clinically.

Hypertension

Thiazide diuretics are usually the diuretic of choice in hypertension because of their long duration of action, especially in black and elderly patients, in whom volume expansion plays an important role in the pathogenesis of their hypertension.

Loop diuretics are more efficacious than thiazides for patients with hypertension and low GFR. Doses of 250 mg to 2,000 mg are often used, but the benefit of such a dosing regimen is unproved and has an increased risk of adverse reactions. They are contraindicated in the presence of chronic anuria, such as occurs in many dialysis patients. High-dose loop diuretics may force a diuresis in an acutely anuric patient. Always exclude prerenal renal failure (dehydration, hypotension, etc.) and urinary obstruction before challenging with high-dose loop diuretics.

Drug Interactions With Loop Diuretics

Nonsteroidal anti-inflammatory drugs decrease renal responsiveness to loop diuretics (presumably by interfering with the formation of vasodilatory prostaglandins). High doses of loop diuretics competitively inhibit the excretion of salicylates that may precipitate salycilate poisoning (tinnitus). Causes of diuretic resistance are listed in Table 2.

Bumetanide

Its site of action and side effects are similar to those of furosemide. The onset of action is less than 30 minutes (peak, 75 to 90 minutes). It may have greater potency and bioavailability than the other loop diuretics in patients with congestive heart failure and "bowel edema." It may also have a lower incidence of ototoxicity and a higher incidence of renal toxicity.

Ethacrynic Acid

This is the only "nonsulfonamide" loop diuretic. It is useful in patients with sulfonamide allergy. Otherwise, it is not widely used. It has a high incidence of ototoxicity.

Thiazide Diuretics

The principal thiazide diuretics are hydrochlorothiazide (Hydrodiuril), chlorothiazide (Diuril), chlorthalidone (Hygroton), and metolazone (Zaroxolyn).

Pharmacology

Thiazide diuretics inhibit the reabsorption of Na^+ and Cl^- in the distal convoluted tubule. This cotransporter is insensitive to loop diuretics. Thus, more sodium reaches the distal tubules to stimulate exchange with potassium, particularly in the presence of an activated renin-angiotensin-aldosterone system. Thiazides also increase active excretion of potassium in the distal renal tubule. They are rapidly absorbed from the gastrointestinal tract. The onset of action

Table 1.—Side Effects of Loop Diuretics

Effect	
Hypokalemia	Increased Na^+ delivery to distal tubule prompts K^+ loss through increased Na^+/K^+ exchange and activation of renin-angiotensin system
Metabolic alkalosis	Increased excretion of H^+ into urine at distal tubule because of hyperaldosteronism, and "contraction alkalosis" due to increased reabsorption of bicarbonate because of intravascular volume depletion
Hyperuricemia	Dose-related due to decreased clearance of uric acid; may precipitate gout
Hyperglycemia	May be due to hypokalemia; correction of decreased K^+ may improve glycemic control
Dyslipidemia	Usually *improves* with chronic use
Hypomagnesemia	Loss of NaCl-dependent magnesium reabsorption in the ascending limb of the loop of Henle; correct *before* hypokalemia
Ototoxicity	Due to electrolyte disturbance of the endolymph; is dose-related and reversible

Note: Although rare, all sulfonamide-derived loop diuretics may precipitate or exaggerate lupus erythematosus or photosensitive skin eruptions or may cause blood dyscrasias.

is 1 or 2 hours depending on the route of administration. The prolonged duration of action is 6 to 36 hours. Thiazides are generally well tolerated.

The major differences compared with loop diuretics include the following:

- Longer duration of action
- Different site of action; thus, thiazides and loop diuretics may be used in combination
- Low ceiling of response, that is, maximal efficacy occurs at lower doses and does not increase with further dose increases
- Decreased efficacy in the presence of renal impairment

Clinical Indications for Thiazides

Hypertension

Thiazides are first-line agents in the absence of specific indications for other antihypertensive agents, e.g., a β-blocker in a patient with concomitant angina (JNC VI). They are particularly efficacious in patients with "volume-dependent" hypertension (the elderly and African-Americans). In the Systolic Hypertension in the Elderly (SHEP) trial, chlorthalidone (12.5 mg) was effective at decreasing systolic blood pressure. Metabolic effects were infrequent. Higher doses were only marginally more effective. A full antihypertensive effect may not be achieved for up to 12 weeks.

Congestive Heart Failure

Thiazides are mostly of benefit in patients with mild chronic congestive symptoms or as additional diuretic agents in

patients who do not have a response to loop diuretics alone (see Metolazone).

Side Effects of Thiazide Diuretics

The side effects of thiazides are similar to those of loop diuretics except 1) there is increased frequency of hyponatremia; 2) serum levels of Ca^{2+} often increase with prolonged use, but this is rarely of clinical significance; and 3) rarely, there is a sulfonamide-type immune effect leading to intrahepatic jaundice, pancreatitis, blood dyscrasias, angiitis, pneumonitis, and interstitial nephritis.

Drug Interactions

- Probenecid (gout) and lithium (bipolar disorders) block thiazide action by preventing thiazide excretion into the urine.
- Lithium toxicity may occur because of impaired renal clearance of lithium.

Other Thiazide-Like Agents

Metolazone

Metolazone is effective in patients with decreased renal function. The duration of action is up to 24 hours. The standard dose for congestive heart failure is 5 to 20 mg and 2.5 to 5.0 mg for hypertension. Metolazone in combination with a loop diuretic may induce profound diuresis. Its side effects are similar to those of other thiazide diuretics.

Indapamide

Indapamide is an effective antihypertensive agent. It acts

Table 2.—Causes of Diuretic Resistance

Cause	Comment
Noncompliance or excessive salt intake	Most common
Globally decreased renal perfusion pressure	Occurs with excessive intravascular volume depletion, e.g., after aggressive diuretic therapy, excessive use of vasodilators, and in presence of decreased cardiac output
Selective decrease in glomerular perfusion pressure	Occurs with use of angiotensin-converting enzyme inhibitors in the presence of bilateral renal artery stenosis or with use of nonsteroidal anti-inflammatory agents
Primary renal dysfunction	Due to cholesterol emboli, renal artery stenosis, drug-induced interstitial nephritis, or obstructive uropathy

primarily as a peripheral vasodilator. The initial dose is 1.25 mg once daily for 4 weeks and is increased as needed to 5 mg. Indapamide has no advantage over other diuretics in patients with congestive heart failure but appears superior to hydrochlorothiazide in inducing regression of left ventricular hypertrophy at equivalent diastolic blood pressure values.

Potassium Supplements

Potassium supplements are unnecessary for most patients taking thiazide diuretics. A diet high in potassium and low in sodium can be achieved with salt substitutes. The addition of a low dose of potassium-sparing diuretic may be more appropriate. The dose of thiazide can then be decreased without any loss in clinical efficacy. For most patients, a liquid form of potassium chloride is the most suitable potassium supplement. Avoid slow-release tablets because of their tendency to cause ulceration of the gastrointestinal tract. Approximately 20 mEq of dietary K^+ daily will avoid potassium depletion. For replacement, prescribe 40 to 100 mEq daily for patients with persistent diuretic-induced hypokalemia.

Potassium-Sparing Diuretics

Pharmacology

Potassium-sparing diuretics antagonize physiologic Na^+ reabsorption in the distal convoluted tubule and cortical collecting system. Because Na^+ exchange at these sites is low, the diuretic action is weak. These diuretics are useful when the likelihood of hypokalemia is high. However, avoid concomitant use of potassium supplements or agents that reduce K^+ excretion, e.g., ACE inhibitors. Potassium-sparing diuretics act through aldosterone-dependent and aldosterone-independent mechanisms.

Aldosterone-Dependent Potassium-Sparing Diuretics

Spironolactone

Spironolactone is a synthetic steroid that inhibits Na^+ reabsorption by competing for the cytoplasmic aldosterone receptor. Hyperkalemia is the most common side effect and is due to impaired K^+ excretion. It is antiandrogenic, which may cause gynecomastia in males and irregular menses in females.

Aldosterone-Independent Potassium-Sparing Diuretics

Triamterene and Amiloride

Triamterene and amiloride are structurally related potassium-sparing diuretics with similar pharmacologic properties. They inhibit Na^+ channels at the level of the distal tubule to diminish the excretion of K^+ and H^+. Triamterene is metabolized by the liver, and the active product is excreted into the proximal tubule. Amiloride is secreted directly into the proximal tubule and appears unchanged in the urine. When combined with a thiazide diuretic, urinary K^+ and Mg^{++} loss is minimized.

Precautions for Use of Diuretics

Avoid overly vigorous diuresis. This is seen most frequently after patients (often noncompliant) are admitted to the hospital and prescribed a regular diuretic regimen. Avoid using diuretics in patients with "restrictive filling" hemodynamics, for example, hypertrophic or restrictive cardiomyopathy or constrictive pericarditis.

Chapter 76

Digoxin

Arshad Jahangir, M.D.

Digitalis compounds have been in use for more than 200 years for the management of congestive heart failure. The digitalis family comprises several active drugs, including digoxin and digitoxin. Digoxin, a cardiac glycoside originally extracted from the leaves of *Digitalis lanata*, is the only positive inotropic agent currently approved for oral use in the U.S.

Pharmacokinetics

The bioavailability of digoxin ranges between 60% and 85% (Table 1). Intestinal microflora may metabolize digoxin in about 10% of patients and reduce bioavailability. For these patients, a higher dose of digoxin is required to achieve therapeutic levels and toxicity may occur with antibiotics that destroy intestinal microflora. Microflora digoxin metabolism is one of the causes of apparent resistance to standard doses of oral digoxin. The elimination half-life of digoxin in patients with normal renal function is 36 to 48 hours, with ~70% of the drug eliminated unchanged through the kidney. This long half-life allows once-a-day dosing. Digoxin has a large (4 to 7 L/kg) apparent volume of distribution mostly bound to skeletal muscle receptors and, thus, is not effectively removed by peritoneal dialysis or hemodialysis. Steady-state blood levels are achieved after 5 half-lives, or about 1 week after the initiation of oral maintenance therapy. Digoxin crosses both the blood-brain barrier and the placenta, with similar levels of drug in maternal and umbilical vein blood.

Digoxin is metabolized hepatically to both active and inactive metabolites with long half-lives (120 to 216 hours), because of extensive serum protein binding. Its duration of action is ~14 days.

- Intestinal microflora may metabolize digoxin in about 10% of patients and reduce bioavailability.

Mechanism of Action

Inotropic Effect
The primary action of digoxin is to inhibit the cell membrane Na^+-K^+-ATPase, which normally maintains the intracellular/extracellular sodium and potassium gradients. Inhibition of the Na^+-K^+ pump increases intracellular sodium, which leads to increased intracellular calcium by Na^+-Ca^{2+} exchanger (Plate 1). Calcium influx is also increased by alteration of the ion selectivity of the membrane voltage-gated sodium channels by a newly described mechanism known as "slip-mode conductance." The increase in intracellular calcium increases the force of myocardial contraction by increasing both the velocity and the extent of sarcomere shortening. The inotropic effect of digoxin is present in both normal and failing atrial and ventricular muscle and results in increased stroke work for a given volume.

- The primary action of digoxin is to inhibit the cell membrane Na^+-K^+-ATPase, which normally maintains

Table 1.—Digoxin Pharmacokinetics

Feature	Value
Bioavailability	75%
Serum half-life	36 hr
Steady state blood level	1 wk (5 half-lives)
Therapeutic serum level	1-2 ng/mL
Volume of distribution*	4-7 L/kg
Renal excretion	70%
Microintestinal floral metabolism	~10% of patients
Crosses blood-brain barrier and placenta	

*Bound to muscle receptors and not removed by dialysis.

the intracellular/extracellular sodium and potassium gradients.

- The inotropic effect of digoxin is present in both normal and failing myocardium and results in increased stroke work for a given volume.

Effect on Vascular Smooth Muscle and Autonomic Nervous System

In normal subjects, digoxin may increase peripheral resistance and venous tone by increasing intracellular calcium in vascular smooth muscle. This effect is not apparent in patients with heart failure, probably because of an increased basal level of autonomic activation.

Digoxin increases parasympathetic activity, resulting in a slowing of sinus impulses and conduction through the atrioventricular (AV) node (Plate 2). In heart failure, digoxin generally has a sympathoinhibitory effect, believed to be mediated through the central nervous system, that results in a decrease in heart rate, sympathetic nervous activity, and plasma norepinephrine concentration. Renin release is decreased because of inhibition of the renal sodium pump; this leads to a natriuretic effect and vasodilatation that may offset the direct vasoconstrictor effect of digoxin. Digoxin may also improve impaired baroreceptor sensitivity through a direct effect on the receptors or indirectly by improvement in blood pressure and cardiac filling pressures. Improved sensitivity of baroreceptors, in turn, decreases sympathetic outflow from the central nervous system.

- Digoxin increases parasympathetic activation, resulting in a slowing of sinus impulses and conduction through the AV node.

Electrophysiologic Actions

Digoxin has direct and indirect effects, which are mediated by the autonomic nervous system (parasympathetic activation and sympathetic inhibition), on cardiac electrophysiology. In the sinoatrial and AV nodal tissues, digoxin at therapeutic plasma concentrations decreases automaticity and conduction velocity, mainly by its vagotonic effect. At higher (toxic) concentrations, sinus bradycardia or sinus arrest and prolongation or block of AV conduction may occur. At therapeutic concentrations, the maximal diastolic resting membrane potential, predominantly in atrial and AV nodal tissues, is increased and the action potential duration may be decreased in atrial tissue—effects mediated by an increase in vagal tone and a decrease in sympathetic nervous system activity. At higher concentration, digoxin enhances automaticity in atrial tissue and the His-Purkinje system by a shift in resting membrane potential to more depolarized values, increasing phase 4 depolarization. Calcium loading in patients with digoxin toxicity leads to enhanced automaticity, delayed afterdepolarization, and triggered activity, resulting in complex arrhythmias.

The major electrocardiographic (ECG) effects of digoxin are PR prolongation and nonspecific ST-segment changes at rest and false-positive ST-T changes during exercise testing.

Therapeutic Uses of Digoxin

Arrhythmias

Paroxysmal Supraventricular Tachycardia

Digoxin, through its effects on sinoatrial and AV nodal tissue, is effective in terminating or preventing sinus node reentry or AV node-dependent supraventricular tachycardia, such as AV nodal reentrant tachycardia and orthodromic AV reentrant tachycardia.

Atrial Fibrillation and Flutter

Digoxin is the drug most commonly used to control a rapid ventricular response in chronic atrial fibrillation. Its predominant effect is mediated by enhancing the vagal effect over the AV node, thus slowing resting heart rate. This vagally mediated effect is easily overcome by catecholamines, and in conditions with high sympathetic tone (during exercise, active young patients, thyrotoxicosis, chronic lung disease), digoxin is only marginally effective in slowing ventricular rate. Therefore, digoxin should not be used alone as the first-line drug for ventricular rate control and should be used concomitantly with verapamil, diltiazem, or a β-blocker. In patients with congestive heart failure and chronic atrial fibrillation, digoxin is particularly useful because of its inotropic effect. Intravenously administered digoxin slows the ventricular response; however, there is a delay (~30 to 60 minutes) in the onset of this effect, with the full effect delayed for up to 4 to 6 hours.

In paroxysmal atrial fibrillation and flutter, digoxin is not efficacious in controlling ventricular rate during recurrence and is ineffective in terminating or preventing recurrence of tachycardia after cardioversion. In some cases, digoxin may make paroxysmal atrial fibrillation worse, by prolonging the duration of atrial fibrillation. Digoxin should not be used in patients with Wolff-Parkinson-White syndrome and atrial fibrillation, because it can enhance anterograde conduction over the accessory pathway and could precipitate ventricular tachycardia or ventricular fibrillation.

- The vagally mediated effect of digoxin is easily overcome by catecholamines, and in conditions with high sympathetic tone, digoxin is only marginally effective in slowing ventricular rate during vigorous exercise in patients with atrial fibrillation.

Congestive Heart Failure
The inotropic action of digoxin, with an increase in cardiac output, improves symptoms and hemodynamics in patients with congestive heart failure. The role of digoxin in treating heart failure and atrial fibrillation has been accepted, but its use in sinus rhythm is controversial. Several recent studies have clarified the efficacy of digoxin in symptomatic ventricular dysfunction and sinus rhythm (Table 2). Although digoxin does not reduce mortality among patients with chronic heart failure, it improves hemodynamics, symptoms, exercise capacity, and quality of life, with a significant reduction in hospitalizations for heart failure. The withdrawal of digoxin, after chronic use in patients with mild to moderate heart failure (New York Heart Association [NYHA] functional class II and III) with systolic ventricular dysfunction and sinus rhythm, is associated with clinical deterioration and increased hospitalizations, as shown in prospective trials: Prospective Randomized Study of Ventricular Failure and the Efficacy of Digoxin (PROVED) and Randomized Assessment of Digoxin on Inhibitors of the Angiotensin-Converting Enzyme (RADIANCE) (Fig. 1).

The only prospective randomized, placebo-controlled trial of digoxin that assessed morbidity and mortality among patients in sinus rhythm with heart failure is the Digitalis Investigation Group (DIG) study. Although in this trial a substantial decrease was seen in hospitalizations and deaths due to worsening heart failure, the overall mortality was not affected by digoxin when added to diuretics and angiotensin-converting enzyme (ACE)

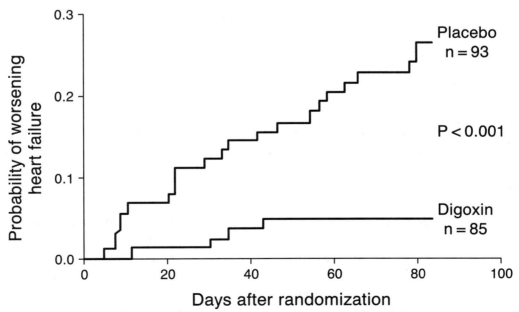

Fig. 1. Kaplan-Meier analysis of the cumulative probability of worsening heart failure in patients continuing to receive digoxin and those whose treatment was switched to placebo. The patients in the placebo group had a higher risk of worsening heart failure throughout the 12-week study (relative risk, 5.9; 95% confidence interval, 2.1 to 17.2). (From *N Engl J Med* 329:1-7, 1993. By permission of the Massachusetts Medical Society.)

Table 2.—Digoxin in Heart Failure: Three Recent Prospective, Randomized, Placebo-Controlled Clinical Trials

	PROVED		RADIANCE		DIG	
	Placebo (n = 46)	Digoxin* (n = 42)	Placebo (n = 93)	Digoxin* (n = 85)	Placebo (n = 3,403)	Digoxin (n = 339)
Mean age, yr	64	64	59	61	63	63
Male, % of patients	80	90	82	71	77	78
LVEF, %	29	27	28	26	28	29
NYHA functional class, % of patients						
II	83	83	75	71	55	53
III	15	17	25	29	31	31
IV	--	--	--	--	2	2
IHD, % of patients	67	60	56	65	70	71
ACE inhibitor treatment, % of patients	0	0	100	100	95	94
Mean follow-up, mo	3		3		37	
Progression/worsening of heart failure, % of patients	39	19	25.0	4.7		
Change in exercise time from baseline, s	-96	+4.5 (P = 0.003)	-26	+17 (P = 0.033)		
Change in body weight, kg	+0.5	-0.9 (P = 0.044)	+1	-1 (P < 0.001)		
Change in LVEF, %	-3	+2 (P = 0.016)	-4	-1 (P < 0.001)		
Hospital admission for worsening heart failure, % of patients	13	7	10	2	34.7	26.8

ACE, angiotensin-converting enzyme; DIG, Digitalis Investigation Group; IHD, ischemic heart disease; LVEF, left ventricular ejection fraction; NYHA, New York Heart Association; PROVED, Prospective Randomized Study of Ventricular Failure and the Efficacy of Digoxin; RADIANCE, Randomized Assessment of Digoxin on Inhibitors of the Angiotensin-Converting Enzyme.
*Withdrawal.

inhibitor therapy (Fig. 2). Patients most likely to benefit from digoxin are those at highest risk for clinical deterioration. Thus, patients with more severe heart failure with a worse functional class (NYHA class III/IV), lower left ventricular ejection fraction (< 25%), and a greater cardiothoracic ratio (> 0.50) had the greatest benefit from digoxin therapy (Fig. 3). It has been suggested that a balance between a reduction in deaths due to worsening heart failure and an increase in deaths from other causes, such as arrhythmia or myocardial infarction, may occur in these patients. Thus, although digoxin may not improve overall survival, it appears to be "safe" for long-term use in patients with heart failure in comparison with other positive inotropic agents, which appear to have a detrimental effect on overall survival. In the DIG trial, digoxin toxicity was infrequent and did not increase hospitalizations or discontinuation with adequate monitoring of patient serum

levels of digoxin. The reduction in risk of worsening heart failure between patients with relatively well preserved left ventricular function and those with impaired left ventricular function was not statistically different, thus alleviating concern about the use of digoxin in patients with heart failure due to diastolic dysfunction. Patients with heart failure due to amyloid heart disease or restrictive cardiomyopathy respond poorly to treatment with digoxin.

- Digoxin therapy in patients with heart failure due to systolic ventricular dysfunction results in reduction in hospitalizations and deaths from worsening heart failure; however, overall mortality is not affected.

Digoxin is recommended as an American College of Cardiology/American Heart Association (ACC/AHA) class I indication in the treatment of patients with heart

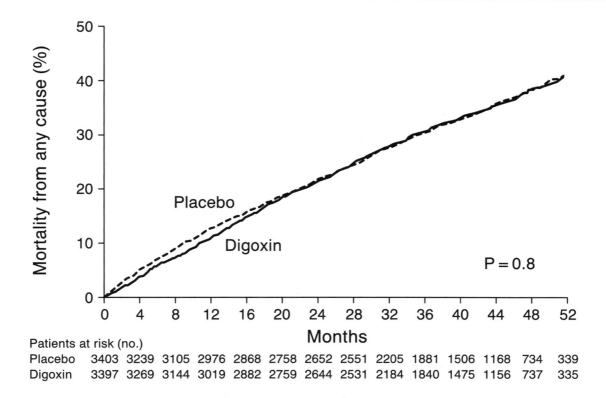

A

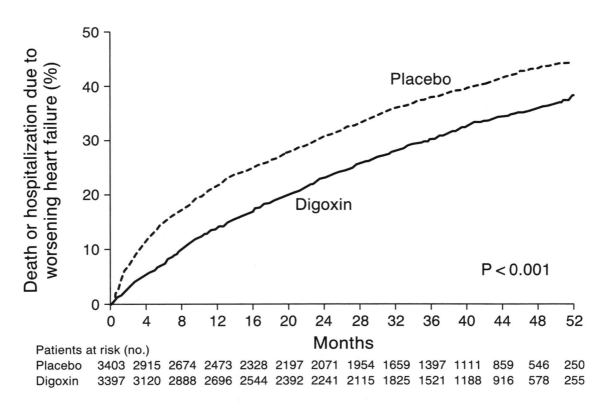

B

Fig. 2. *A*, Mortality and, *B*, incidence of death or hospitalization due to worsening heart failure in digoxin and placebo groups. The number of patients at risk at each 4-month interval is shown in each panel. (From *N Engl J Med* 336:525-533, 1997. By permission of the Massachusetts Medical Society.)

Table 3.—Major Manifestations of Digoxin Toxicity

Cardiac (vagal and direct effects)
    Sinoatrial node—sinus bradycardia, sinoatrial arrest or exit block
    Atrium—paroxysmal atrial tachycardia, vagally induced atrial fibrillation
    Atrioventricular node—Wenckebach, 2° and 3° AV block, junctional rhythm
    His-Purkinje system—Junctional ectopy, escape or accelerated rhythm, nonparoxysmal junctional tachycardia
    Ventricle—Premature beats (bigeminy or trigeminy, unifocal or multifocal), fascicular or bidirectional ventricular tachycardia
Gastrointestinal
    Anorexia, nausea, vomiting (50%-80% of patients) (chemoreceptors in the area postrema of the medulla)
    Vasoconstrictive effect (mesenteric ischemia)
Central nervous system
    Headeache, fatigue, malaise, neuralgic pain, agitation/anxiety, disorientation, confusion, delirium, and seizures
Visual symptoms
    Scotomas, flickering, halos, change in color perception (yellow/green vision)
Other
    Allergic skin reactions
    Gynecomastia in men
    Sexual dysfunction

failure due to systolic dysfunction not adequately responsive to ACE inhibitors and diuretics and in patients with atrial fibrillation and rapid ventricular response. For all other symptomatic patients with heart failure due to left ventricular systolic dysfunction, digoxin has an ACC/AHA class II indication. The primary benefit of digoxin in heart failure is to improve the clinical status, with attenuation of symptoms and reduction in hospitalizations for heart failure. However, because there is no evidence that digoxin decreases mortality, it may not be needed in patients who are asymptomatic after treatment with ACE inhibitors, diuretics, and β-blockers.

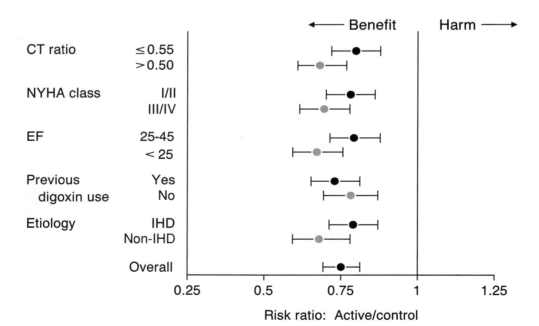

Fig. 3. The effect of digoxin on congestive heart failure mortality or related hospitalization: subgroup analysis of the Digitalis Investigation Group (DIG) trial. Patients with ejection fraction (EF) < 25%, nonischemic congestive heart failure, cardiomegaly on chest radiography (cardiothoracic ratio [CT] > 0.50), and New York Heart Association (NYHA) functional class III/IV symptoms appeared to derive the most benefit from digoxin therapy. IHD, ischemic heart disease. (From Coats A [editor]: *Controversies in the Management of Heart Failure.* Churchill Livingstone, 1997, p 92. By permission of Pearson Professional.)

Table 4.—Factors Altering Digoxin Sensitivity

Hypokalemia, hypomagnesemia (diuretic use, gastrointestinal disease, diabetes mellitus, nutritional status, congestive heart failure with prolonged secondary aldosteronism)

Hyperkalemia, hyponatremia

Hypercalcemia (thiazide)

Acid-base imbalance

Acute hypoxemia (enhanced digitalis sensitivity)

Chronic lung disease (hypoxia, hypercapnia, acidosis, sympathetic activation)

Renal insufficiency

Hypothyroidism or hyperthyroidism

Low lean body mass (decreased binding to skeletal muscle)

Enhanced sympathetic tone (Ca^{2+} loading, afterdepolarization)

Enhanced vagal tone (bradyarrhythmias, pauses, heart block)

Drugs with negative chronotropic and dromotropic properties (class II, IV, amiodarone)

Type and severity of underlying cardiac disease (sinus node disease, atrioventricular conduction disease, amyloidosis [binding], rheumatic or viral myocarditis, immediately post-myocardial infarction?)

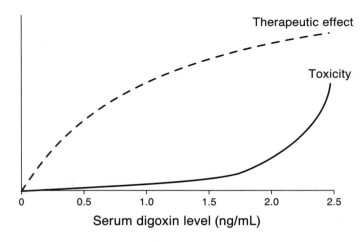

Fig. 4. Relationship between the therapeutic and toxic effects of digoxin and the serum digoxin level. Above a level of 1.5 ng/mL, the additional therapeutic effect is minimal and the frequency of toxicity increases substantially. (From Leier CV [editor]: *Cardiotonic Drugs: A Clinical Survey.* Marcel Dekker, 1987, p 85. By permission of the publisher.)

Side Effects and Toxicity

Digoxin has a narrow therapeutic-toxic margin, and toxicity can develop readily if not carefully monitored. The toxic effects increase markedly with digoxin levels greater than 2.0 ng/mL, without any significant additional therapeutic effect (Fig. 4). The common side effects with a chronic overdose of digoxin are gastrointestinal (anorexia, nausea, vomiting, diarrhea) and visual effects (colored halos around a light) and arrhythmias. Central nervous system effects (malaise, fatigue, confusion, insomnia, and vertigo) and gynecomastia may also occur (Table 3). Adverse effects may occur even with therapeutic serum levels, especially in the presence of hypokalemia and hypomagnesemia, which can independently increase ventricular automaticity and lower the threshold for digoxin-induced cardiac arrhythmias. Because of the direct arterial vasoconstrictive effects of digoxin, intravenous administration can be deleterious in patients with severe atherosclerosis; the precipitation of both coronary and mesenteric ischemia has been reported. Use of digitalis in the setting of cardiac ischemia, for example, after myocardial infarction, has been suggested to be associated with increased mortality. Recent experimental evidence also suggests that inhibition of Na^+-K^+-ATPase activity with digoxin may prevent the infarct size-limiting effect of ischemic preconditioning.

Digoxin toxicity could result from overdosage, decreased excretion, or other factors that may increase the sensitivity of tissue to digoxin even at "therapeutic" serum levels (Table 4). Disturbances of cardiac conduction, impulse formation, or both may occur with digoxin toxicity (Fig. 5). Because of its effect on the shortening of atrial repolarization and increase in dispersion of refractoriness, digoxin has profibrillatory effects on atrial tissue and may prolong the duration of atrial fibrillation. Also, with overdose, intracellular calcium loading, delayed afterdepolarization, and triggered activity may occur in atrial, junctional, and Purkinje tissue. This may result in atrial, junctional, and ventricular tachyarrhythmias, such as accelerated junctional rhythm, paroxysmal atrial tachycardia with AV block (with increased vagal tone), frequent premature ventricular complexes, and fascicular or bidirectional ventricular tachycardia. Ventricular fibrillation may also occur. Factors associated with poor prognosis in patients with digitalis toxicity are summarized in Table 5. With severe intoxication, hyperkalemia due to

Table 5.—Digoxin Toxicity: Poor Prognostic Factors

Advanced age

Male sex

Initial hyperkalemia (degree of Na^+-K^+-ATPase poisoning)

Underlying heart disease (cardiomyopathy, conduction disease)

Advanced atrioventricular block

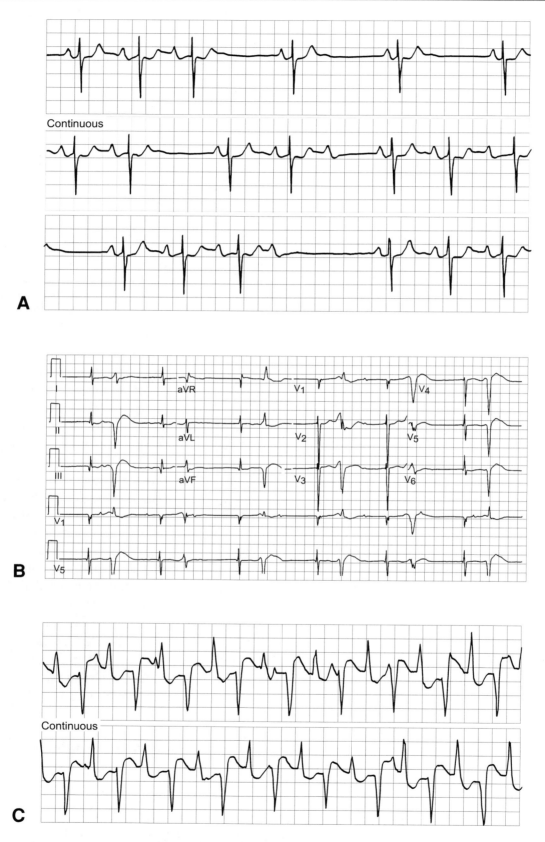

Fig. 5. Cardiac rhythm abnormalities due to digitalis toxicity. *A,* Second-degree sinoatrial block and Mobitz I second-degree atrioventricular block. *B,* Complete atrioventricular block, junctional rhythm, and premature ventricular complexes. *C,* Bidirectional ventricular tachycardia. (*A* and *C* from Chou T-C, Knilans TK: *Electrocardiography in Clinical Practice: Adult and Pediatric.* Fourth edition. WB Saunders Company, 1996, pp 508; 512. By permission of the publisher.)

Table 6.—Management of Digoxin Toxicity

Early recognition and withdrawal of digoxin
Correction of underlying abnormalities (electrolytes, hypoxemia)
Electrocardiographic monitoring and treatment of
    Symptomatic bradycardia
        Atropine or temporary pacemaker (with hyperkalemia, failure to capture may occur)
        Digoxin-specific Fab antibody
    Unstable supraventricular tachycardia
        DC shock (low energy; risk of asystole or ventricular arrhythmias is present)
    Ventricular arrhythmias
        Digoxin-specific Fab antibody (watch for K^+, may need to supplement)
        Lidocaine, phenytoin, propranolol
Subsequent adjustment of dosage schedule to prevent recurrences (goal serum level, ~1.0 ng/mL > 6 hours after last dose)

Na^+-K^+-ATPase poisoning and profound bradyarrhythmias may occur and may be unresponsive to pacing therapy. If digoxin toxicity is suspected, elective cardioversion for atrial fibrillation should be delayed. If urgent cardioversion is required, the energy level should be minimized.

Management of digoxin toxicity is summarized in Table 6. The key to successful treatment is early recognition of digoxin intoxication. For mild manifestations, such as gastrointestinal symptoms or "benign" dysrhythmia (such as occasional ectopy, excessive slowing of conduction in the AV node with atrial fibrillation), temporary withdrawal of digoxin and ECG monitoring is sufficient. In severe bradycardia or heart block associated with hemodynamic impairment, atropine or temporary ventricular pacing may be needed. For frequent ectopic atrial, junctional, or ventricular rhythms, potassium and magnesium supplementation is often helpful, especially if hypokalemia is present.

Digoxin-specific antisera can rapidly reverse potentially life-threatening digoxin toxicity with severe heart block, hyperkalemia, or ventricular arrhythmias. The digoxin-specific Fab fragments are administered intravenously and have a rapid onset of action, large volume of distribution, and rapid clearance. Doses of Fab are calculated using a formula based on either the total body digoxin burden or the estimated dose of drug ingested and are given intravenously in saline over 30 to 60 minutes. Serum levels of digoxin remain abnormal after Fab fragment administration and are not useful clinically to monitor recovery from toxicity. Hemodialysis is ineffective in the treatment of digoxin toxicity because of the large volume of distribution of digoxin.

● Hemodialysis is ineffective in the treatment of digoxin toxicity because of the large volume of distribution of digoxin.

Contraindications to Digoxin Use

1. Digoxin should not be used in patients with Wolff-Parkinson-White syndrome and atrial fibrillation because it may accelerate anterograde conduction over the accessory pathway and could precipitate ventricular fibrillation.
2. In patients with hypertrophic obstructive cardiomyopathy, digoxin should not be used because the inotropic effect may worsen the outflow gradient.
3. Digoxin should be used very cautiously in all conditions (summarized in Table 4) that increase digoxin sensitivity.
4. In patients with preexisting sinus node dysfunction and conduction disease, slowing of the heart rate and symptomatic pauses may occur, causing hemodynamic compromise. Ventricular regularization with atrial fibrillation

Table 7.—Digoxin: Drug Interactions

Decreased serum level	Increased serum level
Decreased absorption	Increased absorption
Antacids	Atropine
Cathartics	Propantheline
Kaolin-pectin	Decreased clearance
Cholestyramine	Amiodarone
Colestipol	Quinidine
Metoclopramide	Flecainide
Neomycin	Propafenone
Phenytoin	Diltiazem
Sulfasalazine	Verapamil
Increased clearance	Cimetidine
Thyroxine	Spironolactone
	Macrolides
	Tetracycline
	Benzodiazepines
	Indomethacin

in a patient taking digoxin suggests toxicity, with AV block and junctional rhythm.

Drug Interactions

Antiarrhythmics and other drugs affecting digoxin concentration are summarized in Table 7. Antacids, cholestyramine, metoclopramide, prednisone, and sulfasalazine decrease the serum concentration of digoxin, whereas benzodiazepines, spironolactone, and ACE inhibitors may increase the concentration. Cimetidine reduces the metabolism of digoxin and renal clearance of the drug, thus potentiating toxicity. Patients taking medications that decrease the absorption of digoxin could develop digoxin toxicity when the concurrent treatment is stopped.

Dosing

Intravenous and oral preparations of digoxin are available. An initial loading dose may be required for an urgent indication, such as slowing of a rapid ventricular response in atrial fibrillation in patients who are in heart failure. A loading regimen of 0.5 mg, followed by 0.25 mg every 4 to 6 hours to a total dose of 1 to 1.5 mg, is usual for a 70-kg patient, with the maintenance dose (0.125 to 0.375 mg/day) adjusted to maintain a concentration of 0.5 to 2 ng/mL.

Loading doses of digoxin generally are not needed solely for inotropic effect in heart failure with a well-controlled ventricular rate. Patients with reduced renal function or baseline cardiac conduction abnormality or those who are elderly or have small stature should start treatment with 0.125 mg/day or less and the dose titrated to an adequate serum level of digoxin. Steady state will be reached in approximately 1 week in patients with normal renal function, although 2 to 3 weeks may be needed for those with renal impairment. Dosing is guided by efficacy, tolerance, and serum concentration (the level should be measured 6 to 8 hours after the last oral dose).

The sensitivity of the patient to digoxin effect may be altered by various factors (Table 4), and clinical judgment should be used to reduce the dose if toxicity is suspected despite apparent "therapeutic serum digoxin levels." The value of regularly determining the serum level of digoxin is uncertain, but it is probably reasonable to check the level once yearly after a steady state has been achieved. Possible interactions with digoxin should be considered whenever treatment is started with a new medication that interacts with digoxin, and the serum level of digoxin should be measured approximately 1 week after the addition of the new drug.

Suggested Review Reading

1. David D, Segni ED, Klein HO, et al: Inefficacy of digitalis in the control of heart rate in patients with chronic atrial fibrillation: beneficial effect of an added beta adrenergic blocking agent. *Am J Cardiol* 44:1378-1382, 1979.

2. The Digitalis Investigation Group: The effect of digoxin on mortality and morbidity in patients with heart failure. *N Engl J Med* 336:525-533, 1997.

3. Falk RH, Leavitt JI: Digoxin for atrial fibrillation: a drug whose time has gone? *Ann Intern Med* 114:573-575, 1991.

4. Ferguson DW, Berg WJ, Sanders JS, et al: Sympathoinhibitory responses to digitalis glycosides in heart failure patients. Direct evidence from sympathetic neural recordings. *Circulation* 80:65-77, 1989.

5. Gheorghiade M, Ferguson D: Digoxin. A neurohormonal modulator in heart failure? *Circulation* 84:2181-2186, 1991.

6. Goldsmith SR, Simon AB, Miller E: Effect of digitalis on norepinephrine kinetics in congestive heart failure. *J Am Coll Cardiol* 20:858-863, 1992.

7. Guidelines for the evaluation and management of heart failure. Report of the American College of Cardiology/American Heart Association Task Force on Practice Guidelines (Committee on Evaluation and Management of Heart Failure). *J Am Coll Cardiol* 26:1376-1398, 1995.

8. Hinderling PH, Hartmann D: Pharmacokinetics of digoxin and main metabolites/derivatives in healthy humans. *Ther Drug Monit* 13:381-401, 1991.

9. Indolfi C, Piscione F, Russolillo E, et al: Digoxin-induced vasoconstriction of normal and atherosclerotic epicardial coronary arteries. *Am J Cardiol* 68:1274-1278, 1991.

10. Kelly RA, Smith TW: Recognition and management of digitalis toxicity. *Am J Cardiol* 69:108G-118G, 1992.

11. Leor J, Goldbourt U, Behar S, et al: Digoxin and mortality in survivors of acute myocardial infarction: observations in patients at low and intermediate risk. *Cardiovasc Drugs Ther* 9:609-617, 1995.

12. Lindenbaum J, Rund DG, Butler VP Jr, et al: Inactivation of digoxin by the gut flora: reversal by antibiotic therapy. *N Engl J Med* 305:789-794, 1981.

13. Lynch JJ, Simpson PJ, Gallagher KP, et al: Increase in experimental infarct size with digoxin in a canine model of myocardial ischemia-reperfusion injury. *Am Heart J* 115:1171-1182, 1988.

14. Matsuda M, Matsuda Y, Yamagishi T, et al: Effects of digoxin, propranolol, and verapamil on exercise in patients with chronic isolated atrial fibrillation. *Cardiovasc Res* 25:453-457, 1991.

15. Nawada R, Murakami T, Iwase T, et al: Inhibition of sarcolemmal Na^+,K^+-ATPase activity reduces the infarct size-limiting effect of preconditioning in rabbit hearts. *Circulation* 96:599-604, 1997.

16. Marcus FI, Opie LH, Sonnenblick EH, et al: Digitalis and other inotropes. In *Drugs for the Heart*. Fourth edition. Edited by LH Opie. Philadelphia, WB Saunders Company, 1997, pp 145-173.

17. Packer M, Gheorghiade M, Young JB, et al: Withdrawal of digoxin from patients with chronic heart failure treated with angiotensin-converting-enzyme inhibitors. RADIANCE Study. *N Engl J Med* 329:1-7, 1993.

18. Ribner HS, Plucinski DA, Hsieh AM, et al: Acute effects of digoxin on total systemic vascular resistance in congestive heart failure due to dilated cardiomyopathy: a hemodynamic-hormonal study. *Am J Cardiol* 56:896-904, 1985.

19. Santana LF, Gomez AM, Lederer WJ: Ca^{2+} flux through promiscuous cardiac Na^+ channels: slip-mode conductance. *Science* 279:1027-1033, 1998.

20. Smith TW: Digitalis. Mechanisms of action and clinical use. *N Engl J Med* 318:358-365, 1988.

21. Uretsky BF, Young JB, Shahidi FE, et al: Randomized study assessing the effect of digoxin withdrawal in patients with mild to moderate chronic congestive heart failure: results of the PROVED trial. *J Am Coll Cardiol* 22:955-962, 1993.

Questions

Multiple Choice (choose the one best answer)

1. Cardiac glycosides enhance cardiac contractility primarily by
   a. Stimulation of sarcolemmal Na^+-K^+-ATPase
   b. Inhibition of sarcolemmal Na^+-K^+-ATPase
   c. Activation of phospholamban
   d. Opening of sarcolemmal calcium channels
   e. Release of calcium from the sarcoplasmic reticulum

2. Digoxin may have all the following effects *except*:
   a. Increase in intracellular Ca^{2+}
   b. Reduction in sympathetic activity in patients with severe congestive heart failure
   c. Increased automaticity and conduction velocity of the atrioventricular node
   d. Increased automaticity of atrial and His-Purkinje tissue

3. All the following statements about the effect of digoxin on cardiac conduction and refractory periods are true *except*:
   a. The refractory period of the atrioventricular node is prolonged
   b. The atrial refractory period and action potential duration are prolonged
   c. Sinoatrial conduction is depressed
   d. The PR and AH intervals on electrograms are prolonged
   e. It has parasympathomimetic and sympatholytic actions

4. In the pressure-volume curve shown in the accompanying Figure, the top curve represents normal cardiac function and HF represents heart failure; match the curves to the response to the given interventions.
   a. Intravenous digoxin
   b. Infusion of dopamine
   c. Intravenous verapamil in patients with left ventricular dysfunction
   d. Use of disopyramide

5. In which one of the following randomized trials has digoxin been shown to improve survival among patients with congestive heart failure?
   a. PROVED
   b. RADIANCE
   c. DIG study
   d. All the above
   e. None of the above

6. Digoxin-induced automaticity is further enhanced by:
   a. Hypernatremia
   b. Hypokalemia
   c. Hypermagnesemia
   d. Hypocalcemia

7. The following arrhythmia(s) is (are) associated with digoxin toxicity:
   a. Sinoatrial block
   b. Atrioventricular junctional tachycardia
   c. Atrial tachycardia
   d. Ventricular tachycardia
   e. All the above

8. A 70-year-old woman with a history of chronic

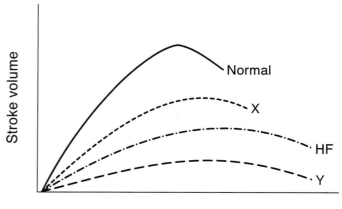

Question 4

obstructive pulmonary disease, congestive heart failure, and paroxysmal atrial fibrillation has anorexia, nausea, fatigue, and an irregular heartbeat. On examination, she has basilar crackles, jugular venous pulse at 9 cm H_2O, and ventricular bigeminy. She is taking digoxin 0.25 mg and thiazide diuretics, and ibuprofen was added a week ago for degenerative joint disease. A week ago, the digoxin level was 1.5 ng/mL. What should be the next step?
   a. Addition of quinidine
   b. Addition of amiodarone
   c. Intravenous furosemide (Lasix)
   d. Hold digoxin
   e. Start lidocaine

9. Quinidine may aggravate digoxin-induced arrhythmias because it:
   a. Blocks the sodium channels at the atrioventricular (AV) node, causing AV block
   b. Increases calcium influx into the cells, causing calcium overload
   c. Increases excretion of digoxin
   d. Displaces digoxin from the binding site

10. Digibind (digoxin immune Fab) is used to
    a. Potentiate the electrophysiologic effects of digoxin
    b. Treat digoxin toxicity by removing digoxin from its binding site in tissue
    c. Treat digoxin toxicity by binding with Na^+-K^+-ATPase to decrease digoxin effect
    d. Check digoxin level in the blood

Answers

1. Answer b

The primary mechanism of action of cardiac glycosides is the inhibition of the sarcolemmal Na+-K+-ATPase. This leads to intracellular accumulation of sodium and, subsequently, calcium by the sodium-calcium exchanger, resulting in increased velocity and extent of sarcomere shortening and increased contractility.

2. Answer c

Digoxin decreases automaticity and conduction velocity in sinoatrial and atrioventricular nodal tissue both by its vagotonic and direct effects.

3. Answer b

Digoxin decreases atrial action potential duration and refractoriness by enhancing vagal tone and increasing outward K+ conductance via the muscarinic K+ channel. With decreased refractoriness, digitalis can promote atrial reentry and atrial fibrillation. The direct and indirect (vagomimetic and sympatholytic) effects of digoxin on sinoatrial and atrioventricular nodal tissue decrease conduction and result in ventricular response slowing with atrial fibrillation and decrease the recurrence of sinus node and atrioventricular nodal reentrant tachycardia.

4. Answer a = X; b = X; c = Y, d = Y

The normal heart has a curvilinear stroke volume–end-diastolic pressure relationship. The top curve represents a normal-functioning left ventricle. In curve B, the shift to the right reflects decreased contractility that could occur with myocardial depressant drugs, such as verapamil or disopyramide, or ventricular systolic dysfunction due to ischemia. In curve A, the shift to the left reflects increased contractility with inotropic agents, such as dopamine and other catecholamines or digitalis. In a patient with ventricular systolic dysfunction, the inotropic agents will shift the curve HF to the left, close to curve A.

5. Answer e

The only randomized, placebo-controlled, prospective trial of digoxin that has reported mortality in patients with congestive heart failure is the Digitalis Investigator Group (DIG) study. None of the digitalis trials have shown any significant beneficial effect on overall or cardiovascular mortality. Digoxin, however, is the only inotropic agent that has been shown to be safe, without a deleterious effect on long-term survival.

6. Answer b

Hypokalemia enhances automaticity in cardiac tissue and could result in digitalis toxicity, even in the presence of "therapeutic digoxin serum levels."

7. Answer e

Almost any arrhythmia may occur with digoxin toxicity. Sinus bradycardia, sinoatrial block, and atrioventricular conduction delay or block probably result from the combination of vagal effects and diminished sympathetic tone as well as the direct effects of digitalis. Enhanced diastolic (phase 4) depolarization can result in atrioventricular junctional tachycardia. Increased automaticity of the Purkinje fibers can result in ventricular tachycardia. Calcium loading and oscillation can cause delayed afterdepolarization and triggered activity.

8. Answer d

Elderly patients are very susceptible to digoxin intoxication, even at a relatively low dose and with apparently normal serum levels. Comorbid conditions and other factors, such as hypoxemia, hypokalemia, hypomagnesemia, and hypercalcemia, could further exacerbate this. The use of nonsteroidal anti-inflammatory drugs may affect renal function and increase the serum level of digoxin. Thiazide diuretics can cause hypercalcemia, whereas potent loop diuretics may result in hypokalemia and hypomagnesemia and should be given cautiously and after checking for electrolyte disturbance and adequate replacement of K and Mg. Quinidine and amiodarone can increase the serum level of digoxin, thereby resulting in toxicity. This patient's symptoms could be the result of digoxin toxicity. Treatment with digoxin should be stopped, and serum electrolytes and renal function should be checked.

9. Answer d

Quinidine displaces digoxin from its binding sites, reducing its volume of distribution; quinidine also decreases the renal clearance of digoxin, resulting in increased serum levels.

10. Answer b

Digibind, the antidigoxin antibody, binds with digoxin, mobilizing it from tissue stores, thereby preventing its effect. The bound digoxin is then excreted through the kidneys.

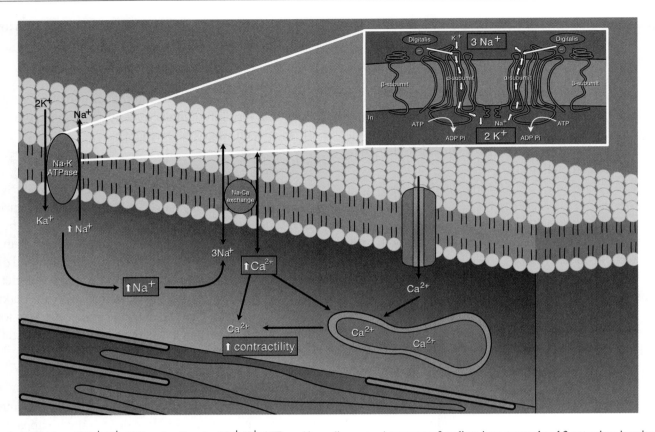

Plate 1. Inhibition of Na^+-K^+-ATPase by digoxin. Na^+-K^+-ATPase (the sodium pump) transports 3 sodium ions outward and 2 potassium ions inward. Inhibition of the Na^+-K^+ pump increases intracellular sodium, which leads to increased intracellular calcium by Na^+-Ca^{2+} exchanger. The increased intracellular calcium increases the force of myocardial contraction by increasing both the velocity and extent of sarcomere shortening. *Inset*, the proposed structure of Na^+-K^+ ATPase, consisting of 2 α-subunits and 2 surrounding β-subunits. The α-domain contains the ionic channel, the external digoxin binding site, the external potassium binding site, the internal sodium binding site, and the ATP hydrolysis site. (*Inset* from Opie LH: *The Heart: Physiology, From Cell to Circulation*. Third edition. Lippincott-Raven Publishers, 1998, p 108. By permission of the author.)

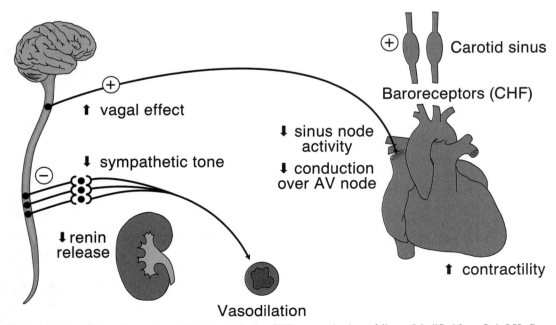

Plate 2. Digoxin effect on neurocardiovascular system. AV, atrioventricular; CHF, congestive heart failure. (Modified from Opie LH: *Drugs for the Heart*. Fourth edition. WB Saunders Company, 1995, p 146. By permission of the publisher.)

Chapter 77

Intravenous Inotropic Drugs

Joseph G. Murphy, M.D.
Arshad Jahangir, M.D.

Intravenous inotropic agents work through either the stimulation of adrenergic (isoproterenol, epinephrine, norepinephrine, terbutaline, albuterol, and dobutamine) or dopaminergic receptors (dopamine) to increase intracellular cyclic adenosine monophosphate (AMP) or the inhibition of phosphodiesterase III enzyme (PDE III) to inhibit cyclic AMP breakdown. Increased intracellular cyclic AMP in turn increases intracellular Ca^{2+}, which interacts directly with the contractile mechanism. β-Receptors are located on the exterior of the myocyte sarcolemma membrane and span the thickness of the membrane to reach the interior of the cell via the G protein system: G_s stimulates and G_i inhibits the adenylate cyclase system. This in turn activates protein kinases, which leads to an increase in intracellular levels of Ca^{2+} through protein phosphorylation. $β_1$ Receptors are found primarily in the atria, ventricles, and atrioventricular (AV) node and are responsible for positive inotropic and chronotropic effects on the heart and augmented AV node conduction. $β_2$ Receptors occur in the arteries, arterioles, veins, and bronchioles and are responsible for peripheral vasodilatation. $α_1$ Receptors are located on arterioles and mediate vasoconstriction, and $α_2$ receptors inhibit norepinephrine release from sympathetic nerve endings. Dopaminergic DA_1 receptors are present in the renal and mesenteric vascular beds and promote vasodilatation and natriuresis.

- $β_1$ Receptors are responsible for the positive inotropic and chronotropic effects on the heart.

- $β_2$ Receptors are responsible for peripheral vasodilatation.
- $α_1$ Receptors mediate vasoconstriction
- $α_2$ Receptors—feedback loop to inhibit norepinephrine release from sympathetic nerve endings

Isoproterenol

Isoproterenol is a pure β-receptor stimulant ($β_1 > β_2$). It has strong positive inotropic and chronotropic effects ($β_1$ effects) and is a weak vasodilator ($β_2$ effect). Also, isoproterenol may precipitate cardiac arrhythmias. It has no effect on α or dopaminergic receptors. The usual starting dose is 0.5 µg/min, increasing to 5 µg/min depending on the hemodynamic and heart rate response. It exacerbates myocardial ischemia and increases heart rate and is arrhythmogenic. Its primary use is to stimulate myocardial contraction after heart surgery.

- Isoproterenol is a pure β-receptor stimulant.

Epinephrine

Epinephrine at high dose stimulates $β_1$ and $β_2$ receptors and α receptors. It is used primarily in the setting of cardiac arrest, because of its powerful inotropic and chronotropic effect in combination with a vasoconstrictor effect, to increase blood pressure. The usual dose in the case of cardiac arrest is 1 mg intravenous bolus every 3 to 5 minutes, but a considerably higher dose of 0.1 mg/kg intravenous bolus every 3 to 5 minutes may also be used (high-dose epinephrine protocol). The intravenous dose in acute shock is 1 to 4 µg/min.

- Epinephrine at high dose stimulates β_1 and β_2 receptors and α receptors.

Norepinephrine

Norepinephrine lacks the vasodilator β_2-receptor effects of epinephrine but has stronger α-receptor stimulating effects. Thus, it is a potent vasoconstrictor with fewer inotropic and chronotropic effects than isoproterenol or epinephrine. It is used primarily to increase arterial blood pressure in severe hypotension, particularly in the setting of septicemic shock accompanied by abnormal vasodilatation (warm shock). The dose is 2 to 20 µg/min intravenously.

Dopamine

Dopamine is a naturally occurring endogenous catecholamine that is administered intravenously in pharmacologic doses in the treatment of severe heart failure, hypotension, and cardiogenic shock. Dopamine stimulates many cardiac and vascular receptors, and its predominant hemodynamic effect depends on the administered dose. It causes a vasodilatory response by direct stimulation of dopaminergic DA_1 postsynaptic and DA_2 presynaptic receptors in the peripheral vasculature and renal tubular cells. Dopamine causes selective vasodilatation of the splanchnic, coronary, cerebral, and renal arterial beds at doses less than 2 µg/kg per minute. The main benefit in this dose range is increased renal blood flow and maintenance of glomerular filtration in patients in incipient renal failure or in those who have become relatively refractory to diuresis.

At intermediate (2 to 8 µg/kg per minute) infusion rates, dopamine enhances norepinephrine release from vascular sympathetic neurons, resulting in increased β-adrenergic receptor activation in the heart. At higher infusion rates (> 8 to 20 µg/kg per minute), peripheral vasoconstriction occurs through direct α-adrenergic receptor stimulation. The hemodynamic response to dopamine may vary among patients because of 1) differences in lean body mass for the same body weight, 2) overlap between the response ranges of the three receptors, and 3) norepinephrine depletion in advanced heart failure that may lessen the adrenergic response to dopamine. Tachycardia and arrhythmias are more pronounced with dopamine than with dobutamine. Dopamine is administered by continuous intravenous infusion and has a half-life of several minutes.

Dopamine is contraindicated in patients taking monoamine oxidase inhibitors and in those with a significant ventricular arrhythmia, hypertrophic cardiomyopathy, severe aortic stenosis, or pheochromocytoma.

- < 2 µg/kg per minute—vasodilator effect
- 2 to 8 µg/kg per minute—adrenergic effect
- > 8 to 20 µg/kg per minute—vasoconstrictor effect

Dobutamine

Dobutamine is a sympathomimetic amine that stimulates both β_1- and β_2-adrenergic receptor subtypes but does not activate α-adrenergic receptors or cause the release of norepinephrine. Although it has mild effects on blood pressure and heart rate, dobutamine increases cardiac output and reduces left ventricular end-diastolic filling pressures. A lower dose of dobutamine results in a positive inotropic effect, predominantly through a β_1-adrenergic effect. Dobutamine does not stimulate dopaminergic receptors and, unlike dopamine, does not selectively alter renal blood flow. Dobutamine does not increase myocardial infarct size or cause significant ventricular arrhythmias.

Dobutamine also has a vasodilator effect, and it reduces aortic impedance and systemic vascular resistance, thus reducing afterload. In contrast, dopamine either has no effect or may increase ventricular afterload by increasing systemic vascular resistance. Dobutamine is preferred to dopamine for most patients with advanced heart failure who have not had an adequate response to conventional treatment. Dobutamine infusions are initiated at 2 µg/kg per minute and titrated up according to hemodynamic response of the patient (the usual maximal dose is 20 µg/kg per minute, based on estimated lean body weight).

No controlled trials have demonstrated the efficacy and safety of "renal-range" dopamine infusion in patients with heart failure and declining renal function who are receiving vasodilators. There is no good evidence that "renal-range" dopamine preserves renal function or promotes significant natriuresis, although it is frequently used for this indication.

For outpatients, dobutamine is administered via a portable

infusion pump through a central venous catheter; it may have symptomatic benefit for those with advanced heart failure and symptoms refractory to conventional drugs used to treat heart failure. No prospective controlled studies have been conducted on this form of therapy for severe heart failure.

- Dobutamine stimulates both β_1- and β_2-adrenergic receptor subtypes.

Milrinone

Milrinone is a relatively selective inhibitor of the cyclic guanosine monophosphate-inhibited, cyclic AMP PDE III enzyme. It causes vasodilatation, with a decrease in systemic vascular resistance in addition to a powerful positive inotropic effect. Intravenous milrinone is approved for short-term hemodynamic support in advanced heart failure. In a longer term prospective trial of oral milrinone in class IV heart failure, mortality increased in spite of an acute hemodynamic benefit (PROMISE Trial). Milrinone may be used in combination with other oral or intravenous drugs for short-term treatment of severe heart failure due to systolic ventricular dysfunction or for patients after bypass.

Milrinone is started with a typical loading dose of 50 µg/kg over 10 minutes and an infusion rate from 0.25 to 1.0 µg/kg per minute. Clinically significant thrombocytopenia was a problem with amrinone, a PDE III inhibitor that preceded milrinone; however, thrombocytopenia is rare with milrinone.

- Milrinone is a relatively selective inhibitor of PDE III enzyme.

Summary of the Properties of Common Adrenergic Inotropic Agents

Agent	Inotropic	Chronotropic	Vasoconstriction	Arrhythmogenic	Receptor stimulated			
					β_1	β_2	α_1	Dopamine
Isoproterenol	+++	+++	0	+++	+++	+++	0	0
Epinephrine	+++	++	++ (high dose)	+++	+++	++	+++	0
Norepinephrine	+	+	++	+	+++	0	+++	0
Dobutamine	++	+	+	+	+++	+	++	0
Dopamine	++	+	++ (high dose)	+	++	+	+++	+++

Questions

Multiple Choice (choose the one best answer)

1. A 50-year-old man is admitted to the hospital with acute inferior myocardial infarction. After 12 hours, he becomes hypotensive and oliguric. He is lying comfortably on his back, blood pressure is 90/60 mm Hg, heart rate is 60 beats/min, and jugular venous pressure is about 15 cm H_2O. The heart sounds are regular without gallop, murmur, or rub, and the lungs are clear to auscultation. The next step should be to give:
   a. Intravenous furosemide
   b. Intravenous fluids
   c. Digoxin
   d. Norepinephrine
   e. Dopamine
   f. Intra-aortic balloon pump

2. Desensitization to catecholamines may be caused by all the following *except*:
   a. Receptor phosphorylation
   b. Receptor internalization
   c. Increased production of cyclic adenosine monophosphate
   d. Alteration of G proteins
   e. Alterations in cyclic nucleotide phosphodiesterase

3. All the following statements about adrenergic drugs are true *except*:
   a. Isoproterenol stimulates α receptors when administered in high doses
   b. Dobutamine does not stimulate dopaminergic receptors
   c. Norepinephrine does not stimulate β_2 receptors
   d. Dopamine stimulates β_1, β_2, and α_1 receptors
   e. Epinephrine is more arrhythmogenic than dobutamine

Answers

1. Answer b

This patient probably has an inferior wall infarction complicated by right ventricular involvement. The cardiac output is probably depressed because of low left-heart filling pressure secondary to right ventricular infarction. The initial treatment should be administering fluids intravenously.

2. Answer c

Chronic exposure to catecholamine leads to desensitization of its effect as a result of modification of adrenergic receptor and postreceptor changes that include phosphorylation of the receptors, internalization and modification of the G proteins, and G-protein-receptor interaction. Increased production of cyclic adenosine monophosphate would heighten the adrenergic effect.

3. Answer a

Isoproterenol is a pure β-agonist and has no significant α receptor stimulation properties. Dobutamine, despite the similarity of its name to dopamine, does not stimulate dopaminergic receptors. Norepinephrine does not stimulate β_2 receptors, whereas dopamine stimulates all adrenergic receptors.

Chapter 78

Nitrates

Peter A. Brady, M.D.

Nitrates exert their antianginal effects by supplying exogenous nitric oxide (NO) to vascular smooth muscle cells, thereby dilating coronary epicardial arteries and arterioles (> 100 µm in diameter) and thus improving myocardial perfusion.

Pharmacology of Organic Nitrates

Organic nitrates are prodrugs and, thus, must undergo a biotransformation before they can have a therapeutic effect. Nitrates are rapidly absorbed from the skin, mucous membranes, and gastrointestinal tract. Both nitroglycerin and isosorbide dinitrate undergo extensive first-pass liver metabolism when taken orally. Liver and intravascular metabolism of nitroglycerin and isosorbide dinitrate yield biologically active dinitrate metabolites with half-lives longer than those of the drug. Isosorbide-5-mononitrate does not undergo first-pass metabolism and is almost 100% bioavailable.

Mechanism of Action

Nitrates relax vascular smooth muscle through an endothelial-independent pathway. The proposed mechanism involves conversion of administered nitrate to NO at or near the plasma membrane (Fig. 1). In turn, NO activates guanylate cyclase to produce cyclic guanosine monophosphate (cGMP). Intracellular accumulation of cGMP causes vasodilation. This mechanism is similar to the vasodilation induced by sodium nitroprusside and endogenous endothelial-derived NO.

Intracoronary, intravenous, and sublingual nitrates dilate coronary arteries and arterioles greater than 100 µm in diameter. Epicardial coronary and arteriolar vasodilation increases blood flow from the epicardial to the endocardial regions and relieves coronary spasm, leading to better perfusion of ischemic myocardium. In contrast to nitrates, vasodilators such as dipyridamole may worsen angina because they may divert blood from the ischemic area to a nonischemic area ("coronary steal phenomenon"). When nitrates are taken orally, they marginally *decrease* overall coronary blood flow. In this circumstance, antianginal effects are due primarily to venodilation, which reduces preload and end-diastolic volume, thus reducing myocardial wall tension. Consequently, myocardial oxygen demand decreases. However, the benefit of decreased myocardial wall tension may be offset by a reflexive increase in heart rate and contractility.

Nitrates improve angina and myocardial ischemia by:
- Dilation of coronary epicardial vessels
- Dilation of arterioles > 100 µm in diameter
- Preload reduction
- Afterload reduction
- Redistribution of blood from the epicardium to the endocardium
- Relief of spontaneous and exercise-induced coronary spasm

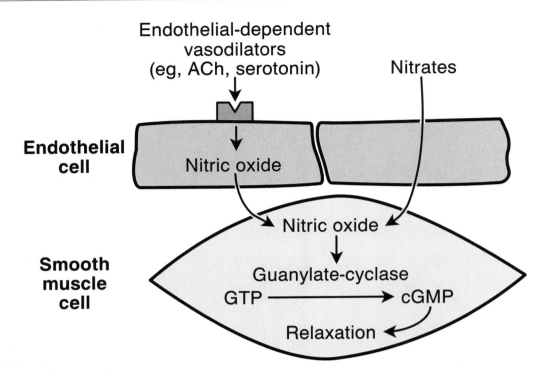

Fig. 1. Mechanism of action of nitrates on vascular smooth muscle cells. ACh, acetylcholine.

Clinical Indications for Nitrate Therapy

Myocardial Infarction

Nitrates appear to limit infarct size and to favorably alter ventricular remodelling. However, these benefits appear to be limited to patients with decreased left ventricular function and are lost after drug treatment is discontinued. Nitrates also have antiplatelet activity, although its clinical significance is not known. The effect of nitrates on long-term mortality after myocardial infarction is unclear. Pooled data from several randomized trials conducted in the prethrombolytic era suggest that intravenous nitroglycerin, given within 24 hours after the onset of symptoms, reduces mortality. More recently, the International Study of Infarct Survival (ISIS)-4 and Gruppo Italiano per lo Studio della Streptochinasi nell' Infarto Miocardio (GISSI)-3 examined the impact of nitrates on mortality among patients who had reperfusion therapy at the time of myocardial infarction. ISIS-4 reported on outcomes of patients randomly assigned within 24 hours after myocardial infarction to 1 month of controlled release mononitrate (30 mg daily initially, titrated to 60 mg daily if tolerated) or placebo. Of these patients, 94% received antiplatelet therapy and 70% received thrombolysis. However, 60% in the placebo group also received nitrates during initial hospitalization. Early (5 weeks) and late (1 yr) mortality were not significantly different between the two groups. Use of mononitrates was associated with a significantly higher incidence of hypotension.

GISSI-3 randomly assigned patients within 24 hours after myocardial infarction to placebo or early intravenous nitrates, followed by transdermal nitroglycerin, providing 10 mg of nitroglycerin daily. Principal outcomes were all-cause mortality and the combined end point of death plus clinical congestive heart failure or asymptomatic left ventricular dysfunction (ejection fraction < 35% by echocardiography). Similar to ISIS-4, GISSI-3 patients were treated with thrombolysis (72%), β-blockade (31%), and aspirin (84%). At 6 weeks, mortality as well as the combined end point of death or heart failure was nonsignificantly lower among patients who received nitrates than among controls. Currently, data from ISIS-4 and GISSI-3 *do not* support routine use of nitrates in addition to standard therapy for acute myocardial infarction.

Indications for Nitrate Therapy Following Myocardial Infarction

- Persistent ischemic pain
- Congestive heart failure and pulmonary edema
- Sustained hypertension

Unstable Angina

Intravenous nitroglycerin, which allows rapid titration of dosage, is most useful in unstable angina. Tolerance usually develops within 24 hours after starting the medication but can be overcome in the short term (24 to 72 hours) by dose increases. Intermittent treatment with intravenous nitrates, to avoid tolerance in patients with unstable angina, is not recommended because of rebound ischemia. Nitrate rebound may be avoided by starting treatment with oral nitrates before discontinuing intravenous nitrates.

Stable Angina

Continuous 24-hour treatment with nitrates is not recommended because of nitrate tolerance. Therefore, regimens that allow for nitrate-free periods are preferable. Intermittent use of nitrate patches, providing a daily nitrate-free interval of 12 hours (at night), is often most effective, if an adequate patch size (delivering at least 7.5 mg of nitroglycerin per 12 hours) is used. However, patients are not protected at night or during the early morning hours. Alternative regimens include twice-a-day isosorbide-5-mononitrate, with the first dose administered in the morning and the second dose 7 hours later. This appears effective for 12 to 14 hours and is not associated with rebound phenomenon. Once-a-day treatment with 120 or 240 mg of slow-release isosorbide-5-mononitrate may also be used.

Congestive Heart Failure

Acutely, nitrates reduce pulmonary capillary wedge pressure, left ventricular end-diastolic pressure, and ventricular volumes. These beneficial effects are lost with more prolonged treatment, because of tolerance. Despite the loss of hemodynamic effects because of tolerance, long-term treatment with high doses of isosorbide dinitrate (30 to 40 mg four times daily) plus hydralazine improved survival compared with placebo and prazosin treatment, but it was inferior to treatment with the angiotensin-converting enzyme (ACE) inhibitor enalapril (Veterans Administration Heart Failure Trial [V-HeFT] II). African-American patients appeared to benefit more from the combination of nitrates and hydralazine than from an ACE inhibitor.

Side Effects of Nitrates

The side effects of nitrates are related mostly to vasodilation and include:
- Headache

- Postural hypotension, which may lead to syncope (especially in the elderly)
- Nausea
- Dermal erythema and inflammation (with nitrate patches)
- Methemoglobinemia after prolonged nitrate use; this is due to oxidation of hemoglobin to methemoglobin by nitrate ions; patients rarely may have severe hypoxia.
- Pulmonary hypoxemia in patients with chronic obstructive pulmonary disease, because of worsening of ventilation-perfusion mismatch by nitrates.

Special Problems With Nitrate Use

Nitrate Tolerance

Nitrate tolerance is defined as loss of the hemodynamic and antianginal effects during sustained therapy and represents a major limitation of the clinical use of nitrates. The precise pathophysiologic mechanism of nitrate tolerance is unknown, but it is not due to altered drug pharmacokinetics, because with chronic nitrate therapy plasma drug concentrations are similar to, or higher than, those during initial therapy. Several hypotheses have been suggested:

1. **Sulfhydryl-depletion hypothesis**—suggests that tolerance is due to depletion of reduced sulfhydryl groups (SH) necessary for the intracellular biotransformation of nitrate to NO. However, addition of sulfhydryl groups in vitro fails to prevent tolerance.

2. **Neurohormonal hypothesis**—based on the observation that long-term nitrate use is associated with increased catecholamines, renin, endothelin, and other vasoactive hormones that lead to reflex vasoconstriction and antagonize the vasodilating effect of nitrates. However, this effect has not been found consistently.

3. **Plasma-volume expansion hypothesis**—chronic use of nitrates induces plasma volume expansion. This hypothesis suggests that nitrate-induced plasma volume expansion offsets the beneficial action of nitrates to reduce ventricular preload. The mechanism of plasma volume expansion is unknown, but it is not due to sodium retention and persists for several days despite the development of hemodynamic tolerance. Attempts to prevent tolerance with diuretics generally have not been successful.

4. **Free radical hypothesis**—suggests tolerance may be due to formation of superoxide anions, which inactivate NO. This is supported by the finding that nitrate tolerance may be reversed, at least in some cases, by antioxidant therapy. The mechanism by which nitrates increase superoxide anions

is unclear but is believed to involve angiotensin II. Of interest, hydralazine, which inhibits formation of superoxide anions, together with nitrates has a beneficial effect on mortality in patients with heart failure despite use of a nitrate-dosing regimen known to induce tolerance. Hydralazine increases renal perfusion, counteracting renal hypoperfusion, another possible mechanism of nitrate tolerance.

5. **Low-affinity and high-affinity nitrate receptors**—receptors with different affinities for nitrates may be present and the high-affinity receptors are downgraded by high levels of nitrate.

The only widely accepted method of preventing nitrate tolerance is to use a dosing strategy that provides a nitrate-free interval of 8 to 12 hours during each 24-hour period.

Nitrate Rebound

Although intermittent nitrate use reduces tolerance, it may also result in nitrate rebound. This often presents as worsening ischemia or myocardial infarction in patients with stable or unstable angina or as worsening symptoms in patients with heart failure during the nitrate-free period. The mechanism is unknown, but it may be due to heightened responsiveness of the vasculature to "constrictor" substances that are increased during nitrate therapy.

Nitrate Resistance

Some patients do not have any hemodynamic response even to very high doses of nitrates given intravenously. Many of these patients have no previous exposure to nitrates and, thus, nitrate tolerance is not an issue. Most of the patients with nitrate resistance have severe heart failure or acute myocardial infarction, both conditions known to cause intense activation of the renin-angiotensin system.

Nitrate Preparations

Commonly used nitrate preparations are listed in Table 1.

Table 1.—Commonly Used Nitrate Preparations

Drug	Usual dose	Duration of action
Short-acting nitrates		
Amyl nitrite	2-5 mg	1-5 min
Nitroglycerin (sublingual)	0.3-0.6 mg	10-30 min
Isosorbide dinitrate		
(sublingual)	2.5-5.0 mg	10-60 min
NTG spray	0.4 mg/metered dose	10-30 min
Long-acting nitrates		
NTG, 2% ointment	1-1.5 in./4 hr	3-6 hr
NTG, slow-release, transdermal	10-25 mg/24 hr	8-10 hr
Isosorbide dinitrate, oral	10-60 mg/4-6 hr	4-6 hr
Isosorbide dinitrate, chewable	5-10 mg/2-4 hr	2-3 hr
Isosorbide mononitrate, oral	20 mg/24 hr	6-10 hr
Intravenous nitrates		
NTG	5-200 μg/min for up to 48 hr	Short

NTG, nitroglycerin

Suggested Review Reading

1. Mahmarian JJ, Moye LA, Chinoy DA, et al: Transdermal nitroglycerin patch therapy improves left ventricular function and prevents remodeling after acute myocardial infarction: results of a multicenter prospective randomized, double-blind, placebo-controlled trial. *Circulation* 97:2017-2024, 1998.

Chapter 79

Calcium Channel Blockers

Arshad Jahangir, M.D.

Calcium channel blockers are potent vasodilators with antihypertensive, antianginal, and, in some cases, antiarrhythmic effects. All clinically approved calcium channel blockers block only L-type channels at therapeutic concentrations. Mibefradil (Posicor), a recently withdrawn calcium channel blocker, blocks both L-type and T-type calcium channels but has a greater selectivity for T-type channels.

Pharmacology

Most calcium channel blockers have high first-pass liver metabolism and high plasma protein binding (Table 1). Their metabolites also may be biologically active and have additional calcium channel blocking properties. Plasma drug concentrations are not routinely measured during therapy.

- All clinically approved calcium channel blockers block only L-type channels at therapeutic concentrations.

Pharmacodynamics

Calcium channel blockers bind to specific receptors on the voltage-gated calcium channels on cardiac myocytes and vascular smooth muscle cells in a voltage-dependent manner (Plate 1). This results in marked reduction in calcium influx into the cells, leading to decreased excitability and contractility. This causes four effects: 1) a relaxation of vascular smooth muscle cells, 2) decreased contractility of the myocardium, 3) a reduction in the sinoatrial node discharge rate, and 4) a reduction in atrioventricular (AV) node conductivity (Plate 2). Calcium channel blockers belonging to the dihydropyridine group (nifedipine, amlodipine) are more selective for vascular smooth muscle cells and are potent vasodilators with less cardiac depressant effect and less electrophysiologic properties than verapamil or diltiazem (Table 2); however, in the presence of myocardial disease and β-adrenergic blockers, dihydropyridines also can have significant cardiac depressant effects. Short-acting calcium channel blockers may cause an abrupt fall in blood pressure, resulting in the reflex activation of the sympathetic nervous system, an effect that is avoided with the long-acting agents.

- Calcium channel blockers bind to specific receptors on the voltage-gated calcium channels in a voltage-dependent manner. This results in marked reduction in calcium influx into the cells, leading to decreased excitability and contractility.

Clinical Use in Cardiovascular Medicine (Table 3)

General Effect in Arrhythmias
Verapamil and diltiazem are class IV (Vaughan-Williams classification) antiarrhythmic agents, whereas dihydropyridines

Table 1.—Pharmacokinetics of Oral Calcium Channel Blockers

Calcium channel blocker	Bioavailability	Protein binding	Onset of action after oral intake, hours	Time to peak concentration, hours	Plasma half-life, hours	Route of major elimination
Verapamil	Low	High	1	1-2	5-12	Renal, hepatic
Diltiazem	Moderate	High	1	1-3	5-7	Hepatic
Amlodipine	High	High	1-2	6-12	35-50	Hepatic
Felodipine	Low	High	1-2	2-5	11-16	Hepatic, renal
Isradipine	Low	High	0.5	1-2	8	Hepatic, renal
Nicardipine	Low	High	0.5	1-2	9	Hepatic, renal
Nifedipine (SR)	Moderate	High	0.5	2-6	6-11	Hepatic
Nimodipine	Low	High	0.5	1	8-9	Hepatic
Bepridil	Moderate	High	2-3	8	24-60	Hepatic

have no clinically useful antiarrhythmic effect. In the sino-atrial and AV nodes, blockade of the slow inward calcium current results in a decreased rate of automatic discharge. AV node conduction and refractoriness are prolonged, thus forming the basis for the antiarrhythmic benefit in AV node-dependent reentrant tachycardias and ventricular rate slowing in atrial tachyarrhythmias. In addition to the sinoatrial and AV node, other tissues dependent on the slow inward calcium current may be affected by class IV drugs. Class IV agents have no significant effect on intra-atrial, intraventricular, or His-Purkinje conduction or refractoriness.

- AV node conduction and refractoriness are prolonged by calcium blockers, thus forming the basis of antiarrhythmic benefit in AV node-dependent reentrant tachycardias and ventricular rate slowing in atrial tachyarrhythmias.

Paroxysmal Supraventricular Tachycardia (PSVT)

In supraventricular tachycardia requiring conduction through the AV node as part of the arrhythmia circuit, such as AV node reentrant or orthodromic AV reentrant tachycardia, verapamil and diltiazem are effective for terminating and suppressing the tachycardia (efficacy, 65% to 100%). Intravenous verapamil and diltiazem are comparable in safety and efficacy to intravenous adenosine for terminating AV node-dependent arrhythmias. Although the effect of adenosine in this situation is more rapid than that of verapamil, it is short-lived, and in cases in which the arrhythmia recurs after initial termination, verapamil is more effective for controlling the rhythm. Oral calcium channel blockers are less effective when used for the prevention of PSVT recurrence than when used intravenously for acute PSVT conversion.

Table 2.—Effects of Calcium Channel Blockers on Left Ventricular Function, Sinus Rate, and Surface and Intracardiac Electrograms

Calcium channel blocker	Clinical effects			Electrocardiograph, interval			Intracardiac electrogram*	
	Ventricular contractility	Vasodilatation	Sinus rate	PR	QRS	QT	AH	HV
Verapamil	↓↓↓	↑	↓↓	↑↑	↔	↔	↑↑	↔
Diltiazem	↓↓	↑	↓	↑	↔	↔	↑	↔
Dihydropyridines	↔↓	↑↑	↑†	↔	↔	↔	↔	↔
Bepridil	↔↓	↑	↓	↑		↑	↑	

↔, no effect; ↓, decreased; ↑, increased.
*Conduction time.
†With short-acting formulations.

Table 3.—Therapeutic Uses of Calcium Channel Blockers

Cardiovascular
  Cardiac arrhythmias
    Supraventricular arrhythmias
      Inappropriate sinus tachycardia
      Sinus node reentrant tachycardia
      AV node reentrant tachycardia
      AV reentrant tachycardia
      Atrial tachycardia, flutter, or fibrillation with rapid
        ventricular response
    Ventricular arrhythmias
      Idiopathic right ventricular outflow tract
        tachycardia
      Idiopathic left ventricular tachycardia
  Ischemic heart disease
    Stable angina pectoris
    Silent ischemia
    Vasospastic angina
  Systemic hypertension
  Primary pulmonary hypertension (second-line agent)
  Diastolic ventricular dysfunction
  Hypertrophic obstructive cardiomyopathy (second-line
    agent)
  Cerebral vasospasm after subarachnoid hemorrhage
    (nimodipine)
Noncardiovascular
  Migraine headache
  Raynaud phenomenon
  Renal protection in hypertensive diabetics

AV, atrioventricular.

With increased use of catheter-based ablation of supraventricular tachycardia circuits (which effectively cures these arrhythmias, in most cases), the prophylactic use of drugs, including calcium channel blockers or β-blockers, to prevent recurrences has decreased markedly.

● Recurrence of PSVT after termination with adenosine is best treated with verapamil or diltiazem given intravenously.

Atrial Tachyarrhythmias

In supraventricular tachycardia not dependent on the AV node, calcium channel blockers have a minor role in preventing recurrence, with the exception of multifocal atrial tachycardia or atrial tachycardia due to digitalis toxicity (probable triggered arrhythmias). In these tachycardias, verapamil may slow the ventricular response by slowing AV node conduction.

Calcium channel blockers have no significant role in converting atrial fibrillation or flutter to sinus rhythm or in maintaining sinus rhythm after it is restored by DC cardioversion. However, verapamil and diltiazem are effective for controlling rapid ventricular response with atrial fibrillation either at rest or during activity.

● Calcium channel blockers have no significant role in converting atrial fibrillation or flutter to sinus rhythm or in maintaining sinus rhythm after it is restored electrically.

Ventricular Arrhythmias

Currently, the role of calcium channel blockers in ventricular arrhythmias is limited to the small subset of patients with idiopathic ventricular tachycardia arising from the right ventricular outflow tract or near the posterior Purkinje fascicle in the left ventricle. This usually occurs in a structurally normal heart, and both β-blockers and verapamil are effective in most cases for terminating and preventing arrhythmia recurrence. No trials comparing the two antiarrhythmic classes have been published, nor are data available about the impact of these agents on survival of this subset of patients.

In triggered arrhythmias due to early and delayed afterdepolarization, even though oscillation of cellular calcium has been suggested to underlie the ventricular arrhythmias, the therapeutic role of calcium channel blockers in suppressing these arrhythmias is not clear.

● The role of calcium channel blockers in ventricular arrhythmias is limited to a small subset of patients with idiopathic right ventricular outflow tract or left ventricular fascicular tachycardia.

Ischemic Heart Disease

Effort and Vasospastic Angina

All calcium channel blockers are potent coronary vasodilators and inhibit exercise-induced coronary vasoconstriction. In addition, verapamil and diltiazem decrease myocardial contractility, heart rate, and ventricular wall stress, reduce cardiac afterload, and decrease myocardial oxygen requirements. A decreased heart rate increases diastolic filling time and increases coronary blood flow, thus limiting myocardial ischemia. Calcium channel blockers not only improve angina but also objectively decrease myocardial ischemia (on exercise test and ambulatory electrocardiographic monitoring), increase coronary artery blood flow, and improve ventricular dysfunction due to myocardial ischemia. Calcium channel blockers are also very effective for relieving and preventing coronary artery spasm, such as in vasospastic angina.

Limited animal and human studies also suggest that calcium channel blockers may have a direct antiatherosclerotic action, limiting the progression of coronary atherosclerosis; however, the extent and clinical importance of this effect have yet to be established.

Myocardial Infarction
Despite well-established anti-ischemic properties, calcium channel blockers do not reduce mortality during or after myocardial infarction (Table 4). Several clinical trials and meta-analyses of short-acting calcium channel blockers in patients with cardiovascular disease have indicated a detrimental effect on long-term survival. One study reported that in patients with coronary artery disease, the use of short-acting nifedipine may increase overall mortality. Several explanations for this apparent detrimental effect of short-acting dihydropyridines on survival have been advanced, including hypotension with a reduction in coronary perfusion pressure, disproportionate dilatation of the coronary arteries adjacent to the ischemic area (so-called steal), and reflex tachycardia and a consequent increase in myocardial oxygen demands due to reflex activation of the sympathetic nervous system. Whether a similar detrimental effect occurs with second-generation sustained-release long-acting dihydropyridine preparations is not known. Several long-term prospective trials are currently ongoing to assess the long-term safety and efficacy of calcium channel blockers.

In patients with non–Q-wave or Q-wave myocardial infarction without complicating pulmonary congestion or ventricular dysfunction, a nonsignificant reduction in the incidence of reinfarction and the combined end point of reinfarction and death has been observed with the heart rate-slowing calcium channel blocker diltiazem or verapamil. However, in patients who have heart failure or bradyarrhythmia, these drugs have a detrimental effect on survival.

Despite the lack of evidence of a beneficial effect on survival, calcium channel blockers have been used frequently in patients with acute myocardial infarction. According to the current guidelines of the American College of Cardiology and American Heart Association (ACC/AHA) (Table 5), calcium channel blockers are not recommended for routine treatment or secondary prevention after acute myocardial infarction; if used, they should be reserved only for patients without heart failure, ventricular dysfunction, or AV block in whom β-blockers are ineffective or contraindicated for relief of ongoing ischemia or control of a rapid ventricular response with atrial fibrillation. Only the heart rate-slowing calcium antagonists diltiazem or verapamil are acceptable, and short-acting nifedipine is contraindicated.

● Calcium channel blockers are not recommended for routine treatment or secondary prevention after acute myocardial infarction; if used, they should be reserved only for patients without heart failure, ventricular dysfunction, or AV block in whom β-blockers are ineffective or contraindicated for relief of ongoing ischemia or control of a rapid ventricular response with atrial fibrillation.

Hypertension

All calcium channel blockers are effective for lowering blood pressure in hypertensive patients, including elderly and African-American patients. Sustained-release or longer-acting calcium channel blockers are more appropriate for controlling hypertension because they provide smoother blood pressure control and cause less adrenergic activation and reflex tachycardia. Calcium channel blockers may be used as monotherapy in patients with other indications for calcium channel blockers, such as supraventricular tachycardia, angina pectoris, or Raynaud phenomenon.

Short-acting dihydropyridines such as nifedipine have been associated with a dose-related increased risk of myocardial infarction and mortality in patients with ischemic heart disease, and their use is contraindicated in acute ischemic syndromes. Long-acting formulations and newer calcium channel blockers may not cause the adverse effects associated with older drugs of this class; however, their long-term safety in patients with documented coronary disease are currently being assessed in several large prospective clinical trials.

● Short-acting dihydropyridines may result in a dose-related increased risk of myocardial infarction and mortality in patients with ischemic heart disease, and they are contraindicated in acute ischemic syndromes.

Congestive Heart Failure

Systolic Dysfunction
The role of calcium channel blockers in congestive heart failure due to systolic dysfunction remains uncertain, and

Table 4.—Meta-Analyses of Randomized Trials of Drug Therapy Given During and After Myocardial Infarction

Drug class and time administered	No. of trials	No. of patients	Relative risk of death (95% CI)	P value	Strength of evidence*
β-Adrenergic antagonists					
During MI	29	28,970	0.87 (0.77-0.98)	0.02	A
After MI	26	24,298	0.77 (0.70-0.84)	< 0.001	A
ACE inhibitors					
During MI†	15	100,963	0.94 (0.89-0.98)	0.006	A
After MI, patients with left ventricular dysfunction	3	5,986	0.78 (0.70-0.86)	< 0.001	A
Nitrates (during MI)	22	81,908	0.94 (0.90-0.99)	0.03	B
Calcium channel blockers (during and after MI)	24	20,342	1.04 (0.95-1.14)	0.41	A
Antiarrhythmic drugs					
Lidocaine (during MI)‡	14	9,155	1.38 (0.98-1.95)	> 0.05	C
Class I drugs (after MI)§	18	6,300	1.21 (1.01-1.44)	0.04	A
Amiodarone (after MI)	9	1,557	0.71 (0.51-0.97)	0.03	C
Magnesium (during MI)	11	61,860	1.02 (0.96-1.08)	> 0.05	A

ACE, angiotensin-converting enzyme; CI, confidence interval; MI, myocardial infarction.

*The strength of the evidence in each meta-analysis was graded as follows: A indicates that a randomized trial of adequate size supports the meta-analysis; B, that data from one or more randomized trials of adequate size do not support the meta-analysis; and C, that no large randomized trial was conducted.

†This study evaluated short-term therapy (mean, 5 weeks).

‡This study evaluated prophylaxis administered during and immediately after acute myocardial infarction.

§This study evaluated long-term oral therapy after acute myocardial infarction.

From *N Engl J Med* 335:1660-1667, 1996. By permission of the Massachusetts Medical Society.

Table 5.—Recommendations for Therapy With Calcium Channel Blockers in Acute Myocardial Infarction

Class I

    None

Class IIa

    1. Verapamil or diltiazem may be given to patients in whom β-adrenoceptor blockers are ineffective or contraindicated (i.e., bronchospastic disease) for relief of ongoing ischemia or control of a rapid ventricular response with atrial fibrillation after acute myocardial infarction in the absence of congestive heart failure, left ventricular dysfunction, or atrioventricular block

Class IIb

    1. In non–ST-elevation infarction, diltiazem may be given to patients without left ventricular dysfunction, pulmonary congestion, or congestive heart failure. It may be added to standard therapy after the first 24 hours and its use continued for 1 year

Class III

    1. Nifedipine (short-acting) is generally contraindicated for the routine treatment of acute myocardial infarction because of its negative inotropic effects and the reflex sympathetic activation, tachycardia, and hypotension associated with its use

    2. Diltiazem and verapamil are contraindicated in patients with acute myocardial infarction and associated left ventricular dysfunction or congestive heart failure

From *J Am Coll Cardiol* 28:1328-1428, 1996. By permission of the American College of Cardiology.

their use should be avoided in this condition until their role is further clarified by randomized clinical trials. Calcium channel blockers, with their anti-anginal and vasodilatory properties, appear to have desirable effects for some patients with heart failure; however, their negative inotropic effect and activation of the neurohormonal systems are detrimental and may cause clinical deterioration. Recent data from clinical trials in selected patients with nonischemic cardiomyopathy using the second-generation dihydropyridines amlodipine and felodipine, however, suggest that these agents may be safe and well tolerated and have a favorable effect on survival and perhaps deaths due to arrhythmia (with amlodipine) when used with angiotensin-converting enzyme (ACE) inhibitors, digoxin, and diuretics. This finding is being further evaluated in the Prospective Randomized Amlodipine Survival Evaluation (PRAISE) II trial.

In the recent ACC/AHA guidelines for the treatment of heart failure, calcium channel blockers are not recommended (class III indication) in the absence of coexistent angina or hypertension. If calcium blockers are used, agents with strong negative inotropic effects should be avoided and those with minimal negative inotropic effects should be used, such as amlodipine or felodipine.

- The role of calcium channel blockers in congestive heart failure due to systolic dysfunction remains uncertain, and their use should be avoided in this condition until their role is further clarified by randomized clinical trials.

Diastolic Dysfunction
Calcium channel blockers have been proposed to improve diastolic dysfunction by augmenting ventricular relaxation and improving ventricular compliance, but only limited data are available to support the theory that these mechanisms are clinically relevant. In patients with diastolic ventricular dysfunction, verapamil or diltiazem may be beneficial for reducing symptoms of heart failure by slowing the heart rate and improving ventricular filling and stroke volume. Calcium channel blockers are currently recommended as a class II indication for patients with heart failure due to diastolic dysfunction.

Hypertrophic Cardiomyopathy
β-Blockers are the preferred agent in hypertrophic cardiomyopathy, but in refractory cases, verapamil may improve clinical symptoms, exercise performance, and diastolic function and also reduce left ventricular outflow gradient.

However, because of peripheral vasodilatation, verapamil may cause hemodynamic collapse in patients with significant resting left ventricular outflow obstruction and thus should be used with great care. Negative inotropic agents such as disopyramide or β-blockers without vasodilating properties are preferred in this case.

- Verapamil may cause hemodynamic collapse in patients with hypertrophic cardiomyopathy because of peripheral vasodilatation.

Other Indications
Cerebral vasospasm may occur *after subarachnoid hemorrhage.* Nimodipine (which has a high affinity for cerebral blood vessels) has been shown to reduce morbidity and improve outcome and is recommended by the AHA for the management of this condition.

In severe *aortic regurgitation*, nifedipine reduces (delays) the need for valve replacement compared with standard management.

In selected patients with *primary pulmonary hypertension*, use of calcium channel blockers in high doses appears to be beneficial. The dose needs to be increased cautiously and the patient needs to be observed for hypotension or heart failure. Epoprostenol (Flolan), a prostaglandin, is more effective in primary pulmonary hypertension and is generally considered the drug of choice.

Calcium channel blockers reduce microalbuminuria and preserve kidney function in patients with diabetes and, when used in combination with angiotensin-converting enzyme inhibitors, may have an additive beneficial effect on protein excretion in *diabetic nephropathy.* The usual dosages of calcium channel blockers are given in Table 6.

Side Effects

Adverse effects due to calcium channel blockers are mainly the result of vasodilatation (dizziness, headache, flushing, and ankle swelling) and a decrease in heart rate and blood pressure (fatigue and lassitude). Constipation is also common with verapamil. Occasionally, skin reaction and gingival swelling may occur. These effects are mild and dose-dependent.

Calcium channel blockers should be avoided or used cautiously in conditions summarized in Table 7. In patients with underlying sinus node or conduction system disease, verapamil and diltiazem may cause profound slowing of

Table 6.—Usual Daily Dosage of Calcium Channel Blockers

Blocker	Usual dosage*
Verapamil	240-480 mg/day†‡ For PSVT: 5-10 mg intravenously over 2 min, repeat in 10 min; then 0.005 mg/kg per minute for 30-60 min
Diltiazem	120-360 mg/day For PSVT: 0.25 mg/kg intravenously over 2 min, then 0.35 mg/kg over 2 min; then 5-15 mg/h infusion
Amlodipine	5-10 mg once/day
Felodipine SR	5-10 mg once/day
Isradipine	2.5-10 mg every 12 h
Nicardipine (sustained-release)	30-60 mg twice/day IV 5-15 mg/h
Nifedipine (sustained release)	30-90 mg/day†
Nimodipine	60 mg every 4 hr for 21 days (for subarachnoid hemorrhage)
Mibefradil	50-100 mg once/day
Bepridil	200-400 mg once daily

PSVT, paroxysmal supraventricular tachycardia.
*All dosages are for oral preparation, unless indicated.
Reduce dose in patients with advanced renal † or hepatic ‡ disease.

Table 7.—Relative Contraindications for Use of Calcium Channel Blockers

Overt ventricular failure
Severe sinus node dysfunction
Severe conduction system disease
Wolff-Parkinson-White syndrome
Wide complex tachycardia of unknown cause
History of serious ventricular arrhythmias or prolonged QT interval (bepridil)
Digitalis toxicity
Severe aortic stenosis
Hypertrophic obstructive cardiomyopathy (dihydropyridines)
Hypotension
Severe constipation (verapamil)
Known hypersensitivity
Pregnancy
Post-myocardial infarction or angina at rest (especially short-acting dihydropyridines in the absence of β-adrenergic blockade)

the heart rate and heart block, which may be exacerbated by the concomitant use of digoxin or β-blockers.

In patients with significant ventricular systolic dysfunction, calcium channel blockers can precipitate heart failure and should be avoided. With intravenous administration, hypotension is common and can be severe. Short-acting nifedipine has been reported to increase the incidence of myocardial infarction.

In patients with wide complex tachycardia not definitively known to be supraventricular in origin, calcium channel blockers are contraindicated because they may precipitate hemodynamic collapse in patients with ventricular tachycardia or Wolff-Parkinson-White syndrome. Right ventricular outflow tract idiopathic tachycardia is a rare exception to this rule and may be treated with calcium channel blockers. In patients with atrial fibrillation in the setting of Wolff-Parkinson-White syndrome, calcium channel blockers are ineffective for blocking conduction over the accessory pathway and may accelerate conduction, resulting in hypoten-

sion or cardiac arrest.

In patients with digitalis toxicity, verapamil is contraindicated because it can increase the blood level of digoxin and lead to complete heart block.

Concerns have been raised in some studies about a possible link between the use of calcium channel blockers and carcinoma. Critical review of these studies and additional studies in which no association was found between therapy with calcium channel blockers and carcinoma suggests that the initial reported association is most likely due to selection bias or chance.

Overdose and Toxicity

In life-threatening situations due to overdose or toxicity of calcium channel blockers, intravenous calcium gluconate (1 to 2 g) or calcium chloride (0.5 to 1 mg) should be used. Managing combined myocardial depression and hypotension with calcium channel blockers is difficult. Positive inotropic agents (dobutamine, dopamine), vasoconstrictive catecholamines (norepinephrine, dopamine), or glucagon (5-10 mg for hypotension) with repeated doses of calcium may be necessary. Intravenous atropine or isoproterenol and a temporary pacemaker might be needed for AV block.

Drug Interactions

Verapamil increases the concentration of digoxin when used concomitantly. Cimetidine increases the bioavailability of calcium channel blockers. Carbamazepine, cyclosporine, and theophylline levels are increased by calcium channel blockers, whereas lithium levels may decrease.

Sinus and AV node slowing agents (digoxin and β-blockers) and negative inotropic agents (disopyramide, β-blockers) may increase the negative chronotropic, dromotropic, and inotropic effects of verapamil and diltiazem and may result in symptomatic bradycardia, heart block, and congestive heart failure. Concomitant calcium administration may prevent the hypotensive response to intravenous calcium channel blockers.

Unique Calcium Channel Blockers

Bepridil is unrelated structurally to any other calcium channel blocker and has additional sodium and potassium channel blocking properties (class IA and III antiarrhythmic effects). It blocks both voltage- and receptor-operated calcium channels in the myocardium and vascular smooth muscle and inhibits calcium binding to calmodulin. It has direct negative chronotropic, inotropic, and vasodilatory actions that reduce myocardial oxygen consumption and increase coronary blood flow, leading to a significant anti-ischemic and antianginal effect in the absence of reflex tachycardia. In contrast to other calcium channel blockers, bepridil produces only modest peripheral vasodilatation and displays weak antihypertensive activity. It is indicated in patients with stable effort angina who are intolerant of conventional antianginal medication or in whom this medication has failed. Bepridil has class I anti-arrhythmic properties and can induce new arrhythmias, including ventricular tachycardia and ventricular fibrillation. Because of its ability to prolong the QT interval, bepridil can cause torsades de pointes, especially in the presence of hypokalemia. Agranulocytosis also has been reported.

Mibefradil is a long-acting nondihydropyridine calcium channel blocker that blocks both the T-type and the L-type calcium channels. Because of its vasodilating activity, ability to lower heart rate without negative inotropic effects, and long duration of action, it was thought to be promising for the management of hypertension and chronic stable angina and was released in the United States in 1997. Postmarketing surveillance, especially in elderly patients, revealed serious interactions between mibefradil and β-blockers, digoxin, verapamil, diltiazem, and dihydropyridine calcium channel blockers, resulting in refractory bradycardia and cardiogenic shock. The manufacturer voluntarily withdrew mibefradil in June 1998.

Suggested Review Reading

1. Boden WE, Ziesche S, Carson PE, et al: Rationale and design of the Third Vasodilator-Heart Failure Trial (V-HeFT III): felodipine as adjunctive therapy to enalapril and loop diuretics with or without digoxin in chronic congestive heart failure. *Am J Cardiol* 77:1078-1082, 1996.

2. Buring JE, Glynn RJ, Hennekens CH: Calcium channel blockers and myocardial infarction. A hypothesis formulated but not yet tested. *JAMA* 274:654-655, 1995.

3. DiMarco JP, Miles W, Akhtar M, et al: Adenosine for paroxysmal supraventricular tachycardia: dose ranging and comparison with verapamil. Assessment in placebo-controlled, multicenter trials. *Ann Intern Med* 113:104-110, 1990.

4. Dougherty AH, Jackman WM, Naccarelli GV, et al: Acute conversion of paroxysmal supraventricular

tachycardia with intravenous diltiazem. *Am J Cardiol* 70:587-592, 1992.

5. Ellenbogen KA, Dias VC, Plumb VJ, et al: A placebo-controlled trial of continuous intravenous diltiazem infusion for 24-hour heart rate control during atrial fibrillation and atrial flutter: a multicenter study. *J Am Coll Cardiol* 18:891-897, 1991.

6. Feigen VL, Rinkel GJ, Algra A, et al: Calcium antagonists in patients with aneurysmal subarachnoid hemorrhage: a systematic review. *Neurology* 50:876-883, 1998.

7. Furberg CD, Psaty BM, Meyer JV: Nifedipine. Dose-related increase in mortality in patients with coronary heart disease. *Circulation* 92:1326-1331, 1995.

8. Gobel EJ, Hautvast RW, van Gilst WH, et al: Randomised, double-blind trial of intravenous diltiazem versus glyceryl trinitrate for unstable angina pectoris. *Lancet* 346:1653-1657, 1995.

9. Held PH, Yusuf S: Effects of beta-blockers and calcium channel blockers in acute myocardial infarction. *Eur Heart J* 14 (Suppl F):18-25, 1993.

10. Hollingshead LM, Faulds D, Fitton A: Bepridil. A review of its pharmacological properties and therapeutic use in stable angina pectoris. *Drugs* 44:835-857, 1992.

11. Howes LG, Edwards CT: Calcium antagonists and cancer. Is there really a link? *Drug Saf* 18:1-7, 1998.

12. January CT, Riddle JM: Early afterdepolarizations: mechanism of induction and block. A role for L-type Ca^{2+} current. *Circ Res* 64:977-990, 1989.

13. Kenny J: Treating overdose with calcium channel blockers. *BMJ* 308:992-993, 1994.

14. Lerman BB, Stein KM, Markowitz SM: Adenosine-sensitive ventricular tachycardia: a conceptual approach. *J Cardiovasc Electrophysiol* 7:559-569, 1996.

15. Littler WA, Sheridan DJ: Placebo controlled trial of felodipine in patients with mild to moderate heart failure. *Br Heart J* 73:428-433, 1995.

16. Materson BJ, Reda DJ, Cushman WC, et al: Single-drug therapy for hypertension in men. A comparison of six antihypertensive agents with placebo. *N Engl J Med* 328:914-921, 1993.

17. Mayberg MR, Batjer HH, Dacey R, et al: Guidelines for the management of aneurysmal subarachnoid hemorrhage. A statement for healthcare professionals from a special writing group of the Stroke Council, American Heart Association. *Circulation* 90:2592-2605, 1994.

18. McGovern B, Garan H, Ruskin JN: Precipitation of cardiac arrest by verapamil in patients with Wolff-Parkinson-White syndrome. *Ann Intern Med* 104:791-794, 1986.

19. Messerli FH: Case-control study, meta-analysis, and bouillabaisse: putting the calcium antagonist scare into context. *Ann Intern Med* 123:888-889, 1995.

20. Mullins ME, Horowitz BZ, Linden DH, et al: Life-threatening interaction of mibefradil and beta-blockers with dihydropyridine calcium channel blockers. *JAMA* 280:157-158, 1998.

21. The Multicenter Diltiazem Postinfarction Trial Research Group: The effect of diltiazem on mortality and reinfarction after myocardial infarction. *N Engl J Med* 319:385-392, 1988.

22. Opie LH, Frishman WH, Thadani U: Calcium channel antagonists (calcium entry blockers). In *Drugs for the Heart*. Fourth edition revised. Edited by LH Opie. Philadelphia, WB Saunders Company, 1997, pp 50-82.

23. Packer M, O'Connor CM, Ghali JK, et al: Effect of amlodipine on morbidity and mortality in severe chronic heart failure. *N Engl J Med* 335:1107-1114, 1996.

24. Parving HH, Tarnow L, Rossing P: Renal protection in diabetes—an emerging role for calcium antagonists. *Cardiology* 88 (Suppl 3):56-62, 1997.

25. Psaty BM, Heckbert SR, Koepsell TD, et al: The risk of myocardial infarction associated with antihypertensive drug therapies. *JAMA* 274:620-625, 1995.

26. Rich S, Kaufmann E, Levy PS: The effect of high doses

of calcium-channel blockers on survival in primary pulmonary hypertension. *N Engl J Med* 327:76-81, 1992.

27. Ryan TJ, Anderson JL, Antman EM, et al: ACC/AHA guidelines for the management of patients with acute myocardial infarction. A report of the American College of Cardiology/American Heart Association Task Force on Practice Guidelines (Committee on Management of Acute Myocardial Infarction). *J Am Coll Cardiol* 28:1328-1428, 1996.

28. Scognamiglio R, Rahimtoola SH, Fasoli G, et al: Nifedipine in asymptomatic patients with severe aortic regurgitation and normal left ventricular function. *N Engl J Med* 331:689-694, 1994.

29. Schroeder JS, Gao SZ, Alderman EL, et al: A preliminary study of diltiazem in the prevention of coronary artery disease in heart-transplant recipients. *N Engl J Med* 328:164-170, 1993.

30. Singh BN: Beta-blockers and calcium channel blockers as antiarrhythmic drugs. In *Cardiac Electrophysiology: From Cell to Bedside*. Second edition. Edited by DP Zipes, J Jalife. Philadelphia, WB Saunders Company, 1995, pp 1317-1330.

31. Taylor SH: Usefulness of amlodipine for angina pectoris. *Am J Cardiol* 73:28A-33A, 1994.

32. Teo KK, Yusuf S, Furberg CD: Effects of prophylactic antiarrhythmic drug therapy in acute myocardial infarction. An overview of results from randomized controlled trials. *JAMA* 270:1589-1595, 1993.

33. Yusuf S: Calcium antagonists in coronary artery disease and hypertension. Time for reevaluation? *Circulation* 92:1079-1082, 1995.

Questions

Multiple Choice (choose the one best answer)

1. All of the following statements regarding calcium channel blockers are correct *except*:
   a. They have greater vasodilatory effects on arterial than venous vessels
   b. They have a negative inotropic effect on the myocardium
   c. They suppress rapid upstroke (phase 0) of the action potential in the atrial and ventricular myocardium
   d. They decrease upstroke of the action potential in the atrioventricular node

2. All of the following statements regarding short-acting dihydropyridine calcium channel blockers are true *except*:
   a. They are potent vasoconstrictors
   b. They decrease myocardial contractility by inhibiting calcium current
   c. They cause relaxation of vascular smooth muscle
   d. They increase heart rate in vivo by reflex sympathetic activation

3. For each of the following phrases, choose the calcium channel blocker that most likely has the listed effect:
   i. Produces marked slowing of heart rate
   ii. Is associated with constipation, especially in the elderly
   iii. May be associated with survival benefit in patients with non-ischemic cardiomyopathy
   iv. Has a high affinity for cerebral blood vessels
   v. Is associated with poor survival outcome in patients with unstable coronary syndromes

a. Mibefradil
b. Nimodipine
c. Verapamil
d. Amlodipine
e. Short-acting nifedipine

4. Verapamil controls the ventricular rate in atrial tachyarrhythmias by:
   a. Increasing the duration of the action potential
   b. Decreasing sinoatrial automaticity
   c. Decreasing conduction time within the ventricle
   d. Decreasing conduction velocity within the atrioventricular node

5. Calcium channel blockers are of therapeutic use in all the following *except*:
   a. Vasospastic angina
   b. Supraventricular tachycardia
   c. Idiopathic ventricular tachycardia
   d. Hypertrophic obstructive cardiomyopathy with severe left ventricular outflow tract gradient
   e. Hypertension

6. A 35-year-old woman with Wolff-Parkinson-White syndrome comes to the emergency department with palpitation, shortness of breath, and chest discomfort. She has mild light-headedness with a blood pressure of 90/60 mm Hg and heart rate of 200 beats/min with wide QRS complexes. Which of the following treatments is appropriate at this time?
   a. Intravenous digoxin to slow the heart rate
   b. Intravenous diltiazem
   c. Intravenous esmolol
   d. Direct-current countershock
   e. Quinidine orally

7. Which of the following drugs is recommended for the management of cerebral vasospasm after subarachnoid hemorrhage?
   a. Nifedipine

b. Nimodipine
c. Diltiazem
d. Verapamil
e. Propranolol

8. Which of the following drugs is helpful in calcium overdose?
   a. Calcium gluconate
   b. Dopamine
   c. Glucagon
   d. Norepinephrine
   e. All of the above

9-14. **True or false**

9. Amlodipine at therapeutic doses is a potent T-type calcium channel blocker

10. Dihydropyridine calcium channel blockers are as effective as adenosine for terminating and preventing recurrences of atrioventricular node reentrant tachycardia

11. In the sinoatrial and atrioventricular nodes, blockade of the sodium current by β-blockers results in a decreased rate of automatic discharge and atrioventricular node conduction slowing

12. Calcium channel blockers are effective for converting atrial flutter to sinus rhythm and for maintaining sinus rhythm after it is restored electrically

13. The American College of Cardiology and American Heart Association recommend calcium channel blockers as a class I indication for routine treatment and secondary prevention after myocardial infarction

14. Mibefradil, a T-type calcium channel blocker, has a better safety profile than an L-type calcium channel blocker when used in combination with β-blockers or nitrates

Answers

1. Answer c

Calcium channel blockers do not significantly influence the action potential in myocardial cells, but in contrast they have a significant effect in specialized conducting tissue.

2. Answer a

All calcium channel blockers are vasodilators.

3.
   i. **Answer a**
  ii. **Answer c**
 iii. **Answer d**
 iv. **Answer b**
  v. **Answer e**

4. Answer d
The predominant effect of verapamil is on the atrioventricular node.

5. Answer d
All drugs with strong vasodilatory properties should be avoided in patients with hypertrophic obstructive cardiomyopathy with severe left ventricular outflow tract gradient. Decrease in afterload can further increase left ventricular outflow obstruction and can result in hemodynamic collapse.

6. Answer d
Patients with known preexcitation syndrome can have either orthodromic reciprocating tachycardia with antegrade conduction over the atrioventricular node and retrograde conduction over the accessory pathway or antegrade reciprocating tachycardia with antegrade conduction over the accessory pathway and retrograde over the atrioventricular node. Orthodromic reciprocating tachycardia usually has narrow QRS complexes (unless there is aberrant conduction over the Purkinje system), whereas antegrade reciprocating tachycardia has wide QRS complexes. Verapamil and digoxin do not slow and can enhance conduction over the bypass tract, leading to rapid ventricular response, ventricular tachycardia, or ventricular fibrillation, and so should be avoided. Direct-current cardioversion should terminate the tachycardia; quinidine also may be of use in slowing conduction over the accessory pathway but will not be effective acutely. Intravenous procainamide could be used if the patient remains hemodynamically stable.

7. Answer b
Cerebral vasospasm may occur after intracranial hemorrhage. Nimodipine, which has a high affinity for cerebral blood vessels, has been shown to reduce morbidity and improve outcome and is recommended by the American Heart Association for the management of cerebral vasospasm after subarachnoid hemorrhage.

8. Answer e
In life-threatening situations due to calcium channel blocker toxicity, intravenous calcium gluconate (1 to 2 g) or calcium chloride (0.5 to 1 mg) should be used. Positive inotropic agents (dobutamine, dopamine), vasoconstrictive catecholamines (norepinephrine, dopamine), or glucagon (5-10 mg for hypotension) with repeated doses of calcium may be necessary. Intravenous atropine or isoproterenol and a temporary pacemaker might be needed for atrioventricular block.

9. False

10. False

11. False

12. False

13. False

14. False

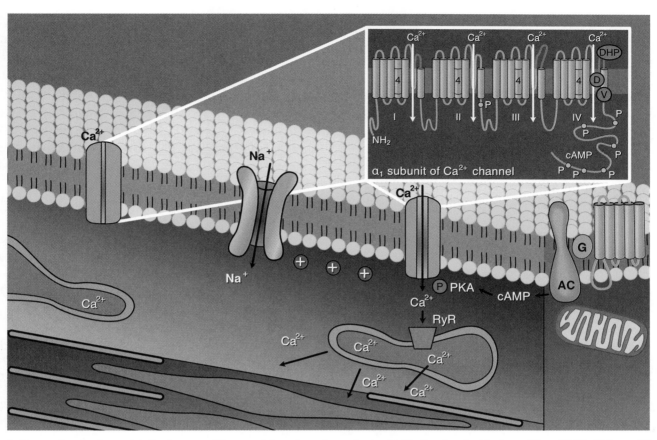

Plate 1. Proposed molecular model of voltage-gated L-type calcium channel α_1 subunit with binding sites for dihydropyridines (DHP), diltiazem (D), and verapamil (V). Calcium ions enter through the pore region between segments 5 and 6 of each of the four transmembrane domains. AC, adenylate cyclase; cAMP, cyclic adenosine monophosphate; G, G protein; P, phosphorylation sites; PKA, protein kinase A; RyR, ryanodine receptors.

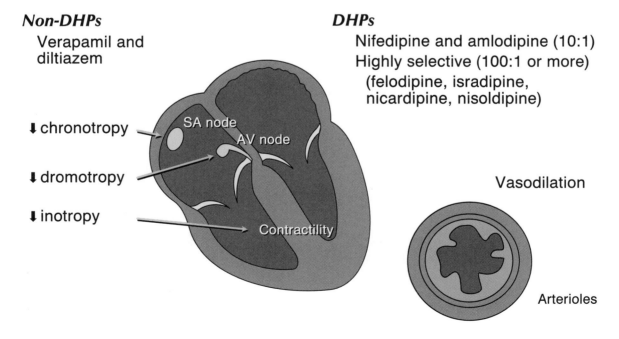

Plate 2. Cardiovascular effects of nondihydropyridines (non-DHP) and dihydropyridine (DHP) calcium channel blockers. AV, atrioventricular; SA, sinoatrial.

Notes

β-Adrenoceptor Blockers

Arshad Jahangir, M.D.

β-Adrenergic Receptor Antagonists

All β-blockers competitively inhibit catecholamine effects at β-adrenergic receptors. The L-isomer is the active β-blocking moiety. For almost all β-blockers, the D-isomer is inert, except for sotalol and propranolol. D-sotalol has additional class III antiarrhythmic properties, whereas D-propranolol has quinidine-like membrane-stabilizing (class I antiarrhythmic) effects at high dosage.

Pharmacokinetics

The pharmacokinetics of various β-adrenergic antagonists are summarized in Table 1. More than 30 β-blockers have been developed, but only a few are commonly used. Most of the drugs are well absorbed after oral administration, with peak concentration occurring 1 to 3 hours after ingestion. β-Blockers exhibit different degrees of lipid solubility (Table 2). More lipid-soluble β-blockers, such as propranolol and metoprolol, are metabolized mainly by the liver and tend to have relatively short plasma half-lives. More water-soluble β-blockers, such as atenolol and nadolol, are cleared by the kidney and tend to have relatively longer plasma half-lives. The elimination half-life of β-blockers varies from 9 minutes for esmolol to 24 hours for nadolol.

- Lipid-soluble β-blockers are metabolized largely by the liver and have relatively short plasma half-lives,

whereas water-soluble β-blockers are cleared by the kidney and have relatively longer plasma half-lives.

Pharmacodynamics of β-Blockers

Classically, β-receptors are divided into β_1-receptors (found mainly in the heart), β_2-receptors (found in vascular and bronchial smooth muscles and myocardium), and β_3-receptors (found in adipocytes). At lower concentration, β-blockers exhibit various degrees of cardiac selectivity (i.e., affinity for β_1 versus β_2 receptor) (Table 2). However, β_1 and β_2 selectivity is relative and can be overcome if large doses are used. Most β-blocking drugs in clinical use are pure antagonists; that is, by occupying a β-receptor, these drugs prevent the receptor from being stimulated by agonists but the drugs themselves do not activate the receptor. However, in addition to β-blockade, pindolol and acebutolol also possess intrinsic sympathomimetic activity, which causes weak β-adrenergic activation (partial agonists). Thus, these drugs decrease resting heart rate and cardiac output less than drugs without intrinsic sympathomimetic activity. Furthermore, drugs with sympathomimetic activity prevent the effect of excessive catecholamine release and increased heart rate during exercise, emotional reactions, and other stressful events. Third-generation β-blockers have additional properties (Table 3), such as vasodilatation by α-adrenergic receptor blockade with carvedilol, labetalol, and bucindolol. Bucindolol has additional mild direct vasodilating properties that likely are mediated by a cyclic guanosine monophosphate-dependent mechanism. Carvedilol and several of its

Table 1.—Pharmacokinetics of β-Adrenergic Receptor Antagonists

	Bioavailability, %	Protein binding, %	Time to peak action after oral intake, hr	Elimination half-life, hr	Route of major elimination
Acebutolol	70	25	3-8	3-10	Liver (kidney)
Bucindolol	30	95	0.5-1.6	2-7	Liver
Carvedilol	30	98	1.0-1.5	7-10	Liver
Labetalol	30	50	2-4 (5 min IV)	3-6	Liver (kidney)
Metoprolol	50	10	1-2	3-6	Liver
Timolol	50	10	1-2	4-5	Liver
Propranolol	35	90	1-2	3-5	Liver
Esmolol	(100 IV)	55	(2-5 min IV)	9 min	Blood esterase (kidney)
Betaxolol	80	50	1-4	14-22	Liver (kidney)
Atenolol	50	5	2-4 (10 min IV)	6-9	Kidney
Bisoprolol	80	30	2-4	9-12	Kidney (liver)
Nadolol	30	30	3-4	14-24	Kidney
Pindolol	90	55	1-3	3-4	Kidney (liver)
Sotalol	90	0	2-4	10-15	Kidney

IV, given intravenously.

Table 2.—β-Blockers: Relative Cardioselectivity, Potency, Lipid Solubility, Intrinsic Sympathomimetic Activity, and Membrane-Stabilizing Properties*

	Relative β_1 selectivity	β_1-Blockade potency ratio (propranolol = 1.0)	Lipid solubility	ISA	Class I antiarrhythmic effect
Cardioselective					
Acebutolol	+	0.3	++	+ β_1	+
Atenolol	++	1.0	-		
Betaxolol	++	1.0	++	0	0
Bisoprolol	+	5-10	+		
Esmolol	++	0.03	+		
Metoprolol	++	1.0	++		
Noncardioselective					
Bucindolol[†‡]		3.0	+	+	
Carvedilol[†§]		2-4	+		++
Labetalol*		0.3	++	+ β_2	±
Nadolol		1.0	-		
Pindolol		6.0	++	++	+
Propranolol		1.0	+++		++
Timolol		6.0	+	±	
Sotalol[//]		0.3	-		

ISA, intrinsic sympathomimetic activity.
*+, low; ++, moderate; +++, high.
[†] Also α_1-adrenergic blockade.
[‡] Direct vascular smooth muscle relaxation.
[§] Antioxidant activity.
[//] Additional class III antiarrhythmic activity.

Table 3.—β-Blockers

Generations	Properties	Examples
1st	Nonselective No additional properties	Propranolol, timolol
2nd	β_1-Receptor selective No additional properties	Metoprolol, atenolol, bisoprolol
3rd	Nonselective with additional properties (vasodilatation, etc.)	Carvedilol, bucindolol, labetalol

metabolites are potent antioxidants that may inhibit catecholamine toxicity resulting from the oxidation of norepinephrine and the subsequent formation of toxic intermediates, including the generation of reactive oxygen free radicals. Carvedilol also has an antiproliferative effect and has been suggested to block the expression of several genes involved in myocardial damage and cardiac remodeling and to inhibit free radical-induced activation of transcription factors and programmed cell death (apoptosis). Because some of the clinical effects of individual β-blockers may be due to effects independent of β-adrenergic blockade, these drugs should not be considered interchangeable for all applications.

Mode of Action

All β-blockers counteract the effect of catecholamines at β-adrenergic receptors. This competition decreases catecholamine-receptor interactions, interrupts the production of cyclic adenosine monophosphate, and ultimately inhibits calcium influx across the sarcolemma and calcium release by the sarcoplasmic reticulum (Plate 1). This results in decreased contractility of atrial and ventricular myocardium and decreased heart rate because of reduced automaticity in the sinus node and slowing of conduction in the atrioventricular node (Plate 2).

Cardiovascular Effects of β-Blockers and Clinical Use

Various indications for the use of β-blockers are summarized in Table 4.

Cardiac Arrhythmias

β-Blockers are effective in treating both supraventricular and ventricular tachyarrhythmias. The beneficial antiarrhythmic effects of β-blockade are marked during ischemia. Some of the potential antiarrhythmic mechanisms of β-blockers are summarized in Table 5. β-Blockers antagonize catecholamine effects in the sinoatrial node, atrioventricular (AV) node, His-Purkinje tissue, and atrial and ventricular myocardium, thus inhibiting normal automaticity and decreasing membrane excitability, conductance, and contractility (Plate 2). A decrease in the diastolic depolarization rate and impulse formation by specialized cardiac fibers results in slowing of sinus and ectopic pacemaker rates and conduction over the AV node.

On electrocardiography (ECG), the PR interval is prolonged without any significant effect on the QRS or QT interval. Sotalol, with its additional class III antiarrhythmic effect, results in prolongation of the action potential and QT interval.

Supraventricular Arrhythmias

β-Blockers have been used to slow sinus tachycardia when there is need to control rate (e.g., to reduce ischemia) in patients with hyperthyroidism or in those with inappropriate sinus tachycardia. These drugs are effective in terminating and suppressing AV nodal-dependent tachyarrhythmias, such as AV nodal reentrant tachycardia and orthodromic AV reentrant tachycardias.

Atrial Fibrillation and Flutter

In atrial flutter or fibrillation, β-blockers effectively control ventricular response at rest and during activity, by increasing the AV nodal refractory period. They have no significant effect on conversion to or maintenance of sinus rhythm, except in atrial fibrillation due to a high catecholamine state (e.g., postoperatively), in which they may be helpful. The prophylactic use of β-blockers perioperatively is effective in preventing postoperative atrial fibrillation in some patients.

In patients with tachycardia-bradycardia syndrome associated with episodic tachycardia alternating with periods of bradycardia, β-blockers with intrinsic sympathomimetic activity (pindolol and acebutolol) may be effective in controlling fast ventricular rate without excessively slowing resting heart rate.

Ventricular Arrhythmias

Because of the major antiadrenergic actions of β-blockers, they are likely to be effective in arrhythmias in which adrenergic stimulation has a major role (exercise-related, postoperative states, anesthesia, the "electrical storm" during

Table 4.—Therapeutic Uses of β-Blockers

Cardiovascular

Cardiac arrhythmias
  Supraventricular arrhythmias
    Inappropriate sinus tachycardia, sinus nodal reentrant tachycardia
    AV nodal reentrant tachycardia, AV reentrant tachycardia
    Atrial tachycardia/flutter/fibrillation with rapid ventricular response
  Ventricular arrhythmias
    Symptomatic premature ventricular complexes
    Idiopathic left ventricular tachycardia
  Triggered arrhythmias
    Digitalis-induced ventricular tachycardia/ventricular fibrillation
    Right ventricular outflow tachycardia
Ischemic heart disease
  Angina pectoris
  Silent ischemia
  Myocardial infarction
    Acute phase
    Long-term
Systemic hypertension
Congestive heart failure
  Systolic ventricular dysfunction
  Diastolic ventricular dysfunction
Hypertrophic obstructive cardiomyopathy
Aortic aneurysm (Marfan syndrome)
Aortic dissection
Neurocardiogenic syncope
Mitral valve prolapse
Congenital long QT syndrome

Noncardiovascular

Glaucoma
Hyperthyroidism
Migraine
Essential tremor
Anxiety states (stage fright)
Alcohol withdrawal
Esophageal varices due to portal hypertension

AV, atrioventricular.

the early phase of acute myocardial infarction, thyrotoxicosis, pheochromocytoma, anxiety, and mitral valve prolapse). β-Blockers have been used to treat symptomatic premature ventricular complexes in patients with digitalis overdose, mitral valve prolapse, or hypertrophic car-

diomyopathy. However, no data have been reported that have convincingly documented a decrease in sudden death rate in these conditions. Catecholamine-sensitive ventricular tachycardia, especially in a subset of patients without structural heart disease, that originates from the right ventricular outflow tract is sensitive to β-blockade and calcium channel blockade. This tachycardia occurs in young persons, is usually exercise-related, and can be induced with infusion of isoproterenol but not consistently with programmed stimulation—all of which suggest a non-reentrant mechanism.

The role of β-blockers in patients with structural heart disease and sustained reentrant ventricular tachycardia is not clear. β-Blockers are not very effective in this setting in preventing inducibility of sustained monomorphic ventricular tachycardia during electrophysiologic study. However, in patients in whom isoproterenol infusion facilitates induction of ventricular tachycardia, β-blockers may prevent recurrence of arrhythmia.

β-Blockers are effective in reducing the incidence of ventricular fibrillation and sudden death in patients who have had myocardial infarction, especially in those with a history of congestive heart failure, suggesting that these patients may be more susceptible to catecholamine-facilitated arrhythmias. In patients with recurrent polymorphic ventricular tachycardia and fibrillation, the so-called electrical storm that may occur with recent myocardial infarction and is often unresponsive to standard antiarrhythmic therapy may respond to β-blockers.

The actions of several antiarrhythmic drugs may be attenuated during sympathetic stimulation, thus decreasing their clinical efficacy. β-Blockade might be beneficial in these patients. In the Cardiac Arrhythmia Suppression Trial (CAST), postmyocardial infarction patients with ventricular systolic dysfunction and ventricular arrhythmias who were receiving β-blockers had a lower all-cause and arrhythmia mortality than patients not receiving β-blockers. These findings suggested a possible "anti-proarrhythmic effect" of β-blocker therapy that reversed or prevented proarrhythmia associated with class IC antiarrhythmic agents.

In the Electrophysiologic Study Versus Electrocardiographic Monitoring (ESVEM) trial, sotalol was more effective in preventing recurrence of ventricular arrhythmias than several class I antiarrhythmic agents. β-Blockers also appeared to have a synergistic effect with amiodarone in reducing ventricular arrhythmias and mortality in postinfarction patients with ventricular dysfunction (in the Canadian Amiodarone Myocardial Infarction Arrhythmia Trial [CAMIAT] and the

Table 5.—Antiarrhythmic and Anti-Ischemic Mechanisms of β-Adrenoceptor Blockade

Decreased automaticity (phase 4 depolarization) (sinus/ectopic pacemakers)
Decreased membrane excitability
Decreased membrane conduction
Decrease in electrophysiologic heterogeneity (dispersion of refractoriness, especially in ischemic tissue)
Raise ventricular fibrillation threshold
Preserve normal serum levels of K^+
Anti-ischemic (improved myocardial energetics)
    Decrease O_2 utilization ($\downarrow$ heart rate, contractility, afterload, wall stress)
    Decrease O_2 wastage (myocardial metabolism)
    Increase O_2 supply to myocardium ($\downarrow$ heart rate—$\uparrow$ diastolic perfusion)
Antiplatelet ($\downarrow$ aggregation)
Limit infarct size and recurrence of infarction
Inhibit catecholamine-induced lipolysis with decreased production of arrhythmogenic fatty acids
Prevention of catecholamine toxicity in failing heart (? cellular loss from necrosis and apoptosis)
Improvement in myocardial force-frequency relationship
Improvement in baroreflex function (?)

European Myocardial Infarct Amiodarone Trial [EMIAT]). Therefore, in the absence of specific contraindications, prophylactic treatment with β-blockers is beneficial, especially in high-risk patients with ischemia or structural heart disease.

In patients with familial long QT syndrome with arrhythmias triggered by physical or emotional stress, β-blockers alone or in combination with permanent pacing decrease the incidence of syncope and sudden death. For asymptomatic persons with a prolonged QT interval and for asymptomatic first-degree relatives of patients with familial long QT syndrome and a history of syncope or sudden death, prophylactic treatment with β-blockers has been suggested. In acquired long QT syndrome due to electrolyte abnormalities or drugs, β-blockers are not effective in preventing torsades de pointes.

Ischemic Heart Disease

Chronic Stable Angina

In patients with chronic stable angina, β-blockers decrease the frequency of anginal episodes and improve exercise tolerance. These effects are related to the decrease in cardiac work and oxygen demand, with decreased heart rate, blood pressure (ventricular wall tension), and myocardial contractility. Also, the longer diastolic time resulting from the slow heart rate leads to better myocardial perfusion, with increased time for diastolic coronary blood flow.

In stable angina, β-blockers are superior to long-acting nitrates and calcium channel blockers in reducing anginal symptoms and ischemia. β-Blockers in combination with antiplatelet agents and nitrates constitute the standard therapy for effort and mixed angina. β-Blockers are more effective than calcium channel blockers and nitrates in reducing episodes of silent ischemia. Although effective in reducing anginal aggravation and silent ischemia, β-blockers in the absence of a previous myocardial infarction are not associated with a reduction in new myocardial infarctions or death in patients with chronic stable angina.

In vasospastic angina, β-blockers are not indicated, because they may increase coronary spasm from unopposed α-receptor activity.

- In vasospastic angina, β-blockers are not indicated, because they may increase coronary spasm from unopposed α-receptor activity.

Myocardial Infarction

Early Use of β-Blockers

The early administration of β-blockers during the acute phase of myocardial infarction decreases the risk of sudden cardiac death, reinfarction, and recurrent ischemia. In patients with suspected myocardial infarction, the immediate intravenous administration of a β-blocker, followed by the oral administration of a β-blocker, significantly reduced short-term mortality compared with those given placebo.

The mortality difference between those who received a β-blocker and those who did not was evident early (within 48 hours) and sustained. The mechanism for this is unclear but may be related to the prevention of cardiac rupture and ventricular arrhythmias. In the Thrombolysis in Myocardial Infarction (TIMI)-II trial, patients who received metoprolol intravenously at the time of thrombolytic therapy, followed by oral therapy, had fewer subsequent nonfatal reinfarctions and less recurrent ischemia than patients who received metoprolol on the sixth day. Mortality or ventricular function, however, was not significantly different between the two groups.

The current American College of Cardiology-American Heart Association (ACA/AHA) recommendations for early therapy with β-blockers are summarized in Table 6.

- The early administration of β-blockers during the acute phase of myocardial infarction decreases the risk of sudden cardiac death, reinfarction, and recurrent ischemia.

Long-Term Use of β-Blockers After Myocardial Infarction

The chronic use of β-blockers in high-risk patients surviving myocardial infarction (i.e., those with recurrent ischemia, a large or anterior infarct, ventricular dysfunction, or cardiac arrhythmias) may decrease all-cause mortality, sudden death, and reinfarction (by about 25%) (Fig. 1). Propranolol (80 mg three times daily), timolol (10 mg twice daily), and metoprolol (100 mg twice daily) have been shown to be effective in reducing sudden and nonsudden cardiac death, an effect that is more striking in the setting of reduced left ventricular function. The beneficial effects of β-blockers in postinfarction patients with asymptomatic left ventricular dysfunction appear to be additive to those of angiotensin-converting enzyme inhibitors in reducing the risk of cardiovascular mortality (by 30%) and development of heart failure (by 21%). The benefits of β-blockers are greatest in the first year after myocardial infarction compared with the second and third years with angiotensin-converting enzyme inhibitors. The beneficial survival effect is maintained in postinfarction patients with coexisting diabetes mellitus and heart failure. The nonselective β-blockers without intrinsic sympathomimetic activity appear to have a greater effect on mortality reduction than selective β-blockers. The mechanism of protection by β-blockade in these patients is not clear and may be related to several of the electrophysiologic and anti-ischemic effects summarized in Table 4.

Low-risk patients (those without previous infarction, anterior infarction, advanced age, ventricular arrhythmias, or ventricular dysfunction) have a good long-term progno-

Table 6.—Recommendations for Therapy With β-Blockers in Myocardial Infarction (MI)

Recommendations for early therapy with β-blockers in acute MI

Class I

Patients without a contraindication to β-blocker therapy who can be treated within 12 hr after onset of MI, regardless of administration of concomitant thrombolytic therapy

Patients with continuing or recurrent ischemic pain

Patients with tachyarrhythmias, such as atrial fibrillation with a rapid ventricular response

Class IIb

Non-Q-wave MI

Class III

Patients with moderate or severe ventricular failure or other contraindications to β-blocker therapy

Recommendations for long-term β-blocker therapy in survivors of MI

Class I

All but low-risk patients without clear contraindication to β-blocker therapy; treatment should begin within a few days after event (if not initiated acutely) and continue indefinitely

Class IIa

Low-risk patients without clear contraindication to β-blocker therapy

Class III

Patients with contraindication to β-blocker therapy

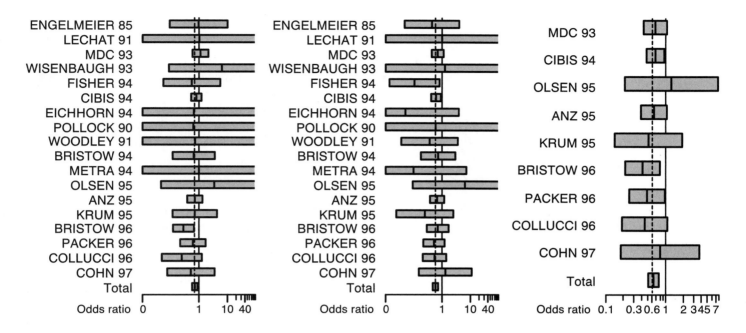

Fig. 1. Effect of β-blockade on, *A*, risk of death, *B*, hospitalization, and, *C*, combined risk of mortality and hospitalizations in chronic heart failure. Effect of β-blockade in each trial (by first author and year of publication) is represented by horizontal bar whose central vertical tick represents point estimate of odds ratio and whose width displays 95% confidence interval of estimate (logarithmic scale). Solid vertical line represents odds ratio of 1 (neutral treatment effect); dotted vertical line represents odds ratio for treatment effect across all trials. Odds ratio <1 indicates lower risk of death with β-blockade, whereas odds ratio >1 indicates higher risk of death with active treatment. Overall, β-blockers reduced risk of death by 31% (*P* = 0.0029) (*A*), hospitalization for heart failure by 41% (*P* < 0.001) (*B*), and death or hospitalization for heart failure by 37% (*P* < 0.001). (From *Circulation* 98:1184-1191, 1998. By permission of the American Heart Association.)

sis, and it is not clear whether adding β-blockers to their therapy improves outcome. Because β-blockers are well tolerated and have several potential beneficial effects, their use in a low-risk patient population is also recommended (Table 6). Despite the proven value of β-blocker use in secondary prevention in postinfarction patients, these agents are still underused and should be considered for all patients after infarction, unless clearly contraindicated (Table 7).

- Long-term use of β-blockers in high-risk patients surviving myocardial infarction (i.e., those with recurrent ischemia, large or anterior infarct, ventricular dysfunction, or cardiac arrhythmias) may decrease all-cause mortality, sudden death, and reinfarction rate.
- Unless contraindicated, β-blockers should be considered for all patients after myocardial infarction.

Congestive Heart Failure

Chronic activation of the adrenergic nervous system is an important component of the pathophysiology of heart failure and is associated with poor long-term outcome. The adverse cardiovascular effects are mediated by various mechanisms triggered by the interaction of epinephrine and norepinephrine with β- and α-adrenergic receptors and can be attenuated with antiadrenergic agents. Despite short-term adverse effects on cardiac contractility, antiadrenergic therapy involving several β-blockers (metoprolol, carvedilol, nebivolol, and bucindolol) has been shown in several clinical trials of patients with heart failure to have long-term beneficial effects (Fig. 2). These beneficial effects include improved hemodynamics, ventricular ejection fraction, symptoms, and quality of life and reduction in the risk of worsening heart failure, with a decrease in death, hospitalization, and the need for heart transplantation (Fig. 3). These effects are thought to occur through the prevention of catecholamine toxicity and improved myocardial energetics. They are more likely to have an effect on patients with severe heart failure who have greater sympathetic activation and a higher resting heart rate than on patients with slower heart rates.

Recent trials with nonselective vasodilating β-blockers have reported a reduction in the risk of mortality. Carvedilol reduced the risk of all-cause mortality in patients with heart

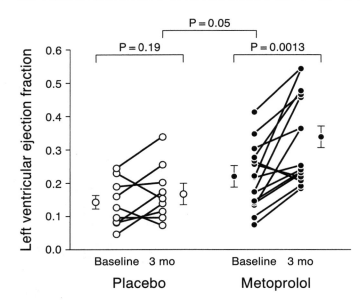

Fig. 2. Changes in left ventricular ejection fraction between baseline and 3 months for placebo and metoprolol groups in patients with dilated cardiomyopathy. A significant increase in ejection fraction was seen only in the metoprolol group. (From *J Am Coll Cardiol* 24:1310-1320, 1994. By permission of the American College of Cardiology.)

Table 7.—Contraindications to β-Blocker Therapy

Absolute
    Severe conduction system disease (sinus node dysfunction
      or high-grade AV block)
    Overt ventricular failure
    Severe asthma or active bronchospasm
    Severe peripheral vascular disease with rest ischemia
    Severe depression
Relative
    PR interval > 0.24 s
    Systolic arterial pressure < 100 mm Hg
    Signs of peripheral hypoperfusion
    Raynaud phenomenon
    Vasospastic angina
    Insulin-dependent diabetes mellitus with frequent
      hypoglycemic reactions
    Mild asthma or severe COPD
    Excessive fatigue
    Hyperlipidemia
    Impotence
    Pregnancy

AV, atrioventricular; COPD, chronic obstructive pulmonary disease.

failure by 65% ($P = 0.001$) (Fig. 4). The mortality reduction with carvedilol was clearer in patients with a baseline heart rate greater than 82 beats/min and was seen in patients in New York Heart Association (NYHA) functional class II as well as in class III or IV and was seen in patients with either ischemic or nonischemic cardiomyopathy. Three major clinical trials of β-blocker use in patients with heart failure are summarized in Table 8. Currently, several β-blocker survival trials are in progress to fully assess the effect of these agents on overall mortality and arrhythmia death.

In a recent meta-analysis of all 18 published double-blinded, placebo-controlled, parallel-group trials of β-blockers in heart failure involving more than 3,000 patients (the majority in NYHA class II or III and < 5% with class IV symptoms), Lechat et al. found that the addition of a β-blocker to conventional therapy was associated with a significant effect on morbidity and mortality: a 32% reduction in the risk of death, a 41% reduction in the risk of being hospitalized for heart failure, and a 37% reduction in the combined risk of morbidity and mortality (Fig. 1). In addition, treatment with a β-blocker produced significant hemodynamic and symptomatic benefits, as indicated by a 29% increase in left ventricular ejection fraction, a 32% increase in the likelihood of functional improvement, and a 30%

decrease in the likelihood of functional deterioration. The reduction of mortality risk was greater for nonselective β-blockers than for β_1-selective agents. The authors estimated that with a mean duration of follow-up of 7 months, 38 patients would need to be treated to avoid one death, 24 patients to avoid one hospitalization for heart failure, and 15 patients to avoid one combined end point.

In the current ACC/AHA guidelines for the treatment of heart failure, β-blocker use is recommended as a class I indication in high-risk patients after an acute myocardial infarction and as a class II indication in patients with dilated cardiomyopathy. β-Blockers should not be used in patients with decompensated heart failure or those dependent on intravenous inotropic agents. Although in controlled clinical trials several β-blockers have been shown to be effective, currently only carvedilol is approved by the U.S. Food and Drug Administration for management of chronic heart failure.

When β-blockers are used, treatment should be started at a low dose and titrated up slowly to the maximal tolerated level (Table 9). The patient should be monitored closely because worsening heart failure, hypotension, or bradycardia could be precipitated during initiation of β-blockade. It

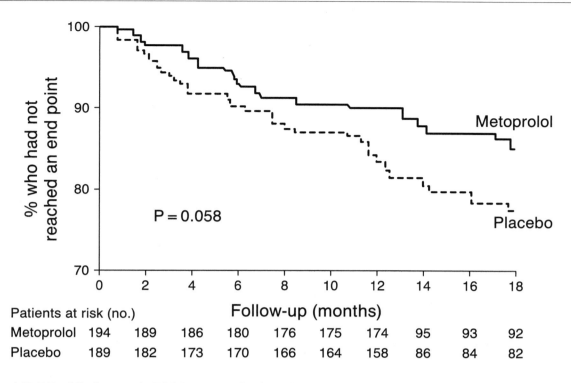

Fig. 3. Metoprolol in Dilated Cardiomyopathy Trial. Percentage of patients who had not reached end point of death or need for cardiac transplantation (211 patients were followed for 12 months and 172 for 18 months). (From *Lancet* 342:1441-1446, 1993. By permission of The Lancet.)

Table 8.—Three β-Blocker Therapy Trials in Heart Failure

Variable	MDC		CIBIS-1		US carvedilol trials	
	Placebo (*n* = 189)	Metoprolol (*n* = 194)	Placebo (*n* = 321)	Bisoprolol (*n* = 320)	Placebo (*n* = 398)	Carvedilol (*n* = 696)
Mean age, yr	49	49	59	60	58	58
Male, %	75	70	83	83	76	77
LVEF, %	22	22	26	25	22	23
NYHA class, %						
II	47	42	0	0	52	54
III	47	51	95	95	44	44
IV	4	4	5	5	3	3
IHD, %	0	0	53	56	47	47
ACE inhibitor treatment, %	82	78	91	89	95	95
Follow-up, mo	16 (median)		23 (mean)		6.5 (median)	
Hospitalization (no. admissions)	83	51 (*P* < 0.04)	90	61 (*P* < 0.01)	19.6%[†]	14.1%[†] (*P* < 0.036)
Mortality, %	11	12	21	17	7.8	3.2*

ACE, angiotensin-converting enzyme; CIBIS I, First Cardiac Insufficiency Bisoprolol Study; IHD, ischemic heart disease; LVEF, left ventricular ejection fraction; MDC, Metoprolol in Dilated Cardiomyopathy Trial; NYHA, New York Heart Association.

*Absolute mortality risk reduction, 4.6%; relative mortality risk reduction, 65% (*P* < 0.001).

[†]Percentage of patients.

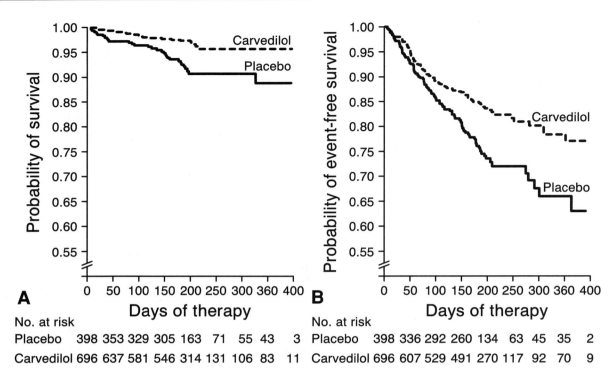

Fig. 4. Kaplan-Meier analysis of, *A*, survival and, *B*, event-free survival (survival without hospitalization for cardiovascular reasons) among patients with chronic heart failure in the placebo and carvedilol groups. Patients in the carvedilol group had a 65% lower risk of death ($P < 0.001$) and a 38% lower risk of death or hospitalization for cardiovascular disease than patients in the placebo group ($P < 0.001$). (From *N Engl J Med* 334:1349-1355, 1996. By permission of the Massachusetts Medical Society.)

may be more than 2 or 3 months before any improvement is noted in symptoms. In case cardiac decompensation occurs in association with only mild to moderate symptoms, the dose up-titration is delayed for 2 to 4 weeks and the dose and schedule of diuretics and angiotensin-converting enzyme inhibitors are adjusted. If severe symptoms result, β-blockers should either be decreased by 50% (for pulmonary edema) or held (for cardiogenic shock) and intravenous inotropes (preferentially milrinone) or vasodilators (nitroprusside or nitroglycerin) used. If β-blocker therapy is discontinued temporarily, it could be started at the previous dose if held for less than 3 days or at one-half the previous dose if held between 3 and 7 days and then resumed and up-titrated as before. If discontinued for more than 7 days, treatment should be resumed at the initial dose and up-titrated as before. An effort should be made to achieve the target dose (Table 9); however, if the target dose is not tolerated, a low dose of β-blocker should be maintained even if the symptoms do not improve, because long-term treatment may reduce the risk of major clinical events. Abrupt withdrawal should be avoided (unless clearly indicated), because it could precipitate clinical deterioration.

In patients with diastolic ventricular dysfunction, β-blockers may be beneficial in reducing symptoms of heart failure by slowing heart rate and improving ventricular filling and stroke volume, as in hypertrophic obstructive cardiomyopathy and hypertensive heart disease. β-Blocker use is recommended as a class II indication for the treatment of heart failure due to diastolic dysfunction.

Hypertension

When β-blockers are given chronically, they lower blood pressure by effects on the heart, blood vessels, the renin-angiotensin system, central nervous system, and perhaps the autonomic nerve terminals. In the vascular system, β-receptor blockade opposes $β_2$-mediated vasodilation and, thus, may result in an initial increase in peripheral resistance from unopposed α-receptor-mediated vasoconstriction; however, with chronic use, peripheral resistance decreases.

As a class, β-blockers have proven efficacy in hypertension and are well tolerated when used alone or in combination with diuretics or vasodilator agents. Together with diuretics, β-blockers are recommended as first-line therapy for hypertension. Control of blood pressure with β-blockers in hypertensive patients results in a reduction in ventricular hypertrophy, stroke, coronary events, and

Table 9.—β-Blocker Dosage Scheme Used in Placebo-Controlled Heart Failure Trials

Titration schedule	Bisoprolol, mg	Carvedilol, mg	Metoprolol, mg
First dose	1.25	3.125	5
Dosing schedule	1.25 qd x 1 wk	3.125 bid x 2 wk	5 bid x 1 wk
	2.5 qd x 1 wk	6.25 bid x 2 wk	7.5 bid x 1 wk
	3.75 qd x 1 wk	12.5 bid x 2 wk	15 bid x 1 wk
	5.0 qd x 4 wk	25.0 bid	25 bid x 1 wk
	7.5 qd x 4 wk	If weight > 75 kg, up to 50.0 bid	37.5 bid x 1 wk
	10.0 qd		50 bid x 1 wk
			75 bid x 1 wk
Target daily dose, mg	10	50	100-150

bid, twice daily; qd, once daily.

mortality. β-Blockers may be less effective in elderly African-Americans than elderly white persons or young African-Americans. Intravenous administration of labetalol, which has both α- and β-adrenergic blocking properties and a rapid onset of action, is recommended for the treatment of hypertensive emergencies and severe hypertension and is well tolerated during pregnancy.

Aortic Dissection and Aneurysm

By reducing the velocity of left ventricular ejection fraction and the propulsive stress on the aortic wall, β-blockers are useful in the acute and long-term management of aortic dissection. In patients with aortic dilatation, such as Marfan syndrome, β-blockers may prevent rapid progression of aortic enlargement.

Neurocardiogenic Syncope

In vasovagal syncope, β-blockers are believed to abort the full syncopal response by suppressing the neurocardiogenic reflex.

Side Effects of β-Blockers

Most of the cardiac side effects of β-blockers are related to their negative chronotropic, dromotropic, and inotropic properties. They may cause sinus slowing, pauses, and heart block in patients with sinus node dysfunction or AV conduction disease. The use of β-blockers with intrinsic sympathomimetic activity in these patients may be better because these agents may reduce profound slowing of heart rate at rest, while preventing excessive heart rate in response to exercise or other stress. Unlike class I and class III antiarrhythmic agents, β-blockers have a remarkable safety record in regard to ventricular proarrhythmia.

In patients with ischemic heart disease, abrupt discontinuation of β-blockers after chronic use should be avoided because of possible rebound hypersensitivity to physiologic adrenergic stimulation (due to "up-regulation" of the number of β-adrenergic receptors) and myocardial ischemia or infarction (withdrawal syndrome).

In patients with severe ventricular systolic dysfunction, congestive heart failure may be precipitated, especially in those in whom cardiac output is dependent on sympathetic drive. In carefully selected patients with moderate-to-severe heart failure, however, the safety of β-blockade with proper dose titration and monitoring has been demonstrated in several recent trials.

Other adverse effects, especially with nonselective β-blockers, include bronchospasm in patients with a history of asthma, fatigue, and central nervous system effects, such as sedation, sleep disturbances, hallucinations, depression, and, rarely, psychotic reactions. The lipid-soluble β-blockers are more prone to affect the central nervous system; however, adverse nervous system effects may occur with any β-blocker used for a long time. Impotence and worsening of symptoms due to severe peripheral vascular or vasospastic disorders may occur. Topical β-blockers (such as timolol) used to treat glaucoma may be absorbed from the eye and have serious adverse effects on the heart (bradycardia and hypotension) and airways in susceptible persons and should be used with caution. Also, the hypoglycemia symptoms may be masked in insulin-requiring diabetic patients. Choosing $β_1$-selective drugs with poor lipid solubility, additional intrinsic sympathomimetic activity, or α-adrenergic blockade may help reduce some of these adverse effects.

The absolute and relative contraindications to β-blocker use are summarized in Table 7.

The safety of β-blocker use during pregnancy has not been established, and the potential benefit should be weighed against the risk to the fetus (low birth weight). β-Blockers may be excreted in breast milk and should be used with caution and only if considered essential.

- In patients with ischemic heart disease, abrupt disconsinuation of β-blockers after chronic use could result in withdrawal syndrome, with rebound hypersensitivity to physiologic adrenergic stimulation, and could lead to myocardial ischemia or infarction.

Overdose

In overdose, β-blockers may cause central nervous system depression and potentiate hypotension, hypoglycemia, and bronchospasm. In a life-threatening situation with β-blocker overdose or toxicity, the adverse cardiac effects of β-blockers may be counteracted with glucagon (100 µg/kg over 1 minute, then 1 to 5 mg/hr), isoproterenol (up to 0.10 µg/kg per minute), or high-dose dobutamine (15 µg/kg per minute) infusion. The intravenous administration of atropine should be tried for symptomatic bradycardia, and a temporary pacemaker may be needed in refractory cases.

Drug Interactions

β-Blockers should be used with caution in conjunction with drugs that slow conduction (digitalis and calcium channel blockers) and those that have negative inotropic effects (calcium channel blockers and disopyramide). The blood levels of β-blockers metabolized in the liver (propranolol, metoprolol, carvedilol, labetalol) are increased by cimetidine, which reduces hepatic blood flow. By decreasing hepatic flow, β-blockers may affect blood levels of drugs such as lidocaine that are metabolized primarily in the liver.

Dosing

All β-blockers have about the same antianginal and antiarrhythmic efficacy at comparable doses, and no one agent is superior to any other at equipotent doses. The usual daily dosages of various β-blockers are summarized in Table 10. The dose should be adjusted to keep the resting heart rate at 55 to 60 beats/min and exertional heart rate less than 100 beats/min in patients with angina or atrial fibrillation. Ancillary properties, such as β_1-adrenergic receptor selectivity, lipid solubility, vasodilatation, intrinsic sympathomimetic activity, longer half-life, and cost, may affect the selection of one agent over others.

Table 10.—Usual Daily Dosage of β-Adrenergic Agents*

	Usual daily dosage, mg	Dose reduction with renal impairment
Acebutolol	200-600 q 12 hr	Yes
Atenolol	50-100 (up to 200) daily	
Bisoprolol	2.5-40 daily (for hypertension)	
Carvedilol	12.5-25 q 12 hr	
Esmolol	IV LD 500 µg/kg over 1 min, then 50-300 µg/kg per min	Yes
Labetalol	100 mg q 12 hr (up to 400 mg twice daily)	
	IV 20 mg over 2 min, add 40 and 80 mg at 10-min intervals	
	Infusion 2 mg/min	
Metoprolol	50-200 q 12 hr, IV 5 mg x 3 at 2-min intervals	
Nadolol	40-80 (up to 240 mg) daily	Yes
Pindolol	2.5-15 q 12 hr	Yes
Propranolol	80-160 q 12 hr (extended release), IV 1 mg/min (up to 6 mg)	
Timolol	10-30 q 12 hr	
Sotalol	80-240 mg q 12 hr (for arrhythmias)	Yes

All doses are for oral preparation unless indicated.

IV, intravenously; LD, loading dose.

Suggested Review Reading

1. Andersson B, Lomsky M, Waagstein F: The link between acute haemodynamic adrenergic beta-blockade and long-term effects in patients with heart failure. A study on diastolic function, heart rate and myocardial metabolism following intravenous metoprolol. *Eur Heart J* 14:1375-1385, 1992.

2. Anonymous: Guidelines for the evaluation and management of heart failure. Report of the American College of Cardiology/American Heart Association Task Force on Practice Guidelines (Committee on Evaluation and Management of Heart Failure). *Circulation* 92:2764-2784, 1995.

3. Australia-New Zealand Heart Failure Research Collaborative Group: Effects of carvedilol, a vasodilator-beta-blocker, in patients with congestive heart failure due to ischemic heart disease. *Circulation* 92:212-218, 1995.

4. The BEST Steering Committee: Design of the Beta-Blocker Evaluation Survival Trial (BEST). *Am J Cardiol* 75:1220-1223, 1995.

5. β-Blocker Heart Attack Study Group: The β-blocker heart attack trial. JAMA 246:2073-2074, 1981.

6. Bristow MR, O'Connell JB, Gilbert EM, et al: Dose-response of chronic beta-blocker treatment in heart failure from either idiopathic dilated or ischemic cardiomyopathy. *Circulation* 89:1632-1642, 1994.

7. Brodsky MA, Chough SP, Allen BJ, et al: Adjuvant metoprolol improves efficacy of class I antiarrhythmic drugs in patients with inducible sustained monomorphic ventricular tachycardia. *Am Heart J* 124:629-635, 1992.

8. Chadda K, Goldstein S, Byington R, et al: Effect of propranolol after acute myocardial infarction in patients with congestive heart failure. *Circulation* 73:503-510, 1986.

9. CIBIS Investigators and Committees: A randomized trial of beta-blockade in heart failure. The Cardiac Insufficiency Bisoprolol Study (CIBIS). *Circulation* 90:1765-1773, 1994.

10. Dahlof B, Lindholm LH, Hansson L, et al: Morbidity and mortality in the Swedish Trial in Old Patients with Hypertension (STOP-Hypertension). *Lancet* 338:1281-1285, 1991.

11. Eichhorn EJ, Heesch CM, Barnett JH, et al: Effect of metoprolol on myocardial function and energetics in patients with nonischemic dilated cardiomyopathy: a randomized, double-blind, placebo-controlled study. *J Am Coll Cardiol* 24:1310-1320, 1994.

12. First International Study of Infarct Survival Collaborative Group: Randomised trial of intravenous atenolol among 16,027 cases of suspected acute myocardial infarction: ISIS-1. *Lancet* 2:57-66, 1986.

13. Gilbert EM, Anderson JL, Deitchman D, et al: Long-term beta-blocker vasodilator therapy improves cardiac function in idiopathic dilated cardiomyopathy: a double-blind, randomized study of bucindolol versus placebo. *Am J Med* 88:223-229, 1990.

14. Heidenreich PA, Lee TT, Massie BM: Effect of beta-blockade on mortality in patients with heart failure: a meta-analysis of randomized clinical trials. *J Am Coll Cardiol* 30:27-34, 1997.

15. Krum H, Sackner-Bernstein JD, Goldsmith RL, et al: Double-blind, placebo-controlled study of the long-term efficacy of carvedilol in patients with severe chronic heart failure. *Circulation* 92:1499-1506, 1995.

16. Lechat P, Packer M, Chalon S, et al: Clinical effects of beta-adrenergic blockade in chronic heart failure: a meta-analysis of double-blind, placebo-controlled, randomized trials. *Circulation* 98:1184-1191, 1998.
A recent meta-analysis of all 18 published double-blinded, placebo-controlled, parallel-group trials of β-blockers in heart failure involving more than 3,000 patients.

17. Mason JW: A comparison of seven antiarrhythmic drugs in patients with ventricular tachyarrhythmias. *N Engl J Med* 329:452-458, 1993.

18. Materson BJ, Reda DJ, Cushman WC, et al: Single-drug therapy for hypertension in men. A comparison of six antihypertensive agents with placebo. *N Engl J Med* 328:914-921, 1993.

19. McTavish D, Campoli-Richards D, Sorkin EM: Carvedilol. A review of its pharmacodynamic and pharmacokinetic properties, and therapeutic efficacy. *Drugs* 45:232-258, 1993.

20. The MIAMI Trial Research Group: Metoprolol in acute myocardial infarction. Patient population. *Am J Cardiol* 56:10G-14G, 1985.

21. Murray KT, Reilly C, Koshakji RP, et al: Suppression of ventricular arrhythmias in man by d-propranolol independent of beta-adrenergic receptor blockade. *J Clin Invest* 85:836-842, 1990.

22. Olsen SL, Gilbert EM, Renlund DG, et al: Carvedilol improved left ventricular function and symptoms in chronic heart failure: a double-blind randomized study. *J Am Coll Cardiol* 25:1225-1231, 1995.

23. Olshansky B, Martins JB: Usefulness of isoproterenol facilitation of ventricular tachycardia induction during extrastimulus testing in predicting effective chronic therapy with beta-adrenergic blockade. *Am J Cardiol* 59:573-577, 1987.

24. Opie LH, Sonnenblick EH, Frishman W, et al: Beta-blocking agents. In *Drugs for the Heart*. Fourth edition revised. Edited by LH Opie. Philadelphia, WB Saunders Company, 1997, pp 1-30.

25. Packer M, Bristow MR, Cohn JN, et al: The effect of carvedilol on morbidity and mortality in patients with chronic heart failure. *N Engl J Med* 334:1349-1355, 1996.

26. Pepine CJ, Cohn PF, Deedwania PC, et al: Effects of treatment on outcome in mildly symptomatic patients with ischemia during daily life. The Atenolol Silent Ischemia Study. *Circulation* 90:762-768, 1994.

27. Roberts R, Rogers WJ, Mueller HS, et al: Immediate versus deferred beta-blockade following thrombolytic therapy in patients with acute myocardial infarction. Results of the Thrombolysis in Myocardial Infarction (TIMI) II-B Study. *Circulation* 83:422-437, 1991.

28. Schwartz PJ, Bonazzi O, Locati E, et al: Pathogenesis and therapy of the idiopathic long QT syndrome. *Ann N Y Acad Sci* 644:112-141, 1992.

29. SHEP Cooperative Research Group: Prevention of stroke by antihypertensive drug treatment in older persons with isolated systolic hypertension. Final results of the Systolic Hypertension in the Elderly Program (SHEP). *JAMA* 265:3255-3264, 1991.

30. Steinbeck G, Andresen D, Bach P, et al: A comparison of electrophysiologically guided antiarrhythmic drug therapy with beta-blocker therapy in patients with symptomatic, sustained ventricular tachyarrhythmias. *N Engl J Med* 327:987-992, 1992.

31. Szabo BM, Crijns HJ, Wiesfeld AC, et al: Predictors of mortality in patients with sustained ventricular tachycardias or ventricular fibrillation and depressed left ventricular function: importance of beta-blockade. *Am Heart J* 130:281-286, 1995.

32. Teo KK, Yusuf S, Furberg CD: Effects of prophylactic antiarrhythmic drug therapy in acute myocardial infarction. An overview of results from randomized controlled trials. *JAMA* 270:1589-1595, 1993.

33. Vantrimpont P, Rouleau JL, Wun CC, et al: Additive beneficial effects of beta-blockers to angiotensin-converting enzyme inhibitors in the Survival and Ventricular Enlargement (SAVE) Study. *J Am Coll Cardiol* 29:229-236, 1997.

34. Viscoli CM, Horwitz RI, Singer BH: Beta-blockers after myocardial infarction: influence of first-year clinical course on long-term effectiveness. *Ann Intern Med* 118:99-105, 1993.

35. Viskin S, Kitzis I, Lev E, et al: Treatment with beta-adrenergic blocking agents after myocardial infarction: from randomized trials to clinical practice. *J Am Coll Cardiol* 25:1327-1332, 1995.

36. Waagstein F, Bristow MR, Swedberg K, et al: Beneficial effects of metoprolol in idiopathic dilated cardiomyopathy. *Lancet* 342:1441-1446, 1993.

Questions

Multiple Choice (choose the one best answer)

1. All except one of the following β-blockers are highly lipid soluble and likely to cross the blood-brain barrier and enter the central nervous system. Which one is least lipid soluble?
   a. Nadolol
   b. Propranolol
   c. Metoprolol
   d. Labetalol
   e. Carvedilol

2. All the following β-blockers have relative selectivity for the β₁-adrenergic receptor *except*:
   a. Acebutolol
   b. Esmolol
   c. Metoprolol
   d. Labetalol
   e. Atenolol

3. After oral administration, propranolol bioavailability is low because it is:
   a. Protein bound
   b. Extensively metabolized in liver
   c. Deposited in adipose tissue
   d. Excreted in urine

4. A 35-year-old woman with hypertrophic cardiomyopathy has chest pain and palpitations with irregular rhythm, heart rate ~155 beats/min, blood pressure 130/80 mm Hg. What is the best initial therapy?
   a. β-Blockers
   b. Intravenous nitroglycerin
   c. Amlodipine
   d. Furosemide
   e. Intravenous digoxin

5-10. For each of the following, select the most appropriate response.

5. At low concentration, activates both β₁- and β₂-adrenergic receptors

6. With overdosage, may cause central nervous system toxicity

7. Could be used in patients with mild asthma

8. Should be used with caution in patients with renal failure

9. Has been shown in clinical trials to reduce mortality
   a. Propranolol
   b. Atenolol
   c. Both
   d. Neither

10. In patients with subacute aortic dissection with hypertension, the following drugs can be used intravenously.
    a. Diazoxide
    b. Labetalol
    c. Hydralazine
    d. Nifedipine
    e. All the above

11. The blood level of which of the following β-blockers is increased by cimetidine?
    a. Nadolol
    b. Atenolol
    c. Metoprolol
    d. Sotalol

12. Of the listed drugs, the first-line drug for β-blocker overdose is:
    a. Glucagon
    b. Phentolamine
    c. Amrinone
    d. Carvedilol
    e. Digoxin

Answers

1. Answer a

β-Blockers exhibit different degrees of lipid solubility. More lipid-soluble β-blockers, such as propranolol and metoprolol, are metabolized largely by the liver and tend to have relatively short plasma half-lives. Because of lipid solubility, these β-blockers are prone to affect the central nervous system and produce adverse effects such as lethargy, sleep disturbance, hallucinations, and depression. However, adverse central nervous system effects may occur with any β-blocker used for a long time. More water-soluble β-blockers, such as atenolol and nadolol, are cleared by the kidney and tend to have relatively longer plasma half-lives.

2. Answer d

At lower concentrations, β-blockers exhibit various degrees of cardiac selectivity (i.e., affinity for β_1- versus β_2-receptor). However, the β_1 and β_2 selectivity is relative and can be overcome if large doses are used. The β_1 (cardioselective)-selective blockers are atenolol, esmolol, acebutolol, and metoprolol. Carvedilol, labetalol, nadolol, pindolol, propranolol, timolol, and sotalol do not have relative β_1 selectivity.

3. Answer b

4. Answer a

β-Blockers decrease both heart rate and the force of ventricular contraction (thus allowing better filling of the ventricles during diastole), improve stroke volume, and decrease myocardial oxygen demand. Digoxin may enhance ventricular contraction and worsen left ventricular outflow gradient, whereas nitroglycerin and furosemide decrease preload, further aggravating ventricular volume. Amlodipine decreases peripheral resistance and may aggravate left ventricular outflow gradient.

5. Answer a

6. Answer c

7. Answer b

8. Answer b

9. Answer c

10. Answer b

In acute and subacute aortic dissection, it is important to reduce the shearing forces on the aorta by reducing cardiac contractility and aortic pressure. A combination of intravenous sodium nitroprusside and a β-blocker such as propranolol is usually effective. Intravenous labetalol, with both α- and β-adrenergic blocking properties, is an effective alternative to the combination of nitroprusside and a β-blocker. In the absence of adequate β-blockade, vasodilators such as nifedipine, hydralazine, and diazoxide are contraindicated, because they can produce reflex sympathetic stimulation, increasing cardiac contractility, and thus may increase the dissection.

11. Answer c

Cimetidine decreases liver blood flow and thus increases blood levels of β-blockers that are metabolized by the liver, such as propranolol, metoprolol, and carvedilol. Renally excreted β-blockers such as nadolol, sotalol, and atenolol are not affected by cimetidine but should be used with caution in patients with renal failure because drug accumulation may occur.

12. Answer a

Because β-adrenergic receptor blockers are competitive inhibitors, infusing a high dose of a β-agonist such as isoproterenol, dobutamine, or epinephrine can counteract their overdose. Glucagon, which activates the cyclic adenosine monophosphate (cAMP) mechanism independently of the β-receptor, is effective in cases unresponsive to a high dose of dopamine or epinephrine. The use of phosphodiesterase inhibitors such as amrinone, which prevents breakdown of cAMP, has also been advocated.

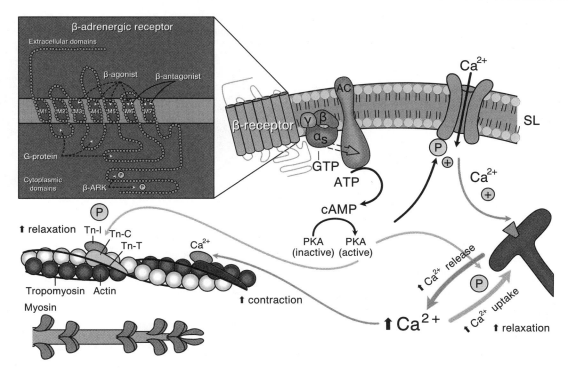

Plate 1. β-Adrenergic signal systems. β-Adrenergic receptor antagonist blocking the catecholamine-mediated increase in rate of contraction and peak force of contraction. Catecholamine activates β-adrenergic receptor, which through stimulatory G protein ($G_{\alpha s}$), activates adenylate cyclase (AC), resulting in increased production of cyclic adenosine monophosphate (cAMP) from adenosine triphosphate (ATP). This in turn activates protein kinases (PKA), leading to phosphorylation of sarcolemmal calcium channel, increased calcium (Ca^{2+}) entry into the cell, calcium-induced calcium release, and increased rate of development of force and peak contraction. *Inset* shows the molecular structure of β-adrenergic receptor. The transmembrane domains (M1-M7) act as a ligand-binding pocket, with domains M6 and M7 more specific for β-antagonists. β-Agonist binding is more diffuse. β-ARK, β-adrenergic receptor kinase; GTP, guanosine triphosphate; SL, sarcolemma; Tn-C, troponin C; Tn-I, troponin I; Tn-T, troponin T. (Modified from Opie LH: *The Heart: Physiology, from Cell to Circulation*. Third edition. Lippincott-Raven Publishers, 1998, pp 173-231. By permission of the publisher.)

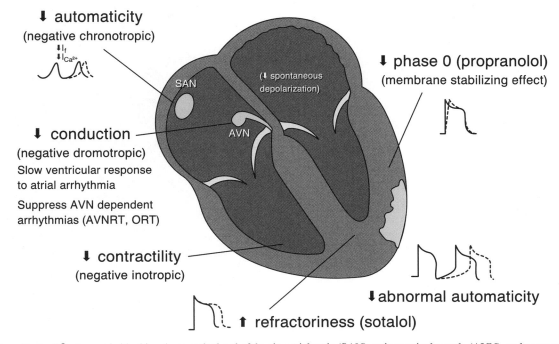

Plate 2. Cardiac effects of β-adrenergic blocking drugs at the level of the sinoatrial node (SAN), atrioventricular node (AVN), and myocardium. AVNRT, atrioventricular nodal reentry tachycardia; $I_{Ca}2+$, inward calcium current; I_f, pacemaker current; ORT, orthodromic reciprocating tachycardia.

Notes

Chapter 81

Platelet Glycoprotein IIb/IIIa Receptor Inhibitors

Yong-Mei Cha, M.D.
Joseph G. Murphy, M.D.
R. Scott Wright, M.D.

Platelets are important in the pathogenesis of atherosclerosis, arterial thrombosis, and acute coronary syndromes and in acute vessel occlusion following percutaneous coronary interventions.

Platelet Physiology

The platelet response to vascular wall injury encompasses the interrelated processes of platelet adhesion, activation, and aggregation, leading to thrombus formation. The loss of vascular endothelial integrity exposes the subendothelial matrix, allowing platelets to adhere passively to the exposed collagen. After adhesion, collagen, adenosine diphosphate (ADP), thromboxane A_2, thrombin, epinephrine, or serotonin activates the platelets. This activation leads to the release of granules by platelets and, thus, the further release of chemical mediators that, in turn, activate nearby platelets and recruit distant platelets to the site of injury. Collagen and thrombin appear to be the most important platelet agonists in this setting. Activated platelets undergo a structural change—from the typical discoid shape to one with pseudopods—that increases the cell surface area and converts the glycoprotein (GP) IIb/IIIa receptors to the activated form that permits fibrinogen binding. This leads to the final step in hemostasis, platelet aggregation (Fig. 1).

- Platelets respond to vascular injury by adhesion, activation, and aggregation, leading to thrombus formation.

Platelet GP IIb/IIIa Receptor

The platelet GP receptor is a transmembrane protein, an "integrin," that consists of two types of subunits (IIb and IIIa) held together by noncovalent bonds (Fig. 2). GP IIb/IIIa receptors are platelet-specific and encoded by separate genes on the long arm of chromosome 17. The two subunits of GP IIb/IIIa receptors are assembled in the megakaryocytes before final expression of platelet receptors. Each platelet has about 50,000 to 80,000 GP IIb/IIIa receptors. These receptors have a high affinity for the peptide sequence arginine-glycine-aspartic acid (RGD)—a sequence in fibrinogen—or the sequence lysine-glycine-aspartic acid (KGD). Fibrinogen crosslinks adjacent platelets to cause platelet aggregation and thrombus formation.

- GP IIb/IIIa receptors are platelet-specific and encoded by separate genes on the long arm of chromosome 17.
- GP IIb/IIIa receptors have a high affinity for the peptide sequence RGD, a sequence in fibrinogen.

GP IIb/IIIa Antagonists

The GP IIb/IIIa receptor is important because it is the final common pathway in platelet aggregation that leads to thrombus formation. The identification of this receptor has led to the development of specific GP IIb/IIIa receptor blockers important in clinical cardiology. Initially, murine antibodies

Platelet physiology

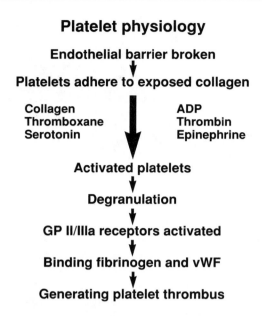

Endothelial barrier broken

↓

Platelets adhere to exposed collagen

Collagen	ADP
Thromboxane	Thrombin
Serotonin	Epinephrine

↓

Activated platelets

↓

Degranulation

↓

GP II/IIIa receptors activated

↓

Binding fibrinogen and vWF

↓

Generating platelet thrombus

Fig. 1. Physiology of platelet activation and aggregation. ADP, adenosine diphosphate; GP, glycoprotein; vWF, von Willebrand factor.

for complement activation and by replacing the constant domain of the Fab by the corresponding human immunoglobulin constant region sequences. Abciximab (ReoPro) is a combined chimeric human-murine c7E3 Fab fragment that blocks GP IIb/IIIa receptors and prevents fibrinogen from binding to platelets.

Naturally occurring GP IIb/IIIa antagonists also exist and include peptides derived from snake venom. Although these natural peptides are potent, they are not suitable for human use because of their high immunogenicity. However, they are excellent templates for the design of synthetic platelet antagonists. Synthetic GP IIb/IIIa antagonists include peptide and nonpeptide mimics, all with specificity for the GP IIb/IIIa receptor. These synthetic peptides typically contain RGD or KGD binding sequences. The nonpeptide synthetic antagonists mimic the spatial and charge conformations of the RGD binding sequence. Eptifibatide is a peptide inhibitor, and tirofiban, lamifiban, and roxifiban are nonpeptide GP IIb/IIIa antagonists (Tables 1 and 2).

against the human GP IIb/IIIa receptor were developed by injecting mice with human platelets and isolating the plasma cell line producing the antibody to the GP IIb/IIIa receptor. The original murine immunoglobulin was modified further by removing the Fc antibody region to avoid the potential

- The GP IIb/IIIa receptor is the final common pathway in platelet aggregation that leads to thrombus formation.
- Abciximab is a combined chimeric human-murine c7E3 Fab fragment that blocks the GP IIb/IIIa receptor and prevents fibrinogen from binding to platelets.

Interaction between fibrinogen and GP IIb/IIIa receptors

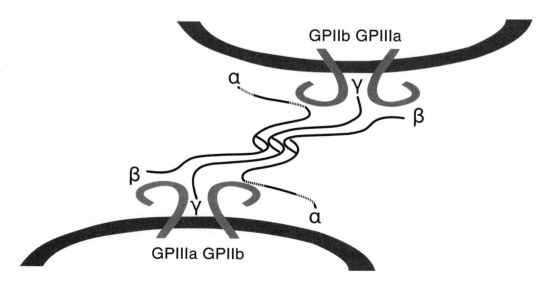

Fig. 2. Fibrinogen crosslinks adjacent platelets. GP, glycoprotein. α, β, γ, polypeptide chains.

Table 1.—Classification of Glycoprotein (GP) IIb/IIIa Inhibitors

Form	Inhibitor
Monoclonal antibody	Abciximab
Natural GP IIb/IIIa antagonist	Snake venom
Synthetic GP IIb/IIIa antagonist	
Peptides	Eptifibatide
Nonpeptides	Tirofiban
	Lamifiban

Table 2.—Differences Between Noncompetitive and Competitive Glycoprotein IIb/IIIa Inhibitors

	Noncompetitive (abciximab)	Competitive (eptifibatide)
Bind to receptor	Irreversible	Reversible
Specificity	Cross-reactivity	High specificity
Biologic half-life	Long (4-6 hr)	Short (30 min to 2 hr)
Duration of anti-platelet effect	2-3 days after medi-cine is stopped	Hours
Bleeding risk	High	Low
Immunogenicity	Significant	Absent

GP IIb/IIIa Clinical Trials

More than a dozen clinical trials of GP IIb/IIIa inhibitors, with more than 30,000 patients participating, have been completed. These inhibitor trials in acute coronary syndromes are listed in Table 3.

GP IIb/IIIa Inhibitors in Coronary Interventions

Platelets play an important role in abrupt vessel closure following coronary interventional procedures.

Abciximab was the first GP IIb/IIIa receptor inhibitor to be tested in a large-scale randomized trial in patients considered at increased risk for abrupt vessel closure after percutaneous transluminal coronary angioplasty (PTCA).

EPIC Trial
In the EPIC (Evaluation of c7E3 in Preventing Ischemic Complications) trial, just over 2,000 patients at high risk for vessel closure after PTCA or directional atherectomy were randomly assigned to one of three treatment groups: no GP IIb/IIIa receptor inhibitor, abciximab bolus (0.25 mg/kg) only, or abciximab bolus followed by a 12-hour infusion (10 µg/min). All patients received aspirin and 10,000 to 12,000 units of heparin.

The significant finding in this study was that, at 30 days, patients who received the abciximab bolus and infusion had a 35% reduction in the frequency of a composite adverse cardiovascular event end point (death, nonfatal myocardial infarction, repeat revascularization, and coronary artery bypass grafting) compared with those not receiving GP IIb/IIIa receptor inhibitor (12.8% vs. 8.3%, $P = 0.008$). The clinical benefit of abciximab was still present at 6 months: a 23% reduction in events (27% vs. 35%). At 3 years, a 13% composite event rate reduction was present (41% vs. 47%).

The conclusion of the EPIC study was that blockade of GP IIb/IIIa receptor with abciximab during high-risk PTCA or directional atherectomy significantly improved short- and long-term clinical outcomes but was associated with a doubling of major bleeding complications that required blood transfusion. To achieve clinical efficacy, an abciximab bolus plus a 12-hour infusion are required.

- The EPIC trial demonstrated that patients who received abciximab at the time of high-risk coronary intervention had a 35% reduction in cardiovascular events at 30 days, a benefit that was maintained to a lesser degree for at least 3 years.

EPILOG Trial
Another study was performed (EPILOG) to try to improve on the results of the EPIC study, in particular to reduce the bleeding complications. The EPILOG study (Evaluation of PTCA to Improve Long-Term Outcome by c7E3 GP IIb/IIIa Receptor Blockade) 1) expanded the enrollment criteria to include patients undergoing an urgent or elective coronary intervention and 2) used a low-dose heparin regimen in conjunction with abciximab to reduce bleeding complications. The trial was terminated at the first interim analysis, with 2,792 of the planned 4,800 patients enrolled. These patients were assigned to one of three treatment arms: standard-dose heparin alone (100 U/kg, additional bolus doses as needed to achieve an activated coagulation time [ACT] > 300 seconds), abciximab (plus

Table 3.—Clinical Trials of Glycoprotein (GP) IIb/IIIa Inhibitors

Coronary intervention	Unstable angina non-Q-wave MI	MI with ST-segment elevation
Evaluation of c7E3 in Preventing Ischemic Complications (EPIC)	Platelet GP IIb/IIIa in Unstable Angina: Receptor Suppression Using Integrilin Therapy (PURSUIT)	Integrilin to Manage Platelet Aggregation to Prevent Coronary Thrombosis in Patients With Acute Myocardial Infarction (IMPACT-AMI)
Evaluation of PTCA to Improve Long-Term Outcome by c7E3 GP IIb/IIIa Receptor Blockade (EPILOG)	Platelet Receptor Inhibition in Ischemic Syndrome Management (PRISM)	Platelet Aggregation Receptor Antagonist Dose Investigation for Reperfusion Gain in Myocardial Infarction (PARADIGM)
Integrilin to Manage Platelet Aggregation to Prevent Coronary Thrombosis (IMPACT) 2	Platelet Receptor Inhibition in Ischemic Syndrome Management in Patients Limited by Unstable Signs and Symptoms (PRISM-PLUS)	Thrombolysis in Myocardial Infarction (TIMI)-14
Randomized Efficacy Study of Tirofiban for Outcomes and Restenosis (RESTORE)	Platelet IIb/IIIa Antagonist for the Reduction of Acute Coronary Syndrome Events in a Global Organization Network (PARAGON)	Global Use of Strategies to Open Occluded Coronary Arteries (GUSTO)-IV
Chimeric 7E3 Fab Antiplatelet Therapy in Unstable Refractory Angina (CAPTURE)		

MI, myocardial infarction; PTCA, percutaneous transluminal coronary angioplasty.

standard-dose heparin as above), or abciximab plus low-dose heparin (70 U/kg plus bolus doses as needed to achieve ACT > 200 seconds). Heparin was discontinued immediately after intervention and the vascular sheaths were removed when ACT was 175 seconds or less. There was a 56% reduction in composite cardiac events (death, myocardial infarction, and urgent revascularization at 30 days) in both abciximab groups compared with the heparin-alone group (5.4%, 5.2%, and 11.7%, respectively). Bleeding was more frequent among patients receiving abciximab with standard-dose heparin. At 6-month follow-up, death, myocardial infarction, and urgent revascularization were significantly reduced in both abciximab groups by 43% (14.7% in the placebo group and 8.3% and 8.4% in the abciximab standard-dose and low-dose heparin groups, respectively, $P < 0.001$).

The conclusion of the EPILOG study was that abciximab plus low-dose heparin was as effective as abciximab plus high-dose heparin for patients at high risk for ischemic complications after coronary intervention but with a lower bleeding risk.

- The EPILOG trial demonstrated that the benefits of abciximab could be sustained without the development of bleeding complications by decreasing the heparin dose at the time of coronary intervention.

CAPTURE Trial

The Chimeric 7E3 Fab Antiplatelet Therapy in Unstable Refractory Angina (CAPTURE) trial was the first major study specifically designed to determine whether abciximab can reduce the risk of ischemic complications in patients with refractory unstable angina undergoing PTCA. In this trial, 1,265 patients were randomly assigned to an infusion of abciximab or to no GP IIb/IIIa receptor blocker for 18 to 24 hours before PTCA and continued for 1 hour afterward. The abciximab group had a 29% reduction in the combined end point of death, acute myocardial infarction, or urgent intervention at 30 days (11.3% vs. 15.9%). Abciximab reduced the incidence of acute myocardial infarction by 71% during the pre-PTCA treatment period (0.6% vs. 2.1%, $P = 0.03$) and by 53% during or within 24 hours after PTCA (2.6% vs. 5.3%, $P = 0.009$).

The CAPTURE study demonstrated that treatment with abciximab 24 hours before PTCA reduces periprocedural complications in patients with refractory unstable angina. At 6 months, there was no statistical difference between the groups for cardiovascular events. It is difficult to reconcile the lack of long-term benefit in the CAPTURE trial with the benefit shown in the EPIC and EPILOG trials; it may be that the infusion of abciximab for a longer time (12 hours) after PTCA in the EPIC and EPILOG trials than in the CAPTURE trial (1 hour) may be important.

- The CAPTURE trial demonstrated a periprocedural benefit of abciximab in patients with refractory unstable angina undergoing PTCA, but no long-term benefit.

IMPACT II Trial

The Integrilin to Manage Platelet Aggregation to Prevent Coronary Thrombosis (IMPACT) 2 trial studied the GP IIb/IIIa competitive peptide inhibitor integrilin (eptifibatide) in nearly 4,000 patients, including both high- and low-risk patients, undergoing coronary intervention. Integrilin has a rapid onset of action, with a short half-life (2 hours). Patients were randomly assigned to 24-hour treatment with either placebo or one of two different doses of integrilin (135 µg/kg bolus plus either 0.50 µg or 0.75 µg/kg per minute infusion). The higher dose arm was intended to maintain platelet inhibition and the lower dose to maximize the safety profile. The composite event rates at 30 days were 11.4% in the placebo group, 9.2% in the lower dose group, and 9.9% in the higher dose group. Although the overall differences between integrilin and placebo were not statistically significant, the trend was toward a reduction in the rate of cardiac events. By treatment-received analysis, the lower dose regimen produced a significant reduction (21%) in the composite events (11.6% vs. 9.1%, $P = 0.035$), but the higher dose regimen produced a less substantial reduction (11.6% vs. 10.0%, $P = 0.18$).

The results of this study were ambiguous, and it was thought that the doses of integrilin studied were at the low end of the efficacy-response curve. Integrilin was not associated with increased risk of major bleeding.

The consensus of the above large-scale, randomized, placebo-controlled clinical trials supports the contention that GP IIb/IIIa antagonists are beneficial at least in high-risk patients undergoing coronary intervention. Although other intravenous GP IIb/IIIa inhibitors have acute periprocedural benefits, abciximab currently provides the most significant long-term benefit. The 30-day composite events of these trials are summarized in Table 4.

Recommendations for use of platelet GP IIb/IIIa inhibitors in coronary interventions:

1. High-risk patients undergoing PTCA unless there are bleeding contraindications

2. Patients with increased risk of thrombosis undergoing stenting, including multiple stents, bypass graft stents, totally occluded vessels, small vessels, etc.

3. Patients undergoing directional coronary atherectomy

4. Abciximab should be administered in a dose of 0.25 mg/kg bolus + 10 µg/min infusion to achieve an 80% platelet GP IIb/IIIa receptor blockade and should be continued for more than 12 hours after the procedure; no data are available about abciximab infusions of longer duration

5. Abciximab should be initiated just before the procedure or the day before and adjunctive heparin should be used in a low dose on a weight-adjusted basis, with a target ACT of 200 seconds. After the procedure, the vascular access sheath should be removed as soon as possible when ACT is < 175 seconds.

GP IIb/IIIa Inhibitors in Unstable Angina/Non-Q-Wave Myocardial Infarction

PURSUIT Trial

The PURSUIT (Platelet GP IIb/IIIa in Unstable Angina: Receptor Suppression Using Integrilin Therapy) trial evaluated the effects of integrilin (eptifibatide) in nearly 11,000 patients who had unstable angina or non-Q-wave myocardial

Table 4.—Thirty-Day Composite Events in Platelet Glycoprotein IIb/IIIa Inhibitor Clinical Trials in Coronary Intervention

| Drug | Trial* | % all events | | % relative reduction | P |
		Placebo	Drug		
c7E3 Fab	EPIC	12.8	8.3	35	0.008
	EPILOG	11.7	5.2	56	0.001
	CAPTURE	15.9	11.3	29	0.012
Eptifibatide	IMPACT-II	11.4	9.2	19	0.06
Tirofiban	RESTORE	12.2	10.3	16	0.16

*The full names of the trials are given in Table 3.

infarction within 24 hours of presentation. Patients were randomly assigned to receive a lower dose or a higher dose of integrilin (a bolus dose of 180 µg/kg, followed by an infusion of 1.3 µg/kg per minute or 2.0 µg/kg per minute) or placebo bolus plus infusion of 72 to 96 hours. The lower dose arm was subsequently stopped because the higher dose had an acceptable safety profile. At 30 days, there was a 9.5% decrease in the composite cardiovascular event rate (death or acute myocardial infarction) in the integrilin group compared with the placebo group (14.2% vs. 15.7%, $P = 0.04$). There was no difference in treatment efficacy for patients whose enrollment diagnosis was non-Q-wave myocardial infarction versus unstable angina.

PRISM Trial

The PRISM (Platelet Receptor Inhibition in Ischemic Syndrome Management) trial evaluated whether tirofiban (a nonpeptide GP IIb/IIIa inhibitor) was superior to standard medical therapy with heparin and aspirin in patients with unstable angina or non-Q-wave myocardial infarction. More than 3,000 patients were randomly assigned to treatment with either intravenous tirofiban or heparin for 48 hours. All patients received aspirin. There was a 36% relative reduction in the primary composite events of death, acute myocardial infarction, and refractory ischemia at 48 hours (5.9% in the heparin group vs. 3.8% in the tirofiban group). The survival benefit afforded by tirofiban was maintained at 30 days (a reduction in death from 3.6% to 2.3%, $P = 0.02$), but the reduction in the combined end points of death and acute myocardial infarction was no longer significant at 30 days (17.1% in the heparin group vs. 15.9% in the tirofiban group, $P = 0.34$). Tirofiban did not increase bleeding events, but there was a higher incidence of reversible thrombocytopenia.

PRISM-PLUS Trial

The PRISM-PLUS (Platelet Receptor Inhibition in Ischemic Syndrome Management in Patients Limited by Unstable Signs and Symptoms) trial compared tirofiban with or without heparin and heparin alone in nearly 2,000 patients with unstable angina. This was a high-risk patient population, and a large proportion (about 30%) of patients had PTCA or coronary artery bypass grafting. The tirofiban-only arm had to be discontinued because of an unacceptably high incidence of death and myocardial infarction at 7 days. The rates of the composite end point in the tirofiban-plus-heparin group were lower than those in the heparin-only group at 30 days (18.5% vs. 22.3%; 23% reduction; $P = 0.03$) and 6

months (27.7% vs. 32.1%; 14% reduction; $P = 0.02$). The benefit was consistent in the various subgroups of patients and in those treated medically as well as those treated with angioplasty. There was no significant difference in major bleeding between the heparin-alone group and the tirofiban-plus-heparin group.

PARAGON Trial

The PARAGON (Platelet IIb/IIIa Antagonist for the Reduction of Acute Coronary Syndrome Events in a Global Organization Network) trial assessed the effect of lamifiban in patients with acute coronary syndromes. A total of 2,282 patients were randomly assigned to a low dose of lamifiban (1 µg/min) with or without heparin, a high dose of lamifiban (5 µg/min) with or without heparin, or heparin alone. Statistically, there were no significant differences between treatment groups for composite events at 30 days. However, at 6 months, patients receiving the low dose of lamifiban plus heparin had a significantly reduced rate of composite events compared with the placebo group (13.7% vs. 17.9%, $P = 0.027$). The combination of a high dose of lamifiban and heparin was associated with a higher rate of major bleeding, but the low dose of lamifiban and heparin group and the control group had similar bleeding rates.

The "4P" trials (PURSUIT, PRISM, PRISM-PLUS, PARAGON) provided a large database for the use of platelet GP IIb/IIIa inhibitors as adjunctive medical treatment for patients with acute coronary syndromes. The findings of these four trials are consistent: in patients with unstable angina/non-Q-wave myocardial infarction, GP IIb/IIIa receptor blockers provide a modest benefit in reducing cardiovascular events. The optimal dosing and duration of treatment have not been fully elucidated. Composite events from the "4P" trials are summarized in Table 5.

GP IIb/IIIa Inhibitors in Acute Myocardial Infarction With ST-Segment Elevation

TAMI-8 Trial

TAMI (Thrombolysis and Angioplasty in Myocardial Infarction)-8 trial was the first clinical assessment of the efficacy of a GP IIb/IIIa inhibitor in combination with thrombolytic therapy. Sequential boluses of abciximab were administered to 60 patients with acute myocardial infarction at 3, 6, and 15 hours after initiation of a 100-mg infusion of recombinant tissue plasminogen activator (tPA).

Table 5.—Platelet Glycoprotein IIb/IIIa Inhibitors in Unstable Angina/Non-Q-Wave Myocardial Infarction

	30-Day events, %			6-Month events, %		
Trial	Placebo	Drug	P	Placebo	Drug	P
PURSUIT	15.7	14.2	0.04	---	---	
PRISM	17.1	15.9	0.34	---	---	
PRISM-PLUS	22.3	18.5	0.03	32.1	27.7	0.02
PARAGON	11.7	10.6	0.67	17.9	13.7	0.02

*The full names of the trials are given in Table 3.

Ten control patients received tPA only. Coronary angiography at 18 to 24 hours after treatment started showed that infarct-related artery patency was achieved in 90% of patients receiving abciximab and in 56% of the control subjects. Patients treated with abciximab did not have excess bleeding complications compared with the control group. It was suggested that combination therapy with a thrombolytic agent and a GP IIb/IIIa receptor blocker might benefit patients with acute myocardial infarction.

IMPACT-AMI Trial

The Integrilin to Manage Platelet Aggregation to Prevent Coronary Thrombosis in Patients With Acute Myocardial Infarction (IMPACT-AMI) study evaluated the combined administration of increasing doses of eptifibatide with front-loaded tPA in 180 patients with acute myocardial infarction. The primary end point was Thrombolysis in Myocardial Infarction (TIMI) grade 3 coronary flow at 90-minute angiography, which was achieved in 66% of patients who received the highest dose of eptifibatide, as compared with only 39% of the rtPA group ($P = 0.006$). However, the addition of eptifibatide did not influence the composite end point of in-hospital death, reinfarction, stroke, revascularization, new heart failure, or pulmonary edema.

The results of the TAMI-8 and IMPACT-AMI trials on the combination of tPA and GP IIb/IIIa inhibitor suggested enhanced myocardial reperfusion, but without definitive evidence of a cardiovascular event. No excess of bleeding complications was documented in any of the active treatment groups.

PARADIGM Trial

The PARADIGM (Platelet Aggregation Receptor Antagonist Dose Investigation for Reperfusion Gain in Myocardial Infarction) trial was another randomized placebo-controlled trial that tested the effect of adding various doses of lamifiban to either tPA or streptokinase in 353 patients with acute myocardial infarction who presented within 12 hours after the onset of symptoms. Lamifiban administered adjunctively to thrombolytic therapy significantly improved the patency of the infarct-related artery at 90 minutes (80% for lamifiban-treated group vs. 62.5% for tPA-alone group, $P = 0.005$). There was no significant benefit for lamifiban vs. tPA alone in reducing clinical end points (30-day mortality rate was 2.1% for patients treated with lamifiban vs. 2.6% for those treated with tPA alone).

TIMI-14 Trial

Recently, the TIMI-14 investigators reported that a full dose of abciximab in combination with thrombolytic therapy improves angiographic outcomes compared with thrombolytic therapy alone. Patients with acute myocardial infarction were randomly assigned to one of five groups: 1) full dose of accelerated tPA, 100 mg, 2) full dose of streptokinase, 1.5 million U, 3) abciximab with a low dose of tPA, 4) abciximab with a low dose of streptokinase, or 5) abciximab alone. The group receiving abciximab with a low dose of tPA (50 mg) had higher coronary artery reperfusion rates than the group receiving tPA alone (79% with TIMI grade 3 flow rate vs. 58%).

The results of the above studies investigating the benefits of GP IIb/IIIa inhibitor after thrombolytic agents have been promising. The patency of the infarct-related artery after administration of GP IIb/IIIa inhibitors in combination with thrombolytics is summarized in Table 6. The incidence and speed of reperfusion were enhanced when GP IIb/IIIa inhibitor was combined with tPA, aspirin, and heparin. Defining the role of GP IIb/IIIa blockade as an adjunct to thrombolytic therapy in preventing coronary reocclusion and enhancing thrombolytic efficacy awaits completion of

Table 6.—Platelet Glycoprotein IIb/IIIa Inhibitors in Anterior Myocardial Infarction With ST-Segment Elevation

Trial*	No. of patients	Treatment groups	Patency of IRA, %	P
PARADIGM	353	Lamifiban 24 h + tPA or streptokinase *or*	80	0.005
		placebo + tPA or streptokinase	63	
IMPACT-AMI	180	Eptifibatide + tPA + heparin *or*	66	0.006
		placebo + tPA + heparin	39	
TIMI-14	219	Abciximab + tPA (60 min) *or*	76	0.001
		tPA alone	57	

IRA, infarct-related artery; tPA, tissue plasminogen activator.
*The full names of the trials are given in Table 3.

ongoing trials. No significantly increased risk of intracranial hemorrhage was reported in the TAMI-8, PARADIGM, IMPACT-AMI, or TIMI-14 trials.

Adverse Effects of GP IIb/IIIa Inhibitors

Bleeding

Bleeding is the most frequent adverse event associated with GP IIb/IIIa inhibitors. In most of GP IIb/IIIa inhibitor trials, bleeding events were classified as "major," "minor," or "insignificant," according to the criteria of the TIMI study group. Major bleeding was an intracranial hemorrhage, a decrease in hemoglobin greater than 5 g/dL, or a decrease in hematocrit greater than 15%. Minor bleeding was blood loss with a decrease in hemoglobin greater than 3 g/dL. The most common bleeding sites were the groin, retroperitoneal sites, or during bypass grafting of the coronary artery.

A matter of greater concern is the combination of GP IIb/IIIa inhibitor with thrombolytic therapy. In the TAMI-8, IMPACT-AMI, and PARADIGM trials, patients who received the combination of thrombolytic and GP IIb/IIIa inhibitor agents did not have an increase in bleeding compared with those who received only thrombolytic agents (Table 7).

Recommendations to reduce bleeding risk:

1. Identify risk factors: acute myocardial infarction, low body weight, older age

2. Contraindications: cerebrovascular accident < 6 months, gastrointestinal hemorrhage < 6 weeks, surgery < 6 weeks, neurosurgery < 6 months, intracranial malignancy, platelets < 100,000

3. In conjunction with lower dose, weight-adjusted heparin

Table 7.—Incidence of Major Bleeding in GP IIb/IIIa Inhibitor Trials

Trial*	Agent	Placebo, % of patients	GP IIb/IIIa inhibitor, % of patients
EPIC	Abciximab	7.0	14.0[†]
EPILOG	Abciximab	3.1	3.5
CAPTURE	Abciximab	1.9	3.8[†]
IMPACT-II	Eptifibatide	4.8	5.2
PURSUIT	Eptifibatide	9.1	10.6[†]
PRISM	Tirofiban	0.4	0.4
PRISM-PLUS	Tirofiban	0.8	1.4
RESTORE	Tirofiban	2.1	2.4

*The full names of the trials are given in Table 3.
[†]P values are significant compared with placebo group.

4. Postprocedure care: discontinue heparin after procedure, early sheath removal

5. Avoid combination treatment with coumadin, INR < 1.5

Thrombocytopenia

The specific mechanisms for this complication are unknown and may differ among the various GP IIb/IIIa inhibitors. A potential mechanism for thrombocytopenia is immune-mediated clearance of platelets. The incidence of thrombocytopenia associated with GP IIb/IIIa inhibitor use may be confused with the thrombocytopenia associated with concomitant heparin therapy. Abciximab-induced thrombocytopenia is reversible, usually occurs rapidly (can be within 24 hours), and responds well to platelet transfusions. After therapy is discontinued, there is a return to normal. Heparin-induced thrombocytopenia usually develops after 5 to 7 days of treatment, does not respond to platelet transfusion, and is associated with both bleeding and thrombosis. The presence of heparin-dependent antibody helps differentiate between the two conditions. Prophylactic transfusion of platelets should be considered if the platelet count is less than 20,000. Platelet count should be maintained above 50,000 if bleeding exists. It would be wise to rule out pseudothrombocytopenia due to platelet clumping by examining a peripheral blood smear. To monitor thrombocytopenia, a platelet count should be performed 2 to 4 hours after initiation of treatment with abciximab and at 24 hours. The incidence of thrombocytopenia in the EPIC, EPILOG, and CAPTURE trials is shown in Figure 3.

Immunogenicity of Abciximab

The GP IIb/IIIa inhibitor abciximab is a modified Fab fragment of a monoclonal antibody to the platelet receptor that is generated partly in mice. This in turn can give rise to human antichimeric antibodies (HACA) that are specific to the murine epitope of the Fab antibody fragment and develop in about 7% of patients receiving abciximab. HACA are IgG antibodies and peak 1 to 4 weeks after abciximab administration and then gradually decline. The clinical significance of HACA is not known; they do not seem to be a major clinical concern.

Practice Guidelines for Use of GP IIb/GP IIIa Inhibitors

The guidelines are given in Tables 8 to 10.

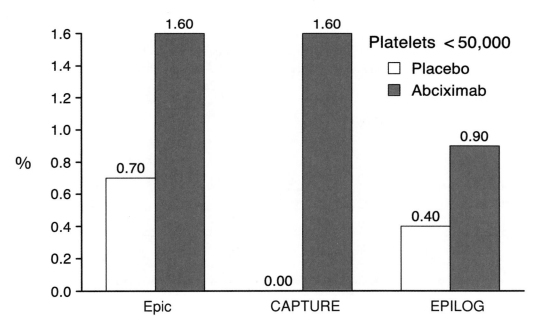

Fig. 3. Thrombocytopenia in glycoprotein IIb/IIIa trials. CAPTURE, Chimeric 7E3 Fab Antiplatelet Therapy in Unstable Refractory Angina; EPIC, Evaluation of c7E3 in Preventing Ischemic Complications; EPILOG, Evaluation of PTCA [Percutaneous Transluminal Coronary Angioplasty] to Improve Long-Term Outcome by c7E3 GP IIb/IIIa Receptor Blockade.

Table 8.—Glycoprotein IIb/IIIa Platelet Inhibitors: Practice Guidelines

Indications

1. Medically refractory unstable angina (recurrent ischemic pain with therapeutic doses of ASA, β-blocker, heparin, and nitrates)
2. High-risk PCI
3. ASA allergy, heparin-induced thrombocytopenia with acute ischemic syndrome

Refractory unstable angina

Abciximab IV—250 µg/kg bolus followed by a continuous infusion of 100 µg/min for 12-24 hr preceding PTCA and continuing for 1 hour after completion of the procedure via infusion pump; add ASA 75-325 mg daily and heparin (aPTT > 60 seconds)

Eptifibatide IV—180 µg/kg before the start of PCI, followed by a continuous infusion of 2 µg/kg per minute; continue for 24-72 hr; add ASA 75-325 mg daily and heparin (aPTT > 60 seconds)

Tirofiban IV—0.4 µg/kg per minute bolus over 30 min before start of PCI, followed by continuous infusion of 0.1 µg/kg per minute for 12-24 hr via infusion pump (if creatinine clearance is < 30 mL/min, use half the infusion rate); continue for 48-108 hr after PCI; add ASA and heparin (aPTT >60 seconds)

End point: symptom resolution

PCI

Abciximab IV—0.25 µg/kg bolus administered 10-60 min before start of PCI, followed by continuous infusion of 0.125 µg/kg per minute (to a maximum of 10 µg/min) for 12 hr via infusion pump; add ASA and heparin (ACT 250-300 in catheterization lab or, on floor, aPTT > 60 seconds)

Eptifibatide IV—180 µg/kg bolus before the start of PCI, followed by continuous infusion of 2 µg/kg per minute (add ASA, 75-325 mg daily, and heparin (ACT 250 to 300 in catherization lab or, on floor, aPTT > 60 seconds)

Tirofiban IV—0.4 µg/kg per minute bolus over 30 min before start of PCI, followed by continuous infusion of 0.1 µg/kg per minute for 12-24 hr via infusion pump (if creatinine clearance is < 30 mL/min, use half the infusion rate); consider ASA and heparin; add ASA and heparin (ACT 250-300 in catheterization lab or, on floor, aPTT >60 seconds)

End point

Continue eptifibatide or tirofiban 12-24 hours after PCI

Contraindications

Platelets < 100,000

Active bleeding

History of stroke/transient ischemic attack

Recent (< 1 mo) major surgery

Allergy to drug

ACT, activated clotting time; aPTT, activated partial thromboplastin time; ASA, acetylsalicylic acid; IV, intravenous; PCI, percutaneous coronary intervention; PTCA, percutaneous transluminal coronary angioplasty.

Consensus recommendation from Coronary Care Unit and Cardiac Catheterization Laboratory groups, Mayo Clinic.

Table 9.—Glycoprotein IIb/IIIa Platelet Inhibitors: Indication, Relative Contraindications, and U.S. FDA Approved Indications

I. Indication—In high-risk unstable angina or non ST-segment elevation MI with ongoing ischemia after receiving optimal medical therapy for ≥ 1 hr

    Consider starting IIb/IIIa inhibitor

               or

    Transfer for cardiac catheterization

II. Relative contraindications

    Bleeding in last 6 weeks

    Intracranial hemorrhage (ever)

    Recent stroke (< 2 years)

    Hypertension (blood pressure > 200/110 mm Hg)

    Surgery ≤ 6 weeks

    Aortic dissection

    Acute pericarditis

    Platelets < 100,000

    Elevated INR

III. U.S. FDA-approved indications

	Unstable	
Drug	Without planned PCI	With planned PCI*
Abciximab (ReoPro)	Not approved	OK
Eptifibatide (Integrilin)	OK	OK
Tirofiban (Aggrastat)	OK	OK

MI, myocardial infarction; PCI, percutaneous coronary intervention; U.S. FDA, United States Food and Drug Administration.

*Within 24 hr.

Table 10.—Glycoprotein IIb/IIIa Platelet Inhibitors: Dosing

Drug	Loading	Maintenance	Duration	AWP, U.S. $*
Abciximab (ReoPro)	0.25 mg/kg	10 µg/min	12-24 hr	1,600-2,200
	Renal insufficiency: no change			
Eptifibatide[†] (Integrilin)	180 µg/kg	2 µg/kg per min	For up to 96 hr (20-24 hr after PCI)	800-1,600
	Creatinine > 2.0: contraindicated			
Tirofiban[†] (Aggrastat)	0.4 µg/kg per min	0.1 µg/kg per min	12-24 hr after PCI	700-1,600
	Creatinine > 2.0: load & infusion reduced by 50%			

aPTT, activated partial thromboplastin time; AWP, average wholesale price; PCI, percutaneous coronary intervention.

*1999 (cost is for a 70-kg patient).

[†]Concomitant heparin is suggested, goal aPTT ~ 60-85 s.

Suggested Review Reading

1. Adgey AA: An overview of the results of clinical trials with glycoprotein IIb/IIIa inhibitors. *Eur Heart J* 19 (Suppl D):D10-D21, 1998.

2. Braunwald E, Maseri A, Armstrong PW, et al: Rationale and clinical evidence for the use of GP IIb/IIIa inhibitors in acute coronary syndromes. *Eur Heart J* 19 (Suppl D):D22-D30, 1998.

3. The CAPTURE Investigators: Randomised placebo-controlled trial of abciximab before and during coronary intervention in refractory unstable angina: the CAPTURE Study. *Lancet* 349:1429-1435, 1997.

4. Chronos N, Vahanian A, Betriu A, et al: Use of abciximab in interventional cardiology. *Eur Heart J* 19 Suppl D:D31-D39, 1998.

5. The EPIC Investigators: Use of a monoclonal antibody directed against the platelet glycoprotein IIb/IIIa receptor in high-risk coronary angioplasty. *N Engl J Med* 330:956-961, 1994.

6. The EPILOG Investigators: Platelet glycoprotein IIb/IIIa receptor blockade and low-dose heparin during percutaneous coronary revascularization. *N Engl J Med* 336:1689-1696, 1997.

7. Ferguson JJ, Kereiakes DJ, Adgey AA, et al: Safe use of platelet GP IIb/IIIa inhibitors. *Eur Heart J* 19 Suppl D:D40-D51, 1998.

8. The IMPACT-II Investigators: Randomised placebo-controlled trial of effect of eptifibatide on complications of percutaneous coronary intervention: IMPACT-II. *Lancet* 349:1422-1428, 1997.

9. Kleiman NS, Ohman EM, Califf RM, et al: Profound inhibition of platelet aggregation with monoclonal antibody 7E3 Fab after thrombolytic therapy. Results of the Thrombolysis and Angioplasty in Myocardial Infarction (TAMI) 8 Pilot Study. *J Am Coll Cardiol* 22:381-389, 1993.

10. Madan M, Berkowitz SD, Tcheng JE: Glycoprotein IIb/IIIa integrin blockade. *Circulation* 98:2629-2635, 1998.

11. Mak KH, Tan AT, Chan C, et al: The clinical impact of platelet glycoprotein IIb/IIIa receptor blockade in cardiovascular medicine. *Jpn Circ J* 62:233-243, 1998.

12. Ohman EM, Kleiman NS, Gacioch G, et al: Combined accelerated tissue-plasminogen activator and platelet glycoprotein IIb/IIIa integrin receptor blockade with Integrilin in acute myocardial infarction. Results of a randomized, placebo-controlled, dose-ranging trial. *Circulation* 95:846-854, 1997.

13. The PARAGON Investigators: International, randomized, controlled trial of lamifiban (a platelet glycoprotein IIb/IIIa inhibitor), heparin, or both in unstable angina. *Circulation* 97:2386-2395, 1998.

14. The Platelet Receptor Inhibition in Ischemic Syndrome Management in Patients Limited by Unstable Signs and Symptoms (PRISM-PLUS) Study Investigators: Inhibition of the platelet glycoprotein IIb/IIIa receptor with tirofiban in unstable angina and non-Q-wave myocardial infarction. *N Engl J Med* 338:1488-1497, 1998.

15. The Platelet Receptor Inhibition in Ischemic Syndrome Management (PRISM) Study Investigators: A comparison of aspirin plus tirofiban with aspirin plus heparin for unstable angina. *N Engl J Med* 338:1498-1505, 1998.

16. The PURSUIT Trial Investigators: Inhibition of platelet glycoprotein IIb/IIIa with eptifibatide in patients with acute coronary syndromes. *N Engl J Med* 339:436-443, 1998.

17. Tan HC: Glycoprotein IIb/IIIa platelet receptor inhibitors: a new dimension in cardiology. *Ann Acad Med Singapore* 26:481-488, 1997.

18. Tcheng JE: Glycoprotein IIb/IIIa receptor inhibitors: putting the EPIC, IMPACT II, RESTORE, and EPILOG trials into perspective. *Am J Cardiol* 78:35-40, 1996.

Chapter 82

The Pathophysiology of Arterial Thrombosis

Robert D. McBane, M.D.

Atherothrombotic disease is now the leading cause of mortality worldwide. This chapter reviews the basic physiology of arterial thrombosis and the risk factors for abnormal thrombogenesis.

The Stages of Arterial Thrombosis

Acute arterial thrombo-occlusive syndromes start with platelet thrombi that form on a newly disrupted arterial plaque. The sequence of events that lead to thrombosis is divided into overlapping stages, which begin with platelet adhesion, followed by coagulation factor activation and amplification and then thrombus propagation, in which resident platelets recruit additional platelets to the growing thrombus mass. Finally, a maturation phase completes the period of platelet residence within the thrombus. Once a white platelet plug has occluded the artery, red fibrin-rich "caps" form at either end, further stabilizing the thrombus.

The four stages of thrombus formation:
- Platelet adhesion
- Coagulation factor activation and amplification
- Thrombus propagation
- Maturation

Platelet Adhesion

The initial step in arterial thrombosis is platelet adhesion, which occurs as the first layer of platelets accretes at the site of vascular injury (Plate 1A). This process is governed by blood flow shear forces and occurs before activation of the coagulation cascade. The vascular endothelial lining normally presents a slippery "nonstick" surface between the vessel wall and circulating cellular elements. Plaque disruption or endothelial denudation exposes various "sticky" arterial wall matrix proteins that bind to specific surface receptors on circulating platelets and thereby provide an anchoring point (Table 1). Platelet adhesion receptors bind to specific type of vascular wall matrix protein dependent on the blood flow shear rate at which each receptor optimally operates.

Under conditions of high blood flow shear rates, glycoprotein Ib-IX (gp Ib-IX) is the principal platelet receptor mediating vascular adhesion by binding von Willebrand factor (vWF) within the arterial wall. vWF, an abundant plasma protein, does not bind to the gp Ib-IX receptor of circulating platelets under normal conditions. Upon exposure to high shear forces, vWF undergoes a structural change that enhances binding (Plate 1A). In contrast, gp Ib-IX requires no "de novo" platelet activation before binding vWF. Once anchored, the platelets spread to cover as much of the injured surface area as possible and then secrete the contents of their intracellular granules. Platelet adhesion contributes only a monolayer of platelets that initiates the thrombotic process. Further thrombus growth requires activation of the coagulation cascade and the recruitment of circulating platelets. The adherent platelet surface provides the phospholipid cell membrane necessary for assembly of coagulation factor activating complexes (Plate 1B).

Table 1.—Platelet Receptors and Shear Stress

Extracellular matrix protein	Platelet receptor	Optimal shear stress
von Willebrand factor	gp Ib-IX	High
Collagen	gp Ia-IIa	Low
	gp VI	
	gp IIb	
Fibronectin	gp Ic-IIa	Low
Laminin	α_6IIa	Low

gp, glycoprotein.

- Plaque disruption or endothelial denudation exposes various "sticky" arterial wall matrix proteins that bind to specific surface receptors on circulating platelets.
- Platelet adhesion contributes only a monolayer of platelets that initiates the thrombotic process.

Coagulation Factor Activation

The second step of arterial thrombosis is "cascade" amplification of the coagulation factors, as activation complexes assemble on the surface of platelets adherent to the vascular wall. The coagulation activation complexes include activating enzymes and proenzymes held in proper alignment by large thrombosis cofactors. Once cleaved to its active form, the coagulation proenzyme becomes the activating enzyme for the next step in the "cascade." Several of these coagulation factors (prothrombin, factors VII, IX, and X) undergo vitamin K-dependent carboxylation after hepatic synthesis. Carboxylation of the amino terminus glutamic acid residues enables these coagulation factors to bind calcium ions, which in turn induces a configurational change that allows the coagulation factor to insert itself into the platelet surface. Inhibition of carboxylation by warfarin or vitamin K depletion impedes the platelet surface-dependent coagulation factor assembly and thereby reduces coagulation factor activation. Calcium sequestration by citrate or EDTA likewise diminishes factor activation by inhibiting the coagulation factor structural changes required for platelet surface binding.

- Once cleaved to its active form, the coagulation proenzyme becomes the activating enzyme for the next step in the "cascade."

Pathways of Coagulation Factor Activation

The two pathways for coagulation factor activation, the extrinsic (or tissue factor-dependent pathway) and the intrinsic (or contact activation pathway), converge at the common end point of factor X and prothrombin activation (Plate 2). Arterial injury exposes blood plasma containing factor VII to tissue factor, a protein particularly abundant in the vascular wall adventitia and in atherosclerotic plaques. Tissue factor enhances the enzymatic activity of factor VIIa for the activation of factors IX and X by several thousand-fold. By activating factor X, this pathway generates small concentrations of thrombin. Thrombin greatly amplifies its own generation by activating cofactors V and VIII in a positive feedback mechanism, appropriately coined the "coagulation vortex." The consequence of this feedback is a rich concentration of thrombin at the site of vascular injury. Thrombin, a potent platelet agonist, greatly enhances platelet recruitment to the growing thrombus.

- The two pathways for coagulation factor activation converge at the common end point of factor X and prothrombin activation.
- Thrombin greatly amplifies its own generation by activating cofactors V and VIII in a positive feedback mechanism.

Thrombus Propagation and the Glycoprotein IIb-IIIa ($\alpha_{2b}\beta_3$) Platelet Receptor

Once platelets have carpeted the site of arterial injury and the coagulation cascade has been fully activated, thrombus propagation occurs as new platelets are incorporated into the growing thrombus mass by platelet-platelet interactions (Plate 3). Unlike adhesion, platelet aggregation requires activation of a second surface receptor, glycoprotein (gp) IIb-IIIa (recently renamed gp $\alpha_{2b}\beta_3$). Once activated, this receptor mediates platelet aggregation by binding fibrinogen as a sort of "glue" that holds adjacent platelets together. Glycoprotein IIb-IIIa is a member of the much larger family of cell adhesion molecules called integrins that are involved in cellular processes ranging from embryogenesis to cancer metastasis. Although broadly distributed, the gp IIb-IIIa integrin is unique to the megakaryocytic cell line. There are approximately 50,000 copies of this receptor per platelet, found either on the cell surface or stored within α granules. Made up of protein dimers of α and β subunits, these receptors, when activated, have the ability to recognize the amino acid sequence RGD (arginine, glycine, aspartic acid) within the adhesion protein to which they bind. Fibrinogen, a large symmetric molecule containing four copies of this RGD sequence, is the ideal "bridging" protein, given its rich plasma concentration and extended configuration. By interacting with gp IIb-IIIa receptors on adjacent platelets, fibrinogen reversibly "glues" platelets together. Other proteins such as vWF contain the RGD sequence and are thus able to support aggregation by the gp IIb-IIIa receptor.

- Platelet aggregation requires activation of a second surface receptor, glycoprotein IIb-IIIa (recently renamed gp $\alpha_{2b}\beta_3$).

Mechanism of Platelet Activation

Platelet activation requires that one of several potential agonists interact with a specific cell membrane receptor to trigger a response (Table 2). Depending on the strength and concentration of the agonist, this response may include arachidonate liberation, gp IIb-IIIa activation, shape change, pseudopodia formation, or granule release. Varying in potency, strong agonists, which include thrombin, thromboxane A_2, and platelet activating factor, initiate platelet activation directly by induction of a second messenger G protein and intracellular phospholipase C pathway (Plate 3). Phospholipase C activity results in mobilization of cytoplasmic calcium and protein kinase C stimulation. These responses lead to protein phosphorylation and signal transduction ultimately responsible for various platelet functions. Weak agonists include collagen, adenosine diphosphate (ADP), epinephrine, serotonin, and vasopressin. These agonists induce the release of arachidonate, which is then converted to prostaglandins and thromboxane A_2 by the cyclooxygenase pathway. Thromboxane A_2 then activates the platelet through the phospholipase C pathway. Thrombin, the most potent platelet agonist, stimulates platelet activation in spite of cyclooxygenase inhibition, whereas ADP- or collagen-induced platelet aggregation can be completely inhibited by aspirin. The in vivo participation of weak agonists in thrombus formation is unclear. The clinical benefit of cyclooxygenase inhibitors and ADP-receptor antagonists in coronary and cerebrovascular disease, however, suggests that these pathways are clinically important.

- Thrombin, the most potent platelet agonist, stimulates platelet activation in spite of cyclooxygenase inhibition.
- ADP- or collagen-induced platelet aggregation can be completely inhibited by aspirin.

Thrombosis Regulation

Growth of an arterial thrombus is a balancing act between two opposing forces: the thrombotic stimulus promoting

Table 2.—Platelet Activation Agonists

Strong agonist	Weak agonist	Physical agonist
Thrombin	ADP	Shear stress
Thromboxane A_2	Epinephrine	(gp Ib-IX receptor)
Platelet-activating factor	Serotonin	

ADP, adenosine diphosphate; gp, glycoprotein.

propagation to occlude the artery and arterial shear forces that erode and undermine the thrombus by shearing off aggregates of platelets. The ultimate outcome depends on the relative magnitude of these opposing forces, and the result may be vessel occlusion, mural thrombus, or clot disaggregation. A complex system of endogenous inhibitors regulates each stage of thrombosis, including tissue factor pathway inhibitor, protein C/protein S, antithrombin III, and the plasminogen/fibrinolytic system. This regulation is of critical importance for both hemostasis and subsequent wound healing regardless of whether the site of injury is coronary plaque rupture or skin laceration. The importance of these pathways may be appreciated in that molecular deficiencies of each of these proteins can lead to thrombophilic states in humans.

Activated factor VIIa has a fairly long circulating half-life. Even with abundant quantities of heparin, factor VIIa is only very slowly inhibited by antithrombin III. Tissue factor pathway inhibitor (TFPI) is a protease inhibitor that serves as a reversible "sink" for factor Xa, factor VIIa, and tissue factor (Plate 4). Synthesized by endothelial cells, TFPI circulates with plasma lipoproteins. Dissociating from the lipoprotein, TFPI forms a complex first with excess factor Xa and then factor VIIa and tissue factor, thus turning off further factor activation. In the setting of vascular injury, TFPI provides a valuable source of factor VIIa to initiate coagulation. Serving as a cofactor for factor VIIa, tissue factor exposure to plasma enhances activation of factor X. Therefore, TFPI serves as an important coagulation regulator, both enabling and limiting the extrinsic (tissue factor) activator pathway. As information accumulates on TFPI physiology, it becomes evident that the original concept of separate intrinsic and extrinsic pathways may have overcomplicated the coagulation activation process. A single, well-integrated system beginning with tissue factor/factor VII and vascular injury seems a more plausible explanation of the commonality of the two pathways.

- TFPI serves as an important coagulation regulator, both enabling and limiting the extrinsic (tissue factor) activator pathway.

Protein C

Protein C, a vitamin K-dependent protein synthesized in the liver, is an important regulator of prothrombin generation. In the "cascade" preceding prothrombin activation, several important cofactors participate by properly aligning the activating enzyme with the subsequent proenzyme. Cofactor VIII and cofactor V are required for the activation of factor X and prothrombin, respectively. Without these cofactors, activation occurs very inefficiently. Thrombin, once generated, may be deposited on a specific endothelial cell receptor called thrombomodulin (Plate 5). Bound to the endothelial thrombomodulin in this fashion, the substrate specificity of thrombin changes from prothrombotic to antithrombotic activity with the activation of protein C. Activated protein C in the presence of protein S behaves as an anticoagulant by proteolytically digesting cofactors Va and VIIIa. Without these cofactors, prothrombin activation is significantly reduced by this negative feedback pathway. While bound to thrombomodulin, thrombin is unable to activate platelets or cleave fibrinogen. Thrombin remains bound to thrombomodulin until scavenged by antithrombin III.

- Activated protein C in the presence of protein S behaves as an anticoagulant by proteolytically digesting cofactors Va and VIIIa.

Antithrombin III

The plasma protein antithrombin III (AT III), in combination with heparin, neutralizes thrombin by forming a stable thrombin-antithrombin (TAT) complex. By altering the protein structure, heparin increases the affinity of AT III for thrombin by a thousand-fold. Heparan sulfate, an endogenous heparin-like molecule with antithrombotic activity produced by endothelial cells and mast cells, serves as a catalyst and cofactor by forming a tertiary intermediate between thrombin and AT III. Once the stable TAT complex has been formed, heparin is free to participate in another thrombin–AT-III coupling. In addition to thrombin, AT III is the major inhibitor of other coagulation factors of the intrinsic pathway, including factors IXa, Xa, XIa, and XIIa. The tertiary intermediate does not appear to be necessary for the inhibition of either factor IXa or Xa.

- The plasma protein antithrombin III (AT III), in combination with heparin, neutralizes thrombin by forming a stable thrombin-antithrombin (TAT) complex.
- Heparin increases the affinity of AT III for thrombin by a thousand-fold.

Fibrinolysis

Endogenous fibrinolytic activity requires the activation of plasminogen to plasmin by one of several activator pathways. Once formed, plasmin degrades fibrin/fibrinogen within the occlusive thrombus, thereby recanalizing the vessel. Plasminogen activation may occur by either the endogenous activator pathway (tissue-type plasminogen activator or urokinase-type plasminogen activator) or surface contact activation (kallikrein, factor XIa, factor XIIa).

Native tPA

Native tissue plasminogen activator (tPA) is synthesized primarily by endothelial cells and is released into the circulation by various agonists, including thrombin, epinephrine, exercise, histamine, bradykinin, and venous occlusion. Once secreted, tPA proteolytically activates plasminogen to plasmin. In the presence of fibrin, this activation is increased several hundred-fold, a property that imparts relative clot specificity to endogenous fibrinolysis. Degraded in the liver, tPA has a circulating half-life of approximately 6 minutes.

- Native tissue plasminogen activator (tPA) is synthesized primarily by endothelial cells.
- tPA proteolytically activates plasminogen to plasmin.

Native Urokinase-Type Plasminogen Activator

This is produced primarily in the kidney as pro-urokinase or single-chain UK (scu-PA). Much like tPA, this form of urokinase has a short half-life (3-6 minutes) and a relative clot specificity. In the face of small concentrations of plasmin, pro-urokinase is converted to two-chain high-molecular-weight urokinase, which further facilitates plasminogen activation. A third form of the enzyme, low-molecular-weight urokinase, has no fibrin specificity yet is an equally efficient plasminogen activator.

Contact Activation

Although not well understood, the contact activation pathway relies on negatively charged surface activation of high-molecular-weight kininogen, which in turn activates prekallikrein and factors XI and XII. Plasminogen activation by this pathway is less efficient than the endogenous activator pathway, and the degree of participation in endogenous fibrinolysis by this pathway is unclear.

Regulation of Fibrinolysis

Like other physiologic processes, fibrinolysis is a finely regulated system of activators and inhibitors. There are three forms of plasminogen activator inhibitor (PAI): PAI-1, PAI-2, and PAI-3. An equally efficient inhibitor of both tPA and urokinase, PAI-1 appears to be the most important regulator of the plasminogen activating system. Synthesized in various cells, PAI-1 exists in high concentrations in platelet α granules, a factor that may contribute to fibrinolytic resistance of some occlusive platelet-rich thrombi. In addition, high plasma levels of PAI-1 have been found to correlate with increased risk of myocardial infarction and stroke. There are two important physiologic inhibitors of plasmin: α_2-antiplasmin and α_2-macroglobulin. More abundant in plasma, α_2-antiplasmin is probably the primary physiologic plasmin inhibitor. These plasmin inhibitors may be cross-linked to fibrin by factor XIIIa, further protecting the thrombus from degradation.

- There are three forms of plasminogen activator inhibitor (PAI): PAI-1, PAI-2, and PAI-3.
- PAI-1 exists in high concentrations in platelet α granules.

Risk Factors for Arterial Thrombosis

More than a century ago, Virchow proposed that atherosclerotic plaque progression resulted from a combination of injury and thrombosis. The variables responsible for plaque disruption include plaque morphology and biochemistry, macrophage activity, and local shear forces. Less mature lipid-rich plaques are probably more vulnerable to disruption and thrombosis than older, calcified lesions, which tend to be more stable. Throughout the arterial tree, atherosclerotic plaques probably are constantly being disrupted on a regular basis. The factors that lead to in situ thrombus formation after plaque disruption are variable and may include inadequate clot lysis, mural thrombus formation, and complete arterial occlusion. The final outcome depends on several variables, including plaque burden and morphology and the "activity" of both circulating platelets and coagulation factors at the time of the injury.

- Less mature lipid-rich plaques are more vulnerable to disruption and thrombosis than older, calcified lesions.

Homocystinuria

Homocystinuria, a rare genetic disorder of impaired homocysteine metabolism, results in high plasma homocysteine levels and severe premature atherosclerosis. Milder increases resulting in hyperhomocysteinemia may account for up to 30% of cases of premature atherosclerosis. Hyperhomocysteinemia may result either from a genetic enzyme deficiency in the conversion pathway of methionine to cysteine or from vitamin B deficiency or renal or hepatic disease. High plasma homocysteine levels significantly increase the risk of acute myocardial infarction and seem to be a stronger predictor for cerebrovascular, peripheral vascular, and coronary disease compared with the more traditional risk factors, including cholesterol level, hypertension, and tobacco use. Proposed pathophysiologic mechanisms include endothelial injury, low-density lipoprotein oxidation, factor V activation, and protein C inhibition. Vitamin B supplementation has been shown to reduce homocysteine plasma levels, but the clinical benefit of this therapy is unproved.

- Hyperhomocysteinemia may result either from a genetic enzyme deficiency in the conversion pathway of methionine to cysteine or from vitamin B deficiency or renal or hepatic disease.

Lp(a)

Lp(a) is a lipoprotein that in high concentrations has been associated with cardiovascular and cerebrovascular disease. Structural similarity to plasminogen has been implicated in its pathophysiology. By competitive inhibition of plasminogen activation, Lp(a) may predispose to thrombosis and atherogenesis. In contrast to other lipoprotein increases, Lp(a) does not respond to fibrate or statin lipid-lowering agents. It may respond to treatment with niacin or hormone replacement therapy in postmenopausal women.

- Lp(a) does not respond to fibrate or statin lipid-lowering agents.

Fibrinogen

Data from the Framingham Heart Study and other investigations have revealed a significant correlation between fibrinogen and coronary artery disease. Fibrinogen levels were closely related to other risk factors, including glucose intolerance, hypertension, and tobacco use. By multivariate analysis, fibrinogen was an independent predictor of coronary artery disease in men. The correlation between high fibrinogen concentration and arterial thrombosis may relate to its impact on blood viscosity, fibrinogen being one of the principal determinants. Increased leukocyte counts and vWF also have been implicated as risk factors for coronary artery and cerebrovascular events. Reduced endogenous fibrinolytic activity has been proposed as an important variable in premature atherosclerosis and thrombosis. Several traditional risk factors have been correlated with decreased fibrinolytic activity, including tobacco use, hyperlipoproteinemia, diabetes, and obesity. Whether causative or epiphenomena, the pathophysiologic participation of each of these hemostatic factors in arterial thrombosis is unclear. These variables may merely reflect their propensity to respond as acute-phase reactants. Likewise, there currently is no meaningful way of modifying these hemostatic variables.

- By multivariate analysis, fibrinogen was an independent predictor of coronary artery disease in men.

Mental Stress

Epidemiologic data point to physiologic stress as a precipitating factor in myocardial infarction. Catecholamines stimulate in vitro platelet aggregation by α_2 subtype receptor activation. In infarction survivors, a mental stress test has been shown to invoke a simultaneous increase in serum epinephrine and norepinephrine levels. This increase in catecholamines was associated with the formation of circulating platelet aggregates and an increase in plasma thromboxane B_2 levels. Population-based studies have shown a diurnal variation in both nonfatal and fatal myocardial infarction, with most events occurring between 6 AM and midday. This variation has been attributed to activation of the sympathetic nervous system and platelet hyperreactivity and aggregability. This diurnal variation was blocked by the use of β-blocker therapy in the Intravenous Streptokinase in Acute Myocardial Infarction (ISAM) study, suggesting an important role for catecholamines in this process.

- Catecholamines stimulate in vitro platelet aggregation by α_2 subtype receptor activation.
- Population-based studies have shown a diurnal variation in both nonfatal and fatal myocardial infarction, with most events occurring between 6 AM and midday.

Smoking

The mechanism by which smoking promotes atherogenesis is probably multifactorial. Tobacco has been shown to enhance platelet reactivity and may alter prostaglandin metabolism. Platelet survival is significantly reduced in chronic smokers, possibly because of tobacco-induced endothelial injury. There is also evidence that tobacco may increase circulating catecholamine levels, thereby further stimulating platelet activation.

Suggested Review Reading

Platelet Adhesion

1. Clemetson KJ: Platelet GPib-V-IX complex. *Thromb Haemost* 78:266-270, 1997.

2. Lopez JA, Dong JF: Structure and function of the glycoprotein Ib-IX-V complex. *Curr Opin Hematol* 4:323-329, 1997.

3. Williams MJ, Du X, Loftus JC, et al: Platelet adhesion receptors. *Semin Cell Biol* 6:305-314, 1995.

Platelet Activation

1. Coughlin SR: Thrombin receptor structure and function. *Thromb Haemost* 70:184-187, 1993.

2. Coughlin SR, Vu TK, Hung DT, et al: Characterization of a functional thrombin receptor. Issues and opportunities. *J Clin Invest* 89:351-355, 1992.

3. Gachet C, Hechler B, Leon C, et al: Activation of ADP receptors and platelet function. *Thromb Haemost* 78:271-275, 1997.

Platelet Aggregation

1. Braunwald E, Maseri A, Armstrong PW, et al: Rationale and clinical evidence for the use of GP IIb/IIIa inhibitors in acute coronary syndromes. *Am Heart J* 135:S56-S66, 1998.

2. Du X, Ginsberg MH: Integrin alpha IIb beta 3 and platelet function. *Thromb Haemost* 78:96-100, 1997.

3. Naik UP, Parise LV: Structure and function of platelet alpha IIb beta 3. *Curr Opin Hematol* 4:317-322, 1997.

Risk Factors for Coronary Artery Disease

1. Duell PB, Malinow MR: Homocyst(e)ine: an important risk factor for atherosclerotic vascular disease. *Curr Opin Lipidol* 8:28-34, 1997.

2. Gensini GF, Comeglio M, Colella A: Classical risk factors and emerging elements in the risk profile for coronary artery disease. *Eur Heart J* 19 (Suppl A):53-61, 1998.

3. Watts GF, Burke V: Lipid-lowering trials in the primary and secondary prevention of coronary heart disease: new evidence, implications and outstanding issues. *Curr Opin Lipidol* 7:341-355, 1996.

Questions

Multiple Choice (choose the one best answer)

1. Which of the following platelet functions is inhibited by aspirin?
   a. Activation
   b. Aggregation
   c. Secretion
   d. Pseudopodia formation
   e. All of the above

2. Potential inhibitors of plasmin include all of the following *except*:
   a. α_2-Antiplasmin
   b. Plasminogen activator inhibitor-1
   c. α_2-Macroglobulin
   d. α_1-Antitrypsin
   e. Antithrombin III

3. Physiologic activation of the fibrinolytic system occurs via each of the following *except*:
   a. Tissue plasminogen activator
   b. Urokinase-type plasminogen activator
   c. Streptokinase
   d. High-molecular-weight kininogen

4. Platelet adhesion:
   a. Results in platelet-platelet interaction necessary for thrombus propagation
   b. Progresses as glycoprotein IIb-IIIa interacts with von Willebrand factor of the arterial wall
   c. Requires platelet activation by the G-protein second messenger system
   d. Is a shear-dependent process
   e. Is abnormal in afibrinogenemic patients

5. Thrombin activity may include all the following *except*:
   a. Cofactor VII activation
   b. Cleaving of fibrinogen to fibrin
   c. Chemotaxis for monocytes
   d. Mitogenesis for smooth muscle cells
   e. Anticoagulation

6. The following statements regarding hyperhomocysteinemia are true *except*:
   a. It predisposes the affected patient to premature atherosclerosis
   b. It may occur in association with chronic renal failure
   c. It is a known risk factor for deep vein thrombosis
   d. It may coincide with pernicious anemia
   e. Treatment with B complex vitamins (B_6, B_{12}, folate) reduces the risk of future arterial occlusive events

Answers

1. Answer e

Platelet activation is required for each of the functions listed. In fact, the only platelet process that does not require activation is adhesion. Depending on the agonist, aspirin may or may not be an effective platelet antagonist. Those agonists utilizing the cyclooxygenase pathway of arachidonate metabolism will be inhibited. Strong agonists (thrombin, platelet activating factor, and thromboxane A_2), however, are largely unaffected by either aspirin or ticlopidine.

2. Answer b

In vitro studies have shown that plasmin activity is blocked by several inhibitors, including α_2-antiplasmin, α_2-macroglobulin, α_1-antitrypsin, antithrombin III, C1 esterase inhibitor, and protease nexin. The most important physiologic inhibitor of these is α_2-antiplasmin, a plasma protein synthesized by the liver and also found in α granules of platelets. Plasminogen activator inhibitor (PAI-1) is a very important inhibitor of plasminogen activation, but not of plasmin. Like α_2-antiplasmin, PAI-1 is found in greatest abundance within the α granules of platelets.

3. Answer c

Each of the listed proteins may participate in plasminogen activation. Of the four, streptokinase is the only protein not involved in endogenous or physiologic plasminogen activation. Urokinase and tissue plasminogen activator are important endogenous activators of plasminogen. The degree to which the contact activator pathway (high-molecular-weight kininogen) participates in endogenous plasminogen activation is unclear. Unlike the other proteins, streptokinase is not an enzyme. Plasminogen activation by streptokinase occurs through its ability to bind plasminogen in such a way as to expose a plasminogen-active site. This exposure allows the plasminogen-streptokinase complex to activate a second molecule of plasminogen to plasmin.

4. Answer d

Platelet adhesion is governed by shear forces and provides an initial layer of platelets covering the arterial injury site. The principal platelet receptor involved in this process is glycoprotein Ib-IX, which binds von Willebrand factor within the injured vessel wall. The glycoprotein Ib-IX receptor does not require prior platelet activation for adhesion to occur normally. In that fibrinogen is not a primary ligand in this process, afibrinogenemic patients have normal platelet adhesion.

5. Answer a

Thrombin is the most potent endogenous procoagulant enzyme known, with many targets, including fibrinogen, platelets, and factor XIII. Thrombin activates cofactors V and VIII, thereby enhancing its own conversion from prothrombin. It has been shown in vitro to have both chemotactic and mitogenic activity, properties that have been invoked in the process of restenosis after percutaneous transluminal coronary angioplasty. When bound to thrombomodulin, thrombin becomes a potent stimulus for anticoagulation by changing substrate activity. In this setting, its only action is that of activating protein C, a potent endogenous anticoagulant. Thrombin is not known to activate factor VII.

6. Answer e

Hyperhomocysteinemia is a known risk factor for both arterial and venous thrombotic occlusive disorders. Among the causes of hyperhomocysteinemia are vitamin B complex deficiency and liver and renal disease. Although vitamin B complex supplementation reduces homocysteine levels, there are as yet no data with regard to alteration of the disease's natural history.

Arterial Injury

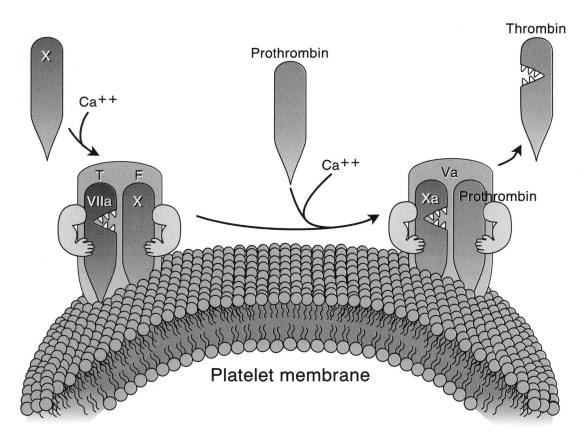

Plate 1. After plaque disruption and exposure to high shear forces, von Willebrand factor (vWF) bound to the subendothelium undergoes a structural change that enhances adhesion of circulating platelets (PLT) via receptor glycoprotein (gp) Ib-IX (*A*). Calcium-dependent activation of the coagulation system occurs as activation complexes assemble on the surface of these adherent platelets (*B*). Initial activation occurs by the tissue factor pathway, where tissue factor (TF) and cofactor Va serve as cofactors properly aligning the activating enzyme with the proenzyme.

Coagulation Vortex

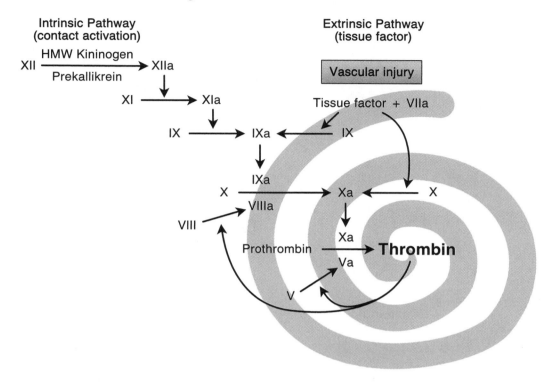

Plate 2. Coagulation activation after arterial injury occurs via the extrinsic (tissue factor) pathway. Once small amounts of thrombin have been generated, its activation is greatly amplified by incorporation of the intrinsic (contact activation) system. HMW, high-molecular-weight.

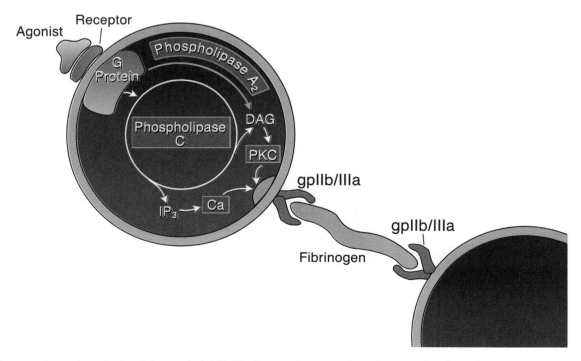

Plate 3. Platelet aggregation requires activation of glycoprotein (gp) IIb-IIIa via a second messenger G-protein system. One of several potential agonists may trigger this activation, which results in a configuration change of gp IIb-IIIa, allowing it to bind fibrinogen. Fibrinogen is the "bridging" protein that anchors one platelet to another by binding gp IIb-IIIa receptors of two adjacent platelets. DAG, diacylglycerol; IP_3, inositol-1,4,5-triphosphate; PKC, protein kinase C.

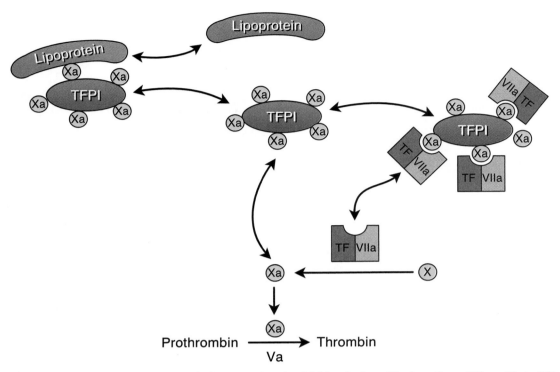

Plate 4. Tissue factor pathway inhibitor (TFPI) serves as both a reservoir and an inhibitor for factor Xa, tissue factor (TF), and factor VIIa, thereby finely regulating coagulation activation at the site of arterial injury. This reversible "sink" provides tissue factor and activated factors X and VII to initiate coagulation and then inhibits the process once factor Xa is in excess.

Anticoagulant Activity of Protein C/Protein S

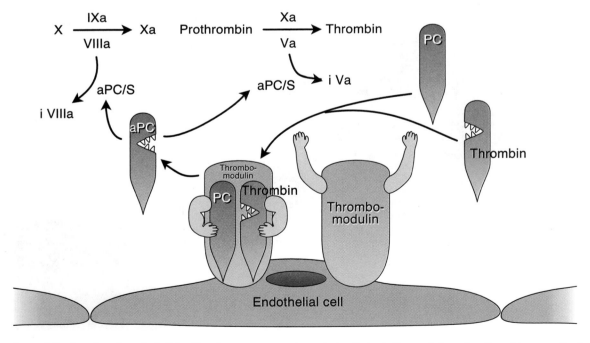

Plate 5. Thrombomodulin, found on the endothelial cell surface, serves as an important cofactor in the regulation of prothrombin generation by providing a site for protein C (PC) activation. Thrombin bound to thrombomodulin no longer participates in prothrombotic activity yet is able to activate protein C. Once activated, protein C in the setting of protein S (S) degrades cofactors VIIIa and Va, thereby terminating further prothrombin activation.

Chapter 83

Treatment and Prevention of Arterial Thrombosis

Robert D. McBane, M.D.

Current antithrombotic therapy targets three of the four stages of thrombus formation: platelet activation, platelet aggregation, and the coagulation factor cascade. Currently, no effective means exist to prevent initial platelet adhesion (the initial stage in thrombus formation) to either the injured vascular wall or to an intravascular prosthetic surface such as a prosthetic valve or intracoronary stent.

Platelet Inhibitors

Antiplatelet therapy is effective in preventing and treating atherothrombotic arterial events. Large clinical trials have documented a morbidity and mortality benefit in both myocardial infarction and stroke. The four major classes of antiplatelet agents are cyclooxygenase inhibitors, adenosine diphosphate (ADP) receptor antagonists, thrombin inhibitors, and platelet glycoprotein (gp) IIb/IIIa (recently renamed "gp $\alpha_{IIb}\beta_3$") receptor inhibitors. Cyclooxygenase inhibitors block platelet activation by agonist inhibition, whereas the gp IIb/IIIa receptor inhibitors block the final common pathway of platelet aggregation (Table 1). Because cyclooxygenase inhibitors and ADP receptor antagonists are relatively weak platelet inhibitors, they are better suited for secondary prevention of thrombotic events or as

adjuvant therapy when combined with the more powerful thrombolytic agents in the management of acute myocardial infarction and thrombotic stroke. Thrombin inhibitors and gp IIb/IIIa inhibitors are effective in acute arterial thrombosis and in the unstable coronary syndromes but are associated with bleeding complications (Table 2).

Platelet Activation

Cyclooxygenase Inhibitors

Weak agonists of platelet aggregation induce arachidonic acid conversion to thromboxane by the cyclooxygenase pathway in the platelet. After thromboxane is produced, it triggers platelet activation. Aspirin, by irreversibly acetylating cyclooxygenase, inhibits thromboxane synthesis and platelet aggregation by ADP and collagen. In healthy subjects, a single aspirin results in 98% inhibition of thromboxane production within 1 hour after ingestion. With discontinuation of aspirin use, cyclooxygenase recovery occurs as new platelets enter the circulation. Because the average life span of platelets is 9 to 11 days, sensitive assays of platelet aggregation may be abnormal for up to 10 days after a single dose of aspirin. A low dose of aspirin is effective antithrombotic prophylaxis for myocardial infarction

---

The acronyms and names of clinical trials mentioned in the text are listed in the Appendix.

Table 1.—Glycoprotein IIb/IIIa Inhibitors

Abciximab
Eptifibatide
Lamifiban
Roxifiban
Tirofiban
Xemilofiban

and stroke; yet alone, it is insufficient antithrombotic treatment for acute thrombotic events. Because gp IIb/IIIa receptor activation by strong agonists is not limited to the cyclooxygenase pathway, platelet activation by other agonists such as thrombin is relatively unaffected by aspirin.

Aspirin Trials

One low dose of aspirin, 81 mg/day, provides effective chronic cyclooxygenase inhibition for thrombotic prophylaxis. In acute coronary syndromes, a higher aspirin dose (162 mg or 325 mg) generally is used, as in the ISIS-2 myocardial infarction trial.

A primary prevention trial with aspirin was the Physicians Health Study, in which more than 22,000 physicians were assigned randomly to receive either 325 mg of aspirin every other day or placebo. At 5-year follow-up, those taking aspirin had a 44% risk reduction for both fatal and nonfatal myocardial infarction. This was at the expense of a non-statistically significant increase in the risk of stroke. In a substudy of physicians with chronic stable angina, aspirin did not affect the severity of angina but did significantly decrease the incidence of first myocardial infarction. Other studies have shown that aspirin not only reduces the risk of future myocardial infarction but attenuates the severity when it does occur. A similar aspirin prevention study performed in the United Kingdom in 5,139 physicians failed to show a statistically significant reduction in fatal or nonfatal coronary events, but the total of overall cardiovascular events was smaller than predicted. Transient ischemic attacks were decreased in frequency by 50%; however, stroke was non-statistically increased in aspirin users.

The United Kingdom-TIA aspirin study compared 300 mg or 1,200 mg of aspirin daily with placebo in patients who had a transient ischemic attack or minor stroke. Aspirin therapy resulted in an 18% decrease in major stroke, myocardial infarction, or death. There was no difference in outcome between the lower and the higher dose of aspirin, but

the incidence of gastrointestinal side effects was significantly greater in the higher dose group.

At least four well-designed clinical trials are studying the efficacy of aspirin in unstable angina. Aspirin has been shown consistently to reduce the risk for both myocardial infarction and death, in comparison with placebo.

A theoretic disadvantage of aspirin is nonselective arachidonate pathway inhibition, blocking not only thromboxane but also prostacyclin production. Prostacyclin is a potent vasodilator and an endogenous inhibitor of platelet aggregation. In contrast to platelets, which lack protein synthetic machinery, endothelial cell production of prostaglandins recovers within several hours after aspirin administration as new unacetylated cyclooxygenase is synthesized. Other nonaspirin nonsteroidal anti-inflammatory drugs reversibly inhibit cyclooxygenase, with the duration of inhibition depending on the dose, serum level, and half-life of the drug.

More specific prostaglandin antagonists include the thromboxane synthase inhibitors (ridogrel) and receptor blockers (ifetroban, vapiprost). These agents not only limit thromboxane production and activity but also cause an accumulation of prostacyclin precursors. Early clinical experience with ridogrel has failed to show superiority over aspirin in fibrinolytic therapy.

Ticlopidine/Clopidogrel

ADP, a weak but important agonist of platelet activation, is abundant in platelet storage granules and activates platelets by a specific cell surface receptor. Ticlopidine and clopidogrel irreversibly inhibit the platelet ADP receptor. Full

Table 2.—Inhibitors of Platelet Activation

Agonist	Inhibitor
Thrombin	Argatroban
	Danaparoid
	Heparin
	Hirudin
	Low-molecular-weight heparin
	Warfarin
ADP	Clopidogrel
	Ticlopidine
Thromboxane A_2	Aspirin
	Ifetroban
	Ridogrel
	Vapiprost

ADP, adenosine diphosphate.

platelet inhibition requires 3 to 5 days of therapy and persists until platelet turnover has generated a new population of platelets.

Ticlopidine has been shown to be effective in secondary prevention trials of myocardial infarction and may be superior to aspirin in stroke. Compared with warfarin plus aspirin, combined antiplatelet therapy with ticlopidine and aspirin after coronary artery stenting reduced the incidence of myocardial infarction and stent thrombosis and the need for repeat percutaneous transluminal coronary angioplasty (PTCA), with fewer vascular access and hemorrhagic complications. This benefit observed at 30 days appears to be durable throughout the first year after the procedure. The STIMS trial compared ticlopidine with placebo in 687 patients with intermittent claudication and found a relative risk reduction of 30% for all-cause mortality and a 50% reduction of fatal vascular events. Ticlopidine significantly improves long-term patency of saphenous vein bypass grafts to the lower extremity compared with placebo. Diarrhea and neutropenia are potential adverse effects, which require close monitoring and discontinuation of treatment in 2% and 1% of patients, respectively.

Clopidogrel, a newer agent of the same class as ticlopidine, does not cause neutropenia. The CAPRIE trial compared clopidogrel with aspirin in 19,185 patients who had a recent stroke, myocardial infarction, or symptomatic peripheral arterial occlusive disease. After nearly 2 years of follow-up, there was an 8.7% relative risk reduction in favor of clopidogrel for the composite end points of stroke, myocardial infarction, and vascular death. Other clinical investigations of this drug are under way. The combined clinical data for ticlopidine and clopidogrel underscore the importance of ADP as an in vivo platelet agonist.

GP IIb/IIIa Inhibitors

The final common pathway between platelet aggregation and coagulation factor activation is the binding of fibrinogen to activated gp IIb/IIIa receptors on numerous adjacent platelets. Receptor blockade, by inhibiting fibrinogen binding, prevents platelet aggregation regardless of the initiating agonist (Plates 1 and 2). The inhibitors of gp IIb/IIIa receptors can be subdivided into anti-gp IIb/IIIa monoclonal antibodies, viper venoms, RGD (arginine, glycine, aspartic acid), and peptide and nonpeptide analogs.

Abciximab (ReoPro), previously known as "c7E3," is the chimeric Fab fragment of a murine monoclonal antibody against the activated gp IIb/IIIa receptor. Infusion of this antibody produces prolonged and extensive receptor blockade, with marked inhibition of platelet aggregation and bleeding times. Successful treatment with abciximab requires that most (90%) gp IIb/IIIa receptors be occupied by the antibody. Clinical efficacy has been documented in unstable angina, with a significant reduction in ischemic events and angiographic improvement of the coronary lesions. In combination with recombinant tissue plasminogen activator (rt-PA) for the treatment of acute myocardial infarction, abciximab improved patency rates.

EPIC and EPILOG Trials

Two abciximab trials, the EPIC and EPILOG trials, involved patients undergoing high-risk angioplasty and comprise the largest clinical experience with this drug. Abciximab, given as a bolus plus a 12-hour infusion, resulted in a 35% reduction in ischemic complications, especially in patients with unstable coronary syndromes. Abciximab was given in conjunction with standard doses of heparin and aspirin and resulted in significantly increased bleeding complications and transfusion requirements. The subsequent EPILOG study included patients who were undergoing urgent or elective PTCA, and concomitant heparin therapy was reduced significantly to improve clinical safety. Abciximab in combination with a reduced dose of heparin resulted in a 68% decrease in 30-day mortality and myocardial infarction, with the rate of bleeding complications similar to that of placebo.

Six-month follow-up data from the EPIC trial suggested that treatment with abciximab decreases the rate of clinical restenosis. The mechanism behind this is unclear but may be related to the antibody cross-reactivity with a second receptor, $\alpha_v\beta_3$, the vitronectin receptor. Platelets, in addition to providing a scaffold for coagulation factor assembly, contain storage granules rich in growth factors. By limiting platelet aggregation at the site of vascular injury, abciximab may decrease the release of these platelet growth factors and the generation of thrombin, both of which have been implicated in the pathogenesis of restenosis.

The CAPTURE study assessed the efficacy of abciximab in patients with refractory unstable angina who were undergoing PTCA. More than 1,200 patients were assigned randomly to receive abciximab intravenously or placebo for 18 to 24 hours before PTCA and for 1 hour after PTCA. At 30 days, ischemic events were reduced significantly in the abciximab group. After 6 months of follow-up, however, death, myocardial infarction, or need for repeat intervention was equivalent in the two treatment groups.

Nonpeptide GP IIb/IIIa Receptor Inhibitors

The gp IIb/IIIa receptor recognition of the amino acid sequence RGD (arginine, glycine, aspartic acid) on the fibrinogen molecule permits binding of the receptor to this protein. By occupying these receptor sites, synthetic RGD peptides competitively inhibit fibrinogen platelet receptor interaction and thereby prevent aggregation. Several RGD nonpeptide mimetics including lamifiban, tirofiban, xemilofiban, and roxifiban are bioavailable in both intravenous and oral formulations, an important feature when considering long-term platelet inhibition for thrombotic syndromes.

In a study of 2,139 patients with acute coronary syndromes undergoing PTCA, the RESTORE investigators assessed the efficacy of tirofiban in the reduction of composite end points, including all-cause mortality and recurrent ischemic events. Within 2 days after intervention, a highly significant 38% relative risk reduction of composite end points was noted in the tirofiban group. By 7 days, the relative reduction was 27% and at 30 days, 16%, still in favor of tirofiban although no longer statistically significant. The rate of major bleeding was not different between the two groups.

In the Canadian Lamifiban Trial, 365 patients with unstable angina were randomly assigned to one or four doses of lamifiban or placebo given intravenously for 72 to 120 hours. The combined lamifiban groups reduced the risk of death, myocardial infarction, or revascularization by 69% over placebo at 1 month follow-up.

Eptifibatide (Integrilin) is a cyclic heptapeptide containing a modified KGD sequence in which arginine (R) is replaced by lysine (K). This short-acting inhibitor was modeled after the venom of the southeastern pygmy rattlesnake. The lysine substitution provides greater inhibition specificity for gp IIb/IIIa than for other integrins containing the RGD sequence. The IMPACT-II trial compared two doses of eptifibatide with placebo in 4,010 patients undergoing elective, urgent, or emergent coronary intervention. The lower of the two doses reduced rates of early abrupt closure and ischemic events at 30 days compared with placebo. This effect was not significantly (statistically) better at the higher dose of eptifibatide.

These trials stress the importance of platelets in acute arterial syndromes and suggest that gp IIb/IIIa inhibitors are effective in reducing adverse outcomes during high-risk angioplasty and in the initial treatment of unstable angina or myocardial infarction. More studies are needed to determine their long-range efficacy and the role of oral gp IIb/IIIa inhibitors in chronic platelet suppression.

Thrombin Inhibitors

Hirudin, Hirugen, Hirulog

Thrombin, the most potent platelet agonist known, is directly involved in both platelet aggregation and thrombus propagation. Thrombin has two sites important for enzymatic activity: the exosite, which provides substrate recognition and interaction, and the catalytic active site, which cleaves the substrate. Hirudin, a specific and irreversible thrombin inhibitor derived from leach saliva, wraps around the thrombin molecule and inhibits both of these sites. Inhibition of thrombin by hirudin blocks platelet aggregation and limits platelet deposition to a monolayer at the site of injury. This finding led to the development of many thrombin inhibitors, of which hirudin is the reference standard. Unlike heparin, hirudin does not require antithrombin III or other cofactors for inhibitory activity. Clot-bound thrombin, an important thrombotic risk factor inaccessible to the antithrombin III–heparin complex, is effectively inhibited by hirudin. Hirudin therapy can be monitored with standard activated partial thromboplastin time (aPTT) clotting assays. Immunogenicity of this agent is low, with no reported associated allergic phenomena. Several hirudin analogues have been developed, including hirulog and hirugen. Hirulog (bivalirudin), similar to its parent compound, binds both the active site and the anion exosite. Hirugen, or "hirudin tail," inhibits only the exosite, leaving the active site unoccupied. The efficacy of hirugen underscores the importance of this exosite in normal thrombin-substrate interactions. Although highly effective antithrombotic agents, recent fibrinolytic trials with hirudin were stopped prematurely because of unacceptable rates of bleeding complications, including intracranial hemorrhage.

Three trials, the OASIS pilot study, GUSTO IIb, and TIMI 9B, compared hirudin with heparin in patients with either unstable angina or myocardial infarction. Within the first week after randomization, the results were promising in favor of hirudin therapy; however, the benefits did not persist in either the TIMI 9B or the GUSTO IIb trials. Moderate bleeding was more common in the hirudin-treated patients of the OASIS and GUSTO trials.

The Helvetica trial compared heparin with hirudin in the prevention of restenosis following coronary angioplasty. Hirudin resulted in a significant reduction in early cardiac events; however, at 6 months there was no difference in angiographic restenosis rates. Similar results were reported for hirulog in a separate trial of PTCA for unstable or post-infarction angina. Whether the modest clinical benefit of hirudin will justify the risk of hemorrhage is not known; however, the potential risk has limited the enthusiasm for this family of inhibitors. Other synthetic thrombin inhibitors such as argatroban have similar hemorrhagic side effects.

Heparin

Heparin is the mainstay of therapy for most thrombotic disorders. Its anticoagulant properties are mediated through its interaction with antithrombin III. By inducing a conformational change in antithrombin III, heparin potentiates the affinity of antithrombin III for thrombin by about 1,000-fold. Once formed, the thrombin-antithrombin III complex is essentially irreversible. Heparin is a highly negatively charged proteoglycan extracted from either porcine or bovine intestinal mucosa. Nonspecific binding to various cells and plasma proteins neutralizes its anticoagulant activity. Unfractionated heparin preparations are heterogeneous and contain heparin chains of various lengths and molecular weights, ranging from 5,000 to 50,000 kd. Unpredictable volume of distribution and elimination kinetics require that therapy with unfractionated heparin be strictly monitored by serial aPTT for safety and efficacy. With a weight-adjusted nomogram, only 82% of patients will reach the therapeutic range within 24 hours, with a 5% to 7% risk of major hemorrhage. Despite these imperfections, the efficacy of heparin in acute arterial occlusive syndromes is well established. Compared with placebo, unfractionated heparin markedly reduces acute myocardial infarction, refractory angina, and mortality in patients with unstable angina. In the prethrombolytic era, unfractionated heparin decreased both the rate of reinfarction and mortality after acute myocardial infarction. As an adjuvant to thrombolytic therapy, heparin improves early patency and may improve survival.

Low-Molecular-Weight Heparin

Low-molecular-weight heparin (LMWH) is produced by depolymerizing unfractionated heparin with either chemical or enzymatic methods. This yields a preparation of small heparin fragments of a more uniform molecular weight (4,000 to 6,000 kd). LMWH requires antithrombin III for activity; yet, unlike its parent compound, it has a higher specificity for factor Xa than thrombin. Because of its uniformity of size and less negative charge, LMWH has much less nonspecific binding to plasma proteins, improved bioavailability, and more predictable pharmacokinetics. Dosing of LMWH is based on patient body weight, and aPTT monitoring is neither required nor useful. Several potential anticoagulant advantages also favor LMWH over unfractionated heparin. First, platelet factor 4 secreted by activated platelets blocks the interaction between antithrombin III and heparin but not LMWH. Second, factor Xa bound to the platelet surface within the prothrombin activation complex is inaccessible to heparin-antithrombin III, whereas LMWH-antithrombin III can inhibit factor Xa under these circumstances.

The greatest experience with LMWH has been with prophylaxis for deep vein thrombosis following orthopedic procedures. In this setting, LMWH has been shown to be safe, effective, and convenient. More recent studies have provided efficacy data for the treatment of deep vein thrombosis, pulmonary embolism, and arterial thrombosis.

In the ESSENCE study, 3,171 patients with unstable angina or non-Q-wave myocardial infarction received treatment with either LMWH (enoxaparin) or unfractionated heparin. Enoxaparin therapy resulted in a significant reduction of angina, myocardial infarction, or death compared with unfractionated heparin, with fewer bleeding complications. This benefit persisted for 30 days, with fewer patients in the enoxaparin group requiring revascularization. In contrast, the FRIC study, which compared LMWH (dalteparin) with unfractionated heparin in patients with unstable angina, showed no difference between the two groups for composite cardiac end points. The different outcomes of these two trials is difficult to explain and may reflect differences in efficacy of the two LMWH preparations. Nonetheless, LMWH is at least as effective as standard heparin in managing arterial occlusive syndromes. The dose of LMWH is weight-adjusted, given once or twice daily subcutaneously depending on the formulation, and does not require laboratory monitoring.

LMWH in Deep Vein Thrombosis

Two large studies evaluated the safety and efficacy of LMWH compared with standard heparin in the treatment of acute proximal deep vein thrombosis. The difference between the groups in recurrent thrombosis, major bleeding, or mortality was not significant. The mean hospital stay was significantly shorter in the LMWH group, with up to 50% of patients treated entirely on an outpatient basis. The investigators concluded that patients with acute proximal deep vein thrombosis can be treated safely and effectively with LMWH at home and not require hospitalization during the initiation of warfarin therapy.

LMWH in Pulmonary Embolism

Two studies considered LMWH in the treatment of pulmonary embolism. In these studies, 1,633 patients were randomly assigned to LMWH or heparin while warfarin therapy was being initiated. The primary end points of recurrent venous thromboembolism, major hemorrhage, and mortality were not statistically different between the two groups in either trial. It was concluded that LMWH is a safe and effective treatment of pulmonary embolism and deep vein thrombosis.

Heparin-Induced Thrombocytopenia

Heparin-induced thrombocytopenia (HIT) or heparin-induced thrombocytopenia with thrombosis (HITT) is an immune response to heparin-platelet factor-4 complex. Immunoglobulins induced by these complexes may activate platelets directly by binding to the platelet FcII receptors or indirectly by inducing cytokine production and complement activation. In patients receiving heparin, heparin-induced thrombocytopenia should be suspected when the platelet count decreases to less than 100,000/µL or decreases by more than 40% from the basal platelet count. This occurs in 1.3% of patients receiving therapeutic doses of porcine heparin. Heparin-induced thrombocytopenia is more common with bovine heparin and less common with prophylactic doses or LMWH preparations. The diagnosis is confirmed by in vitro testing either directly by identifying the antibody or indirectly by documenting platelet aggregation induced by mixing heparin and donor platelets with the patient's plasma. Thrombocytopenia may occur 3 to 15 days after the initiation of heparin therapy. In patients previously exposed to heparin, however, platelet counts can begin to decrease within hours after treatment. The incidence of thrombosis in heparin-induced thrombocytopenia ranges from 0.2% to 20%, may involve the arterial or venous circulation, and results in mortality rates as high as 30%. Treatment includes discontinuation of heparin, which results in a return of the platelet count to baseline within 4 days. Prolonged thrombocytopenia of 1 to 2 weeks has been observed. Acceptable alternative anticoagulants include the heparinoid compound danaparoid or other thrombin inhibitors such as the hirudin analogues or argatroban. Because of significant cross-reactivity, LMWH is not an acceptable alternative for these patients.

Warfarin

Warfarin blocks the hepatic carboxylation of vitamin K-dependent coagulation factors, thus inhibiting the activation of the proenzyme to the enzyme. Carboxylation is required for the calcium binding and shape reconfiguration necessary for incorporation of the protein into activation complexes on the phospholipid bilayer. With either the inhibition of carboxylation or calcium sequestration (with citrate, EDTA, etc.), coagulation factor activation is brought to a standstill.

The clinical efficacy of warfarin in venous thromboembolism and atrial fibrillation is universally acknowledged. Its role in the treatment of acute and chronic coronary arterial occlusive syndromes is less clear. In the prethrombolytic era, several post-myocardial infarction studies documented a significant reduction in recurrent myocardial infarction, stroke, and mortality in those receiving warfarin anticoagulation. The ASPECT trial randomly assigned patients with a recent myocardial infarction to warfarin at a goal prothrombin-time international normalized ratio (INR) of between 2.8 and 4.8 or to placebo. At 37-month follow-up, the decrease in the rate of recurrent myocardial infarction and stroke was statistically significant; however, no mortality benefit was shown between the two groups. The ATACS study compared warfarin plus aspirin with aspirin alone in 214 patients with unstable angina or non-Q-wave myocardial infarction. At the end of the trial, there was a trend favoring the warfarin-aspirin group in the reduction of recurrent angina, myocardial infarction, or death. The CARS investigators hypothesized that the addition of a small fixed dose of warfarin added to aspirin would add the benefit of an antithrombotic agent to an antiplatelet agent without increasing either the risk of bleeding or the complexity of the treatment regimen. The study was stopped prematurely by the Data and Safety Monitoring Committee because of the similar efficacy of treatment strategies. In summary, the role of warfarin anticoagulation in the secondary prevention of acute coronary syndromes is unclear and still a matter of controversy.

Bleeding complications have limited the enthusiasm for warfarin therapy, especially in elderly patients. In the SPAF II study, at an approximate prothrombin-time INR of between 2.0 and 4.5, major hemorrhage occurred at a rate of 2.3% per year, compared with 1.1% per year for aspirin. Age, increasing number of prescribed medications, and intensity of anticoagulation were independent risks for bleeding. In patients younger than 75 years, the rate of major hemorrhage was 1.7% per year, compared with 4.2% per year in older patients. Other variables associated with excessive anticoagulation include advanced malignancy, potentiating medications such as antibiotics or acetaminophen, anorexia, and diarrheal illnesses.

Fibrinolytic Agents

The mainstay of medical treatment for acute arterial thrombosis, including myocardial infarction, massive pulmonary embolus, and thrombotic stroke, is the plasminogen activating agents: streptokinase, rt-PA, urokinase, and their derivatives. Unlike endogenous fibrinolysis, which is marked by clot specificity, pharmacologic plasminogen activation is indiscriminate in substrate preference and degrades fibrin, fibrinogen, platelet receptors, and coagulation factors. Streptokinase, uniquely among the plasminogen activators, is not an enzyme and, thus, cannot directly activate plasminogen. Purified from β-hemolytic streptococci, streptokinase promotes fibrinolysis by inducing a conformational change of the plasminogen molecule and exposing the enzymatic active site. The streptokinase-plasminogen complex then cleaves a second plasminogen molecule to active plasmin. Although streptokinase does not have a fibrin-binding site, this process is accelerated in the presence of fibrin and is somewhat clot specific.

Anisolated plasminogen streptokinase activator complex (APSAC) is a complex of streptokinase already bound to plasminogen. This complex has increased specificity for fibrin and is not inhibited by endogenous inhibitors of plasminogen systems. APSAC has a plasma half-life 2 to 3 times longer (70 minutes) than that of streptokinase (25 minutes) and, thus, can be given as a single bolus rather than as a prolonged infusion. Because streptokinase and APSAC are foreign proteins, neutralizing antibodies develop and limit the efficacy of repetitive use of these agents.

Staphylokinase, a protein produced by *Staphylococcus aureus*, activates plasminogen similarly to streptokinase. Staphylokinase is fibrin-specific and is less inhibited by α_2-antiplasmin. Although staphylokinase is effective in the treatment of acute myocardial infarction, it has been associated with the induction of high titers of neutralizing antibody formation. Thus, like streptokinase, its use is limited to a single infusion.

Purified and recombinant forms of endogenous plasminogen activators have become widely used for local delivery and systemic fibrinolysis in many arterial and venous thrombotic disorders. These endogenous agents, including rt-PA, urokinase, single-chain urokinase (scu-PA or pro-urokinase), act directly on plasminogen. Agent superiority and clinical indication are debated; however, in vivo plasminogen activation is likely comparable, with minimal differences in clot specificity between agents. In contrast to bacterial proteins, these agents are nonimmunogenic and, thus, can be reinstituted. Although effective in thrombolysis, endogenous inhibitors of plasminogen activation such as plasminogen activator inhibitor-1 (PAI-1) are abundant in platelet α-granules. With platelet activation, PAI-1 is released from α-granules, thereby inhibiting local plasminogen activation. This may explain the 20% to 40% failure rate of pharmacologic fibrinolytic therapy.

Stroke and Thrombolysis

One of the most devastating complications of thrombolytic therapy is stroke. The overall risk in the GUSTO trial was 1.4% and was lower in patients receiving streptokinase (1.19%) than in those receiving rt-PA (1.55%). Of all strokes, 45% were fatal and 31% were disabling. Primary intracranial hemorrhage occurred in 45% of the strokes and resulted in a 60% mortality. Hemorrhagic conversion of a cerebral infarct into a hemorrhagic stroke occurred in only 10% of the other stroke patients, with a 32% case fatality rate. Advanced age, previous cerebrovascular disease, and hypertension were significant predictors of intracranial hemorrhage. Severe or life-threatening hemorrhage, defined as either intracranial hemorrhage or hemodynamic compromise requiring treatment, occurred in 0.3% to 0.5% of patients and was similar in all groups. Moderate hemorrhage occurred with an overall frequency of 5% to 6% and was statistically less frequent for patients treated with rt-PA.

Suggested Review Reading

Aspirin

1. Willard JE, Lange RA, Hillis LD: The use of aspirin in ischemic heart disease. *N Engl J Med* 327:175-181, 1992.

Ticlopidine/Clopidogrel

1. Anonymous: A randomised, blinded, trial of clopidogrel versus aspirin in patients at risk of ischaemic events (CAPRIE). CAPRIE Steering Committee. *Lancet* 348:1329-1339, 1996.

2. Balsano F, Rizzon P, Violi F, et al: Antiplatelet treatment with ticlopidine in unstable angina. A controlled multicenter clinical trial. The Studio della Ticlopidina nell'Angina Instabile Group. *Circulation* 82:17-26, 1990.

3. Berger PB, Bell MR, Grill DE, et al: Frequency of adverse clinical events in the 12 months following successful intracoronary stent placement in patients treated with aspirin and ticlopidine (without warfarin). *Am J Cardiol* 81:713-718, 1998.

4. Hass WK, Easton JD, Adams HP Jr, et al: A randomized trial comparing ticlopidine hydrochloride with aspirin for the prevention of stroke in high-risk patients. *N Engl J Med* 321:501-507, 1989.

Hirudin/Hirulog/Hirugen

1. Antman EM: Hirudin in acute myocardial infarction. Thrombolysis and Thrombin Inhibition in Myocardial Infarction (TIMI) 9B trial. *Circulation* 94:911-921, 1996.

2. Bittl JA, Strony J, Brinker JA, et al: Treatment with bivalirudin (Hirulog) as compared with heparin during coronary angioplasty for unstable or postinfarction angina. *N Engl J Med* 333:764-769, 1995.

3. The Global Use of Strategies to Open Occluded Coronary Arteries (GUSTO) IIb Investigators: A comparison of recombinant hirudin with heparin for the treatment of acute coronary syndromes. *N Engl J Med* 335:775-782, 1996.

4. Organization to Assess Strategies for Ischemic Syndromes (OASIS) Investigators: Comparison of the effects of two doses of recombinant hirudin compared with heparin in patients with acute myocardial ischemia without ST elevation: a pilot study. *Circulation* 96:769-777, 1997.

5. Serruys PW, Herrman JP, Simon R, et al: A comparison of hirudin with heparin in the prevention of restenosis after coronary angioplasty. *N Engl J Med* 333:757-763, 1995.

Heparin/LMW Heparin

1. Cohen M, Demers C, Gurfinkel EP, et al: A comparison of low-molecular-weight heparin with unfractionated heparin for unstable coronary artery disease. *N Engl J Med* 337:447-452, 1997.

2. The Columbus Investigators: Low-molecular-weight heparin in the treatment of patients with venous thromboembolism. *N Engl J Med* 337:657-662, 1997.

3. Fragmin during Instability in Coronary Artery Disease (FRISC) Study Group: Low-molecular-weight heparin during instability in coronary artery disease. *Lancet* 347:561-568, 1996.

4. Hirsh J: Heparin. *N Engl J Med* 324:1565-1574, 1991.

5. Hirsh J, Levine MN: Low molecular weight heparin. *Blood* 79:1-17, 1992.

6. Levine M, Gent M, Hirsh J, et al: A comparison of low-molecular-weight heparin administered primarily at home with unfractionated heparin administered in the hospital for proximal deep-vein thrombosis. *N Engl J Med* 334:677-681, 1996.

7. McCrae KR, Cines DB: Drug induced thrombocytopenias. In *Thrombosis and Hemorrhage*. Edited by J Loscalzo, AI Schafer. Boston, Blackwell Scientific Publications, 1994, pp 552-558.

8. Theroux P, Ouimet H, McCans J, et al: Aspirin, heparin, or both to treat acute unstable angina. *N Engl J Med* 319:1105-1111, 1988.

GP IIb/IIIa Inhibitors

1. Anonymous: Randomised placebo-controlled trial of abciximab before and during coronary intervention in refractory unstable angina: the CAPTURE Study. *Lancet* 349:1429-1435, 1997.

2. Anonymous: Randomised placebo-controlled trial of effect of eptifibatide on complications of percutaneous coronary intervention: IMPACT-II. *Lancet* 349:1422-1428, 1997.

3. The EPILOG Investigators: Platelet glycoprotein IIb/IIIa receptor blockade and low-dose heparin during percutaneous coronary revascularization. *N Engl J Med* 336:1689-1696, 1997.

4. Lincoff AM, Califf RM, Anderson KM, et al: Evidence for prevention of death and myocardial infarction with platelet membrane glycoprotein IIb/IIIa receptor blockade by abciximab (c7E3 Fab) among patients with unstable angina undergoing percutaneous coronary revascularization. *J Am Coll Cardiol* 30:149-156, 1997.

5. The RESTORE Investigators: Effects of platelet glycoprotein IIb/IIIa blockade with tirofiban on adverse cardiac events in patients with unstable angina or acute myocardial infarction undergoing coronary angioplasty. *Circulation* 96:1445-1453, 1997.

6. Theroux P, Kouz S, Roy L, et al: Platelet membrane receptor glycoprotein IIb/IIIa antagonism in unstable angina. The Canadian Lamifiban Study. *Circulation* 94:899-905, 1996.

Warfarin

1. Cohen M, Adams PC, Parry G, et al: Combination antithrombotic therapy in unstable rest angina and non-Q-wave infarction in nonprior aspirin users. Primary end points analysis from the ATACS trial. *Circulation* 89:81-88, 1994.

2. Coumadin Aspirin Reinfarction Study (CARS) Investigators: Randomised double-blind trial of fixed low-dose warfarin with aspirin after myocardial infarction. *Lancet* 350:389-396, 1997.

3. Smith P, Arnesen H, Holme I: The effect of warfarin on mortality and reinfarction after myocardial infarction. *N Engl J Med* 323:147-152, 1990.

4. Stroke Prevention in Atrial Fibrillation Investigators: Warfarin versus aspirin for prevention of thromboembolism in atrial fibrillation: Stroke Prevention in Atrial Fibrillation II Study. *Lancet* 343:687-691, 1994.

Fibrinolytic Agents

1. Collen D, Lijnen HR: Molecular basis of fibrinolysis, as relevant for thrombolytic therapy. *Thromb Haemost* 74:167-171, 1995.

2. The GUSTO Angiographic Investigators: The effects of tissue plasminogen activator, streptokinase, or both on coronary-artery patency, ventricular function, and survival after acute myocardial infarction. *N Engl J Med* 329:1615-1622, 1993.

3. The GUSTO Investigators: An international randomized trial comparing four thrombolytic strategies for acute myocardial infarction. *N Engl J Med* 329:673-682, 1993.

Appendix

Acronyms and Names of Clinical Trials Mentioned in the Text

ASPECT	Anticoagulants in the Secondary Prevention of Events in Coronary Thrombosis
ATACS	Antithrombotic Therapy in Acute Coronary Syndromes
CAPRIE	Clopidogrel Versus Aspirin in Patients at Risk of Ischaemic Events
CAPTURE	c7E3 Fab Antiplatelet Therapy in Unstable Refractory Angina
CARS	Coumadin Aspirin Reinfarction Study
EPIC	Evaluation of 7E3 for the Prevention of Ischemic Complications
EPILOG	Evaluation in PTCA to Improve Long-Term Outcome With Abciximab GP IIa/IIIb Blockade
ESSENCE	Efficacy and Safety of Subcutaneous Enoxaparin in Non-Q-Wave Coronary Events
FRIC	Fragmin in Unstable Coronary Artery Disease Study
FRISC	Fragmin During Instability in Coronary Artery Disease
GUSTO	Global Use of Strategies to Open Occluded Coronary Arteries
IMPACT	Integrilin to Minimise Platelet Aggregation and Coronary Thrombosis
ISIS	International Study of Infarct Survival
OASIS	Organization to Assess Strategies for Ischemic Syndromes
RESTORE	Randomized Efficacy Study of Tirofiban for Outcomes and Restenosis
SPAF	Stroke Prevention in Atrial Fibrillation
STIMS	Swedish Ticlopidine Multicenter Study
TIMI	Thrombolysis and Thrombin Inhibition in Myocardial Infarction

Questions

Multiple Choice (choose the one best answer)

1. Which of the following platelet functions can be inhibited by the new class of antagonist, gp IIb/IIIa inhibitors?
   a. Adhesion
   b. Activation
   c. Aggregation
   d. Secretion
   e. Pseudopod formation

2. Hirudin and its derivatives hirulog and hirugen exert antithrombotic activity through the inhibition of:
   a. Thrombin
   b. Platelet activation
   c. Platelet aggregation
   d. Fibrinogen cleavage
   e. All the above

3. Therapy with low-molecular-weight heparin can best be monitored by which of the following coagulation assays?
   a. Activated partial thromboplastin time (aPTT)
   b. Prothrombin time INR
   c. Russell's viper venom time
   d. Activated clot time
   e. Anti-factor Xa activity

4. Correct statements about the thienopyridine class of platelet antagonists (ticlopidine, clopidogrel) include:
   a. Ticlopidine and clopidogrel therapy both are associated with a significant risk of neutropenia
   b. In the CAPRIE trial, ticlopidine was superior to aspirin for the composite end point of stroke, myocardial infarction, or vascular death
   c. This class of drug fully inhibits platelet activity within hours after ingestion
   d. Platelet inhibition occurs through irreversible blockade of the ADP receptor
   e. Reversibility of platelet inhibition is temporally related to the half-life of the parent molecule

5. True statements about heparin-induced thrombocytopenia (HIT) include all of the following *except*:
   a. The incidence of HIT is higher in bovine heparin preparations compared with porcine preparations
   b. The diagnosis of HIT should be considered in patients treated with heparin whose platelet count decreases to below 100,000
   c. In patients with documented HIT, reasonable alternative therapy includes low-molecular-weight heparin
   d. Normalization of the platelet count despite ongoing heparin therapy does not alleviate the risk of thrombotic complications
   e. HIT may occur after trivial heparin exposure (i.e., heparin flushes)

6. Anticoagulation with warfarin
   a. Blocks synthesis of coagulation factors by the liver
   b. Inhibits post-translational hepatic glycosylation of coagulation factors
   c. Limits coagulation factor calcium binding
   d. Inhibits the active site of the cleaving enzyme as it participates in the platelet-bound activation complex

7. True statements about platelet gp IIb/IIIa receptor and its inhibitors include:
   a. GP IIb/IIIa inhibition has been shown to be effective therapy in the acute setting of unstable angina and high-risk angioplasty
   b. These inhibitors work by effective blockade of platelet adhesion
   c. Use of these inhibitors provides effective inhibition of platelet activation
   d. Following myocardial infarction, prolonged therapy with oral gp IIb/IIIa inhibitors has been shown to reduce risk of reinfarction, death, or need for revascularization compared with placebo

Answers

1. Answer c

The only platelet function listed that requires normal gp IIb/IIIa activity is aggregation or thrombus propagation. Platelet adhesion is a gp Ib/IX receptor-mediated activity and is not affected by gp IIb/IIIa antagonists. Once adherent to the injured vessel wall, platelet spreading likely involves both gp Ib/IX and gp IIb/IIIa receptors. Platelet activation, secretion, and pseudopod formation are not gp IIb/IIIa-mediated processes.

2. Answer e

Hirudin is a specific inhibitor of thrombin. Originally, it was derived from leach saliva but now is available in a recombinant form. To date, no cross-reactivity of inhibition has been reported with any other enzyme. In that thrombin is the most potent platelet agonist known, inhibition with hirudin similarly produces potent platelet antagonism. By inhibiting thrombin, hirudin effectively blocks the cleavage of fibrinogen to fibrin. A potent antithrombotic agent, hirudin has great potential, especially in situations of heparin contraindication such as heparin-induced thrombocytopenia.

3. Answer e

Unlike its parent compound, therapy with low-molecular-weight heparin has predictable pharmacokinetics and, thus, does not require laboratory monitoring for either safety or efficacy. Because it is insensitive to the aPTT or prothrombin time, if monitoring is necessary, the most reliable assay is anti-factor Xa activity. For prophylactic measures against deep vein thrombosis, 0.4 to 0.7 anti-factor Xa unit appears sufficient. For full anticoagulant activity, 0.7 to 1.0 is the effective range.

4. Answer d

Both ticlopidine and clopidogrel are inactive until they undergo extensive first-pass metabolism in the liver. Platelet inhibition occurs when the active metabolite irreversibly binds to the platelet ADP receptor. Platelet activity returns to normal only after new platelets are released into the circulation from the bone marrow. Unlike ticlopidine, clopidogrel, studied in the CAPRIE trial, does not cause significant neutropenia.

5. Answer c

Although the in vitro testing with low-molecular-weight heparin may not induce spontaneous platelet aggregation, this is not an acceptable alternative therapy in patients with documented HIT. Treatment must include discontinuation of all heparin products and initiation of alternative anticoagulants such as danaparoid. Danaparoid, a heparinoid, has cross-reactivity with standard heparin of approximately 20%.

6. Answer c

By inhibiting vitamin K-dependent carboxylation, coagulation factors (VII, IX, X, and prothrombin) are unable to bind calcium. Ionized calcium allows the "Gla domain" to undergo a protein structural change that enables incorporation of the factors onto a platelet phospholipid surface necessary for proenzyme activation. Without this ability, the activation of coagulation factors occurs at an unacceptably slow rate. Protein synthesis is not limited by warfarin nor is post-translational glycosylation. The enzymatic active site is unaffected by the vitamin K-dependent carboxylation process.

7. Answer a

This class of inhibitors blocks neither platelet adhesion nor activation but rather targets the final common pathway of platelet aggregation. Although attractive in principle, no data are available about the safety or efficacy of prolonged therapy with orally bioavailable gp IIb/IIIa inhibition following acute myocardial infarction.

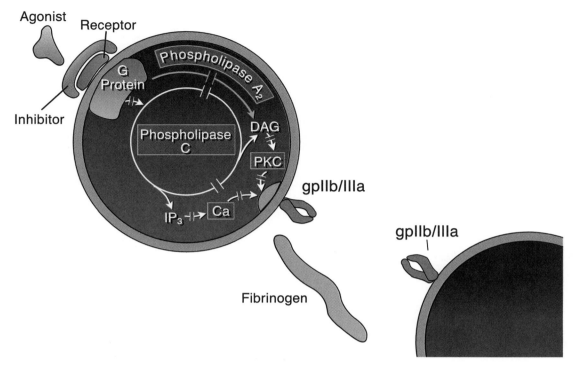

Plate 1. Inhibition of platelet activation. Arterial thrombus propagation requires platelet activation by one of a variety of potential agonists. When the platelet becomes activated, the glycoprotein (gp) IIb/IIIa receptor undergoes a conformational change permitting platelet-platelet interactions and platelet aggregation. Inhibition of platelet activation prevents activation of gp IIb/IIIa, and thrombus propagation is limited. DAG, diacylglycerol; IP_3, inositol 1,4,5-triphosphate; PKC, protein kinase C.

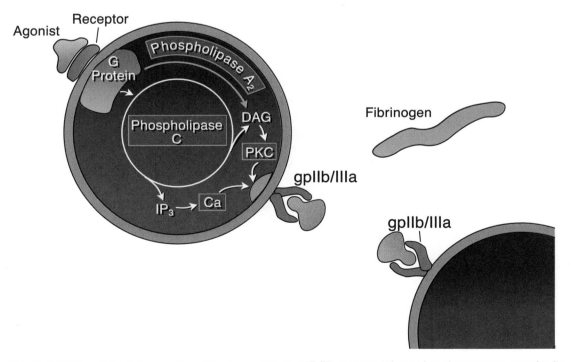

Plate 2. Inhibition of platelet aggregation. The glycoprotein (gp) IIb/IIIa receptor, when activated, supports aggregation by binding fibrinogen as a sort of "glue" that holds adjacent platelets together. By inhibiting this receptor, platelets are no longer capable of aggregating, and thrombus propagation is limited or potentially reversed. DAG, diacylglycerol; IP_3, inositol 1,4,5-triphosphate; PKC, protein kinase C.

Notes

Chapter 84

Lipid-Lowering Agents

R. Scott Wright, M.D.
Thomas E. Kottke, M.D.
Gerald T. Gau, M.D.

The principal pharmacologic agents used in the treatment of hyperlipidemia include resins, niacin, statins, and the fibric acid derivatives.

Resins: Bile Acid-Binding Sequestrants

The anionic resins, or bile acid-binding sequestrants (cholestyramine, Questran; colestipol, Colestid), are both safe and moderately effective in the therapy for hyperlipidemia. These agents reduce total cholesterol and low-density lipoprotein (LDL) cholesterol levels by binding positively charged bile acids in the gut to interrupt the enterohepatic circulation of bile acids. This stimulates new bile acid production and a secondary increase in hepatic LDL receptors, which in turn remove LDL cholesterol from the circulation. Resins usually have no significant effect on high-density lipoprotein (HDL) or triglyceride levels, but, paradoxically, they may increase triglycerides dramatically in some patients.

As expected from their mode of action, the major side effects associated with the resins are gastrointestinal intolerance with gas, bloating, constipation, nausea, and esophageal reflux. They are sufficient to cause about 50% of patients to discontinue therapy at 1 year. These agents work well to lower LDL cholesterol, and if the dose is slowly incremented, they can be reasonably tolerated by many patients. They are excellent agents in severe hyperlipidemia, used alone or in combination with statins or nicotinic acid. They are relatively contraindicated in hypertriglyceridemia.

A problem with resins is their effect on the absorption of vitamin K, especially in patients receiving warfarin. Resins also inhibit the absorption of digoxin, warfarin, thyroxine, statins, and diuretics if given concomitantly with these agents.

Plant Stanol Esters

Plant sterols and stanols derived from wood pulp and vegetable oils lower total and LDL cholesterol by inhibiting cholesterol absorption from the intestine. Plant stanols are virtually unabsorbable, which makes them more ideal hypocholesterolemic agents than plant sterols. The esterification of plant stanols has allowed their incorporation into various foods such as margarine without changing the taste and texture. Two to 3 grams a day of plant stanol esters reduces LDL cholesterol by 10% to 15% without side effects. Serum cholesterol is reduced with sitostanol-ester margarine in mild hypercholesterolemia. Thus, plant stanol esters appear to be a helpful adjunct to a prudent diet for lowering cholesterol. Also, they appear to have a synergistic effect for lowering cholesterol when used in combination with lipid-lowering agents that act at other steps of lipid metabolism. The combination of 3 g/day of plant stanol ester with 10 to 20 mg of simvastatin reduces total and LDL cholesterol by an additional 11% to 16%, respectively.

Nicotinic Acid

Nicotinic acid (niacin) is also a widely used, inexpensive, water-soluble B complex vitamin in the treatment of hyperlipidemia. Niacin lowers total cholesterol, LDL cholesterol, and triglyceride values and increases the HDL cholesterol level by a poorly defined mechanism, and it is probably the most potent agent for increasing a low HDL value. It also reduces lipoprotein (a) and small, dense LDL. This is the most economical of all lipid-lowering agents and is a nonprescription drug. The major side effects of nicotinic acid are pruritus, flushing, gastrointestinal distress, glucose intolerance, rash, provocation of gout, and liver toxicity. Aspirin taken 30 to 60 minutes before nicotinic acid can reduce the flushing. There is a rare occurrence of atrial arrhythmia or maculopathy. Nicotinic acid increases the risk of myopathy when used concomitantly with a statin. Patient tolerability of niacin is increased by using a sustained-release formulation (Niaspan).

Statins

The statin agents (HMG Co-A reductase enzyme inhibitors) are the most commonly used and most potent agents to reduce LDL cholesterol. These agents act by inhibiting the synthesis of cholesterol in the liver and promote increased uptake and degradation of LDL cholesterol from the blood. Most patients with hypercholesterolemia can be managed with monotherapy with a statin agent. These drugs are safe and cost-effective and reduce both coronary-related and total mortality in patients with coronary artery disease. The most common side effects in patients treated with statins are muscle cramps, myositis, and asymptomatic increase of hepatic transaminase enzyme values. These side effects are largely reversible with discontinuation of use of the medication but necessitate periodic monitoring of hepatic transaminase enzyme levels. The statins are the best tolerated of the currently available agents used for treating hyperlipidemia.

Fibric Acid Derivatives

The fibric acid derivatives include clofibrate, fenofibrate, gemfibrozil, and benzafibrate.

Clofibrate, the original fibric acid derivative, is now rarely used and has been supplanted in the treatment of hypertriglyceridemia and mixed hyperlipidemias by the newer fibric acid derivatives. Benzafibrate is a new agent that has been available in Europe and Canada for some time.

Gemfibrozil is widely used in the treatment of mixed hyperlipidemias, which are characterized by an increase in both serum triglyceride and LDL cholesterol, a common occurrence in diabetic patients. The major side effect is gastrointestinal, with a possible increased risk of cholelithiasis.

Fenofibrate is an agent recently approved for the treatment of hypertriglyceridemia. It is available commercially in the micronized form (Tricor) and is structurally similar to clofibrate and gemfibrozil. Fibric acid derivatives stimulate lipoprotein lipase activity, which results in enhanced triglyceride clearance. They also activate peroxisome proliferator-activated receptors, nuclear hormone receptors that modify expression of several genes responsible for lipoprotein expression. Fibric acid derivatives also result in the shift of small, dense LDL particles into less dense LDL particles that are considered less atherogenic. Fenofibrate also has been reported to lower lipoprotein (a) and fibrinogen levels, although it is not approved by the Food and Drug Administration for the treatment of these entities. Fenofibrate has been compared with pravastatin and simvastatin in the treatment of hyperlipidemia. It lowered LDL cholesterol less than pravastatin or simvastatin, but it increased HDL cholesterol level more than either statin agent, and it also lowered triglyceride levels (30%-50%) more effectively than simvastatin or pravastatin. Fenofibrate also has been tested against atorvastatin. Similarly, atorvastatin was more effective than fenofibrate for lowering LDL cholesterol, but less effective for increasing HDL cholesterol or for lowering triglyceride values. No outcome data are available with regard to primary or secondary prevention of coronary artery disease. The dosage of fenofibrate is 200 mg taken once daily in the morning. One small trial also suggests that fenofibrate is well tolerated when used in combination with simvastatin or pravastatin, but the risk of myopathy is increased. The major side effects have included rash and gastrointestinal upset. Similar to niacin, fibrates potentiate the effects of warfarin by decreasing protein binding.

Tables 1 and 2 provide information on the effects of lipid-lowering agents and their interactions and side effects.

Primary Prevention of Cardiac Disease

There is strong clinical evidence that treatment of hypercholesterolemia reduces future cardiac events in persons without clinically evident ischemic heart disease.

Table 1.—Drug Treatment of Hyperlipidemia

Agent	Dosage per day	Typical expected effects		
		Cholesterol effect		Triglyceride effect, %
		↓ LDL, %	↑ HDL, %	
Cholestyramine	12-24 g	15-20	0-2	5-10 ↑
Colestipol	15-30 g	15-20	0-2	5-10 ↑
Sitosterol esters	1.5-3.3 g	10	0-2	4-8 ↓
Niacin	1.5-6 g	20-30	20	30-40 ↓
Gemfibrozil	600-1,200 mg	10	20	50-60 ↓
Fenofibrate	67-200 mg	10-15	5-20	40-50 ↓
Lovastatin	20 mg	25-30	0-10	0-6 ↓
	80 mg	35-40	0-10	25 ↓
Cerivastatin	0.4 mg	35	0-10	35
Pravastatin	20 mg	25-30	0-7	10-15 ↓
	40 mg	25-35	0-12	25 ↓
Simvastatin	10 mg	25-30	0-10	0-5 ↓
	80 mg	40-50	0-16	25-40 ↓
Atorvastatin	10 mg	35-40	0-10	20 ↓
	40 mg	40-60	0-10	35 ↓
	80 mg	60	0-10	35-45
Fluvastatin	40 mg	20-25	0-5	10-20 ↓

N/A, not available.

The West of Scotland Prevention Study (WOSCOP)

Hypothesis: That primary prevention with pravastatin would reduce mortality and nonfatal infarctions in patients with hyperlipidemia who have not had a prior myocardial infarction

Study type: Randomized, multicenter study of pravastatin (Pravacol, 40 mg/day) versus placebo

Study patients: Nearly 6,600 middle-aged men (45-64 years old) with hypercholesterolemia without a prior history of myocardial infarction but with fasting LDL cholesterol values more than 252 mg/dL who failed to respond adequately to diet after 4 weeks (LDL, >155 mg/dL)

Follow-up period: > 32,000 patient-years

Drug effect: LDL cholesterol reduced by 26% with pravastatin, no effect with placebo

Study results

Pravastatin reduced:

1. The all-cause mortality risk by 22% ($P = 0.05$)
2. All coronary events by 31% ($P < 0.001$)
3. The risk of nonfatal myocardial infarction by 31% ($P < 0.001$)
4. The risk of death from all cardiovascular causes by 33% ($P = 0.033$)
5. The need for myocardial revascularization (bypass and angioplasty) by 37%

In addition:

There was no increase in noncardiac mortality

Study weaknesses

No female patients were included in the study

78% of patients were smokers or ex-smokers

Study conclusion: Primary prevention treatment with pravastatin in middle-aged men with significantly increased serum cholesterol values decreases the risk of cardiovascular events by about a third and death by a fifth in the following 5 years.

The Lipid Research Clinics (LRC) Coronary Primary Prevention Trial and the Helsinki Heart Study both examined the benefit of lipid-lowering therapy on primary prevention. The LRC study used a combination of cholestyramine and dietary intervention to reduce the serum cholesterol level. It found a 19% reduction in nonfatal myocardial infarction and a 24% reduction in deaths from

Table 2.—Interactions and Side Effects of Lipid-Lowering Agents

Agent	Interactions and side effects
Cholestyramine and colestipol	Other medications should be given 1 hour before or 4-6 hours after resin agent. May impair absorption of vitamins A, D, E, and K and cause vitamin K deficiency. May alter absorption of digoxin, warfarin, thiazide diuretics, propranolol, tetracycline, penicillin G, estrogens and progestins, and thyroid supplements. May produce or worsen constipation, nausea, abdominal pain, flatulence, vomiting, and anorexia
Niacin	Patients may experience flushing, itching, tingling, feelings of warmth, headache, rash, upset stomach, hypotension. May worsen fasting hyperglycemia and cause atrial arrhythmias
Gemfibrozil	Contraindicated in renal failure (creatinine > 2.0 mg/dL), hepatic dysfunction (including primary biliary cirrhosis), and preexisting gallbladder disease. Incidence of rhabdomyolysis is increased when agent is used with lovastatin
Fenofibrate	Contraindicated in renal failure (creatinine clearance < 50 mL/min), hepatic dysfunction. Doses of warfarin must be reduced and prothrombin time monitored frequently. Dose may need to be adjusted when given with cyclosporine. May increase risk of gallbladder disease
	Coadministration with statin agent is not yet approved by the Food and Drug Administration, but small studies with pravastatin and simvastatin have shown efficacy and safety over a short time
All statins	May increase aspartate aminotransferase. Monitor at initiation of therapy and with any change in dose. Rarely associated with myositis and rhabdomyolysis. Should not be used in pregnant or nursing women. Should not be used with oral or intravenous antifungal agents. May be used with bile acid-binding resins. No effect on β-adrenergic blockers, angiotensin-converting enzyme inhibitors, and diabetic agents
Lovastatin	Should not be used with gemfibrozil. May cause rhabdomyolysis when used with cyclosporine plus itraconazole, or with erythromycin. Widely studied, with good primary and secondary prevention data
Cerivastatin	A new, potent agent available only in low-dose formulation as yet
Pravastatin	Most widely studied agent, with good primary and secondary prevention data. Little evidence of myopathy when used with cyclosporine, niacin, or gemfibrozil
Simvastatin	Widely studied, with good secondary prevention data. Very efficacious. Dose should be decreased when given with cyclosporine. May potentiate effect of digoxin and warfarin
Atorvastatin	A very efficacious agent with a good side-effect profile. Results of long-term mortality studies are pending

cardiovascular disease. These reductions were of borderline statistical significance, and there was no decrease in overall mortality.

- In the Lipid Research Clinics Primary Prevention Trial, there was a trend toward a reduction in nonfatal myocardial infarctions and cardiovascular deaths but no statistically significant decrease in overall mortality.

The Helsinki Heart Study used gemfibrozil for the treatment of hyperlipidemia, which resulted in a 34% reduction in the combined end points of death, fatal myocardial infarction, and nonfatal myocardial infarction. Overall mortality was not reduced, and there was some statistically significant increase in noncardiovascular mortality in the gemfibrozil-treated group.

- In the Helsinki Heart Study primary prevention trial, there was a trend toward a reduction in the composite end points of cardiac death and cardiac events but no statistically significant decrease in overall mortality.

Finally, the recent Air Force/Texas Coronary Atherosclerosis Prevention Study (AFCAPS/TexCAPS) trial has extended the benefit of primary prevention to patient populations with "average" cholesterol values. The investigators randomized just over 6,600 patients without coronary artery disease to lovastatin or placebo for a mean period of 5.2 years. Treatment with lovastatin decreased total cholesterol by 18%, decreased LDL cholesterol by 25%, and increased HDL cholesterol by 6% in the population studied. The investigators observed a 37% risk reduction in the occurrence of the composite end point of fatal or nonfatal myocardial infarction, sudden death, or unstable angina. They also found a risk reduction of 33% in the need for coronary revascularization, 32% in the occurrence of unstable angina, and 40% in the occurrence of a fatal or nonfatal myocardial infarction. All of the observations favored the group treated with lovastatin. The AFCAPS/TexCAPS investigators demonstrated for the first time a treatment benefit favoring statin therapy in a population without known coronary artery disease and with previously identified "average" cholesterol values. Together, the WOSCOP and AFCAPS/TexCAPS data demonstrate the powerful effect of statin-based treatment of hyperlipidemia with regard to primary prevention of coronary artery disease.

Secondary Prevention of Cardiac Disease

The Scandanavian Simvastatin Survival Study (4S) clearly established the benefit of lipid-lowering therapy for secondary prevention of coronary artery disease.

The Scandinavian Simvastatin Survival Study (4S)

Hypothesis: That secondary prevention with simvastatin would reduce mortality and nonfatal infarctions in patients with hyperlipidemia

Study type: Randomized, multicenter study of simvastatin (Zocor, 20 mg/day) versus placebo. The simvastatin dosage was increased to 40 mg/day if needed

Study patients: 4,444 patients (35-70 years old) with documented coronary artery disease and total cholesterol values between 200 and 300 mg/dL. Excluded patients were those with congestive heart failure, who had a myocardial infarction within 6 months of enrollment, or who were considered likely to need revascularization (coronary artery bypass grafting or angioplasty).

Follow-up period: median 5.4 years

Drug effect: Simvastatin decreased total cholesterol

by 25% and LDL cholesterol by 35%, with a modest (~10%) increase in HDL and a decrease in triglyceride values

Study results

Simvastatin reduced:

1. The all-cause mortality by 30%
2. Coronary events by 34%
3. The risk of coronary death by 42%
4. The need for myocardial revascularization (bypass and angioplasty) by 37%

In addition:

There was no increase in noncardiac mortality

Study comment

1. Postmenopausal female patients were included in the study
2. The sickest patients with coronary artery disease were excluded from the study

Study conclusion: There is a clear benefit to secondary prevention treatment with simvastatin for patients with hypercholesterolemia

The most striking finding in the 4S study was a 30% decrease by simvastatin in all-cause mortality. The 4S study was the first major randomized trial to demonstrate an actual reduction in overall mortality in patients undergoing treatment for hyperlipidemia. This observation removed the questions regarding a mortality benefit from cholesterol lowering by the LRC and the Helsinki Heart Study.

The mortality in the placebo group for women was less than 50% of the mortality for men; thus, the study was underpowered to draw statistical conclusions regarding the mortality benefit of lipid lowering in women. However, women had a decrease in major coronary events that directly paralleled that in men, who showed a mortality benefit. Patients older than 60 years had both improved all-cause survival and a decreased incidence of major coronary events, similar to those that occurred in patients younger than 60 years.

The Program on the Surgical Control of Hyperlipidemia (POSCH) examined the benefits of partial ileal bypass surgery plus dietary intervention on reductions of mortality in 838 patients with hyperlipidemia. There was a 27% reduction in cardiovascular mortality and a 35% reduction in cardiac events in the surgically treated group. The relative risk reductions were similar to those in the 4S trial. There is no need to consider ileal bypass in patients with hyperlipidemia because pharmacologic agents can achieve a similar benefit.

The Cholesterol and Recurrent Events (CARE) Study

Hypothesis: That secondary prevention with pravastatin would reduce mortality and cardiac events in patients with "average" cholesterol levels
Study type: Randomized, multicenter study of pravastatin (Pravacol, 40 mg/ day) versus placebo
Study patients: Nearly 4,200 patients (21–75 years old) who had had a myocardial infarction at least 3 months previously, had a total cholesterol value less than 240 mg/dL, LDL value between 115 and 174 mg/dL, and triglyceride value of 350 mg/dL. Excluded patients were those with symptomatic congestive heart failure and low ejection fractions (< 25%)
Follow-up period: median 5.0 years
Drug effect: Pravastatin decreased LDL cholesterol by 32%
Study results
Pravastatin reduced:

1. The all-cause mortality by 9% (not statistically significant)
2. Coronary events by 24%
3. Nonfatal myocardial infarction by 23%
4. The risk of coronary death by 19%
5. Stroke by 31%
6. The need for myocardial revascularization (bypass and angioplasty) by 27%

In addition:
There was no increase in noncardiac mortality
Study comment
1. Female patients were included in the study
2. Women benefited from pravastatin more than men
3. Breast carcinoma was statistically ($P < 0.01$) more common in women receiving pravastatin but the total numbers affected were low. This finding is of uncertain significance
Study conclusion: There is a clear nonmortality benefit to secondary prevention treatment with pravastatin in patients with average cholesterol levels

It is of interest that women had a more dramatic reduction in fatal and nonfatal myocardial infarction with pravastatin than men (45% versus 19%) in the CARE study. Overall, the CARE study showed no significant decrease in all-cause mortality, and no other significant benefit (mortality or otherwise) occurred in the patient subgroup

with a baseline LDL cholesterol of 125 mg/dL or less.

A plot of the degree of LDL cholesterol lowering in the LRC, CARE, WOSCOP, and 4S trials versus the decreased coronary artery disease relative risk shows a clear treatment outcome finding. The greater the degree of LDL cholesterol lowering, the greater the decrease in cardiovascular events (Fig. 1).

Atorvastatin Versus Revascularization Treatment (AVERT)

Hypothesis: That secondary prevention with atorvastatin compared with angioplasty would reduce ischemic events in patients with stable coronary artery disease and, at most, moderate angina, all of whom had initially been recommended for angioplasty
Study type: Open-label, randomized, multicenter study of atorvastatin (Lipitor, 80 mg/day) versus angioplasty combined with usual care, including lipid-lowering therapy
Study patients: 341 patients with angiographically proven coronary artery disease with stenosis of 50% or more in at least one vessel recommended for angioplasty. LDL value was 115 mg/dL or more, and angina was class I or II. There was no electrocardiographic evidence of ischemia at less than 4 minutes on a Bruce protocol treadmill test
Follow-up period: 18 months
Drug effect: LDL cholesterol was reduced by 46% in the atorvastatin-treated arm and by 18% in the angioplasty/usual-care arm.
Study results

1. 36% reduction in ischemic events in the atorvastatin arm compared with angioplasty ($P = 0.045$)
2. Patients receiving atorvastatin who had a 40% or more reduction in LDL cholesterol had significantly fewer ischemic events than those with less than 40% reduction
3. 87% of the patients receiving atorvastatin were able to remain on medical therapy for 18 months without an ischemic event

Study comment: Angioplasty and aggressive lipid reduction should be complementary rather than competitive strategies for the treatment of coronary artery disease. LDL lowering beyond current goals of the National Cholesterol Education Program may be beneficial, and this hypothesis will be tested in the upcoming TNT (Towards New Targets) trial.

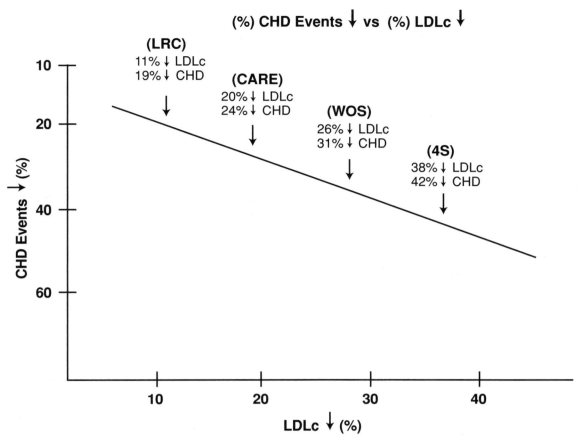

Fig. 1. Management of hyperlipidemia. CARE, Cholesterol and Recurrent Events study; CHD, coronary heart disease; LDLc, LDL cholesterol; LRC, Lipid Research Clinics trial; 4S, Scandinavian Simvastatin Survival Study; WOS, West of Scotland Study.

The Long-Term Intervention with Pravastatin in Ischemic Disease (LIPID) trial examined 9,014 patients with known coronary artery disease who were randomized to treatment with pravastatin or placebo and followed for 6.1 years. Death from coronary artery disease was reduced from 8.3% in the placebo group to 6.4% in the pravastatin group (*P* < 0.001). All-cause mortality was reduced from 14.1% to 11.0% (*P* < 0.001). In addition, the risk reduction was 19% for stroke, 20% for coronary revascularization, and 29% for myocardial infarction.

In summary, clear and compelling evidence now demonstrates that the rate of nonfatal cholesterol events and deaths from cardiovascular disease and total mortality can be reduced with aggressive lipid lowering in patients with known coronary artery disease. This is especially important in patients who have recently had a myocardial infarction, in that the CARE study demonstrated benefit in as little as 2 months after initiation of treatment.

Coronary Artery Regression Studies

Several coronary angiographic trials have examined the effect of lipid lowering on the regression of coronary artery disease lesions. These angiographic trials used aggressive lipid management, reducing the LDL cholesterol value by 25% to 40%, and overall in these trials the relative decrease in myocardial infarction and coronary mortality was 25% to 45%. Some evidence of coronary disease regression was demonstrated in 14% to 20% of the patients, but perhaps the most significant finding was that coronary disease progression can be reduced by about 50%. The Multicenter Anti-Atheroma Study (MAAS, simvastatin versus placebo), the Regression Growth Evaluation Statin Study (pravastatin versus placebo), and the Pravastatin Limitation of Atherosclerosis in the Coronary Arteries I Study (PLAC-I, pravastatin versus placebo) all demonstrated significant reductions in the rate of progression of coronary disease for patients in whom treatment lowered serum cholesterol values. The reductions in coronary events and death that were observed in the WOSCOP study, the 4S study, and the CARE study all occurred more quickly than would have been predicted if coronary atherosclerotic regression was the only mechanism possible. New evidence suggests that the primary mechanism of action of lipid-lowering therapy is in plaque stabilization when cholesterol is removed.

Antioxidant Therapy

Antioxidants, particularly vitamin E, vitamin C, β-carotene, and probucol, have been looked at with greater interest in the past 2 or 3 years. Observational data from the Nurses' Heart Study have indicated that nurses who took vitamin E as a supplement had a significant reduction in the myocardial infarction event rate compared with those who did not. The data on vitamin E are currently the most compelling, and the Cambridge Heart Anti-Oxidant Study (CHAOS) has given a further boost to the use of antioxidants (vitamin E) for the treatment of coronary artery disease. That study randomized patients with known coronary artery disease to treatment with 400 mIU of vitamin E, 800 mIU of vitamin E, or placebo. The relative reduction in the occurrence of the combined end points of cardiovascular death and nonfatal myocardial infarction was 47% in the trial. Nonetheless, there was no reduction in overall mortality. Further studies are pending.

Probucol
Probucol is a weak LDL cholesterol-lowering agent but a powerful antioxidant that protects LDL and lipoprotein (a) from oxidation. It was withdrawn because of its tendency to prolong the QT interval with resultant ventricular arrhythmias.

Fish Oils
Fish oils contain omega-3 fatty acids, which can significantly reduce elevated triglyceride levels. Their cardiovascular benefit, although much promoted, is scientifically unproved. Fish oils appear to be particularly beneficial in the treatment of retinoid (Accutane)-induced increase of serum triglyceride levels, a drug commonly used in the treatment of severe cystic acne.

Combination Therapy in Refractory Hyperlipidemia or Mixed Hyperlipidemia

Combination therapy is frequently necessary to treat refractory hyperlipidemia, often allows lower drug doses, and may reduce the incidence of side effects. Combination therapy can often lower LDL cholesterol, increase HDL cholesterol, and lower triglyceride values very effectively.

Statin + Resin
The combination of a statin agent and a bile acid-binding resin is very effective when either agent alone fails to reduce the LDL cholesterol to the target goal. The combination of a statin agent and a bile acid-binding agent is particularly effective for lowering LDL cholesterol in type II-A hyperlipidemia. Careful upward titration of the resin dose often avoids the gastrointestinal side effects frequently observed with resins.

Statin + Fibric Acid Derivative
The combination of pravastatin and gemfibrozil is excellent for lowering both triglyceride and LDL cholesterol levels, but at an increased risk of myositis. One approach to treatment of mixed hyperlipidemia is to estimate the percentage reduction needed to bring the LDL and triglyceride values into the desired target range.

Monotherapy with high-dose simvastatin or atorvastatin reduces triglyceride values 25% to 40% and LDL cholesterol values by 30% to 60%. One should consider combination therapy with a statin and fenofibrate or gemfibrozil if the need to lower the triglyceride value exceeds that typically obtained with statin monotherapy. Fenofibrate should be used if a 10% to 20% reduction in LDL cholesterol is desired. If a greater reduction in LDL cholesterol is the goal, then combination therapy of gemfibrozil plus a statin is necessary. The use of fibrates alone occasionally is associated with myopathy. The combined use of a statin with a fibrate increases the risk of myopathy, and combination therapy must be instituted at low doses of both agents, with careful upward titration until the desired lipid lowering is achieved.

Treatment of an Isolated Low HDL
An isolated low HDL cholesterol value may be difficult to treat. Niacin, gemfibrozil, and fenofibrate will all increase an isolated low HDL value by 10% to 15%, whereas most statins will increase the HDL level by 5% to 8%. Simvastatin may increase HDL up to 16%. Niacin, fenofibrate, and gemfibrozil will all effectively treat the combination of a low HDL

level and an increased triglyceride level. This pattern is often found in patients with diabetes mellitus or obesity with insulin resistance. Combination therapy with a statin plus niacin, gemfibrozil, or fenofibrate effectively treats a low HDL and high LDL pattern without increased triglycerides, which may occur in patients with advanced coronary artery disease.

Side Effects and Drug Interactions of Lipid-Lowering Drugs

The two most serious side effects of statins and fibrates are myositis and an increase in hepatic transaminase enzymes. Both of these are uncommon ($\leq 1\%$) and disappear when the drug therapy is discontinued. There are few clinical data to support a carcinogenic role for statins in humans except for a slight statistical increase in breast cancer noted in the CARE study. This finding was not seen in other large statin trials and will need to be evaluated further. There is also a reported increased incidence of myositis in patients receiving statin agents and high-dose niacin. The use of cyclosporine in combination with statins may increase serum concentrations of statins and increase the incidence of drug-related side effects. It is appropriate to reduce the dose of statin by 50% when a patient is starting treatment with cyclosporine. The dose of statin may be slowly increased with time if the serum cholesterol values necessitate upward titration. Pravastatin may be the best statin to use with cyclosporine because of less drug-drug interaction.

Common Pitfalls in Lipid Treatment

A major pitfall in the treatment of patients with hyperlipidemia is a failure to achieve the desired LDL cholesterol target goal, despite a maximal dose of the administered drug. This is often the result of patient non-adherence to pharmacologic and, more frequently, nonpharmacologic treatment strategies (diet and exercise). Consider an exacerbation of a coexisting illness such as diabetes mellitus, hypothyroidism, renal failure, or excess alcohol consumption. Additionally, we instruct patients to take their lipid-lowering agent at bedtime, because the liver synthesizes cholesterol predominantly during the sleep cycle.

There are several possible treatment strategies for a persistently increased LDL cholesterol despite seemingly adequate lipid-lowering therapy.
1. Check the lipoprotein (a) value to be certain there is no interaction from this lipoprotein fraction.
2. Switch to a more effective statin, such as atorvastatin or simvastatin. Both simvastatin and atorvastatin can be used safely at high doses (80 mg/day) with additional lipid-lowering benefit.
3. A bile acid-binding resin can be added to the statin.
4. Consider the addition of fenofibrate or gemfibrozil to potentiate the effect of triglyceride lowering plus additional LDL lowering.
5. Consider referral to a specialized center that performs LDL apheresis for the persistently increased LDL cholesterol value despite maximal pharmacologic therapy. LDL apheresis removes apo-B–containing lipoproteins directly from the blood by extracorporeal circulation through adsorption columns and is indicated in the treatment of refractory hypercholesterolemia despite the use of maximally tolerated lipid-lowering drug therapy and intense dietary modification.

LDL apheresis reduces the following:
- LDL cholesterol by 50% to 75%
- HDL cholesterol by about 15%
- Triglycerides by about 50%
- Lipoprotein (a) by about 60%

LDL apheresis is approved by the Food and Drug Administration for refractory hypercholesterolemia:
- LDL > 200 mg/dL with coronary disease
- LDL > 300 mg/dL without coronary disease

LDL apheresis may be beneficially combined with high-dose statin therapy (simvastatin, 160 mg/day; atorvastatin, 80 mg/day) in some patients with homozygous familial hypercholesterolemia to achieve a further 30% reduction in LDL levels.

Special Populations With Hyperlipidemia

Women With Heart Disease
Heart disease is the leading cause of death in women, although it develops in women at an older age than in men, in general. The benefit of aggressive lipid-lowering therapy with statin agents in women is now well established from recent trials. The role of estrogen replacement therapy remains controversial. Although there is clear benefit from estrogen replacement therapy for some noncardiac diseases such as osteoporosis, the benefit of estrogen replacement on secondary prevention of cardiac events is less clear. Several observational studies have established a potential epidemiologic link between estrogen use and

benefit with either primary and secondary prevention. Estrogen therapy lowers cholesterol and lipoprotein (a) values. The recent Heart and Estrogen/Progestin Replacement Study (HERS) examined the role of daily conjugated equine estrogen plus medroxyprogesterone acetate (progestin) on the occurrence of nonfatal myocardial infarction or coronary heart disease-related death. A total of 2,763 women were randomized to combination therapy or placebo. There was no apparent benefit from combination therapy with regard to nonfatal infarction, coronary heart disease-related death, need for coronary revascularization, development of unstable angina, congestive heart failure, stroke or transient ischemic attack, and peripheral vascular disease. These results were surprising to many investigators because of the lack of apparent benefit even in secondary coronary prevention. Additional trials are in progress, but for now the data on estrogen/progestin therapy are mixed in that a benefit has been demonstrated by observational studies and a lack of benefit has been shown by a single randomized trial. In most women, other issues either substantiate (osteoporosis) or preclude (history of breast cancer) the use of estrogen replacement therapy.

Elderly Patients

The data regarding treatment of hyperlipidemia in the elderly has been controversial, and no one study clearly demonstrates a benefit with primary prevention in this age group. The Established Populations for Epidemiological Studies in the Elderly (EPESE) study investigated 6,566 elderly patients without documented coronary artery disease. The mean age was 79.2 years at the time of analysis. The EPESE investigators demonstrated a linear increase in the risk of development of coronary artery disease in subjects with hyperlipidemia. Elderly patients with total cholesterol values more than 240 mg/dL had a relative risk of coronary artery disease development of 1.57. Elderly patients with a total cholesterol less than 160 mg/dL had a relative risk of 0.83. The EPESE investigators also found an association between a low HDL cholesterol value and increased risk of development of coronary artery disease. An HDL cholesterol value less than 35 mg/dL had a relative risk of 2.17, whereas an HDL cholesterol value more than 60 mg/dL had a relative risk of 1.0. Although no trial has shown a reduction in mortality and morbidity from coronary artery disease with regard to primary prevention in the elderly, the data from the EPESE investigation strongly suggest that treatment

of the elderly with hyperlipidemia is warranted, because they are at greatest risk of death from coronary artery disease and thus stand to gain the most from pharmacologic intervention.

The 4S trial also has data regarding secondary prevention in coronary artery disease. The 4S investigators demonstrated similar reduction in morbidity and mortality from coronary artery disease in patients older than 65 years compared with those younger than 65 years who were treated. The observed reductions in cardiovascular death and morbidity occurred independent of age. Thus, the available evidence suggests that elderly patients with hyperlipidemia should be aggressively treated and that withholding lipid-lowering treatment solely on the basis of age is unjustified.

Patients With Diabetes

Diabetes mellitus is an important risk factor for the development of coronary artery disease. Most patients with diabetes die of complications from coronary artery disease or peripheral vascular disease. Recent data report that diabetic patients without known coronary artery disease died of cardiovascular causes at the same rate as patients with known disease, suggesting that most diabetes-associated coronary disease is clinically silent or unrecognized. Hypertriglyceridemia is a strong predictor of coronary artery disease in diabetics. Aggressive primary prevention of coronary artery disease is important in diabetic patients with hyperlipidemia with a goal LDL cholesterol value less than 100 mg/dL, HDL cholesterol value more than 35 mg/dL, and triglyceride value less than 200 mg/dL. Pharmacologic therapy with a statin or combination statin and fibrate should be initiated if nonpharmacologic measures, including strict diabetes control and diet, fail to reach these goals.

No randomized trial has been specifically powered to analyze the impact of treatment of hyperlipidemia on secondary prevention of coronary artery disease. However, post-hoc analyses of the 4S and CARE trials have shown a significant benefit with regard to secondary prevention of coronary heart disease events. The 4S trial found a greater magnitude of benefit for patients with diabetes mellitus than those without diabetes mellitus. In the CARE trial, the magnitude of benefit among diabetic patients was at least equal to that in nondiabetic patients. In both trials, treatment with a statin agent in diabetic subjects was safe and efficacious and reduced future cardiovascular event rates.

Recipients of Organ Transplants

Recipients of heart and other organ transplants often manifest an accelerated form of coronary and peripheral vascular disease (posttransplant vasculopathy) several years after transplantation. The cause of this vasculopathy is probably multifactorial: low-grade transplant rejection, the untoward effects of chronic treatment with immunosuppressive agents (cyclosporine, steroids), hypertension, diabetes, and hypercholesterolemia. Although post-transplantation vasculopathy is not strongly linked to serum LDL cholesterol levels, it is recommended that all transplant patients be treated according to targets established by the National Cholesterol Education Program for patients with known coronary artery disease. This approach will often require pharmacologic therapy with a statin agent. Pravastatin is considered the statin of choice when the anti-rejection drug cyclosporine also is being administered. The use of cyclosporine in conjunction with a statin increases the risk of myopathy significantly, but probably less so with pravastatin than with the other potent statins. Simvastatin, although noted to increase plasma cyclosporine levels, has been evaluated in a small trial of patients after orthotopic heart transplantation who were receiving triple immunosuppression, including cyclosporine. The group randomized to simvastatin had a reduction in graft vessel disease and no significantly increased incidence of myositis.

Statins and the Vulnerable Atherosclerotic Plaque

The ultimate target of all lipid-lowering therapy is the vulnerable atherosclerotic plaque. Coronary plaque rupture is the final common pathway for all the unstable coronary syndromes. Experimental data suggest that statin therapy, in addition to its effect on LDL cholesterol metabolism, can stabilize the vulnerable atherosclerotic plaque and convert lipid-rich plaques that are at high risk of rupture into more stable fibrotic plaques. The reduction in cardiovascular events found in all the statin trials occurred earlier than would be expected from coronary plaque regression alone due to lipid lowering. This suggests an additional beneficial mechanism by statins on vulnerable plaques. Statin therapy may stabilize the vulnerable plaque through reduction in macrophages and extracellular lipid accumulation in the plaque region, by an increase in the collagen content of the extracellular plaque matrix, by reduced calcification and neovascularization in the intima of the plaque, and through an inhibitory role on the coagulation and inflammatory cascades that promote plaque rupture.

Suggested Review Reading

1. Anonymous: The Lipid Research Clinics Coronary Primary Prevention Trial results. I. Reduction in incidence of coronary heart disease. *JAMA* 251:351-364, 1984.

2. Anonymous: The Lipid Research Clinics Coronary Primary Prevention Trial results. II. The relationship of reduction in incidence of coronary heart disease to cholesterol lowering. *JAMA* 251:365-374, 1984.

3. Anonymous: Randomised trial of cholesterol lowering in 4444 patients with coronary heart disease: the Scandinavian Simvastatin Survival Study (4S). *Lancet* 344:1383-1389, 1994.

4. Brown BG, Hillger L, Zhao ZQ, et al: Types of change in coronary stenosis severity and their relative importance in overall progression and regression of coronary disease. Observations from the FATS Trial. Familial Atherosclerosis Treatment Study. *Ann N Y Acad Sci* 748:407-417, 1995.

5. Buchwald H, Varco RL, Matts JP, et al: Effect of partial ileal bypass surgery on mortality and morbidity from coronary heart disease in patients with hypercholesterolemia. Report on the Program on the Surgical Control of the Hyperlipidemias. *N Engl J Med* 323:946-955, 1990.

6. Frick MH, Elo O, Haapa K, et al: Helsinki Heart Study: primary-prevention trial with gemfibrozil in middle-aged men with dyslipidemia. Safety of treatment, changes in risk factors, and incidence of coronary heart disease. *N Engl J Med* 317:1237-1245, 1987.

7. Goldman L, Garber AM, Grover SA, et al: 27th Bethesda Conference: matching the intensity of risk factor management with the hazard for coronary disease events. Task Force 6. Cost effectiveness of assessment and management of risk factors. *J Am Coll Cardiol* 27:1020-1030, 1996.

8. Gylling H, Radhakrishnan R, Miettinen TA: Reduction of serum cholesterol in postmenopausal women with previous myocardial infarction and cholesterol malabsorption induced by dietary sitostanol ester margarine: women and dietary sitostanol. *Circulation* 96:4226-4231, 1997.

9. Hulley S, Grady D, Bush T, et al: Randomized trial of estrogen plus progestin for secondary prevention of coronary heart disease in postmenopausal women. *JAMA* 280:605-613, 1998.

10. Jones P, Kafonek S, Laurora I, et al: Comparative dose efficacy study of atorvastatin versus simvastatin, pravastatin, lovastatin, and fluvastatin in patients with hypercholesterolemia. *Am J Cardiol* 81:582-587, 1998.

11. The Long-Term Intervention with Pravastatin in Ischaemic Disease (LIPID) Study Group: Prevention of cardiovascular events and death with pravastatin in patients with coronary heart disease and a broad range of initial cholesterol levels. *N Engl J Med* 339:1349-1357, 1998.

12. Miettinen TA, Puska P, Gylling H, et al: Reduction of serum cholesterol with sitostanol-ester margarine in a mildly hypercholesterolemic population. *N Engl J Med* 333:1308-1312, 1995.

13. Nguyen TT, Dale LC, von Bergmann K, et al: Cholesterol-lowering effect of stanol ester in a US population of mildly hypercholesterolemic men and women: a randomized control trial. *Mayo Clin Proc* 74:1198-1206, 1999

14. Pedersen TR, Berg K, Cook TJ, et al: Safety and tolerability of cholesterol lowering with simvastatin during 5 years in the Scandinavian Simvastatin Survival Study. *Arch Intern Med* 156:2085-2092, 1996.

15. Pedersen TR, Kjekshus J, Boccuzzi SJ, et al: Clinical and resource utilization benefits of the Scandinavian Simvastatin Survival Study (4-S) applied to the U.S. population (abstract). *Circulation* 92 (Suppl 1):I-521, 1995.

16. Pedersen TR, Kjekshus J, Pyörälä K, et al: Effect of simvastatin on survival and coronary morbidity in coronary heart disease patients 65 or older (abstract). *Circulation* 92 (Suppl 1):I-672, 1995.

17. Rosenson RS, Tangney CC: Antiatherothrombotic properties of statins: implications for cardiovascular event reduction. *JAMA* 279:1643-1650, 1998.

18. Sacks FM, Pfeffer MA, Moye LA, et al: The effect of pravastatin on coronary events after myocardial infarction in patients with average cholesterol levels. *N Engl J Med* 335:1001-1009, 1996.

19. Scandinavian Simvastatin Survival Study Group: Baseline serum cholesterol and treatment effect in the Scandinavian Simvastatin Survival Study (4S). *Lancet* 345:1274-1275, 1995.

20. Shepherd J, Cobbe SM, Ford I, et al: Prevention of coronary heart disease with pravastatin in men with hypercholesterolemia. *N Engl J Med* 333:1301-1307, 1995.

21. Stampfer MJ, Hennekens CH, Manson JE, et al: Vitamin E consumption and the risk of coronary disease in women. *N Engl J Med* 328:1444-1449, 1993.

22. Stephens NG, Parsons A, Schofield PM, et al: Randomised controlled trial of vitamin E in patients with coronary disease: Cambridge Heart Antioxidant Study. *Lancet* 347:781-786, 1996.

23. Wright RA, Flapan AD: Scandinavian simvastatin study (4S) (letter to the editor). *Lancet* 344:1765, 1994.

Questions

Multiple Choice (choose the one best answer)

1. Increases of the serum fibrinogen value have been associated with an increased risk for development of coronary artery disease in some studies. Which of the commonly available lipid-lowering drugs has been shown to lower the serum fibrinogen level?
   a. Atorvastatin (Lipitor)
   b. Simvastatin (Zocor)
   c. Lovastatin (Mevacor)
   d. Fenofibrate (Tricor)
   e. Fluvastatin (Lescol)

2. Which of the following drugs would be first-line therapy for a patient without documented heart disease who has the following lipid profile:

   low-density lipoprotein = 138 mg/dL
   high-density lipoprotein = 20 mg/dL
   triglycerides = 964 mg/dL

   a. Atorvastatin (Lipitor)
   b. Simvastatin (Zocor)
   c. Lovastatin (Mevacor)
   d. Gemfibrozil (Lopid)
   e. Fluvastatin (Lescol)

3. Which of the following drugs or combinations is not indicated for the treatment of mixed hyperlipidemia?
   a. Atorvastatin
   b. Simvastatin
   c. Pravastatin + gemfibrozil
   d. Niacin + lovastatin

4. Which of the following lipid-lowering agents may worsen glycemic control in patients with borderline fasting hyperglycemia?
   a. Simvastatin
   b. Atorvastatin
   c. Niacin
   d. Gemfibrozil
   e. None of the above

5. Which of the following Food and Drug Administration-approved drugs has been shown to reduce lipoprotein (a), Lp(a)?
   a. Estrogen
   b. Fenofibrate
   c. Atorvastatin
   d. Simvastatin
   e. Both a and b

6. Which of the following is the recommended treatment of hyperhomocystinemia?
   a. Atorvastatin
   b. Pravastatin
   c. Vitamin B_{12}
   d. Folic acid, vitamin B_6, + vitamin B_{12}
   e. Vitamin E

7. A 49-year-old man who received a living-related donor kidney transplant 2 years ago is referred to you after an inferior myocardial infarction, which was successfully treated with streptokinase. His lipid profile is as follows:

   total cholesterol = 300 mg/dL
   high-density lipoprotein cholesterol = 45 mg/dL
   low-density lipoprotein cholesterol = 216 mg/dL
   glucose = 120 mg/dL
   triglycerides = 195 mg/dL
   Lp(a) = 8 mg/dL
   homocysteine = 8 mmol/L
   fibrinogen = 245 mg/dL

   His renal allograft function is normal and he is maintained on prednisone, cyclosporine, and study drug B, a novel antilymphocyte agent.

7A. Which of the following drugs is the best choice for this patient?
   a. Simvastatin
   b. Atorvastatin
   c. Niacin
   d. Pravastatin
   e. Fluvastatin

7B. What would the target low-density lipoprotein cholesterol level be in this patient?
   a. 130 mg/dL
   b. 100 mg/dL
   c. 110 mg/dL
   d. 125 mg/dL
   e. 150 mg/dL

8. A 49-year-old chief executive officer of a Fortune 500 company presents to your cardiovascular health clinic as part of an executive physical examination program. He runs 15 miles three times per week, was an Olympic athlete during his college years, and is a devout Mormon. He recently invested $50,000 in Heart Check America, and as part of the investment he received a complimentary coronary computed tomography scan. He was told he had moderate calcifications in the right coronary artery, but little of significance overall. He has a normal electrocardiogram, a normal thyroid profile, and no evidence of fasting hyperglycemia. His father died of heart disease at age 88, and his mother is alive at age 92. His lipid profile is as follows:

total cholesterol = 260 mg/dL
triglycerides = 100 mg/dL
high-density lipoprotein cholesterol = 85 mg/dL
low-density lipoprotein cholesterol = 155 mg/dL

Which of the following approaches to "preventive cardiology" is recommended by the recent American Heart Association guidelines?
a. Reassure him that he is free of any coronary artery disease
b. Send him for an exercise thallium stress test
c. Start therapy with pravastatin, 20 mg nightly
d. Start therapy with niacin, 1 g daily
e. Start therapy with atorvastatin, 10 mg nightly

9. A 55-year-old father of six children is concerned about his lipid profile. His father and mother both died of myocardial infarctions at age 51 and 58, respectively. He is healthy, does not smoke, and exercises daily by swimming for 45 minutes. He comes to you for counseling regarding primary prevention. He follows a low-fat diet but does not take any medications. His blood chemistry profile and blood pressure are as follows:

total cholesterol = 220 mg/dL
triglycerides = 125 mg/dL
glucose = 95 mg/dL
high-density lipoprotein cholesterol = 65 mg/dL
low-density lipoprotein cholesterol = 130 mg/dL
blood pressure = 110/75 mm Hg

Which of the following is appropriate for this patient and supported by outcomes data?

a. Send him for exercise echocardiography
b. Send him for exercise thallium scanning
c. Pravastatin 20 mg nightly, aspirin 162 mg daily
d. Vitamin E 400 IU daily, vitamin C 500 mg daily, aspirin 162 mg daily
e. Aspirin 162 mg daily

10. A 71-year-old retired schoolteacher comes for an annual cardiovascular examination. She had an inferolateral myocardial infarction 3 years ago and was treated with primary percutaneous transluminal coronary angioplasty. She has normal left ventricular function. She takes aspirin daily and follows a low-fat diet. She exercises four times per week at the local YMCA. Her blood chemistry values are as follows:

total cholesterol = 195 mg/dL
triglycerides = 150 mg/dL
Lp(a) = 8 mg/dL
high-density lipoprotein cholesterol = 45 mg/dL
fibrinogen = 385 mg/dL
glucose = 125 mg/dL

She recently started estrogen replacement therapy with an estrogen patch. Exercise echocardiography is negative for ischemia at an excellent workload (155% predicted functional aerobic capacity). Which of the following recommendations in her management is not supported by recent clinical trials?
a. Simvastatin, 10 mg nightly
b. Change from estrogen patch to an oral estrogen
c. Vitamin E, 400 IU daily
d. Atorvastatin, 10 mg nightly

11. A 58-year-old orthopedic surgeon comes to your office for advice about her hyperlipidemia. She has been taking pravastatin (40 mg nightly) for 6 months and strictly adheres to a low-fat diet. She does not have a family history of coronary artery disease, but she does have recently diagnosed diabetes mellitus and has started therapy with glyburide (5 mg daily). She has an abnormal exercise thallium scan with a reversible apical perfusion defect that occurs without angina at a moderate workload (75% predicted functional aerobic capacity). Her lipid profile and blood pressure are as follows:

total cholesterol = 240 mg/dL
high-density lipoprotein cholesterol = 30 mg/dL

blood pressure = 145/95 mm Hg
homocysteine = 12 mmol/L
triglycerides = 350 mg/dL
glucose = 145 mg/dL
fibrinogen = 215 mg/dL
Lp(a) = 12 mg/dL

She takes oral estrogen daily and has been taking vitamins A, C, E, and B$_{12}$ for 5 years. She also uses garlic on an every-other-day basis and recently started taking CoEnzyme Q 10. Which of the following alternatives would you advise for her hyperlipidemia?

a. Switch from pravastatin to cerivastatin, 0.3 mg nightly
b. Switch from pravastatin to simvastatin, 40 mg, or atorvastatin, 20 mg, nightly
c. Add cholestyramine 1 g daily and continue taking pravastatin
d. Add nicotinic acid (Slo-Niacin), 1,000 mg twice a day over 8 weeks
e. Reduce the intake of fresh fruit and fats to attempt to lower her triglyceride level

12. A 44-year-old police officer was brought to the hospital with an out-of-hospital cardiac arrest due to an acute anterolateral myocardial infarction. He had quit smoking the day before the acute infarction. He received tissue plasminogen activator and "rescue" percutaneous transluminal coronary angioplasty and stenting to the proximal left anterior descending coronary artery. His ejection fraction was 45% on the fifth day of hospitalization. One of your associates started therapy with atorvastatin, 10 mg nightly. He comes today for a 6-week examination after completion of cardiac rehabilitation. He has lost 25 pounds and feels "great." His blood chemistry values and blood pressure are as follows:

total cholesterol = 165 mg/dL
high-density lipoprotein cholesterol = 35 mg/dL
fibrinogen = 285 mg/dL
blood pressure = 128/82 mm Hg
triglycerides = 85 mg/dL
low-density lipoprotein cholesterol = 113 mg/dL
glucose = 120 mg/dL
aspartate aminotransferase = 21 U/L

Which of the following recommendations do you implement in this patient's management?
a. Increase atorvastatin to 20 mg nightly
b. Switch to fluvastatin, 40 mg nightly
c. Add niacin, 500 mg twice a day
d. Recheck lipid and aspartate aminotransferase values in 3 months

Answers

1. Answer d

Fenofibrate is a new lipid-lowering agent that lowers the serum fibrinogen level. Some early reports suggested that atorvastatin may increase the serum fibrinogen level, but these reports were contradicted by later studies. Simvastatin, pravastatin, and fluvastatin have not been reported to increase the serum fibrinogen value.

2. Answer d

Gemfibrozil is the most potent triglyceride-lowering agent among the possible answers. Gemfibrozil reduces plasma triglycerides by 40% to 55%, usually within a month of onset of therapy. Lovastatin and fluvastatin do not appreciably alter the plasma triglyceride values. There is a 25% to 40% decrease in triglycerides with either simvastatin or atorvastatin.

3. Answer d

Niacin lowers the triglyceride values appreciably, but it is not indicated for the treatment of mixed hyperlipidemia in combination with a statin drug because of the increased risk of rhabdomyolysis. All of the other agents or agent combinations can be safely used in the treatment of mixed hyperlipidemia.

4. Answer c

Niacin worsens fasting hyperglycemia in some patients. Gemfibrozil and simvastatin reduced coronary event rates (including death) in patients with non-insulin-dependent diabetes mellitus in the Helsinki Heart Study and Simvastatin Scandinavian Survival Study, respectively. There are few data on cardiac event outcome with atorvastatin as yet, but the TNT (Towards New Targets) Study will evaluate the effect of atorvastatin (10 mg and 80 mg) on cardiac events in a large randomized study.

5. Answer e

Both estrogen and fenofibrate reduce Lp(a). Niacin also reduces Lp(a). Atorvastatin and simvastatin do not affect Lp(a) appreciably. There are epidemiologic data implicating Lp(a) as a strong risk factor for development of cardiovascular disease, but there are no current clinical data demonstrating a treatment-induced reduction in cardiovascular disease event rates and cardiovascular disease-associated mortality in patients with increased Lp(a) values.

6. Answer d

Folic acid lowers increased plasma homocysteine values. Vitamins B_6 and B_{12} are recommended so that treatment with folic acid will not mask the development of pernicious anemia and dementia due to vitamin B_{12} deficiency. There have been reports of dementia developing in patients with B_{12} deficiency who were receiving folic acid supplements.

7A. Answer d

Pravastatin is the preferred choice of statin among the listed drugs. This patient has known cardiovascular disease and should be aggressively treated with a statin agent. He has glucose intolerance, and niacin may worsen his fasting hyperglycemia. The high-density lipoprotein cholesterol value is not "low," and thus the risk of niacin outweighs its potential benefit of high-density lipoprotein elevation. Simvastatin use has been associated with the development of rhabdomyolysis in patients taking cyclosporine. Atorvastatin has not been adequately tested in patients with transplants and should be avoided in patients taking cyclosporine until further data are available. Fluvastatin is also untested in patients taking cyclosporine and is a much less potent statin than pravastatin.

7B. Answer b

This patient has coronary artery disease and should be aggressively treated with pravastatin to achieve a low-density lipoprotein cholesterol value of 100 mg/dL or less.

8. Answer c

This patient has a high probability of having at least nonobstructive coronary artery disease, as documented by coronary calcification on his coronary computed tomography scan. He is asymptomatic, and the degree of stenosis in the right coronary artery is not quantified. He fits the profiles of the West of Scotland and CARE studies. He should be treated for secondary prevention of atherosclerotic heart disease and primary prevention of ischemic heart disease.

9. Answer e

This patient does not have any evidence of ischemic heart disease or atherosclerotic heart disease. His low-density lipoprotein cholesterol value meets the guidelines of the American Heart Association. Aspirin is the only indicated agent with proven outcomes data. Vitamins E and C are not proved by outcomes data to prevent the development of cardiovascular disease but may reasonably be recommended pending further studies.

10. Answer d

This patient has known coronary artery disease but is currently asymptomatic. Her low-density lipoprotein cholesterol calculated from the data given is 120 mg/dL. She should be more aggressively treated for her hyperlipidemia according to recent American Heart Association guidelines. She fits the 4S study population with regard to secondary prevention. She may benefit from vitamin E for secondary prevention. She may get additional lipid lowering from a switch from transdermal estrogens to oral estrogens. Atorvastatin has not been tested for primary or secondary coronary prevention, although it is widely used in the United States for this patient population and is a very effective drug for lowering low-density lipoprotein cholesterol level.

11. Answer b

This patient has coronary artery disease with a reduced exercise tolerance and a reversible perfusion defect on thallium scintigraphy. She is taking a maximal dose of pravastatin, and her low-density lipoprotein cholesterol level remains above the recommended target for someone with known coronary artery disease. Switching to cerivastatin would probably not bring the low-density lipoprotein cholesterol into range. Adding cholestyramine would worsen the hypertriglyceridemia. Adding nicotinic acid would worsen the glucose intolerance and could potentially interact with pravastatin to cause myositis. Reducing the intake of fresh fruit and fat might help the hypertriglyceridemia, but most likely it would not reduce the low-density lipoprotein cholesterol appreciably. Treatment with simvastatin or atorvastatin would further reduce the low-density lipoprotein cholesterol and would also reduce her plasma triglyceride value.

12. Answer a

This patient has coronary artery disease, and the low-density lipoprotein cholesterol value does not meet target guidelines. Increasing the atorvastatin would most likely reduce the low-density lipoprotein cholesterol further. Switching to fluvastatin would most likely provide less effective control of the low-density lipoprotein cholesterol than the current dose of atorvastatin. Adding niacin might worsen the glucose intolerance that is present in this patient. Rechecking the lipid and aspartate aminotransferase values in 3 months is a good idea after the atorvastatin dosage is doubled.

Veterans Affairs High-Density Lipoprotein Cholesterol Intervention Trial (VA-HIT)

Rubins HB, Robins SJ, Collins D, et al: Gemfibrozil for the secondary prevention of coronary heart disease in men with low levels of high-density lipoprotein cholesterol. *N Engl J Med* 341:410-418, 1999

Hypothesis: Secondary prevention with gemfibrozil to increase HDL cholesterol and decrease triglycerides reduces cardiac mortality and nonfatal myocardial infarction in patients with low HDL cholesterol.

Study type: Randomized, multicenter study of gemfibrozil (Lopid), 1,200 mg/day versus placebo.

Study patients: 2,531 men (< 74 years old) with documented coronary artery disease and HDL cholesterol 40 mg/dL or less, cholesterol 140 mg/dL or less, and triglycerides 300 mg/dL or less

Follow-up period: median, 5.1 years

Drug effect: Mean baseline HDL cholesterol, triglycerides, and LDL cholesterol were 32, 166, and 113 mg/dL, respectively. Gemfibrozil increased HDL cholesterol by 6%, decreased triglycerides by 31%, and did not change LDL cholesterol

Study results: Gemfibrozil reduced:
1. Nonfatal myocardial infarction by 22%
2. The risk of coronary death by 23% ($P = 0.07$)
3. All-cause mortality by 11% (not statistically significant)

Study comment:
1. Female patients were not included in this study
2. Gemfibrozil use was not associated with any major adverse events. Most common side effect was dyspepsia
3. Beneficial effect did not become apparent until about 2 years after randomization

Study conclusion: Gemfibrozil is effective for the prevention of myocardial infarction and coronary death in patients with coronary heart disease whose primary lipid abnormality is a low HDL cholesterol level

Preliminary results from another fibrate secondary prevention trial, the Bezafibrate Infarction Prevention Trial (Goldbourt U, Behar S, Reicher-Reiss H, et al: Rationale and design of a secondary prevention trial of increasing serum high-density lipoprotein cholesterol and reducing triglycerides in patients with clinically manifest atherosclerotic heart disease [the Bezafibrate Infarction Prevention Trial]. *Am J Cardiol* 71:909-915, 1993), showed no significant reduction in fatal or nonfatal myocardial infarction and sudden death in 3,000 patients, although increases in HDL cholesterol appeared to predict benefits. Thus the secondary prevention trials with fibrates have not yet demonstrated benefits as consistent as the trials with statins.

Chapter 85

Concise Review of Principles, Adverse Effects, and Interactions of Cardiac Drugs

Lance J. Oyen, Pharm.D.
Joseph G. Murphy, M.D.

"Primum non nocere": first, do no harm. Most drug interactions and side effects can be prevented by a careful review of the patient's characteristics, including age, ventricular function, conduction system function, liver and kidney function, presence of associated diseases, and the patient's other medications. Adverse drug reactions are often dose-dependent, and correct dosing minimizes patient risk.

Principles of Drug Therapy

Drug side effects and interactions can occur for pharmacokinetic or pharmacodynamic reasons.

Pharmacokinetics refers to the time course and quantity of drug absorption into the bloodstream, distribution to the site of drug action, metabolism to an inactive form, and final elimination. The half-life of an active drug in the body (time for half of the administered and absorbed dose of the drug to be inactivated or eliminated) depends not only on drug clearance but on volume of distribution as well. As the volume of distribution increases, the clearance of the drug is decreased. For example, when using procainamide to treat severe congestive heart failure, increased body water can double the volume of distribution.

Renal or liver failure can markedly decrease the clearance of a drug. As a result, increasing the loading dose (for increased volume of distribution) and decreasing the maintenance dose (for decreased clearance) optimizes procainamide therapy.

Pharmacodynamics refers to the effect of the drug at the site of action (cell membrane or receptor). Coadministered drugs, advanced age, and disease may affect drug dynamics. For example, β-blockers exert a lesser pharmacologic effect in the elderly than in the young, but when doses are titrated, the clinical benefit can be the same regardless of age. More often, drugs have a heightened effect in the elderly and initiation at half the normal starting doses is prudent.

- Pharmacokinetics refers to the absorption, distribution, metabolism (bioconversion), and elimination of drugs.
- Pharmacodynamics refers to the effect of the drug at the cellular level.

The *therapeutic index* (Fig. 1) is the ratio of the toxic concentration to the minimally effective concentration. When this ratio is low (i.e., 2 or 3 or less, as with digoxin), small changes in pharmacokinetics can push the drug into the toxic range or pull the drug down and out of the therapeutic window.

- Therapeutic index = $\dfrac{\text{Toxic Effect Concentration}}{\text{Minimal Effective Concentration}}$

Liver and Kidney Function and Drug Therapy

Liver or kidney failure can result in decreased metabolism and elimination of specific drugs. For instance, the use of two class Ia antiarrhythmic agents without allowing adequate

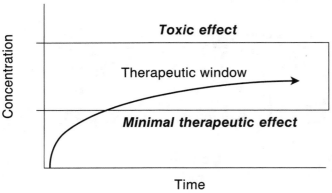

Fig. 1. Therapeutic window.

- Two important formulas:

$$\text{Creatinine Clearance (Cl}_{Cr}) = \frac{140 - \text{Age}}{72} \times \frac{\text{Ideal Body Weight in kg}}{\text{Serum Creatinine in mg/dL}}$$

(For females, answer of above formula multiplied by 0.85.)

Ideal Body Weight (IBW) = [(Height {in inches} - 60) x (2.3)] + # kg

\# = 45 kg for females

\# = 50 kg for males

drug washout (at least 5 half-lives) increases the risk for torsades de pointes (Fig. 2). With renally eliminated drugs, the drug half-life and, consequently, the wash-out period are longer in patients with renal failure.

Renal dose adjustments and patient surveillance minimize the potential for toxic accumulation of drugs and metabolites (Table 1). The initiation of sotalol in a patient with renal dysfunction at routine doses may be well tolerated initially, but drug accumulation may result in torsades de pointes several days later as the concentration increases (Fig. 3).

Renal clearance of drugs eliminated primarily through the kidney is based on correlating drug clearance to the glomerular filtration rate (GFR). Assuming the drug clearance is largely via filtration without active secretion or reabsorption from the renal tubules, an estimated creatinine clearance is as follows:

Drug substitution in renal insufficiency should be by drugs not metabolized by the kidney and therapeutically equivalent. An example would be the use of metoprolol instead of atenolol. Atenolol is eliminated primarily by the kidneys and metoprolol is not, yet both drugs are pharmacologically and clinically equivalent.

Generally, calcium channel blockers, most β-blockers, statins, and anticoagulants have little dependence on renal elimination. Diuretics, angiotensin-converting enzyme (ACE) inhibitors, fibrinic acids, phosphodiesterase inhibitors, and digoxin are all dependent on renal clearance. Cardiac drugs that are potentially nephrotoxic include ACE inhibitors, aspirin, hydralazine, methyldopa, diuretics, and thrombolytics as well as the hypotensive potential of many antihypertensives that may exacerbate prerenal renal failure.

Liver function may be important in drug metabolism for two reasons:

1) Drug elimination depends on bioconversion to inactive

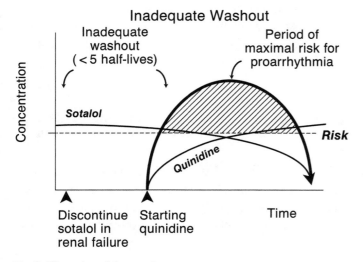

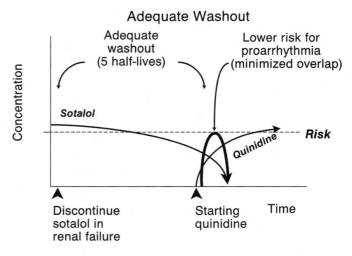

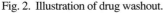

Fig. 2. Illustration of drug washout.

Table 1.—Adjustments of Renally Eliminated Cardiovascular Agents

Drug	Clearance[*] 30-50 mL/min[†]	Clearance 10-30 mL/min[†]	Clearance < 10 mL/min[†]	Dialysis
Acebutolol	↓↓	↓↓↓	↓↓↓	HD
Amiloride	↓↓	↓↓↓	Avoid	
Amrinone			↓↓ – ↓↓↓	
Atenolol	(< 35, max 50 mg)	↓↓ (< 15)	↓↓	HD
Benazepril		↓↓ (max dose 40 mg/day)		HD
Bisoprolol	↓↓ (< 40)	↓↓ (max dose 10 mg/day)		
Bretylium	↓ - ↓↓	↓ - ↓↓	Avoid	
Captopril	↓ (35-75)	↓	↓↓	HD
Carteolol	↓↓ (20-60)	↓↓ (20-60)	↓↓↓ (< 20)	
Clofibrate	↓	↓↓ (10-15)	Avoid	
Digoxin‡	Loading dose = 10 µg/kg (15 µg/kg for AFib); daily dose (µg/day) = [(14 + creatinine clearance/5) ÷ 100] x loading dose			
Disopyramide‡	↓ (30-40)	↓↓ (15-30)	↓↓↓ (< 15)	
Enalapril		↓↓	↓↓	HD, PD
Fenofibrate	Avoid			
Flecainide‡		Initial dose 100 mg/day	↓ - ↓↓ (< 20)	
Fosinopril			↓	
Hydralazine	↓	↓	↓↓ - ↓↓↓	
Lisinopril		↓↓	↓↓↓	HD
Low-molecular-weight heparins			May need to reduce dose	
Magnesium‡	Monitor levels and watch for clinical signs of toxicity			
Milrinone	↓	↓↓	↓↓ - ↓↓↓	
Morphine	↓	↓	↓↓ (use caution)	
Nadolol	↓↓	↓↓	↓↓↓	HD
Nitroprusside	Monitor thiocyanate levels and cyanide toxicity; risk: proportional to dosing rate, duration; inversely proportional to creatinine clearance			HD, PD
Procainamide‡§	↓	↓↓§	↓↓§	HD
Propranolol	↓↓ (10-40)	↓↓	↓↓↓	
Quinapril	↓↓	↓↓↓	↓↓↓ (use caution)	
Quinidine‡			↓	HD
Ramipril	↓ - ↓↓ (max initial dose 5 mg/day)		↓↓ – ↓↓↓	HD
Sotalol	↓↓ (30-60)	↓↓↓	↓↓↓ Close monitoring	HD, PD
Spironolactone	↓↓	↓↓	Avoid	
Thiazide diuretics	Avoid; loop diuretics are preferred for diuresis in renal failure			
Tocainide‡		↓↓	↓↓	HD
Verapamil			↓ - ↓↓	

AFib, atrial fibrillation; HD, hemodialysis removes significant amount; PD, peritoneal dialysis removes significant amount; assess additional doses.

[*]Dose adjustment: ↓ = 25%, ↓↓ = 50%, and ↓↓↓ = 75% empiric dose reduction required from usual dose or frequency (total daily dose).

[†](mL/min numbers) = altered estimated creatinine clearance from category.

[‡]Follow drug levels.

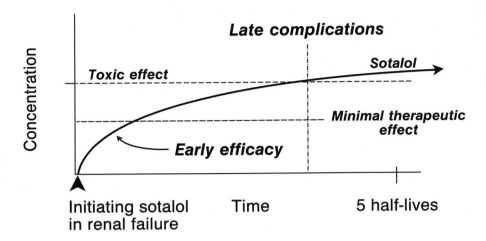

Fig. 3. Drug accumulation.

metabolites (many antiarrhythmics). Conversely, some drugs (enalapril) require conversion by the liver to their active metabolite (enalaprilat).

2) Many cardiac drugs have significant drug-drug interactions by competing for liver enzyme metabolism. Drug bioconversion occurs rapidly with some drugs when administered orally, called the "first-pass effect" (Fig. 4).

With oral intake of a drug, drug absorption occurs via the portal circulation and the drug is immediately subject to liver clearance (Fig. 4). Enzymatic clearance also may occur with cytochrome P-450 (CYP450) enzymes in the small intestine. Both of these degradations yield substantially lower levels of some drugs when given orally instead of intravenously, necessitating much lower doses when given parenterally (Table 2). Lidocaine cannot be given orally because of the rapid elimination of first-pass clearance. Even when given intravenously, lidocaine clearance diminishes markedly in liver insufficiency. When administering lidocaine in cardiogenic shock after myocardial infarction, presumed liver insufficiency necessitates a 50% dose reduction, with close monitoring of toxicity and drug levels.

Estimation or calculation of liver drug clearance is not as convenient as with estimating renal drug clearance. A method used to modify hepatically cleared drugs is to decrease doses when liver enzymes exceed three times normal. In general, most cardiac drugs have some degree of liver clearance, and drugs to absolutely avoid in liver failure include amiodarone, statins, niacin, hydralazine, methyldopa, nifedipine, salicylates, and verapamil. Dose adjustments may be required in liver failure for many "high

first-pass" drugs as well as drugs that are cleared by the kidney and liver, such as flecainide, digoxin, and procainamide. Drug levels are valuable for assessing drug therapy for patients with multiorgan disorders.

● Safe drug therapy depends on appropriate dosing based on patient-specific organ function and individual drug pharmacokinetics.
● Liver metabolism may change the drug from active to inactive (e.g., lidocaine), to another active form (e.g., acebutolol), or from an inactive drug (e.g., enalapril) to an active drug (enalaprilat).

Adverse Reactions to Cardiac Drugs

Most drug side effects are dose-related. Much less frequent are idiosyncratic reactions, which often are immunogenically mediated. Although *all* adverse drug effects may be important, prioritizing surveillance for the most toxic specific side effects simplifies monitoring. The following tables summarize many adverse effects in a manner to simplify your risk-benefit assessment (Tables 3-9).

Cardiac Drugs in Pregnancy

The United States Food and Drug Administration risk factor rating system of drug use in pregnancy is as follows:

Category A—Safe for use during pregnancy.

Category B—No evidence of toxicity but not proven safe.

Category C—Evidence of toxicity in animals but no controlled human studies. Drugs should be given only if the

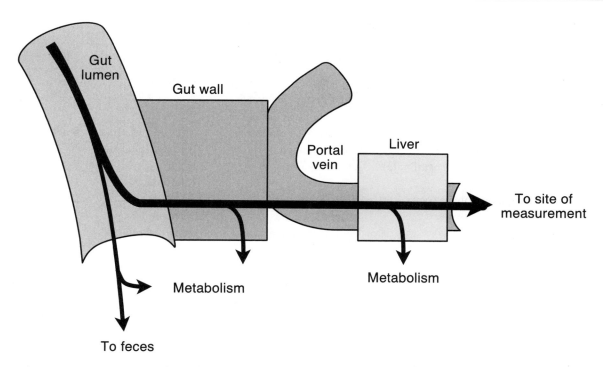

Fig. 4. A drug, given as a solid, encounters several barriers and sites of loss in its sequential movement during gastrointestinal absorption. Dissolution, a prerequisite to movement across the gut wall, is the first step. Incomplete dissolution or metabolism in the gut lumen or by enzymes in the gut wall is a cause of poor absorption. Removal of drug as it first passes through the liver further reduces absorption. (From Rowland M, Tozer TN: *Clinical Pharmacokinetics: Concepts and Applications*. Second edition. Lea & Febiger, 1989, p 114. By permission of Lippincott, Williams & Wilkins.)

potential benefit justifies the potential risk to the fetus.

Category D—There is evidence of human fetal risk, but the benefits from use in pregnant women may be acceptable despite the risk.

Category X—Contraindicated during pregnancy because of proven teratogenicity.

Drug-Drug Interactions

Drug-drug interactions are summarized in Table 10. Clinically significant interactions may be difficult to predict because of many variables, including the pharmacology and therapeutic index of each drug, mechanism of drug

Table 2.—Cardiac Drugs With High First-Pass Liver Clearance

Analgesics	All calcium channel blockers
Meperidine, morphine	Varying degrees between agents
Antiarrhythmics	All HMG-CoA reductase inhibitors ("statins")
Amiodarone	Miscellaneous
Disopyramide, quinidine	Azosemide, clofibrate, warfarin, estrogen, fenoldopam,
Encainide, flecainide, lorcainide	pimobendan, salicylamide
Moricizine, propafenone	Vasodilators
Lidocaine, mexiletine, tocainide	Guanabenz
Angiotensin-converting enzyme inhibitors*	Hydralazine
Enalapril, perindopril, spriapril, trandolapril	Losartan
Most β-blockers	Nicorandil, pinacidil, trapidil
Except atenolol, nadolol, sotalol	Nitrates

*Metabolized to active drug form.

Table 3.—Adverse Effects of Lipid-Lowering Drugs

Drug	Toxic side effect	General side effects	Hypersensitivity	Safe use in pregnancy
Binding resins	None	GI, increase triglycerides, vitamin deficiency (fat-soluble vitamins)	Possible	May bind fat-soluble vitamins (B)
Fibrates	Rhabdomyolysis (rare) Hepatitis (rare) Renal failure (benzafibrate)	GI, diuretic (clofibrate), leukopenia, cholecystitis, cholelithiasis, rash (photosensitivity)	Arthritis, vasculitis; Stevens-Johnson syndrome (clofibrate)	Safety is unknown (C)
HMG-CoA reductase inhibitors	Rhabdomyolysis (rare) Hepatitis (rare) Pancreatitis	GI, CNS, myositis, myalgia, increased serum transaminases (liver), conjunctivitis	LLS; rash (lichenoid eruption), arthralgia, thrombocytopenia	Do not use: reports of birth defects (X)
Nicotinic acid derivatives	Hepatitis Rhabdomyolysis (rare) Coronary steal Hypotension Lactic acidosis	Ocular changes, decreased vision, rash (itching and flushing, acanthosis nigricans, exfoliation, brown pigmentation), GI, CNS, hyperglycemia	Rash (not determined to be allergic-mediated)	(A), Not "toxic" in usual doses for lipid therapy

A, B, C, X, refer to pregnancy class warnings; ANA, antinuclear antibodies; CNS, central nervous system effects; GI, gastrointestinal effects; LDL, low-density lipoprotein; LLS, lupus-like syndrome.

clearance, gastrointestinal function and metabolism, disease states, serum protein status and drug protein binding qualities, and route of administration of the drug (Fig. 5).

- Patients with certain cardiovascular diseases, including arrhythmias, hypertension, renovascular disease, congestive heart failure, and hyperlipidemia, are more susceptible to drug interactions.

Assessing the time course of drug effects depends largely on the half-life of the drugs involved and any active metabolite. Drug interactions may be due to additive or synergistic cellular effects between drugs (pharmacodynamic interactions) or caused by drugs altering the time course of another drug in the body (pharmacokinetic interactions). For example, the half-life of amiodarone averages about 1 month and the drug also has an active metabolite that may further prolong its action. Some pharmacodynamic interactions, such as atrioventricular nodal effects, may occur relatively early in the course of therapy when used with other atrioventricular nodal drugs such as β-blockers, causing exaggerated bradycardia. The metabolic inhibition of amiodarone on warfarin metabolism correlates better with the half-life of the drug and may occur weeks or months after the initiation

of treatment with the combination of the two drugs.

- Amiodarone–warfarin drug interaction is a good example of a serious delayed interaction.

Torsades de Pointes

Torsades de pointes is a side effect that may occur with high doses of a single drug, including many antiarrhythmic agents, or, more likely, may be the result of drug-drug interactions. Torsades de pointes can be idiosyncratic or dose-dependent.

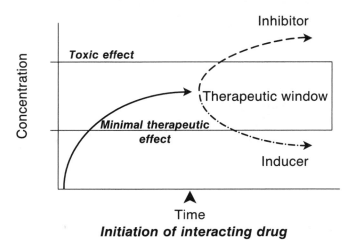

Fig. 5. Clinically significant pharmacokinetic drug interactions.

Table 4.—Cardiac Drug Side Effects

Drug	Toxic side effects	General side effects	Hypersensitivity	Safe use in pregnancy
Angiotensin II antagonists	Hypotension	Headache	Hepatitis, angioedema (rare, cross reaction with ACE inhibitor)	No (D)
ACE inhibitors	Renal failure, hypotension, hyperkalemia, hepatitis	Cough, skin rashes, taste disturbance	Angioedema, skin rash, bone marrow suppression, hepatitis, and alveolitis	No (D)
β-Blockers	Bronchospasm, hypotension, heart failure	Raynaud phenomenon, impotence, increased serum glucose/lipid levels	None	Yes (B, C)*
Calcium channel antagonists†	Proarrhythmia, hypotension, end-organ ischemia ("steal syndrome")—nifedipine IR	Dizziness, flushing, peripheral edema, constipation, postural hypotension, taste disturbances	Verapamil, nifedipine, diltiazem: skin eruption, liver and kidney function defects, fever, eosinophilia, lymphadenopathy, maculopapular rash	Unknown (C)
Centrally acting vasodilators (clonidine and methyldopa)	Withdrawal response, hypotension, proarrhythmias, hepatitis, (methyldopa)	CNS frequent, sexual dysfunction	Methyldopa: Coombs positive (rarely hemolytic anemia), hepatitis, fever, eosinophilia, rash. Clonidine: skin reactions	Unknown (C), methyldopa regarded as safe in pregnancy (JNC VI)
Digoxin	Cardiovascular (heart block, ectopic proarrhythmias, ventricular extra beats, ventricular tachycardia, paroxysmal supraventricular tachycardia)	GI (anorexia, nausea, vomiting, diarrhea) CNS (drowsiness, dizziness, confusion, vision abnormalities, photophobia) with toxicity	Rare: thrombocytopenia, rash	May be used therapeutically for fetal arrhythmias, ouabain drug of choice (B)
Hydralazine	Hypotension, hepatitis, neuropathy	Flushing	LLS; blood dyscrasias and necrotizing vasculitis (rare)	Yes (C)
Loop diuretics	Dehydration, pancreatitis, jaundice, deafness (high dose), thrombocytopenia	Dizziness, postural hypotension, hyponatremia, hypokalemia	Interstitial nephritis, skin reactions (erythema multiforme, Stevens-Johnson syndrome, tissue necrosis)	Use with caution (C)
Nitrates	Syncope, transient ischemic attacks, peripheral edema	Headache, flushing, palpitation	Contact irritation, allergic contact dermatitis	Unknown (C)
Potassium-sparing diuretics‡	Hyperkalemia, dehydration	Rashes, gynecomastia (men) and breast enlargement/soreness (women)‡	Skin reactions	Unknown, amiloride (B)
Thiazide diuretics	Dehydration and, rarely, thrombocytopenia, cholestatic jaundice, pancreatitis, hepatic encephalopathy (in patients with cirrhosis)	Dizziness, gout, increased serum glucose/lipid, orthostasis, hypokalemia/hypomagnesemia, hypercalcemia	Skin rashes, allergic vasculitis	No (D)

ACE, angiotensin-converting enzyme; B, C, D, pregnancy class warning; CNS, central nervous system effects; GI, gastrointestinal effects; IR, immediate release; JNC VI, recommendations of the Sixth Joint National Committee on Hypertension; LLS, lupus-like syndrome.

*Metoprolol, atenolol, and labetalol may be used in late pregnancy (JNC VI).

†Unproven association with internal malignancy.

‡Possible association with breast carcinoma and antiandrogenic effect.

Table 5.—Side Effects of Hematologically Active Agents Used in Cardiology

Drug	Toxic side effects	General side effects	Hypersensitivity	Safe use in pregnancy
Aspirin	Reye syndrome, bleeding, GI ulceration, renal toxicity, pulmonary edema, blood dyscrasias	Tinnitus and hearing changes, minor bleeding, hemolytic anemia, gastritis	Bronchospasm, urticaria, angioedema, vasomotor rhinitis, anaphylaxis, shock, purpura, hemorrhagic vasculitis, erythema multiforme, Stevens-Johnson syndrome, Lyell syndrome	Yes (C) - no increased risk in large cohort studies
Abciximab	Bleeding (intra-abdominal, retroperitoneal), thrombocytopenia, hypotension	Pain, sweating	Unknown (none reported with chimeric form); rare with reexposure	Unknown (C)
Clopidogrel	Hemorrhage, skin reactions, gastric ulceration	Gastritis (similar to aspirin), fatigue, flu-like syndrome, myalgias (all similar to aspirin)	Allergic reactions (necrosis, ischemic)	Unknown (B)
Danaparoid	Very low risk for type II HIT (vs. heparin), hemorrhage	Injection site pain, GI (nausea, constipation), fever, rash, pain	Rash and fever; low cross-reactivity with type II HIT (no cases)	Unknown (B)
Dipyridamole	Bleeding, myocardial infarction, chest pain, partial seizure	ST-segment abnormalities, GI, dizziness, rash, dyspnea, syncope	Allergic reactions reported (skin)	Unknown (C)
Heparin, unfractionated (UFH)	HIT type I (mild) and type II (severe), syndrome of thrombohemorrhagic complications (see Hypersensitivity), hypotension; spontaneous arterial emboli	Delayed wound healing, osteoporosis (chronic therapy), minor bleeding, hypoaldosteronism, priapism	Urticaria, conjunctivitis, rhinitis, asthma, cyanosis, tachypnea, feeling of oppression, fever, angioneurotic edema, and anaphylactic shock Rarely—hemorrhagic skin necrosis, vasospastic reactions DIC Anaphylaxis (rare)	Chronic administration: osteopenia for mother (B)
Eptifibatide	Hemorrhage, hypotension	Minor bleeding; others rare		Unknown (B)
Low-molecular-weight heparin	Hemorrhage, thrombocytopenia (type I [mild] and type II [severe] but lower incidence than UFH; cross-reactive with UFH-induced events)	Same as for UFH	Same as for UFH	Yes (B)
Protamine	Noncardiogenic pulmonary edema	Hypotension (with too rapid infusion rates)	Flushing, urticaria, wheezing, angioedema and hypotension, anaphylaxis, bronchospasm or shock (IgE or IgG), pulmonary vasoconstriction, anaphylactoid	Unknown (C)
Ticlopidine	Hemorrhage, hematologic disorders (leukopenia, agranulocytosis, thrombocytopenia and pancytopenia [reversible], thrombotic thrombocytopenia (some lethal cases), hepatitis	Skin rashes, severe chronic diarrhea	Rashes (immunogenically mediated unknown)	Unknown (B)

Table 5 (continued)

Drug	Toxic side effects	General side effects	Hypersensitivity	Safe use in pregnancy
Tirofiban	Hemorrhage, bradycardia, dissection of coronary artery	Mild bleeding, edema, pain, CNS	Not reported, no repeat exposure information available	(B)
Thrombo- lytics	Hemorrhage, transient hypotensive reactions with streptokinase, embolic phenomena (acute renal failure, cholesterol emboliza- tion), reperfusion arrhythmias	Phlebitis at site (strepto- kinase)	Most associated with streptokinase and anistrep- lase (history of prior exposure to *Streptococcus* spp), Guillain-Barré, hemolysis, anaphylactic shock, pyrexia, skin rash, angioedema, bronchospasm, ARDS	Yes (urokinase) (B), others unknown (C)
Warfarin	Hemorrhage, hemorrhagic skin necrosis, fetal toxicity Rare—cholestatic hepatitis	Vasodilatation, cholesterol embolization ("purple toe or glove syndrome")	Maculopapular rashes, pruritic purpuritic skin eruptions	No (D) (warfarin, embryopathy)

ARDS, acute respiratory distress syndrome; B, C, pregnancy class warning; CNS, central nervous system effects; DIC, disseminated intravascular coagu- lation; GI, gastrointestinal effects; HIT, heparin-induced thrombocytopenia; LLS, lupus-like syndrome.

Table 6.—Antiarrhythmic Drug Side Effects

Drug	Toxic side effects	General side effects	Hypersensitivity	Safe use in pregnancy
Adenosine	Chest pain, ischemia, bronchoconstriction, increased ICP, VF (infant)	Dyspnea, dizziness, epi- gastric pain, flushing, GI, headache	Not reported	Unknown (C)
		Type I antiarrhythmic agents		
Cibenzoline	Hypertension, proarrhyth- mias, hypotension, heart failure, hepatotoxicity	GI, CNS, muscle pain, hypo- glycemia, hyperkalemia, pruritus, taste disturbances, foul-smelling sweat	Not reported	Unknown
Disopyramide	Heart failure, proarrhyth- mias	Hypoglycemia, anticho- linergic syndromes	Angioedema (rare)	Uterine contractions (C)*
Flecainide	Proarrhythmias, hypo- tension (IV), heart failure	CNS, GI, neutropenia, urinary retention, ankle edema	Not reported	Unknown (C)
Lidocaine	Coma, seizures, respiratory depression, proarrhythmias	CNS (nystagmus is early sign of toxicity)	Not reported	Unknown (C)

Table 6 (continued)

Drug	Toxic side effects	General side effects	Hypersensitivity	Safe use in pregnancy
Mexiletine	Proarrhythmias	CNS, cholestasis, GI, rash	Thrombocytopenia, ANA	Unknown (C)
Procainamide	Proarrhythmias, hypotension, worsened myocardial contractility, neutropenia	CNS, rash, cholestasis, Raynaud phenomenon	Lupus-like syndrome, ANA, fever, hematologic (neutropenia, pancytopenia, pure red cell aplasia, Achilles tendinitis, Coombs'-positive hemolytic anemia)	Unknown (C)*
Propafenone	Proarrhythmias, bronchospasm and dyspnea, heart failure	SIADH, neutropenia, GI, CNS (including peripheral neuropathy), impotence, taste disturbance	ANA, LLS	Unknown (C)
Quinidine	Proarrhythmias, heart failure, hypotension	GI (most common), CNS, cinchonism, esophagitis, anticholinergic syndrome	Fever, rash, thrombocytopenia, neutropenia, hemolytic anemia, hepatitis, Coombs'-positive lupus anticoagulant, asthma, anaphylaxis Rarely, LLS	Unknown (C)*
Tocainide	Interstitial pneumonitis, pulmonary fibrosis, blood dyscrasias (1 in 300), hepatitis, proarrhythmias	CNS, GI, night sweats	Rash, eosinophilia, LLS, ANA	Unknown (C)
		Type III antiarrhythmic agents		
N-acetylprocainamide (NAPA)	Proarrhythmias (especially if level > 30 µg/mL)	GI, CNS	Not reported	Unknown (C)
Amiodarone	Hypothyroid, hyperthyroid, hepatitis, pulmonary (pneumonitis, fibrosis, bronchiolitis obliterans, organizing pneumonia), IV administration—AV block and hypotension, proarrhythmias	Corneal microdeposits, GI, photosensitivity and blue skin, rashes, neuropathy	Interstitial pneumonitis may be hypersensitivity reaction	Neonatal thyroid effects (C)
Bretylium	Hypotension, proarrhythmias	GI, hypertension, hyperthermia	Not reported	Unknown (C)
Sotalol	Proarrhythmias, bronchospasm, hypotension	CNS, GI, reduced peripheral vascular perfusion, impotence, increased serum glucose/lipid, fatigue	Not reported	Unknown (C)

ANA, antinuclear antibodies; AV, atrioventricular; C, pregnancy class C warning; CNS, central nervous system effects; GI, gastrointestinal effects; ICP, intracranial pressure; IV, intravenous; LLS, lupus-like syndrome; SIADH, syndrome of inappropriate antidiuretic hormone; VF, ventricular fibrillation.
*Drugs with anticholinergic effects have been found to cause neonatal meconium ileus.
Anticholinergic syndrome: dry mouth, dysuria/increased urinary retention, increased intraocular pressure/blurred vision, flushing, agitation/psychosis/dementia, sinus tachycardia.

Table 7.—Electrocardiographic (ECG) Effects of Cardiac Drugs

Drug	ECG effects	Toxic effects
N-acetylprocainamide (NAPA)	↑ QRS, QT interval	Torsades de pointes; ventricular proarrhythmias
Adenosine	↑ PR interval, ↓ HR	AVB, sinus bradycardia, ventricular extra beats
Amiodarone	↑ PR and QT interval ↑ QRS (may), ↓ HR	Sinus bradycardia, AVB, infra-His block, asystole refractory to DC cardioversion; torsades de pointes, VF
β-Blockers	↓ PVCs, ↑ PR interval ↓ HR	Sinus bradycardia, AVB, alternating sinus rhythm with intermittent sinoatrial block
Bretylium	↑ QT	Ventricular proarrhythmias
Calcium channel antagonists (verapamil, diltiazem, bepridil, mibefradil)	↑ PR interval, ↑ QT (bepridil), ↓ HR	Mobitz type I AVB, 3rd-degree AVB, sinus bradycardia, junctional escape, accelerated junctional rhythm
		If sick sinus: AVB, sinoatrial block, sinus arrest or sinus bradycardia
		If WPW: rapid ventricular response, VT or VF
Centrally acting agents (clonidine and methyldopa)	↑ PR interval	AVB and 3rd-degree AVB (clonidine and methyldopa) Wenckebach (clonidine)
Digoxin	↑ PR, ↓ QT interval, ↓ HR	Any proarrhythmia possible, AVB, asymmetrical T-wave inversion, L or R BBB, PSVT with block, paroxysmal atrial tachycardia and bigeminy
Disopyramide	↑ QRS, QT interval, ↑ or ↓ HR	Torsades de pointes; tachycardia with BBB or conversion to SVT (anticholinergic effects)
Flecainide	↑ QRS, PR, QT interval	Torsades de pointes (rare), ↓ atrial-His conduction, bradycardia, sinus node dysfunction, BBB, atrial or ventricular proarrhythmias
Hydralazine	None or ↑ HR	Reflex tachycardia
Ibutilide	↑ QRS and QT interval	Torsades de pointes, ventricular extrasystoles, nonsustained monomorphic VT, SVT, BBB, AVB, sinus bradycardia
Lidocaine	↓ QTc or none Toxicity may ↑ PR and QRS	Sinus bradycardia, sustained ventricular tachycardia, asystole in severe AVB
Loop diuretics	None	Hypokalemia related
Mexiletine	↑ QRS interval or none	Sinus arrest, bradycardia, AV dissociation, heart block
Phenytoin	↑ PR interval, ↓ QT interval or none	AVB, sinus bradycardia, ventricular proarrhythmias
Procainamide	↑ or ↓ PR, QRS, or QT interval	Torsades de pointes, bradycardia, heart block
Propafenone	↑ QRS width, ↑ PR interval, ↓ HR	Sinus bradycardia, sinus arrest, AVB, BBB, atrial proarrhythmias, VT, VF
Quinidine	↑ or ↓ PR, ↑ QT interval, ↑ QRS, ↑ HR	AVB, sinus bradycardia, sinus dysfunction, BBB, atrial fibrillation, VT, VF, "quinidine syncope"
Sotalol	↑ QRS, QT interval, ↓ HR	Torsades de pointes, ventricular proarrhythmias, AVB
Thiazide diuretics	None	Hypokalemia-related
Tocainide	↑ QRS interval or none	Sinus bradycardia, sinus arrest with sinoatrial block, may worsen VT, VF

AV, atrioventricular; AVB, atrioventricular block; BBB, bundle branch block; HR, heart rate; PVST, paroxysmal supraventricular tachycardia; SVT, supraventricular tachycardia; VF, ventricular fibrillation; VT, ventricular tachycardia; WPW, Wolff-Parkinson-White syndrome.

Table 8.—Risk Factors for Complications With Cardiac Drugs

Drug	Risk factors
Adenosine	Drug interaction with dipyridamole
Angiotensin II antagonists	(See entry below for ACE inhibitors, "for Renal Failure" in ACE-Inhibitor section, Pregnancy)
ACE inhibitors	Pregnancy; for renal failure: low sodium or volume status (high renin activation), diuretic use, collagen vascular disease, renal disease (bilateral renal artery stenosis), prior angioedema, severe heart failure, diabetes mellitus
β-Blockers	Severe LV dysfunction, 2nd/3rd-degree AVB, bronchial asthma, IDDM, renal impairment (atenolol/nadolol/sotalol), anaphylaxis, withdrawal (hypertensive crises), rapid dose titration
Calcium channel antagonists	LV dysfunction and severe post-AMI or CAD, CV disease with non-slow drug formulations, HOCM (increased proarrhythmias), WPW, SSS, severe LV heart failure (especially verapamil, diltiazem, bepridil), portal hypertension (nifedipine—may increase variceal hemorrhage risk)
Centrally acting agents	Withdrawal reactions: clonidine and methyldopa—hypertension, tachycardia, tremors, sweating
Fibrates	Renal failure, hypothyroidism (myopathy), liver failure or cirrhosis, biliary cirrhosis/gallstones
Digoxin	Liver and renal failure, electrolyte imbalance, ischemic cause of disease, normal ejection fraction plus no heart failure
HMG-CoA reductase inhibitors	Liver failure, drug interactions, elderly
Hydralazine	Ischemic patient without rate-controlling agent
Loop diuretics	Severe hepatic insufficiency, premature infants
Nitrates	Withdrawal, severe myocardial infarction, CAD, prior cardiac disease may predispose to steal syndrome; hypotension, reflex tachycardia and bradycardia
Potassium-sparing diuretics	Elderly and renal insufficiency
Thiazide diuretics	Heart failure, compensated hepatic cirrhosis with secondary hyperaldosteronism
Type I antiarrhythmic agents	Use with other QT-prolonging drug, ischemic disease, electrolyte imbalances
Disopyramide	Heart failure, benign prostatic hypertrophy, glaucoma, myasthenia gravis, etc. (anticholinergic effects), liver or renal failure
Flecainide	Heart failure, liver disease, routine use after MI
Lidocaine	CHF, liver and renal failure, severe AVB, seizure history, routine use after MI
Mexiletine	Blood dyscrasias, liver failure
Phenytoin	Drug interactions, severe AVB, liver failure
Procainamide	CHF, renal or liver failure, fast infusion (hypotension), sinus disease, long-term use (> 6 mo) associated risk of lupus-like syndrome
Propafenone	Bronchospastic disease, heart failure, liver failure, structural heart disease, rapid dose titration
Quinidine	Anticholinergic effects (benign prostatic hypertrophy, glaucoma, myasthenia gravis, etc.), liver failure or severe renal failure
Tocainide	Blood dyscrasias, renal or liver failure
Type III antiarrhythmic agents	Use with other QT-prolonging drugs, electrolyte imbalances
N-acetylprocainamide (NAPA)	Renal failure
Amiodarone	Elderly, dose > 400 mg/d, thyroid, lung, eye, or liver dysfunction; fast IV infusion (hypotension), low ejection fraction ($\uparrow$ hepatitis)
Ibutilide	Electrolyte imbalances, torsades de pointes risk factors
Bretylium	Fast infusion (hypotension)
Sotalol	Renal failure, dose-related torsades de pointes/proarrhythmia

ACE, angiotensin-converting enzyme; AMI, acute myocardial infarction; AVB, atrioventricular block; CAD, coronary artery disease; CHF, congestive heart failure; CV, cardiovascular; HOCM, hypertrophic obstructive cardiomyopathy; IDDM, insulin-dependent diabetes mellitus; LV, left ventricular; MI, myocardial infarction; SSS, sick sinus syndrome; WPW, Wolff-Parkinson-White syndrome.

Table 9.—Metabolic Effects of Cardiac Drugs

Agent	Total cholesterol	LDL	HDL	TG	Insulin sensitivity
High-dose thiazides	↑	↑	↔	↑	↓
Low-dose thiazides	↔	↔	↔	↔	↔
β-Blockers	↔	↔	↓	↑	↓
α-Blockers	↓	↔	↑	↔	↑
ACE inhibitors	↔	↔	↔	↔	↑
Calcium channel blockers	↔	↔	↔	↔	↔

ACE, angiotensin-converting enzyme; HDL, high-density lipoproteins; LDL, low-density lipoproteins; TG, triglycerides.

Table 10—Drug Interactions[*†]

Type	Drug affected (column 1)	Effect on (column 1 by 3)	Caused by (column 3)	Action required
Antiarrhythmics	Ia antiarrhythmics	Risk	AV blockers Type I and III anti-arrhythmic agents	Enhanced AV node effects, monitor ECG, use of Ia with III agents increases risk for torsades de pointes
	Disopyramide Quinidine Mexiletine (phenytoin, phenobarbital) Propafenone (phenytoin, phenobarbital)	↓	**Antiepileptics**	Initial dose increase may be necessary, monitor drug levels and effects Antiepileptics: phenytoin, carbamazepine, phenobarbital are enzyme inducers
	Disopyramide Quinidine Mexiletine Propafenone	↓	**Rifampin**	Initial dose increase necessary, monitor drug levels and effects
	Disopyramide Lidocaine Mexiletine	↑	**Protease inhibitors (HIV antivirals)**	Decrease initial dose 50%, monitor drug levels (do not stop protease inhibitor) Protease inhibitors: ritonavir, indinavir, saquinavir, nelfinavir
	Lidocaine Quinidine Procainamide N-acetylprocainamide	↑	Cimetidine	Cimetidine: monitor drug levels and clinical effects or use alternative H_2 antagonist

Table 10 (continued)

Type	Drug affected (column 1)	Effect on (column 1 by 3)	Caused by (column 3)	Action required
	Quinidine	↑	Azole antifungals Metronidazole Verapamil	Monitor QRS closely, progressive increase in levels possible Verapamil: initiate at 50% quinidine dose
			Azole antifungals, ketoconazole, itraconazole, miconazole (IV), fluconazole	
	Lidocaine Quinidine Propafenone	↑	Propranolol Metoprolol	β-blockers: monitor closely for increased AV effect and increased drug levels (lidocaine)
	Quinidine Disopyramide	↑	Macrolides	Monitor QT closely, reports of increased levels
			Macrolides: erythromycin, clarithromycin, troleandomycin	
	Flecainide Mexiletine Propafenone	↑	**SSRIs** **Quinidine**	Avoid combination with SSRIs because of risks of ↑ levels, quinidine may increase levels (consider initial dose ↓ 50%)
			SSRIs: fluvoxamine, fluoxetine, sertraline, paroxetine	
	Procainamide Quinidine Flecainide Mexiletine Propafenone	↑	**Amiodarone**	↑ Levels and ↑ risks, reduce initial dose 30%-50% when using with amiodarone, monitor QT and toxic effects closely
	Adenosine	↑	Dipyridamole β-Blockers	Reduce dose used
		↓	Theophylline	Increased dose may be required
	Amiodarone	↓	Phenytoin	Phenytoin may ↓ amiodarone and amiodarone may ↑ phenytoin, monitoring levels of each may be required
ACE inhibitors		Risk	**Allopurinol** **Diuretics** **NSAIDs** α-Antagonists	Increased risk of hypersensitivity (allopurinol), renal toxicity (diuretics, NSAIDs), and orthostatic hypotension (α-antagonists)

Table 10 (continued)

Type	Drug affected (column 1)	Effect on (column 1 by 3)	Caused by (column 3)	Action required
Anticoagulants	Warfarin (Always check drug package inserts for interactions with warfarin; this table is not all-inclusive)	↑	**Amiodarone** **Allopurinol** **Azole antifungals**‡ **Erythromycin** Omeprazole Quinolones‡	Antagonize metabolism: Amiodarone—delayed effect, initiate warfarin with 50% anticipated dose; others decrease initial dose 25% Initiate amiodarone and follow PT closely for chronic increase, most occur in days to weeks
			Cimetidine SSRIs‡ Metronidazole Chloramphenicol **Phenylbutazone** Penicillins‡ Leukotriene agents‡ Cephalosporins‡ **Sulfonamides**‡ **Cotrimoxazole**	Alternative agents within classes may be less causative, monitor INR frequently Azole antifungals: ketoconazole, itraconazole, miconazole (IV), fluconazole Increased effect: NSAIDs (select)—displacement from plasma protein binding site or platelet effect plus erosive tissue effect (GI)
			Anabolic steroids **Thyroid drugs**‡ NSAIDs‡ **Propafenone** **Quinidine** **Clofibrate** Chemotherapy‡ **Anticonvulsants**‡ (inhibitors/ displacers)	Cephalosporins inhibit vitamin K synthesis
		↓	**Rifampin** **Anticonvulsants**‡ (inducers) **Resin-binding cholesterol agents** Haloperidol Oral contraceptives Sucralfate Nafcillin/dicloxacillin **Vitamin K**	The use of oral contraceptives may be procoagulant, use with oral anticoagulants may be contrabeneficial Follow INR/PT very closely or avoid combination Vitamin K: maintain diet as consistent as possible
	Anticoagulants	↑	**Aspirin** **Clopidogrel** **Ticlopidine** **NSAIDs** **Glycoprotein IIb/ IIIa inhibitors** **Thrombolytics**	Platelet effect: increased risk of bleeding due to antiplatelet effects, assess risk and benefits carefully

Table 10 (continued)

Type	Drug affected (column 1)	Effect on (column 1 by 3)	Caused by (column 3)	Action required
Antiplatelet agents	Dipyridamole (IV)	↑	**AV blockers**	Monitor for excessive bradycardia due to enhanced AV blockade
	Glycoprotein IIb/IIIa inhibitors	↑	**Heparin**	May need to reduce dose of heparin to ~40% of normal targeted aPTT range (Abciximab-EPILOG trial), monitor closely for bleeding
	Phenytoin	↑	**Ticlopidine** **Clopidogrel**	Phenytoin levels may double, necessitating frequent check of phenytoin levels
Calcium channel antagonists	Amlodipine Felodipine Isradipine Mibefradil Nicardipine Nifedipine Nimodipine Nisoldipine Verapamil	↑	Erythromycin Azole antifungals Protease inhibitors Cimetidine Grapefruit juice	Reduce initial doses up to 50% and monitor for clinical toxicity (side effects), titrate doses upward as tolerated Grapefruit juice interaction may require large amounts ingested (≥ 200 mL/d) for effect Protease inhibitors: ritonavir, indinavir, saquinavir, nelfinavir Azole antifungals: ketoconazole, itraconazole, IV miconazole, fluconazole
		Risk	Phenytoin	Phenytoin may ↓ CCBs or CCBs may ↑ Phenytoin levels: avoid CCBs if possible
		↓	Rifampin/rifabutin Phenobarbital	May need increased doses, monitor clinical effect, phenobarbital with nifedipine
	Nifedipine Felodipine Verapamil	↑	Ethanol	Increased toxicity because of elevated levels if alcohol is consumed with chronic therapy
	Verapamil Diltiazem Mibefradil Bepridil	↑	**AV blockers** **Adenosine** **Dipyridamole**	Increased AV antagonism; monitor for excessive AVB or bradycardia and avoid as appropriate
Antihyperlipidemic agents	Fibrates Niacin	Risk	**Statins** Furosemide	Increased risk of myositis and rhabdomyolysis Furosemide has ↑ risk with bezafibrate

Table 10 (continued)

Type	Drug affected (column 1)	Effect on (column 1 by 3)	Caused by (column 3)	Action required
	HMG-CoA reductase inhibitors ("statins")	↑	**Macrolides** **Mibefradil** **Azole antifungals** **Cyclosporine** **Nefazodone** **Protease inhibitors**	Monitor for toxic side effects (myopathy, rhabdomyolysis), addition of antivirals requires 50% dose reduction and therapeutic monitoring for toxicity
			Protease inhibitors: ritonavir, indinavir, saquinavir, nelfinavir	
			Azole antifungals: ketoconazole, itraconazole, miconazole (IV), fluconazole	
	Oral drugs (general)	↓	**Cholestyramine** **Colestipol**	Reduced absorption of many drugs, check interactions with other drugs
	Statins	↑	**Nicotinic acid** **Fibrates**	Increased risk of myositis and rhabdomyolysis (all statins potential)
Antihypertensive agents	All antihypertensive agents	↓	**Bretylium** NSAIDs **Aspirin** (high dose)	Reduce use of offending agents when appropriate, alternative agents include acetaminophen (paracetamol) or opiate analgesics
	Clonidine	↑	**AV blockers**	Enhanced AVB effect
β-Blockers	General	↑	**Dipyridamole (IV)** **Adenosine** **AV blockers**	Increased AV antagonism, monitor for excessive AVB or bradycardia and avoid as appropriate
	Bisoprolol Labetalol Metoprolol Pindolol Propranolol Timolol	↑	Ritonavir SSRIs‡ **Mibefradil** **Amiodarone**	Monitor for toxic side effects and reduce dose of β-blocker as appropriate, amiodarone has affected metoprolol and may include others that are cleared by liver
		↓	Rifampin	May need larger initial doses; monitor for effect
Diuretics	General	Risk	**Digoxin** **Antiarrhythmic agents**	Follow potassium levels closely; may increase toxicity of digoxin and antiarrhythmics

Table 10 (continued)

Type	Drug affected (column 1)	Effect on (column 1 by 3)	Caused by (column 3)	Action required
			TdP drugs **ACE inhibitors**	TdP = (torsades) drugs: see Table 11 Diuretic therapy may increase risk of initiating ACE inhibitors, encourage supine while initiating ACE inhibitors if taking diuretics chronically
	Loop diuretics	↑	**Aminoglycosides** **Cisplatin**	Increased ototoxicity, reduce rate of administration (loop diuretics) or avoid agent
	Potassium-sparing	Risk	**Potassium supplements** **ACE inhibitors**	Avoid potassium supplement, increase frequency of serum potassium level measurements
Digitalis Glycosides	Digoxin	↑	**Amphotericin B** **Amiodarone** **Calcium supplements** **CCBs** Cyclosporine Erythromycin **Flecainide** **Itraconazole** **Mibefradil** Neuromuscular blockers Omeprazole **Propafenone** **Quinidine** Quinine **Reserpine** Tetracycline	May increase digoxin as much as 50%-75%, assess digoxin levels more frequently Amiodarone, verapamil, propafenone, quinidine: initiate at 50% starting dose Neuromuscular blockers may cause increased proarrhythmias CCBs: those affected include verapamil, diltiazem, and nifedipine
		↓	**Cholestyramine** **Colestipol** Antacids Metoclopramide Sulfasalazine	Avoid coadministration, consider effective alternative therapy if difficult to use
Vasodilators	Nitroglycerin	↓	Ergotamines	Vasoconstriction antagonizes effects, avoid use together

ACE, angiotensin-converting enzyme; aPTT, activated partial thromboplastin time; AV, atrioventricular; CCBs, calcium channel blockers; ECG, electrocardiogram; HIV, human immunodeficiency virus; INR, international normalized ratio; IV, intravenous; NSAID, nonsteroidal anti-inflammatory drug; PT, prothrombin time; SSRI, selective serotonin reuptake inhibitor.

*Boldface type signifies more prevalent or severe interactions.

†In patients taking the drug in column 1, the addition of the drug in column 3 causes the effect in column 2 on drug 1.

‡Check for specific agents before use.

The proarrhythmias caused by class Ia antiarrhythmic agents are not directly dose-related, but risk increases with serum concentrations. Most other drug causes of torsades de pointes appear dose-related. Table 11 describes drug and other reported causes of torsades de pointes. Table 12 highlights the most important interactions.

Torsades de pointes drug interactions may be classed as pharmacodynamic or pharmacokinetic. As mentioned above, quinidine plus sotalol share cellular mechanisms for potentially triggering torsades de pointes. Drug antagonism of hepatic cytochrome P-450 isoenzyme metabolism may cause torsades de pointes, whereas antagonism of gut enzymes would prevent absorption. Table 12 describes two of the most common isoenzymes, CYP2D6 and CYP3A4, that account for the metabolism of most drugs that cause torsades de pointes. When the isoenzymes are inhibited, the concentrations of torsades de pointes drugs increase, which increases proarrhythmic risks. For example, the combination of erythromycin and astemizole may cause torsades de pointes.

Table 11.—Acquired Forms of Torsades de Pointes*

Drug-induced
  Antiarrhythmic agents
Type Ia, Ic	Erythromycin	Fenoxidil
Type III	Quinine	Pentamidine
Terfenadine	Diuretics (potassium related)	Pimozide
Astemizole	Probucol	Prenylamine
Haloperidol (IV)	Bepridil	Lidoflazine
Cisapride	TMP-SMX	Pirmenol
Phenothiazines	Ketanserin	Corticosteroids
Tricyclic anti-depressants	Amantadine	Chloroquine
Tetracyclic anti-depressants	Chloral hydrate	Atropine

Toxin-induced—organophosphates, arsenic, cocaine
Disease-induced—subarachnoid hemorrhage, cerebrovascular accident, encephalitis, head injury, myocarditis, hypothyroidism, hyperparathyroidism, pheochromocytoma, hyperaldosteronism, severe bradycardia
Electrolyte-induced—hypomagnesemia, hypokalemia, hypocalcemia
Nutritional disorders—liquid protein diets, starvation

TMP-SMX, trimethoprim-sulfamethoxazole.
*Italics indicates higher frequency of reports.

Table 12.—Potential and Documented Drug-Drug Interactions for Torsades de Pointes*

	CYP2D6[†]		CYP3A4[†]	
Substrates (drugs reported to cause torsades de pointes)	Chlorpromazine	Imipramine	**Astemizole**	**Erythromycin**
	Cyclobenzaprine	Mexiletine	Amitriptyline	Imipramine
	Desipramine	Perphenazine	**Cisapride**	**Quinidine**
	Encainide	Propafenone	Chlorpromazine	**Quinine**
	Flecainide	Thioridazine	Cyclobenzaprine	**Terfenadine**
	Haloperidol	Trimipramine		
Inhibitors (drugs inhibiting metabolism of above drugs and precipitating torsades de pointes)	Amiodarone	Paroxetine	**Cimetidine**	Metronidazole
	Cimetidine	Perphenazine	**Cisapride**	Mibefradil
	Clomipramine	Propafenone	**Clarithromycin**	Miconazole
	Clotrimazole	Quinidine	**Erythromycin**	Nefazodone
	Delaviridine	Ranitidine	**Itraconazole**	Nelfinavir
	Dextropropoxyphene	Ritonavir	**Ketoconazole**	Nevirapine
	Doxorubicin	Sertindole	**Troleandomycin**	Omeprazole
	Fluoxetine[‡]	Sertraline	Anastrozole	Paroxetine
	Fluvoxamine	Thioridazine	Cyclosporine	Quinidine
	Fluphenazine	Venlafaxine	Danazol	Ranitidine
	Haloperidol	Vinblastine	Delavirdine	Ritonavir
	Lomustine	Vinorelbine	Diltiazem	Saquinavir
	Mibefradil		Fluconazole	Sparfloxacin
			Fluoxetine[‡]	Sertindole
			Fluvoxamine	Troglitazone
			Grapefruit drink	Verapamil
			Indinavir	Zafirlukast

*Boldface type signifies documented cases of interactions causing torsades de pointes.
[†]CYP2D6 and CYP3A4 are cytochrome enzyme systems.
[‡]Metabolite inhibits in addition to drug.

Suggested Review Reading

1. Briggs GG, Freeman RK, Yaffe SJ: *Drugs in Pregnancy and Lactation: A Reference Guide to Fetal and Neonatal Risk*. Fifth edition. Baltimore: Williams & Wilkins, 1998.
A definitive source of information about drug effects in pregnancy and lactation.

2. Dukes MNG (editor): *Meyler's Side Effects of Drugs*. Thirteenth edition. Amsterdam: Elsevier Science BV, 1996.
One of the most comprehensive and up-to-date reference texts on drug side effects. Citing all drug-induced disorders and including a description of the event, the text serves as an integral drug information source.

3. Hansten PD, Horn JR: *Hansten and Horn's Drug Interactions, Analysis and Management*. Vancouver, Washington: Applied Therapeutics, 1997.
This reference is one of the "gold standard" updated references on drug interactions.

4. Joint National Committee on Prevention, Detection, Evaluation, and Treatment of High Blood Pressure: The sixth report of the Joint National Committee on Prevention, Detection, Evaluation, and Treatment of High Blood Pressure. *Arch Intern Med* 157:2413-2446, 1997.
As a clinical guideline to the management of hypertension, this document provides rationale for using antihypertensive agents and delineates many key issues in using these agents when contraindications or drug interactions occur in the treatment of hypertension.

5. Koren G, Pastuszak A, Ito S: Drugs in pregnancy. *N Engl J Med* 338:1128-1137, 1998.
Excellent summary of drugs safe to use in pregnancy.

6. Kowey PR: Pharmacological effects of antiarrhythmic drugs. Review and update. *Arch Intern Med* 158:325-332, 1998.
This concise, comprehensive review article is an up-to-date discussion of antiarrhythmic therapy, emphasizing pharmacology, pharmacokinetics, and the role disease states play in using antiarrhythmics.

7. Michalets EL: Update: clinically significant cytochrome P-450 drug interactions. *Pharmacotherapy* 18:84-112, 1998.
Excellent review chapter on cytochrome P-450 (CYP450) enzymatic drug interactions.

8. Rowland M, Tozer TN: *Clinical Pharmacokinetics: Concepts and Applications*. Third edition. Baltimore: Williams & Wilkins, 1995.
A user-friendly textbook integrating pharmacokinetic concepts with clinical decision-making.

9. Tan HL, Hou CJ, Lauer MR, et al: Electrophysiologic mechanisms of the long QT interval syndromes and torsade de pointes. *Ann Intern Med* 122:701-714, 1995.
This review summarizes theoretical electrophysiologic mechanisms of long QT syndrome and torsades de pointes, covers pharmacologic rationale for drugs implicated, and discusses therapy of both disorders.

Questions

Multiple Choice (choose the one best answer)

1. The *clinical* significance of a drug-drug interaction is likely to be most dependent on:
   a. Method of administration
   b. Therapeutic index (narrow versus wide)
   c. Volume of distribution
   d. Half-life of metabolite

2. High first-pass metabolism is important for many reasons *except*:
   a. Oral medications require significantly lower doses compared with intravenous doses
   b. Impaired liver perfusion decreases dosing requirement
   c. Some medications do not achieve therapeutic effectiveness when given orally
   d. Lidocaine dosing is dependent on first pass

3. When initiating amiodarone therapy in a patient stabilized with warfarin, you would need to:
   a. Decrease the amiodarone dose 50%
   b. Increase the amiodarone dose 50%
   c. Follow prothrombin time for acute changes
   d. Follow prothrombin time for chronic progressive changes

4. Torsades de pointes can result from all *except*:
   a. Cisapride when taken with erythromycin
   b. Grapefruit juice when taken with cyclosporine
   c. Haloperidol intravenous push given in high doses
   d. Sotalol in renal insufficiency

5. Most complications of cardiac drugs can be classed generally as:
   a. Dose-dependent
   b. Immunologically mediated
   c. Dose-independent
   d. Drug-drug interactions

6. Renal clearance is important with all the following β-blockers *except*:
   a. Nadolol
   b. Metoprolol
   c. Sotalol
   d. Acebutolol

7. Toxic side effects limiting the dose of procainamide typically include all the following *except*:
   a. Excessive (> 50% over baseline) prolongation of QRS
   b. Hypotension
   c. Hypertension
   d. Ventricular tachycardia

8. The risk of myositis, myopathy, or rhabdomyolysis is greatest with which drug combination?
   a. Gemfibrozil plus pravastatin while taking digoxin
   b. Gemfibrozil plus pravastatin while taking itraconazole
   c. Gemfibrozil plus ketoconazole
   d. Pravastatin plus β-carotene while taking itraconazole

Answers

1. Answer b

The therapeutic index is the most important predictor of the options listed for the clinical significance of a drug-drug interaction.

2. Answer a

Oral doses require much higher doses than intravenous ones with high first-pass metabolism drugs.

3. Answer d

The interaction is a metabolic effect of amiodarone on warfarin, correlating best with the half-life of amiodarone. The interaction is a chronic progressive one, often inducing little effect when amiodarone is started. It may take weeks to months for full effects to develop.

4. Answer b

Grapefruit juice does not prolong the QT interval itself; it is an inhibitor of the CYP3A4 enzyme system that in turn may cause increased levels of other drugs, which can prolong QT and induce torsades de pointes. Cyclosporine also requires CYP3A4 metabolism, but it is not a potent inhibitor.

All the other choices could predispose a patient to torsades de pointes.

5. Answer a

Drug side effects may be dose-dependent or immunologically mediated. Most commonly, they are concentration- or dose-dependent.

6. Answer b

Metoprolol does not have any significant renal elimination.

7. Answer c

Hypertension is not a typical dose-limiting effect of procainamide. Hypotension may occur while a patient is taking procainamide, but often this is not significant enough to preclude its use.

8. Answer b

The risk of myopathy is present with gemfibrozil and pravastatin individually, the risk is enhanced when they are used together, and even greater risk is possible when the metabolism of pravastatin is inhibited by a CYP3A4 inhibitor such as itraconazole (a very potent inhibitor).

Chapter 86

Cardiac Emergencies

Arshad Jahangir, M.D.
Joseph G. Murphy, M.D.

> The management of cardiac emergencies is an important topic to review for the Cardiology Examinations. This chapter outlines the general principles of managing cardiac emergencies, but it is deliberately not an exhaustive discussion of the topic.

Pulmonary Edema

1. Identify and treat precipitating factors if possible.
2. Place the patient in a sitting position to improve lung function.
3. Give supplemental oxygen by mask or nasal cannula to maintain $PO_2 > 60$ mm Hg.
4. Intubate and mechanically ventilate the patient if hypoxia and/or hypercapnia cannot be corrected adequately.
5. Give morphine sulfate, 2 to 5 mg intravenously; repeat every 10 to 25 minutes if needed (as tolerated).
6. Give a loop diuretic such as furosemide, 20 to 80 mg intravenously.
7. Start an infusion of nitroglycerin.
   Nitroglycerin is a venodilator that predominantly affects cardiac preload. (Initiate at 5 µg/min and increase 5 to 10 µg/min every 3 to 5 minutes to a maximum of 200 µg/min, as tolerated.)
   Nitroprusside is a mixed arterial and venous vasodilator that decreases both cardiac preload and afterload.

Nitroprusside is indicated specifically in pulmonary edema due to systemic hypertension and acute mitral or aortic insufficiency. Start at 0.3 µg/kg per minute, and titrate up to 10 µg/kg per minute as needed.
8. Inotropic agents (dopamine, dobutamine) may be helpful in pulmonary edema due to hypotension and cardiogenic shock. Dopamine, 0.5 to 10 µg/kg per minute; dobutamine, 2 to 15 µg/kg per minute.
9. An intra-aortic balloon pump may be valuable in selected patients.

Aortic Dissection

1. Dissection of the ascending aorta should be treated surgically if possible.
2. Dissection of the descending aorta may be treated medically or surgically.
3. Systemic systolic blood pressure should be lowered to 100 to 120 mm Hg or the lowest possible blood pressure that permits adequate organ perfusion. Administer nitroprusside intravenously (start with 0.3 µg/kg per minute and increase up to 10 µg/kg per minute) combined with esmolol intravenously (start with 500 µg/kg for 1 minute and titrate to 250 to 300 µg/kg per minute) to achieve a target heart rate of 60 to 70 beats/min.
4. In dissection of the ascending aortic arch, watch for acute

aortic valve incompetence, inferior myocardial infarction due to extension of the dissection into the right coronary artery, neurologic signs due to dissection into the arch vessels, and ischemia of the upper limbs.

Pericardial Tamponade

1. The treatment of choice for nontraumatic cardiac tamponade is pericardiocentesis under echocardiographic guidance.
2. The treatment of choice for traumatic cardiac tamponade and tamponade due to aortic dissection is emergency thoracotomy.
3. Volume expansion with saline, blood, or plasma is valuable pending pericardiocentesis or surgery.
4. Avoid mechanical ventilation and β-blockade.
5. Diuretics and nitrates are contraindicated.

Ventricular Tachycardia

1. Synchronized DC cardioversion if the patient is hemodynamically unstable.
2. Treat pharmacologically if the patient is hemodynamically stable.

   Lidocaine, 1 to 1.5 mg/kg intravenously, followed by infusion at 1 to 4 mg/min, supplemented by boluses of 0.5 to 0.75 mg/kg every 5 to 10 minutes to a maximum of 3 mg/kg (in older patients and those with congestive heart failure or liver dysfunction, the infusion rate should be reduced to avoid lidocaine toxicity) *or*

   Procainamide, 1 g intravenously over 30 minutes, followed by 1 to 2 mg/min (lower infusion rates for patients with renal insufficiency), *or*

   Amiodarone, 150 mg intravenously over 10 minutes, followed by 360 mg intravenously over 6 hours, then 0.5 mg/min infusion.
3. Elective synchronized DC cardioversion for hemodynamically stable patients (starting at 100J) who do not have conversion to sinus rhythm pharmacologically (brief anesthesia is necessary).
4. A rapid blow to the sternum may also be effective for hemodynamically unstable patients.
5. Correct precipitating factors for ventricular tachycardia, including myocardial ischemia and electrolyte and acid-base imbalance.

Ventricular Fibrillation or Pulseless Ventricular Tachycardia

1. Cardiopulmonary resuscitation until defibrillator is available.
2. Defibrillate up to three times at 200J, 300J, and 360J.
3. Resume cardiopulmonary resuscitation and intubate.
4. Epinephrine, 1 mg intravenously (1:10,000), and defibrillate with 360J.
5. Repeat step 4 every 3 to 5 minutes.
6. For recurrent or refractory ventricular fibrillation or ventricular tachycardia, give lidocaine (1 to 1.5 mg/kg intravenously, then 1 to 4 mg/min) or procainamide (30 mg/min [up to a total of 1 g] followed by 1 to 2 mg/min intravenously) or intravenous amiodarone (150 mg over 10 minutes, then 1 mg/min for 6 hours, followed by 0.5 mg/min), or bretylium (5 mg/kg intravenously initially and, at 10 mg/kg, repeat at 15-minute intervals to a total dose of 30 mg/kg).
7. Precipitating factors such as myocardial ischemia and electrolyte and acid-base disturbance should be corrected.

Asystole

1. Cardiopulmonary resuscitation until defibrillator is available.
2. Defibrillate if there is any possibility that the rhythm is other than asystole (fine ventricular fibrillation).
3. Intubate.
4. Epinephrine, 1 mg intravenously every 3 to 5 minutes.
5. Atropine, 1 mg intravenously every 3 to 5 minutes up to 3 mg.
6. Continously monitor rhythm for ventricular fibrillation and defibrillate if appropriate.
7. High dose of epinephrine, 2 to 5 mg intravenously every 3 to 5 minutes.
8. Sodium bicarbonate, 1 mEq/kg intravenously, followed by 0.5 mEq/kg every 10 minutes for documented acidosis not due to hypoventilation.
9. Immediate transcutaneous ventricular pacing.
10. Emergency echocardiography to check for tamponade and to assess ventricular function.

Torsades de Pointes

Torsades de pointes is a specific type of polymorphic ventricular tachycardia in which there is a gradual change in the QRS amplitude and axis that appears to swing around a point. It is associated with a prolonged QT interval that is either congenital in origin (Romano-Ward and Jervell and Lange-Nielsen syndromes) or acquired, such as drug-induced or with electrolyte abnormalities. Common predisposing factors include marked bradycardia and electrolyte disturbances (hypokalemia, hypomagnesemia).

1. Unsynchronized DC cardioversion if the patient is hemodynamically unstable, starting at 200J, followed by 300J and 360J.
2. Stop treatment with all potentially provocative agents.
   Antiarrhythmics: quinidine, procainamide, disopyramide, flecainide, propafenone, sotalol, ibutilide, amiodarone (rarely)
   Antipsychotics: haloperidol, thioridazine, droperidol
   Antibiotics: erythromycin
   Antivirals and antiprotozoals: amantidine, pentamidine
   Antifungal agents: ketoconazole, itraconazole
   Antihistamines: terfenadine, astemizole
   Propulsive agents: cisapride
   Hypolipidemic agents: probucol
3. Correct underlying electrolyte abnormalities such as hypokalemia and hypomagnesemia.
4. Give 1 to 2 g of magnesium sulfate by intravenous bolus even if the serum level of magnesium is within normal limits.
5. Shorten the QT interval and eliminate triggering long-short RR interval by increasing the heart rate to 100 to 120 beats/min with isoproterenol infusion (start at 1 µg/min up to 20 µg/min) *or*
   Temporary pacemaker.
6. β-Blockers may be effective in preventing torsades de pointes in the setting of congenital long QT syndromes.
7. Polymorphic ventricular tachycardia (PVT) that morphologically resembles torsades de pointes in the setting of a normal QT interval can be treated with standard antiarrhythmic agents (lidocaine, preferably). Drug-refractory sustained PVTs ("electrical storm") have been reported in rare cases of acute MI and may be related to uncontrolled ischemia and increased sympathetic tone and may be managed with intravenous β-blocker, intravenous amiodarone, intra-aortic balloon pump, or emergency revascularization.

Paroxysmal Supraventricular Tachycardia

1. Vagal maneuvers.
2. Adenosine, 6 to 12 mg intravenously, *or*

3. Verapamil, 5 to 10 mg intravenously and repeat once, *or*
4. Diltiazem, 0.25 to 0.3 mg/kg intravenously over 2 minutes and then infuse at 5 to 15 mg/hr, *or*
5. Esmolol, 500 µg/kg over 1 min, then 50 to 200 µg/kg per minute intravenously, *or*
6. Digoxin, 0.25 mg intravenously and repeated every 4 to 6 hours to a total dose of 1.0 to 1.5 mg.
7. Elective DC cardioversion.

Atrial Flutter or Atrial Fibrillation With Rapid Ventricular Response

To control rapid ventricular response:
1. Verapamil, 5 to 10 mg intravenously and repeat once, *or*
2. Diltiazem, 0.25 to 0.3 mg/kg intravenously, then 5 to 15 mg/hr, *or*
3. Esmolol, 500 µg/kg over 1 min, then 50-200 µg/kg per minute intravenously *or* intravenous atenolol 2.5 to 5.0 mg over 2 min to a total of 10 mg in 10 to 15 min *or* intravenous metoprolol 2.5 to 5.0 mg every 2 to 5 min to a total of 15 mg over 15 minutes.
4. Digoxin, 0.25 mg intravenously and repeated every 4 to 6 hours to a total dose of 1.0-1.5 mg.

To restore sinus rhythm:
1. Procainamide, 1 g intravenously over 30 minutes followed by infusion at 1 to 2 mg/min, *or*
2. Ibutilide, 1 mg over 10 minutes, repeat once after 10 minutes; watch for torsades de pointes.
3. Synchronized DC cardioversion.
4. Rapid atrial or esophageal pacing for type I atrial flutter.
5. Adenosine is not effective therapy for atrial fibrillation or atrial flutter.

Heparin should be given to patients who are not anticoagulated and anticoagulation continued after cardioversion. To prevent recurrence, an antiarrhythmic agent such as propafenone, sotalol, or amiodarone should be considered.

Reciprocating Tachycardia Complicating Wolff-Parkinson-White Syndrome

1. Synchronized DC cardioversion if the patient is hemodynamically unstable.
2. Avoid diltiazem, verapamil, and digoxin because they

may accelerate anterograde conduction over the bypass tract and increase the tachycardia rate.

3. If the patient is hemodynamically stable, with orthodromic conduction (narrow complex QRS), give adenosine intravenously (watch for conversion from reciprocating tachycardia to atrial fibrillation). Atrial fibrillation with a rapid ventricular response may require emergency synchronized DC cardioversion.

4. Procainamide, 1 g intravenously over 30 minutes followed by 1 to 2 mg/min (watch for hypotension).

5. If pharmacologic therapy fails in a hemodynamically stable patient, consider DC cardioversion.

6. For atrial fibrillation that complicates Wolff-Parkinson-White syndrome, adenosine is contraindicated and may require DC cardioversion or procainamide given intravenously.

Pulseless Electrical Activity (Electromechanical Dissociation)

1. Cardiopulmonary resuscitation.
2. Intubate.
3. Emergency echocardiography to look for tamponade and to assess ventricular function.
4. Look for secondary causes of electromechanical dissociation, and correct if possible.
   Cardiac tamponade
   Tension pneumothorax, massive pulmonary embolism
   Hypothermia
   Hyperkalemia
   Acidosis
   Hypovolemia, hypoxia
5. Epinephrine, 1 mg intravenously every 3 to 5 minutes.
6. Atropine, 1 mg intravenously every 3 minutes up to 3 mg.
7. High dose of epinephrine, 2 to 5 mg intravenously every 3 to 5 minutes.
8. Sodium bicarbonate, 1 mEq/kg intravenously, followed by 0.5 mEq/kg every 10 minutes for documented acidosis not due to hypoventilation.

Multifocal Atrial Tachycardia

1. Treat the underlying disease (frequently, lung disease and hypoxemia).
2. Stop treatment with provocative agents such as β-agonists or theophylline.

3. Avoid β-blockers if there is underlying bronchospastic lung disease.

4. Magnesium or potassium given intravenously may be effective even if the serum levels of magnesium and potassium are normal (magnesium sulfate 1 to 2 g intravenously over 10 minutes, then 1 to 2 g/hr over 5 hours).

5. Verapamil given orally or intravenously is usually the drug of choice (5 to 10 mg intravenously, repeat 5 to 10 mg for a total of 20 mg).

6. Digoxin is not effective in treating this arrhythmia.

7. In paroxysmal atrial tachycardia with block, always suspect digoxin toxicity and treat accordingly.

Digoxin Toxicity and Overdose

Specific cardiac arrhythmias include ventricular tachycardia (especially bidirectional ventricular tachycardia), sinus bradycardia, heart block, and paroxysmal atrial tachycardia with block.

Nausea, vomiting, and drowsiness may occur.

1. Induce emesis or perform gastric lavage in digoxin overdose and administer charcoal to decrease further absorption of the drug.

2. Give digoxin-immune Fab: give 10 μg to test for hypersensitivity initially, then give up to 20 vials (dose per calculated digoxin body load if known) through a 0.22-μm membrane filter for
   Ventricular tachycardia or fibrillation
   High-grade atrioventricular block not responding to atropine or hyperkalemia
   Acute ingestion of 10 mg or more
   Serum level of 10 ng/mL or greater or severe hyperkalemia

3. Digoxin overdose may cause severe hyperkalemia. Treat in the usual way with insulin, glucose, and bicarbonate but avoid calcium gluconate because it potentiates digoxin toxicity.

4. Treat high-grade atrioventricular block with atropine and temporary pacing if needed.

5. Treat ventricular arrhythmias with lidocaine, phenytoin (100 mg intravenously over 5 minutes and repeat 100 mg over 5 minutes until a full loading dose of 18 mg/kg), esmolol (500 μg/kg intravenously, then 50 to 200 μg/kg per minute intravenously), or magnesium (1 to 2 g intravenously over 10 minutes). If hemodynamically

unstable, synchronized DC cardioversion beginning at 10J, increasing by 10J to 50J, then 100J, 200J, 300J, and 360J if necessary.
6. Correct hypokalemia or hypomagnesemia.

β-Blocker Overdose

Emergency care to stabilize the airway, breathing, and circulation is the priority. Patients should have ECG monitoring.
1. Perform gastric lavage and administer charcoal, but avoid emesis because of vagal side effects.
2. Treat hypotension with saline and isoproterenol given intravenously, at 2 to 20 µg/min initially and increase up to 200 µg/min.
3. Glucagon (50 to 150 µg/kg over 1 minute, then 1 to 5 mg/hr in 5% dextrose solution). Calcium chloride or calcium gluconate (10 mL of 10% solution over 10 minutes) given intravenously may be useful for myocardial depression.
4. Treat bronchospasm with β-adrenergic agonists administered systemically or by inhalation or with theophylline.
5. Treat heart block with atropine (up to 2 mg intravenously) or temporary pacing.
6. Treat hypoglycemia with glucose and glucagon given intravenously if needed.
7. Sotalol overdose may cause torsades de pointes.

Calcium Channel Blocker Overdose

As with β-blocker overdose, the goal of treatment is to decrease absorption of the drug and increase perfusion to the critical organ system.
1. Perform gastric lavage and administer charcoal, but avoid emesis because of vagal side effects.
2. Treat hypotension and bradycardia with saline infusion and intravenous calcium chloride, 1-g bolus (10 mL of 10% solution over 10 minutes), followed by a continuous infusion (20 to 50 mg/kg per hour). For patients taking digoxin, caution should be used because calcium may have deleterious effects.
3. Treat high-grade heart block with atropine (up to 2 mg) given intravenously or temporary pacing.
4. Glucagon (50 to 150 µg/kg intravenously over 1 minute followed by 1 to 5 mg/hr) may also be helpful for hypotension and heart block.

5. Dobutamine or dopamine should be used for heart failure and norepinephrine for hypotension.

Hypertensive Emergencies

1. Nitroprusside, start treatment with 0.3 µg/kg per minute and titrate up to 10 µg/kg per minute.
2. Nitroglycerin, 10 to 400 µg/minute.
3. Esmolol, start treatment with 200 µg/kg for 1 minute and follow with 25 to 300 µg/kg per minute.
4. Labetalol, start treatment with 20 mg given intravenously and repeat with 20 to 40 mg every 10 minutes or 0.5 to 2.0 mg/min continuous infusion up to 300 mg.
5. Captopril, 6.25 to 50 mg orally at hourly intervals or enalapril at 0.625 to 1.25 mg intravenously every 6 hours.
6. Nitroprusside should be administered only in an intensive care setting and with intra-arterial blood pressure monitoring.
7. Nitroprusside is the drug of choice for hypertensive encephalopathy, cerebral hemorrhage, clonidine withdrawal syndrome, and aortic dissection (in combination with a β-blocker).
8. Captopril or nitroglycerin is the drug of choice after myocardial infarction and in left ventricular failure.
9. Labetalol or phentolamine is the drug of choice for an adrenergic crisis (cocaine overdose, monoamine oxidase inhibitor-induced hypertensive crisis, pheochromocytoma).

Pacemaker-Mediated Tachycardia

Pacemaker-mediated tachycardia occurs in DDD pacemakers when a ventricular depolarization retrogradely activates the atrium and is sensed by the atrial lead, which then initiates a paced ventricular beat that repeats the sequence, resulting in incessant tachycardia at or near the upper rate limit of pacemakers.
1. Apply a magnet to disable atrial tracking.
2. Vagal maneuvers.
3. Program DVI or VVI.

Unstable Angina

1. Nitroglycerin given intravenously (5 to 10 µg/min, increase by 10 µg/min every 3 to 5 minutes to a maximal dose of 200 µg/min).

2. Heparin given intravenously (5,000 to 10,000 units bolus, then 1,000 to 1,500 units/hr to keep aPTT around 60 to 70).
3. Give aspirin orally (325 mg).
4. β-Blocker given orally or intravenously unless contraindicated (metoprolol [Lopressor], 5 mg intravenously [repeat times 3] and then 50 to 100 mg orally twice daily, or esmolol, 500 μg/kg per minute initially and then titrate to 50 to 200 μg/kg per minute).
5. Avoid calcium channel blockers in unstable angina if possible.
6. Oxygen (by nasal cannula or face mask).
7. Sedation and analgesia.
8. Intra-aortic balloon pump for selected patients to stabilize before coronary artery bypass graft or percutaneous transluminal coronary angioplasty.
9. Emergency coronary angiography and angioplasty for refractory unstable angina.

Myocardial Infarction

1. Give aspirin orally (325 mg).
2. Nitroglycerin given sublingually and followed by nitroglycerin infusion (5 to 10 μg/min intravenously initially, increase by 10 μg/min every 3 to 5 minutes to a maximum of 200 μg/min). Avoid systolic blood pressure less than 90 mm Hg.
3. Thrombolysis or emergency percutaneous transluminal coronary angioplasty.
   Streptokinase 1.5 million IU over 1 hour.
   rtPA, 15-mg bolus, followed by 0.75 mg/kg (up to 50 mg) over 30 minutes, then 0.5 mg/kg (up to 35 mg) infusion over 1 hour.
   Anistreplase, 30 IU over 2 minutes.
4. β-Blocker given orally or intravenously unless contraindicated (metroprolol, 5 mg intravenously, repeat 3 times, then 50 mg and, next, 100 mg orally twice daily as tolerated).
5. Oxygen (by nasal cannula or face mask).
6. Sedation and analgesia (morphine sulfate, 2 to 4 mg every 5 to 10 minutes as tolerated).
7. Inotropic agents for cardiogenic shock.
   Dobutamine, 2 to 15 μg/kg per minute.
   Dopamine, 0.5 to 10 μg/kg per minute (increases renal blood flow at less than 2 μg/kg per minute only).
   Amrinone, 0.75 mg/kg followed by 5 to 10 μg/kg per minute.

8. Intra-aortic balloon pump for selected patients with hypotension.
9. Fluids given intravenously for right ventricular infarction. (Avoid nitroglycerin or diuretics.)
10. Lidocaine for ventricular arrhythmias but not for prophylaxis.
11. Avoid calcium channel blockers.
12. Magnesium sulfate for patients with low serum levels of magnesium.
13. Angiotensin converting enzyme inhibitor unless contraindicated. Captopril orally, start with 6.25 mg and increase to 50 mg twice daily as tolerated.
14. Emergency PTCA for cardiogenic shock.

Right Ventricular Ischemia or Infarction

1. Maintain right ventricular preload with volume loading (intravenous saline). Avoid nitrates and diuretics because they decrease preload. Maintain atrioventricular synchrony, and initiate atrioventricular pacing for symptomatic high-grade atrioventricular block unresponsive to atropine. Prompt cardioversion is important for hemodynamically significant supraventricular tachycardia (atrial fibrillation may occur in up to one-third of patients).
2. Inotropic support—Start intravenous dobutamine if cardiac output fails to improve after infusion of 1 to 2 L of saline solution.
3. Decrease afterload in patients with left ventricular dysfunction with an intra-aortic balloon pump and/or arterial vasodilatation (sodium nitroprusside).

Pulmonary Thromboembolism

1. Supplemental oxygen.
2. Anticoagulation with heparin given intravenously (bolus 7,500 to 10,000 U, maintenance at 20 U/kg per hour to keep aPTT around 60 to 80).
3. Thrombolytic given intravenously for hemodynamically unstable or profoundly hypoxemic patient with evidence of massive pulmonary embolism even without overt hemodynamic compromise (unless contraindicated, e.g., postoperative state).
   Streptokinase, bolus 250,000 U, maintenance 100,000 U/hr for 24 to 72 hours.
   Urokinase, bolus 2,000 U/lb, maintenance 2,000 U/lb per hour for 24 to 72 hours.

rtPA, bolus 15 mg, then 50 mg over 30 minutes, then 35 mg over next hour.

Full-dose heparin anticoagulation should be started along with infusion of a lytic agent.

4. Aggressive fluid resuscitation and inotropic or pressor agents if hypotension develops.
5. Surgical thrombectomy (only with severe hemodynamic compromise, when thrombolytic therapy is contraindicated or unsuccessful).

Hyperkalemia

1. Continuous ECG monitoring.
2. Calcium gluconate or calcium chloride (10 mL of 10% solution over 10 minutes).
3. Glucose with insulin (50 mL of 50% dextrose intravenously, with 5 to 10 U regular insulin).
4. Sodium bicarbonate.
5. β_2-Adrenergic agonists (albuterol by inhalation or intravenously).
6. Sodium polystyrene sulfonate (Kayexalate) (20 to 30 g orally with equal amount of sorbitol) or retention enema (50 to 100 g in 200 mL of water and sorbitol).
7. Correction of underlying defect (renal failure, potassium-sparing diuretics, or adrenal insufficiency).
8. Dialysis may be required for persistent hyperkalemia.

Notes

Index

Page numbers in *italics* indicate figures. Page numbers followed by "P" indicate plates. Page numbers followed by "t" indicate tables.

Abbreviated Table of Contents